Female Genitourinary and Pelvic Floor Reconstruction

Francisco E. Martins •
Henriette Veiby Holm •
Jaspreet S. Sandhu •
Kurt A McCammon
Editors

Female Genitourinary and Pelvic Floor Reconstruction

Volume 1

With 422 Figures and 78 Tables

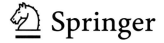

Editors
Francisco E. Martins
University of Lisbon
Lisbon, Portugal

Henriette Veiby Holm
University of Oslo
Oslo, Norway

Jaspreet S. Sandhu
Memorial Sloan Kettering Cancer Center
New York, NY, USA

Kurt A McCammon
Eastern Virginia Medical School
Norfolk, VA, USA

ISBN 978-3-031-19597-6   ISBN 978-3-031-19598-3 (eBook)
https://doi.org/10.1007/978-3-031-19598-3

© Springer Nature Switzerland AG 2023

This work is subject to copyright. All rights are solely and exclusively licensed by the Publisher, whether the whole or part of the material is concerned, specifically the rights of translation, reprinting, reuse of illustrations, recitation, broadcasting, reproduction on microfilms or in any other physical way, and transmission or information storage and retrieval, electronic adaptation, computer software, or by similar or dissimilar methodology now known or hereafter developed.

The use of general descriptive names, registered names, trademarks, service marks, etc. in this publication does not imply, even in the absence of a specific statement, that such names are exempt from the relevant protective laws and regulations and therefore free for general use.

The publisher, the authors, and the editors are safe to assume that the advice and information in this book are believed to be true and accurate at the date of publication. Neither the publisher nor the authors or the editors give a warranty, expressed or implied, with respect to the material contained herein or for any errors or omissions that may have been made. The publisher remains neutral with regard to jurisdictional claims in published maps and institutional affiliations.

This Springer imprint is published by the registered company Springer Nature Switzerland AG.
The registered company address is: Gewerbestrasse 11, 6330 Cham, Switzerland

Paper in this product is recyclable.

First, I would like to thank my co-editors for their outstanding and tireless contribution, and support with this book. I would also like to express my appreciation and gratitude to my several surgical mentors, my countless good colleagues, and my dedicated fellows and residents who have taught, supported, and encouraged my vocation in the field of male and female urologic reconstruction. To all the patients that I had the privilege to treat, care for, learn from, and who teach me daily the meaning of dignity in the face of adversity, my sincere thanks. To the ones I will always love, most especially my recently departed wife and colleague Natasha and our children Filipe, Daniela, and Tomás for the unswerving inspiration, strength, love, unconditional support, and sacrifice they shared with me for the long hours dedicated to this project and life in general. This book is my humble dedication to them. I certainly would never have made it without them.

Francisco E. Martins

Foreword

It was with pleasure that I accepted the invitation from Professor Martins to write a Foreword for this most impressive textbook, which covers virtually all aspects of lower urinary, genital, and pelvic floor abnormalities in women and their relevant anatomy, physiology, pathophysiology, and management. The co-editors are all experts with sub-specialization in various areas of such as pathology and dysfunction and have chosen their individual chapter authors with great care. The chapter authors are all experts in their own right with a history of referenced experience in the areas of their particular contributions. The book covers all the major subjects described in its title and, in addition, various subjects such as the history, basic science, epidemiology, and diagnostic evaluation in this field. Besides topics strictly related to genitourinary and pelvic floor reconstruction, readers will find within the 65 chapter, the topics of lower urinary tract storage and emptying disorders, fecal incontinence, and defecatory dysfunction. Genitourinary and pelvic trauma, congenital defects, and genital-affirming surgery are covered as well. The book should find a place in the libraries of urologists, urogynecologists, pelvic surgeons, and trauma surgeons and should stand the test of time quite well.

Emeritus Founders Professor   Alan J. Wein, MD, PhD (hon), FACS
Chief of Urology and Program Director
Department of Surgery
Perelman School of Medicine at the
University of Pennsylvania
Philadelphia, Pennsylvania

Foreword

Gender medicine is quite a young discipline and historically evolved from the International Women's Movement in the 1960s and 1970s. In 2001, the American Institute of Medicine published its report "Exploring the biological contributions to human health: does sex matter?" [1], representing a starting point of gender-specific medicine, which since then steadily evolved to the present date. Against this background, embracing female genitourinary and pelvic floor reconstruction in one book is a perfect contribution to personalized medicine for females. I would like to thank and congratulate the editors Francisco Martins, Henriette V. Holm, Jaspreet Sandhu, and Kurt McCammon for their commitment to further improve health care in women by this book.

Including 65 chapters the book covers the history, anatomy, physiology, and all areas of specific problems. It starts with the historical milestones in genitourinary and pelvic floor reconstruction and gives an insight on the embryology and development of congenital anomalies in females. Pelvic floor disorders and incontinence are increasing with age. Taking the demographic changes in industrial countries into consideration, a significant rise can be expected with a major socioeconomic impact and burden to the healthcare systems. Thus, there is an urgent need for established standards with respect to diagnostics, treatments, and follow-up. Consequently, a large part of the book focusses on the evaluation and management (conservative and surgical) of the underlying disorders and diseases. For reconstruction, minimal invasive techniques are addressed as well as open surgical procedures. In addition, there is a focus on possible and common complications and their management. Besides common diseases and disorders, rare conditions such as urethral strictures or diverticula are also addressed. Solutions are offered for challenging conditions as for trauma, bladder pain syndrome, or severe irradiation damage. In principle, all types of urinary diversion can be used in females but some, such as neobladders, might have a different functional outcome compared to males – a topic also addressed in the book. Gender-assigning surgery has become an increasing part of genitourinary reconstructions in males as well as females, another actual and important subject covered. Moreover, a chapter on stem cells and tissue engineering provides a careful look into potential future treatment. Even though the same principles for reconstruction of the genitourinary tract are used in males and females, there are significant differences in the surgical approach and steps. In this book, the surgical techniques for reconstruction are described in detail by well-known and experienced surgeons. The editors succeeded in bringing together experts from all over the world as authors, thus guaranteeing a sophisticated and global perspective.

It always needs someone to take the initiative for such a contribution, which means a tremendous amount of work in addition to our daily routine and patient care. I would like to thank my colleague and dear friend Francisco Martins for taking this step. It undermines his dedication to the field of reconstructive urology and his active role in the international community of reconstructive urologists.

I highly recommend this book to everyone interested in reconstructive urology.

Professor of Urology   Margit Fisch, M.D., FEAPU, FEBU
Past President ESGURS
Past President GURS
Past President DGU

References

1. Wizemann TM, Mary-Lou P, Hrsg. Exploring the biological contributions to human health: Does sex matter? Washington: National Academies Press; 2001.

Preface

This book on female genitourinary and pelvic floor reconstruction is the end-result of the work of an international panel of renowned experts in the field, who kindly lent their time, efforts, and patience to make this project a on historical perspectives, innovations, challenges, and controversies in the field of female genitourinary and pelvic floor disorders.

As the human population lives longer and general health has improved, the prevalence of these genitourinary and pelvic floor problems has also been on the rise. The term female pelvic medicine has been adopted recently to incorporate a broad array of inter-related clinical conditions that range from lower urinary tract dysfunctions and disorders, pelvic organ prolapses and anatomical anomalies, urinary voiding dysfunctions, defecatory dysfunction, sexual dysfunction, to several chronic pelvic pain problems. It has been reported and estimated that more than half of the adult females will suffer from one or more of these problems for some period in their lifetimes and about 11% will undergo surgical treatment for genitourinary and pelvic floor problems by 80 years of age. Financial costs and global healthcare burden associated with genitourinary and pelvic floor disorders result in huge adverse psychosocial impact, which ultimately reflects on quality of life. Both the increase and demand for healthcare services related to these problems will, at least, double the growth rate of the world population over the next 40 years.

Research in genitourinary and pelvic floor disorders is based on and supported by a few principles. The first principle is to increase knowledge on pathophysiology of the specific disorders, a principle that is transversal to other medical specialties. Clinical research to enhance patient outcomes is another important principle. A third principle, critical and unique to reconstructive surgery, deals with advances in wound healing, an essential component for the success of any reconstructive surgery as well as the optimization of overall clinical management.

International interest in genitourinary and pelvic floor disorders of the female patient has promoted awareness of the high prevalence of these health problems in an increasingly ageing population. A widespread need for education and training in the field of genitourinary and pelvic floor disorders and reconstructive surgery is critical as demands are on the rise and both quantity and quality of life have become an increasingly relevant issue.

This book includes 65 chapters divided into 10 sections. Section 1 includes chapters 1 through 6 and features a historical perspective of the field, dating millennia back in time, as well as its basic science and epidemiology. Section 2 includes chapters 7 through 11 and features clinical diagnosis and essential diagnostic tools needed for the various disorders included. Section 3 includes chapters 12 through 27 and features disorders of bladder storage and emptying. Section 4 includes chapters 28 through 38 and features pelvic organ prolapse disorders. Section 5 groups chapters 39 through 49 and describes urethral reconstruction associated with fistulae, diverticula, and urethral strictures. Section 6 includes chapters 50 and 51 that deal with ureteral injuries and their surgical reconstruction. Section 7 includes chapters 52 through 54 and discusses chronic pelvic pain, irritative voiding disorders, and female sexual dysfunction. Section 8 comprises chapters 55 and 56 and discusses fecal incontinence and defecatory prolapse and dysfunction. Section 9 covers chapters 57 through 59 and deals with the use of bowel in genitourinary and pelvic reconstruction. Section 10 includes chapters 60 and 61 that cover genitourinary and pelvic trauma inflicted iatrogenically, by obstetric trauma and by genital mutilation, an unfortunate procedure still perpetrated in some parts of the globe in the twenty-first century. Finally, section 11 includes chapters 62 through 65 that discuss topics related to vaginoplaty, neovagina construction due to congenital anomalies and trauma, and gender-affirming surgery. All authors in this book are hand-picked experts that have detailed the best approaches and thoughts on these challenging disorders and their respective reconstructions. We could not feel more grateful and proud. We hope that this book will be a valuable resource and an important reference text to help improve scientific knowledge and standards of clinical practice of all involved with genitourinary and pelvic floor reconstruction to take better care of their patients.

Lisbon, Portugal	Francisco E. Martins
Oslo, Norway	Henriette Veiby Holm
New York, USA	Jaspreet S. Sandhu
Norfolk, USA	Kurt A McCammon
October 2023	Editors

Acknowledgments

The editors would like to thank all contributors of this book for their hard efforts, precious time, inexhaustible patience, and kind help devoted to this challenging project and for making it a reality. We would also like to thank the Springer editorial staff, especially Monika Conji, for the tremendous volume of administrative collaboration, support, and exemplary work, including an enormous, tireless, overzealous, and prompt assistance with this project. All these generous attributes facilitated this project immensely.

Finally, a word of appreciation and enormous gratitude to all our family members and friends for their patience, understanding, and encouragement.

Francisco E. Martins
Henriette Veiby Holm
Jaspreet S. Sandhu
Kurt A McCammon

Contents

Volume 1

Part I   History, Basic Science, and Epidemiology 1

1   Historical Milestones in Female Genitourinary and Pelvic Floor Reconstruction 3
Francisco E. Martins, Natalia Martins, and Liliya Tryfonyuk

2   Embryology and Development of Congenital Anomalies of the Pelvis and Female Organs 29
Vishen Naidoo, Ejikeme Mbajiorgu, and Ahmed Adam

3   Neuroanatomy and Neurophysiology 49
John T. Stoffel

4   Pathophysiology of Female Micturition Disorders 71
Alex Gomelsky, Ann C. Stolzle, and William P. Armstrong

5   The Epidemiology and Socioeconomic Impact of Female GU and Pelvic Floor Disorders 85
Gabriela Gonzalez and Jennifer T. Anger

6   Measurement of Urinary Symptoms, Health-Related Quality of Life, and Outcomes of Treatment of Genitourinary and Pelvic Floor Disorders 97
Ly Hoang Roberts, Annah Vollstedt, Priya Padmanabhan, and Larry T. Sirls

Part II   Diagnostic Evaluation 111

7   Clinical Evaluation of the Female Lower Urinary Tract and Pelvic Floor 113
Stephanie Gleicher and Natasha Ginzburg

8   Ultrasound Imaging of the Female Lower Urinary Tract and Pelvic Floor 125
Lewis Chan, Vincent Tse, and Tom Jarvis

9   Electrophysiologic Evaluation of the Pelvic Floor 139
Simon Podnar and David B. Vodušek

**10   Urodynamic Evaluation: Traditional, Video, and
Ambulatory Approaches** 157
Miguel Miranda and Ricardo Pereira e Silva

11   Endoscopic Evaluation 179
Francisco E. Martins, Natalia Martins, Liliya Tryfonyuk, and
José Bernal Riquelme

Part III   Bladder Storage and Emptying Disorders 195

12   Idiopathic Urinary Retention in the Female 197
Abdulghani Khogeer, Lysanne Campeau, and
Mélanie Aubé-Peterkin

**13   Overview of Diagnosis and Pharmacological Treatment
of Overactive and Underactive Bladder Disorders** 207
S. Saad, N. Osman, O. A. Alsulaiman, and C. R. Chapple

**14   Behavioral Modification and Conservative
Management of Overactive Bladder and Underactive
Bladder Disorders** 221
Alain P. Bourcier and Jean A. Juras

**15   Bladder Dysfunction and Pelvic Pain: The Role of Sacral,
Tibial, and Pudendal Neuromodulation** 255
Ly Hoang Roberts, Annah Vollstedt, Jason Gilleran, and
Kenneth M. Peters

16   Voiding Dysfunction After Female Pelvic Surgery 275
Shirin Razdan and Angelo E. Gousse

17   Bladder Augmentation and Urinary Diversion 301
Henriette Veiby Holm

**18   Pathophysiology and Diagnostic Evaluation of Stress
Urinary Incontinence: Overview** 323
Helal Syed and Matthias Hofer

**19   Pudendal Nerve Entrapment Syndrome: Clinical Aspects
and Laparoscopic Management** 333
Renaud Bollens, Fabienne Absil, and Fouad Aoun

**20   Retropubic Suspension Operations for Stress Urinary
Incontinence** 361
Jennifer A. Locke, Sarah Neu, and Sender Herschorn

**21   Sling Operations for Stress Urinary Incontinence and Their
Historical Evolution: Autologous, Cadaveric, and Synthetic
Slings** 371
Felicity Reeves and Tamsin Greenwell

22	**Complications of Stress-Urinary Incontinence Surgery**	395
	Bilal Chughtai, Christina Sze, and Stephanie Sansone	
23	**Artificial Urinary Sphincter for Female Stress Urinary Incontinence**	407
	Amélie Bazinet, Emmanuel Chartier-Kastler, and Stéphanie Gazdovich	
24	**Urethral Bulking Agents**	437
	Quentin Alimi, Béatrice Bouchard, and Jacques Corcos	
25	**Laparoscopic Burch**	449
	Tamara Grisales and Kathryn Goldrath	
26	**Management of Urinary Incontinence in the Female Neurologic Patient**	457
	Oluwarotimi S. Nettey, Katherine E. Fero, and Ja-Hong Kim	
27	**Stem Cell and Tissue Engineering in Female Urinary Incontinence**	487
	Elisabeth M. Sebesta and Melissa R. Kaufman	

Part IV Pelvic Organ Prolapse **505**

28	**Etiology, Diagnosis, and Management of Pelvic Organ Prolapse: Overview**	507
	Connie N. Wang and Doreen E. Chung	
29	**Transvaginal Repair of Cystocele**	519
	Rita Jen, Atieh Novin, and David Ginsberg	
30	**Laparoscopic Paravaginal Repair**	533
	Nikolaos Thanatsis, Matthew L. Izett-Kay, and Arvind Vashisht	
31	**Minimally Invasive Approaches in the Treatment of Pelvic Organ Prolapse: Laparoscopic and Robotic**	551
	Justina Tam, Dena E. Moskowitz, Katherine A. Amin, and Una J. Lee	
32	**Complications of the Use of Synthetic Mesh Materials in Stress Urinary Incontinence and Pelvic Organ Prolapse**	569
	Michelle E. Van Kuiken and Anne M. Suskind	
33	**Vaginal Vault Prolapse: Options for Transvaginal Surgical Repair**	593
	Michele Torosis and Victor Nitti	
34	**Role of Vaginal Hysterectomy in the Treatment of Vaginal Middle Compartment Prolapse**	607
	Luiz Gustavo Oliveira Brito, Cassio Luis Zanettini Riccetto, and Paulo Cesar Rodrigues Palma	

35 Minimally Invasive Sacrocolpopexy 617
Priyanka Kancherla and Natasha Ginzburg

36 Open Abdominal Sacrocolpopexy 631
Frederico Ferronha, Jose Bernal Riquelme, and
Francisco E. Martins

**37 Management of Vaginal Posterior Compartment
Prolapse: Is There Ever a Case for Graft/Mesh?** 643
Olivia H. Chang and Suzette E. Sutherland

38 Vaginal Surgery Complications 657
Jamaal C. Jackson and Sarah A. Adelstein

Volume 2

**Part V   Urethral Reconstruction: Fistulae, Diverticula,
and Strictures** 675

**39 Overview, Epidemiology, and Etiopathogenetic
Differences in Urogenital Fistulae in the Resourced
and Resource-Limited Worlds** 677
Heléna Gresty, Madina Ndoye, and Tamsin Greenwell

40 Urethrovaginal Fistula Repair 693
Christopher Gonzales-Alabastro, Bailey Goyette, and
Stephanie J. Kielb

**41 Reconstruction of the Absent or Severely
Damaged Urethra** 707
Elisabeth M. Sebesta, W. Stuart Reynolds, and Roger R.
Dmochowski

**42 Vesicovaginal Fistula Repair: Minimally
Invasive Approach** 731
Caroline A. Brandon and Benjamin M. Brucker

43 Vesicovaginal Fistula Repair: Vaginal Approach 761
Annah Vollstedt, Ly Hoang Roberts, and Larry T. Sirls

44 Vesicovaginal Fistula Repair: Abdominal Approach 785
F. Reeves and A. Lawrence

45 Rectovaginal Fistula 805
Christine A. Burke, Jennifer E. Park, and Tamara Grisales

46 Ureterovaginal Fistula Repair 821
Kelsey E. Gallo, Michael W. Witthaus, and Jill C. Buckley

47 Female Urethral Reconstruction 829
Ignacio Alvarez de Toledo

48	**Surgical Reconstruction of Pelvic Fracture Urethral Injuries in Females**	841
	Pankaj M. Joshi, Sanjay B. Kulkarni, Bobby Viswaroop, and Ganesh Gopalakrishnan	
49	**Surgical Repair of Urethral Diverticula**	857
	S. Saad, N. Osman, O. A. Alsulaiman, and C. R. Chapple	

Part VI Ureteral Reconstruction ... 869

50	**Surgical Reconstruction of Ureteral Defects: Strictures, External Trauma, Iatrogenic, and Radiation Induced**	871
	Gillian Stearns and Jaspreet S. Sandhu	
51	**Techniques of Ureteral Reimplantation**	885
	Andrew Lai, Rabun Jones, Grace Chen, and Diana Bowen	

Part VII Pelvic Pain, Irritative Voiding Disorders, and Female Sexual Dysfunction ... 907

52	**Pathophysiology and Clinical Evaluation of Chronic Pelvic Pain**	909
	Elise J. B. De and Jan Alberto Paredes Mogica	
53	**Bladder Pain Syndrome: Interstitial Cystitis**	931
	Francisco Cruz, Rui Pinto, and Pedro Abreu Mendes	
54	**Female Sexual Dysfunction**	959
	Francisco E. Martins, Farzana Cassim, Oleksandr Yatsina, and Jan Adlam	

Part VIII Fecal Incontinence and Defecatory Dysfunction ... 995

55	**Pathophysiology, Diagnosis, and Treatment of Defecatory Dysfunction**	997
	Amythis Soltani, Domnique Malacarne Pape, and Cara L. Grimes	
56	**Management of Fecal Incontinence, Constipation, and Rectal Prolapse**	1013
	Johannes Kurt Schultz and Tom Øresland	

Part IX Use of Bowel in Genitourinary and Pelvic Reconstruction and Other Complex Scenarios ... 1031

57	**Indications and Use of Bowel in Female Lower Urinary Tract Reconstruction: Overview**	1033
	Warren Lo and Jun Jiet Ng	

58 Options for Surgical Reconstruction of the Heavily Irradiated Pelvis 1063
Jas Singh, Margaret S. Roubaud, Thomas G. Smith III, and O. Lenaine Westney

59 Use and Complications of Neobladder and Continent Urinary Diversion in Female Pelvic Cancer 1099
Bastian Amend, Kathrin Meisterhofer, Jens Bedke, and Arnulf Stenzl

Part X Genitourinary and Pelvic Trauma: Iatrogenic and Violent Causes (War and Civil Causes) 1127

60 Surgical Reconstruction of the Urinary Tract Following Obstetric and Pelvic Iatrogenic Trauma 1129
Farzana Cassim, Jan Adlam, and Madina Ndoye

61 Female Genital Mutilation/Cutting 1163
Madina Ndoye, Serigne Gueye, Lamine Niang, Farzana Cassim, and Jan Adlam

Part XI Vaginoplasty and Neovagina Construction in Congenital Defects, Trauma, and Gender Affirming Surgery 1183

62 (Neo) Vaginoplasty in Female Pelvic Congenital Anomalies 1185
Manuel Belmonte Chico Goerne, David Bouhadana, Mohamed El-Sherbiny, and Mélanie Aubé-Peterkin

63 Genital Reconstruction in Male-to-Female Gender Affirmation Surgery 1209
Marta R. Bizic, Marko T. Bencic, and Mirosav L. Djordjevic

64 Complications of Gender-Affirmation Surgery 1227
Silke Riechardt

65 Functional and Aesthetic Surgery of Female Genitalia 1235
S. Pusica, B. Stojanovic, and Mirosav L. Djordjevic

Index 1253

About the Editors

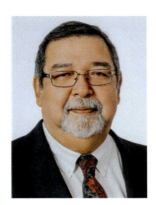

Francisco E. Martins is a Consultant Urologist with specialization on male and female genitourinary reconstruction, focusing on the complications of the treatments of pelvic malignancies, minimally invasive treatment options for penile and urethral cancers, and andrology. He obtained his Medical Degree from the Faculty of Medicine, University of Lisbon, in 1983. He was conferred the title Specialist in Urology by the Portuguese Medical Association, College of Urology, in 1993. He did temporary Urology residency training at the Brigham and Women's Hospital, Harvard University in Boston (International Exchange Urology Residency Program, September–December 1991), and a research and clinical fellowship at the University of Southern California in Los Angeles (1993–1994). His areas of major clinical and research interest are in Genito-urethral and Pelvic Trauma Reconstruction, Vesicovaginal and Rectovaginal Fistula, Female Pelvic Medicine, Erectile Dysfunction, Urinary Diversion, and Penile and Urethral Cancer. He has been Consultant Urological Surgeon at Santa Maria University Hospital (2008–present).

In May 2017, he was elected to the GURS Board of Directors (Genitourinary Reconstructive Surgeons). In October 2017, September 2018, and March 2021, he was awarded Honorary Membership of the Hungarian Urological Association (HUA), the South African Urological Association (SAUA), and the Philippine Society of Genitourinary Reconstructive Society, respectively. In May 2019, he was elected President of the GURS (Society of Genito-Urinary Reconstructive Surgeons). He is a member of several national and international societies and associations, including the Portuguese Urological Association, European Association of Urology (EAU), American Urological Association, Société Internationale d'Urologie (SIU), Canadian Urological Association (CUA), Hungarian Urological Society (HUA), and Society of Urodynamics and Functional Urology (SUFU).

He is a member of the first EAU Guidelines Panel for Urethral Strictures and a peer reviewer for several journals, including *Actas Urológicas Españolas*, *Advances in Urology*, *Biomed Research International*, *British Journal of Medicine and Medical Research*, *European Urology*, *International Urology and Nephrology*, *Journal of Men's Health*, *Journal of Surgery*, *World Journal of Urology and Journal of Urology*, and *Urology Video Journal*. He has presented and lectured at numerous national and international meetings, conferences, and congresses and has published and co-authored over 80 articles in peer-reviewed journals and 7 book chapters and has edited 4 books on erectile dysfunction, penile cancer, and male, as well as female, genitourethral reconstruction. He has also published four special issues for *Advances in Urology*, *Biomed Research International*, *Translational Andrology and Urology*, and *Journal of Clinical Medicine*.

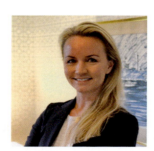

Henriette Veiby Holm is a consultant urological surgeon with specialization on female and male genitourinary reconstruction. She has a special focus on the complications of the treatments of pelvic lower urinary tract disorders, both benign and malignant, and other pelvic disorders. Female and male urethral surgery, urological implants, and andrological surgery are among her specialities. She also specializes in neurogenic dysfunction of the lower urinary tract and offers minor and major reconstructive urological surgery.

Holm obtained her medical degree from the Faculty of Medicine, Semmelweis University in Budapest, in 2004 and her Ph.D. from the Faculty of Medicine, University of Oslo, in 2015. She was conferred the title Specialist in Urology by the Norwegian Medical Association in 2020. She currently works as consultant urological surgeon at the Section of Reconstructive Urology and Neurourology, Department of Urology, Oslo University Hospital Rikshospitalet, Norway. She is member of several national and international societies and associations, including the Norwegian Urological Association, Nordic Urological Association, European Association of Urology (EAU), Société Internationale d'Urologie (SIU), and Society of Genito-Urinary Reconstructive Surgeons (GURS).

Holm is chair of the Nordic Urological Association Collaboration Group on Lower Urinary Tract Disorders and is a member of the editorial board of the *Scandinavian Journal of Urology*. She is a peer reviewer for several international journals including the *British Journal of Urology International*, *Journal of Urology*, *Neurourology and Urodynamics*, and *Scandinavian Journal of Urology*. She is a member of the Nordic Implanter Advisory Board and a former member of the Nordic Advisory Board on Botulinumtoxin in Urology.

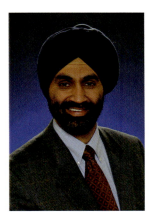

Jaspreet S. Sandhu is an Attending Urologist within the Department of Surgery (Urology Service) at Memorial Sloan Kettering Cancer Center. His primary interest is to understand, predict, prevent, and treat voiding dysfunction caused by cancer or its treatments, with a focus on the treatment of male and female incontinence and urinary tract/pelvic reconstruction. In addition, Dr. Sandhu has a strong interest in the surgical treatment of benign prostatic hyperplasia and voiding dysfunction caused by advanced cancers. He has been active, serving on committee and as faculty for annual meetings, in the American Urological Association; the Society of Urodynamics, Female Pelvic Medicine, and Urogenital Reconstruction; the Society of Genitourinary Reconstructive Surgeons; and the Society for International Urology. Dr. Sandhu has authored over 200 peer-reviewed manuscripts, review articles, and book chapters.

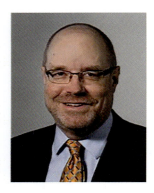

Kurt A McCammon is the Devine Chair in Genitourinary Reconstructive Surgery and Chairman and Professor of the Department of Urology at Eastern Virginia Medical School. He is the Program Director of the Urology Residency Program and also the Program Director of the Adult and Pediatric Genitourinary Reconstructive Surgery Fellowship Program at Eastern Virginia Medical School. He received his medical degree from the Medical College of Ohio and then went on to do his urology residency at Eastern Virginia Medical School (EVMS) followed by a 2 year fellowship in genitourinary reconstructive surgery also at EVMS. He received the Distinguished Alumnus Award from the University of Toledo in October 2011.

Dr. McCammon is past president of the Society of Genitourinary Surgeons and is the Chair of the Board of IVUmed. He is a member of the American Urological Association (AUA) and currently is the Mid-Atlantic representative to the AUA. He is also a member of the American College of Surgeons, the IVUmed, and Société Internationale d'Urologie. He is Diplomate of the American Board of Urology.

Dr. McCammon lectures both nationally and internationally on the topics of male and female reconstruction and has also authored numerous chapters and publications on pelvic reconstruction. His clinical interests include female urology, pelvic reconstruction, urethral reconstruction, and male incontinence.

Contributors

Fabienne Absil Gynaecology, Epicura Hospital, Ath, Belgium

Ahmed Adam Division of Urology, University of the Witwatersrand, Johannesburg, South Africa

Sarah A. Adelstein Rush University Medical Center, Chicago, IL, USA

Jan Adlam Department of Obstetrics and Gynaecoogy, Stellenbosch University/Tygerberg Hospital, Cape Town, South Africa

Quentin Alimi Department of Urology, McGill University, Jewish General Hospital, Montreal, QC, Canada

O. A. Alsulaiman Department of Urology, Sheffield Teaching Hospitals NHS Foundation Trust, Sheffield, UK

Ignacio Alvarez de Toledo Buenos Aires British Hospital, University of Buenos Aires, Buenos Aires, Argentina

Bastian Amend Department of Urology, University Hospital of Tuebingen, Eberhard Karls University, Tuebingen, Germany

Katherine A. Amin Department of Urology, University of Miami Miller School of Medicine, Miami, FL, USA

Jennifer T. Anger Department of Urology, University of California, San Diego School of Medicine, La Jolla, CA, USA

Fouad Aoun Urology, Hôtel Dieu de France, Université Saint Joseph, Beyrouth, Lebanon

William P. Armstrong LSU Health Shreveport School of Medicine, Shreveport, LA, USA

Mélanie Aubé-Peterkin Department of Surgery/Urology, McGill University Health Center and Lachine Hospital, Montreal, QC, Canada

Amélie Bazinet Department of Urology, Maisonneuve-Rosemont Hospital, University of Montreal, QC, Canada

Jens Bedke Department of Urology, University Hospital of Tuebingen, Eberhard Karls University, Tuebingen, Germany

Manuel Belmonte Chico Goerne Sexual Medicine and Genitourinary Reconstructive Surgery, McGill University Health Center, Montreal, QC, Canada

Marko T. Bencic Department of Urology, Faculty of Medicine, University of Belgrade, Belgrade, Serbia

Belgrade Center for Urogenital Reconstructive Surgery, Belgrade, Serbia

Marta R. Bizic Department of Urology, Faculty of Medicine, University of Belgrade, Belgrade, Serbia

Belgrade Center for Urogenital Reconstructive Surgery, Belgrade, Serbia

Renaud Bollens Urology, Centre Hospitalier de Wallonie Picarde, Tournai, Belgium

Urology Department, Catholic University of North of France, Lille, France

Béatrice Bouchard Department of Urology, McGill University, Jewish General Hospital, Montreal, QC, Canada

David Bouhadana McGill University, Montreal, QC, Canada

Alain P. Bourcier Centre d'Imagerie Médicale Cardinet, International Committee of Postpartum Management, Paris, France

Diana Bowen Department of Urology, Northwestern University Feinberg School of Medicine, Chicago, IL, USA

Caroline A. Brandon New York University School of Medicine, New York, NY, USA

Luiz Gustavo Oliveira Brito Division of Gynecological Surgery, Department of Obstetrics and Gynecology, Faculty of Medical Sciences, State University of Campinas – UNICAMP, Campinas, Brazil

Benjamin M. Brucker New York University School of Medicine, New York, NY, USA

Jill C. Buckley UC San Diego Health, San Diego, CA, USA

Christine A. Burke University of California Los Angeles, Los Angeles, CA, USA

Lysanne Campeau Department of Urology, Jewish General Hospital, Montreal, QC, Canada

Farzana Cassim Division of Urology, Stellenbosch University/Tygerberg Hospital, Cape Town, South Africa

Lewis Chan Department of Urology, Concord Repatriation General Hospital and University of Sydney, Sydney, NSW, Australia

Olivia H. Chang Division of Female Urology, Voiding Dysfunction and Pelvic Reconstructive Surgery, Department of Urology, University of California Irvine, Irvine, CA, USA

C. R. Chapple Department of Urology, Sheffield Teaching Hospitals NHS Foundation Trust, Sheffield, UK

Emmanuel Chartier-Kastler Department of Urology, Sorbonne Université, Academic Hospital Pitié-Salpêtrière, Paris, France

Grace Chen Department of Urology, University of Illinois at Chicago, Chicago, IL, USA

Bilal Chughtai Department of Urology, Weill Cornell Medicine/New York Presbyterian, New York, NY, USA

Department of Obstetrics and Gynecology, Weill Cornell Medicine/New York Presbyterian, New York, NY, USA

Doreen E. Chung Department of Urology, Columbia University Irving Medical Center, New York, NY, USA

Jacques Corcos Department of Urology, McGill University, Jewish General Hospital, Montreal, QC, Canada

Francisco Cruz Department of Urology, Faculty of Medicine of University of Porto, Hospital São João, I3S Institute for Investigation and Innovation in Health, Porto, Portugal

Elise J. B. De Massachusetts General Hospital, Boston, MA, USA

Mirosav L. Djordjevic Belgrade Center for Urogenital Reconstructive Surgery, Belgrade, Serbia

Roger R. Dmochowski Department of Urology, Vanderbilt University Medical Center, Nashville, TN, USA

Mohamed El-Sherbiny Department of Surgery and Pediatric surgery, McGill University Health Center and Montreal Children's Hospital, Montreal, QC, Canada

Katherine E. Fero Department of Urology, David Geffen School of Medicine at UCLA, Los Angeles, CA, USA

Frederico Ferronha Centro Hospitalar e Universitário Lisboa Central, Lisbon, Portugal

Kelsey E. Gallo UC San Diego Health, San Diego, CA, USA

Stéphanie Gazdovich Department of Urology, Maisonneuve-Rosemont Hospital, University of Montreal, QC, Canada

Jason Gilleran William Beaumont School of Medicine, Beaumont Hospital, Oakland University, Royal Oak, MI, USA

David Ginsberg USC Institute of Urology, Los Angeles, CA, USA

Natasha Ginzburg Department of Urology, SUNY Upstate Medical University, Syracuse, NY, USA

Stephanie Gleicher Department of Urology, Vanderbilt University Medical Center, Nashville, TN, USA

Kathryn Goldrath University of California Los Angeles, Los Angeles, CA, USA

Alex Gomelsky Department of Urology, LSU Health Shreveport, Shreveport, LA, USA

Christopher Gonzales-Alabastro Department of Urology, Northwestern University Feinberg School of Medicine, Chicago, IL, USA

Gabriela Gonzalez Department of Urology, University of California, Davis School of Medicine, Sacramento, CA, USA

Ganesh Gopalakrishnan Vedanayagam Hospital, Coimbatore, India

Angelo E. Gousse Department of Urology, Larkin Hospital Palm Springs Teaching Hospital, Miami, FL, USA

Bailey Goyette Division of Urology, Department of Surgery, University of MIssouri, Columbia, USA

Tamsin Greenwell University College London Hospitals, London, UK

Heléna Gresty University College London Hospitals, London, UK

Cara L. Grimes Departments of Obstetrics and Gynecology and Urology, New York Medical College, Valhalla, NY, USA

Tamara Grisales University of California Los Angeles, Los Angeles, CA, USA

Serigne Gueye Cheikh Anta Diop University/Hospital General Idrissa Poueye, Dakar, Senegal

Sender Herschorn Sunnybrook Health Sciences Centre, Toronto, ON, Canada

Ly Hoang Roberts William Beaumont School of Medicine, Beaumont Hospital, Oakland University, Royal Oak, MI, USA

Matthias Hofer Urology San Antonio, San Antonio, TX, USA

Henriette Veiby Holm Section of reconstructive urology and neurourology, Department of Urology, Oslo University Hospital Rikshospitalet, Oslo, Norway

Matthew L. Izett-Kay Department of Urogynaecology, The John Radcliffe Hospital, Oxford University Hospitals, Oxford, UK

Nuffield Department of Women's and Reproductive Health, Women's Centre, Oxford University, Oxford, UK

Jamaal C. Jackson Rush University Medical Center, Chicago, IL, USA

Tom Jarvis Department of Urology, Prince of Wales Hospital and University of NSW, Randwick, NSW, Australia

Rita Jen USC Institute of Urology, Los Angeles, CA, USA

Rabun Jones Department of Urology, University of Illinois at Chicago, Chicago, IL, USA

Pankaj M. Joshi UROKUL, Pune, India

Jean A. Juras Centre d'Imagerie Médicale Cardinet, Paris, France

Priyanka Kancherla Department of Urology, SUNY Upstate Medical University, Syracuse, NY, USA

Melissa R. Kaufman Department of Urology, Vanderbilt University Medical Center, Nashville, TN, USA

Abdulghani Khogeer Department of Surgery, Faculty of Medicine, Rabigh, King Abdulaziz University, Jeddah, Saudi Arabia

Stephanie J. Kielb Department of Urology, Northwestern University Feinberg School of Medicine, Chicago, IL, USA

Ja-Hong Kim Division of Pelvic Medicine and Reconstructive Surgery, David Geffen School of Medicine at UCLA, Los Angeles, CA, USA

Department of Urology, David Geffen School of Medicine at UCLA, Los Angeles, CA, USA

Michelle E. Van Kuiken Department of Urology, University of California, San Francisco, CA, USA

Sanjay B. Kulkarni UROKUL, Pune, India

Andrew Lai Department of Urology, University of Illinois at Chicago, Chicago, IL, USA

A. Lawrence Counties Manukau and Auckland Hospital, Auckland, New Zealand

Una J. Lee Section of Urology and Renal Transplantation, Virginia Mason Franciscan Health, Seattle, WA, USA

Warren Lo Urology, Hospital Kuala Lumpur, Kuala Lumpur, Malaysia

Jennifer A. Locke Sunnybrook Health Sciences Centre, Toronto, ON, Canada

Francisco E. Martins Department of Urology, Reconstructive Urology Unit, School of Medicine, Hospital Santa Maria, CHULN, University of Lisbon, Lisbon, Portugal

Natalia Martins Urology Division, Armed Forces Hospital, Lisbon, Portugal

Ejikeme Mbajiorgu School of Anatomical Sciences, University of the Witwatersrand, Johannesburg, South Africa

Kathrin Meisterhofer Department of Urology, University Hospital of Tuebingen; Eberhard Karls University, Tuebingen, Germany

Pedro Abreu Mendes Department of Urology, Faculty of Medicine of University of Porto, Hospital São João, I3S Institute for Investigation and Innovation in Health, Porto, Portugal

Miguel Miranda Urology Department, Centro Hospitalar Universitário Lisboa Norte, Lisbon, Lisboa, Portugal

Dena E. Moskowitz Department of Urology, University of California Irvine, Irvine, CA, USA

Vishen Naidoo Division of Urology, University of the Witwatersrand, Johannesburg, South Africa

Madina Ndoye Department of Urology, Cheikh Anta Diop University/Hospital General Idrissa Poueye, Dakar, Senegal

Oluwarotimi S. Nettey Scott Department of Urology, Baylor College of Medicine, Houston, Texas, USA

Sarah Neu Sunnybrook Health Sciences Centre, Toronto, ON, Canada

Jun Jiet Ng Urogynecology, Hospital Kuala Lumpur, Kuala Lumpur, Malaysia

Lamine Niang Cheikh Anta Diop University/Hospital General Idrissa Poueye, Dakar, Senegal

Victor Nitti Division of Female Pelvic Medicine and Reconstructive Surgery, Departments of Urology and Obstetrics and Gynecology, David Geffen School of Medicine at UCLA, Los Angeles, CA, USA

Atieh Novin USC Institute of Urology, Los Angeles, CA, USA

Tom Øresland Faculty of Medicine University of Oslo, Oslo, Norway

N. Osman Department of Urology, Sheffield Teaching Hospitals NHS Foundation Trust, Sheffield, UK

Priya Padmanabhan Oakland University William Beaumont School of Medicine, Beaumont Hospital, Royal Oak, MI, USA

Paulo Cesar Rodrigues Palma Department of Surgery, Faculty of Medical Sciences, State University of Campinas – UNICAMP, Campinas, Brazil

Domnique Malacarne Pape Departments of Obstetrics and Gynecology and Urology, New York Medical College, Valhalla, NY, USA

Jan Alberto Paredes Mogica Anahuac University, Mexico City, Mexico

Jennifer E. Park University of California Los Angeles, Los Angeles, CA, USA

Ricardo Pereira e Silva Urology, Faculdade de Medicina, Universidade de Lisboa; Centro Hospitalar Universitário Lisboa Norte, Lisbon, Portugal

Kenneth M. Peters William Beaumont School of Medicine, Beaumont Hospital, Oakland University, Royal Oak, MI, USA

Rui Pinto Department of Urology, Faculty of Medicine of University of Porto, Hospital São João, I3S Institute for Investigation and Innovation in Health, Porto, Portugal

Simon Podnar Division of Neurology, University Medical Centre Ljubljana, Ljubljana, Slovenia

S. Pusica Belgrade Center for Urogenital Reconstructive Surgery, Belgrade, Serbia

Shirin Razdan Department of Urology, Icahn School of Medicine at Mount Sinai Hospital, New York, NY, USA

F. Reeves Department of Urology, The Royal Melbourne Hospital, Melbourne, Australia

Felicity Reeves Addenbrookes Hospital, Cambridge, UK

W. Stuart Reynolds Department of Urology, Vanderbilt University Medical Center, Nashville, TN, USA

Cassio Luis Zanettini Riccetto Division of Female Urology, Department of Surgery, Faculty of Medical Sciences, State University of Campinas – UNICAMP, Campinas, Brazil

Silke Riechardt Department of Urology, University Hospital Hamburg-Eppendorf, Hamburg, Germany

Jose Bernal Riquelme Urology Division, Hospital Sotero Del Rio, Santiago, Chile

Margaret S. Roubaud Department of Plastic Surgery, Division of Surgery, The University of Texas MD Anderson Cancer Center, Houston, TX, USA

S. Saad Department of Urology, Sheffield Teaching Hospitals NHS Foundation Trust, Sheffield, UK

Jaspreet S. Sandhu Memorial Sloan Kettering Cancer Center, New York, NY, USA

Stephanie Sansone Department of Urology, Weill Cornell Medicine/New York Presbyterian, New York, NY, USA

Department of Obstetrics and Gynecology, Weill Cornell Medicine/New York Presbyterian, New York, NY, USA

Johannes Kurt Schultz Department of GI Surgery, Akershus University Hospital, Lørenskog, Norway

Elisabeth M. Sebesta Department of Urology, Vanderbilt University Medical Center, Nashville, TN, USA

Jas Singh Department of Urology, Division of Surgery, The University of Texas MD Anderson Cancer Center, Houston, TX, USA

Larry T. Sirls Oakland University William Beaumont School of Medicine, Beaumont Hospital, Royal Oak, MI, USA

Thomas G. Smith III Department of Urology, Division of Surgery, The University of Texas MD Anderson Cancer Center, Houston, TX, USA

Amythis Soltani Department of Obstetrics and Gynecology, Westchester Medical Center, Valhalla, NY, USA

Gillian Stearns Carolinas Medical Center, Charlotte, NC, USA

Arnulf Stenzl Department of Urology, University Hospital of Tuebingen; Eberhard Karls University, Tuebingen, Germany

John T. Stoffel University of Michigan, Ann Arbor, MI, USA

B. Stojanovic Belgrade Center for Urogenital Reconstructive Surgery, Belgrade, Serbia

School of Medicine, University of Belgrade, Belgrade, Serbia

Ann C. Stolzle LSU Health Shreveport School of Medicine, Shreveport, LA, USA

Anne M. Suskind Department of Urology, University of California, San Francisco, CA, USA

Suzette E. Sutherland UW Medicine Pelvic Health Center, Department of Urology, University of Washington School of Medicine, Seattle, WA, USA

Helal Syed Division of Urology, Department of Surgery, Children's Hospital Los Angeles | University of Southern California Keck School of Medicine, Los Angeles, CA, USA

Christina Sze Department of Urology, Weill Cornell Medicine/New York Presbyterian, New York, NY, USA

Justina Tam Section of Urology and Renal Transplantation, Virginia Mason Franciscan Health, Seattle, WA, USA

Urogynecology, Stony Brook Medicine, Stony Brook, NY, USA

Nikolaos Thanatsis Urogynaecology and Pelvic Floor Unit, University College London Hospital, London, UK

Michele Torosis Division of Female Pelvic Medicine and Reconstructive Surgery, Departments of Urology and Obstetrics and Gynecology, David Geffen School of Medicine at UCLA, Los Angeles, CA, USA

Liliya Tryfonyuk Urology Division, Rivne Regional Hospital, Rivne, Ukraine

Vincent Tse Department of Urology, Concord Repatriation General Hospital and University of Sydney, Sydney, NSW, Australia

Arvind Vashisht Urogynaecology and Pelvic Floor Unit, University College London Hospital, London, UK

Bobby Viswaroop Vedanayagam Hospital, Coimbatore, India

David B. Vodušek Institute of Clinical Neurophysiology, Division of Neurology, University Medical Centre Ljubljana, Ljubljana, Slovenia

Annah Vollstedt Department of Urology, University of Iowa Hospitals and Clinics, Iowa City, IA, USA

Connie N. Wang Department of Urology, Columbia University Irving Medical Center, New York, NY, USA

O. Lenaine Westney Department of Urology, Division of Surgery, The University of Texas MD Anderson Cancer Center, Houston, TX, USA

Michael W. Witthaus UC San Diego Health, San Diego, CA, USA

Oleksandr Yatsina Department of Urological Surgery, National Cancer Institute, Kyiv, Ukraine

Part I

History, Basic Science, and Epidemiology

Historical Milestones in Female Genitourinary and Pelvic Floor Reconstruction

1

Francisco E. Martins, Natalia Martins, and Liliya Tryfonyuk

Contents

Introduction 4

Antiquity 4

Medieval Era 6

The Renaissance 7

The Seventeenth Century 10

The Eighteenth Century 11

The Nineteenth Century Before Asepsia 11

The Nineteenth Century: The Birth of Asepsia 13

The Twentieth and Twenty-First Centuries: The Evolution of a Specialty 18

Conclusion 25

References 25

Abstract

The history of female genitourinary and pelvic floor reconstruction dates back to the earliest

F. E. Martins (✉)
Department of Urology, Reconstructive Urology Unit, School of Medicine, Hospital Santa Maria, CHULN, University of Lisbon, Lisbon, Portugal
e-mail: faemartins@gmail.com

N. Martins
Urology Division, Armed Forces Hospital, Lisbon, Portugal

L. Tryfonyuk
Urology Division, Rivne Regional Hospital, Rivne, Ukraine

days of recorded medical history. Throughout this time, pelvic organ prolapse, urinary incontinence, and vesicovaginal fistula are among the conditions that have undergone significant evolution in terms of both pathophysiology and treatment. Lack of anesthesia, ignorance of asepsis, defective suture materials, poor instrumentation, and deficient exposure hampered any consistent success until the mid-nineteenth century.

The evolution of the female pelvic surgery from the Hippocratic age to the antiseptic period has fascinated many physicians involved with the treatment of these pelvic conditions in the female, often leading to original concepts and

© Springer Nature Switzerland AG 2023
F. E. Martins et al. (eds.), *Female Genitourinary and Pelvic Floor Reconstruction*,
https://doi.org/10.1007/978-3-031-19598-3_1

theories occasionally to fell from favor only to be resuscitated and popularized by subsequent generations. Pelvic organ prolapse was one of these conditions to be first described in the dawn of recorded medical history in the Ebers Papyrus in 1500 BC. The condition has remained a common and debilitating pelvic floor disorder in women leading to significant impact on quality of life. Pelvic organ prolapse has evolved from rudimentary pessaries and herbal medicines into modern robotic repair procedures. Both ancient anatomists and, more recently, advances in modern technology have followed the path of progress in surgical treatment. Moreover, with the significant increase of the post-menopausal population with life expectancy doubling through the twentieth century, there has been a growing demand for better quality of life and management of genitourinary and pelvic floor disorders. The objective of this chapter is to attempt to highlight the milestones that occurred along this long path and to honor the pioneers who significantly contributed to shape a specialty and upon whose shoulders we stand.

Keywords

History · Female · Genitourinary · Pelvic medicine · Reconstruction · Pelvic organ prolapse · Ancient civilization · Papyrus

Introduction

The entrance into the new millennium with all the many advances in genitourinary and pelvic floor reconstructive surgery, it would be appropriate to focus on the achievements of past and to make new suggestions for the future. The post-menopausal population has significantly expanded which has been paralleled by a growing demand for better quality of life and management of genitourinary and pelvic floor conditions.

Although factors such as childbearing and persistent and sudden increases in intra-abdominal pressure are known to contribute to pelvic organ prolapse, only recently has there been rising interest and demand to deal with the resulting problems. In the industrialized world, urinary incontinence has become the most common cause of admission to long-term institutionalized centers with billions of government budgets spent diapers and pad products to "palliate" the discomfort, as these measures do not treat the underlying problem of incontinence.

Since the beginning of the medical written history, gynecological and urological conditions have been described. Disorders of the female urinary bladder can be found in the Kahun Papyrus approximately 2000 years BC. A disease classification by systems and organs can be found in the Ebers Papyrus, 1500 BC.

Enormous progress has been made in the diagnosis and treatment of pelvic floor disorders and urinary incontinence in the last century leading to the creation of a new, burgeoning subspecialty termed as female urology by urologists, urogynecology by gynecologists, and also involving colorectal surgeons in this competing political feud. Nonetheless, in the ultimate best interest of the patient, this challenge should be solved by providing the best women's healthcare and quality of life possible through a multidisciplinary approach to manage genitourinary and pelvic floor disorders, including urinary incontinence, fecal incontinence, genital and anal prolapse, urogenital aging, conservative treatment, and reconstructive pelvic surgery [1].

Antiquity

The first sources dealing briefly with female genitourinary and pelvic floor disorders are Egyptian manuscripts dating back to the second millennium BC (1500 BCE), specifically the Ebers Papyrus and the Smith Papyrus [2–4]. The Ebers Papyrus is a collection of around 900 recipes to remedy a wide diversity of poorly defined problems. Among these remedies, some were aimed at "to remove the urine too often" and "to remove constant running of urine" [2, 5, 6]. In its 31st case, Smith Papyrus described urinary incontinence resulting from spinal cord injury in a man. "A dislocation of a cervical vertebra should cause a state of quadriplegia, while the phallus would be erect, and urine would drop persistently without notice." This was the 31st description in the Smith Papyrus [3, 7].

Uterine prolapse is a condition that has likely affected women for always as it is documented in the oldest medical literature. In fact, uterine prolapse and its potential treatment is mentioned in the Ebers Papyrus, considered the oldest documental medical literature, where it is written "of a woman whose posterior, belly, and branching of her thighs are painful, say thou as to it, it is the falling of the womb" (Kahun papyrus ca. 1835 BCE) [8]. The Ebers Papyrus goes on to recommend "to correct a displaced womb: with oil of earth (petroleum) with fedder (manure) and honey; rub the body of the patient" (Ebers Papyrus ca. 1550 BCE) [9].

For more than one thousand years later, during Hippocrates' epoch (c. 460–377 BCE) and the subsequent generations that he influenced, an animalistic concept prevailed in the medical thought comparing the uterus to a wild animal that would act aggressively unto itself when deprived of male semen. This animalistic concept would lead to treatments such as fumigation; the pleasant ones would be placed at a woman's head and the wicked ones near her prolapsed womb to cause retreat of the uterus. Hippocrates and Polybus (his son-in-law) provided the earliest description in their noted text "On Diseases of Women" of a pessary with the application of an astringent to the womb and placement of a vinegar-soaked sponge or pomegranate to reduce uterine prolapse. If these treatments failed, women would be subjected to the practice of hanging a woman upside down tied by her feet to a fixed bar and bouncing her continually until her prolapse reduced then leaving her bound to her bed for 3 days with her legs tied together. This procedure was called succussion (Fig. 1) [10, 11].

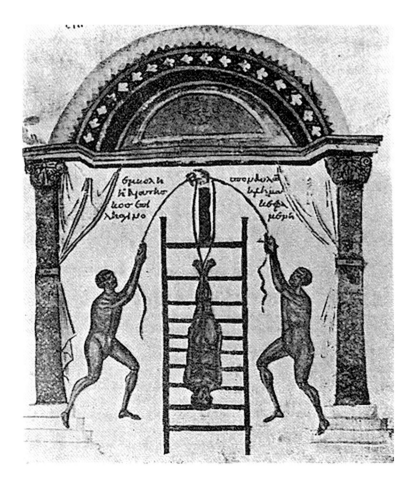

Fig. 1 Illustration from a medieval book describing treatment of prolapse by Hippocrates. Succussion treatment – the practice of tying a woman upside down by her feet to a fixed frame and bouncing her repeatedly until her prolapse reduced then leaving her bedbound for 3 days with her legs tied together [9]

A gradual shift in medical perception began to take place at the end of the Hippocratic era. Medicine slowly began to drift away from rituals and magic, with the doctrine of Common Era (CE) replacing the animalistic theory. By the first century of CE, Soranus of Ephesus (98–138 CE), considered the most notable gynecologic authority of antiquity, rejected Hippocrates' approach to treating uterine prolapse, considering them nonsensical, useless, and physically unbearable. He described the uterus based on human cadaver dissection and performed hysterectomy for uterine prolapse. However, he also described medical treatments such as "...bathing the prolapsed part of the uterus with much lukewarm olive oil, and making a woolen tampon corresponding in shape and diameter to the vagina and wrapping it in very thin clean linen... then dipping it briefly in vinegar... acacia juice... or wine, and then applying it to the uterus and moving the whole prolapsed part, forcing it up gently until the uterus has been reverted to its proper place and the whole mass of wool being left in the vagina" [12]. Soranus' writings set the foundations for gynecologic texts until the seventeenth century. Yet, despite Soranus' contribution to therapeutic advances, old-fashioned, preconceived concepts about the uterus would linger. As late as the second century CE, prominent Greek physician Aretaeus the Cappadocian, in his "Causes and Indications of Acute and Chronic Diseases," still described the uterus as "an animal within an animal" [13].

Despite Soranus's vast knowledge of obstetrics and gynecology, female pelvic anatomy persisted imperfectly understood. Physicians of that time commonly referred to the uterus as mater (Latin for mother) or hystera (Greek for womb) in the plural form, believing the uterus consisted of several compartments [10]. Unfortunately, Rome's prohibition on the use of human cadavers hindered Claudius Galen's work (129–201 AD) to advance the knowledge of the female genital anatomy and led him to extrapolate his understanding of human anatomy from dissections and vivisections of lower animals in which the finding of uterine horns was commonplace [10].

In contrast to other more frequent diseases such as bladder stones, urinary retention, and urinary fistula, urinary incontinence is rarely mentioned in ancient medical writings. The first descriptions date back to Egyptian Papyri from the second millennium BC. However, these Egyptian manuscripts already mention devices for the collection of urine in men and pessaries in women.

Upon examination of the mummy Henhenit (circa 2050 BC), D. E. Derry in 1935 revealed a large vesicovaginal fistula with laceration of the perineum, which was most likely caused by birth trauma [4, 14].

The outstanding work of Hippocrates (460–377 BC) dominated Greek medicine of his time and beyond. He wrote extensively on the diseases of the urinary tract, specifically on perineal lithotomy and the management of urinary incontinence [6].

Claudius Galen from Pergamon was one of the first physicians to carry out physiological experiments on the lower urinary tract and postulated that micturition occurs by contraction of the abdominal muscles. He also clinically divided the causes of urinary retention into paralysis of the bladder due to spinal injury and bladder outlet obstruction due to bladder stones [6, 15].

Medieval Era

The Dark Ages and Medieval Period (476–1453) spanned from the fall of the Western Roman Empire to the Goths to the fall of Constantinople to the Ottomans in 1453. This era was characterized by a return to Theurgy and a regression of medicine. It was often referred to as the "Age of Faith" or "Era of Monastic Medicine" in which confidence in human deeds and achievements were replaced by divine faith. The Middle Ages were prodigal in bizarre concepts regarding female genitourinary and pelvic anatomy. The seven cells doctrine was an example of such concept which stated that the uterine cavity consisted of seven compartments, three on each side and one in the middle whereby male embryos developed on the right, the female on the left, and hermaphrodites in the middle [16]. Additionally, old beliefs from the Hippocratic period reemerged and as late as 1603. Rodrigo de Castro (c. 1546–1627), a Portuguese medical author, of Jewish origin, who was exiled in Hamburg after escaping persecution by the Inquisition, wrote "De Universa Mulierum Medicina" (1603). In one of his texts, he advised a drastic treatment for uterus prolapse "with a red-hot iron as if to burn, consequently causing fright to force the prolapsed part to retreat into the vagina" [10]. Another example came from Saint Benedict, founder of the Benedictine Order, who encouraged his monks to care for the sick but prohibited any official medical education. Most of their work was exclusively to care for patients with leprosy, plagues, prostitution, and poverty, without any investment in medical knowledge. Many of these medical practitioners were itinerant quacks and charlatans. Therefore, from the standpoint of medical science, the Medieval Era stands for a dark period for Europe, in which the ideas of Greek and Roman authors were maintained and supported by Arabian medicine as exemplified by the writings of Avicenna (930–1037 AD), until they were ultimately revived by the European Renaissance scientists.

anatomy. Artists of that time participated in private anatomic dissections to further their training, something physicians needed to perform in a rational and persistent fashion [10]. However, with some exceptions, important drawings by master artists of that time, particularly Leonardo da Vinci, did not capture the physicians' attention. In the early sixteenth century, an Italian physician, Jacopo Berengario da Carpi (c. 1460–c. 1530), published a book titled *Isagoge Breves* in 1522 that made him the most important anatomist before Andreas Vesalius (Fig. 2). He was also credited as producing the first authenticated description of vaginal hysterectomy in 1521 based on two cases, one performed by himself and the other by his father [18]. He was later appointed *Maestro nello Studio* at the University of Bologna, an institution of high prestige with scholars of considerable reputation. Berengario made several important advances in anatomy through dissection of human cadavers. He also denied some of Galenic anatomy, including the existence of Galen's *rete mirabile* based on his vast personal work in dissection, thereby leaving a significant legacy in medicine.

Leonardo da Vinci (1452–1519), contemporary of Berengario da Carpi, was the founder of

The Renaissance

This period of European history, initiated in Florence, marked the transition from the Medieval Era to modern age and covers the fifteenth and sixteenth centuries. It was characterized by the rebirth of a culture of individual thinking, free enterprise, and independence from authoritarian rule. A group of artists and intellectuals began to center their attention on the achievements and fashions of the classical age. This brought about a renewed awareness of the beauty of nature and human form based on humanism, the intellectual basis of the Renaissance period [17].

The Renaissance period was marked by the emergence of academic life, universities, printing press, as well as self-education that fostered the medical field to a superior level and promoted an improved understanding of female genitourinary

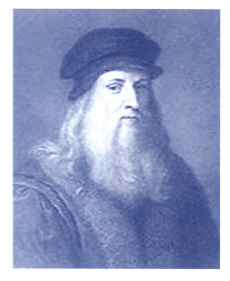

Fig. 2 Giacomo Berengario Da Carpi (1470–1550). An Italian physician and anatomist, who gave the first authenticated report of vaginal hysterectomy in 1521

iconographic and physiologic anatomy, responsible for the basis of modern anatomic illustration. In his highly impressive studies and numerous dissections of the human body over more than 25 years, he produced a vast anatomical portfolio, particularly of the lower urinary tract. He depicts an open and funnel-shaped bladder neck in his drawings of the bladder and pelvic cavity with detailed definition of the bladder neck and internal urinary sphincter structures (Fig. 3). He also gives the first accurate descriptions of the fetus in utero. However, he was not aware of the contraction capacity of the detrusor muscle and does not mention the problem of urinary incontinence. Unfortunately, as Leonardo da Vinci did not finish his work and failed to publish them as a textbook on anatomy, his drawings were considered only of medico-legal interest and did not impact the scientific progress at his time [19].

Ambroise Paré (1510–1590) was a French barber and later a renowned military surgeon, who served as a barber for the French kings Henry II, Francis II, Charles IX, and Henry III. He was considered the most famous surgeon of the Renaissance period and one of the pioneers of surgery and modern forensic medicine. He described the changes leading to bladder outlet obstruction and perceived the mechanism of synchronized detrusor contraction and sphincter relaxation during micturition. He introduced innovative surgical techniques such as vascular ligatures for hemostasis in lieu of cautery and in the battlefield medicine, especially in the treatment of wounds. However, the use of ligatures did not gain popularity for the ensuing three centuries until Sir Joseph Lister (1827–1912) introduced a longer-lasting aseptic type of suture in the mid-nineteenth century.

Andreas Vesalius (1514–1564) was a Dutch-born anatomist, physician, and author of one of the most authoritative books on human anatomy, titled *De Humani Corporis Fabrica Libri Septem* (on the fabric of the human body in seven books) (Fig. 4). He is often referred to as the founder of modern human anatomy. He became a professor at the University of Padua (1537–1542) and later physician to Emperor Charles V. In 1542, Vesalius met Jan van Calcar, a famous illustrator and

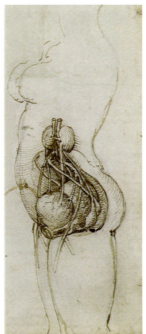
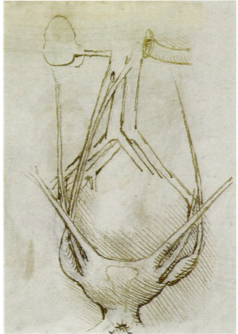

Fig. 3 Leonardo da Vinci (Vinci 1452-Amboise 1519). Recto: The vulva and anus. Verso: The male and female reproductive systems c.1508. Royal Collection Trust. [19]

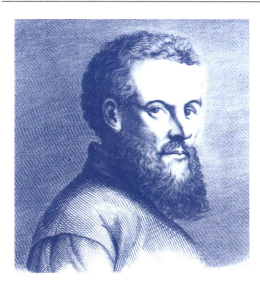 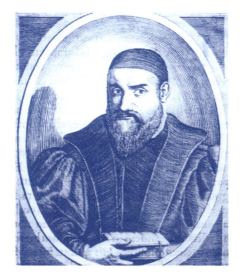

Fig. 4 Andreas Vesalius (1514–1564). Father of modern anatomy

Fig. 5 Gabriele Falloppio (1523–1562) and the Fallopian tube (oviduct) | (SpringerLink)

student of Titan, with whom he published his first and famous anatomical illustrations *Tabulae Anatomicae Sex* in 1583 [20]. He was one of the first of his time to challenge the unassailable teachings of Claudius Galen of Pergamon, asserting that any physician must perform cadaver dissection before learning his art. Consequently, Vesalius converted human cadaver dissection into a feasible and reputable profession, considering hands-on direct observation the only reliable source of learning and evidence. Vesalius illustrated accurately the entire female genitourinary tract and its vasculature, highlighting for the first time the fact that the left ovarian vein drained directly into the left renal vein as well as an accurate description of the suspensory ligaments of the uterus [16]. Vesalius produced distinguished students such as Gabriele Falloppio (1523–1562), an Italian Catholic priest and one of the most distinguished anatomists of the sixteenth century, who first accurately reported the human oviduct, naming it Fallopian tube, and described the clitoris as a vasomuscular structure (Fig. 5). Matthaeus Realdus Columbus (1484–1559), a professor of anatomy and surgeon also from Italy, was the first to employ the term *labia*, which he considered essential to protect the uterus from dust, cold, and air. Bartolomeo Eustachio (1520–1574), an Italian anatomist and one of the founders of human anatomy as a science, outlined accurately the uterine cavity and cervical canal. However, he is best known for his studies on the internal ear, giving his name to a tube in the internal ear anatomy.

Wilhelm Fabricius Hildanus (1560–1634), often considered the "Father of German Surgery," produced a modified urinal for the treatment of urinary incontinence which consisted either of a glass or the bladder of a pig that was secured to the genitals by straps for females and a penile clamp for males which was removed before micturition [4].

Caspar Stromayr, although mainly a German ophthalmologist and hernia surgeon, produced a book titled *Practica Copiosa* in 1559 that contains beautifully executed watercolors illustrating diseases of the genitourinary tract, including examination of uterine prolapse and placement of a pessary consisting of a sponge bound by twine, sealed with wax, and dipped in butter (Fig. 6). However, despite the many advances in pelvic anatomy during the Renaissance era, the clinical approach to most female genitourinary problems showed negligible progress compared to the classical period.

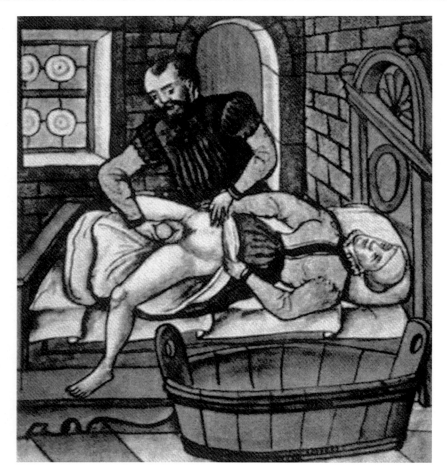

Fig. 6 Examination of uterine prolapse and placement of a pessary, sixteenth century. (From Stromayr C. Die Handschrift des Schnitt-und Augenarzles Caspar Stromayr, Lindau Munscript, 1559)

The Seventeenth Century

From the seventeenth century onward, a wealth of human knowledge shed light on science, specifically on physiology, anatomy, and human reproduction. Reinier de Graaf (1641–1673), a Dutch physician, physiologist, and anatomist, made fundamental discoveries, including the description of ovarian follicles and uterine fibroids as well as provided the first accurate account of the ovary's gross morphology, anatomic relations, and function (Fig. 7). He was the first to develop a syringe to inject dye into human reproductive organs for an accurate understanding of their structure and function. De Graaf may have been the first to realize the reproductive function of the Fallopian tube, to report the hydrosalpinx, relating its development to female infertility. Although De Graaf admitted he was not the first to describe the ovarian follicles, he described their development and recognized their reproductive significance, thereby being eponymously termed Graafian follicles [21, 22].

Johannes Scultetus (1595–1645), a German anatomist and surgeon, authored a book on pelvic surgery and surgical instruments with the title *Armamentarium Chirurgicum* shortly before his death. He was credited as being the first to utilize a series of drawings to detail surgical procedures in a stepwise fashion, and, therefore, this was considered the first textbook of surgery, describing the common surgical procedures and instruments

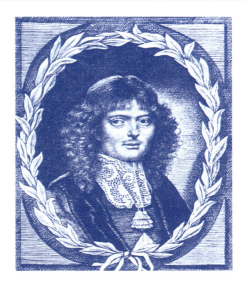

Fig. 7 Reinier de Graaf (1641–1673) provides the first accurate account of the female reproductive system and ovarian follicles ("de Graaf's follicles") [21]

at the time in words and illustrations in encyclopedical format, granting him the reputation of one of the most relevant surgeons of his century [23]. A few examples of these procedures were treatment of imperforate hymen, hematocolpos, clitoral hypertrophy, and the use of a T-binder after vaginal surgery [24].

The Eighteenth Century

A constant conflict between old and new ideas regarding female pelvic anatomy, pathology, and treatment characterized the eighteenth century. Although some relevant contributions were made in the fields of biology, physics, and microscopy, relatively sporadic advances took place in medicine. Surgery began to evolve beyond the isolated skills of an individual surgeon and coincided with the foundation of surgical societies and publication of medical journals. Remarkable achievements were made toward the understanding of pelvic anatomy during this period. Physicians remained, however, under close scrutiny from the public community, especially popular medical caricaturists.

In 1737, James Douglas (1675–1742), a famous anatomist, gynecologist, and an excellent botanist and zoologist, was the first to describe accurately the peritoneum. In his book titled *The Description of the Peritoneum, and of that part of the Membrane Cellularis which lies on its outside, with an Account of the True Situation of All the Abdominal Viscera*, he also was responsible for the description of important anatomical landmarks such as the "pouch of Douglas" and the "ligaments of Douglas" (Fig. 8a, b). The achievements of such utmost importance helped pave the way to retroperitoneal surgery and the concomitant decline in peritonitis that was a highly frequent and lethal complication of abdominal surgery of the era. Later, William Hunter (1718–1783), a disciple of Douglas, concluded his colossal work titled *Anatomy of the Gravid Uterus* in 1774. After Hunter's death, his collections were transferred to Glasgow University, forming the basis of the Hunterian Library and Museum. This collection also included manuscripts by James Douglas which most of them remain unpublished [24–26]. Jan van Rymsdyk lent his great artistic talent to this book which led many to regard this work as the best atlas of anatomy ever produced.

Vaginal specula continued to evolve with some modifications for better vaginal examinations and differential diagnosis between various "vaginal hernias," apparently different types of vaginal prolapse as already described by Ricci [10].

The Nineteenth Century Before Asepsia

Prior to the nineteenth century, any surgical attempt at treating pelvic organ prolapse, especially uterine, and concomitant cervical disease, was mostly limited to cervical amputation. Conrad Langenbeck (1776–1851), a German surgeon, ophthalmologist, and anatomist, performed the first elective and successful vaginal hysterectomy, alone and without anesthesia (Fig. 9). As Baskett wrote in 1996, "at one-point Langenbeck was left clutching the bleeding area in one hand and holding one end of the ligature in his teeth while tying the other end with his right hand" [24].

Several advances were made in America during the first half of the nineteenth century.

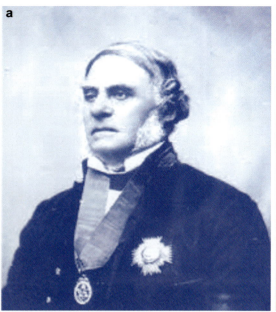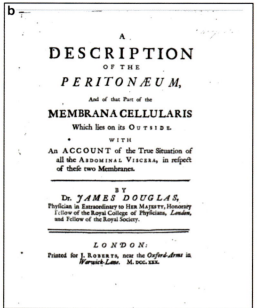

Fig. 8 (**a**) James Douglas (1675–1742) gave the first adequate description of the peritoneum. (**b**) The cover page of the famous book by James Douglas published in 1730. In this book, for the first time, is recorded the famous "pouch of Douglas." Public domain, Cureus. 2019 Jan; 11(1): e3919. Published online 2019 Jan 19 [26]

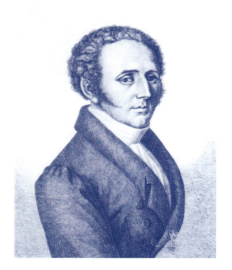

Fig. 9 Konrad Johann Martin Langenbeck (1776–1851) performed the first planned and successful vaginal hysterectomy [24]

However, the most widely known and reported was apparently performed by James Marion Sims (1813–1883), also known as the "father of modern gynecology." He described the surgical treatment of vesicovaginal fistula as a complication of obstructed labor. In the twenty-first century, however, he was criticized for developing his surgical procedures based on his improper medical ethics, such as operating without anesthesia on vulnerable, enslaved black women [27]. Marion Sims is also known for inventing the Sims' vaginal speculum, and the Sims' position used for examination of vaginal wall prolapse. John Peter Mettauer (1787–1875), a Virginia gynecologist, was credited with the first successful vesicovaginal fistula repair in 1883. He used lead suture in his surgical procedure. However, unaware of Mettauer's success, George A. Hayward (1791–1863) practicing at the Massachusetts General Hospital published the first report of an acceptable outcome approximately 1 year later. Hayward used silk suture for his procedure.

Surgical instruments used during the pre-aseptic era, which ended around 1890, were quite remarkable and extraordinary in variety and beauty. James M. Edmonson, PhD and Curator of the Dittrick Museum of Medical History, provided in his work entitled "American Surgical Instruments: The History of Their Manufacture and a Directory of Instrument Makers to 1900" a meticulous analysis of the medical, surgical, and dental instrument trades in America during a period from the late eighteenth century to early twentieth century. He also noted that surgical instruments manufactured prior to 1890 displayed high standards of workmanship, detail, and overall artistry, in many instances incorporating rare and beautiful materials that were later abandoned in the production of aseptic instruments [28]. The vaginal speculum was one of the most remarkable specimens that underwent continuous evolution through multiple modifications by their inventors in an attempt to improve exposure. In 1838, Joseph Charrière (1803–1876), a Swiss-born French manufacturer of surgical instruments, introduced an original shape of vaginal speculum that could be used as bivalve, trivalve, or quadrivalve device (Fig. 10). Charrière is currently best known for inventing a system to measure the size of the outer diameter of a catheter and other urological instruments such as endoscopes. In 1870, Edward Gabriel Cusco (1819–1894) introduced the more familiar "duckbill"-shaped speculum which remains in use by clinicians today (Fig. 11). However, in 1878 Cusco's speculum was replaced by the bivalved speculum designed by Thomas W. Graves.

In 1845, Sims (1813–1883) initiated his surgical experiments on slaves in his own hospital in Montgomery, Alabama, that he established for black slaves that he owned or rented and kept on his property. He called this facility "the first woman's hospital in history" (Fig. 12). These women suffered from vesicovaginal fistula, a condition Sims had not seen before, although common in those days. After multiple failed attempts at fistula repair, during 6 years of experimental work, without the use of anesthesia, he was the first to develop a consistently successful operation to cure vesicovaginal fistula. One of his patients underwent 30 operations before the repair was considered a success [29]. His success resulted from the use of silver sutures and the speculum of his own design that he used for exposure with the patient in his knee-chest position (Fig. 13).

Although Sims was not the first to use silver sutures in surgical procedures, most would agree that he popularized one of the first crucial changes in pelvic surgery. Soon after Sims' achievement, Washington Lemuel Atlee and Walter Burnham performed a myomectomy in 1844 and the first successful abdominal hysterectomy in 1853, respectively. Unfortunately, many of these operations were plagued by deadly, septic complications.

The Nineteenth Century: The Birth of Asepsia

The second half of the nineteenth century opened a new avenue of "more suitable" principles for more satisfactory surgery. These included anesthesia, antisepsis, and adequate suture materials. From mid-nineteenth century onward, female pelvic surgery began to accelerate its pace leading to

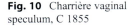

Fig. 10 Charrière vaginal speculum, C 1855

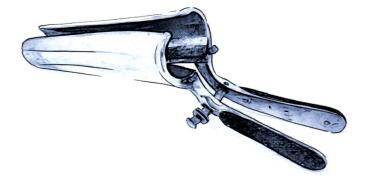

Fig. 11 Cusco Vaginal Speculum

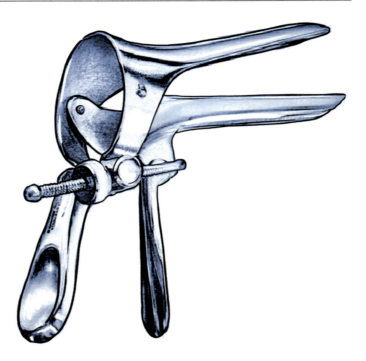

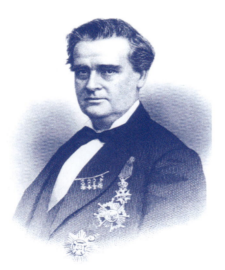

Fig. 12 James Marion Sims (1813–1883), American surgeon, known as the "father of gynecology"

unprecedented advances in gynecology in the entire domain of medicine. The remarkable achievement in transforming an essentially medical gynecology into a surgical specialty was quite impressive considering that this specialty remained stagnant for more than 2000 years.

This rapid growth of successful surgery became possible due to the introduction of effective anesthesia in 1846, Joseph Lister's work on asepsis in 1867, as well as the introduction of aseptic suture in 1869 which consisted of silk soaked in carbolic acid. Several individuals contributed to the evolution of the modern concept of asepsis. Ignaz Philipp Semmelweis (1818–1865), a German-Hungarian physician and scientist, became known as a pioneer of antisepsis and the "savior of mothers" (Fig. 14). He discovered that puerperal fever, a common problem in mid-nineteenth-century hospitals, could be drastically reduced to less than 1% if physicians disinfected their hands with chlorinated lime solutions in 1847 in Vienna General Hospital's First Obstetrical Clinic. Semmelweis' observations conflicted with the established scientific and medical opinions of the time. As a result, his ideas were ridiculed and rejected by the medical community. A few additional minor factors may also have played a role to this disbelief. Some doctors were offended at the suggestion that they should wash their hands, feeling that their social status as gentlemen was inconsistent with the idea that their hands could be unclean. Unfortunately, Semmelweis' results

Fig. 13 Sims' double-bladed vaginal speculum

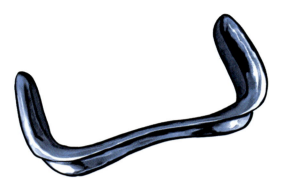

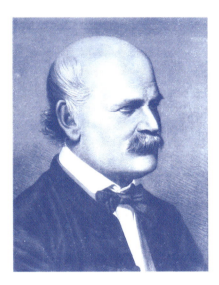

Fig. 14 Ignaz P. Semmelweis, a pioneer of antisepsis and known as "the savior of mothers"

lacked scientific foundation at the time. That became possible only in the 1860s and 1870s, when Louis Pasteur, Joseph Lister, and others further developed the germ theory of disease. Semmelweis' hypothesis of uncleanliness as the only cause was extreme at the time and was largely ignored, rejected, or ridiculed. He was dismissed from the hospital for political reasons and harassed by the medical community in Vienna, being eventually forced to move to Budapest.

Louis Pasteur (1822–1895) was a French chemist and microbiologist who became famous for his discoveries of the principles of vaccination, bacterial fermentation, and a process of food sterilization through heat (usually below 100 °C/ 212 °F) called pasteurization (Fig. 15). His research in chemistry and microbiology led to significant breakthroughs in the etiology and prevention of diseases, thereby laying the foundations of hygiene, public health, and much of modern medicine [30]. He was also considered the "father of bacteriology" [31].

Joseph Lister is also considered a pioneer of antiseptic surgery and preventive medicine, successfully introducing and championing the use of carbolic acid, also known as phenol, in the sterilization of surgical instruments and cleaning wounds. Lister's work led to a reduction in postoperative infections and made surgery safer for patients, distinguishing him as the "father of modern surgery" (Fig. 16) [32].

William Stewart Halsted (1852–1922), surgeon at the Johns Hopkins Hospital in Baltimore, Maryland, is considered a pioneer of everything from operating room uniforms to surgical gloves, implementing a no-street clothes policy in the operating room (Fig. 17). This helped to prevent infection of open wounds. He also enforced a rigorous hand-washing ritual with strong chemicals like permanganate and mercury bichloride solution and scrubbing with stiff brushes. However, William Halsted is likely best known in the surgical field by the introduction of several new operations, especially the radical mastectomy for breast cancer.

An astonishing variety of surgical procedures were performed in the nineteenth century are splendidly illustrated in *Traité Complet de l'Anatomie de l'Homme Comprenant la Médicine*

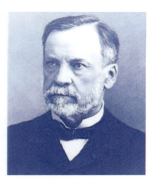

Fig. 15 Louis Pasteur, French chemist and microbiologist [30]

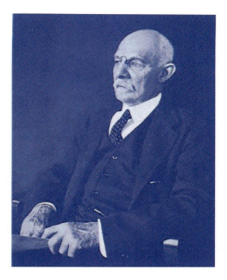

Fig. 17 William Stewart Halsted (1852–1922) a pioneer in surgical therapy and father of modern breast surgery

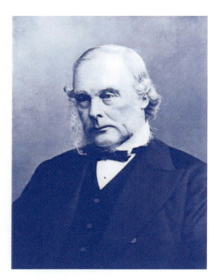

Fig. 16 Joseph Lister, a British surgeon, medical scientist, experimental pathologist and a pioneer of antiseptic surgery and preventative medicine [32]

Opératoire by Jean-Baptiste Marc Bourgery and Nicolas Henri Jacob. This work of 749 hand-colored lithographs was considered unrivaled in technical detail and beauty in the entire literature of medicine in the nineteenth century.

The second half of the nineteenth century was marked by several notable additions to pelvic surgery and a refined understanding of the anatomy of the pelvic cavity. Anders Adolf Retzius (1796–1860), a Swedish physician, professor of anatomy and a supervisor at the Karolinska Institute, defined the limits of the prevesical space in 1849 which is named after him. Léon Clement Le Fort (1829–1893), a French surgeon, is best remembered for his work on uterine prolapse, including the description of partial colpocleisis that is also known as Le Fort's operation, useful and simple alternative treatment of uterine prolapse in the high-risk patient. Alwin Mackenrodt (1859–1925), a German gynecologist, reported on the etiology and cure of uterine prolapse in 1895 and produced an accurate description of the pelvic connective tissue including the transverse cervical or cardinal ligaments, also known as Mackenrodt's ligaments (Fig. 18).

About the same time, William Fothergill (1865–1926) and Archibald Donald (1840–1908), two obstetric/gynecologists from Manchester, developed the Manchester operation for uterine prolapse and cystocele consisting of cervical amputation, uniting, or plicating, parametric and paravaginal tissues including Mackenrodt's ligaments to one another in front of the cervix, followed by anterior colporrhaphy and posterior colpoperineorrhaphy, thus allowing women to keep their uterus, if desirable. This procedure was a good alternative to the use of a pessary in young women.

Although the first radical hysterectomy operation is credited to John G. Clark at the Johns Hopkins Hospital in 1895, Ernst Wertheim

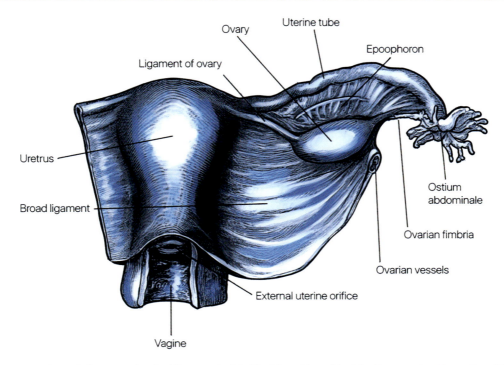

Fig. 18 Mackenrodt ligaments (cardinal ligaments). (Modified from Henry Vandyke Carter et al. – Henry Gray (1918) *Anatomy of the Human Body*: Gray's Anatomy)

(1864–1920), an Austrian gynecologist, introduced important modifications and ultimately popularized the radical abdominal hysterectomy operation for cervical cancer in 1898 [33]. This operation involved removal of the uterus, parametrium, paravaginal tissues, and pelvic lymph nodes, but leaving the ovaries in place. In 1944, Meigs "re-popularized" the surgical technique introducing an additional modification characterized as removal of all pelvic lymph nodes. This surgical procedure became known as Wertheim-Meigs operation.

Pessaries are manual devices that are inserted into the vagina to help support and reposition descended pelvic organs. Their use for the treatment of female pelvic prolapse dates back to before Hippocrates and was documented in early Egyptian papyruses. The term "pessary" derives from the Ancient Greek word "*pessós*," meaning round stone used for games [34]. The use of pessaries to treat pelvic prolapse became more established by the end of the sixteenth century, when the first purpose-made pessaries appeared due to the creativity of Ambroise Paré [34]. Surprisingly, the popularity of pessaries started to grow only during the second half of the nineteenth century as practitioners became apprehensive with anatomical misplacement of the uterus (Fig. 19). Hugh Hodge of Philadelphia (1796–1873) was a major proponent of pessary use apparently related to his belief that certain diseases were induced by uterine retroversion. Sharing the sentiments of many of his American fellow gynecologists, in 1860, he declared pessary use to be the "sine qua non" for the treatment of uterine displacements [35]. One of the ideal qualities for a pessary was the incorruptible nature of the material used for its manufacture, that is, material that resisted decomposition, besides maintaining a normal uterine position, allowing for normal movement, and neither causing pain nor infection or bleeding [36]. These qualities

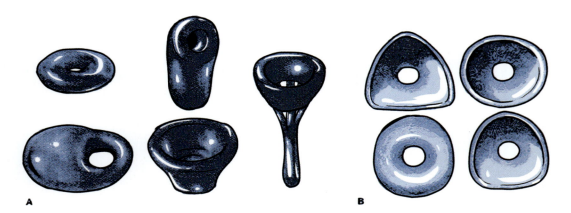

Fig. 19 A. Baskett T.F. (2006) The History of Passaries for Uterovaginal Prolapse. Modified from Farell S.A. (eds) Pessaries in Clinical Practice. Springer, London. B. Some nineteenth-century vaginal pessaries. From Bourgery JM. Traité Complet de l'Anatomie de L'Homme Comprenant la Médicine Opératoire. *Paris: Guerin*, 1866–1868

fostered an explosion in the number and varieties of pessaries in the market as well as fortune made by gynecologists who prescribed them and those who removed them (something like the use of vaginal mesh recently) [36].

However, not everyone in the medical profession was so keen on pessary use. In 1866, during his satirical presidential address to the New Hampshire State Medical Society, W. D. Buck commented: "I do think that this filling the vagina with such traps, making a Chinese toy-shop of it, is outrageous" [37]. Despite this negative sentiment, pessaries would remain popular throughout the nineteenth century. The introduction of asepsis by Lister and anesthesia by Morton, coupled with advances in suture materials and surgical instruments, would lead surgery to replace the pessary as the prevailing method of treatment of uterine prolapse. Nonetheless, modern-day pessaries can be used as an interim option for women who wish to have children, those women awaiting surgery, or as a definitive option if surgery is contraindicated.

Maximilian Nitze (1848–1906) (Fig. 20), a German urologist, is credited with the invention of the modern, electrically illuminated cystoscope in 1877 in collaboration with Joseph Leiter (1830–1892), an instrument maker from Vienna.

The Twentieth and Twenty-First Centuries: The Evolution of a Specialty

The rapid growth of knowledge, technology, and innovative procedures in the field of gynecology and urology persisted into the twentieth century. It is acknowledged that Marion Sims, in the USA, was among the first to establish the association between urology and gynecology. Howard Atwood Kelly (1858–1943), considered the first professor of gynecology at the Johns Hopkins Medical School, was credited as establishing as a specialty by describing innovative surgical procedures for gynecologic diseases (Fig. 21). He was also responsible for other medical innovations, including his air cystoscope in 1893, and surgical instruments such as Kelly's clamp, Kelly's speculum, and Kelly's forceps. He believed that gynecology and urology were so closely interconnected that a physician could not master one and ignore the other. He was the first physician to perform ureteric catheterization under direct vision. Guy LeRoy Hunner (1868–1957), Kelly's disciple and successor, described Hunner's ulcer, a type of bladder lesion which today is associated with interstitial cystitis [38]. Houston Spencer Everett (1900–1975), Kelly's and Hunner's successor, contributed to link the urinary tract to cervical cancer. These

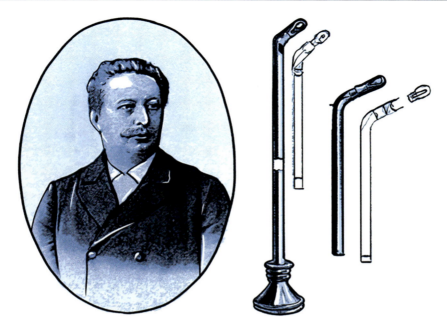

Fig. 20 Maximilian Carl-Friedrich Nitze (1848–1906) and Nitze endoscope

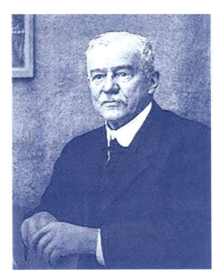

Fig. 21 Howard Atwood Kelly (1858–1943), American gynecologist at the Johns Hopkins Hospital and Medical School and promotor of Gynecology as a separate specialty

three physicians were responsible for a golden era in the dawn of Johns Hopkins Hospital urogynecology as a specialty.

In 1900, David Gilliam (1844–1923) introduced a new method of the round ligament ventrosuspension of the uterus for treatment of uterine prolapse. This operation consisted of mobilizing the proximal round ligament through the peritoneum and attach it to the posterior rectus sheath just lateral to the rectus muscle [39]. His innovative procedure was soon followed by other authors such as John Montgomery Baldy (1860–1934) and John Clarence Webster (1863–1959) who independently introduced slight modifications to his procedure. Hermann Johannes Pfannenstiel (1862–1909), a German gynecologist, introduced his low transverse abdominal incision to minimize postoperative herniation, for which he remained best remembered [40]. Frederick Foley (1891–1966), an American urologist, was the first to introduce a self-retaining urethral balloon catheter in 1929 that still bears his name. The main purpose of this catheter was to achieve hemostasis after endoscopic prostatectomy and provide continuous drainage of the bladder through an indwelling catheter [41]. However, Foley developed a novel technique to treat hydronephrosis resulting from strictures of the ureteropelvic junction which became known as Foley Y-V pyeloplasty [42]. Alexis Moschcowitz (1865–1933), a Columbia University graduate, proposed the pathogenesis of rectal prolapse as a type of sliding hernia in 1912. He described a surgical procedure to address this problem by placing silk sutures circumferentially at the level of the cul-de-sac (pouch of Douglas). Later, gynecologists used the operation to prevent or correct enterocele concurrently with abdominal hysterectomy. In 1942, Latzko reported a technique of vesicovaginal fistula repair based on an operation devised by Gustav Simon (1824–1876), a German surgeon, who developed his own technique after returning to Germany after observing Antoine J. J. de Lamballe's operative treatment of genitourinary fistulae in Paris in early 1850s. Gustav Simon's technique is also known as "German method." Latzko's operation basic steps include denuding the vaginal epithelium within the circumscribed area, followed by placement of a double row of imbricating suture layers, and overclosure of the vaginal epithelium. In the 1890s, Friedrich Trendelenburg (1844–1924) published the first vesicovaginal fistula repair using the transvesical approach. In the same article, he introduced the operating position that still carries his name until our days [43].

Throughout the twentieth century, treatment of female urinary incontinence underwent significant progress. By the turn of the century, there were four main treatments for stress (or sphincter weakness) urinary incontinence: (1) intraurethral injection of paraffin, (2) massage and electrical shock, (3) torsion of the urethra, and (4) advancement of the external urethral meatus. In 1913, Howard A. Kelly outlined in his landmark article the following operations for urinary incontinence in women: (1) placement a suprapubic catheter, (2) closure of the urethra and creation of a vesico-abdominal fistula, (3) closure of the vagina and creation of a rectovaginal fistula, (4) compression of the urethra with an anterior colporrhaphy, (5) periurethral injection of paraffin, and (6) advancement of the urethral meatus to the clitoris [44]. In 1913, Kelly reported initially a success rate of 80% with his suture plication procedure, which was not confirmed by further reports, stating a failure rate of 60% [45]. Karl Pawlik (1849–1914), an Austro-Hungarian obstetrician and gynecologist, suggested apposition of the urethral walls by flattening the distal end of the

urethra by drawing the external urethral orifice forward to the clitoris and sharply to each side and fixing it in that position with sutures [4]. Robert Gersuny (1844–1924), an Austrian surgeon, performed the first torsion of the urethra 1888 having published his technique as an improvement of Pawlik's procedure [46]. Comparable methods of urethral torsion and transfer of the urethral meatus toward the clitoris were practiced later by Alfred Pousson (1853–1940) and by Joaquin Albarran (1860–1912) [47]. Howard A. Kelly introduced the first surgical technique that persisted as a routine clinical procedure until our days. It consisted of anterior colporrhaphy and plication of the bladder neck with mattress sutures. He presented his initial results and follow-up on 20 patients, which was considered to be a milestone in the history of female pelvic medicine and standard of care for the following six decades [47, 48].

Sling procedures were pioneered in the early 1990s by three German physicians, namely, R. Goebell, Paul Frankenheim (1876–1934), and Walter Stoeckel (1871–1961). However, the earliest described sling procedure was by Giordano in 1907, using the gracilis muscle wrapped around the urethra [49, 50]. In 1911, Squier reported the use of the levator ani muscles for placement between the urethra and the vagina [51]. In 1910, Goebell first described the suburethral placement of freed pyramidalis muscle. In 1914, Frangenheim modified Goebell's technique, employing fascial attachments of the pyramidalis muscles and the recommendation for use of the rectus abdominis muscles if the pyramidalis muscles were insufficient. The final modification to this technique was performed by Stoeckel in 1917, who combined anterior colporrhaphy with sphincter muscle plication at the bladder neck with great success. This became known as the Goebell-Fragenheim-Stoeckel sling technique [49, 52–54]. In 1923, further modifications of the sling procedure were reported by Thompson, recommending the use of strips of rectus muscle and fascia that should be passed in front of the pubic bones and around the urethra, and later in 1929 by Martius, using bulbocavernosus muscle and its surrounding fatty pad to be grafted suburethrally which became predominantly useful in genitourinary fistula surgery [55, 56]. All these sling procedures used different autologous grafts. Muscle sling grafts were later abandoned secondary to difficulty in maintaining an adequate vascular and neural supply and therefore a viable graft. In 1942, Albert H. Aldrich (1894–1984), a New York gynecologist and Professor at Columbia University, described yet another modification of the sling operation using bilateral strips of the external oblique muscle aponeurosis through a transverse suprapubic incision, resembling the modern fascial sling. In his procedure, Aldridge maintained the medial attachment of the two fascial strips and passed the lateral arms inferiorly to be sutured suburethrally at the level of the vesicourethral junction. In the same report, Aldridge discussed the advantages of autologous fascia lata over abdominal wall fascia [57]. In 1968, John Chassar Moir (1900–1977), a Scottish Professor of Gynecology and Obstetrics, introduced the concept of the gauze hammock procedure based on a modification of the original Aldrich's technique (Fig. 22) [58]. Chassar Moir acknowledged the fact that "operations of this type do no more than support the bladder neck and urethrovesical junction and so prevent the undue descent of parts when the woman strains or coughs." Chassar Moir also defined the characteristics and medical benefits of ergometrine (an ergot alkaloid), a drug credited with saving hundreds of thousands of women's lives worldwide [59]. The Aldrich and other similar fascial sling procedures became standard treatment for recurrent sphincter weakness urinary incontinence for the next five decades.

In 1923, William F. Victor Bonney (1872–1953), known as a prominent British gynecologist in the period between the world wars, recognized that urinary incontinence depended upon a sudden and abnormal descent of the urethral and urethrovesical junction immediately behind the symphysis pubis [60]. This was followed by a description of a similar observation from B. P Watson (1880–1976), a Scottish obstetrician and gynecologist, that the failure of the anatomic structures that normally support the base and neck of the bladder in maintaining its normal position, allowing their hypermobility will cause incontinence and, therefore, anterior colporrhaphy was not a satisfactory operation for stress incontinence. He further stated that "so far as the incontinence of urine is concerned, the important sutures are those placed at the level of the bladder neck and overlapping the fascia and so restore the urethrovesical junction to its normal position" [61].

In 1949, Victor F. Marshall (1913–2001), a New York urologist and Professor at Cornell University, together with Andrew A. Marchetti (1901–1970), a gynecologist, and Kermit E. Krantz (1923–2007), a Gynecology resident, developed an operation to treat urinary incontinence in both male and female patients, still in use today and known as the Marshall-Marchetti-Krantz bladder suspension procedure [62]. A retropubic approach was used to suspend the bladder and bladder neck by placing interrupted sutures to the periurethral tissues on both sides of the vesicourethral junction and fix them to the periosteum of the symphysis and posterior rectus sheath. A landmark in female genitourinary surgery, the Marshall-Marchetti-Krantz operation remained standard for at least half a century since its implementation. Shortly thereafter, in

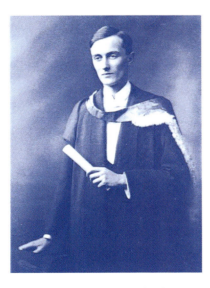

Fig. 22 Chassar Moir at his graduation in 1922. (Credit: Wellcome Library [58])

1950, H.H. Fouracre Barns, a British obstetrician and gynecologist, described the round ligament sling procedure for treatment of stress incontinence, drawing attention to the possibility of using the round ligaments of the uterus to alleviate stress urinary incontinence [63].

In 1961, John Christopher Burch (1900–1977), a Professor of Obstetrics and Gynecology at Vanderbilt University Medical School, USA, was unable to secure sutures into the retropubic periosteum while performing the Marshall-Marchetti-Krantz operation, he found that support he needed in Cooper's ligaments bilaterally (Fig. 23) [64]. Given its reasonably high therapeutic efficacy, Burch colposuspension is still used today and has been adopted over time for laparoscopy, and modifications of the original technique, such as use of synthetic mesh to secure the paraurethral support, have been introduced [65–67].

Although vaginal hysterectomy dates back to ancient times, there is a reference of vaginal hysterectomy being performed by Themison of Athens in 50 BC [68]. Soranus of Ephesus also in Greece, and later in Rome, performed this procedure in 120 AD, by removing an inverted gangrenous uterus, and the many reports of its use in the medieval era were almost exclusively for the removal of an inverted and gangrenous uterus with a high mortality rate [68]. Early, usually fatal, attempts at vaginal hysterectomy were recorded from the sixteenth century. Indeed, most physicians in the eighteenth century held a strong opinion that a woman was 90% unlikely to survive a hysterectomy [69]. In 1813, Konrad J. M. Langebeck (1776–1851), Professor at Göttingen University, Germany, performed the first planned vaginal hysterectomy associated with uterine prolapse in 1813 but was criticized by his peers and did not receive any credit for his achievement [70]. In 1822, Sauter of Baden performed one of the earliest planned vaginal hysterectomies on a woman without prolapse, but for cervical cancer [71]. The patient survived the operation but was complicated by vesicovaginal fistula and died 6 months later. In 1829, Joseph Récamier, a gynecologist from Paris (1774–1852), performed the first successful hysterectomy for cervical cancer, deliberately ligating the uterine arteries and broad ligaments, finishing the operation in 20 min. The patient died later due to spread of the cancer. Récamier is also acknowledged by the popularization of some gynecologic instruments, such as the curette, vaginal speculum, and uterine sound. In 1829, he was the first to use the term "metastasis" for the dissemination of cancer. Curettage of the uterus is also known as "Récamier's operation."

In 1934, Nobel Sproat Heaney (1880–1955), a Chicago gynecologist, was one of the most vigorous proponents of vaginal hysterectomy. He reported a series of 627 vaginal hysterectomies performed for benign conditions with only three deaths [71]. Heaney was encouraged by the lower mortality rate of vaginal hysterectomy compared to its abdominal counterpart. However, because of improved surgical instrumentation, anesthesia and antisepsis, the mortality rate dropped from 15% in 1886 to 2.5% in 1910 [71].

Fig. 23 (**a**) John Christopher Burch (1900–1977); (**b**) Burch colposuspension [64]

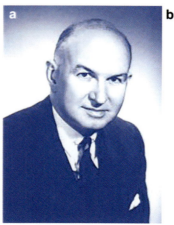
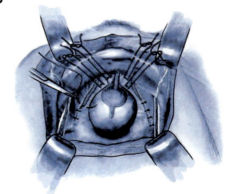

In 1957, Milton Lawrence McCall (1911–1963), described a surgical technique, that he termed culdoplasty, to address the development of enterocele, a common complication of vaginal hysterectomy. It consists of a relatively simple procedure that is performed following the removal of the uterus and cervix from the vaginal apex wherein the vaginal angles are sutured to the uterosacral ligaments and the open cul-de-sac is surgically obliterated for postoperative support, thereby incorporating these supporting ligaments into the closure of the peritoneum and upper vagina [72].

The first deliberate opening of the abdominal cavity to remove an ovarian mass was conducted by Ephraim McDowell (1771–1830), a surgeon of Danvile, Kentucky, USA, who removed a 10.2 kg ovarian mass successfully without anesthesia from Jane Todd Crawford, in 1809 [70, 73]. Mrs. Crawford made an uneventful recovery and returned home 25 days after the operation to live another 32 years [74]. Conscious that all attempts at abdominal exploration before 1809 had resulted in peritonitis and death, he reinforced the importance of acting as "clean, neatly and scrupulously as possible," and in a honest and humble posture he declared "I can only say that the blessing of God has rested on my efforts" [75]. He waited until he had performed two additional similar surgeries, both successful, before publishing his work in 1817. His publication included surgical details such as the removal of blood from the peritoneal cavity and bathing of the intestines with warm water. He performed 13 similar operations in his career [74].

In 1843, Charles Clay (1801–1893), an English surgeon, performed the first recorded abdominal hysterectomy in Manchester, England. Unfortunately, the patient died of a massive hemorrhage in the immediate postoperative period [70]. The following year, Charles Clay performed a second similar operation successfully and was almost the first to claim a surviving patient from this operation; however, the woman died 15 days later after accidentally being dropped on the floor while the nurses were changing the bed clothes [71]. In fact, these were subtotal hysterectomies

for huge uterine fibroids. In 1846, John Bellinger (1804–1860), a US surgeon, descendent of an old English family, performed the first planned subtotal hysterectomy for uterine fibroids. The patient succumbed to sepsis 5 days postoperatively [71]. In 1853, Walter Burnham (1808–1883) did the first abdominal hysterectomy, by accident, through an incision extending from the sternum to the pubis without anesthesia. An unplanned hysterectomy had to be performed as the patient extruded a huge myomatous uterus. Unable to return it to its original place inside the peritoneal cavity, he proceeded with removal of the gigantic uterus, ligating both uterine arteries [68]. Twelve of his 15 patients died of peritonitis, hemorrhage, or exhaustion [70].

All these early hysterectomies were subtotal procedures, usually performed without anesthesia, and with a high mortality rate ranging from 70% to 90%, even as late as the 1880s [68]. Abdominal hysterectomy received formal disapproval by the Academy of Medicine in Paris in 1872 because of its high mortality rate [70]. However, this dismal scenario was improved with the advent of anesthesia, adequate surgical instrumentation, and antisepsis by the end of the nineteenth century.

In 1929, Richardson (1911–2010), a urologist at Johns Hopkins University and Hospital, conducted the first total abdominal hysterectomy (which he termed as "abdominal panhysterectomy"), recommending the excision of the cervix to avoid cervical stump carcinoma [76]. Despite Richardson's recommendation, subtotal hysterectomy continued to be the most popular surgical operation up until the late 1940s. The most likely reasons were to avoid peritonitis due to contamination of the peritoneal cavity with vaginal bacterial and fungal flora and the decreased risk of bladder and ureteric injury [68]. Nonetheless, the advent of antibiotics, blood transfusion, modern anesthesia methods, awareness of cancer growth in the cervical stump, and better surgical procedures toward the 1940s motivated surgeons to do total hysterectomy which became the standard of care for the next 20 years. The only additional change in the total abdominal hysterectomy procedure was the nearly universal adoption of the low transverse incision introduced by Johannes Pfannenstiel, in 1900, which offers a better cosmetic appearance with less complications. These beneficial features significantly fostered the number of procedures performed to a point that hysterectomy is now the second most common operation performed on women after cesarean section [77].

Radical abdominal hysterectomy was developed in the nineteenth century for the treatment of cervical cancer and upper vagina. John G. Clark, H. Rumpf, and E. Ries performed independently the operation for the first time in 1895 and 1897 without removing the parametrium together with the lymph nodes in all his 12 patients [78, 79]. Hence, Ernst Wertheim is credited for developing and perfecting the basic technique of radical hysterectomy, including the routine removal of pelvic lymph nodes and the parametrium (Fig. 24) [33, 80]. This subject has already been mentioned above and, therefore, will not be discussed further at this stage. Karl A. Schuchardt (1856–1901), a Göttingen gynecologist, developed a more radical extension of vaginal hysterectomy [81]. However, Friedrich Schauta (1849–1919), an Austrian gynecologist, introduced radical vaginal hysterectomy in 1901 and reported a lower operative mortality rate compared to the abdominal counterpart [82, 83].

Because small invasive cervical cancer has become more frequent and is often diagnosed in younger women who desire to maintain fertility and childbearing potential, there has been a trend toward a more conservative surgical approach to overcome this management dilemma. In 1977, Burghardt and Holzer acknowledged that it was not necessary to remove the entire uterus and adnexa to successfully treat small-volume cervical cancer [84]. However, Aburel, a Romanian gynecologist was the first to propose a conservative approach for the surgical management of cervical cancer, a procedure he called "subfundic radical hysterectomy" [85, 86]. However, the procedure did not achieve popularity. In 1986, Daniel Dargent (1937–2005), a Professor of Gynecology at the University of Lyon, France, is credited with performing the first successful systematic conservative surgical approach for invasive cervical cancer, a procedure they called "vaginal radical trachelectomy." Radical trachelectomy was designed to preserve the functions of the uterus by combining laparoscopic pelvic lymphadenectomy and transvaginal trachelectomy including removal of distal uterine third. He published his technique later in 1994 [86]. Currently, both abdominal and vaginal fertility-preserving approaches have been described and approved by the gynecologic oncology community [84]. The procedure is also known as "Dargent's operation" [87].

In 1988, Harry Reich performed the first laparoscopic hysterectomy in Pennsylvania, USA. The whole procedure was performed using only laparoscopic techniques and was published 1 year later [88]. Although familiar with other laparoscopic procedures such as laparoscopic appendectomy performed by him in 1981, it was not until 1991 that Kurt Semm (1927–2003) in Kiel, Germany, reported the first laparoscopic subtotal hysterectomy which he termed "CASH" (Classic Abdominal Semm Hysterectomy) [89]. It never became popular because of technical difficulties.

The advent of laparoscopy marked a critical change in the evolution of surgery. Since its dawn nearly a 100 years ago, the procedure has witnessed groundbreaking changes in the 1960s and 1980s from a purely diagnostic tool into a separate and autonomous surgical field.

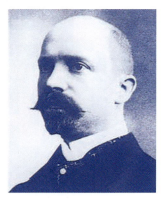

Fig. 24 Ernst Wertheim (1864–1920), Austrian gynecologist, performed the first radical abdominal hysterectomy for cervical cancer in 1898 [80]

The main advantage of laparoscopy is to avoid a large laparotomy wound. Laparoscopy has become a routine approach in the twenty-first century, only to be supplanted more recently by the robot-assisted surgery.

Conclusion

The evolution of female genitourinary pelvic surgery from antiquity to modern times has undergone distinct historical stages over thousands of years, including Hippocratic Age, through the Dark Ages and Medieval Era (Fifth till Fifteenth Centuries), from the Renaissance to the Nineteenth Century prior to the Aseptic Age (Fifteenth to Early Nineteenth Centuries), and then through the Dawn of Aseptic Age (Mid-Nineteenth to Twenty-First Centuries), all of these with their own specific and fascinating historical features and landmarks. Theories and beliefs that were once considered unquestionably dogmatic would soon fall from favor only to be revived/regenerated and generalized by future generations. Many women have suffered from these conditions affecting the genitourinary tract and pelvic floor and many physicians have attempted to treat. The slow historical progress of this field of medicine combined with the challenges and barriers that our ancestors faced in dealing with these problems inspired by a blend of creativity, skill, and art reflect the genuine complexities of these disorders that simultaneously captivate and perplex our minds. At present, physicians devoted to female pelvic medicine both realize the long way and benefits derived from the historical advances throughout generations, as well as the refinements achieved by modern, innovative, and sophisticated technology. Although the current, accumulated evidence provides us with a better etiopathogenetic understanding of these disorders, as well as improved modern therapeutic tools to treat them, more multi-institutional research is needed to appreciate the long-term efficacy and outcomes of our discoveries.

References

1. Nager CW, Kumar D, Kahn M, Stanton SL. Management of the pelvic floor dysfunction. Lancet. 1997; 350:1751. https://doi.org/10.1016/S0140-6736(05) 63575-1.
2. Joachim H. Papyrus Eber. Berlin: G. Reimer; 1890. (Cited in ref. 4 – Eur Urol. 2000;38(3):352–62).
3. Breasted JH. Edwin Smith surgical papyrus in facsimile and hieroglyphic transliteration and commentary. Chicago: University of Chicago Oriental Institute; 1930. (Cited in ref. 4 – Eur Urol. 2000;38(3):352–62).
4. Schultheiss D, Höfner K, Oelke M, Grünewald V, Jonas U. Historical aspects of treatment of urinary incontinence. Eur Urol. 2000;38(3):352–62. https://doi.org/10.1159/000020306.
5. Brothwell D, Sandison AT. Diseases in antiquiry. Springfield: Charles C. Thomas; 1969.
6. Murphy LJT. The history of urology. Springfield: Charles C. Thomas; 1972.
7. Hanafy HM, Saad SM, Al-Ghorab MM. An ancient Egyptian medicine. Urology. 1974;4:114–20.
8. McKay WJS. The history of ancient gynaecology. London, UK: Balliere, Tindal and Cox; 1901.
9. Bryan CP. Ancient Egyptian medicine: the Papyrus Ebers. Chicago: Ares Publishers; 1974.
10. Ricci JV. The genealogy of gynaecology: history of the development of gynaecology throughout the ages, 2000 BC–1800 AD. Philadelphia: The Blakiston Company; 1950. (Cited in ref. 11 – Obstet Gynecol Int. 2012;2012:649459).
11. Downing KT. Uterine prolapse: from antiquity to today. Obstet Gynecol Int. 2012;2012:649459. https://doi.org/10.1155/2012/649459.
12. Soranus TO. Soranus' gynecology. Baltimore: Johns Hopkins University Press; 1991.
13. Adams F. The extant works of Aretaeus. Cappadocian: Nabu Press; 2010. (Cited in ref. 11 – Obstet Gynecol Int. 2012;2012:649459).
14. Derry DE. Note on five pelves of women of the eleventh dynasty in Egypt. J Obstet Gynecol Br Emp. 1935;42:490.
15. Bloom DA, Milen MT, Heininger JC. Claudius Galen: from 20th century genitourinary perspective. J Urol. 1999;161:12–9.
16. Speert H. Iconographia Gyniatrica; a pictorial history of gynecology and obstetrics. Philadelphia: F. A. Davis; 1973.
17. Gombrich EH. A little history of the world. New Haven: Yale University Press; 2005.
18. Emge LA, Durfee RB. Pelvic organ prolapse: four thousand years of treatment. Clin Obstet Gynecol. 1966;9:997.
19. Schultheiss D, Grünewald V, Jonas U. Urodynamic aspects in the work of Leonardo da Vinci (1452–1519). World J Urol. 1999;17:137–44.

20. "Vesalius at 500". The Physician's Palette. Archived from "the original" on 10 December 2014. https://web.archive.org/we/20141210143700/http://thephysicianspalette.com/2014/12/01/vesalius-at-500/
21. Ankum WM, Houtzager HL, Bleker OP. Reinier De Graaf (1641–1673) and the fallopian tube. Hum Reprod Update. 1996;2(4):365–9. https://doi.org/10.1093/humupd/2.4.365. PMID 9080233.
22. Jocelyn HD, Setchell BP. Regnier de Graaf on the human reproductive organs. An annotated translation of Tractatus de Virorum Organis Generationi Inservientibus (1668) and De Mulierub Organis Generationi Inservientibus Tractatus Novus (1962). J Reprod Fertil Suppl. 1972;17:1–222. PMID 4567037.
23. Anneliese S. Johannes Scultetus and his work. Biography and glossary. Supplement to the reprint of the "Wund-Artzneyisches Zeug-Haus" by the Merckle company. Stuttgart: Kohlhammer in Commission; 1974.
24. Tizzano AP, Muffly TM. Historical milestones in female pelvic surgery, gynecology, and female urology. In: Walters MD, Karram MM, editors. Urogynecology and reconstructive pelvic surgery, 4th ed. Philadelphia: Elsevier Saunders; 2015. p. 3–15.
25. Thomas BK. James Douglas of the pouch, 1675–1742. Br Med J. 1960;1:1649–50.
26. Cooke TJND, Gousse AE. A historical perspective on cystocele repair – from honey to pessaries to anterior colporrhaphy: lessons from the past. J Urol. 2008;179: 2126–30.
27. Spettel S, White MD. The Portrayal of J. Marion Sims' Controversial surgical legacy. J Urol. 2011;185(6): 2424–7.
28. Edmonson JM. American surgical instruments: the history of their manufacture and a directory of instrument makers to 1900. 1st ed. San Francisco: Jeremy Norman & Co; 1997.
29. Ojunga D. The medical ethics of the 'Father of Gynaecology', Dr J Marion Sims. J Med Ethics. 1993;19(1): 28–31.
30. Ligon BL. Biography: Louis Pasteur: a controversial figure in a debate on scientific ethics. Semin Pediatr Infect Dis. 2002;13(2):134–41.
31. Adam P. Louis Pasteur: Father of bacteriology. Can J Med Technol. 1951;13(3):126–8.
32. Pitt D, Aubin JM. Joseph Lister: father of modern surgery. Can J Surg. 2012;55(5):E8–9.
33. Wolfson AH, Varia MA, Moore D, Rao GG, Gaffney DK, Erickson-Wittmann BA, Jhingran A, Mayr NA, Puthawala AA, Small W, Yashar CM, Yuh W, Cardenes HR. ACR Appropriateness Criteria® role of adjuvant therapy in the management of early-stage cervical cancer. Gynecol Oncol. 2012;125(1):256–62.
34. Oliver R, Thakar R, Sultan AH. The history and usage. Reprod Biol. 2011;156(2):125–30.
35. Hodge HL. On diseases peculiar to women, including displacements of the uterus. Philadelphia, Blanchard and Lea, 1860. Am J Obstet Gynecol. 1972;112(8): 1129.
36. Speert H. Obstetric and gynecologic milestones: essays in eponymy. New York: Macmillan; 1958.
37. Buck WD. A raid on the uterus. N Y Med J. 1867;5: 464.
38. Meijlink JM. Interstitial cystitis and the painful bladder: a brief history of nomenclature, definitions and criteria. Int J Urol. 2014;21:4–12. https://doi.org/10.1111/iju.12307. Wiley Online Library. PMID 24807485.
39. Gilliam DT. Round ligament ventrosuspension of the uterus: a new method. Am J Obstet Dis Women Child. 1900;41:299–303.
40. Pfannenstiel HJ. On the advantages of the symphyseal transverse fascial incision for gynecological caliotomies as well as the contribution to the surgical indications. Samml Klin Vortr. 1900;268:1735–56.
41. Foley FEB. Cystoscopic prostatectomy: a new procedure: preliminary report. J Urol. 1929;21(3):289–306.
42. Foley FE. A new plastic operation for stricture at the uretero-pelvic junction. Report of 20 operations. J Urol. 1937;6(38):643–72.
43. Thiery M. Friedrich Trendenlenburg (1844–1924) and the Trendelenburg position. Gynecol Surg. 2009;6: 295–7. https://doi.org/10.1007/s10397-009-0499-x.
44. Kelly HA. Incontinence of the urine in women. Urol Cutan Rev. 1913;17:291.
45. Bergman A, Elia G. Three surgical procedures for genuine stress urinary incontinence: five-year follow-up of a prospective randomized study. Am J Obstet Gynecol. 1995;173(1):66–71.
46. Gersuny R. Eine neue Operation zur Heilelung der Incontinentia urinae. Zentralbl Chir. 1889;16(25): 433–7. (Cited in ref. 4 – Eur Urol. 2000;38(3):352–62).
47. Kelly HA, Dumm WM. Urinary incontinence in women, without manifest injury to the bladder. Surg Gynecol Obstet. 1914;18:444–50.
48. Kelly HA, Dumm WM. Classical article in urogynecology – urinary incontinence in women, without manifest injury to the bladder. Int Urogynecol J. 1998;9: 158–64.
49. Schultz JA, Drutz HP, Robertson JR. History of urogynecology and female urology, Chap 1. In: Cardozo L, Staskin D, editors. Textbook of female urology and urogynecology, vol. 1. CRC Press; 2017.
50. Giordano D. Twentieth congress. Franc. de Chir. 1907;20:506. (Cited in ref. 49).
51. Squier JB. Postoperative urinary incontinence. Med Rec. 1911;79:868.
52. Goebell R. Zur operative Besierigung der angeborenen Incontinentia vesical. Z Gynäk Urol. 1910;2:187.
53. Frankenheim P. Zentral Verhandl, d, Deutsch. Geseusch Chir. 1914;43:149.
54. Stoeckel W. Über die Verwändung der Musculi Pyramidales bei der opeutinen Behandlung der Incontinentia Urinae. Zentralbl Gynäkol. 1917;41:11.
55. Thompson R. A case of epispadias associated with complete incontinence treated with rectus transplantation. Br J Dis Child. 1923;20:146–51.

56. Martius H. Sphincter und Harndöurenplastic aus dem Musicailus Bulbocavernosus. Chirurgie. 1929;17:769.
57. Aldridge AH. Transplantation of fascia for the relief of urinary stress incontinence. Am J Obstet Gynecol. 1942;44:398–411.
58. Chasser MJ. The gauze hammock operation (a modified Aldrich sling operation). J Obstet Gynaecol Br Commonw. 1968;75:1–9.
59. Moir JC. From 'St. Anthony's Fire' to the isolation of its active principle, ergometrine. Am J Obstet Gynaecol St Louis. 1974;120(2):290–6.
60. Bonney V. On diurnal incontinence of urine in women. J Obstet Gynecol Br Emp. 1923;30:358–65.
61. Watson BP. Imperfect urinary control following childbirth and its surgical treatment. Br Med J. 1924;11:566.
62. Marshall VF, Marchetti AA, Krantz KE. The correction of stress incontinence by simple vesicourethral suspension. Surg Gynecol Obstet. 1949;88(4):509–18.
63. Barns HHF. Round ligament sling operation for stress incontinence. J Obstet Gyanecol Br Emp (currently BJOG). 1950;57(3):404–7.
64. Burch JC. Urethrovaginal fixation to Cooper's ligament for correction of stress incontinence, cytoscele and prolapse. Am J Obstet Gynecol. 1961;81:281–90.
65. Ross J. Two techniques of laparoscopic Burch repair for stress incontinence: a prospective, randomized study. J Am Assoc Gynecol Laparosc. 1996;3:351–7.
66. Valpas A, Kivela A, Penttinen J, et al. Tension-free vaginal tape and laparoscopic mesh colposuspension in the treatment of stress urinary incontinence: immediate outcome and complications–a randomized clinical trial. Acta Obstet Gynecol Scand. 2003;82:665–71.
67. Cutner A, Smith AR. Laparoscopic colposuspension. Curr Opin Obstet Gynecol. 2001;13:533–7.
68. Sutton C. Past, present and future of hysterectomy. J Minim Invasive Gynecol. 2010;17(4):421–35.
69. Sparic R, Hudelist G, Berisavac M, Gudovic A, Buzadzic S. Hysterectomy through history. Acta Chir Iugosl. 2011;58(4):9–14.
70. Sutton C. Hysterectomy: a historical perspective. Baillieres Clin Obstet Gynaecol. 1977;11:1–22.
71. Baskett TF. Hysterectomy: evolution and trends. Best Pract Res Clin Obstet Gynaecol. 2005;19:295–305.
72. McCall ML. Posterior culdoplasty: surgical correction of enterocele during vaginal hysterectomy; a preliminary report. Obstet Gynecol. 1957;10(6):595–602.

73. Rutkow IM. The history of surgery in the United States, 1775–1900, vol. 2. Norman Publishing; 1988. p. 90. ISBN 9780930405489.
74. Toledo-Pereyra LH. Ephraim McDowell. Father of abdominal surgery. J Investig Surg. 2004;17:237–8.
75. Othersen HB. Ephraim McDowell: the qualities of a good surgeon. Ann Surg. 2004;239(5):648–50. https://doi.org/10.1097/01.sla.0000124382.04128.5a.
76. Richardson EH. A simplified technique for abdominal panhysterectomy. Sur Gynecol Obstet. 1929;47:248–56.
77. ACOG. Choosing the route of hysterectomy for benign disease. ACOG Committee opinion no. 444. Obstet Gynecol. 2009;114:1156–8.
78. Hoskins WJ, Ford JH, Lutz MH, et al. Radical hysterectomy and pelvic lymphadenectomy for the management of early invasive cancer of the cervix. Gynecol Oncol. 1976;4:278–90.
79. Mikuta JJ. A history of the centennial of the first radical hysterectomy and its developer, Dr. John Clark. J Pelvic Surg. 1995;1:3–7.
80. Ballon SC. The Wertheim hysterectomy. Surg Gynecol Obstet. 1976;142:920–4.
81. Schuchardt K. Eine neue Methode der Gerbärmutterexstirpation. Zentralbl Chir. 1893;20:1121–6.
82. Schauta F. Die erweiterte vaginal totalexstirpationbeim des Uterus bei Kollumkarzinom. Leipzig: J Safar; 1908.
83. Roy M, Plante M. Place of Schauta's radical vaginal hysterectomy. Best Pract Res Clin Obstet Gynecol. 2011;25(2):227–37.
84. Shepherd JH, Milken DA. Conservative surgery for carcinoma of the cervix. Clin Oncol. 2008;20:395400.
85. Aburel E. Colpohisterectomia largita subfundica. In: Sirbu P, editor. Chirurgica gynecologica. Bucharest: Editura Medicala Pub; 1981. p. 714–21.
86. Dargent D, Martin X, Sacchetoni A, Mathevet P. Laparoscopic vaginal radical trachelectomy: a treatment to preserve the fertility of cervical carcinoma patients. Cancer. 2000;88:1877–81.
87. Roy M, Querleu D. In memoriam of Prof Daniel Dargent. Gynecol Oncol. 2005;99:1–2.
88. Reich H, DeCaprio J, McGlynn F. Laparoscopic hysterectomy. J Gynecol Surg. 1989;5:213–6.
89. Semm K. Hysterectomy via laparotomy or pelviscopy. A new CASH method without colpotomy. Geburtshilfe Frauenheilkd. 1991;51:996–1003. https://doi.org/10.1055/s-2008-1026252. (In German).

Embryology and Development of Congenital Anomalies of the Pelvis and Female Organs

2

Vishen Naidoo, Ejikeme Mbajiorgu, and Ahmed Adam

Contents

Introduction	30
The Early Zygote and Embryogenesis	30
Cloacal Division	30
Primitive Mullerian Duct Development	30
Development of the Genital Ducts	31
Development of the Uterus and Vagina	31
Sexual Differentiation	32
The Array of Relevant Anomalies Which May Present in the Clinical Setting	32
Vaginal and Uterine Anomalies	32
Ureteric Bud Anomalies	37
Gartner's Duct Cyst (GDC)	41
Mayer–Rokitansky–Küster–Hauser syndrome (MRHK)	42
McKusick-Kaufman Syndrome (MKKS)	43
Pelvic Anomalies	44
Conclusion	45
References	45

Abstract

A sound understanding and appreciation underlying embryology is paramount in the management of the complex anomalies that may result. The embryology and development of the female reproductive system is an intricate and complex cascade of time-specific inter-related events. This process is inter-related with the renal system and the Wolffian

V. Naidoo · A. Adam (✉)
Division of Urology, University of the Witwatersrand, Johannesburg, South Africa
e-mail: ahmed.adam@wits.ac.za

E. Mbajiorgu
School of Anatomical Sciences, University of the Witwatersrand, Johannesburg, South Africa
e-mail: Ejikeme.Mbajiorgu@wits.ac.za

© Springer Nature Switzerland AG 2023
F. E. Martins et al. (eds.), *Female Genitourinary and Pelvic Floor Reconstruction*,
https://doi.org/10.1007/978-3-031-19598-3_2

tract. Its initial phase begins with the formation and establishment of the genital ridge. This unravelling has the occasional anomaly in the relation to the pelvis, the internal and external female structure, and resultant function. An overview of this relationship is presented in this chapter.

Keywords

Embryology · Female · Anomalies

Introduction

This chapter will outline the basic fundamental steps in the development of the female reproductive system and the pelvis. The related clinical anomalies associated with these embryological steps are expanded at the latter end of this chapter.

The Early Zygote and Embryogenesis

The nephrogenic cords grow posteriorly and develop three prominent structures: the pronephros (rudimentary and non-functional), which develops in the cervical region during week 3 post-fertilization and later degenerates at about week 5, the mesonephros forms the primitive or embryonic urinary system between 4 and 8 weeks, and the metanephros which forms the functional permanent kidney. Though the pronephros and mesonephros are temporary structures but very essential to the formation of the metanephros. The mesonephros develops at the thoracic region in the 4th week as the embryonic urinary system. The mesonephros is drained by the paired mesonephric ducts (Wolffian duct) into the cloaca. During week 12 of development, in females the mesonephros and mesonephric ducts become highly convoluted but the epoophoron, para-oophoron, and Gartner's duct which are non-function persist [1].

The development of the urinary and reproductive systems begins as two separate but intertwined processes arising from the intermediate mesoderm. Intermediate mesoderm forms a longitudinal elevation along the dorsal body wall on each side of dorsal aorta/dorsal mesentery of gut. The medial part (genital/gonadal ridge) forms the genital system (gonads) and lateral part forms the nephrogenic cord which gives rise to the urinary system. The genital ridges initially are devoid of germ cells [1, 2].

Cloacal Division

The cloacal membrane arises in week 3 under the umbilical cord. The lower abdominal wall is noted to be formed when the cloacal membrane migrates more caudally displaced by adjacent proliferating mesenchyme. By week 5, the cloacal membrane is surrounded laterally by the cloacal folds which join anteriorly to give rise to the genital tubercle which is formed in week 4. The cloacal membrane remains imperforate at this time. In week 4, the genital tubercle results from mesenchymal proliferation and a protophallus anterior to the cloacal membrane starts to develop. During week 6, the urethral groove and anal pit form resulting in focal depressions along the cloacal membrane. The primary urogenital folds surround the primary urethral groove. The genital or labioscrotal swellings form lateral to the urethral folds [1, 2].

During week 7, the cloacal membrane involutes and the primary urethral groove becomes continuous with the definitive urogenital sinus. The secondary urethral groove forms as a result of widening and deepening of the primary urethral groove in week 8. The external genitalia begin display sexual differentiation during week 10 [2].

Primitive Mullerian Duct Development

In females the paramesonephric (Müllerian) ducts come from the mesoderm which is lateral to the mesonephric ducts in week 7. The paramesonephric ducts grow caudally, and its path is lateral to the urogenital ridges. In week 8, the paired paramesonephric ducts are situated medial to the mesonephric ducts. The paramesonephric ducts join to form a common structure. This process is known as Müllerian organogenesis and is the first stage in the development of the upper two-thirds of the vagina, the cervix, uterus, and both fallopian tubes. The cranial portion of the fused ducts becomes the future uterus which contains mesoderm that will form the uterine endometrium and myometrium. The unfused cranial ends of the paramesonephric ducts conform to a funnel shape and stay open to the future peritoneal cavity as the fimbrial portions of the fallopian tubes. The caudal end of the fused ducts will form the upper two-thirds of the vagina. Lateral fusion of the paramesonephric ducts occurs between weeks 7 and 9 when the lower segments of the paramesonephric ducts fuse. A midline septum is present in the uterine cavity; this usually degenerates at around week 20 but can persist. Vertical fusion occurs in week 8 when the lowermost fused paramesonephric ducts fuse with the ascending endoderm of the sinovaginal bulb. The lower third of the vagina is formed as the sinovaginal bulb canalizes [2, 3].

Development of the Genital Ducts

During week 7 of development, post-fertilization, the undifferentiated genital system comprises two pairs of ducts: the mesonephric (Wolffian) and paramesonephric (Mullerian) ducts. The paramesonephric ducts arise from the fusion of the edges of a groove on the lateral surface of the urogenital ridge, with its cranial ends opening into the coelomic cavity. In the absence of the testis-determining factor (TDF), testosterone from the Leydig cells, and Müllerian-inhibiting substance (MIS) or Mullerian-inhibiting substance (MIS), secreted by the Sertoli cells at 8–10th weeks, the indifferent gonad differentiates to an ovary and therefore female phenotype (uterine or fallopian tubes, the vagina, cervix, and uterus) from paramesonephric ducts which process is completed by the end of first trimester. The uterine endometrium is derived from simple epithelium covering the lumen while myometrium and perimetrium develop from surrounding

mesenchyme. The presence of estrogen is crucial in the development of female external genitalia, whereas testosterone (secreted by Leydig cells beginning at week 9) allows the formation of male reproduction structures (epididymis, vas deferens, ejaculatory duct, and seminal vesicles) and male external genitalia (penis and scrotum).

In males, the paramesonephric ducts degenerate under the influence of anti-Mullerian hormone (AMH) produced by Sertoli cells starting at weeks 8–10. The uterine endometrium is derived from simple epithelium covering the lumen while myometrium and perimetrium develop from surrounding mesenchyme [2].

Development of the Uterus and Vagina

The genital system remains indifferent up until weeks 5 and 6 of fetal life. Two pairs of genital ducts are present at this time, the mesonephric (Wolffian duct) and paramesonephric (Mullerian duct). In females, the absence of anti-Mullerian hormone (AMH) and SRY gene conditions the regression of Wolff ducts and further differentiation of Mullerian ducts. The upper third of the vagina, cervix, both fallopian tubes, and the uterus arise from the paramesonephric ducts [4]. During week 7, paired paramesonephric ducts stem from focal invaginations of the coelomic epithelium that is noted on the upper part of each mesonephros. Not so long after this process, the Mullerian ducts grow caudally and laterally to the urogenital ridges [5].

Vertical fusion of paramesonephric ducts occurs during week 8. The fused cranial end gives rise to the left and right parts of what will eventually become the uterus. This configuration contains mesoderm that will give rise to the endometrium and myometrium. The unfused cranial ends of the Mullerian ducts will form into the fallopian tubes. The fimbrial end of the fallopian tubes arises from the tip of this configuration that remains open and takes on a funnel shape. The caudal end of the fused ducts will become the upper third of the vagina [6]. During this time, a midline septum is present along these structures and within the uterine cavity. This septum normally resorbs completely around 20 weeks; however it can persist and create a septate uterus [4]. The gubernaculum and undifferentiated mesenchymal tissue give rise to the uterine ligaments; the round ligament and the ovarian ligament is attached to the ovary in the female fetus. The round ligament must attach to both the ovary and uterus for the ovary to be in place [7]. By the end of the first trimester, development of the uterus and the other structures derived from the Mullerian ducts is complete [4].

The primary function of the uterus is reproductive. The principal elements of uterine physiology are the endometrium and myometrium. The uterus accepts the ovum after fertilization and holds and provides nutrients and oxygen for the fetus and during birth, and it contracts to cause delivery. The uterus is a hormone-sensitive organ: differentiation, proliferation, exfoliation of the endometrium, and contraction during childbirth get regulated by the interaction between itself and the hypothalamus, pituitary gland, and ovaries [8].

Most congenital anomalies of the female reproductive tract are due to disruptions of normal morphogenetic sequences and the underlying molecular pathways. Most human female reproductive tract malformations are due to abnormalities of the Müllerian duct (MD) growth; however these anomalies are rare. Some are spontaneous in occurrence, while others are precipitated by endocrine-interrupting substances, in essence, mostly those that have estrogenic activity. The administration of diethylstilbestrol (DES) to pregnant women is the best example of estrogen-induced malformation of the human female reproductive tract. It was prescribed from the 1940s to 1971 thereafter the Food and Drug Administration (FDA) banned its use. The anomalies ranged from malformations of the uterine tubes, uterine corpus, cervix, and vagina, which included T-shaped uterotubal junctions, malformed and incompetent cervix, abnormally shaped endometrial cavity, vaginal adenosis (presence of glandular epithelium in the vagina where normally stratified squamous epithelium should reside) as well as clear cell adenocarcinoma of the vagina [9].

Sexual Differentiation

The fetus has bipotential sexual development for the first 3 months of life. The phenotype depends on the presence of sex chromosomes and the prevailing biochemical and hormonal profile. The default sex phenotype is female in the presence of 2 X-chromosomes. Under the influence of 2 X-chromosomes, the cortex of the indifferent gonad is better developed in the female embryo than the male. The cortex gives rise to the secondary sex cords. These extend from the surface epithelium to the mesenchyme. The secondary sex cords maintain and regulate the ovarian cortical follicular development. The undifferentiated gonads persist until around week 10, the ovaries first become identifiable at this time. A male fetus will develop in the presence of a Y-chromosome which translates the SRY protein. The SRY protein allows for testicular differentiation and for the production of androgens including testosterone. The medulla of the indifferent gonad in males differentiates into the testis, and the cortex regresses and gives rise to vestigial remnants. In addition to the SRY protein and androgens, another factor is needed in order for male development. This is anti-Müllerian hormone (AMH). AMH prevents female genital ductal differentiation. An immature female will develop in the absence of these three factors. Development of the immature female is dependent on the effect of estrogens [1–3].

The Array of Relevant Anomalies Which May Present in the Clinical Setting

Vaginal and Uterine Anomalies

In females, the reproductive organs are divided into three main areas. They are the gonads, reproductive ducts, and external genitalia. The female reproductive system is derived from four origins, namely, the mesoderm, primordial germ cells, coelomic epithelium, and mesenchyme. The uterus is developed during Mullerian organogenesis and is accompanied by the development of the upper third of the vagina, the cervix, and both fallopian tubes [10, 11].

Mullerian anomalies can be clinically asymptomatic and can be missed in routine gynecological examinations; however they may also manifest with infertility and amenorrhea during puberty.

The American fertility classified these anomalies into seven categories [12]:

- Class 1: Hypoplasia/uterine hypoplasia
- Class 2: Unicornuate uterus
- Class 3: Uterus didelphys
- Class 4: Bicornuate uterus
- Class 5: Septate uterus
- Class 6: Arcuate uterus
- Class 7: T-shaped uterus resulting from the exposure to Diethylstilbestrol (DES) in fetal life

Class 1

Congenital cervical atresia occurs in 1 in 80,000–1,000,000 women [13] and is associated with total or partial aplasia of the vagina and renal anomalies. The uterus and fallopian tubes can be extensively dilated due to the menstrual blood that has no outflow and in extreme cases can lead to an acute abdomen due to rupture. Early diagnosis and treatment is imperative due to its significant morbidity and mortality.

Class 2

Unicornuate uterus accounts for 0.3–4% of the uterine anomalies and occurs in 1 in 5400 women, and 74–90% are associated with a rudimentary horn [14, 15]. This occurs when one of the Müllerian ducts does not migrate to its correct place, there is failure in the unilateral development. The single uterine horn can be different to normal development. When there is complete agenesis of one of the Müllerian ducts, or accompanied by another rudimentary uterine horn, which could be of three types. The structure can be without a cavity, cavitated, or cavitated with non-communicating horn. The endometrium in the latter undergoes hormonal stimulation and its

cavity increases progressively in volume due to the retention of menstrual blood as it has no way of flowing out. This causes pain and abdominal distension due to the progressively distending uterus. Patients with a unicornuate uterus have poor reproductive prognosis and can have obstetrical complications such as premature labor, miscarriages, and intrauterine growth restriction.

The presence of only one uterine artery and lack of the contralateral arterioles compromises the blood supply and reduces the muscular mass of the organ. Unicornuate uterus will only require surgical correction if there is a cavitated non-communicating rudimentary uterine horn. This needs resection due to the pain that is caused from the disruption of menstrual flow. In some cases, its muscle mass is reduced and thus causes isthmus-cervical incompetence and there might be the necessity of cervical cerclage in a future pregnancy [15].

Class 3

Uterus didelphys occurs when there is complete failure of coming together and fusion of the Müllerian ducts; their development will continue individually. This then gives rise to two uterine cavities, two cervices, and two vaginas which are separated by a longitudinal septum and with normal menstrual flow. The septum can be vertical or oblique. If oblique, it may obstruct one of the vaginas and cause menstrual flow obstruction of that hemi-uterus causing pelvic and lumbar pain, hematometra, hematocolpos, vaginal discomfort, and hematosalpinx. When there is ipsilateral renal agenesis associated with this anomaly, it is called the Herlyn-Werner-Wunderlich (HWW) syndrome. It accounts for 3–4% of the Müllerian malformations. The obstetric prognosis is good and there are reported cases of pregnancies with twins with a fetus in each uterus [16]. Uterus didelphys only needs surgical correction in cases of HWW syndrome, due to one of the vaginas being obliterated and the septum between them needs to be resected to drain the hematocolpos and hematometra. It also allows for the outflow of normal menstrual flow [16]. Uterus didelphys has a good reproductive prognosis.

Class 4

Bicornuate uterus occurs when there is a failure in the fusion of the two Müllerian structures that ends with having two uterine horns and only one cervix. Varying degrees of deficiency of the fusion will allow the bicornuate uterus to be complete or partial. The cavities can be separated up to the internal orifice of the cervix and are not linked or partially linked when there is some connection. This malformation accounts for around 10% of the Müllerian malformations. It is asymptomatic in most cases and can cause miscarriage or premature birth [17]. Bicornuate uterus accounts for recurrent miscarriage in the 2nd trimester of pregnancy and premature birth and not really is not a cause of difficulty conceiving. When no other cause can be identified, a Strassman's metroplasty can be done. These show good results and a 90% rate of full pregnancy [18].

Class 5

Septate uterus is the result of incomplete reabsorption of the median septum post fusion of the Müllerian structures. The septum can be complete or partial depending on the moment when the failure occurred. The external contour of the uterus is always normal. The structure of the septum can be muscular or fibrous, and this diagnosis is important in terms of treatment options. It accounts for 55% of the malformations and is associated with recurrent miscarriage and premature birth. It is one of the malformations with the worst obstetric outcomes with regard to reproducing [17, 19]. The management of choice is hysteroscopy and metroplasty. These have been shown to have good outcomes [19].

Class 6

Arcuate uterus is thought of as a variant of the normal uterus, and it only presents an isolated curvature on the bottom of the uterus. It has no clinically significant differences [20]. It occurs due to the failure in the final stage of reabsorption of the inter-Müllerian septum and does not need intervention.

Class 7

T-shaped uterus is induced by diethylstilbestrol (DES); it is noted as a T-shaped uterus detected in daughters of women who used this drug during pregnancy. The uterine cavity is irregular and hypoplastic. There is poor outcomes for pregnancy and has a high risk of miscarriage or ectopic pregnancy [21]. It is an increasingly rare anomaly as diethylstilbestrol was discontinued in 1971.

Transverse vaginal septum results from the failure of canalization of the vaginal plaque, where the urogenital sinus meets the Müllerian duct. It is not associated with other malformations. It can be perforated or not and be of different thicknesses and area along the vagina. Women with a perforated septum are more difficult to diagnose as they menstruate normally and there are few symptoms. The thickness and area along the vagina is important to outline the treatment options. The lower, the thinner and if its perforated have better outcomes, while the higher and the thicker ones have high chances of complication such as rectovaginal fistula and hysterectomy. Its occurrence is estimated to be between 1/2100 and 1/72000 women [22]. Transverse vaginal septum should be managed with surgical resection and anastomosis of the proximal and distal vaginas. The choice of the technique depends on its localization and thickness. This is diagnosed during physical exam, sonar, and MRI. Surgery can be done vaginal or laparoscopic. The lowest, the thinnest and the perforated ones have the best results, and the main complications are dyspareunia, stenosis, re-obstruction, and psychological difficulties. Vaginal dilatation is said to have beneficial outcomes after surgery to improve the result [22, 23].

Performing a gynae exam on every patient with suspected genital malformations is of paramount importance. In any patient with primary amenorrhea, it is vital to examine the distal vagina. However, many cases may not solely be diagnosed via clinical examination and may require further assessment with radiological imaging. The initial diagnostic method is 2D sonar of the pelvis and pelvic organs, but 3D sonar, MRI, hysterosalpingo-contrast-sonography, X-ray hysterosalpingography, hysteroscopy, and laparoscopy are also used. The main advantages and disadvantages of these diagnostic methods are as noted. Sonar is the initial tool used because it is simple, noninvasive, and low cost; it is usually available and provides good information. Drawbacks being that it is highly dependent on the experience of the examiner [24–26].

3D sonar has good reproducibility and provides additional and more reliable images and allows for the visualization of the cervix and the vagina, the drawbacks being that it is less available and requires more comprehensive training as compared to a 2D sonar [24–27].

MRI is noted to be the gold standard. It offers good 3D images and information regarding the genitals and perineum as well as surrounding structures. It can be used in all cases of suspected malformations, including obstructive malformations. The drawbacks mainly being cost, it is more expensive and less available than the sonar and needs a radiologist to interpret the results [24, 28–30].

Hysterosalpingo-contrast-sonography is a minimally invasive method, is low cost, and provides good information about the cervix and uterine cavity. However it is highly dependent on the examiner, and the distention of the uterine cavity can change its inner shape which can generate false-negative images [26, 33].

X-ray hysterosalpingography is able to assess the uterine cavity and fallopian tubes. It is used mostly in cases of infertility. It is an invasive, painful examination. It does not evaluate the external shape or irregularities. For example, it will not differentiate the septate uterus from the bicornuate one, cannot diagnose the non-communicating uterine horn, and cannot be used in vaginal and cervical obstructions [24, 31].

Hysteroscopy is minimally invasive and gives good images and provides valuable information about the vagina, cervical canal, and the uterine cavity, although it does not evaluate the external contours or the thickness of the uterine wall and does not differentiate the septate uterus from the bicornuate one [24].

Laparoscopy is the exam of choice used to evaluate the external contour and irregularities of the uterus and the surrounding structures as well as intra peritoneal organs. It is an invasive exam and does not evaluate the thickness of the uterine wall and completely depends on the experience and evaluation of the examiner who is performing the procedure. It will also need anesthetic and one must consider anesthetic risks, respectively [24].

Some Müllerian malformations are healed with surgery and the success of the treatment depends on accurate diagnosis and the choice of the best technique [32].

Vaginal agenesis can be treated with dilatation as mentioned prior or vaginoplasty, and since 2002, the ACOG has recommended dilatation as the first choice given the high rate of success and lack of complications [33]. When the dilatation is unsuccessful, vaginoplasty could be done by various techniques [34], the recommended one being that in which the surgical team has more experience. The best anatomical results with the lowest rates of complications are in patients that perform dilatation through coitus. The McIndoe vaginoplasty has the highest rate of complications, the most common of which are the shrinkage and stenosis of the neovagina [35]. The choice for the best treatment for vaginal agenesis continues to be controversial, primarily due to the lack of comparative studies. The uncommonness of the disease makes the surgical teams always use the same technique.

Congenital cervical and vaginal atresia is debated in terms of treatment. There are no set guidelines or randomized studies that point to the best surgery and outcomes. It is a gynecological urgency with many risks and hysterectomy is the first option for management. Several sources mention this, specifically due to its many benefits [35]. Zhang Y et al. [13] in 2015 did a study on four patients diagnosed with cervical and vaginal atresia who had been treated with robotic-assisted reconstruction of the cervix and vagina. This was done using SIS graft. All of them recovered after the surgery and had regular menstruations without periodic pelvic pain. Average follow-up was 12 months with average vaginal length being 8.9 ± 0.3 cm, vaginal width was 2.9 ± 0.1 cm, and there were no re-admissions for any post-surgery complications.

There are multiple anomalies that may occur, and rectoperineal fistula is the simplest of all the defects. The rectum opens in a small, stenotic orifice which is located anterior to the center in relation to sphincter. Most of these patients have intact sphincter control, with the rectum and vagina usually well separated [36]. Rectovestibular fistula is the most common female defect, evident on examination as a normal external urethral opening and vagina, with a third hole in the vestibule which is noted to be the rectum [37]. 10% of cases have two hemivaginas [38]. Rectovaginal fistula is rare and accounts for <1% of cases [37]; it is regularly misdiagnosed as vestibular fistula or cloaca. Vaginal agenesis (absent vagina), is due to absence of Müllerian duct formation. It is a rare disorder that is also often associated with absence of the cervix and uterus [39]. Septate vaginal abnormalities occur from failure of septal regression after the fusion of the Müllerian ducts. Fusion is thought to progress in a caudal to cephalad direction, and combined anomalies, such as completely divided uterine, cervical, and vaginal canals, should be most severe when the vagina is involved, as this is the most distal structure [40]; however more recent literature has shown exceptions to this rule and have proposed that Müllerian duct fusion starts at the uterus, with fusion proceeding caudally and cephalad to this area [41–44]. A septate vaginal canal regularly occurs in the presence of other septate structures such as the cervix and uterus. Imperforate hymen is relatively uncommon and occurs in 1 in 1000 newborn females. This anomaly is generally sporadic but has been seen in families with both dominant and recessive modes of inheritance which suggests multiple genes may be involved [45, 46]. Vaginal adenosis is abnormal or excessive mucus-secreting cervico-vaginal glands and has been noted to occur exclusively under diethylstilboestrol (DES) exposure in utero. It is associated with increased risk of developing adenocarcinoma.

Anorectal malformations (ARM) include a wide variety of diseases and involve the distal rectum and anus which is in an abnormal anatomical position. The prevalence of imperforate anus in newborns is 1 in 4000–5000 [46]. The incidence of imperforate anus without fistula is noted at 5%. Half are diagnosed to have Down's syndrome. 38% of these patients have associated genitourinary defects [37]. Rectal atresia or stenosis prevails in 1% of all cases [37]. It is the only disease in this spectrum with normal anal canal and sphincter mechanisms. The most multifaceted female ARM is the persistent cloaca. This is when the rectum, vagina, and urinary tract confluence in a single common cloaca (CC) and the length range is 1–7 cm. CC >3 cm are normally associated with complex defects. Clinically, a single perineal orifice can be appreciated. In roughly 50% of these patients, the vagina is abnormally distended by secretions from the cervix. 50% of cloaca patients have a high incidence of Mullerian anomalies. Understanding and identification of such anomalies during the main repair allows for reconstruction to occur before puberty.

The significant finding of having a sacral deformity is regularly associated with ARM. Often, one or more sacral vertebrae are missing, with poor signs for lack of bowel function. The presence of a pathological cord is associated with a poor prognosis in terms of urofecal continence. High urological malformations can also be associated with ARM.

In the management of ARM, it is vital to know the level at which the anomaly is occurring as well as the nature of the anomaly. In terms of operative treatment in the neonatal period, surgical repair is rarely urgent. Most patients tolerate lower bowel obstruction without any symptoms for more than 24 h if the upper gastrointestinal tract is decompressed.

Female reconstructions of ARM can be repaired using the posterior sagittal approach. This is performed via laparotomy/laparoscopy. The procedure can be performed at 1–2 months of age. During this procedure, the rectum is separated from the UGS, and the vagina is separated from the urethra; this is to try to place each structure in its correct anatomical position. 30% cloacal anomalies cannot be operated using the posterior sagittal approach, this is if the CC is >3 cm and abdominal approach is needed. For the other 70%, the standard approach is the posterior sagittal operation.

Ureteric Bud Anomalies

Ureteric bud is also known as the metanephrogenic diverticulum and is a protrusion of the mesonephric duct. It will eventually form the urinary collecting system. This is the abnormal position of the ureteric bud and results in renal dysplasia as well as a refluxing system due to abnormal position of the ureteric orifice in the bladder [47].

Renal fusion anomalies were first noted by Wilmer in 1938, with the topic being expanded by McDonald and McClellan in 1957 [48]. Classification is based on characteristics such as crossed or uncrossed and fused or unfused. They may be further subdivided noted below.

Pelvic kidney includes a range of anatomical anomalies when the kidney fails to rise from the pelvis in its metanephros stage during development. Majority of patients are asymptomatic; however, they are sometimes associated with greater risk of injury from trauma, renal calculi, urinary tract infections, and other urological issues. They may complicate other surgeries due to anatomical situation, such as for aortic aneurysms repairs.

Congenital renal anomalies are extremely common type of birth deformities. They are only surpassed by cardiac and skeletal defects [48]. Of all the various renal fusion anomalies, the horseshoe kidney is the most common, while a pancake or lump kidney is the least common occurrence [49].

Ectopic kidneys' blood supply is not consistent. They may receive vascular supply and drainage from a variety of vessels as the fetal blood supply can be retained. Multiple vascular sources may supply the ectopic kidney. These range from the iliac arteries or direct branches from the aorta or midsacral vessels, or the hypogastric arteries have all been noted to supply the ectopic kidneys [50]. A good knowledge as to the blood supply would be important prior to performing any surgery on these patients with ectopic kidney.

Ectopic kidneys are also linked with numerous other congenital anomalies. These may involve pelvic organs, such as Mullerian agenesis or unicornuate uterus in females [51, 52]. Ectopic kidney can also be a feature of multifacet congenital syndromes such as CHARGE syndrome (coloboma, heart disease, atresia choanae, retarded growth, genital hypoplasia, and ear anomalies) or VACTERL malformations (vertebral, anal, cardiac, tracheal, esophageal, renal, and limb anomalies) [53, 54].

During kidney development between weeks 6 and 8, the embryologic kidney arises from the pelvis into the lumbar region in week 9. If the kidney fails to pass above the fork of the umbilical arteries, the blood supply degenerates. There may be other factors preventing renal migration; if this happens, then the kidney fails to rise to its normal anatomical place and instead lies ectopic [55, 56].

The precise location can be different in each patient, majority of cases being in the contralateral pelvis. In the cases of crossed renal ectopia, both of the kidneys can be on the same side of the spine or, more rarely, the kidney can be outside of the pelvis or outside of the retroperitoneal space. It can even be located within the chest cavity. This is usually associated with a diaphragmatic hernia [57, 58].

There are six anatomical subtypes of crossed fused ectopic kidneys that are noted [59].

- Superior ectopia. The anatomically normal kidney's superior pole is fused with the inferior pole of the ectopic kidney.
- Inferior ectopia. The ectopic kidney is lying inferiorly to the anatomically normal kidney.
- Sigmoid which is also known as S-shaped.
- Pancake which is also known as lump.
- Disk-shaped.

There has been an additional subtype termed "Y type" by Zhuo Yin et al. (2014) and has fusion of the ureters [60].

Ectopic kidney is normally a unilateral condition; however, there are cases noted with bilateral ectopic kidneys [61, 62]. This is different from a horseshoe kidney in which the inferior poles of both kidneys are fused together and they are usually within the retroperitoneal space [63].

A pancake kidney is a rare subset of fused ectopic kidneys and occurs when there is a fusion of the kidneys along their medial aspects leading to a round discoid kidney. There may be cases where a central hole (donut kidney) occurs or if the medial portion fuses entirely [64]. Despite this, there will normally still two separate collecting systems with an anterior, medial lying renal pelvis that does not communicate with each other. Pancake kidneys are mostly found in men as opposed to women (2.5,1) with the most common age for detection being between 30 and 60 years [65].

The incidence noted is inconsistent but is roughly 1 in 1000 births. A retrospective study of 13,701 antenatal scans in Turkey found an incidence of 1 in 571 of pelvic kidneys. However, this study only included scans with normal amniotic fluid volumes [66]. A Taiwanese study of 132,000 schoolchildren were screened and found a lower incidence of only 1 in 5000 [67].

Even in asymptomatic patients, the ectopic kidney generally has diminished renal function as compared to the contralateral normal kidney [62]. Since most patients with ectopic kidneys are asymptomatic as noted previously, they are diagnosed incidentally, if diagnosed at all. This is while investigating other pathology or on routine antenatal ultrasonography. However, some may be symptomatic, and urinary tract complications can arise. Patients can present with a variety of pathologies, including higher reports of urinary tract infections, uretero-pelvic junction obstruction in the ectopic kidney, or increased risk of renal calculi. Most commonly associated abnormality is vesicoureteric reflux and which occurs in 30% of patients with simple renal ectopia [62].

Pancake kidneys are often associated with other congenital anomalies such as undescended testes, tetralogy of Fallot, vaginal agenesis, sacral agenesis, spina bifida, and strabismus. They are more likely to develop hydronephrosis, renal trauma reflux, and calculi as compared with normal kidneys.

Primary, continuous urinary incontinence in a female can be attributed to a small or even tiny ectopic pelvic kidney; however this is rare. It may sometimes be too small to be seen by ultrasound alone and may require a renal nuclear scan or MRI with contrast to identify the associated hydroureter-nephrosis and tiny ectopic renal tissue. Thus, a high degree of suspicion should accompany any female patient with primary, continuous incontinence. There may even be compensatory hypertrophy of the contralateral kidney [68, 69]. Surgical management option is by removal of the ectopic pelvic kidney, usually laparoscopically or robotically [69].

On antenatal ultrasound, an empty renal fossa would be seen, and an ectopic kidney would be the most common cause of this finding, especially if the amniotic fluid is normal.

Workup and evaluation of pelvic kidneys differ somewhat depending on the center. Of note however, ectopic kidneys should always have an initial, postnatal imaging to assess for hydronephrosis and to visualize the anatomy of the contralateral kidney – if normal. If there are no further positive radiological findings, such as hydronephrosis and normal renal biochemistry (creatinine), further action may not be necessary. There is thought that mentions serial ultrasounds to monitor renal growth as well as for the early detection of hydronephrosis and calculi [70].

If there is significant radiological finding of severe hydronephrosis or urinary tract infections, a voiding cystourethrogram (VCUG) can be indicated. If this is normal, further evaluation with a mercaptoacetyltriglycine-3 (MAG-3) or diethylenetriamine penta-acetic acid (DTPA) renal nuclear scan imaging should be considered, especially if the serum creatinine is elevated which indicates a possible obstruction is likely. In contrast, if there is only mild to moderate hydronephrosis, a follow-up review in 3 to 6 months is advised, to decide if there is a progression in the hydronephrosis and satisfactory renal tissue growth is recommended. If abnormal progression is found, further imaging and nuclear scans should be done to investigate for a ureteric obstruction.

If the contralateral kidney is anatomically abnormal as well or if there is impaired renal biochemistry (creatinine), then the differential renal function should be assessed with a DMSA scan and specialist advice sought. Guardino et al. found that in 82 cases of a simple ectopic kidney, 74 exhibited lower renal function in the ectopic kidney as compared to the contralateral kidney on DMSA imaging [62]. In that same case series published by Guardino, the incidence of simultaneous pathology was found to be high with an ectopic kidney.

In uncomplicated pelvic kidneys that are asymptomatic, no intervention is mandatory. If there are complications such as renal calculi, the distorted anatomy may make the condition more difficult to manage. It is thus imperative to recognize the anatomy and vasculature of pelvic kidneys [50].

If a patient with ectopic kidney develops renal calculi in the ectopic pelvic kidney, surgical intervention is much more complex than in an anatomically normal urinary tract; this is due to the different location of the ureters [71]. Laparoscopic-assisted percutaneous transperitoneal nephrolithotomy has been used to treat stones too large for shockwave lithotripsy of which is more effective in renal stones under 2 cm in diameter. This procedure may need the surgeon to mobilize the colon. There is a risk of urine leak into the abdomen, but it is an option if the stone is not contained within the renal pelvis and calyces [72]. Mobilization of the bowel may not be required if the surgeon performs a transmesocolic pyelolithotomy or with robot-assisted surgery. This has the additional benefit of being able to remain within the retroperitoneal space which reduces the risk of an intra-abdominal urine leak and urinoma formation [73–75].

Specific problems with ectopic kidneys can be operated on if needed; however a fused renal mass does not yield great outcomes due to the potential for vascular injury, renal infarction, tissue necrosis, and decreased renal function [76].

Taking into consideration, the outcomes of surgery performed on ectopic kidneys or complications that arise as a result are generally poor and hence operative management discouraged in ectopic kidneys except for specific problems and most cases can be managed conservatively. Percutaneous access to relieve an obstruction or for percutaneous nephrolithotomy may be more complex or even impossible in some cases depending on the individual anatomy, and this needs to be taken into consideration. A 24-h urine testing as well as urine microscopy and culture for renal calculus prophylaxis is recommended in patients that have had renal calculus with ectopic kidneys due to the increased complexity of kidney stone surgery in these individuals and the risk of loss of renal function as well as treating urinary infection if need be.

Unilateral renal agenesis [62]. In ectopic renal and unilateral renal agenesis, one renal fossa will be empty on the sonar examination. However, in the case of renal agenesis, the kidney fails to form entirely as contrasting to ectopia where it is forming but failing to reach its normal anatomical position.

Horseshoe kidney [62]. In horseshoe kidneys, the renal system may not be located in their normal anatomical position. Rather than being a defect of only one kidney, both kidneys are fused, forming one single U-shaped mass in the lower abdomen. This is normally located easily on ultrasound and other abdominal imaging studies.

If there is no other pathology, ectopic kidneys are not commonly associated with renal dysfunction or hypertension. Van den Bosch et al. (2010) published a series of 41 patients, all of whom underwent VCUG investigation with 13 displaying vesicoureteric reflux. The relative function of the ectopic kidney was 38% on DMSA scan, and 88% had an eGFR >90. These findings were consistent in both simple and crossed ectopic kidneys [77].

In contrast, when there is malrotation and related extrarenal calyces, these types of patients are at increased risk of recurrent urinary tract infection and hydronephrosis [78]. Their incidence of vesicoureteric reflux and renal failure is also higher than the general population [62].

Like other ectopic kidneys, pancake kidneys are usually asymptomatic but are also associated with an increased risk of recurrent urinary tract infection and stone formation [63]. This increased risk of renal calculus in ectopic kidney is due to reduced urinary flow through a more tortuous ureter and the vascular anomalies that are associated with the condition [79].

A review of crossed fused ectopic kidney published in 2019 found only 35 documented cases of stones and 30 cases of malignancy associated with the condition [59]. The function of the kidney was sufficient to use them as donor organs for renal transplant [80]. While renal ectopia is not completely without complications nor harmless condition, the overall prognosis is usually good.

Most patients with pelvic kidneys have a good prognosis and are asymptomatic however due to the abnormal anatomy of their ureters, this can impair urinary flow. This follows that they are associated with an increased incidence of vesicoureteric reflux and renal calculi formation. Vesicoureteric reflux, in turn, is associated with recurrent urinary tract infection and chronic kidney disease.

Vesicoureteric Reflux

Ectopic kidneys are linked with abnormal ureteric anatomy. The course of the ureter can be more tortuous and the point of insertion can be higher in the kidney which impairs the flow of urine through the urinary tract [81]. This may lead to the back-flow of urine, causing vesicoureteric reflux (VUR) or dilatation of the renal pelvis and calyces, resulting in hydronephrosis. The incidence of these complications is variable with most of the studies showing they don't regularly occur. Hydronephrosis can be diagnosed with sonography imaging; however vesicoureteric reflux requires further investigation such as voiding cystourethrography (VCUG) which is the gold standard. Vesicoureteric reflux is associated with recurrent urinary tract infections and renal impairment.

Calisti et al. [82] published a series including 50 patients with a single ectopic kidney, none of whom had significant concomitant pathology [82]. However, there are reports where the incidence of pathology is higher. Gleason et al. [83] published a series of 77 patients with 82 ectopic kidneys from the Mayo Clinic. They found 56% had hydronephrosis, and 26% had vesicoureteric reflux [83].

Renal Calculi

Due to distorted anatomy and compromised urinary flow rates, these patients are predisposed to develop urinary calculi. The exact incidence of renal calculi in pelvic kidneys is unknown but is thought to be higher than the general population. The altered anatomy does have important implications in the surgical management of renal calculi. The risk of vascular injury is higher as compared to the general population [81].

Malignancy

Malignancy in pelvic kidneys is not common. The risk of malignancy is not normally thought to be notably higher than anatomically normal kidneys [84]. However, there have been some documented cases. It has been proposed that patients with ectopic fused renal anomalies are more probable to develop Wilms tumor or renal cell carcinoma as compared with the general population [85]. Patients with horseshoe kidneys are twice as likely to develop Wilms tumor than age-matched cohorts with normal anatomy. Special consideration should be taken given the inconstant nature of the renal blood supply if such patients require surgery.

Ectopic ureter is a ureter which opens anywhere outside of the bladder trigone and will constitute a displaced ureteral bud. Buds that develop low along the mesonephric duct will be situated in a laterocranial ectopic position – with significant vesicoureteric reflux (VUR). If the bud develops high along the mesonephric duct, it bypasses the trigone and inserts in the urethra or vagina. 70% of ectopic ureter are associated with a duplicated system, despite a single ectopic ureter being able to drain a single system. Complete ureteral duplication arises when there are two separate buds that arise independently from the mesonephric duct. A duplex kidney is a result of these two buds confluencing at the metanephric blastema. Workup of these patients includes a voiding cysto-urethrogram, which would show refluxing into the ectopic ureter in 70–80% of the cases. CT intravenous pyelogram may be performed to delineate the duplicated system as well as showing a dilated system [47, 86].

Treatment varies from ureteroureterostomy in duplex systems, or upper pole resections with or without ureterectomy, or ureteroneocystostomy, or nephroureterectomy [87].

Gartner's Duct Cyst (GDC)

This is a remnant of the Wolffian duct and can be located in the lateral vaginal wall. This may have clinical significance if they become swollen or become infected. They may rupture, and if there is a poorly functioning renal system associated, this may present as continuous incontinence.

Garner duct cyst are the cystic remnants of the Wolffian (mesonephric) duct and account for roughly 11% of all vaginal cysts [88]. They occur as a result of incomplete regression of the mesonephric or Wolffian duct during fetal development [89]. They are located sub-mucosally along the anteromedial wall of the vagina [89, 90]. They are normally solitary, however may be multiple [89, 91]. The cysts are small and are usually less than 2 cm in diameter. There have been reported giant cysts which are even rarer [91]. The cyst wall is lined with a non-mucin-secreting, cuboidal epithelium [3]. The fluid within the cyst is white, thick, and viscous [3]. Mucoid fluid rules out a mesonephric cyst [88].

The incidence of diagnosing GDC in pediatric group is very low and other diagnosis should be considered [92]. The differential diagnosis of Gartner cyst in a neonate is vast [90]. It includes imperforate hymen, which is the most common, paraurethral Skene's duct cyst, urethral prolapse, prolapsed ectopic ureterocele, urethral polyp, congenital lipoma, vaginal prolapse, and rhabdomyosarcoma of the vagina [93, 94]. Vaginal cysts and Bartholin gland cysts are normally diagnosed later in the third and fourth decades and not in neonates [89].

Accurate diagnosis requires a thorough understanding of differential diagnosis and a systemic examination [90]. Physical examination is the most useful in diagnosing the certain pathology [88]. The patient should be placed in "frog-leg position," and the labia majora should be gently grasped and pulled inferiorly and laterally enabling visualization of the introitus and vagina [93]. The size of the clitoris, hymen assessment (possible imperforate), urethral location, and the

site and character of the mass can be appreciated and documented [90]. Placement of a small feeding tube through the urethral orifice can aid in the urogenital examination [90]. Abdominal ultrasound is a good aid in diagnosing related renal pathology [90].

Histology gives an accurate diagnosis on the embryological origin [94]. The vagina is derived from the paramesonephric (Mullerian) duct, the mesonephric (Wolffian) ducts, and the urogenital sinus [94]. The vaginal cysts are lined with stratified squamous epithelium as they originate from the Mullerian duct. Gartner duct cysts are lined with cuboidal epithelium (mesonephric/Wolffian origin) [94]. Transitional epithelium in the cyst wall shows the origin to be in the urinary tract (paraurethral cysts, urethral prolapse, Skene's ducts cysts, ureterocele prolapse, and ectopic ureter) and requires a full renal workup to be carried out [94–96].

Association of GDC with ipsilateral renal agenesis or dysplasia is rare and is caused by the abnormal development of the ureter [97, 98]. The presence of ureteric ectopia associated with GDC has been reported to be caused by the failure of separation of the ureteric bud from the mesonephric duct, which leads to persistence of Gartner's duct, frequently with cystic dilation [97, 98]. Presentation with sepsis or non- or poorly functioning renal tissue is an indication for ureterectomy or nephroureterectomy on the affected side [97].

Management options are aspiration, deroofing, marsupialization, and complete excision [93–99]. A recent study by Rios et al. involving four women has shown that conservative treatment can be a safe option for asymptomatic patients with vaginal GDCs [100]. In a study involving 15 patients by Abd-Rabbo et al., aspiration and injection sclerotherapy with tetracycline has been reported as one of the management options [101]. This technique has been reported as an ideal, safe, and effective simple office procedure for management of symptomatic Gartner cysts. However, its application in neonates is unknown. The long-term prognosis is good [99].

Mayer–Rokitansky–Küster–Hauser syndrome (MRHK)

A female genital malformation syndrome known as Mayer-Rokitansky-Kuster-Hauser (MRKH) occurs in 1 in 4000 live births. Interrupted embryonic development of the Mullerian ducts during week 5 can be attributed to the defects noted in this syndrome [102]. The defects consist of atresia of the upper part of the vagina which is reduced to a less deep vaginal dimple (2–7 cm). Aplasia of the upper part of the vagina and uterus correspond to Type 1 MRKH. MRKH Type 2 consist of any malformations noted in the upper urinary tract, skeleton and heart. Patients during puberty have primary amenorrhea and inability to have penetrative vaginal intercourse and primary sterility; these issues occur despite having normal development of secondary sexual characteristics, external genitalia, level of gonadotrophins, ovarian function, and 46XX karyotype.

Pillars of treating MRKH patients are aimed at creating better quality of life for these patients. Surgical treatment consists of allowing MRKH patients to have sexual intercourse by creating a neovagina. Non-surgical techniques have been proposed for patients who are suitable candidates; these involve vaginal dilators which was introduced by Frank in 1938. They are the most commonly used non-surgical procedure, which progressively increases the length and diameter of the vagina.

Davydov procedure is one of many different surgical techniques which have been proposed for the correction of vaginal agenesis [103]. The peritoneal vaginoplasty adopted the use of peritoneum to line a newly created vaginal space but is complicated with the risk of bladder and ureteric injuries and vesicovaginal fistula. Banister and McIndoe [104] proposed the use of split-thickness skin grafts, but these are compromised and complicated by scarring at the donor site as well as risks of graft failure as well as graft loss.

Williams' vaginoplasty [105] involves the use of a vulval flap to create a vaginal canal. This procedure is complicated by local scarring but also by formation of an abnormal vaginal angle. Sigmoidal colpoplasty seems to be an efficient procedure; however complete adequacy for coital function requires prolonged care and support [106].

The Vecchietti procedure involves placement of plastic olives in the vaginal dimple, connected by a traction device attached to the abdomen. Continuous and increasing tension is applied to the vaginal wall to lengthen the vagina [106]. This is performed open or laparoscopically. The literature suggests that it is the optimal surgical technique for MRKH patients in terms of safety, anatomical outcomes, and patient satisfaction.

Imaging investigations are important in valuation of the anatomy and function of pelvic organs in patients with congenital abnormalities. MRI allows for accurate evaluation of the uterine aplasia, as well as a clear visualization of the rudimentary horns and ovaries in MRKH syndrome [107]. Magnetic resonance imaging (MRI) is acknowledged to provide the most accurate evaluation of soft tissue. Dynamic MRI of the pelvic floor also permits the delineation of continence organ function.

Computerized tomography (CT) with 3D reconstruction has also been shown to be a useful diagnostic tool for soft tissue abnormalities. It provides a better understanding of the pelvic floor anatomy in BE. However, MRI has the highest soft tissue resolution and therefore better anatomical assessment as well as functional assessment of continence organs without ionizing radiation used for CT scan. MRI therefore is the most appropriate imaging modality despite the cost and lengthy examination time performed to perform the study.

The use of minimally invasive surgery is becoming more popular due to the need to improve cosmetic outcomes in reconstructive surgery for urinary and fecal incontinence in children and adolescents. To improve cosmesis and decrease future adhesions, laparoscopy is utilized [108].

A laparoscopic modification of Vecchietti's procedure for MRKH syndrome is often preferred and leads to comparable results. A recent study by Bianchi et al. [109] compared Vecchietti's and Davydov's laparoscopic techniques for the creation of a neovagina in MRKH patients. Anatomical and functional outcomes were comparable at

12-month follow-up, and the only significant difference was the greater length of the neovagina achieved by Davydov's approach.

McKusick-Kaufman Syndrome (MKKS)

The syndrome was first described by McKusick in 1964 and was seen in 2 Amish siblings [110]. Recent count of the MKKS phenotype revealed only around 90 individual cases, but the true incidence of MKKS still remains unknown [110].

McKusick-Kaufman syndrome is a rare, autosomal recessive inherited disorder characterized by a triad of post axial polydactyly (PAP), congenital heart disease, and hydrometrocolpos (HMC) in women and genital anomalies in men. These include hypospadias, cryptorchidism, and chordee. In both women and men, no features of overlapping syndromes such as the Bardet-Biedl syndrome (BBS) should be present [110].

MKKS is sometimes known as HMC-polydactyly syndrome. These are usually clinically apparent at an early stage in diagnosis [111]. Vaginal agenesis or atresia can be possible causes for HMC or a transverse vaginal septum which results in vaginal and uterine dilatations secondary to the accumulation of cervical secretions stimulated by maternal estrogen secretion [110]. An imperforate hymen remains the most common obstructive anomaly of the lower female genital tract even though it has an incidence of 0.1% in female babies. It results from incomplete canalization of the endoderm of the urogenital sinus [112]. In the neonatal period, HMC may present with ascites or acute kidney injury. This is due to the obstructive uropathy and manifest with dilation of the renal pelvicalyceal system which is appreciated as hydronephrosis with or without hydroureter on sonar [113]. Patients may also present with bowel obstruction which is due to a large pelvic cystic mass on examination [30]. Other complications which may arise are inferior vena caval obstruction or respiratory distress due to diaphragmatic elevation [114]. Teenagers may present with primary amenorrhea, constipation, menstrual pain, lower back pain, or even acute urinary retention [113].

Once the diagnosis of HMC is confirmed, management of MKKS is multimodal and aimed at addressing the manifestations of the disorder and preventing secondary complications. Definitive management to drain the accumulated fluid and creating a communication between the vaginal canal and vulva is also advocated [115]. A perineal approach is indicated for patients with an imperforate hymen and low vaginal atresia, whereas an abdominoperineal approach is preferred for high vaginal atresia. Treatment may involve a simple cruciate-shaped hymenectomy which is indicated for isolated imperforate hymen. Major surgery is performed for more complex urogenital anomalies [116]. Children without a mucocele and who are asymptomatic can undergo delayed definitive treatment/delayed drainage, in puberty, before the occurrence of hematocolpos or hematometra. This is to reduce anesthetic risk that may occur with children [116]. Polydactyly is managed as per hands unit. Sound clinical examination, electrocardiogram, and echocardiography should be adequate in detecting congenital cardiac defects. If patient has any cardiac anomalies, referral to the cardiologist is imperative for initiation of treatment and further management by cardiothoracic surgeon if needed.

Clinical findings are the cornerstone in diagnosing MKKS. Most cases are detected by sound clinical acumen and a high index of suspicion [116]. BBS, Pallister-Hall syndrome, and Ellis-van Creveld syndrome are among the differential diagnosis for MKKS [115]. BBS exhibits the closest phenotypic overlap with MKKS and represents a spectrum of genetically heterogeneous autosomal recessive disorders. The defining features for BBS are the triad for MKKS as well as retinitis pigmentosa, retinal dystrophy, obesity, renal abnormalities or nephropathy, hypogonadism in men, and cognitive impairment [116, 117]. BBS can mostly only be diagnosed in older children or teenagers when the additional features become evident whereas MKKS is normally diagnosed in young children [111].

Surveillance involves monitoring of blood pressure, ophthalmological assessment, renal sonar, and renal function in patients who have renal dysfunction or any anatomical abnormality, and growth and developmental monitoring. If manifestations or complications are identified early, these renal abnormalities can be referred appropriately and managed [110, 118].

Parents who have an affected child have a 25% risk in future pregnancies for MKKS. They should be referred for genetic counselling. Carrier testing is possible for at-risk relatives [110, 118].

Pelvic Anomalies

Premature rupture of the cloacal membrane causes an array of abnormalities, one of which is bladder exstrophy (BE). It is a complex and severe pelvic malformation and is seen in 1 in 40,000 newborns. Incidence is equal in males and females [119, 120].

A defect in the anterior pelvic floor gives rise to BE, it involves the urogenital diaphragm and the surrounding musculoskeletal structures (levator ani muscles – LAM). The pelvic bones are not fused at the pubic symphysis and the bladder lies between the two pubic rami. The sacroiliac joints and the anterior and posterior pelvis are rotated externally [121, 122]. A change in the elliptical shape of the levator ani muscles occurs. 70% of the levator mass is located posterior to the rectum and 30% lies anterior to the rectum which results in a flattened pelvic floor. The anterior aspect of the pelvic diaphragm becomes thickened, and the remaining portion of the pelvic diaphragm lies completely posterior to the exstrophic bladder. The internal surface of the posterior part of the bladder lies in the central part of the abdomen. The bladder mucosa is continuous with the skin, and the ureteral ostia lie in the inferior part of the exstrophic plaque and do not have any sphincters.

Multidisciplinary approach is required to fully manage and treat this disorder. Surgically, a complex approach involving several steps is required to achieve aesthetic and functional level of urinary continence and reconstruction of the external genitalia. Surgery involves primary closure of the bladder, with or without iliac osteotomies which assists to help close the pelvic ring. In newborns, if operated on within 48 h of birth, a primary closure of the exstrophic plaque can be performed without pelvic osteotomy. If the bladder is non-functional or procedure cannot adequately correct abnormalities, functional and anatomically, the mucosa must be removed in order to prevent recurrent infections or risk of carcinoma.

Outcomes of surgical correction appear to depend on initial bladder size and the bladder neck tissue quality. Woodhouse et al. [123] commented on 101 patients born with BE. Closure of the bladder and bladder neck area, performed between 6 and 18 months, was attempted in 62 children.

Once bladder capacity improves, the bladder neck is reconstructed for continence to be achieved. Bilateral ureteric reimplantation is performed to prevent reflux.

Urinary diversion is necessary if it is not possible to perform a primary closure of the bladder or if continence is not achieved after this procedure. The ureters are implanted in the sigmoid colon with a non-refluxing type of anastomosis (ureterosigmoidostomy). This allows the patient to maintain continence and to evacuate urine through the anus and avoids a cutaneous diversion. Long-term complications with this surgical procedure can include pyelonephritis, nephrolithiasis, and colon adenocarcinoma.

Reconstruction of the external genitalia is needed in female patients with BE. This is normally performed during infancy or childhood. Procedures which are performed are vulvo-plasty, which involves joining the two halves of the clitoris and fusing the posterior ends of the labia to create a fourchette. Vaginoplasty allows opening the introitus to achieve an adequate vaginal diameter and monsplasty. Flaps of skin and fat are used to cover the midline defect; however it is not usually possible to move the vagina posteriorly into the correct position. Eight BE patients (average age 18.1 years) had undergone vulvovaginoplasty and clitoral repair. Only one subsequently experienced dyspareunia post surgery and required revision [124].

Conclusion

The outline and overview of these embryological events help in the understanding of these associated conditions. Although the minor anomalies may not have a significant clinical correlation, the same cannot be said for all, whose surgery and reconstructive management has repercussions which in some instances may be lifelong.

References

1. Baker TG. A quantitative and cytological study of germ cells in the human ovaries. Proc R Soc Lond Ser B. 1963;158:417–33.
2. Bardo DM, Black M, Schenk K, Zaritzky MF. Location of the ovaries in girls from newborn to 18 years of age: reconsidering ovarian shielding. Pediatr Radiol. 2009;39:253–9.
3. Moore KL, Persaud TVN. The urogenital system. In: Moore KL, Persaud TVN, editors. The developing human. Clinically oriented embryology. 6th ed. Philadelphia: WB Saunders; 1998. p. 303–47.
4. Robbins JB, Broadwell C, Chow LC, Parry JP, Sadowski EA. Müllerian duct anomalies: embryological development, classification, and MRI assessment. J Magn Reson Imaging. 2015;41(1):1–12.
5. Guioli S, Sekido R, Lovell-Badge R. The origin of the Mullerian duct in chick and mouse. Dev Biol. 2007;302(2):389–98.
6. Warne GL, Kanumakala S. Molecular endocrinology of sex differentiation. Semin Reprod Med. 2002;20(3):169–80.
7. Chaudhry SR, Chaudhry K. StatPearls [Internet]. Treasure Island StatPearls Publishing; Jul 26, 2021. Anatomy, Abdomen and Pelvis, Uterus Round Ligament.
8. de Ziegler D, Pirtea P, Galliano D, Cicinelli E, Meldrum D. Optimal uterine anatomy and physiology necessary for normal implantation and placentation. Fertil Steril. 2016;105(4):844–54.
9. Chandler TM, Machan LS, Cooperberg PL, Harris AC, Chang SD. Mullerian duct anomalies: from diagnosis to intervention. Br J Radiol. 2009;82(984):1034–42.
10. Kobayashi A, Behringer RR. Developmental genetics of the female reproductive tract in mammals. Nat Rev Genet. 2003;4(12):969–80.
11. Witschi E. Embryology of the uterus: normal and experimental. Ann N Y Acad Sci. 1959;09(75):412–35.
12. Troiano RN, McCarthy SM. Mullerian duct anomalies: imaging and clinical issues. Radiology. 2004;233(1):19–34.
13. Zhang Y, Chen Y, Hua K. Outcomes in patients undergoing robotic reconstructive uterovaginal anastomosis of congenital cervical and vaginal atresia. Int J Med Robot Comput Assist Surg. 2017;13:e1821.
14. Letterie GS. Management of congenital uterine abnormalities. Reprod BioMed Online. 2011;23(1):40–52.
15. Reichman D, Laufer MR, Robinson BK. Pregnancy outcomes in unicornuate uteri: a review. Fertil Steril. 2009;91:1886–94.
16. Kapczuk K, Friebe Z, Iwaniec K, Kedzia W. Obstructive Müllerian anomalies in menstruating adolescent girls: a report of 22 cases. J Pediatr Adolesc Gynecol. 2018;31(3):252–7.
17. Yoo R-E, Cho JY, Kim SY, Kim SH. A systematic approach to the magnetic resonance imaging-based differential diagnosis of congenital Müllerian duct anomalies and their mimics. Abdom Imaging. 2014;40(1):192–206.
18. Papp Z, Mezei G, Gavai M, Hupukizi P, Urbancsek J. Reproductive performance after transabdominal metroplasty: a review of 157 consecutive cases. J Reprod Med. 2006;51:544–52.
19. Valle RF, Ekpo GE. Hysteroscopic metroplasty for the septate uterus: review and meta-analysis. J Minim Invasive Gynecol. 2013;20(1):22–42.
20. American Fertility Society. The American Fertility Society classification of adnexal adhesions, distal tubal occlusion secondary or tubal ligation, tubal pregnancies, Mullerian anomalies and intrauterine adhesions. Fertil Steril. 1988;49(6):944–55.
21. Kaufman RH, Adan E, Binder GL, Gerthoffer F. Upper genital tract changes and pregnancy outcome in offspring exposed in uterus to diethylstilbestrol. Am J Obstet Gynecol. 1980;137:299.
22. Williams CE, Nakhal RS, Hall-Craggs MA, Wood D, Cutner A, Pattison SH, et al. Transverse vaginal septae: management and long-term outcomes. BJOG. 2014;121:1653–9.
23. Davies MC, Creighton SM, Woodhouse CRJ. The pitfalls of vaginal construction. BJU Int. 2005;95:1293–8.
24. Grimbizis GF, Di Spiezio Sardo A, Saravelos SH, Gordts S, Exacoustos C, Van Schoubroeck D, et al. The Thessaloniki ESHRE/ESGE consensus on diagnosis of female genital anomalies. Hum Reprod. 2016;31(1):2–7.
25. Nicolini U, Bellotti M, Bonazzi B, Zamberletti D, Candiani GB. Can ultrasound be used to screen uterine malformations? Fertil Steril. 1987;47:89–93.
26. Woodward PJ, Sohaey R, Wagner BJ. Congenital uterine malformations. Curr Probl Diagn Radiol. 1995;24:178–97.
27. Raga F, Bonilla-Musoles F, Blanes J, Osborne NG. Congenital Müllerian anomalies: diagnostic accuracy of three-dimensional ultrasound. Fertil Steril. 1996;65:523.

28. Troiano RN, McCarthy SM. Mullerian duct anomalies: imaging and clinical issues. Radiology. 2004;233:19.
29. Pellerito JS, McCarthy SM, Doyle MB, Glickman MG, DeCherney AH. Diagnosis of uterine anomalies: relative accuracy of MR imaging, endovaginal sonography, and hysterosalpingography. Radiology. 1992;183:795.
30. Olpin JD, Moeni A, Willmore RJ, Heilbrun ME. MR imaging of Müllerian fusion anomalies. Magn Reson Imaging Clin N Am. 2017;25(3):563–75.
31. Vahdat M, Sariri E, Kashanian M, Najmi Z, Mobasseri A, Marashi M, et al. Can combination of hysterosalpingography and ultrasound replace hysteroscopy in diagnosis of uterine malformations in infertile women? Med J Islam Repub Iran. 2016;30:352.
32. Edmonds DK. Congenital malformations of the genital tract and their management. Best Pract Res Clin Obstet Gynaecol. 2003;17(1):19–40.
33. ACOG Committee on Adolescent Health Care. ACOG Committee opinion Number 274. Nonsurgical diagnosis and management of vaginal agenesis. Obstet Gynecol. 2002;100(2002):213–6.
34. Karim RB, Hage JJ, Dekker JJ, Schoot CM. Evolution of the methods of neovaginoplasty for vaginal aplasia. Eur J Obstet Gynecol Reprod Biol. 1995;58(1):19–27.
35. Herlin M, Bay Bjørn AM, Jørgensen LK, Trolle B, Petersen MB. Treatment of vaginal agenesis in Mayer-Rokitansky-Küster-Hauser in Denmark: a Nationwide comparative study of anatomical outcome and complications. Fertil Steril. 2018;110(4):746–53.
36. Levitt M, Pena A. Anorectal malformations. Orphanet J Rare Dis. 2007;26:2–33.
37. Pena A, Hong A. Advances in the management of anorectal malformations. Am J Surg. 2000;180:370–6.
38. Levitt MA, Peña A. Outcomes from the correction of anorectal malformations. Curr Opin Pediatr. 2005;17:394–401.
39. Robson S, Oliver GD. Management of vaginal agenesis: review of 10 years' practice at a tertiary referral centre. Aust N Z J Obstet Gynaecol. 2000;40:430–3.
40. Crosby WM, Hill EC. Embryology of the Müllerian duct system. Obstet Gynecol. 1962;20:507–15.
41. Hundley AF, Fielding JR, Hoyte L. Double cervix and vagina with septate uterus: an uncommon Müllerian malformation. Obstet Gynecol. 2001;98:982–5.
42. Musset R, Muller P, Netter A, et al. Study of the upper urinary tract in patients with uterine malformations. Study of 133 cases. Presse Med. 1967;75:1331–6.
43. McBean JH, Brumsted JR. Septate uterus with cervical duplication: a rare malformation. Fertil Steril. 1994;62:415–7.
44. Hyatt SW. Imperforate hymen: review of the literature and report of four additional cases. Am Pract Dig Treat. 1960;11:1016–21.
45. Lim YH, Ng SP, Jamil MA. Imperforate hymen: report of an unusual familial occurrence. J Obstet Gynaecol Res. 2003;29:399–401.
46. Peña A. Preface: advance in anorectal malformations. Semin Pediatr Surg. 1997;6:165–9.
47. Ahmed S, Barker A. Single-system ectopic ureters: a review of 12 cases. J Pediatr Surg. 1992;27(4):491–6.
48. Bakshi S. Incidentally detected pancake kidney: a case report. J Med Case Rep. 2020;14(1):129.
49. Glodny B, Petersen J, Hofmann KJ, Schenk C, Herwig R, Trieb T, Koppelstaetter C, Steingruber I, Rehder P. Kidney fusion anomalies revisited: clinical and radiological analysis of 209 cases of crossed fused ectopia and horseshoe kidney. BJU Int. 2009;103(2):224–35.
50. Eid S, Iwanaga J, Loukas M, Oskouian RJ, Tubbs RS. Pelvic kidney: a review of the literature. Cureus. 2018 Jun;10(6):e2775.
51. D'Alberton A, Reschini E, Ferrari N, Candiani P. Prevalence of urinary tract abnormalities in a large series of patients with uterovaginal atresia. J Urol. 1981;126(5):623–4.
52. Fedele L, Bianchi S, Agnoli B, Tozzi L, Vignali M. Urinary tract anomalies associated with unicornuate uterus. J Urol. 1996;155(3):847–8.
53. Pagon RA, Graham JM, Zonana J, Yong SL. Coloboma, congenital heart disease, and choanal atresia with multiple anomalies: CHARGE association. J Pediatr. 1981;99(2):223–7.
54. Evans JA, Stranc LC, Kaplan P, Hunter AG. VACTERL with hydrocephalus: further delineation of the syndrome(s). Am J Med Genet. 1989;34(2):177–82.
55. Bush KT, Vaughn DA, Li X, Rosenfeld MG, Rose DW, Mendoza SA, Nigam SK. Development and differentiation of the ureteric bud into the ureter in the absence of a kidney collecting system. Dev Biol. 2006;298(2):571–84.
56. Gokalp G, Hakyemez B, Erdogan C. Vascular anomaly in bilateral ectopic kidney: a case report. Cases J. 2010;05(3):5.
57. Murphy JJ, Altit G, Zerhouni S. The intrathoracic kidney: should we fix it? J Pediatr Surg. 2012;47(5):970–3.
58. Dretler SP, Olsson C, Pfister RC. The anatomic, radiologic and clinical characteristics of the pelvic kidney: an analysis of 86 cases. J Urol. 1971;105(5):623–7.
59. Cao Y, Zhang Y, Kang W, Suo N, Cui Z, Luo Y, Jin X. Crossed-fused renal ectopia with renal calculi: two case reports and a review of the literature. Medicine (Baltimore). 2019;98(48):e18165.
60. Yin Z, Yang JR, Wei YB, Zhou KQ, Yan B. A new subtype of crossed fused ectopia of the kidneys. Urology. 2014;84(6):e27.
61. Meizner I, Barnhard Y. Bilateral fetal pelvic kidneys: documentation of two cases of a rare prenatal finding. J Ultrasound Med. 1995 Jun;14(6):487–9.
62. Guarino N, Tadini B, Camardi P, Silvestro L, Lace R, Bianchi M. The incidence of associated urological

abnormalities in children with renal ectopia. J Urol. 2004;172(4 Pt 2):1757–9. discussion 1759

63. Kirkpatrick JJ, Leslie SW. StatPearls [Internet]. Treasure Island: StatPearls Publishing; 2021. Horseshoe Kidney.

64. Tiwari AK, Choudhary AK, Khowal H, Chaudhary P, Arora MP. Pancake kidney: a rare developmental anomaly. Can Urol Assoc J. 2014;8(5–6):E451–2.

65. Chavis CV, Press HC, Gumbs RV. Fused pelvic kidneys: case report. J Natl Med Assoc. 1992;84(11): 980–2.

66. Yuksel A, Batukan C. Sonographic findings of fetuses with an empty renal fossa and normal amniotic fluid volume. Fetal Diagn Ther. 2004;19(6):525–32.

67. Sheih CP, Liu MB, Hung CS, Yang KH, Chen WY, Lin CY. Renal abnormalities in schoolchildren. Pediatrics. 1989;84(6):1086–90.

68. Gupta NP, Goel A, Kumar P, Aron M. Laparoscopy in diagnosis and management of urinary incontinence caused by small ectopic dysplastic kidney. Int Urogynecol J Pelvic Floor Dysfunct. 2002;13(5): 332–3.

69. Challacombe B, Kelleher C, Sami T, Scott H, Chandra A, O'Brien T, Dasgupta P. Laparoscopic nephroureterectomy for adult incontinence caused by functioning ectopic pelvic kidney draining into vagina. J Endourol. 2004 Jun;18(5):447–8.

70. Bhoil R, Sood D, Singh YP, Nimkar K, Shukla A. An ectopic pelvic kidney. Pol J Radiol. 2015;80:425–7.

71. Bozkurt IH, Cirakoglu A, Ozer S. Retroperitoneal laparoscopic pyelolithotomy in an ectopic pelvic kidney. JSLS. 2012;16(2):325–8.

72. Holman E, Tóth C. Laparoscopically assisted percutaneous transperitoneal nephrolithotomy in pelvic dystopic kidneys: experience in 15 successful cases. J Laparoendosc Adv Surg Tech A. 1998;8(6):431–5.

73. Gupta NP, Yadav R, Singh A. Laparoscopic transmesocolic pyelolithotomy in an ectopic pelvic kidney. JSLS. 2007;11(2):258–60.

74. Nayyar R, Singh P, Gupta NP. Robot-assisted laparoscopic pyeloplasty with stone removal in an ectopic pelvic kidney. JSLS. 2010;14(1):130–2.

75. Kumar S, Bishnoi K, Panwar VK, Kumar A, Sharma MK. Stone in ectopic pelvic pancake kidney: a surgical challenge overcome by robotic surgery. J Robot Surg. 2018;12(1):181–3.

76. Hollis HW, Rutherford RB, Crawford GJ, Cleland BP, Marx WH, Clark JR. Abdominal aortic aneurysm repair in patients with pelvic kidney. Technical considerations and literature review. J Vasc Surg. 1989;9(3):404–9.

77. van den Bosch CM, van Wijk JA, Beckers GM, van der Horst HJ, Schreuder MF, Bökenkamp A. Urological and nephrological findings of renal ectopia. J Urol. 2010;183(4):1574–9.

78. Gencheva R, Gibson B, Garugu S, Forrest A, Sakthi-Velavan S. A unilateral pelvic kidney with variant vasculature: clinical significance. J Surg Case Rep. 2019;2019(11):rjz333.

79. Ganesamoni R, Sabnis RB, Mishra S, Desai MR. Microperc for the management of renal calculi in pelvic ectopic kidneys. Indian J Urol. 2013 Jul;29(3):257–9.

80. Lee SK, Mwipatayi BP, Abbas M, Narayan S, Sieunarine K. Transplantation of crossed fused renal ectopia. Asian J Surg. 2007;30(1):82–4.

81. Cinman NM, Okeke Z, Smith AD. Pelvic kidney: associated diseases and treatment. J Endourol. 2007;21(8):836–42.

82. Calisti A, Perrotta ML, Oriolo L, Ingianna D, Miele V. The risk of associated urological abnormalities in children with pre and postnatal occasional diagnosis of solitary, small or ectopic kidney: is a complete urological screening always necessary? World J Urol. 2008 Jun;26(3):281–4.

83. Gleason PE, Kelalis PP, Husmann DA, Kramer SA. Hydronephrosis in renal ectopia: incidence, etiology and significance. J Urol. 1994 Jun;151(6): 1660–1.

84. Alokour RK, Ghawanmeh HM, Al-Ghazo M, Lafi TY. Renal cell carcinoma in ectopic-pelvic kidney: a rare case with review of literature. Turk J Urol. 2018 Sep;44(5):433–6.

85. Walther A, Cost NG, Garrison AP, Geller JI, Alam S, Tiao GM. Renal rhabdomyosarcoma in a pancake kidney. Urology. 2013;82(2):458–60.

86. Fernbach SK, Feinstein KA, Spencer K, et al. Ureteral duplication and its complications. Radiographics. 1997;17(1):109–27.

87. Avni FE, Nicaise N, Hall M, et al. The role of MR imaging for the assessment of complicated duplex kidneys in children: preliminary report. Pediatr Radiol. 2001;31(4):215–23.

88. Bats A-S, Metzger U, Le Frere-Belda M-A, Brisa M, Lecuru F. Malignant transformation of Gartner cyst. Int J Gynecol Cancer. 2009;19:1655–7.

89. Delmore J. Glob. Benign neoplasms of the vagina. Libr. Women's Med. 2008. ISSN: 1756-2228.

90. Rink R-C, Kaefer M, Wein AJ. Campbell-Walsh urology. 9th ed. Philadelphia: WB Saunders; 2007. Surgical management of disorders of sexual differentiation, cloacal malformation, and other abnormalities of external genitalia in girls. p. 3629–66.

91. Vlahovic A, Stankovic Z-B, Djuricic S, Savic D. Giant Gartner duct cyst and elevated CA-125. J Pediatr Adolesc Gynecol. 2014;27(6):e137–8.

92. Paradies G, Zullino F, Caroppo F, Orofino A, Lanzillotto M-P, Leggio S. Gartner's duct cyst: report of three cases (in Italian). Pediatr Med Chir. 2011;33: 247–52.

93. Molina ER, Navas Martinez M-C, Castillo O-A. Vaginal Gartner cysts: clinical report of four cases and a bibliographic review. Arch Esp Urol. 2014;67(2): 181–4.

94. Moralioğlu S, Bosnalı O, Celayir A-C, Sahin C. Paraurethral Skene's duct cyst in a newborn. Urol Ann. 2013;5(3):204–5.

95. Bergner DM. Paraurethral cysts in the newborn. South Med J. 1985;78:749–50.

96. Kimbrough HM, Vaughan ED. Skene's duct cyst in a newborn: case report and review of the literature. J Urol. 1977;117:387–8.

97. Holmes M, Upadhyay V, Pease P. Gartner's duct cyst with unilateral renal dysplasia presenting as an introital mass in a new born. Pediatr Surg Int. 1999;15:277–9.

98. Dwyer PL, Rosamilia A. Congenital urogenital anomalies that are associated with the persistence of Gartner's duct: a review. Am J Obstet Gynecol. 2006;19:354–9.

99. Binsaleh S, Al-Assiri M, Jednak R, El-Sherbiny M. Gartner duct cyst simplified treatment approach. Int Urol Nephrol. 2007;39(2):485–7.

100. Rios SS, Pereira LCR, Santos CB, Chen ACR, Chen JR, Vogt MB. Conservative treatment and follow-up of vaginal Gartner's duct cysts: a case series. J Med Case Rep. 2016;10:147.

101. Abd-Rabbo MS, Atta MA. Aspiration and tetracycline sclerotherapy: a novel method for management of vaginal and vulval Gartner cyst. Int J Gynecol Obstet. 1991;35:235–7.

102. Oppelt P, Renner SP, Kellermann A, et al. Clinical aspects of Mayer–Rokitansky–Kuester–Hauser syndrome: recommendations for clinical diagnosis and staging. Hum Reprod. 2006;21:792–7.

103. Davydov SN. Colpopoeisis from the peritoneum of the uterorectal space. Akush Ginekol (Mosk). 1969;45(12):557. Banister JB, McIndoe AH. Congenital absence of the vagina, treated by means of an indwelling skin-graft. Proc R Soc Med. 1938;31(9):1055–6.

104. Williams EA. Congenital absence of the vagina: a simple operation for its relief. J Obstet Gynaecol Br Commonw. 1964;71:511–2.

105. Louis-Sylvestre C, Haddad B, Paniel BJ. Creation of a sigmoid neovagina: techniques and results in 16 cases. Eur J Obstet Gynecol Reprod Biol. 1997;75:225–9.

106. Vecchietti G. The neovagina in the Robitansky-Kuster-Hauser syndrome. Rev Med Suisse Romande. 1979;99(9):593–601.

107. Carrington BM, Hricak H, Nuruddin RN, Secaf E, Laros RK Jr, Hill EC. Mu̇llerian duct anomalies: MR imaging evaluation. Radiology. 1990;176:715–20.

108. López PJ, Mushtaq I, Curry JI. Laparoscopic inguinal herniotomy in bladder exstrophy: a new solution to an old problem? J Pediatr Urol. 2007;3:28–31.

109. Bianchi S, Frontino G, Ciappina N, Restelli E, Fedele L. Creation of a neovagina in Rokitansky syndrome: comparison between two laparoscopic techniques. Fertil Steril. 2011;95(1098–100):e1–3.

110. McKusick VA, Bauer RL, Koop CE, et al. Hydrometrocolpos as a simply inherited malformation. JAMA. 1964;189:813–6.

111. Slavotinek AM. McKusick-Kaufman syndrome, gene reviews. 2015. Available at: https://www.ncbi.nlm.nih.gov/books/NBK1502/. Accessed 20 Nov 2016.

112. David A, Bitoun P, Lacombe D, et al. Hydrometrocolpos and poly-dactyly: a common neonatal presentation of Bardet-Biedl and McKusick-Kaufman syndromes. J Med Genet. 1999;35:599–603.

113. Awad EE, El-agwany A, Dayem TMA, El-habashy AM. Imperfo- rate hymen as an unusual cause of non-urological urine retention – a case report. Afr J Urol. 2015;21:72–5.

114. Ayrim AA, Gozdemir E, Turhan N, et al. Acute urinary retention associated with an imperforate hymen and haematocolpos. Gynecol Obstet Reprod Med. 2016;15:105–7.

115. Hatti RB, Badakali AV, Vanaki RN, et al. McKusick-Kaufman syndrome presenting as acute intestinal obstruction. J Neonatal Surg. 2013;2:7.

116. Sharma D, Murki S, Pratap O, et al. A case of hydrometrocolpos and polydactyly. Clin Med Insigh Paediat. 2015;9:7–11.

117. Yewalkar SP, Yadav VK, Khadse GJ. The McKusick-Kaufman hydrometrocolpos-polydactyly syndrome: a rare case report. Indian J Radiol Imaging. 2013;2:183–5.

118. Slavotinek A, Biesecker LG. Phenotypic overlap of McKusick- Kaufman syndrome with Bardet-Biedl syndrome: a literature review. Am J Med Genet. 2000;95:208–15.

119. Gearhart JP. Exstrophy, epispadias, and other bladder anomalies. In: Walsch PC, editor. Campbell's urology. 8th ed. Philadelphia: WB Saunders; 2002.

120. Nelson CP, Dunn RL, Wei JT. Contemporary epidemiology of bladder exstrophy in the United States. J Urol. 2005;173:1728–31.

121. Stec AA, Pannu HK, Tadros YE, Sponsellor PD, Fishman EK, Hearhart JP. Pelvic floor anatomy in classic bladder exstrophy using 3-dimensional computerized tomography: initial insights. J Urol. 2001;166:1444–9.

122. Stec AA, Pannu HK, Tadros YE, et al. Evaluation of the bony pelvis in classic bladder exstrophy by using 3D-CT: further insights. Urology. 2001;58:1030–5.

123. Woodhouse CRJ, Ransley PG, Williams DI. The patient with exstrophy in adult life. Br J Urol. 1983;55:632–5.

124. Damario MA, Carpenter SE, Jones HW Jr, Rock JA. Reconstruction of the external genitalia in females with bladder exstrophy. Int J Gynecol Obstet. 1994;4:245–53.

Neuroanatomy and Neurophysiology

3

John T. Stoffel

Contents

Introduction	50
Bladder Biomechanics	51
Bladder Architecture	51
Neuropharmacology of Bladder Storage and Emptying	56
Peripheral Nervous System	59
Afferent Communication	60
Sympathetic/Parasympathetic/Somatic Efferent Coordination	61
Therapeutics	62
Central Nervous System	64
Storage	64
Voiding	65
Knowledge Gap: Cell Replacement	66
Conclusion	66
References	66

Abstract

The bladder has only two simple tasks, to store and empty urine. However, the regulation of these tasks requires strong coordination of afferent and communication between the bladder and the brain, known as the spino-bulbo-spinal reflex arc. As more urine is stored in the bladder, the urothelium is stretched, and afferent neurons are activated. For urinary storage and emptying, information is carried through the pelvic and pundendal nerves to the sacral

spinal cord and then to the periaqueductal gray region in the midbrain. Input from the cortex initially shifts the bladder to storage. The sympathetic nervous system is stimulated through the hypogastric nerve, and the detrusor muscle relaxes and the bladder outlet tightens to facilitate storage of urine and avoid leakage per urethra. Once a volume threshold is met, the periaqueductal gray region releases inhibition of the pontine micturition complex. Bladder voiding is now initiated by parasympathetic stimulation of the detrusor through the pelvic nerves. Coordination between this change between storage and voiding can be disrupted

J. T. Stoffel (✉)
University of Michigan, Ann Arbor, MI, USA
e-mail: jstoffel@med.umich.edu

© Springer Nature Switzerland AG 2023
F. E. Martins et al. (eds.), *Female Genitourinary and Pelvic Floor Reconstruction*,
https://doi.org/10.1007/978-3-031-19598-3_3

by neurologic diseases or injuries to the central or peripheral nervous system.

Keywords

Bladder · Physiology · Neuro-urology

Introduction

A functioning urinary system is a critical need for any organism. It has two basic functions – storage and emptying of urine. In an intact, functional urinary system, the bladder will allow near continuous drainage of urine from the kidneys and store the urine until evacuation is initiated. As the human bladder fills, a person will detect first a sense of bladder fullness followed by an urge to empty as the bladder volume continues to increase. An intact system will protect against urine leakage by closing the bladder outlet, but still maintain low bladder pressures to avoid damaging the bladder wall or the upper tracts. Once a functional capacity is reached and a volitional desire to void is initiated, the bladder will empty with a coordinated contraction, while the bladder outlet remains open and relaxed.

The coordination of this urine storage and emptying is complex and requires a dynamic nervous system that continuously samples volumes in the bladder and can quickly and efficiently change the bladder from storage to emptying and then back again to storage. From a neurologic perspective, this is a spino-bulbo-spinal reflex arc where local information is afferently communicated to the brainstem/midbrain region and a motor response is then provoked [1]. Injuries to the bladder can impact this communication as can neurologic conditions. Although the term neurogenic bladder is defined as any change in bladder function due to an underlying neurologic condition, this is somewhat of a nonspecific term. Disrupting function at different parts of the coordinated feedback loop can result in different urinary symptoms. For example, a cervical spinal cord injury usually results in failure to store urine, whereas a pelvic fracture with sacral involvement usually results in failure to empty. Figure 1 demonstrates that a neurogenic bladder can, in fact, be from a pathology affecting the peripheral nervous system, the spinal cord, or the brain.

This chapter will review the neuroanatomy and neurophysiology of bladder storage and emptying with specific focus on how neurologic disruption of the system can lead to different urinary symptoms. It will also discuss how this can impact on upper tract safety and quality of life. However, an important caveat is while that much is known about bladder physiology, the neurologic regulation of the urinary tract remains less clear. Some information presented is extrapolated from animal

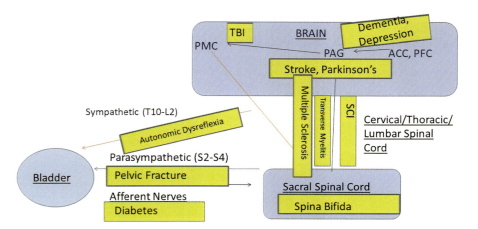

Fig. 1 Different presentations of neurogenic bladder symptoms and physiology can be caused by pathology (Yellow) affecting the peripheral nervous system, spinal cord, and brain

models, and the findings may not be directly replicated in humans. When applicable, this chapter will also highlight knowledge gaps between animal models and human physiology.

Bladder Biomechanics

The human bladder can be roughly divided into the following layers (starting at bladder lumen): the urothelium, lamina propria/submucosa, detrusor muscle, and the serosa [2] (Fig. 2). Distension or irritation of the bladder will communicate sensory information, particularly wall pressure/tension, pain, and temperature, to the central nervous system. Adrenergic stimulation facilitates bladder relaxation, outlet tightening, and urine storage. Cholinergic stimulation causes detrusor contraction, blockage of outlet tightening, and urine emptying.

Bladder Architecture

Urothelium

The urothelium is the first structure to contact urine. It covers the renal pelvis, ureters, bladder, and proximal urethra. This chapter will focus on bladder urothelium. The transitional epithelial lining consists of three layers of cells oriented from bladder lumen to basement membrane: the superficial (umbrella), intermediate, and basal cells. The superficial umbrella cells are polarized and particularly malleable in shape to adjust to bladder volume. They appear cuboidal in shape in the unfilled bladder but become flat and squamous in appearance as the bladder fills [3] (Fig. 3). The urothelium is highly impermeable, and there are tight junctions between the umbrella cells which prevent diffusion of solutes. The superficial cells are also covered by a glycosaminoglycan layer (GAG) consisting of hyaluronic acid, heparin sulfate, and chondroitin sulfate [4]. Barrier and occluding proteins, such as uroplakins, reinforce the layer and prevent irritation from urine solutes or pathogens to structures beneath. Changes to the GAG layer have been observed in people with chronic interstitial cystitis [5], which has led to the development of intravesical treatments aimed at replenishing or repairing this region [6].

However, the urothelium is not simply a passive barrier to urine, and there is a dynamic relationship between bladder volume and urothelium. This superficial layer is postulated to sample the urine through a process of apical endocytosis which then informs remodeling of the biomembrane to adapt to bladder capacity [7]. The urothelium also triggers the initial event of sensory signaling in the bladder. There are a multitude of receptors/ion channels embedded in the urothelium, such as P2X3 purinergic receptors, adrenoreceptors, muscarinic and nicotinic

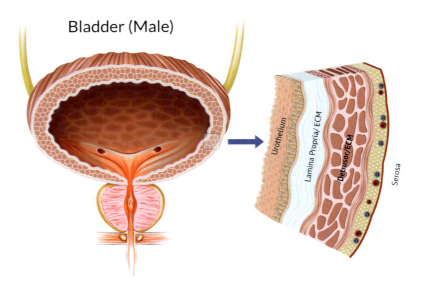

Fig. 2 Architectural layers of the bladder. Although a male bladder is pictured here, the layers are identical between sexes

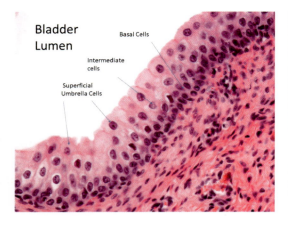

Fig. 3 Human urothelium examined under high power microscopy. Note the different cuboidal shape of the umbrella cells of the most superficial layer compared the flatter shape deeper within the layer

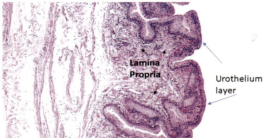

Fig. 4 Human bladder examined under high power microscopy. Note how the lamina propria supports the "fjord" like projections of the superficial layers

cholinergic receptors, and transient receptor potential (TRP) channels [8, 9]. These receptors, when triggered by mechanical, thermal, or chemical stimulation can initiate Adenosine Triphosphate (ATP), prostaglandins, nitric oxide/GMP, calcium, and others, to initiate communication of afferent sensation. Initiation of afferent signaling pathways has been found in both umbrella and intermediate urothelial cells [4, 8, 10, 11].

In addition to sensory capabilities, the urothelium layer has been demonstrated to have immunologic properties and can stimulate immunoglobin, cytokine, interleukin, neutrophils, and lymphocyte release in response to bacteria or injury [12]. Research suggests that urothelial receptors, such as the calcium-activated voltage-gated potassium channel on the urothelium, BK, may be of particular interest in regulating the effect of inflammation. A mouse model shows that BK activity is increased in response to lipopolysaccharides commonly seen on bacterial endotoxins. This increased BK activity then leads to increased macrophage activity [13, 14]. Certain urothelial cancer therapies such as Bacillus Calmette-Guérin are effective because they trigger a cytokine release in the urothelium which induces necrotic cell death in some cancer cells [15]. Other modifications at the urothelial receptor level are being explored as treatment for urothelial malignancies [16].

There is also great interest in better understanding how alterations of the urinary biome impact inflammation and cell signaling in the bladder. New discoveries suggest that urine is not sterile. The most common organisms found in a healthy microbiome include Lactobacillus, *Streptococcus*, and *Corynebacterium*, although there is some variation between men and women [17, 18] Changes in concentrations of *Lactobacillus* species may alter the steady-state storage environment and trigger inflammatory responses leading to increased sensation or ultimately detrusor contractions. It has been postulated that an alteration in the biome could be a mechanism for conditions such as recurrent urinary tract infections, interstitial cystitis, and overactive bladder [18, 19].

Lamina Propria

The lamina propria is a submucosal layer that lies between the detrusor muscle and basal cell layer of the urothelium. It contains multiple different types of cells, many of which the function has not been fully identified (Fig. 4). It is known that interstitial cells (ITC) are found in the lamina propria, and these are of particular interest regarding bladder signaling. It is postulated that ITC are stimulated by ATP generated by stimulation of the urothelial layer, and ITC in turn stimulate afferent nerves that communicate with the CNS via the spinal cord [20] (Fig. 5). ITC cells may also coordinate detrusor contraction. Studies suggest that during emptying, IC cells may promote intercellular communication via connexin calcium channels among ITC cells to

3 Neuroanatomy and Neurophysiology

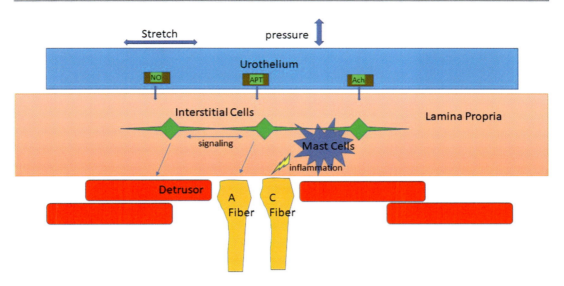

Fig. 5 Interstitial cells receive signaling from urothelium via nitric oxide (NO), APT, and acetylcholine (Ach). Information is communicated to afferent A and C fibers and to detrusor

coordinate initiation of detrusor contractions. It is proposed that they act as "pacemaker" cells for the bladder in a similar way as ITC cells of Cajal function in the gastrointestinal tract [10, 21]. There is clinical support for the bladder pacemaker hypothesis given that increased ITC connexin channels have also been associated with detrusor overactivity/overactive bladder in people [21, 22]. It is not conclusive, however, since other researchers have suggested that ITC cells also can act in the opposite function and provide a cellular "braking mechanism" and inhibit detrusor contractility during bladder filling [23].

The lamina propria appears to have a role in mediating cell growth, regeneration, and inflammatory responses in the bladder. At least ten different growth factors, including those from the VEGF, TGF, and EGF families, have been found in the lamina propria region [24]. It has been studied as a donor material as a tissue matrix for reconstructive urologic procedures. Two different models have been reported on using porcine acellular matrix [25] and submucosa [26, 27]. Ingrowth of bladder mucosa was noted in animal models, but wide-scale application for use in urologic reconstructions in humans has not been established.

Activated mast cells and the presence of inflammatory infiltrates have also been found in this region among IC patients, suggesting that the layer participates in inflammatory responses [28, 29]. This is best evidenced in a feline interstitial cystitis model in which the IC felines showed normal urothelium in the bladder and urethra but degranulated mast cells and increased cyclooxygenase expression. Additionally, electron microscopy showed neovascularization and alterations in the extracellular matrix suggesting that the inflammation was provoking tissue remodeling [30]. Studies such as these suggest a possible mechanism for bladder/urethral pain as well as the reduced bladder capacity and fibrosis that some IC patients experience.

Detrusor

There are three layers of overlapping detrusor muscle in the body of the bladder (above the trigone). The inner and outer layers are arranged longitudinally, and the middle layer is horizontally oriented. In each layer, the detrusor muscle cells are grouped in bundles which stretch and contract to give the bladder capacity during storage and coordinated luminal pressure during emptying [31]. The muscle layers are thicker near the base of the bladder and become thinner toward the bladder dome. There are differing views on whether the detrusor muscles extend down into the bladder neck to form an internal sphincter, although there appears to be some histological evidence for this [32].

Through mechanisms described above, the urothelium and extracellular matrix communicate sensory information which informs the detrusor muscle configuration for storage or emptying. There is some controversy on how coordination of the detrusor is regulated. Most smooth muscles in the body function via "single-unit" contraction. This means that the muscle cells communicate through tight junction ion channels which allows a signal to propagate between individual cells and stimulate a coordinated contraction along a whole layer of muscle. Researchers have demonstrated that detrusor muscle cells do communicate through connexin-regulated channels arranged at tight cell-to-cell junctions and the bladder has some single-unit contraction properties [33, 34]. However, there is also evidence that the detrusor may also utilize a "multi-unit" contraction pattern. Here, groups of muscle cells act independently and require individual stimulation to initiate contraction rather than respond to a larger propagated signal. This "multi-unit" contraction pattern has been postulated to be active in overactive bladder models [22, 31, 33, 34].

Two different types of detrusor contractions have been observed. Phasic contractions are large, coordinated contraction of the bladder body used to evacuate urine. This is stimulated by parasympathetic input and is discussed below. The second type of contractions are spontaneous contractions which are not neurologically mediated. They are typically small, uncoordinated contractions in sections of the bladder wall. The mechanism is not fully understood, but voltage-gated calcium channels on the detrusor have been observed to cause these spontaneous contractions, particularly when the bladder is close to capacity. It is hypothesized that these spontaneous contractions may help the detrusor muscles readjust its length in preparation for contraction [35]. Spontaneous contractions have been observed more commonly in overactive bladder models [36] (Fig. 6).

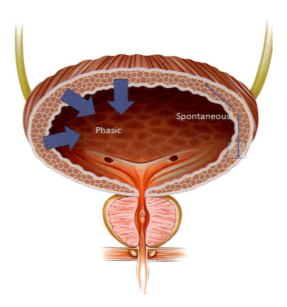

Fig. 6 The detrusor muscle has two types of contraction patterns. Phasic – coordinated contractions that generate pressure toward the bladder lumen for voiding. Spontaneous – small, non-coordinated contractions possibly designed to reshape the bladder during filling

Extracellular Matrix

The bladder extracellular matrix is a scaffold of proteins that provides structural support as the bladder stretches and contracts. It is composed of mostly collagen (type 1 > type 3), metalloproteinases, and elastin. These are woven among the urothelium, lamina propria, and detrusor smooth muscle. Some consider the laminal propria and extracellular matrix to be the same structure, and it is characterized occasionally as this in the literature. The matrix is continuously remodeled via metalloproteinases adjusting the collagen/elastin cross-linked patterns and communicates to other bladder cells in the urothelium via receptors such as integrins in response to local stimulation. As the bladder distends and the detrusor relaxes, the collagen in the extracellular matrix stretches to help equally dissipate pressure within the bladder lumen. It has been postulated that folds in the bladder urothelium/lamina propria allow reversible recruitment of collagen to facilitate the stretching [37]. This allows the bladder to maintain some rigidity and support but minimizes luminal pressures. When the bladder contracts, the elastin fibers in the extracellular matrix allow the bladder to recoil into a smaller shape [38, 39] (Fig. 7).

The extracellular matrix is integral to bladder compliance (defined as change in volume/change in detrusor pressure). When filling, a healthy bladder maintains high compliance, or low intraluminal pressures at high volumes (Fig. 8). Low bladder compliance, notable for high intraluminal resting pressure and low bladder volumes, is associated with increased risk of hydronephrosis, renal function, and urinary tract infections (Fig. 9). Loss of bladder compliance is directly related to extracellular matrix remodeling. In animal models and human tissue studies, low compliance bladders have replacement of type 1 collagen with type 3 collagen in the extracellular matrix and loss of detrusor smooth muscle [40, 41]. The collagen-type change results in permanent recruitment of collagen into a configuration which results in loss of folds [39]. Clinically, loss of bladder compliance can be seen in radiation cystitis, bladder outlet obstruction, and neurogenic bladder pathologies. Currently, there are no effective treatments for fibrosis in the bladder. However, inhibiting growth factor receptors like VEGF inhibited the progression of collagen change and bladder fibrosis in a mouse spinal cord injury model which suggests there could be some potential future therapeutic options [42].

Other extracellular matrix changes other than collagen type could also contribute to loss of bladder compliance. Loss of elastin has also been observed in low bladder compliance, but other studies suggest that loss of elastin may be more associated with reduced bladder contractility than compliance changes [43]. Changes in metalloproteinase concentrations have also been observed in low bladder compliance models. In a

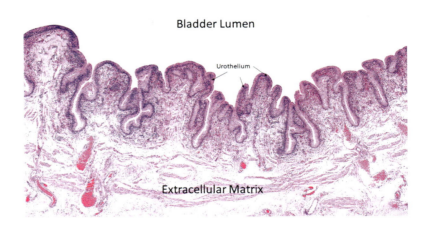

Fig. 7 Human bladder examined under high power microscopy. The extracellular matrix supports the lamina propria and urothelium by maintaining some rigidity to structure during filling

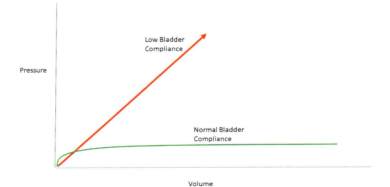

Fig. 8 This figure shows the difference between low and high bladder compliance. Note that low bladder compliance has high pressure increases for small changes in volume

40-spina-bifida-patient study, abnormal urine concentration of matrix metalloprotein 2 (MMP-2) and tissue inhibitor metalloproteiniase 2 (TIMP-2) were noted in people with low bladder compliance. TIMP-2 was also elevated in people with upper tract changes [44].

Neuropharmacology of Bladder Storage and Emptying

Adrenergic Stimulation: Storage

Adrenergic receptors facilitate detrusor smooth muscle relaxation and bladder outlet tightening (Fig. 10). There are multiple subtypes of adrenergic receptors, but only alpha1, alpha 2, and beta have been identified in the bladder. The receptors are stimulated by norepinephrine via the hypogastric nerve in the sympathetic nervous system, which in turn initiates from the T12–L2 region of the spinal cord [45, 46].

The alpha 1 adrenergic receptor is a postsynaptic receptor with three subtypes, 1A, 1B, and 1D. They have been studied in multiple animal models, and the 1A subtype mRNA has been found in high concentration at the bladder neck in all studied models except in pigs. Interestingly, humans are unique in having a higher ratio of 1D subtype when compared to rats. However, stimulation of 1A subtype is primarily responsible for bladder neck and urethral constriction in most species [46–48]. There is little alpha 1A expression in the bladder body, although a small amount has been detected in some assays at the bladder dome [49]. Alpha 1A is found also in the prostatic stroma in men, and blockade of this results in reduction of smooth muscle contractility in the prostatic urethra. Additionally, alpha 1A is the only alpha adrenoreceptor subtype found in the remainder of the urethra [50]. The spinal cord also has alpha 1 receptors, but D is found in greater concentration than A. A clinical trial has demonstrated that adrenoceptor blockade with terazosin resulted in improved bladder

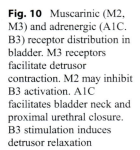

Fig. 9 This is CT imaging of hydronephrosis causes by low bladder compliance. High bladder pressure caused significant upper tract changes

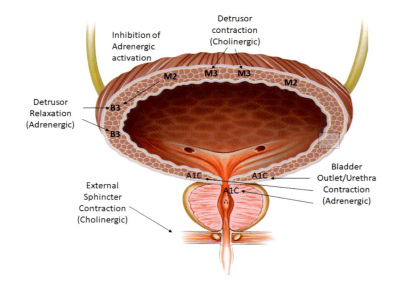

Fig. 10 Muscarinic (M2, M3) and adrenergic (A1C. B3) receptor distribution in bladder. M3 receptors facilitate detrusor contraction. M2 may inhibit B3 activation. A1C facilitates bladder neck and proximal urethral closure. B3 stimulation induces detrusor relaxation

compliance which raises the question as to whether spinal alpha D adrenoceptors have a direct impact on bladder wall tension [51]. Side effect of alpha adrenoceptor blockade therapy can be hypotension due to alpha adrenoceptors' presence in the vascular endothelium.

Alpha 2 adrenergic receptors are, in general, a presynaptic receptor and are also present in the bladder and urethra. In some animal models, they demonstrate a weak contractile effect in the urethra, but this has not been demonstrated in humans. The importance of alpha 2 receptors is not fully understood in human bladder physiology [46].

There are three beta adrenogenic receptor subtypes, B1,B2, and B3. PCR studies have shown that B3 subtype accounts for more than 95% of human bladder B subtypes. B3 are located in the detrusor throughout the bladder but with less density in the bladder neck and trigone [52]. Other animal models such as rats, mice, and pigs have a mixture of B2 and B3 receptors which facilitate relaxation [53]. In humans, sympathetic stimulation causes direct myocyte relaxation through B3 mediation. In rats, overexpression of B3 adrenoreceptors cause underactive bladder symptoms, which suggests a possible model for studying chronic urinary retention [54]. Side effects of B3 agonist therapy for OAB includes possible hypertension due to vasoconstriction of peripheral blood vessels.

Cholinergic Stimulation

Bladder emptying is initiated through lumbrosacral parasympathetic cholinergic stimulation of muscarinic receptors on the detrusor myocyte. There has been some evidence showing muscarinic receptor presence in the urothelium, but it is difficult to determine receptor density in this location, and the role of muscarinic receptors here is less clear. There are five muscarinic receptor subtypes (M1–M5) with M2 and M3 localized to the detrusor. Roughly 80% of muscarinic receptors in the bladder are M2, 20% are M3. M2 stimulation does not appear to directly cause bladder contraction, but it may be linked to inhibition of adrenergic B3-mediated detrusor relaxation [55]. The M3 subtype is more directly linked to

detrusor contraction. Research has shown that M3 stimulation leads to the activation of L-type calcium channels and a rise on intracellular calcium. This leads to the activation of the rho kinase pathway and modulation of myosin light chain phosphorylation and ultimately contributes to smooth muscle contraction. Atropine administration on the bladder strip in general inhibits detrusor muscle contractions, confirming the importance of muscarinic receptor [56, 57].

The external urethral sphincter and pelvic floor also respond to cholinergic stimulation. These somatic muscles have nicotinic receptors and are stimulated by acetylcholine release from the pudendal nerve. This initiates a muscle contraction which increases closure pressure on the urethra [31] (Table 1).

As noted above, muscarinic receptors are highly prevalent in other organ systems. Consequently, the use of anticholinergic medications for the management of overactive bladder is associated with concomitant side effects such as dry mouth, constipation, and cognitive changes. Tolterodine, trospium, solifenacin, and darifenacin have less affinity for muscarinic receptors in the salivary glands compared to oxybutynin [56]. The potential for anticholinergic medications to penetrate the central nervous system (CNS) was also investigated in a rat model by comparing brain and plasma drug concentration ratios. Oxybutynin showed the greatest CNS penetration. Tolterodine and solifenacin also showed significant CNS penetration, but not as great as oxybutynin. Darifenacin and trospium chloride displayed the lowest brain:plasma ratio [58]. Table 2 summarizes receptor subtype selectivity of commonly used bladder medications.

Table 1 Location of muscarinic receptor subtype in the human body

Subtype	Location
M1	Brain
M2	**Bladder/gut**
M3	**Bladder/brain**
M4	Forebrain
M5	Brain

Table 2 Target receptors in bladder/proximal urethra for overactive bladder and bladder outlet obstruction medications [50, 56, 58]

Nonspecific muscarinic antagonists
Oxybutynin (slight M3 > M2 selectivity, but also M1 and M4 stimulation)
Tolterodine (no selectivity)
Trospium chloride (no selectivity)
M3 muscarinic selective antagonists
Solifenacin (M3 > M2, but also some M1 stimulation)
Darifenacin
Fesoterodine
B3 adrenergic agonists
Mirabegron
Vibegron
Alpha adrenergic antagonists
Tamsulosin (A1 specific)
Alfuzosin (A1 specific)
Silodosin (A1 specific)
Prazosin
Doxazosin
Terazosin
Alternative
Imipramine – serotonin (5-T) reuptake inhibitor. Mechanism on bladder detrusor not fully understood

Urinary Symptoms/Signs Associated with Signaling Changes in the Bladder

There is mounting evidence that targeting the additional receptions/proteins other than adrenergic and cholinergic muscarinic receptors may yield therapeutic benefit for some urinary conditions (Table 3). To this end, research has demonstrated that completely inhibiting the muscarinic receptors with atropine does not always block detrusor contractions. However, a direct relationship between urothelial signaling changes and conditions such as IC or OAB has yet to be established in humans.

It has been postulated that stimulation of purine receptors, possibly in the urothelium or detrusor, may be an alternative, non-cholinergic pathway for bladder contraction in pathologic states such as bladder outlet obstruction [45, 59]. Inhibiting the P2X7R receptor for 2 weeks in a spinal cord-injured rat model decreased the risk of developing neurogenic OAB [60]. P2X3 has been identified as a potential target for treating chronic pain. It is known that inhibition of P2X3 decreases neuroinflammation. Mice deficient in P2X3 receptors exhibit decreased bladder contractility and pain-related behavior [61, 62]. Eliapixant (BAY 1817080), a selective P2X3 inhibitor, is currently undergoing phase 2 and 3 clinical trials for overactive bladder, diabetic neuropathic pain, and endometriosis [63].

Phosphodiesterase 5 inhibitors (PDE5I) have been investigated for patients with lower urinary symptoms and/or partial bladder outlet obstruction. Phosphodiesterase 5 is part of the nitric oxide/cyclic guanosine monophosphate (NO/cGMP) intracellular pathway and is found in the bladder neck, prostate, and pelvic vasculature. As noted above, the NO/cGMP pathway is present in the urothelium, possibly concentrating in the intermediate urothelial cell layer [10]. Nitric oxide facilitates cGMP production which then causes smooth muscle relaxation. Since phosphodiesterase 5 increases the breakdown of cGMP, inhibiting this reaction could promote more smooth muscle relaxation and help improve overactive bladder and bladder outlet obstruction symptoms [66]. Data has demonstrated efficacy in men, although data in women is lacking. In a study of 581 men with lower urinary tract symptoms and erectile dysfunction, the PDE5i tadalafil treatment demonstrated significant improvement in urinary quality of life on the total International Prostate Symptom Score compared to placebo (-4.7 at 20 mg vs -2.1 placebo, $p < 0.05$). However, post-void residual and maximum voiding velocity (Qmax) was not significantly different [67]. Other cyclic nucleotide (cAMP) modulators have also been postulated as potential therapeutics.

TRP channels have also been investigated for treating both overactive bladder and DO. A number of these channels, including TRPV1, TRPV4, TRPM8, TRPA1, and TRPM4, are actively being investigated in animal models [68]. Idiopathic detrusor overactivity has also been noted in rats overexpressing TRPM8, a receptor part of the TRP superfamily expressed throughout the urothelium [69]. Since there is TRP expression in other parts of the nervous system which impede clinical trial implementation, there are not robust data currently to gage efficacy in humans.

Table 3 Conditions potentially associated with signaling changes in the urothelium/lamina propria

Condition	Symptoms	Associated changes
Interstitial cystitis	Bladder pain Urinary frequency	Loss of GAG layer [64] Abnormal umbrella cell polarity [64] Activated mast cells in lamina propria [29]
Overactive bladder	Urinary frequency Urinary urgency Incontinence	Increased P2X3 and TRP expression Increased connexin channels [22]
Underactive bladder and bladder outlet obstruction	Urinary retention Urinary hesitancy Incomplete emptying	Decreased P2X3 expression Increased B3 receptor Decreased Muscarinic receptors Decreased ATP signaling [65]
Spinal Cord Injury	Overactive bladder	Increased P2X7 expression [60]

GAG: glycosaminoglycan, P2X3: purinergic receptor P2X3, TRP: transient receptor potential, ATP: Adenosine triphosphate, B3: adrenoreceptor B3, P2X7: purinergic receptor P2X7

Potassium channel blockers have long-held fascination as a potential target for treating overactive bladder. Given the high reception/ion channel presence within the urothelium and detrusor, it has been hypothesized that blocking potassium signaling in the urothelium or detrusor may decrease smooth muscle overactivity. Animal and human trials have studied BK and SK channel blockers iberiotoxin and apamin, respectively, as potential therapeutic agents. To date, most potassium channel blocker intervention have been unsuccessful outside of muscle strip trials in reducing detrusor overactivity. There has also been concern of potential cardiac toxicity in future human trials due to cross-reactivity with cardiac tissue [70].

Knowledge Gap: Animal Models for Bladder Biomechanics

The most common animal models for studying bladder physiology include mice, rats, guinea pigs, cats, dogs, and pigs. Each model has been cited as having particular strengths regarding similarity to specific aspects of human anatomy of physiology [71, 72]. However, it should be stated that there is no ideal animal model for studying all of bladder physiology because of inherent differences between humans and other animals. From an anatomic standpoint, bipedal locomotion of humans causes different physiologic stress on the bladder and outlet compared to quadruped locomotion. When comparing rat bladder models to human bladders, one must thus account for the looser abdominal wall of the rat giving less

pressures on the bladder. A rat will also have different orientation of pelvic floor muscles compared to humans which will also yield different urethral and bladder pressure modeling during filling and emptying [72]. Another limitation of animal models is that humans can void in a selected place and at a specific time which differs from the voiding patterns of many animals. Mice, rats, guinea pigs, and rabbits do not have the ability to select time and place to void, but cats do have this ability. This is particularly important when studying the brain regions responsible for inhibiting voiding and when investigating overactive bladder physiology. Further confounders include experimental design when studying animal models. In particular, space limitation in cages may also negatively affect the animal's ability to normally void and thus alter interpretations of physiologic storing and emptying. Given these and other differences, care must be taken before extrapolating bladder physiology findings in animals into humans.

Peripheral Nervous System

After the urothelium is activated, afferent nerves in the pelvis carry sensory information to the spinal cord which is then communicated to the brain. After processing, bladder contraction and relaxation is stimulated through the pelvic nerve (parasympathetic) and hypogastric nerve (sympathetic), respectively. When filling, sympathetic/somatic stimulation through the pudendal nerve

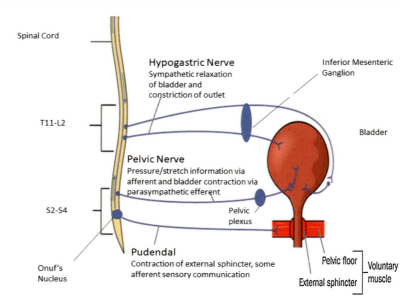

Fig. 11 Pelvic, pudendal, and hypogastric innervation of the bladder

increases proximal urethral pressure to maintain continence. During emptying, somatic and sympathetic stimulation is inhibited so the bladder empties through an unobstructed outlet (Fig. 11).

Afferent Communication

Anatomy

The majority of sensory/afferent nerve endings originate in the detrusor muscle (~80%), and a smaller subset (~20%) originate in the urothelium and lamina propria. The urethra also has a similar distribution but with some afferent terminals extending to the lumen. They are differentiated by immunoreactivity for calcitonin-gene-related peptide (CGRP), pituitary adenylate cyclase-activating polypeptide (PACAP), and substance P (SP) and are distributed throughout the bladder wall. The density of nerve terminals in the urinary tract is low, compared to other sensory organs. Radiolabeling studies have demonstrated that less than 3% of nerves in a dorsal nerve root are bladder or urethral afferent nerves [73, 74].

Bladder afferent nerve fibers in the pelvic nerve have been best studied. Histochemistry studies have shown that the greatest pelvic afferent nerve terminals have been found in the muscle (63%), lamina propria (14%), and urothelium (14%) layers [22]. As the bladder fills, afferent Aδ and C nerves carry sensory information mostly through the bilateral pelvic, pudendal, and, to a lesser extent, hypogastric nerves. The afferent fibers of the pelvic and pudendal nerves coalesce in the sacral dorsal nerve root ganglion (S2–4). There can be some variation on nerve root origin. Shafif et al. performed pudendal nerve dissection in 13 cadavers and found that the nerve partially originated from S1 in five and S5 in one [75].

Aδ and C Fibers

In a rat bladder model, approximately one third of the afferent nerves were Aδ as stained by neurofilament staining [76]. These myelinated Aδ fibers are sensitive to wall tension, bladder pressure, and strain to give information on bladder fullness. It has been reported that human bladders experience fullness at pressures of 5–15 mmHg/200 ml and urgency at pressures above 20 mm Hg/500 ml, although there is considerable variation [77]. Many Aδ afferent fibers are considered "in-series" and fire proportionally with bladder pressure and wall tension [78]. A smaller amount of Aδ fibers are not "in series" with detrusor contractility and report only on wall tension and may be volume threshold dependent [79].

In contrast, two thirds of afferent nerves in a rat model were C fibers [76]. These unmyelinated C fibers are sensitive to nociceptive stimulation such as high bladder pressure, inflammation, or injury. They also inform, to a lesser degree, on bladder volume [80]. C fibers have been detected in the proximal urethral and activation leads to contraction of the external sphincter. C fiber upregulation may contribute to increased urinary symptoms such as frequency, urgency, and bladder pain. It has been shown that TRP receptors (TRPV1) on bladder afferent C fibers are pathologically activated in overactive bladder and bladder pain syndromes. Ultrasensitive TRP vanilloid agonists, such as capsaicin and resiniferatoxin, have been studied as possible treatment for interstitial cystitis by desensitizing bladder C fibers [81]. Physiologic testing using ice water challenges has also demonstrated upregulation of C fiber signaling after neurologic injury [22] such as spinal cord injury and multiple sclerosis which could, in part, explain the urinary symptoms seen with these conditions. Constant stimulation of C fibers could potentially lead to a central sensitization pattern, seen in chronic pain. Here, the spinal neurons stimulated by C fibers become hypersensitized and develop lower activation thresholds with greater evoked responses. This would result in greater sensation from smaller stimulation. Hypersensitized spinal neurons are also triggered by normal Aδ at lower thresholds [82].

Sympathetic/Parasympathetic/Somatic Efferent Coordination

Sympathetic

As noted above, efferent, sympathetic stimulation facilitates bladder relaxation. Sympathetic stimulation originates from the T11 to the L2 dorsal nerve root ganglion, passes through the sympathetic chain and inferior mesenteric ganglions and hypogastric nerve, and reaches the bladder through a pelvic plexus surrounding the bladder. The hypogastric afferent fibers run through the superior hypogastric plexus and synapse in the lumbar dorsal root ganglion. There can be some anatomic variation in the location of superior hypogastric plexus and nerve root origin, and a unilateral accessory hypogastric nerve has been

found in 25% of people in a cadaver series [83]. Norepinephrine is released with sympathetic stimulation, and it activates B3 adrenoreceptors to relax the detrusor smooth muscle.

Pudendal

The somatic pudendal nerve fibers innervate EUS function and directly originate in Onuf's nucleus, located on the ventral part of the anterior horn in the spinal cord, between S2 and S4. Discovered by the scientist Bronislaw Onufrowicz (Onuf) in 1899 [84], it is found on the ventral horn of the upper sacral segment including S2–S3. It innervates not only the external urethral sphincter though the pudendal nerve but also the external anal sphincter, bulbocavernosus muscles, and the levator ani. In females, the external urethral sphincter is a striated muscle consisting of a compressor urethrae muscle, sphincter urethrae muscle, and urethrovaginal sphincter. In men, the external sphincter is a distinct structure surrounding the membranous urethra.

Parasympathetic

The innervation for the bladder originates from splanchnic nerves (S2–S4). The presynaptic fibers run through the anterior/ventral region of the spinal nerve roots, into the pelvic nerves bilaterally, and join a pelvic plexus or synapse into the bladder wall. Stimulation of the parasympathetic nervous system causes a release of acetylcholine and activation of the muscarinic M3 receptors which causes the detrusor to contract. It is significant that there are postganglionic nerves both in the pelvic plexus and directly in the bladder wall. This means that the bladder may still have parasympathetic innervation even if the pelvic plexus is injured. In the urethra, parasympathetic activation causes smooth muscles in the urethra to relax in some species. Activation of M2 muscarinic receptors in response to acetylcholine causes a suppression of norepinephrine release from adrenergic nerves in human bladder strips [85], indicating coordination between parasympathetic and sympathetic stimulation of the bladder.

Bladder Outlet Coordination

Coordinated sympathetic and pudendal nerve stimulation is needed for urethral closure during urine storage. As the bladder fills, adrenergic hypogastric stimulation of the bladder neck's alpha 1A receptors and pudendal stimulation of the external sphincter complex progressively raise urethral pressure through a process termed "the guarding reflex" which promotes continence [86, 87]. The resting detrusor pressure required to leak urine through this urethral tone is called the detrusor leak point pressure during urodynamic testing. High detrusor leak point pressures are considered dangerous because it means the bladder is storing at a high resting pressure without leaking per urethra. In people with normal bladder compliance and neurologic signaling, a detrusor leak point pressure is never reached because the bladder continue to actively relax and maintain low storage pressures. If the bladder continues to fill to high volumes, afferent signaling indicates a full bladder to initiate a voiding reflex.

External pressure is applied to the bladder through cough laugh, an activity which requires active recruitment of the external urinary sphincter. Rat models have demonstrated increased sphincteric EMG activity, mediated by pudendal nerve stimulation, in response to changes in abdominal pressure [88]. The abdominal/cough pressures during urodynamic testing that are required to cause leakage of urine per urethra are called valsalva/cough leak point pressures and can be a proxy measurement of external sphincter urethral functionality (Fig. 12). It has been suggested that some types of urinary stress incontinence, specifically, intrinsic sphincter deficiency, represent neurologic loss of a guarding reflex due to lack of sympathetic and pudendal nerve functioning. An open bladder neck seen on cystogram in some spina bifida and lumbar/sacral spinal cord injury people is thought to follow this model (Fig. 13).

Therapeutics

The afferent nervous system has also been targeted for treating overactive bladder and painful bladder. Trials of intravesical capsaicin and resiniferatoxin instillations have been published. Oliveira et al. instilled resiniferatoxin in the bladders of spinal cord-injured rats during the spinal shock period and noted a significant decrease in

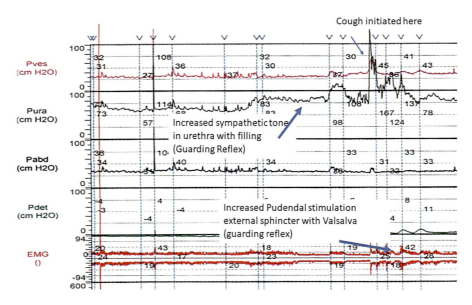

Fig. 12 Guarding reflex on urodynamic testing. pUra on the tracing represents a urethral sensor on catheter located at the external sphincter. Rising volumes cause increased urethral closure, as noted as increased urethral pressure. The electromyograph (EMG) tracing shows active recruitment of external muscle fibers in response to a cough (Valsalva). Note the increased pelvic floor activity in response to this

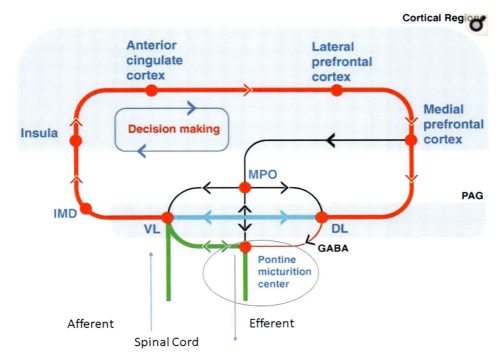

Fig. 13 Functional model of urinary continence as regulated by brain. PAG = periaqueductal gray (VL = ventrolateral region, DL = dorsolateral region), MPO = (median pre-optic nucleus of hypothalamus). (Modified from Zare et al. [89])

the incidence of neurogenic overactive bladder. These findings could suggest pathologic activation of C fibers as a source of neurogenic OAB after an injury [90]. Less promising results were reported in a double-blinded, placebo-controlled trial of resiniferatoxin instillation for the treatment of interstitial cystitis. In this 163 person study, RTX was not effective in improving urinary symptoms [91].

Treating the afferent nervous system directly through neuromodulation has yielded significantly better results for overactive bladder and urinary retention. Sacral neuromodulation is performed by stimulating the S3 dorsal nerve which carried sensory information from the pelvic and pudendal nerve. A meta-analysis of 21 studies comprising of 881 patients revealed an 82% success rate for the treatment of overactive bladder [92]. Posterior tibial nerve stimulation stimulates the same dorsal S3 nerve root via stimulation of the posterior tibial nerve near the medial malleolus. Showing similar outcomes to sacral neuromodulation, a meta-analysis of 28 posterior tibial nerve stimulation studies comprising of 2461 patients demonstrated significant reductions in urgency(-2.2 episodes), nocturia(-1.6 episodes/night), and incontinence(-1.4 episodes/day) [93]. Given what is now known about afferent signaling, it is reasonable to postulate that neuromodulation's effectiveness may stem in part from the upregulation of Aδ fiber and downregulation of C fiber signaling. Upregulation of Aδ may then decrease reflexive parasympathetic stimulation. Researchers have also published on peroneal, pudendal, and dorsal clitoral stimulation as additional options for treatment of OAB. However, more research is needed to better understand the therapeutic mechanism of neuromodulation and the optimal stimulation site.

Knowledge Gap: Peripheral Neurologic Assessment for Understanding Bladder Physiology

Bladder physiology is routinely assessed through urodynamic pressure flow studies. However, detailed knowledge about neurologic signaling to and from the bladder is lacking from these assessments. Although first sensation, first desire, and strong desire are measured as part of good urodynamic practices, this yields little information about potential pathologic alteration in Aδ and C fiber activation. Interesting research is being performed to assess afferent bladder function by selectively depolarizing different subpopulations of afferent nerves to determine a current perception threshold as a quantitative measure. By directly measuring activation, researchers could better potentially differentiate symptoms related to nociceptive sources. It may also give more objective assessment for the efficacy of therapeutic treatments [94].

Understanding the neurologic pathway of DSD may open more elegant treatment options and improve both safety and quality of life. Detrusor sphincter dyssynergia (DSD) is a condition that results from injury to the central nervous system, such as multiple sclerosis, cervical spinal cord injury, and spina bifida. It occurs when the detrusor contracts against a poorly relaxing external sphincter. It can cause significant morbidity, including urinary retention, urinary tract infections, and loss of bladder compliance [95]. It is speculated that it occurs because of a disruption between the PMC and Onuf's nucleus that results in high continued stimulation of the pudendal nerve [96]. However, this mechanism is poorly understood, particularly in how the condition can occur in both high cervical spinal cord injuries and sacral dysraphism. Some data suggest that lack of GABA stimulation in the lumbosacral spinal cord increases risk of DSD and intrathecal injection of GABA into spinal cord-injured rats was noted to reduce DSD [97, 98]. Other animal model studies report improvement of DSD through gene therapy replacement of the GABA synthesis enzyme glutamic acid decarboxylase (GAD) [99]. Until the neurologic pathway of DSD is better defined, this lack of knowledge ultimately limits therapeutic options to denervating the external sphincter with either on a botulinum toxin or surgical ablation or inhibiting detrusor contractility such that the bladder is manually emptied via a catheter. Understanding the neurologic pathway of DSD may open more elegant treatment options and improve both safety and quality of life.

Central Nervous System

The central nervous system coordinates urinary storage and emptying through the periaqueductal gray region (PAG) in the midbrain and the pontine micturition center (PMC) in the brain stem. These two areas are the central components of the spino-bulbo-spinal micturition reflex pathway. The PAG receives afferent information from the bladder and facilitates storage by inhibiting the PMC [100, 101]. This causes sympathetic stimulation which results in detrusor relaxation and urethral tightening. Once a volume threshold is reached in the bladder as signaled by the afferent nerves, the PAG releases inhibition on the PMC. Sympathetic stimulation is then inhibited, and parasympathetic-induced emptying occurs through relaxation of the urethra and contraction of the bladder.

Storage

PAG

The PAG can be considered as a "control center" in the brain for coordinating urine storage and emptying. It is located in the midbrain and also plays a major role in the processing of autonomic stimulation of respiration and cardiac function, pain, and defensive behavior such as fear, anger, and aversion. It has two distinct columns involved in micturition regulation, the ventrolateral and dorsolateral. The ventrolateral region first receives the afferent input. It has been shown that stimulation of the bladder of rats in a frequency below voiding threshold causes an increase in the caudal ventrolateral PAG activity [102]. The ventrolateral region communicates with the PMC and to anterior cingulate cortex which then communicates with the dorsolateral PAG (Fig. 13). The dorsolateral PAG inhibits the PMC through GABA-mediated stimulation which negates the ventrolateral PAG stimulation [103]. It suspected that incontinence in infants is from lack of development of the cortex and lack of inhibitory stimulation of the dorsolateral PAG. This allows continuous stimulation of the ventrolateral PAG on the PMC and the lack of bladder control visualized in infants. The importance of the PAG is also seen in neurologic conditions where the

PAG is affected, such as multiple system atrophy and Alzheimer's. When affected in these conditions, urinary incontinence is usually prevalent because of the lack of inhibitory signaling from the cortex on the dorsal PAG.

ACC

PAG activation from bladder filling stimulates the dorsal anterior cingulate cortex (ACC) [104]. The ACC is thought to be involved in regulating attention, mood, and other cognitive functions. People with frontal lobe pathology that affects the ACC, such as injury or tumor, have been shown to develop urgency and urge incontinence, likely from disruption of regulating the PAG-PMC pathway. In one study from the 1960s, 32 of 34 people with frontal lobe lesions had refractory overactive bladder. The ACC in the anterior-medial part of the frontal lobe was commonly affected in these people [105]. Subsequent studies of stroke patients also demonstrated a high prevalence of urge incontinence when the frontal lobe was affected [106]. Other conditions that affect the frontal lobe, such as depression, are also noted to be prevalent among women with overactive bladder symptoms [107, 108]. Based on these and other studies, it is likely that a functional ACC is needed for effective urinary storage.

Prefrontal Cortex

The prefrontal cortex is also thought to be involved in activating dorsolateral PAG suppression of the PMC. Studies have shown that the prefrontal cortex is involved in regulating spontaneous behavior, internally driving decision-making, and free choice. It is unclear how the prefrontal cortex gives input on continence, but it may inhibit decision-making, particularly regarding ability to suppress urinary urge. Pang and Liao performed resting-state functional near-infrared spectroscopy on ten people with interstitial cystitis/painful bladder syndrome and found that the functional connectivity of prefrontal cortex with other brain regions was low compared to non-IC people [109]. As with the ACC, the prefrontal cortex is likely working within a functional connectivity network within the brain to drive bladder storage. This is best demonstrated by an fMRI evaluation of 12 women both before and after neuromodulation for overactive bladder. Successfully treated women showed decreased brain activity in the left anterior cingulate cortex, the bilateral insula, the left dorsolateral prefrontal cortex, and the bilateral orbitofrontal cortex [110].

The prefrontal cortex also has connections with a region in the hypothalamus that has sleep active inhibiting neurons [111, 112]. This is relevant because nocturia is highly prevalent in conditions like Parkinson's disease which can affect the hypothalamus, among other brain regions. Loss of hypothalamus regulation might thus explain a mechanism for neurogenic nocturia.

Voiding

PMC

The release of inhibition of the pontine micturition center (PMC) changes the bladder intent from storage to emptying. The PMC was first discovered by Barrington in 1925 when he observed that injuring a region in the dorsal pons of a cat would cause urinary retention [113]. Although the mechanism is not clearly elucidated, research suggests that micturition is activated when dorsolateral PAG releases inhibition of a specific region in the PMC called Bar. Bar has excitatory neurotransmitters such as glutamine and neurons from this region projecting to the sacral spinal cord [114]. Once activated, the parasympathetic pelvic nerves are activated, the sympathetic hypogastric nerves are inhibited, the stimulation of Onuf's nucleus and the pudendal nerve decreases (Fig. 14) [105].

Locus Coeruleus

The PMC may not be the only central nervous system region responsible for stimulating micturition. The locus coeruleus (LC) is a region in the pons near the amygdala and is thought to influence response to stress or anxiety. Recent research demonstrated that ablation of this region led to overflow incontinence whereas stimulation caused a voiding contraction. It is speculated that neurons from the LC also synapse in the lumbosacral region. Ablating noradrenergic neurons in the lumbosacral region resulted in loss of detrusor and external sphincter coordination.

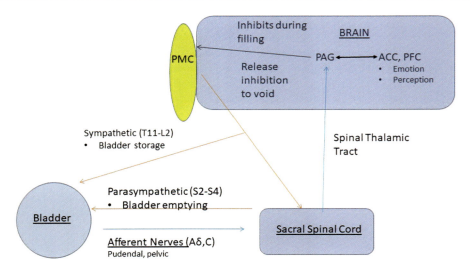

Fig. 14 Pontine micturition center function in urinary continence and voiding. PMC= pontine micturition complex, PAG = periaqueductal gray, ACC = anterior cingulate cortex, PFC = prefrontal cortex

Knowledge Gap: Cell Replacement

A significant gap in knowledge relates to how the nervous system can be repaired. The central nervous system appears to have limited ability to initiate repairs once injured and relies on redundant pathways for function after an injury. Examples of the include spinal cord injuries, Parkinson's disease, and Alzheimer's disease. Damaged neurons do not repair themselves in animal models, as evidenced by lack of new production of myelin or glial scars [115]. Researchers have suggested that cell replacement therapy may lead to viable neuron replacement. One possible mechanism is to use stem cells which then differentiate into mature neuron cells. Potential sources of stems cells have been discussed including pluripotent embryonic stem cells and autologous neural cells created from patient-specific somatic cells like dermal fibroblasts [116]. Stem cell therapy is being actively investigated for treatment of multiple sclerosis with interest in storing lost organ system function [117]. Another mechanism is to target cells in vivo, such as for reprogramming via gene therapy. There has been some limited success in vitro demonstrating that astrocytes can be reprogrammed into neurons and peripheral glial cells can become myelin-producing central glial cells with targeted gene therapy [116]. Gene therapy trials have been investigated for diseases such as Huntington's disease and ALS but with limited long-term data to discuss.

Conclusion

Successful storage and emptying of urine needs careful coordination. First, it requires a functional urothelium and a bladder that is malleable to stretch and compression. Second, it requires an intact peripheral nervous system to transmit information on bladder volume and pressure to the central nervous system and message back to the bladder to facilitate either urine storage or emptying. Finally, successful storage and emptying requires a functional midbrain, cortex, and pons in the central nervous system and an intact spinal cord to communicate with the peripheral nervous system. Injury or deficits in any part of these subsystems will impact bladder coordination.

References

1. Merchant SH, Vial F, Leodori G, Fahn S, Pullman SL, Hallett M. A novel exaggerated "spino-bulbo-spinal like" reflex of lower brainstem origin. Parkinsonism Relat Disord. 2019;61:34–8.

2. Lewis SA. Everything you wanted to know about the bladder epithelium but were afraid to ask. Am J Physiol Renal Physiol. 2000;278(6):F867–74.

3. Khandelwal P, Abraham SN, Apodaca G. Cell biology and physiology of the uroepithelium. Am J Physiol Renal Physiol. 2009;297(6):F1477–501.

4. Birder LA, Kanai AJ, Cruz F, Moore K, Fry CH. Is the urothelium intelligent? Neurourol Urodyn. 2010;29 (4):598–602.

5. Hauser PJ, Dozmorov MG, Bane BL, Slobodov G, Culkin DJ, Hurst RE. Abnormal expression of differentiation related proteins and proteoglycan core proteins in the urothelium of patients with interstitial cystitis. J Urol. 2008;179(2):764–9.

6. Cvach K, Rosamilia A. Review of intravesical therapies for bladder pain syndrome/interstitial cystitis. Transl Androl Urol. 2015;4(6):629–37.

7. Arrighi S. The urothelium: anatomy, review of the literature, perspectives for veterinary medicine. Ann Anat. 2015;198:73–82.

8. Birder LA, Ruggieri M, Takeda M, van Koeveringe G, Veltkamp S, Korstanje C, et al. How does the urothelium affect bladder function in health and disease? ICI-RS 2011. Neurourol Urodyn. 2012;31(3):293–9.

9. Everaerts W, Vriens J, Owsianik G, Appendino G, Voets T, De Ridder D, et al. Functional characterization of transient receptor potential channels in mouse urothelial cells. Am J Physiol Renal Physiol. 2010;298(3):F692–701.

10. Gillespie JI, Markerink-van Ittersum M, de Vente J. cGMP-generating cells in the bladder wall: identification of distinct networks of interstitial cells. BJU Int. 2004;94(7):1114–24.

11. Neuhaus J, Gonsior A, Cheng S, Stolzenburg JU, Berger FP. Mechanosensitivity is a characteristic feature of cultured suburothelial interstitial cells of the human bladder. Int J Mol Sci. 2020;21(15):5474.

12. Uehling DT, Johnson DB, Hopkins WJ. The urinary tract response to entry of pathogens. World J Urol. 1999;17(6):351–8.

13. Yeh J, Lu M, Alvarez-Lugo L, Chai TC. Bladder urothelial BK channel activity is a critical mediator for innate immune response in urinary tract infection pathogenesis. Am J Physiol Renal Physiol. 2019;316 (4):F617–F23.

14. Acevedo-Alvarez M, Yeh J, Alvarez-Lugo L, Lu M, Sukumar N, Hill WG, et al. Mouse urothelial genes associated with voiding behavior changes after ovariectomy and bladder lipopolysaccharide exposure. Neurourol Urodyn. 2018;37(8):2398–405.

15. Shah G, Zhang G, Chen F, Cao Y, Kalyanaraman B, See WA. The dose-response relationship of bacillus Calmette-Guerin and urothelial carcinoma cell biology. J Urol. 2016;195(6):1903–10.

16. Saito R, Smith CC, Utsumi T, Bixby LM, Kardos J, Wobker SE, et al. Molecular subtype-specific immunocompetent models of high-grade urothelial carcinoma reveal differential neoantigen expression and response to immunotherapy. Cancer Res. 2018;78 (14):3954–68.

17. Lewis DA, Brown R, Williams J, White P, Jacobson SK, Marchesi JR, et al. The human urinary microbiome; bacterial DNA in voided urine of asymptomatic adults. Front Cell Infect Microbiol. 2013;3:41.

18. Josephs-Spaulding J, Krogh TJ, Rettig HC, Lyng M, Chkonia M, Waschina S, et al. Recurrent urinary tract infections: unraveling the complicated environment of uncomplicated rUTIs. Front Cell Infect Microbiol. 2021;11:562525.

19. Govender Y, Gabriel I, Minassian V, Fichorova R. The current evidence on the association between the urinary microbiome and urinary incontinence in women. Front Cell Infect Microbiol. 2019;9:133.

20. Wu C, Sui GP, Fry CH. Purinergic regulation of guinea pig suburothelial myofibroblasts. J Physiol. 2004;559(Pt 1):231–43.

21. Kanai A, Fry C, Hanna-Mitchell A, Birder L, Zabbarova I, Bijos D, et al. Do we understand any more about bladder interstitial cells?-ICI-RS 2013. Neurourol Urodyn. 2014;33(5):573–6.

22. Kanai A, Andersson KE. Bladder afferent signaling: recent findings. J Urol. 2010;183(4):1288–95.

23. Andersson KE, McCloskey KD. Lamina propria: the functional center of the bladder? Neurourol Urodyn. 2014;33(1):9–16.

24. Chun SY, Lim GJ, Kwon TG, Kwak EK, Kim BW, Atala A, et al. Identification and characterization of bioactive factors in bladder submucosa matrix. Biomaterials. 2007;28(29):4251–6.

25. Liu Y, Bharadwaj S, Lee SJ, Atala A, Zhang Y. Optimization of a natural collagen scaffold to aid cell-matrix penetration for urologic tissue engineering. Biomaterials. 2009;30(23-24):3865–73.

26. Davis NF, Mooney R, Piterina AV, Callanan A, McGuire BB, Flood HD, et al. Construction and evaluation of urinary bladder bioreactor for urologic tissue-engineering purposes. Urology. 2011;78(4): 954–60.

27. Shaikh FM, O'Brien TP, Callanan A, Kavanagh EG, Burke PE, Grace PA, et al. New pulsatile hydrostatic pressure bioreactor for vascular tissue-engineered constructs. Artif Organs. 2010;34(2):153–8.

28. Liu HT, Shie JH, Chen SH, Wang YS, Kuo HC. Differences in mast cell infiltration, E-cadherin, and zonula occludens-1 expression between patients with overactive bladder and interstitial cystitis/bladder pain syndrome. Urology. 2012;80(1):225 e13–8.

29. Sant GR, Kempuraj D, Marchand JE, Theoharides TC. The mast cell in interstitial cystitis: role in pathophysiology and pathogenesis. Urology. 2007;69 (4 Suppl):34–40.

30. Kullmann FA, McDonnell BM, Wolf-Johnston AS, Lynn AM, Giglio D, Getchell SE, et al. Inflammation and tissue remodeling in the bladder and urethra in feline interstitial cystitis. Front Syst Neurosci. 2018;12:13.

31. Andersson KE, Arner A. Urinary bladder contraction and relaxation: physiology and pathophysiology. Physiol Rev. 2004;84(3):935–86.

32. Stolzenburg JU, Schwalenberg T, Do M, Dorschner W, Salomon FV, Jurina K, et al. Is the

male dog comparable to human? A histological study of the muscle systems of the lower urinary tract. Anat Histol Embryol. 2002;31(4):198–205.

33. Zhou F, Li H, Zhou C, Lv H, Ma Y, Wang Y, et al. Structural and functional changes in gap junctional intercellular communication in a rat model of overactive bladder syndrome induced by partial bladder outlet obstruction. Exp Ther Med. 2016;11(6):2139–46.

34. Phe V, Behr-Roussel D, Oger-Roussel S, Roupret M, Chartier-Kastler E, Lebret T, et al. Involvement of connexins 43 and 45 in functional mechanism of human detrusor overactivity in neurogenic bladder. Urology. 2013;81(5):1108 e1–6.

35. Hypolite JA, Malykhina AP. Regulation of urinary bladder function by protein kinase C in physiology and pathophysiology. BMC Urol. 2015;15:110.

36. Fry CH, Vahabi B. The role of the mucosa in normal and abnormal bladder function. Basic Clin Pharmacol Toxicol. 2016;119(Suppl 3):57–62.

37. Kim SJ, Kim J, Na YG, Kim KH. Irreversible bladder remodeling induced by fibrosis. Int Neurourol J. 2021;25(Suppl 1):S3–7.

38. Rosenbloom J, Koo H, Howard PS, Mecham R, Macarak EJ. Elastic fibers and their role in bladder extracellular matrix. Adv Exp Med Biol. 1995;385:161–72; discussion 79–84.

39. Aitken KJ, Bagli DJ. The bladder extracellular matrix. Part I: architecture, development and disease. Nat Rev Urol. 2009;6(11):596–611.

40. Inaba M, Ukimura O, Yaoi T, Kawauchi A, Fushiki S, Miki T. Upregulation of heme oxygenase and collagen type III in the rat bladder after partial bladder outlet obstruction. Urol Int. 2007;78(3):270–7.

41. Bellucci CHS, Ribeiro WO, Hemerly TS, de Bessa J Jr, Antunes AA, Leite KRM, et al. Increased detrusor collagen is associated with detrusor overactivity and decreased bladder compliance in men with benign prostatic obstruction. Prostate Int. 2017;5(2):70–4.

42. Kwon J, Lee EJ, Cho HJ, Jang JA, Han MS, Kwak E, et al. Antifibrosis treatment by inhibition of VEGF, FGF, and PDGF receptors improves bladder wall remodeling and detrusor overactivity in association with modulation of C-fiber afferent activity in mice with spinal cord injury. Neurourol Urodyn. 2021;40(6):1460–9.

43. Landau EH, Jayanthi VR, Churchill BM, Shapiro E, Gilmour RF, Khoury AE, et al. Loss of elasticity in dysfunctional bladders: urodynamic and histochemical correlation. J Urol. 1994;152(2 Pt 2):702–5.

44. Peyronnet B, Richard C, Bendavid C, Naudet F, Hascoet J, Brochard C, et al. Urinary TIMP-2 and MMP-2 are significantly associated with poor bladder compliance in adult patients with spina bifida. Neurourol Urodyn. 2019;38(8):2151–8.

45. Clemens JQ. Basic bladder neurophysiology. Urol Clin North Am. 2010;37(4):487–94.

46. Michel MC, Vrydag W. Alpha1-, alpha2- and beta-adrenoceptors in the urinary bladder, urethra and prostate. Br J Pharmacol. 2006;147(Suppl 2):S88–119.

47. Scofield MA, Liu F, Abel PW, Jeffries WB. Quantification of steady state expression of mRNA for alpha-1 adrenergic receptor subtypes using reverse transcription and a competitive polymerase chain reaction. J Pharmacol Exp Ther. 1995;275(2):1035–42.

48. Yono M, Foster HE Jr, Shin D, Takahashi W, Pouresmail M, Latifpour J. Doxazosin-induced up-regulation of alpha 1A-adrenoceptor mRNA in the rat lower urinary tract. Can J Physiol Pharmacol. 2004;82(10):872–8.

49. Walden PD, Durkin MM, Lepor H, Wetzel JM, Gluchowski C, Gustafson EL. Localization of mRNA and receptor binding sites for the alpha 1a-adrenoceptor subtype in the rat, monkey and human urinary bladder and prostate. J Urol. 1997;157(3):1032–8.

50. Schwinn DA, Roehrborn CG. Alpha1-adrenoceptor subtypes and lower urinary tract symptoms. Int J Urol. 2008;15(3):193–9.

51. Swierzewski SJ 3rd, Gormley EA, Belville WD, Sweetser PM, Wan J, McGuire EJ. The effect of terazosin on bladder function in the spinal cord injured patient. J Urol. 1994;151(4):951–4.

52. Nomiya M, Yamaguchi O. A quantitative analysis of mRNA expression of alpha 1 and beta-adrenoceptor subtypes and their functional roles in human normal and obstructed bladders. J Urol. 2003;170(2 Pt 1):649–53.

53. Yamazaki Y, Takeda H, Akahane M, Igawa Y, Nishizawa O, Ajisawa Y. Species differences in the distribution of beta-adrenoceptor subtypes in bladder smooth muscle. Br J Pharmacol. 1998;124(3):593–9.

54. Jiang YH, Kuo HC. Urothelial barrier deficits, suburothelial inflammation and altered sensory protein expression in detrusor underactivity. J Urol. 2017;197(1):197–203.

55. Yamanishi T, Chapple CR, Yasuda K, Chess-Williams R. The role of M(2)-muscarinic receptors in mediating contraction of the pig urinary bladder in vitro. Br J Pharmacol. 2000;131(7):1482–8.

56. Hegde SS. Muscarinic receptors in the bladder: from basic research to therapeutics. Br J Pharmacol. 2006;147(Suppl 2):S80–7.

57. Schneider T, Hein P, Michel MC. Signal transduction underlying carbachol-induced contraction of rat urinary bladder. I. Phospholipases and Ca2+ sources. J Pharmacol Exp Ther. 2004;308(1):47–53.

58. Callegari E, Malhotra B, Bungay PJ, Webster R, Fenner KS, Kempshall S, et al. A comprehensive non-clinical evaluation of the CNS penetration potential of antimuscarinic agents for the treatment of overactive bladder. Br J Clin Pharmacol. 2011;72(2):235–46.

59. Vanneste M, Segal A, Voets T, Everaerts W. Transient receptor potential channels in sensory mechanisms of the lower urinary tract. Nat Rev Urol. 2021;18(3):139–59.

60. Munoz A, Yazdi IK, Tang X, Rivera C, Taghipour N, Grossman RG, et al. Localized inhibition of P2X7R at the spinal cord injury site improves neurogenic

60. bladder dysfunction by decreasing urothelial P2X3R expression in rats. Life Sci. 2017;171:60–7.

61. Cockayne DA, Dunn PM, Zhong Y, Rong W, Hamilton SG, Knight GE, et al. P2X2 knockout mice and P2X2/P2X3 double knockout mice reveal a role for the P2X2 receptor subunit in mediating multiple sensory effects of ATP. J Physiol. 2005;567(Pt 2): 621–39.

62. Cockayne DA, Hamilton SG, Zhu QM, Dunn PM, Zhong Y, Novakovic S, et al. Urinary bladder hyporeflexia and reduced pain-related behaviour in P2X3-deficient mice. Nature. 2000;407(6807):1011–5.

63. Davenport AJ, Neagoe I, Brauer N, Koch M, Rotgeri A, Nagel J, et al. Eliapixant is a selective P2X3 receptor antagonist for the treatment of disorders associated with hypersensitive nerve fibers. Sci Rep. 2021;11(1):19877.

64. Slobodov G, Feloney M, Gran C, Kyker KD, Hurst RE, Culkin DJ. Abnormal expression of molecular markers for bladder impermeability and differentiation in the urothelium of patients with interstitial cystitis. J Urol. 2004;171(4):1554–8.

65. Cho KJ, Koh JS, Choi J, Kim JC. Changes in adenosine triphosphate and nitric oxide in the urothelium of patients with benign prostatic hyperplasia and detrusor underactivity. J Urol. 2017;198(6):1392–6.

66. He W, Xiang H, Liu D, Liu J, Li M, Wang Q, et al. Changes in the expression and function of the PDE5 pathway in the obstructed urinary bladder. J Cell Mol Med. 2020;24(22):13181–95.

67. Porst H, McVary KT, Montorsi F, Sutherland P, Elion-Mboussa A, Wolka AM, et al. Effects of once-daily tadalafil on erectile function in men with erectile dysfunction and signs and symptoms of benign prostatic hyperplasia. Eur Urol. 2009;56(4):727–35.

68. Fernandez-Carvajal A, Gonzalez-Muniz R, Fernandez-Ballester G, Ferrer-Montiel A. Investigational drugs in early phase clinical trials targeting thermotransient receptor potential (thermoTRP) channels. Expert Opin Investig Drugs. 2020;29(11):1209–22.

69. Lashinger ES, Steiginga MS, Hieble JP, Leon LA, Gardner SD, Nagilla R, et al. AMTB, a TRPM8 channel blocker: evidence in rats for activity in overactive bladder and painful bladder syndrome. Am J Physiol Renal Physiol. 2008;295(3):F803–10.

70. Skibsbye L, Poulet C, Diness JG, Bentzen BH, Yuan L, Kappert U, et al. Small-conductance calcium-activated potassium (SK) channels contribute to action potential repolarization in human atria. Cardiovasc Res. 2014;103(1):156–67.

71. Kitta T, Kanno Y, Chiba H, Higuchi M, Ouchi M, Togo M, et al. Benefits and limitations of animal models in partial bladder outlet obstruction for translational research. Int J Urol. 2018;25(1):36–44.

72. Shen JD, Chen SJ, Chen HY, Chiu KY, Chen YH, Chen WC. Review of animal models to study urinary bladder function. Biology (Basel). 2021;10(12):1316.

73. de Groat WC, Yoshimura N. Afferent nerve regulation of bladder function in health and disease. Handb Exp Pharmacol. 2009;194:91–138.

74. Morgan C, deGroat WC, Nadelhaft I. The spinal distribution of sympathetic preganglionic and visceral primary afferent neurons that send axons into the hypogastric nerves of the cat. J Comp Neurol. 1986;243(1):23–40.

75. Shafik A, el-Sherif M, Youssef A, Olfat ES. Surgical anatomy of the pudendal nerve and its clinical implications. Clin Anat. 1995;8(2):110–5.

76. Yoshimura N, Erdman SL, Snider MW, de Groat WC. Effects of spinal cord injury on neurofilament immunoreactivity and capsaicin sensitivity in rat dorsal root ganglion neurons innervating the urinary bladder. Neuroscience. 1998;83(2):633–43.

77. Sengupta JN. Visceral pain: the neurophysiological mechanism. Handb Exp Pharmacol. 2009;194:31–74.

78. Zagorodnyuk VP, Costa M, Brookes SJ. Major classes of sensory neurons to the urinary bladder. Auton Neurosci. 2006;126–127:390–7.

79. Sengupta JN, Gebhart GF. Mechanosensitive properties of pelvic nerve afferent fibers innervating the urinary bladder of the rat. J Neurophysiol. 1994;72 (5):2420–30.

80. Habler HJ, Janig W, Koltzenburg M. Activation of unmyelinated afferent fibres by mechanical stimuli and inflammation of the urinary bladder in the cat. J Physiol. 1990;425:545–62.

81. Juszczak K, Ziomber A, Thor PJ. Effect of partial and complete blockade of vanilloid (TRPV1-6) and ankyrin (TRPA1) transient receptor potential ion channels on urinary bladder motor activity in an experimental hyperosmolar overactive bladder rat model. J Physiol Pharmacol. 2011;62(3):321–6.

82. Baron R, Hans G, Dickenson AH. Peripheral input and its importance for central sensitization. Ann Neurol. 2013;74(5):630–6.

83. Aurore V, Rothlisberger R, Boemke N, Hlushchuk R, Bangerter H, Bergmann M, et al. Anatomy of the female pelvic nerves: a macroscopic study of the hypogastric plexus and their relations and variations. J Anat. 2020;237(3):487–94.

84. Marcinowski F. Bronislaw Onuf-Onufrowicz (1863–1928). J Neurol. 2019;266(1):281–2.

85. Rogers MJ, Shen B, Reese JN, Xiao Z, Wang J, Lee A, et al. Role of glycine in nociceptive and non-nociceptive bladder reflexes and pudendal afferent inhibition of these reflexes in cats. Neurourol Urodyn. 2016;35(7):798–804.

86. Fowler CJ. Integrated control of lower urinary tract-clinical perspective. Br J Pharmacol. 2006;147(Suppl 2):S14–24.

87. D'Amico SC, Schuster IP, Collins WF 3rd. Quantification of external urethral sphincter and bladder activity during micturition in the intact and spinally transected adult rat. Exp Neurol. 2011;228(1):59–68.

88. Jiang HH, Salcedo LB, Song B, Damaser MS. Pelvic floor muscles and the external urethral sphincter have different responses to applied bladder pressure during continence. Urology. 2010;75(6):1515 e1–7.

89. Zare A, Jahanshahi A, Rahnama'i MS, Schipper S, van Koeveringe GA. The role of the periaqueductal

gray matter in lower urinary tract function. Mol Neurobiol. 2019;56(2):920–34.

90. Oliveira R, Coelho A, Franquinho F, Sousa MM, Cruz F, Cruz CD. Effects of early intravesical administration of resiniferatoxin to spinal cord-injured rats in neurogenic detrusor overactivity. Neurourol Urodyn. 2019;38(6):1540–50.

91. Payne CK, Mosbaugh PG, Forrest JB, Evans RJ, Whitmore KE, Antoci JP, et al. Intravesical resiniferatoxin for the treatment of interstitial cystitis: a randomized, double-blind, placebo controlled trial. J Urol. 2005;173(5):1590–4.

92. van Ophoven A, Engelberg S, Lilley H, Sievert KD. Systematic literature review and meta-analysis of sacral neuromodulation (SNM) in patients with neurogenic lower urinary tract dysfunction (nLUTD): over 20 years' experience and future directions. Adv Ther. 2021;38(4):1987–2006.

93. Wang M, Jian Z, Ma Y, Jin X, Li H, Wang K. Percutaneous tibial nerve stimulation for overactive bladder syndrome: a systematic review and meta-analysis. Int Urogynecol J. 2020;31(12):2457–71.

94. Fujihara A, Ukimura O, Iwata T, Miki T. Neuroselective measure of the current perception threshold of A-delta and C-fiber afferents in the lower urinary tract. Int J Urol. 2011;18(5):341–9.

95. Stoffel JT. Detrusor sphincter dyssynergia: a review of physiology, diagnosis, and treatment strategies. Transl Androl Urol. 2016;5(1):127–35.

96. Castro-Diaz D, Taracena Lafuente JM. Detrusor-sphincter dyssynergia. Int J Clin Pract Suppl. 2006;151:17–21.

97. Miyazato M, Sugaya K, Nishijima S, Ashitomi K, Hatano T, Ogawa Y. Inhibitory effect of intrathecal glycine on the micturition reflex in normal and spinal cord injury rats. Exp Neurol. 2003;183(1):232–40.

98. Miyazato M, Sugaya K, Nishijima S, Ashitomi K, Ohyama C, Ogawa Y. Rectal distention inhibits bladder activity via glycinergic and GABAergic mechanisms in rats. J Urol. 2004;171(3):1353–6.

99. Miyazato M, Sugaya K, Saito S, Chancellor MB, Goins WF, Goss JR, et al. Suppression of detrusor-sphincter dyssynergia by herpes simplex virus vector mediated gene delivery of glutamic acid decarboxylase in spinal cord injured rats. J Urol. 2010;184(3):1204–10.

100. Griffiths D, Tadic SD. Bladder control, urgency, and urge incontinence: evidence from functional brain imaging. Neurourol Urodyn. 2008;27(6):466–74.

101. Ding YQ, Zheng HX, Gong LW, Lu Y, Zhao H, Qin BZ. Direct projections from the lumbosacral spinal cord to Barrington's nucleus in the rat: a special reference to micturition reflex. J Comp Neurol. 1997;389(1):149–60.

102. Meriaux C, Hohnen R, Schipper S, Zare A, Jahanshahi A, Birder LA, et al. Neuronal activation in the periaqueductal gray matter upon electrical stimulation of the bladder. Front Cell Neurosci. 2018;12:133.

103. An X, Bandler R, Ongur D, Price JL. Prefrontal cortical projections to longitudinal columns in the midbrain periaqueductal gray in macaque monkeys. J Comp Neurol. 1998;401(4):455–79.

104. Griffiths DJ, Tadic SD, Schaefer W, Resnick NM. Cerebral control of the lower urinary tract: how age-related changes might predispose to urge incontinence. NeuroImage. 2009;47(3):981–6.

105. Andrew J, Nathan PW. Lesions on the anterior frontal lobes and disturbances of micturition and defaecation. Brain. 1964;87:233–62.

106. Sakakibara R, Hattori T, Yasuda K, Yamanishi T. Micturitional disturbance after acute hemispheric stroke: analysis of the lesion site by CT and MRI. J Neurol Sci. 1996;137(1):47–56.

107. Stoffel JT, Morgan D, Dunn R, Hsu Y, Fenner D, Delancey J, et al. Urinary incontinence after stress incontinence surgery: a risk factor for depression. Urology. 2009;73(1):41–6.

108. Zhang FF, Peng W, Sweeney JA, Jia ZY, Gong QY. Brain structure alterations in depression: psychoradiological evidence. CNS Neurosci Ther. 2018;24(11):994–1003.

109. Pang D, Liao L. Abnormal functional connectivity within the prefrontal cortex in interstitial cystitis/bladder pain syndrome (IC/BPS): a pilot study using resting state functional near-infrared spectroscopy (rs-fNIRS). Neurourol Urodyn. 2021;40(6):1634–42.

110. Weissbart SJ, Bhavsar R, Rao H, Wein AJ, Detre JA, Arya LA, et al. Specific changes in brain activity during urgency in women with overactive bladder after successful sacral neuromodulation: a functional magnetic resonance imaging study. J Urol. 2018;200 (2):382–8.

111. Hyder F, Phelps EA, Wiggins CJ, Labar KS, Blamire AM, Shulman RG. "Willed action": a functional MRI study of the human prefrontal cortex during a sensorimotor task. Proc Natl Acad Sci U S A. 1997;94(13): 6989–94.

112. Boes AD, Fischer D, Geerling JC, Bruss J, Saper CB, Fox MD. Connectivity of sleep- and wake-promoting regions of the human hypothalamus observed during resting wakefulness. Sleep. 2018;41(9):zsy108.

113. Morrison JF. The discovery of the pontine micturition centre by F. J. F. Barrington. Exp Physiol. 2008;93(6): 742–5.

114. Verstegen AMJ, Vanderhorst V, Gray PA, Zeidel ML, Geerling JC. Barrington's nucleus: neuroanatomic landscape of the mouse "pontine micturition center". J Comp Neurol. 2017;525(10):2287–309.

115. Filbin MT. Myelin-associated inhibitors of axonal regeneration in the adult mammalian CNS. Nat Rev Neurosci. 2003;4(9):703–13.

116. Tso D, McKinnon RD. Cell replacement therapy for central nervous system diseases. Neural Regen Res. 2015;10(9):1356–8.

117. Smith JA, Nicaise AM, Ionescu RB, Hamel R, Peruzzotti-Jametti L, Pluchino S. Stem cell therapies for progressive multiple sclerosis. Front Cell Dev Biol. 2021;9:696434.

Pathophysiology of Female Micturition Disorders

4

Alex Gomelsky, Ann C. Stolzle, and William P. Armstrong

Contents

Introduction 71

Micturition 72
Pelvic Anatomy and Clinical Correlations 72
Neuroanatomy of the Urinary Tract 76
Physiology of Urinary Storage and Emptying (Fig. 8) 77
Physiology of Stress Urinary Continence 78
Pathophysiology of Micturition Dysfunction 79

Conclusion 82

References 83

Abstract

Urinary storage and emptying involve multiple anatomic organs, muscular and fascial support structures, and the autonomic and somatic nervous systems. Urinary storage involves a compliant bladder, closed urinary outlet, and an absent detrusor overactivity. Conversely, urinary emptying involves a coordinated detrusor contraction of appropriate magnitude, the relaxation and opening of the bladder outlet, and an absence of anatomic outflow obstruction. When a woman develops storage or emptying lower urinary tract symptoms, urinary incontinence, or urinary retention, the failure of this complex mechanism can become a challenging problem. The aims of this chapter are to define the normal physiologic adaptations to urinary storage and filling and then to delve further into the possible reasons behind the dysfunction of these interactions.

Keywords

Pathophysiology · Anatomy · Micturition · Urinary storage · Urinary emptying · Incontinence · Lower urinary tract symptoms

A. Gomelsky (✉)
Department of Urology, LSU Health Shreveport, Shreveport, LA, USA
e-mail: alexander.gomelsky@lsuhs.edu

A. C. Stolzle · W. P. Armstrong
LSU Health Shreveport School of Medicine, Shreveport, LA, USA
e-mail: acs002@lsuhs.edu; wpa001@lsuhs.edu

Introduction

Efficient storage and emptying of urine involve multiple anatomic organs, interwoven areas of muscular and fascial support, and the autonomic

© Springer Nature Switzerland AG 2023
F. E. Martins et al. (eds.), *Female Genitourinary and Pelvic Floor Reconstruction*,
https://doi.org/10.1007/978-3-031-19598-3_4

and somatic nervous systems. When all these components are working in concert, micturition is almost effortless and easy to take for granted. However, when a woman develops lower urinary tract symptoms (LUTS), urinary incontinence, or impaired emptying, the failure of this complex mechanism can quickly become a bothersome and embarrassing problem. The aims of this chapter are to define the normal physiologic adaptations to urinary storage and filling and then to delve further into the possible reasons behind the dysfunction of these interactions. We will not address surgical or pharmacologic intervention to treat these individual disorders in detail. Likewise, the discussion of pelvic anatomy is, intentionally, not meant to be exhaustive.

Micturition

Pelvic Anatomy and Clinical Correlations

1. There are **four pelvic bones (sacrum, coccyx, and bilateral innominate bones)**, with the innominate bones composed of the **ilium, ischium, and pubis** (Figs. 1 and 2). The bones have several prominences and locations (e.g., ischiopubic rami, ischial spines, sacral promontory, and pubic symphysis) that serve as anchoring points for ligaments and landmarks for support during surgical repair of incontinence and pelvic organ prolapse.
2. **Fasciae** are sheets of connective tissue that attach, stabilize, enclose, and separate muscles and other internal organs. There are several fasciae that are important in pelvic support.
   2.a. The **rectus fascia** is formed by the aponeuroses of the transversus abdominis, internal oblique, and external oblique muscles and contains the rectus abdominis and pyramidalis muscles. A strip of this fascia may be used for construction of autologous slings and serves as an attachment point for these anti-incontinence procedures.
   2.b. The **pubocervical fascia (PCF)** extends from the cardinal ligament (cranially) to the pubic symphysis (caudally) and is attached to the pelvic sidewall (laterally) and endopelvic fascia at the **arcus tendineus fascia pelvis (ATFP)**. This fascia is fused to the vagina and supports the bladder. Weakness in the midportion of the PCF may contribute to a central defect cystocele, while

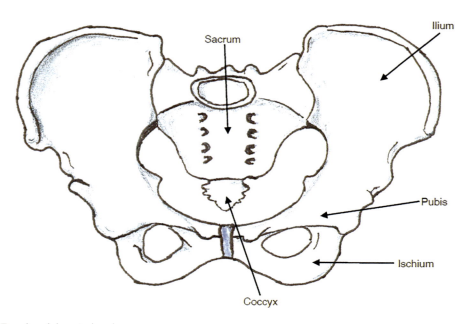

Fig. 1 Female pelvis, anterior view

Fig. 2 Female pelvis, midsagittal view

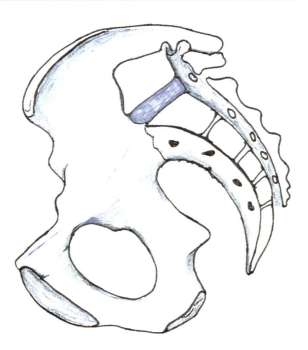

separation of this fascia from the ATFP contributes to a lateral defect cystocele.

2.b.i. Weakness in the midportion of the PCF may contribute to a central defect cystocele, while separation of this fascia from the ATFP contributes to a lateral defect cystocele.

2.b.ii. The distal portion of the PCF supports the urethrovesical junction (bladder neck and proximal urethra) and serves as a supportive structure for compression of the urethral walls during increases in abdominal pressure. Stress urinary incontinence (SUI) may result if this portion of the PCF is attenuated.

2.c. The **endopelvic fascia** is the continuation of the abdominal parietal peritoneum which contributes to the support of the pelvic viscera.

2.d. The **obturator fascia** (also known as the fascia of the obturator internus) covers the pelvic surface of that muscle and piriformis.

2.e. The **ATFP** runs from the ischial spine (proximally) to the pubis (distally) and serves as an important attachment point for other fasciae. As mentioned previously, a separation of the pubocervical fascia from the ATFP contributes to a lateral defect cystocele.

3. **Ligaments** are bands of membranous, connective tissue which connect two bones or cartilages, give stability to joints, support organs, and keep them in position. Several ligaments are prominent in pelvic support (Figs. 3 and 4).

3.a. The **sacrospinous ligament (SSL)** spans from the ischial spine (laterally) to the lateral sacrum (medially), while the **sacrotuberous ligament** connects the ischial tuberosity (laterally) to the same medial attachment point as the SSL. The SSL is an anchoring point for the vaginal apex during an SSL fixation. Both the sciatic and pudendal nerves pass near both ligaments and may incur injury during improper placement of sutures during apical suspension.

3.b. The **pubourethral ligaments (PUL)** are paired structures on either side of the urethra that extend from the bladder neck to the posterior aspect of the pubic symphysis. The Integral theory posits that a competent

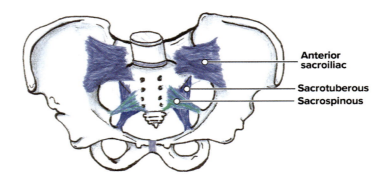

Fig. 3 Pelvic ligaments, anterior view

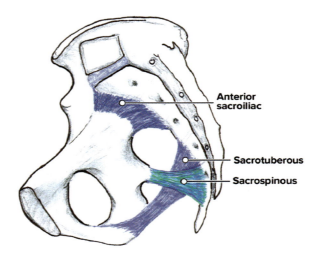

Fig. 4 Pelvic ligaments, midsagittal view

PUL will close off the mid-urethra during increases in intra-abdominal pressure and contribute to stress continence [22].

3.c. **The uterosacral ligaments (USL)** originate from the inferior surface of the ilium and insert into the cervix, uterine isthmus, and vagina medially. The USL are often used for apical suspension at the time of hysterectomy. The ureter lies near the anterior/distal portion of the USL and is at risk for kinking or entrapment during USL suspension.

3.d. The **cardinal ligaments (CL)** originate from the lateral pelvic sidewall and attach to the lateral aspect of the cervix and vagina. Posteriorly, the CL are confluent with the USL and provide uterocervical support prior to hysterectomy.

4. The **pelvic musculature** is analogous to a bowl, albeit a dynamic one where the walls and floor are malleable and adjust their tension and position based on the patient's position, activity, and location of their pelvic organs (Figs. 5 and 6).

4.a. The **piriformis** is part of the posterolateral pelvic wall. It connects the upper part of the sacrum and the greater trochanter of the femur. It passes through the greater sciatic foramen. The coccygeus (ischiococcygeus) is another part of the posterolateral pelvic wall. It passes from the lower part of the sacrum and inserts at the ischial spine. It lies anterior to the SSL and posterior to the levator ani.

4.b. The **obturator internus** makes up a major portion of the lateral pelvic sidewall. It originates on the medial surface of the obturator membrane, the ischium, and the pubic symphysis. It exits the pelvic cavity through the lesser sciatic foramen and inserts onto the greater trochanter of the femur.

4.c. The pelvic floor is composed of the **levator ani**, which is comprised of (distally to proximally) the iliococcygeus, pubococcygeus, and puborectalis muscles (Figs. 5 and 6).

4.c.i. The **iliococcygeus** arises from the inner side of the ischium and from the posterior part of the tendinous arch of the obturator fascia. It is attached to the coccyx medially and the anococcygeal raphe. It sits anterior to the SSL.

4.c.ii. The **pubococcygeus** arises from the back of the pubic symphysis and from the anterior part of the obturator fascia. It attaches to the coccyx and sacrum and runs on either side of the anal canal.

4.c.iii. The **puborectalis** arises from the back of the pubic symphysis and

Fig. 5 Pelvic musculature, superior view

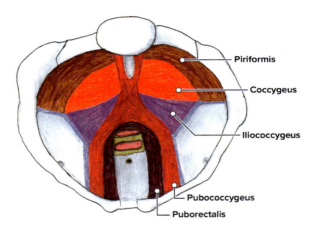

Fig. 6 Pelvic musculature, medial view

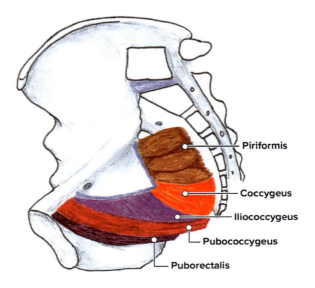

urogenital diaphragm and forms a U-shaped sling that harnesses the anorectal junction to the pubic symphysis.
5. There are two recognized **sphincters** in the urinary tract.
   5.a. The voluntary, striated **external urethral sphincter (EUS)** is composed of two portions. The **intrinsic/intramural** striated sphincter (rhabdosphincter) consists of striated muscle arranged in a circular manner that comprises the outer layer of the urethra in women. It is thickest ventrally and sparse dorsally [16].
      5.a.i. The **inner (paraurethral)** layer of striated muscle is composed of slow-twitch muscle fibers which maintain tonic contraction of the urethra and contribute to passive continence [15, 27].
      5.a.ii. The **outer (periurethral/extramural)** layer consists of fast-twitch fibers and resembles the surrounding levator ani. Voluntary contraction of the fast-twitch fibers produces urethral compression during increases in intra-abdominal pressure [9, 17, 25].
   5.b. The **internal urethral sphincter (IUS)** is composed of smooth muscle and is normally, and statically, closed at rest. The role of the IUS during episodes of increased intra-abdominal pressure is controversial. Some have maintained that proximal urethral closure is essential to maintaining continence [20]; however, there is evidence that up to 50% of continent women may have an open bladder neck at rest and with stress maneuvers [6, 27, 28].
6. The **pelvic organs** can be classified as **urologic** (urethra, bladder, and mid/distal ureters), **gynecologic** (vagina, cervix, uterus, fallopian tubes, and ovaries), and **colorectal** (anus, large and small intestines) (Fig. 7).
7. Arterial blood supply and venous drainage are provided by branches of the **internal iliac arteries and veins**, respectively.

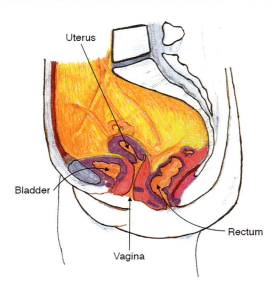

Fig. 7 Pelvic viscera, midsagittal view

8. Lymphatic drainage passes through the **internal iliac lymph nodes**.

Neuroanatomy of the Urinary Tract

1. The pelvic organs have both somatic (sensory and motor function) and autonomic (sympathetic and parasympathetic) innervation. Somatic innervation is voluntary, while autonomic innervation is involuntary.
   1.a. **Somatic innervation** originates in the sacrum. The pudendal nerve arises from S2 to S4, and its branches carry efferent impulses to the muscles of the pelvic floor and afferent signals from the urethra. These nerves act primarily on the EUS, which contracts when stimulated by somatic innervation. EUS relaxation is mediated indirectly by suppressing Onuf's nucleus in the sacral spinal cord.
   1.b. **Sympathetic innervation** (hypogastric) originates from preganglionic fibers at the T10–T12 level and supply the pelvic organs through the hypogastric plexus. Sympathetic innervation serves to promote urinary

storage by inhibiting the detrusor muscle and activating contraction of involuntary IUS.

1.c. **Parasympathetic innervation** through the pelvic nerves originates in the S1–S3 segments and promotes urinary emptying. Parasympathetic nerves activate the detrusor muscle causing it to contract and relax the internal sphincter.

1.d. Higher centers: Micturition is a product of stimulation of the **pontine micturition center (PMC; Barrington's nucleus)**, which leads to detrusor muscle contraction and urethral sphincter relaxation. Suprapontine centers, such as the **periaqueductal gray (PAG)**, have a role in interpreting afferent signaling from the bladder and relaying it to the PMC for action.

Physiology of Urinary Storage and Emptying (Fig. 8)

1. Efficient and safe **urinary storage** involves accommodation, a process of storing urine at a low intravesical pressure during filling. Accommodation should be high during normal bladder filling and can be calculated by change in volume divided by the change in pressure. As the bladder fills with urine, bladder distention activates afferent signaling which communicates with the sacral spinal cord through the pelvic nerve (solid purple line, left side of Fig. 8). In turn, the sympathetic outflow in the thoracolumbar spinal cord is stimulated via the hypogastric nerve (dotted orange line, left side). The hypogastric nerve fibers inhibit detrusor contraction through **β3-adrenoreceptors (β3-ARs)** and stimulates

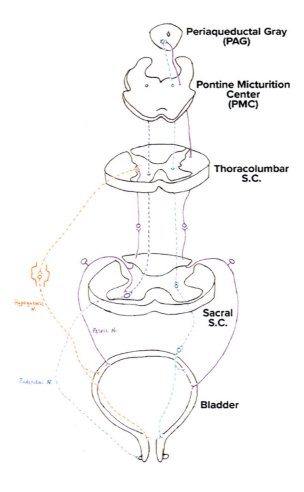

Fig. 8 Neuroanatomy and physiology of micturition. Urinary storage is on the left-hand portion of the figure, and urinary emptying is on the right-hand portion of the figure

the **α1-ARs** in the bladder neck/smooth IUS. Sympathetic outflow also stimulates EUS contraction through the pudendal nerve (dotted dark blue line, left side). These spinal reflex pathways coordinate relaxation of the detrusor and simultaneous contraction at the IUS and EUS, which represents the "guarding reflex." The parasympathetic innervation and PMC are quiescent during urinary storage.

2. During the **voiding phase**, the significant increase in afferent firing in the mechanoreceptors in the bladder wall activates **spinobulbospinal reflex pathways**. In this case, the pelvic nerve communicates with the sacral spinal cord, which, in turn, communicates with the PAG relay center before activating the PMC (solid purple line, right side of Fig. 8). This has been likened to an off/on switch, where the process of urinary storage and accommodation is switched off and voiding is turned on. The PMC shuts off the spinal guarding reflex by halting the sympathetic efferents from the thoracolumbar spinal cord (which were inhibiting the detrusor and contracting the IUS during storage) and the pudendal outflow from the sacral spinal cord (which was responsible for EUS contraction during storage). The PMC also stimulates the parasympathetic outflow from the sacral spinal cord (via the pelvic nerve) to the bladder by stimulating detrusor contraction through the muscarinic (M2 and M3) receptors (dotted light blue line, right side). The pelvic nerve also relaxes the bladder neck by the release of nitric oxide (dotted light blue line, right side). In summary, efficient voiding is achieved by detrusor contraction via parasympathetic innervation, relaxation of the bladder neck, and inhibition of the sympathetic and somatic efferents to the detrusor, IUS, and EUS.

Physiology of Stress Urinary Continence

1. Achieving continence in the neurologically intact female involves the interaction of urethral and bladder neck support, intrinsic properties of the urethra, the urethral sphincter (intrinsic and extrinsic) mechanism, and the pelvic floor musculature. Furthermore, there is input from autonomic and somatic innervation. If the other components cannot compensate for the failure of one, incontinence may result.

2. During a sudden increase in intra-abdominal pressure, a reflex contraction of the levator muscle and urogenital diaphragm increases tension on the ligamentous support of the urethra, thereby elevating and compressing the proximal urethra. Both mid-urethral and urethral closure pressure increase along with the abdominal pressure, and if the urethral support is intact, the increased intra-abdominal pressure is transmitted equally to the bladder and the urethra. The net effect of these changes is increased outlet resistance during stress maneuvers and urinary continence. Conversely, when normal transmission of abdominal pressure to the urethra is lost, incontinence results [12].

3. There are two theories regarding the primary location of urethral support.

   3.a. DeLancey's "hammock hypothesis" postulated that the urethra lies on a supportive layer that is composed of the endopelvic fascia and the anterior vaginal wall, which are attached laterally to the ATFP and levator ani [10]. The anterior and posterior walls of the urethra coapt once compressed against the hammock during increases in intra-abdominal pressure and the urethral lumen is closed. The stability of this sub-urethral layer depends on the intact connection of the vaginal wall and endopelvic fascia to the arcus tendineus fascia pelvis and levator ani. This mechanism may explain the efficacy of a sling placed at the bladder neck.

   3.b. The **Integral Theory** focused on the mid-urethra as the site of maximum intraurethral pressure [22, 31]. The authors defined three opposing muscle forces (vectors) that act on the micturition mechanism: (1) a forward force activated by the pubococcygeus muscle, (2) a backward force activated by the levator ani musculature, and (3) an inferior force controlled by the longitudinal muscle of the anus. During an increase in intra-abdominal pressure, contraction of the pubococcygeus pulls the anterior vaginal wall forward and closes off the urethra. As mentioned previously, this response is contingent on an intact attachment between the anterior vaginal wall and PULs, which act as a fulcrum at the mid-urethra. This theory accounts for the reported effectiveness of the mid-urethral slings which simulate the action of intact PULs.

3.c. **Intrinsic properties of the urethra** also contribute to continence. Starting inside the urethral lumen and proceeding outward, the 4–5-cm-long female urethra is composed of (1) an inner mucosa; (2) submucosa, with loose connective tissue, infiltrating smooth muscle bundles, and extensive vascular plexus; (3) inner longitudinal smooth muscle layer; and (4) outer circular smooth muscle layer [25]. When the vascular plexus fills with blood, the submucosa expands and compresses the mucosa creating a watertight seal [23]. The mucosal seal is further strengthened by contraction of the IUS and EUS, as well as luminal secretions from the periurethral glands. Conditions that decrease the inflow of blood to the urethra (e.g., estrogen deficiency, radiation, or prior surgery) may compromise the mucosal seal and contribute to SUI. Improving coaptation of the urethra via bulking therapy addresses this mechanism.

3.d. In summary, bladder filling requires accommodation of increasing urinary volume at low filling pressure, absence of unstable detrusor contractions, and a closed bladder outlet at rest and with increases in intra-abdominal pressure [29, 30]. Bladder emptying requires a coordinated detrusor contraction of sufficient magnitude with a concomitant lowering of the outlet resistance as well as an absence of anatomic outlet obstruction.

Pathophysiology of Micturition Dysfunction

1. When looking at disorders of micturition, we find that Alan Wein's functional classification is both elegant and efficient [29, 30]. He proposed that all disorders can be separated by failure of either voiding or storage and that each of these could have their origin in the bladder or the outlet. Using this simple classification, disorders can be quickly categorized, and treatment options delivered.

2. **Disorders of urinary storage** (failure to store) include bladder problems, such as detrusor overactivity and impaired compliance, and outlet problems, such as bladder neck incompetence, urethral hypermobility, and ISD. Women will typically present with storage lower urinary tract symptoms (LUTS), such as urgency, frequency, nocturia, and incontinence. Incontinence may be further divided into SUI, urgency urinary incontinence (UUI), and mixed urinary incontinence (MUI).

2.a. **Detrusor Overactivity (DO)**

2.a.i. As mentioned previously, sympathetic outflow relaxes the detrusor and contracts the smooth sphincter, while somatic outflow contracts the striated sphincter. Since storage occurs via spinal reflex pathways, suprapontine centers and the PMC are not engaged during filling. The net effect is storage of an increasing volume of urine at low detrusor pressures against a closed bladder outlet. Normally, little or no change in pressure should occur during this stage nor should any involuntary contraction be initiated [1].

2.a.ii. DO may be idiopathic and neurogenic and may be associated with other coexistent conditions such as bladder outlet obstruction, SUI, and aging [4]. DO is typically associated with the symptom of urgency, but DO demonstrated on urodynamic assessment may not be associated with bothersome symptoms in many women.

2.a.iii. DO has many overlaps with the syndrome of **overactive bladder (OAB)**, defined by the International Continence Society (ICS) as "urinary urgency, with or without UUI, usually with increased daytime frequency and nocturia, if there is no proven infection or other obvious pathology" [11]. The proposed pathophysiology of DO may be summarized as follows: (1) reduced suprapontine inhibition, (2) damaged axonal paths in the spinal cord, (3) damaged axonal paths in the periphery, (4) loss of peripheral inhibition, (5) enhancement of excitatory neurotransmission in the micturition reflex pathway, (6) increased LUT afferent input, and (7) idiopathic [4]. Neurologically, involuntary bladder contractions can occur secondary to any lesion occurring above the sacral spinal cord.

2.a.iv. The AUA/SUFU Guidelines for non-neurogenic OAB provides a framework for evaluation and treatment [14, 19].

2.b. **Impaired (Low) Compliance**

2.b.i. Compliance is the change in volume during a filling cycle divided by the change in intravesical pressure during that cycle. During a normal urinary filling cycle, an increasing volume of urine occurs at low detrusor pressures resulting in a high compliance. Any significant increase in filling pressure may occur toward the end of the cycle just prior to voiding. Elastic and viscoelastic forces allow for stretching of the bladder wall without an increase in tension until the bladder has reached its full capacity [5].

2.b.ii. Impairment of this process occurs when there is an inappropriate rise in detrusor pressure with an increase rise in volume during filling resulting in a failure to store urine. One of the concerns with low compliance is that the buildup of pressure during filling may be transmitted to the upper tracts and impair emptying from the renal pelvises causing renal impairment. Conversely, the pressure may "pop off" through the bladder outlet and contribute to urinary incontinence. Impaired compliance may be caused by functional or neurologic conditions (sacral spinal cord injury) as well as structural problems (connective tissue scarring and fibrosis of the bladder wall resulting from chronic catheterization or chronic UTIs). Bladder wall hypertrophy and idiopathic causes may also lead to increasing amounts of collagen deposition in the stroma.

2.c. **Urethral Hypermobility**

2.c.i. As mentioned previously, there are several theories regarding the anatomical changes that result in SUI [10, 22, 31]. Loss of support, whether ligamentous or fascial, is at the root. Intact urethral and bladder neck support is meant to counteract and oppose changes in intra-abdominal pressure and keep urine from moving from the bladder into the urethra.

2.c.ii. In the absence of adequate support, several adaptations occur that lead to urinary loss after increases in intra-abdominal pressure. The bladder base rotates, and the bladder neck opens, leading to distraction of the anterior and posterior urethral walls. Subsequently, urine enters the urethra and is expelled from the meatus. Slings placed at the bladder neck address the perceived loss of fascial support at that location, while slings placed at the mid-urethra address weakness in the PULs.

2.d. **Intrinsic Sphincter Deficiency (ISD)**

2.d.i. Failure of the urethral mucosal seal may lead to poor coaptation of the urethra during increases in intra-abdominal pressure. This may be caused by intrinsic dysfunction of the urethral smooth muscle or deficiency at the mucosa or submucosa. Etiologies include neurologic origin, consequence of previous surgery or trauma, fibrosis, or idiopathic [3].

2.d.ii. ISD is typically associated with low abdominal or Valsalva leak point pressure and low urethral closure pressure, and, on occasion, the urethra may be open at rest [24]. Bulking therapy augments the urethral mucosal seal and improves coaptation of the urethral walls at rest and with increases in intra-abdominal pressure.

3. **Abnormalities of Urinary Emptying**
   3.a. **Detrusor Underactivity (DUA)**

   3.a.i. DUA is defined as "a contraction of reduced strength and/or duration, resulting in prolonged bladder emptying and/or failure to achieve complete bladder emptying within a normal time span [2]." This concept has been difficult to define due to symptoms that overlap with those of OAB and bladder outlet obstruction (BOO); however, an ICS definition has been accepted [7].

   3.a.ii. Many patients have idiopathic DUA that may develop as an age-related decline in detrusor function. Other reasons may be myogenic, neurogenic, iatrogenic from previous surgery, functional (e.g., Fowler syndrome or dysfunctional voiding), and secondary to certain pharmacotherapeutic interventions (e.g., antimuscarinics, antihistamines, and opioids).

   3.a.iii. Voiding symptoms include slow urinary stream, urinary hesitancy, intermittency, straining to void, and a feeling of incomplete emptying. Storage symptoms may include urgency, frequency, nocturia, and urinary incontinence.

   3.a.iv. The only accepted modality for calculating detrusor function is urodynamic assessment; however, there are no definitive criteria for DUA diagnosis [8].

   3.a.v. The goals of DUA management are to establish efficient and safe bladder emptying, minimize adverse sequelae such as UTIs and incontinence, and improve quality of life. Conservative options include behavioral modification, pelvic floor physiotherapy, and intermittent catheterization. Currently available pharmacotherapeutic interventions such as parasympathomimetics and α-AR antagonists have concerning adverse event profiles. Surgical intervention may be considered for refractory cases or those associated with BOO.

   3.b. **Detrusor External Sphincter Dyssynergia (DESD)**

   3.b.i. The detrusor and EUS work in coordination with one another under brainstem control to allow efficient and safe voiding. The EUS surrounds the proximal urethra and consists of striated muscle. Under normal neurologic control, detrusor contraction and external sphincter relaxation must occur together. However, absence of EUS relaxation during a voluntary or involuntary detrusor contraction leads to DESD. As such, emptying is either absent or incomplete, and detrusor pressure rises in the bladder in response to a closed outlet.

   3.b.ii. True DESD occurs in the background of neurologic disease or injury located between the sacral spinal cord and brainstem PMC [18]. Common causes are spinal cord injuries (cervical lesion more likely), spina bifida, and multiple sclerosis [13]. DESD in the setting of DO represents both a storage and emptying failure and should be treated aggressively to minimize the chance of upper tract deterioration. The EUS may be addressed with indwelling or intermittent catheterization, on a botulinum toxin A injections into the sphincter, or sphincterotomy. Storage may be improved with multiple measures that have been mentioned previously.

3.c. **Bladder Outlet Obstruction (BOO)**

3.c.i. BOO can be functional or anatomic and may have multiple causes. These include bladder neck dysfunction, dysfunctional voiding, urethral stricture, anterior vaginal compartment prolapse, or poor relaxation of the pelvic floor [21]. Each of these may lead to increased outflow resistance and incomplete emptying.

3.c.ii. Urodynamic assessment demonstrating elevated voiding pressures and low flow is definitive; however, a clear-cut urodynamic definition for obstruction in women does not exist. Video-urodynamics are especially helpful in these cases to demonstrate the level of obstruction and any vesicoureteral reflux.

3.c.iii. **Primary bladder neck obstruction** refers to incomplete opening of an anatomically normal bladder neck during voluntary or involuntary voiding, and the cause of this uncommon reason for BOO is not clearly understood [26].

3.c.iv. **Smooth sphincter dyssynergia** may occur in the setting of autonomic hyperreflexia and DESD, and the smooth sphincter can be competent, but not relaxing, in certain cases of sacral SCI and disk disease [18].

3.c.v. A more common reason for BOO is a **sequela of an anti-incontinence procedure** that overcorrected the weakness in support and produced a static kink in the proximal or mid-urethra. This may present with either typical voiding symptoms or frank urinary retention, or a worsening of, or de novo, urinary storage symptoms. If a temporal relationship exists between the anti-incontinence procedure and the onset of these symptoms, then the surgery is the culprit, and loosening or revision of the surgery contributes to symptom resolution.

3.c.vi. **Anterior vaginal compartment prolapse** (commonly referred to as a cystocele) represents the herniation of the bladder into the vagina through an attenuated pubocervical fascia. As the bladder prolapse is greater than the laxity around the urethra, a relative kink develops at the bladder neck. Unkinking of the bladder neck either with a pessary or surgery will typically lead to resolution of the voiding/storage symptoms. This unkinking may also uncover occult SUI in a woman who was stress continent when the prolapse was unreduced.

3.c.vii. In women with voiding LUTS stemming from **pelvic floor dysfunction**, pharmacotherapy and pelvic floor physiotherapy may help with pelvic relaxation and improve emptying.

Conclusion

Disorders of urinary storage and emptying can originate from deficiencies in the bladder, outlet, or both. In turn, multiple mechanisms (e.g., neurogenic, myogenic, idiopathic) may be responsible for these deficiencies. Detailed knowledge of pelvic anatomy and neurophysiology will be of great help to the clinician diagnosing and treating these disorders.

References

1. Abrams P. Describing bladder storage function: overactive bladder syndrome and detrusor overactivity. Urology. 2003;62(5):28–37. https://doi.org/10.1016/j.urology.2003.09.050.
2. Abrams P, Cardozo L, Fall M, Griffiths D, Rosier P, Ulmsten U, van Kerrebroeck P, Victor A, Wein A, Standardisation Sub-committee of the International Continence Society. The standardisation of terminology of lower urinary tract function: report from the Standardisation Sub-committee of the International Continence Society. Neurourol Urodyn. 2002;21(2):167–78.
3. Boone TB, Stewart JN, Martinez LM. Additional therapies for storage and emptying failure. In: Partin AW, Dmochowski RR, Kavoussi LR, Peters CA, editors. Campbell-Walsh-Wein urology. 12th ed. Philadelphia: Elsevier; 2020. p. 2889–904.
4. Brown ET, Wein AJ, Dmochowski RR. Pathophysiology and classification of lower urinary tract dysfunction: overview. In: Partin AW, Dmochowski RR, Kavoussi LR, Peters CA, editors. Campbell-Walsh-Wein urology. 12th ed. Philadelphia: Elsevier; 2020. p. 2514–24.
5. Brucker BM, Nitti VW. Urodynamic and video-urodynamic evaluation of the lower urinary tract. In: Partin AW, Dmochowski RR, Kavoussi LR, Peters CA, editors. Campbell-Walsh-Wein urology. 12th ed. Philadelphia: Elsevier; 2020. p. 2550–79.
6. Chapple CR, Helm CW, Blease S, Milroy EJG, Rickards D, Osborne JL. Asymptomatic bladder neck incompetence in nulliparous females. Br J Urol. 1989;64(4):357–9. https://doi.org/10.1111/j.1464-410x.1989.tb06042.x.
7. Chapple CR, Osman NI, Birder L, Dmochowski R, Drake MJ, van Koeveringe G, Nitti VW, Oelke M, Smith PP, Yamaguchi O, Wein A, Abrams P. Terminology report from the International Continence Society (ICS) Working Group on Underactive Bladder (UAB). Neurourol Urodyn. 2018;37(8):2928–31.
8. Chapple CR, Osman NI. The underactive detrusor. In: Partin AW, Dmochowski RR, Kavoussi LR, Peters CA, editors. Campbell-Walsh-Wein urology. 12th ed. Philadelphia: Elsevier; 2020. p. 2650–63.
9. DeLancey JO. Structural aspects of the extrinsic continence mechanism. Obstet Gynecol. 1988;72:296–301.
10. DeLancey JOL. Structural support of the urethra as it relates to stress urinary incontinence: the hammock hypothesis. Am J Obstet Gynecol. 1994;170(5):1713–23. https://doi.org/10.1016/s0002-9378(12)91840-2.
11. Drake MJ. Do we need a new definition of the overactive bladder syndrome? ICI-RS 2013. Neurourol Urodynam. 2014;33:622–4.
12. Enhorning G. Simultaneous recording of the intravesical and intraurethral pressure. Acta Obstet Gynecol Scand. 1961;276(Suppl):1–69.
13. Feloney MP, Leslie SW. Bladder sphincter dyssynergia. In: StatPearls [Internet]. Treasure Island: StatPearls Publishing; 2021.
14. Gormley EA, Lightner DJ, Burgio KL, Chai TC, Clemens JQ, Culkin DJ, Das AK, Foster HE Jr, Scarpero HM, Tessier CD, Vasavada SP. Diagnosis and treatment of overactive bladder (non-neurogenic) in adults: AUA/SUFU guideline. J Urol. 2012;188:2455–63.
15. Gosling J. The structure of the bladder and urethra in relation to function. Urol Clin N Am. 1979;6:31–8.
16. Gosling JA. The structure of the female lower urinary tract and pelvic floor. Urol Clin N Am. 1985;12:207–14.
17. Gosling JA, Dixon JS, Critchley HO, Thompson SA. A comparative study of the human external sphincter and periurethral levator ani muscle. Br J Urol. 1981;53:35–41. https://doi.org/10.1111/j.1464-410x.1981.tb03125.x.
18. Kowalik CG, Wein AJ, Dmochowski RR. Neuromuscular dysfunction of the lower urinary tract. In: Partin AW, Dmochowski RR, Kavoussi LR, Peters CA, editors. Campbell-Walsh-Wein urology. 12th ed. Philadelphia: Elsevier; 2020. p. 2600–36.
19. Lightner DJ, Gomelsky A, Souter L, Vasavada SP. Diagnosis and treatment of overactive bladder (non-neurogenic) in adults: AUA/SUFU guideline amendment 2019. J Urol. 2019;202:558–63.
20. McGuire EJ, Woodside JR. Diagnostic advantages of fluoroscopic monitoring during urodynamic evaluation. J Urol. 1981;125:830–4. https://doi.org/10.1016/s0022-5347(17)55223-4.
21. Ong HL, Lee CL, Kuo HC. Female bladder neck dysfunction-a video-urodynamic diagnosis among women with voiding dysfunction. Low Urin Tract Symptoms. 2020;12(3):278–84.
22. Petros PE, Ulmsten UI. An integral theory of female urinary incontinence. Acta Obstet Gynecol Scand. 1990;69(S153):7–31. https://doi.org/10.1111/j.1600-0412.1990.tb08027.x.
23. Raz S, Caine M, Zeigler M. The vascular component in the production of intraurethral pressure. J Urol. 1972;108:93–6.
24. Smith PP, van Leijsen SAL, Heesakkers JPFA, Abrams P, Smith ARB. Can we, and do we need to, define bladder neck hypermobility and intrinsic sphincteric deficiency?: ICI-rs 2011. Neurourol Urodynam. 2012;31(3):309–12. https://doi.org/10.1002/nau.22220.
25. Staskin DR, Zimmern PE, Hadley HR, Raz S. The pathophysiology of stress incontinence. Urol Clin N Am. 1985;12:271–8.
26. Sussman RD, Drain A, Brucker BM. Primary bladder neck obstruction. Rev Urol. 2019;21(2–3):53–62.
27. Versi E, Cardozo LD, Studd J. Distal urethral compensatory mechanisms in women with an incompetent bladder neck who remain continent, and the effect of menopause. Neurourol Urodynam. 1990;9:579.
28. Versi E, Cardozo LD, Studd JW, Brincat M, O'Dowd TM, Cooper DJ. Internal urinary sphincter in

maintenance of female continence. Br Med J (Clin Res Ed). 1986;292:166–7.

29. Wein AJ. Classification of neurogenic voiding dysfunction. J Urol. 1981;125:605–9.

30. Wein AJ, Barrett DM. Voiding function and dysfunction: a logical and practical approach. Chicago: Year Book Medical Publishers; 1988.

31. Westby M, Asmussen M, Ulmsten U. Location of maximum intraurethral pressure related to urogenital diaphragm in the female studied by simultaneous urethrocystometry and voiding urethrocystography. Am J Obstet Gynecol. 1982;144:408–12.

The Epidemiology and Socioeconomic Impact of Female GU and Pelvic Floor Disorders

5

Gabriela Gonzalez and Jennifer T. Anger

Contents

Introduction 86

Pelvic Organ Prolapse 87
Epidemiology 87
Risk Factors 87
Race/Ethnicity 88
Socioeconomic Burden 88

Urinary Incontinence 89

Stress Urinary Incontinence 89
Epidemiology 89
Risk Factors 89
Race/Ethnicity 90
Socioeconomic Impact 90

Overactive Bladder 91
Epidemiology 91
Risk Factors 92
Socioeconomic Impact 92

Mixed Urinary Incontinence 92

Conclusion 93

References 93

G. Gonzalez
Department of Urology, University of California, Davis
School of Medicine, Sacramento, CA, USA
e-mail: gabygonzalez@ucla.edu

J. T. Anger (✉)
Department of Urology, University of California, San
Diego School of Medicine, La Jolla, CA, USA
e-mail: janger@health.ucsd.edu

Abstract

At least 24% of women in the United States suffer from pelvic floor disorders (PFDs), which include urinary incontinence, pelvic organ prolapse, and other lower urinary tract symptoms. PFDs predominantly affect women as they age and can often remain undiagnosed or undertreated. Despite the high prevalence of PFDs, they are not frequently discussed due to patient embarrassment and lack of community

© Springer Nature Switzerland AG 2023
F. E. Martins et al. (eds.), *Female Genitourinary and Pelvic Floor Reconstruction*,
https://doi.org/10.1007/978-3-031-19598-3_5

awareness of these conditions. PFDs have a significant impact on quality of life, negatively affecting one's social life, participation in recreational activities, and emotional health. This chapter will focus on the epidemiology and economic costs of pelvic organ prolapse and urinary incontinence, including stress urinary incontinence, overactive bladder and urge urinary incontinence, and mixed urinary incontinence. Topics to be highlighted include the incidence, prevalence, risk factors, and associations of disease with race and ethnicity. The cost burdens associated with PFDs are complex and include both direct and indirect factors. The demand for medical services to treat these conditions will continue to grow with the aging population.

Keywords

Female urology · Pelvic organ prolapse · Pelvic floor disorders · Urinary incontinence · Stress urinary incontinence · Epidemiology · Health economics

Introduction

According to the International Urogynecological Association (IUGA)/International Continence Society (ICS), pelvic floor disorders (PFDs) include urinary incontinence (UI), pelvic organ prolapse (POP), and other lower urinary tract symptoms related to storage, emptying, and sensory conditions [1]. A US national prevalence study of women included in the 2005–2006 National Health and Nutrition Examination Survey identified that at least 24% of women will report at least one PFD [2].

Although many pelvic floor conditions may fall under the umbrella of PFDs, in this chapter we will focus on UI, stress urinary incontinence (SUI), POP, overactive bladder (OAB), and mixed urinary incontinence (MUI). Briefly, UI relates to loss of bladder control with the inability to control urination. SUI is the leakage of urine associated with cough, laugh, or sneezing. POP is any descent of the vaginal wall(s). OAB is

urinary urgency with or without urge urinary incontinence (UUI) when women have an intense urge to void with involuntary loss of urine. MUI is a combination of SUI and UUI symptoms. Often women have a combination of PFDs that must be comprehensively addressed. However, many do not seek care because of the belief that pelvic disorders are a normal aspect of aging for which no medical treatment is warranted [3].

Burton et al. demonstrated that women suffering from PFDs are unaware of such disorders, despite their high prevalence, and they often rely on prevention and treatment strategies from online sources prior to consulting with a medical professional, which may lead to misinformation [4]. All PFDs mentioned are under-discussed and poorly recognized due to embarrassment and low community awareness of pelvic floor health. In prior qualitative studies addressing lower urinary tract symptoms, women have reported being overburdened with anxiety, toilet mapping, carrying additional clothing and sanitary pads, and difficulty with recreational activities [4–8]. Our recent social media analysis of posts by women with prolapse identified feelings of shame and depression, misconceptions regarding risk factors, and interest in learning more about surgical versus nonsurgical options [6]. Likewise, our analysis of OAB online forum post analysis identified similar emotional burdens and concerns about overlap with interstitial cystitis, medication side effects, and navigating the different tiered treatment options [7].

Herein we will address the epidemiology and the associated socioeconomic costs of UI, SUI, POP, OAB/UUI, and MUI. The prevalence reported in epidemiologic studies may vary based on the type of analysis conducted, demographic factors, presence of comorbidities, the study period, assessment tool(s) used, definitions used, and incorporation of physical examination or diagnostic studies. Although we include data accumulated from various studies, some may not stratify analysis based on subtype of urinary incontinence, race, age, access to healthcare, or geographic analysis, which may significantly impact the findings.

Many of the cost burden study results we present will refer to quality-adjusted life years (QALYs), representing how long one's quality of life improves after treatment. QALYs combine length of life and quality of life into a single index measure. This measure is calculated by multiplying the change in utility value which is provided by a treatment by the expected years of treatment benefit or harm. The utility value represents perceptions of quality of life from 1.0 (perfect health) to 0.0 (death). It is calculated using the average cost difference between treatment modalities (incremental cost) and the average difference in QALYs (incremental effectiveness). The cost-effectiveness ratio is represented by the cost difference per QALY ($/QALY). The cost-effectiveness of a treatment is evaluated based on the following criteria: if it is more effective and less expensive; if it is more expensive, yet the patient assumes the cost difference for a better quality of life; or if it is less effective and less expensive, but the other treatment is more expensive with a quality-of-life improvement that does not justify the additional cost [9].

Pelvic Organ Prolapse

The reported prevalence of POP, which is defined as the descent of one or more of the anterior wall, posterior wall, or apex of the vagina, is 3–6% and up to 50%, when identified by symptom-based surveys and pelvic examination, respectively [1, 10]. Vaginal prolapse represents a complex set of conditions, and definitions vary widely.

The definition used for POP also influences the estimated prevalence. Prolapse above the hymenal ring may develop before patients experience bothersome symptoms, and identifying POP based on self-reported symptoms may be challenging due to the poor sensitivity and specificity associated with symptoms [11]. For example, the prevalence of POP based on reports of a bulging vaginal mass or identification during pelvic examination is between 4% and 12% [12, 13]. However, a bulging mass is likely stage 3 prolapse (1 cm or more beyond the hymen) or greater.

Epidemiology

In a multicenter analysis from private and public outpatient clinics that included 1004 asymptomatic women aged 18–83 years presenting for their annual gynecologic examinations, Swift et al. identified the prevalence of stages 0 (no prolapse) to 3 POP to be 24%, 38%, 35%, and 2%, respectively [14]. This means that stage 2 prolapse is not only common but is *normal*. During pelvic examinations, anterior wall prolapse is most commonly identified at twice and three times the rate of posterior and apical prolapse, respectively [15, 16]. However, apical prolapse usually co-occurs with the high-grade prolapse of other compartments.

The annual incidence of POP surgery is between 1.5 and 1.8 cases per 1000 woman-years [10]. Handa et al., in a subgroup analysis of women enrolled in the Women's Health Initiative Estrogen Plus Progestin Trial, used a standardized pelvic examination and found the incidence of new cystoceles, rectoceles, and uterine prolapse to be 9%, 6%, and 2%, respectively [17].

Risk Factors

Well-established risk factors for prolapse include obesity, age, parity, vaginal delivery, and weight of the largest baby. Often obesity is viewed as one of the most modifiable risk factors, and it has also been shown to be associated with recurrence of anterior wall prolapse after an anterior colporrhaphy (OR 2.5, 95% CI 1.2–5.3) [18]. The incidence and prevalence of prolapse have been consistently demonstrated to increase with age despite variations in POP definitions and assessment tools [12, 19, 20]. Peak surgery rates for POP occur in the seventh decade of life [19]. There is a 20%–40% increased risk of developing POP with either gravidity, parity, vaginal delivery, or increased weight of a vaginally delivered newborn [21]. Women with a history of vaginal delivery have been found to be at a higher risk for undergoing POP surgery (OR 2.9, 95% CI 0.9–10.0) [22]. Compared to women with a history of cesarean delivery, those with a forceps-assisted delivery had a higher risk of having POP surgery (OR 5.4, 95% CI 1.6–18.4) [22]. Additionally, in a nationwide prospective cohort study, a prior history of a hysterectomy or other pelvic surgeries was found to be associated with an increased risk of POP [12]. Vaginal hysterectomy conferred the highest risk for requiring subsequent prolapse surgery compared to controls (HR 3.8, CI 95% 3.1–4.8) [12].

Race/Ethnicity

Unlike other well-established risk factors, race and ethnicity studies have varied results. As previously mentioned, prevalence based on validated questionnaires may lead to different results, especially when considering ethnicity. Dunivan et al. found that Hispanic and Native American women were significantly more bothered by POP stage 2 when compared to non-Hispanic white women, who tended to experience bother at stage 3 [8]. A cross-sectional analysis of women who enrolled in the Women's Health Initiative Hormone Replacement Therapy clinical trial found that, based on pelvic examination, African American women had the lowest risk of prolapse, while Hispanic women had the highest risk after controlling for comorbidities [17, 23]. Adjusted odds ratio for uterine prolapse among Hispanic women was 1.2 (95% CI 1.0–1.5) compared to non-Hispanic white women [23].

Socioeconomic Burden

The rising incidence and prevalence of prolapse with age will continue to increase societal and personal costs due to surgical procedures and negative quality of life associated with decreased productivity. Several qualitative studies have identified well-established personal burdens associated with POP, such as shame, fear, sexual dysfunction, poor access to specialists, and distress about surgical versus nonsurgical management treatment options [4, 6, 8].

In a classic paper from 1997, Olsen et al. identified that about 11% of women in the United States undergo surgery for urinary incontinence or pelvic organ prolapse, while 30% of those women will need a reoperation for recurrence or worsening of their incontinence or prolapse symptoms [19]. These high rates of surgical treatment place a large burden on the healthcare system. Annually, in the United States, the estimated associated cost of POP is 1 billion dollars [10].

Women with POP are at an increased risk of having concomitant or de novo SUI after a surgical prolapse repair without an anti-incontinence procedure, thus affecting both economic and personal costs [24]. Using the 1997 National Hospital Discharge Survey by national average Medicare reimbursement for physician service and hospitalizations, Subak and colleagues calculated the direct cost of POP operations, including anti-incontinence procedures, to be $218 million [25]. In 1997, Subak et al. also calculated the direct costs of prolapse to be $1012 million, including $494 million for vaginal hysterectomy, $279 million for cystocele and rectocele repair, and $135 million for abdominal hysterectomy [25].

Richardson et al. conducted a decision analysis model comparing cost-effectiveness over a 1 year postoperative period to determine the cost associated with placement of a mid-urethral sling to prevent occult SUI when undergoing an abdominal sacrocolpopexy (ASC) for POP [26]. The cost-effectiveness model compared ASC with a deferred option for a mid-urethral sling, ASC with a concomitant mid-urethral sling, and ASC with preoperative urodynamics for selective mid-urethral sling placement. Concomitant mid-urethral sling placement was the most cost-effective ($2867/QALY), while preoperative urodynamics was more expensive [26]. A randomized control trial comparing costs associated with laparoscopic and robotic sacrocolpopexy by Anger and colleagues found that the robotic group had higher initial hospital costs ($19,616 compared with $11,573, $P < 0.001$) [27].

Although surgical management of POP is a durable option, not all patients are surgical candidates or wish to undergo surgery. Vaginal pessaries are nonsurgical treatment options for women who may want an alternative to invasive procedures. Pessaries are flexible rubber intravaginal devices available in different sizes designed to provide pelvic organ support. There is a required initial device fitting with a provider, and they need to be removed and cleaned regularly. Patients or physicians can exchange pessaries on an established routine basis. However, some women do not have exchanges, and others rely on quarterly visits with a provider. Alperin and colleagues used a national dataset to study patterns of pessary use in a cohort of 34,782 women, which also include patients with asymptomatic POP, and determined that only 11.6% of women were treated with a pessary despite its category as a first-line treatment [28]. A cost-utility analysis using a Canadian public payer model estimated a 5 year budget impact of $0.5 million for publicly funded POP pessaries [29].

Urinary Incontinence

Urinary incontinence, defined as involuntary leakage of urine with different subcategories, is a major health problem for women [1]. The prevalence of incontinence increases with age. Approximately 25% of premenopausal women and 40% of postmenopausal women report urinary incontinence [30]. Forde et al. examined the 2009–2010 National Ambulatory Medical Survey and the National Hospital Ambulatory Medical Care Survey databases. They estimated that 6.8 million women were seen for a chief complaint of UI, and yet only 15.3% of those women were treated in the primary care setting [31]. An observational cohort study from 2003 to 2012 of 969 women in a Northern California integrated healthcare system found that patients with a lower level of education and socioeconomic status discuss incontinence symptoms with healthcare providers at lower rates [32]. Despite the low recognition rates of UI, the US estimated direct cost (treatment, diagnosis, and routine care) continues to increase. The estimated cost in 1987 was $10.3 billion, in 1995 it was $16 billion, and in 2000 it was $19.5 billion [33, 34]. Overall, the direct costs

are estimated to be higher for community-dwelling women than institutionalized women [35]. Many prevalence-based cost estimates only stratify the treatment costs according to UI subtype [35]. To better understand the epidemiology of UI, it is important to distinguish between SUI, UUI/OAB, and MUI.

Stress Urinary Incontinence

SUI, defined as the leakage of urine with physical exertion, cough, laugh, or sneeze in the absence of a detrusor contraction by the International Continence Society, is a significant social and economic health problem among women [1]. The etiology of SUI is associated with pelvic floor muscle weakening and thus a loss of urethral support.

Epidemiology

SUI prevalence varies due to the wide range of disease definitions, study designs, utilization of different patient-reported outcome measures (validated surveys, number and size of pads, and pad weights), and diagnostic criteria beyond a physical exam such as urodynamics. The peak incidence of SUI occurs between 45 and 49 years of age; however, 18% of young women between the ages of 25 and 39 are also affected [36, 37]. In the United States, SUI affects between 25% and 50% of women [9]. Hunskaar et al. examined the prevalence of SUI in four European countries conducting a cross-sectional study of 17,080 community-dwelling women and found similar estimates of 41%–44% in France, the United Kingdom, and Germany [26]. A lower prevalence of 23% was found in Spain [38].

Risk Factors

SUI and POP have common established risk factors including age, history of vaginal childbirth, pregnancy, obesity, and race [30, 39–41]. Data demonstrates that obese women (BMI $\geq$ 30) have twice the risk of developing SUI even when controlling for age and parity [30]. Pregnancy, gestational age, and vaginal childbirth are also associated risk factors. SUI prevalence in pregnancy is 40%, although incontinence may resolve after delivery [42]. The odds ratio for experiencing weekly UI was higher (OR 1.47, CI 95% 1.16–1.86) for women with a history of vaginal birth of a large baby (4 kg or more) when compared to women with smaller newborns [43]. A cross-sectional analysis of pre- and postmenopausal women identified that SUI increased with the number of pregnancies and vaginal deliveries; however, an increase in cesarean deliveries did not appear to affect SUI rates. After the first vaginal delivery, the rate of SUI was 7.7%; after the second, it was 25%; after three, it was 31.3%; and after four, it was 15.8% ($P = 0$) [44].

Race/Ethnicity

Differences in the prevalence of SUI based on racial and ethnic variation have been reported. After adjusting for comorbidities, a US population-based, cross-sectional study of middle-aged women found that Hispanics and African American women were 60% less likely to have incontinence compared to non-Hispanic white women [45]. However, the subtype of UI was not identified. The Reproductive Risks for Incontinence Study at Kaiser (RRISK) study was one of the few population-based cohort studies with a diverse study population that did analyze the prevalence of various UI subtypes by race and ethnicity and found contradictory information [46]. In the RRISK study, Thom and colleagues identified that Hispanic women were twice as likely to have daily incontinence and experienced the highest prevalence of weekly incontinence (36%). MUI was also found at a higher rate in Hispanic women, with predominantly stress versus urge symptoms [47]. Additionally, this study revealed that Asian-American women had lower levels of stress and urge urinary incontinence in comparison with Hispanic and non-Hispanic white women [46]. The authors explain the different results from prior studies due to enrollment of varying age groups, a diverse study population

with more representation of Mexican women, and distinct incontinence definitions for subtype classification. Interestingly, in the RRISK study, incontinence was more prevalent in non-Hispanic white women compared to African American women, which is consistent with other population-based studies [48–50]. Our recent work analyzing mid-urethral sling outcomes in an urban Latina population also identified a uniquely high rate of MUI at 72% [51].

Socioeconomic Impact

The actual economic impact of SUI may be challenging to compute given the extensive financial, social, and quality-of-life burdens that contribute to the costs. Additionally, the economic burden of SUI depends on surgical versus nonsurgical treatment options and diagnostic evaluation. Despite the high prevalence of SUI, a US cross-sectional analysis identified that only 47% of women with moderately to extremely bothersome symptoms of SUI consulted a physician for their symptoms, which could lead to underestimating healthcare utilization costs [52].

Studies divide the cost of SUI management into direct (treatment, diagnosis, and routine care) and indirect costs (changes in productivity and lost work days). However, there are more data regarding direct costs than indirect factors, which are harder to quantify [9]. The estimated cost for incontinence in women is over $12 billion, and SUI accounts for 82% of the total cost, with more than 70% considered out-of-pocket expenses [33, 53]. Out-of-pocket costs are largely attributed to pads, diapers, and laundry [33].

Behavioral and lifestyle changes such as weight loss, smoking cessation, a decrease of bladder diet irritants, and improvement of medical comorbidities such as diabetes are some nonsurgical treatment options. Imamura et al. conducted a systematic review and cost analysis in 2010 of nonsurgical management strategies using UK National Health Service (NHS) data [41]. Although it is challenging to calculate lifestyle changes, the authors report a wide range of cost (which we converted to US dollar [USD] using the 2010 US dollar to British pound exchange rate), from $0 for outdoor exercising to $50 for a monthly gym membership, and even thousands of dollars for optimization of comorbid diseases [9, 41]. Beyond lifestyle modifications, other nonsurgical options include sanitary pads, vaginal incontinence pessaries, and pelvic floor muscle therapy (PFMT). About half of the women fitted with a pessary will continue using it for 1–2 years [30]. PFMT is also commonly known as Kegel pelvic muscle exercises which help strengthen urethral sphincter tone.

In the 2010 UK NHS cost analysis, three months of basic PFMT without any biofeedback costs $291(converted from British pounds); however, the duration of the therapy will depend on the patient [41]. Women can also perform self-guided Kegel exercises which is essentially free. It is important to note that the UK cost analysis was from publicly funded healthcare data, and it may now underestimate the actual cost. Incontinence pessary costs range from $40 to $60, but this does not account for the physician fee and routine exchange [9]. A Canadian cost-utility analysis from a public payer perspective estimated a 5 year budget impact of $0.3 million for publicly funded incontinence pessaries [29]. According to the Stress Incontinence Surgical Treatment Efficacy (SISTEr) Trial, the estimated individual cost for women managing SUI was $15 ± $25 per week ($751 ± $1277 annually) and $27 ± $37 weekly for patients with 4.5 daily incontinence episodes [54].

Surgical treatments for SUI can include urethral bulking agents, slings (transvaginal and trans-obturator, mesh and non-mesh), and the Burch colposuspension. Surgical interventions have evolved, as many of the surgeries are now conducted in the outpatient setting. A 1997 retrospective study comparing periurethral bulking agents to fascia lata sling surgery in women with intrinsic sphincter deficiency found that slings were twice costly at $10,382, with the cost of bulking agents at $4996 [55]. Yet, during follow-up at 15 months, 71% of women in the sling group were symptom-free compared to only 26% in the bulking agent group [55]. In more recent 2015 data, Kunkle et al. conducted a decision tree cost analysis over a 1 year horizon of bulking agents versus mid-urethral sling in patients with SUI and no urethral hypermobility. The authors found bulking agents to be the most cost-effective. Yet when a sling procedure costs less than $5132, it becomes a cost-effective treatment [56].

A Swedish cost-analysis study compared the cost of transvaginal slings (TVT), open colposuspension, and laparoscopic colposuspension with respective costs being $1529, $2722, and $2587 [57]. The cost of inpatient TVT procedures with a two-day length of stay ranged from $1140 to $1274 [57]. Outpatient TVT procedures had an estimated cost between $702 and $1274 [57]. Lier et al. conducted a Canadian-based, cost-effectiveness analysis between TVT and trans-obturator (TOT) slings over 12 months [58]. They found a non-statistically significant savings of $1133 in the TOT group without any associated improvement in quality-adjusted life years [58]. The savings were due to more postoperative admissions in the TVT group.

Overactive Bladder

Overactive bladder (OAB) is a symptom syndrome defined as urinary urgency, frequency, and nocturia with or without urgency urinary incontinence, in the absence of urinary infection or other pathology [1]. There are two subtypes of OAB, OAB-wet, which is frequency and urgency associated with urge incontinence, and OAB-dry, which is frequency and urgency without urge incontinence.

Epidemiology

According to the National Overactive Bladder Evaluation (NOBLE) study of 5000 community-dwelling participants in the United States, the prevalence in women is 16.9%, which is surprisingly similar in men [59]. However, OAB-wet tends to be more prevalent in women (9.3% versus 2.6% in men). Men had a higher prevalence of OAB-dry (13.4% versus 7.6% in women). Aging is associated with an increased prevalence, as well as a progression from OAB-dry to OAB-wet/urge urinary incontinence. However, OAB can also be stable overtime with remissions, especially in mild cases and in younger women with predominantly OAB-dry [60, 61].

Race and ethnicity have also been established as predictors of OAB for African American women compared to non-Hispanic white women. Data regarding Latina women is not as well established. African American women have a higher prevalence (39%) and degree of bother compared to non-Hispanic white women (29.4%) and Hispanic women (29%) [62]. Interestingly, a cross-sectional Internet-based study involving a regression analysis controlling for OAB medical comorbidities found that African American women were 3.4 times and Hispanic women were 4.7 times more likely than non-Hispanic white women to develop OAB [63].

Risk Factors

Similar to the other PFDs discussed thus far, age and obesity are also risk factors. OAB also has a higher association with female gender [63]. Though the relationship of obesity and OAB remains unclear, in a meta-analysis investigating the risk factors of OAB, Zhu et al. found that age and BMI were higher in OAB patients compared to controls (standardized mean differences [95% CIs], 0.30 [0.19–0.41] and 0.39 [0.24–0.53]) [64]. There were no significant associations between parity, vaginal delivery, and OAB [64]. Dietary habits and fluid intake can also exacerbate symptoms for some women. Avoiding bladder irritants such as caffeine may reduce symptoms of frequency and urgency [60]. Reducing intake of fluids by at least 25% has demonstrated to improve OAB symptoms [60]. A cross-sectional analysis of ambulatory adults older than 65 found high rates of urinary frequency (81%) in patients taking diuretics [65].

Socioeconomic Impact

In the United States, the total cost of OAB is estimated to be $69.5 billion, of which $51 billion is direct medical expenses that also account for the cost of pads, diapers, gloves, and laundry. Indirect medical expenses related to lost productivity, such as income disparities, account for $14 billion of the total cost [66, 67]. The loss in productivity and quality of life is attributed to the adverse effect on work, sleep, sexual function, and physical and recreational activities [7]. Tiered treatment options include behavioral modifications and incontinence pads; then, it progresses to include pharmacotherapy with anticholinergics or beta-adrenergics and onabotulinumtoxin A injections and implantable sacral nerve stimulation (SNS) devices and percutaneous tibial nerve stimulation (PTNS) for symptoms refractory to medications. A 10 year cost analysis of the different treatment modalities identified that SNS was the costliest therapy at $27,823, PTNS cost was $14,103, and 100 units of onabotulinumtoxin A was $15,059 [68]. Overall, Murray et al. concluded that 100 units of onabotulinumtoxin A was the most cost-effective treatment option with the largest gain in QALYs (7.179) and the lowest incremental cost-effectiveness ratio ($32,680/QALY).

Mixed Urinary Incontinence

A minority of women may experience pure SUI, while a larger proportion will have mixed urinary incontinence (MUI), associated with involuntary urine leakage due to urinary urgency. 40% of women with UI have MUI. Distinguishing if a patient has SUI versus MUI and which symptoms are the most bothersome is important to guide management.

Conservative management usually includes Kegel exercises and fluid restriction, combined with medication when needed. The second-line therapies typically address the more bothersome component (stress versus urge). Unlike in patients with pure SUI, women with MUI are more likely to undergo urodynamics testing prior to sling surgery for the stress component, contributing significantly to the diagnostic cost. MUI accounts for approximately 12% of the total reported UI cost [35]. Homer et al. conducted a randomized control pilot trial with cost-analysis across 7 centers in the United Kingdom of 218 women with a diagnosis of SUI or MUI (stress>urge) to receive urodynamics or no urodynamics before undergoing further treatment. At 6 months, the mean cost difference was equivalent to $186 per women without any gain in QALY [69]. The cost difference was due to 74% of women in the urodynamics group undergoing surgery versus 94% of women in the no urodynamics group.

Conclusion

Pelvic floor conditions including UI, SUI, POP, OAB, and MUI detrimentally affect the health and quality of life of many women. The prevalence, incidence, costs, and growth in demand to treat these conditions will continue to increase over time. In prior studies, women have reported shame, fear, anxiety, and avoidance of sexual intercourse and exercise activities [5, 70, 71]. Despite these quality-of-life burdens, few women seek care. In addition, many primary care providers report feeling unprepared to address UI, with recent retrospective data demonstrating low adherence rates to established indicators for women with urinary incontinence [36, 72]. Overall, there is a need to raise awareness regarding pelvic floor health, risk factors, preventive strategies, and treatment options for both patients and physicians.

References

1. Haylen BT, de Ridder D, Freeman RM, Swift SE, Berghmans B, Lee J, et al. An International Urogynecological Association (IUGA)/International Continence Society (ICS) joint report on the terminology for female pelvic floor dysfunction. Int Urogynecol J. 2010;21(1):5–26.
2. Nygaard I, Barber MD, Burgio KL, Kenton K, Meikle S, Schaffer J, et al. Prevalence of symptomatic pelvic floor disorders in US women. JAMA. 2008;300 (11):1311–6.
3. Mitteness LS. Knowledge and beliefs about urinary incontinence in adulthood and old age. J Am Geriatr Soc. 1990;38(3):374–8.
4. Burton CS, Gonzalez G, Vaculik K, Khalil C, Zektser Y, Arnold C, et al. Female lower urinary tract symptom prevention and treatment strategies on social media: mixed correlation with evidence. Urology. 2021;150:139–45.
5. Gonzalez G, Vaculik K, Khalil C, Zektser Y, Arnold C, Almario CV, et al. Women's experience with stress

urinary incontinence: insights from social media analytics. J Urol. 2020;203(5):962–8.
6. Gonzalez G, Vaculik K, Khalil C, Zektser Y, Arnold C, Almario CV, et al. Using digital ethnography to understand the experience of women with pelvic organ prolapse. Female Pelvic Med Reconstr Surg. 2021;27(2): e363–e7.
7. Gonzalez G, Vaculik K, Khalil C, Zektser Y, Arnold CW, Almario CV, et al. Social media analytics of overactive bladder posts: what do patients know and want to know? Int Urogynecol J. 2021;32(10):2729–36.
8. Dunivan GC, Anger JT, Alas A, Wieslander C, Sevilla C, Chu S, et al. Pelvic organ prolapse: a disease of silence and shame. Female Pelvic Med Reconstr Surg. 2014;20(6):322–7.
9. Chong EC, Khan AA, Anger JT. The financial burden of stress urinary incontinence among women in the United States. Curr Urol Rep. 2011;12(5):358–62.
10. Barber MD, Maher C. Epidemiology and outcome assessment of pelvic organ prolapse. Int Urogynecol J. 2013;24(11):1783–90.
11. Ellerkmann RM, Cundiff GW, Melick CF, Nihira MA, Leffler K, Bent AE. Correlation of symptoms with location and severity of pelvic organ prolapse. Am J Obstet Gynecol. 2001;185(6):1332–7; discussion 7–8.
12. Hunskaar S, Burgio K, Clark A, Lapitan M, Nelson R, Sillen U, et al. Epidemiology of urinary (UI) and faecal (FI) incontinence and pelvic organ prolapse (POP). Incontinence. 2005;1:255–312.
13. Slieker-ten Hove MC, Pool-Goudzwaard AL, Eijkemans MJ, Steegers-Theunissen RP, Burger CW, Vierhout ME. Symptomatic pelvic organ prolapse and possible risk factors in a general population. Am J Obstet Gynecol. 2009;200(2):184.e1–7.
14. Swift S, Woodman P, O'Boyle A, Kahn M, Valley M, Bland D, et al. Pelvic Organ Support Study (POSST): the distribution, clinical definition, and epidemiologic condition of pelvic organ support defects. Am J Obstet Gynecol. 2005;192(3):795–806.
15. Neuman M, Lavy Y. Conservation of the prolapsed uterus is a valid option: medium term results of a prospective comparative study with the posterior intravaginal slingoplasty operation. Int Urogynecol J Pelvic Floor Dysfunct. 2007;18(8):889–93.
16. Inoue H, Sekiguchi Y, Kohata Y, Satono Y, Hishikawa K, Tominaga T, et al. Tissue Fixation System (TFS) to repair uterovaginal prolapse with uterine preservation: a preliminary report on perioperative complications and safety. J Obstet Gynaecol Res. 2009;35(2):346–53.
17. Handa VL, Garrett E, Hendrix S, Gold E, Robbins J. Progression and remission of pelvic organ prolapse: a longitudinal study of menopausal women. Am J Obstet Gynecol. 2004;190(1):27–32.
18. Kawasaki A, Corey EG, Laskey RA, Weidner AC, Siddiqui NY, Wu JM. Obesity as a risk for the recurrence of anterior vaginal wall prolapse after anterior colporrhaphy. J Reprod Med. 2013;58(5–6):195–9.
19. Olsen AL, Smith VJ, Bergstrom JO, Colling JC, Clark AL. Epidemiology of surgically managed pelvic organ

20. Swift SE. The distribution of pelvic organ support in a population of female subjects seen for routine gynecologic health care. Am J Obstet Gynecol. 2000;183(2):277–85.

21. MacLennan AH, Taylor AW, Wilson DH, Wilson D. The prevalence of pelvic floor disorders and their relationship to gender, age, parity and mode of delivery. BJOG. 2000;107(12):1460–70.

22. Moalli PA, Jones Ivy S, Meyn LA, Zyczynski HM. Risk factors associated with pelvic floor disorders in women undergoing surgical repair. Obstet Gynecol. 2003;101(5.1):869–74.

23. Hendrix SL, Clark A, Nygaard I, Aragaki A, Barnabei V, McTiernan A. Pelvic organ prolapse in the Women's Health Initiative: gravity and gravidity. Am J Obstet Gynecol. 2002;186(6):1160–6.

24. Bai SW, Jeon MJ, Kim JY, Chung KA, Kim SK, Park KH. Relationship between stress urinary incontinence and pelvic organ prolapse. Int Urogynecol J Pelvic Floor Dysfunct. 2002;13(4):256–60. discussion 60

25. Subak LL, Waetjen LE, van den Eeden S, Thom DH, Vittinghoff E, Brown JS. Cost of pelvic organ prolapse surgery in the United States. Obstet Gynecol. 2001;98 (4):646–51.

26. Richardson ML, Elliott CS, Shaw JG, Comiter CV, Chen B, Sokol ER. To sling or not to sling at time of abdominal sacrocolpopexy: a cost-effectiveness analysis. J Urol. 2013;190(4):1306–12.

27. Anger JT, Mueller ER, Tarnay C, Smith B, Stroupe K, Rosenman A, et al. Robotic compared with laparoscopic sacrocolpopexy: a randomized controlled trial. Obstet Gynecol. 2014;123(1):5–12.

28. Alperin M, Khan A, Dubina E, Tarnay C, Wu N, Pashos CL, et al. Patterns of pessary care and outcomes for medicare beneficiaries with pelvic organ prolapse. Female Pelvic Med Reconstr Surg. 2013;19(3):142–7.

29. McMartin K, et al. Vaginal pessaries for pelvic organ prolapse or stress urinary incontinence: a health technology assessment. Ont Health Technol Assess Ser. 2021;21(3):1–155.

30. Rogers RG. Urinary stress incontinence in women. N Engl J Med. 2008;358(10):1029–36.

31. Forde JC, Chughtai B, Cea M, Stone BV, Te A, Bishop TF. Trends in ambulatory management of urinary incontinence in women in the United States. Female Pelvic Med Reconstr Surg. 2017;23(4):250–5.

32. Duralde ER, Walter LC, Van Den Eeden SK, Nakagawa S, Subak LL, Brown JS, et al. Bridging the gap: determinants of undiagnosed or untreated urinary incontinence in women. Am J Obstet Gynecol. 2016;214(2):266. e1–e9

33. Wilson L, Brown JS, Shin GP, Luc KO, Subak LL. Annual direct cost of urinary incontinence. Obstet Gynecol. 2001;98(3):398–406.

34. Hu TW, Wagner TH, Bentkover JD, Leblanc K, Zhou SZ, Hunt T. Costs of urinary incontinence and overactive bladder in the United States: a comparative study. Urology. 2004;63(3):461–5.

35. Coyne KS, Wein A, Nicholson S, Kvasz M, Chen CI, Milsom I. Economic burden of urgency urinary incontinence in the United States: a systematic review. J Manag Care Pharm. 2014;20(2):130–40.

36. Hannestad YS, Rortveit G, Sandvik H, Hunskaar S. A community-based epidemiological survey of female urinary incontinence: the Norwegian EPINCONT study. Epidemiology of Incontinence in the County of Nord-Trøndelag. J Clin Epidemiol. 2000;53(11):1150–7.

37. Peyrat L, Haillot O, Bruyere F, Boutin JM, Bertrand P, Lanson Y. Prevalence and risk factors of urinary incontinence in young and middle-aged women. BJU Int. 2002;89(1):61–6.

38. Hunskaar S, Lose G, Sykes D, Voss S. The prevalence of urinary incontinence in women in four European countries. BJU Int. 2004;93(3):324–30.

39. Minassian VA, Stewart WF, Wood GC. Urinary incontinence in women: variation in prevalence estimates and risk factors. Obstet Gynecol. 2008;111(2.1):324–31.

40. Nygaard IE, Heit M. Stress urinary incontinence. Obstet Gynecol. 2004;104(3):607–20.

41. Imamura M, Abrams P, Bain C, Buckley B, Cardozo L, Cody J, et al. Systematic review and economic modelling of the effectiveness and cost-effectiveness of non-surgical treatments for women with stress urinary incontinence. Health Technol Assess. 2010;14(40):1–188. iii–iv

42. Dolan LM, Walsh D, Hamilton S, Marshall K, Thompson K, Ashe RG. A study of quality of life in primigravidae with urinary incontinence. Int Urogynecol J Pelvic Floor Dysfunct. 2004;15(3):160–4.

43. Thom DH, Brown JS, Schembri M, Ragins AI, Creasman JM, van den Eeden SK. Parturition events and risk of urinary incontinence in later life. Neurourol Urodyn. 2011;30(8):1456–61.

44. Findik RB, Unluer AN, Sahin E, Bozkurt OF, Karakaya J, Unsal A. Urinary incontinence in women and its relation with pregnancy, mode of delivery, connective tissue disease and other factors. Adv Clin Exp Med. 2012;21(2):207–13.

45. Nygaard I, Turvey C, Burns TL, Crischilles E, Wallace R. Urinary incontinence and depression in middle-aged United States women. Obstet Gynecol. 2003;101(1):149–56.

46. Thom DH, Brown JS, Schembri M, Ragins AI, Subak LL, van den Eeden SK. Incidence of and risk factors for change in urinary incontinence status in a prospective cohort of middle-aged and older women: the reproductive risk of incontinence study in Kaiser. J Urol. 2010;184(4):1394–401.

47. Leroy LS, Lopes MHBM, Shimo AKK. Urinary incontinence in women and racial aspects: a literature review. Texto e Contexto Enferm. 2012;21:692–701.

48. Fultz NH, Herzog AR, Raghunathan TE, Wallace RB, Diokno AC. Prevalence and severity of urinary incontinence in older African American and Caucasian women. J Gerontol A Biol Sci Med Sci. 1999;54(6): M299–303.

49. Grodstein F, Fretts R, Lifford K, Resnick N, Curhan G. Association of age, race, and obstetric history with urinary symptoms among women in the Nurses' Health Study. Am J Obstet Gynecol. 2003;189(2):428–34.

50. Burgio KL, Matthews KA, Engel BT. Prevalence, incidence and correlates of urinary incontinence in healthy, middle-aged women. J Urol. 1991;146(5):1255–9.

51. Gonzalez G, Arora A, Choi E, Bresee C, Perley J, Anger JT. Outcomes of the Supris sling in an urban Latina population. Urology. 2021;163:3.

52. Fultz NH, Burgio K, Diokno AC, Kinchen KS, Obenchain R, Bump RC. Burden of stress urinary incontinence for community-dwelling women. Am J Obstet Gynecol. 2003;189(5):1275–82.

53. Cortes E, Kelleher C. Costs of female urinary incontinence. Women Health Med. 2005;2:3–5.

54. Subak LL, Brubaker L, Chai TC, Creasman JM, Diokno AC, Goode PS, et al. High costs of urinary incontinence among women electing surgery to treat stress incontinence. Obstet Gynecol. 2008;111(4):899–907.

55. Berman CJ, Kreder KJ. Comparative cost analysis of collagen injection and fascia lata sling cystourethropexy for the treatment of type III incontinence in women [see comments]. J Urol. 1997;157(1):122–4.

56. Kunkle CM, Hallock JL, Hu X, Blomquist J, Thung SF, Werner EF. Cost utility analysis of urethral bulking agents versus midurethral sling in stress urinary incontinence. Female Pelvic Med Reconstr Surg. 2015;21 (3):154–9.

57. Ankardal M, Järbrink K, Milsom I, Heiwall B, Lausten-Thomsen N, Ellström-Engh M. Comparison of health care costs for open Burch colposuspension, laparoscopic colposuspension and tension-free vaginal tape in the treatment of female urinary incontinence. Neurourol Urodyn. 2007;26(6):761–6.

58. Lier D, Ross S, Tang S, Robert M, Jacobs P. Transobturator tape compared with tension-free vaginal tape in the surgical treatment of stress urinary incontinence: a cost utility analysis. BJOG. 2011;118(5):550–6.

59. Stewart W, van Rooyen J, Cundiff G, Abrams P, Herzog A, Corey R, et al. Prevalence and burden of overactive bladder in the United States. World J Urol. 2003;20(6):327–36.

60. Irwin DE, Milsom I, Chancellor MB, Kopp Z, Guan Z. Dynamic progression of overactive bladder and urinary incontinence symptoms: a systematic review. Eur Urol. 2010;58(4):532–43.

61. Heidler S, Mert C, Temml C, Madersbacher S. The natural history of the overactive bladder syndrome in females: a long-term analysis of a health screening project. Neurourol Urodyn. 2011;30(8):1437–41.

62. Coyne KS, Margolis MK, Kopp ZS, Kaplan SA. Racial differences in the prevalence of overactive bladder in the United States from the epidemiology of LUTS (EpiLUTS) study. Urology. 2012;79(1):95–101.

63. Coyne KS, Sexton CC, Bell JA, Thompson CL, Dmochowski R, Bavendam T, et al. The prevalence of Lower Urinary Tract Symptoms (LUTS) and Overactive Bladder (OAB) by racial/ethnic group and age: results from OAB-POLL. Neurourol Urodyn. 2013;32 (3):230–7.

64. Zhu J, Hu X, Dong X, Li L. Associations between risk factors and overactive bladder: a meta-analysis. Female Pelvic Med Reconstr Surg. 2019;25(3):238–46.

65. Ekundayo OJ, Markland A, Lefante C, Sui X, Goode PS, Allman RM, et al. Association of diuretic use and overactive bladder syndrome in older adults: a propensity score analysis. Arch Gerontol Geriatr. 2009;49(1):64–8.

66. Ganz ML, Smalarz AM, Krupski TL, Anger JT, Hu JC, Wittrup-Jensen KU, et al. Economic costs of overactive bladder in the United States. Urology. 2010;75(3):526–32, 32. e1–18.

67. Coyne KS, Sexton CC, Thompson CL, Clemens JQ, Chen CI, Bavendam T, et al. Impact of overactive bladder on work productivity. Urology. 2012;80(1): 97–103.

68. Murray B, Hessami SH, Gultyaev D, Lister J, Dmochowski R, Gillard KK, et al. Cost-effectiveness of overactive bladder treatments: from the US payer perspective. J Comp Eff Res. 2019;8(1):61–71.

69. Homer T, Shen J, Vale L, McColl E, Tincello DG, Hilton P. Invasive urodynamic testing prior to surgical treatment for stress urinary incontinence in women: cost-effectiveness and value of information analyses in the context of a mixed methods feasibility study. Pilot Feasibility Stud. 2018;4:67.

70. Asoglu MR, Selcuk S, Cam C, Cogendez E, Karateke A. Effects of urinary incontinence subtypes on women's quality of life (including sexual life) and psychosocial state. Eur J Obstet Gynecol Reprod Biol. 2014;176:187–90.

71. Wagg AR, Kendall S, Bunn F. Women's experiences, beliefs and knowledge of urinary symptoms in the postpartum period and the perceptions of health professionals: a grounded theory study. Prim Health Care Res Dev. 2017;18(5):448–62.

72. Burton CS, Gonzalez G, Choi E, Bresee C, Nuckols TK, Eilber KS, et al. The impact of provider gender and experience on the quality of care provided for women with urinary incontinence. Am J Med. 2021;135:524.

Measurement of Urinary Symptoms, Health-Related Quality of Life, and Outcomes of Treatment of Genitourinary and Pelvic Floor Disorders

6

Ly Hoang Roberts, Annah Vollstedt, Priya Padmanabhan, and Larry T. Sirls

Contents

Introduction	98
Patient-Reported Outcome (PRO) Data Via Validated Questionnaire	100
How Do we Develop a Questionnaire?	104
Theorization and Item Development	104
Scale Development	104
Scale Evaluation with Psychometric Analysis	104
Ideal Properties of a Validated Questionnaire	104
Validation Via Psychometric Analysis	105
Linguistic and Cultural Validation	108
Grading System	108
Factors to Consider for Research [6]	108
Conclusion	109
Cross-References	109
References	109

Supplementary Information: The online version contains supplementary material available at https://doi.org/10.1007/978-3-031-19598-3_6.

L. Hoang Roberts (✉)
William Beaumont School of Medicine, Beaumont Hospital, Oakland University, Royal Oak, MI, USA
e-mail: hoangrl@ccf.org

A. Vollstedt
Department of Urology, University of Iowa Hospitals and Clinics, Iowa City, IA, USA

P. Padmanabhan · L. T. Sirls
Oakland University William Beaumont School of Medicine, Beaumont Hospital, Royal Oak, MI, USA

Abstract

To conduct high-quality clinical research in the field of pelvic reconstructive surgery, it is vital to capture not only objective but also subjective data, such as the degree of bother from symptoms, the impact on quality of life, and the effectiveness of treatment. This chapter focuses on understanding the value and efficacy of subjective outcome measurement tools in diagnosis, treatment, and follow-up of urinary, gynecological, sexual, and bowel dysfunction. In a comprehensive and easy-to-read manner, we define the different types of

© Springer Nature Switzerland AG 2023
F. E. Martins et al. (eds.), *Female Genitourinary and Pelvic Floor Reconstruction*,
https://doi.org/10.1007/978-3-031-19598-3_6

validated questionnaires relevant to this field, describe the process of questionnaire development, explain psychometric concepts, suggest research considerations, and provide a supplemental tool – a concise compilation of published surveys and their psychometric traits – to assist the researcher in identifying the most appropriate questionnaire for their needs.

Keywords

Questionnaires · Urinary incontinence · Quality of life · Validity · Reliability

Introduction

The field of pelvic reconstructive surgery treats conditions that affect bladder and bowel function, sexual function, pelvic pain, and quality of life. Proper clinical evaluation should include a combination of both objective (physical examination, urodynamics, voiding diary, pad weight tests, etc.) and subjective data (patient questionnaires). Since 1998, there has been an exponential growth in the number of questionnaires developed for pelvic disorders; yet, there is no standardized questionnaire or set of questionnaires used uniformly in clinical trials, making data interpretation for systematic reviews and meta-analysis difficult. For example, one study on stress urinary incontinence (SUI) treatment outcomes looked at 42 randomized controlled trials (RCTs) published from January 2015 to July 2017 and found that 24 different questionnaires were used [1]. Organizations such as the International Consultation on Incontinence (ICI), the National Institute for Health and Clinical Excellence (NICE), and the Scottish Intercollegiate Guidelines Network (SIGN) have routinely evaluated the published literature to grade and recommend select questionnaires based on their psychometric properties [2, 3]. Overall, there is a general consensus that a standardized outcome measure to assess the degree of bother from symptoms, impact on quality of life, and effectiveness of treatment is vital in this field.

Further complicating the issue is the disparity of objective and subjective measurements. For instance, based on the Trial of Mid-Urethral Slings (TOMUS) study, Nager et al. reported no correlation between urodynamic findings (i.e., Valsalva Leak Point Pressure (VLPP), Maximum Urethral Closure Pressure (MUCP), and Functional Urethral Length (FUL)) to any subjective ($r = -0.13$ to 0.04) measurement of severity. However, other objective measurements of severity such as pad weight and incontinence episode frequency on a 3-day voiding diary had moderate correlation with subjective outcomes ($r = 0.06$ to 0.45) [4]. It is clear that both patient-reported outcomes and objective clinical should be used as a composite outcome with each category in order to better understand the clinical picture [5] (Table 1).

This chapter will focus on understanding the value and efficacy of subjective outcome measurement tools in diagnosis, treatment, and follow-up of standard pelvic floor disorders. We begin by defining the terminology and the different types of validated questionnaires along with descriptions of select Grade A questionnaires, which come as "highly recommended" based published evidence of the questionnaire being *valid, reliable, and responsive to change*. Next, the process of developing a novel questionnaire is discussed along with a brief description of psychometric concepts and the ICI grading system. Lastly, we conclude with suggestions on research factors to consider when choosing a questionnaire for a clinical trial. There is an enormous amount of published patient-reported outcome (PRO) instruments for urinary, gynecological, sexual, and bowel dysfunction. Thus, the need to develop a new tool is low. Instead we need to explore and hopefully consolidate the validated tools we have. As a supplemental tool, a comprehensive and concise compilation of published surveys and their psychometric traits is provided to assist the researcher in identifying the most appropriate questionnaire for their needs.

Table 1 Guidelines and recommendation levels for the objective measurement of UI by the AUA/SUFU, EUA, and ICI

Objective measurement	AUA/SUFU	EUA	ICI
Cough Stress Test	Clinical principle Should have objective demonstration of SUI with a comfortably full bladder on initial assessment (any method)	NA	Highly recommended stress test during initial evaluation

Post-Void Residual	Clinical principle
	    Should be included on initial assessment (any method)
		Strong
		    Measure PVR in UI patients with voiding symptoms or complicated UI
		    When measuring PVR, use ultrasound
		    PVR should be monitored in patients receiving treatments that may cause or worsen voiding dysfunction, including surgery for SUI
			Recommended if result is likely to influence management

Urinalysis (UA)	Clinical principle
	    Should be included on initial assessment
		Strong
		    Perform UA as part of initial assessment for UI
		    Do not routinely treat asymptomatic bacteruria in elderly patients to improve UI
		    If a symptomatic UTI is present with UI, reassess after treatment
			Highly recommended during initial evaluation

Voiding Diary (VD)	NA	Strong
		    Ask patients with UI to complete a VD when standardized assessment is needed
		    Use a diary duration of at least 3 days
			Highly recommended in patients with urinary symptoms

Pad Test	NA	Strong
		    Use a pad test of standardized duration and activity protocol
		Weak
		    Use a pad test when quantification of UI is required.
			Optional of 1-h pad test for routine evaluation of urinary incontinence

Urodynamics (UDS)	Conditional; Grade B
	    May omit UDS for index patient desiring treatment when SUI is clearly demonstrated
	    May perform in non-index patient
		Strong
		    Do not routinely perform UDS for uncomplicated SUI
		    Do not use UPP or LPP to grade severity of incontinence
		    When performing UDS adhere to ICS' "Good Urodynamics Practice"
		Weak
		    Perform UDS if findings may change the choice of invasive treatment
			Recommended when results change management or in complicated incontinence

Cystoscopy	Clinical principle Should not perform cystoscopy in index patients to evaluate for SUI unless concerned for urinary tract abnormalities.	NA	Optional in complicated, persistent, or recurrent SUI

(continued)

Table 1 (continued)

Objective measurement	AUA/SUFU	EUA	ICI
Imaging	NA	Strong Do not routinely carry out imaging of upper or lower urinary tract to assess UI	Highly recommended in specific situations

AUA/SUFU grading system based on the AUA nomenclature system (clinical principle, strong, moderate, conditional, and expert opinion). Index patient defined as healthy female with no prior SUI surgery and only low grade prolapse. EUA grading based on Oxford Centre for Evidence-Based Medicine Levels of Evidence (1a/b/c, 2a/b/c, 3a/b, 4, 5) and strength (strong, weak). ICI based on own definition (highly recommended, recommended, optional, not recommended)
ICS International Continence Society, *NA* not assessed

Patient-Reported Outcome (PRO) Data Via Validated Questionnaire

Clinical outcome data are categorized by the method of collection (i.e., clinical test, voiding diary, pad test, questionnaire) and how the information is reported (patient or provider) [6]. Given the subjective nature of pelvic floor conditions, PRO data plays a crucial role in evaluation.

Per the US Food and Drug Administration (FDA), PRO data is any report by the patient regarding their health condition that is not interpreted by someone else [6, 7]. It can be used to screen for a disease, measure the severity and bother factor of a disease, and assess impact on daily activities and on health-related quality of life (HRQL). Additionally, PRO data helps determine treatment risk or benefits and evaluate patient satisfaction after treatment. There are a multitude of questionnaires which have been designed and validated based on these goals.

Screening. Some instruments were specially designed for screening. These tools are self-administered and used to improve the detection of specific symptoms by patients, aiding in physician diagnosis [6]. While screening tools have rigorous validation, they do not utilize longitudinal data and thus do not have the ability to detect changes in disease conditions (responsiveness). The format of screening instruments can range from simple "yes or no" questions, such as the 3 Incontinence Questions (3IQ) to longer score-weighted questionnaires like the Overactive Bladder-Validated 8- question screener (OAB-V8) and the Overactive Bladder Symptom

Score (OABSS) [8]. Both the OAB-V8 and OABSS are Grade A recommended screening questionnaires for OAB, though there are key differences. With OAB-V8, patients are asked to rate how bothered they are by OAB symptoms on a five-point Likert scale with scores ≥ 8 suggesting OAB [9]. OABSS is a four-question, 15-point questionnaire on frequency (2 points), nocturia (3 points), urgency (5 points), and urinary incontinence (5 points) whose total score rates the condition into mild [1–7], moderate [8–12], and severe [10, 13–15]. Table 2 provides a complete list of Grade A recommended screening questionnaires.

MESA (Medical, Epidemiologic, and Social Aspects of Aging) is a commonly used screening tool to confirm the presence and severity of SUI and urge UI and to evaluate which is clinically dominant. There are nine questions on SUI and six on UUI scored from 0 to 3 for answers of "never," "rarely," "sometimes," and "often" for a total maximum score of 27 and 18 in each category, respectively. By dividing the score in each category by its maximum, an index ratio for each category can be obtained and compared to determine the predominant symptom [11].

Symptom Severity. To assess longitudinal data and monitor clinical progression, there are validated questionnaires designed to evaluate the severity of specific condition. An example is the Incontinence Symptom Severity Index (ISS), an eight-item Grade A questionnaire highly correlated with the International Consultation on Incontinence Questionnaire-Urinary Incontinence Short Form (ICIQ-UI SF) which focuses on only urine incontinence symptom severity [12]. The

6 Measurement of Urinary Symptoms, Health-Related Quality of Life, and Outcomes of... 101

Table 2 Grade A recommended questionnaires to **screen** for OAB, UI, LUTS, prolapse, pelvic floor/sexual health, and fecal incontinence

Organization	Urgency	OAB	UI	LUTS	POP	Pelvic floor/sexual health	FI	Comprehensive
ICI		QUID OAB-SS OAB-V8 OAB-V3		B-SAQ				
EUA		OAB-SS OABV8 OABV3 QUID		B-SAQ				

ICIQ-UI SF is highly recommended for future trials given that it is a frequently used four-item Grade A questionnaire validated for both genders that also correlates the highest with objective outcome measures [1]. Some questionnaires also evaluate quality of life in conjunction with severity, such as the International Consultation on Incontinence Questionnaire for Overactive Bladder (ICIQ-OAB), a Grade A four-item instrument with a minimal importance difference (MID, see *Responsiveness* section) of 1 [13–15]. A complete list of Grade A validated questionnaires evaluating symptom severity for different conditions is in Table 3.

Bother. Some instruments assess the bother to the patient of a specific symptom, such as the Urogenital Distress Inventory (UDI-6) on urinary leakage. UDI-6 consists of six Likert scale questions asking "how much are you bothered by..." the symptoms of frequency, urge or stress incontinence, difficulty emptying, or pelvic pain [16]. If administered serially, data from these instruments can be tracked throughout the course of the disease and compared for clinical information. Because of this, validation studies for this type of data includes responsiveness. For example, as a Grade A questionnaire, the UDI-6 has a MID of 11 [17]. However, because it was designed and tested to assess bother, it is not recommended to be used to assess other data such as symptom severity or HRQL. Despite these limitations, the UDI-6 is commonly used and has been shown to correlate with urodynamic findings for stress urinary incontinence (SUI, phi coefficient: 0.51, $p < 0.001$), bladder outlet obstruction (BOO, phi coefficient: 0.38, $p < 0.001$), and detrusor overactivity (DO, phi coefficient: 0.31, $p = 0.002$)

[17]. In other words, the UDI-6 was sensitive enough to predict positive urodynamic findings of SUI (84.8%), BOO (43.9%), and DO (68.6%). See Table 4.

Health-Related Quality of Life (HRQL). For assessment of quality of life (QoL), a HRQL questionnaire should be considered. HRQL is defined as a questionnaire with a multi-domain view of the condition's impact on a patient's physical, psychological, economical, and social well-being [6]. HRQL instruments are useful in calculating quality-adjusted life year (QALY), the measurement of both life quantity (mortality) and quality (morbidity). This is used universally for disease-specific cost-utility analysis [6]. Given the growing interest in cost-effectiveness for healthcare resource allocation, there has been heavy emphasis on HRQL for calculation of economic impact. Specifically for urinary incontinence, various reviews suggested that the top performing instruments are King's Health Questionnaire (KHQ), Incontinence-Quality of Life (I-QOL), and ICIQ-UI SF as they are all Grade A and are most frequently used in prior trials [3]. However, each has its own drawbacks. The KHQ has a complicated scoring system, and the I-QOL has 22 items compared to its shorter counterparts [3]. Table 5 lists all HRQL grade A validated instruments.

Satisfaction. Lastly, there are PRO instruments designed to measure patient satisfaction following treatment. For instance, the Patient Global Impression of Improvement (PGI-I) is a widely used Grade A one-item questionnaire used to assess the response to a specific therapy. It has been applied to treatment satisfaction for urinary incontinence, lower urinary tract symptoms

Table 3 Grade A recommended questionnaires to evaluate **symptom severity** of OAB, UI, LUTS, prolapse, sexual health, fecal incontinence, or comprehensive

Organization	Urgency	OAB	UI	LUTS	POP	Pelvic floor/ sexual health	FI	Comprehensive
ICI	UQUUS IUSS USS PPIUS	ICIQ-OAB OAB-q	ICIQ-UI SF ISS ICIQ-Uqol (I-QOL) PRAFAB UISS LUSQ SUIQQ PGI-S	LUTSS ICIQ-FLUTS ICIQ-MLUTS AUA-7 (AUASS) ICIQ-N DAN-PSS ICSQOL	P-QOL	ICIQ-MLUTSsex ICIQ-FLUTSsex	FIQL BBUSQ-22 Questionnaire for Assessment of Fecal incontinence and Constipation	PFDI-20 PISQ-IR
EUA		OAB-q	ICIQ-UI SF I-QOL ISS PRAFAB UISS PGI-S	ICIQ-FLUTS ICIQ-MLUTS				PFDI-20

Table 4 Grade A recommended questionnaires to evaluate **HRQL** or **bother** of OAB, UI, LUTS, prolapse, pelvic floor/sexual health, and fecal incontinence

Organization	Urgency	OAB	UI	LUTS	POP	Pelvic floor/sexual health	FI	Comprehensive
ICI	UQ	OAB-q OAB-q SF ICIQ-OAB	ICIQ-UI SF IIQ IIQ-7 ICIQ-UqolL (I-OQL) PRAFAB UISS SUIQQ SEAPI-QMM LUSQ	LUTSS N-QOL ICIQ-MLUTS ICIQ-FLUTS ICIQ-LUTSqol Urolife ICIQ-N DAN-PSS ICSQol	P-QOL	ICIQ-MLUTSsex ICIQ-FLUTSsex	ICIQ-B FIQL	KHQ PFID PFID-7 LIS UDI-6 UDI PPBC
EUA	UU Scale	OAB-q OAB-q SF	ICIQ-UI SF IIQ IIQ-7 ICIQ-UqolL (I-OQL) PRAFAB UISS SUIQQ ISS LUSQ	N-QOL ICIQ-MLUTS ICIQ-FLUTS		ICIQ-MLUTSsex ICIQ-FLUTSsex		KHQ PFID PFID-7 LIS UDI-6 UDI PPBC
NICE			ICIQ-UI SF ICIQ-UqolL (I-OQL) SUIQQ UISS SEAPI-QMM ISI	BFLUTS				KHQ

Table 5 Grade A recommended questionnaires to evaluate **treatment satisfaction** of OAB, UI, LUTS, prolapse, pelvic floor/sexual health, and fecal incontinence

Organization	Questionnaires
ICI	PGI-I TBS BSW
EUA	PGI-I TBS BSW OAB-S OABSAT-q

(LUTS), and prolapse surgery [17, 18]. This instrument asks the patient to compare and rate their pretreatment condition to their current from "1-very much better" to "7-very much worse." The Benefit, Satisfaction with Treatment, and Willingness to Continue Treatment (BSW) questionnaire is another grade A tool that not only captures a patient's satisfaction with treatment but also evaluates the patient's perception of treatment benefit and their willingness to continue with treatment [19]. See Table 5.

Other instruments identify patient treatment goals. The Goal Attainment Scale (GAS) assesses patient treatment goals to clarify objectives for the healthcare provider, increase patient's involvement in problem-solving efforts, and improve patient's motivation for self-care. An example is the Self-Assessment Goal Attainment (SAGA) [20, 21], a validated instrument for LUTS and OAB symptoms. It is administered in two parts – before the initial and follow-up visits – with the patient ranking goals such as "reduce the sudden need to rush to the bathroom" and "reduce my urine loss when I have a sudden need to rush to the bathroom" on a five-point Likert scale. Nine prefixed goals are asked, but patients are able to free-text additional goals. They choose their top three goals. After treatment discussion, patients are asked to mark those specific actions (i.e., "change what I eat and drink"; "take medication as prescribed by my doctor") and provide a signature to confirm their commitment. The follow-up visit is similarly conducted, with the slight difference in that they are asked to rate their goal achievements on the Likert scale with 1 being "much worse than expected" and 5 being "much better than expected." This instrument assesses satisfaction and provides a framework to manage patient expectations.

How Do we Develop a Questionnaire?

The proper development of a validated questionnaire is a time-consuming process that demands the meeting of rigorous, scientific standards. There is no specified algorithm, though many have written extensively on this subject. In general, the steps are as follows (adapted [6, 22, 23]):

Theorization and Item Development

First, the topic of interest and purpose of the instrument should be explicitly stated. Is this instrument to be used to measure OAB or pelvic pain? Should this instrument function to screen for the condition or determine the level of treatment satisfaction? Once established, an exhaustive literature review should be performed. It is best to use an established, validated instrument rather than "re-invent the wheel."

If none exist, item development can occur using focus groups, cognitive interviews with patients, expert committees, and literature searches of similar instruments. This is an iterative process that assesses content validity and confirms that items express the desired concept prior to pursuing more intense validation studies.

Scale Development

Once items are generated, questions such as the mode of administration (i.e., patient- vs interviewer-administered; electronic vs hard copy), sample size calculation, total number of instrument questions and responses, etc., may be addressed. Validation of one mode does not mean validation for all modes. Successful instruments must strike a fine balance between being comprehensive yet not too long or burdensome.

Scale Evaluation with Psychometric Analysis

Lastly, the instrument is placed through rigorous psychometric analysis to evaluate quality. Questions asked may include: Is this instrument capable of being completed by the target population (i.e., feasibility)? Can it give reliable answers in variable scenarios (i.e., reliability)? Can it measure accurately what it is supposed to measure (i.e., validity)? Is it clinically useful (i.e., responsiveness)? There are many methods to answer these questions, but a high-quality instrument would answer as many of these questions as possible.

Ideal Properties of a Validated Questionnaire

In designing a validated questionnaire, specific criteria are considered [6, 24]. The instrument should be:

I. Specific to the concept being measured.
II. Based on the end-point model, which diagrams the relationships between subjective and objective measurement (i.e., pad weight test) tools that captures the study's objectives.
III. Have conceptual equivalence, so that it is equally relevant in multiple languages and cultures.
IV. Contain an optimum number of items.
V. Have easy and specific measurement properties so that the target population can easily understand it.
VI. Have proper evidence for the conceptual framework, which defines the concepts (i.e., OAB), domains (i.e., urinary frequency), and items (i.e., how often do you pass urine during the day?") that are measured by the instrument.
VII. Maintain the confidentiality of the patient.
VIII. Be reproducible.

Validation Via Psychometric Analysis

Validation is a multistep, iterative process which seeks to prove that an instrument performs a specific function, using statistical evidence. This is achieved by rigorous examination of the content (i.e., feasibility, internal consistency, reliability) and by determining correlation, or the bidirectional liner association of two variables, to prior standards of similar or dissimilar concepts (i.e., criterion validity, construct validity) [25]. As further evidence is gathered for the studied instrument, the grade of the instrument increases to reflect its quality.

Correlation. An important concept to understand when validating HRQL is correlation. Correlation statistically shows the *linear* relationship of two variables and ranges from −1 to 1, with −1 indicating perfect negative correlation, 0 indicating no correlation, and 1 indicating perfect positive correlation [25]. Of significant importance, correlation does not mean causation, but rather that there is an association between two variables. Different types of correlation coefficients are best suited for different data sets that are being measured.

A comprehensive understanding of the field of psychometric analysis is vast and beyond the scope of this chapter. However, there are basic concepts that any researcher working with patient-reported outcome data should be familiar with. We will describe the most common concepts used.

Feasibility. Feasibility assesses the instrument's ease of use and includes considerations such as the simplicity of format, clarity of questions, percentage of completed response, and length of time to fill out [23]. This can be objectively shown in many ways: the percentage of completed questionnaires, average administration time, or the Flesch-Kincaid Readability score [26]. The latter is an equation which estimates the grade level of the reader and can be used to ensure the appropriateness of the instrument's wording. Higher scores indicate ease of readability at a lower grade level. Both the NIH and American Medical Association recommend a reading level of 7th–eighth grade (score 60–70) or 5th–sixth grade (score of 90–100), respectively [27, 28]. There are other equations to calculate grade levels such as the Simple Measure of Gobbledygook grade level [26], Coleman-Liau Index [27], and the Gunning-Fog Index [28].

For example, Betschart [29] evaluated the readability of 13 urinary questionnaires using the Flesch-Kincaid equation and found them to range from a second to 11th grade reading level (ICIQ-FLUTS-SF = 2.7 y; ICIQ-FLUTS-LF = 2.9 y; ICIQ-MLTS-LF = 2.9 y; ICIQ-MLUTS-SF = 3.3 y; I-WOL = 5.0; Qualiveen = 6.7 y; SF-Qualiveen = 7.3 y; SF-36v2 = 6.8 y; ICSI = 6.5 y; IPSS = 6.4 y; NIH-CPSI = 8.6 y; IIEF = 9.8; IIEF-5 = 11.2 y). Sanchez-Sanchez et al. evaluated the feasibility of Prolapse Quality of Life Questionnaire (P-QOL) in Spanish via administration time and found that it was an average of 10 minutes [30].

Reliability. Reliability asks if the instrument consistently measure what it intends to measure [23]. Hence, it is the ability of an instrument to provide the same answer with different groups (i.e., interobserver reliability), at different time (i.e., reproducibility), and with different items within the instruments (i.e., internal consistency). There are multiple facets to this, yet three are the most common focus:

Interobserver or inter-rater reliability assesses the studied instrument's ability to give the same measurement despite different observers. In other words, if two different observers rated the same situation, would they agree? A robust questionnaire should show strong agreement. To do this, correlation would be calculated among the rater's completed responses via Cohen's k, Pearson product-moment correlation (PPMC), or the intraclass correlation (ICC). Results between 0.8 and 0.9 are considered "strong" for k, and ≥ 0.70 for Pearson's r and ICC is acceptable [17, 19].

For example, Otmani et al. [31] assessed inter-rater reliability by having two different interviewers administer the Moroccan version of the I-QOL to 100 patients. Correlation was then calculated using ICC to show a very strong association for the total score (ICC = 0.99) as well as the subscores (avoidance or limiting behaviors = 0.97; psychological behaviors = 0.99; social embarrassment = 0.97) [31].

Reproducibility assesses the instrument's ability to produce the same result at different times. It is measured using the test-retest method where the same target population completes the instrument initially and then again approximately 1 week later. Correlation is then commonly calculated using ICC.

Internal consistency evaluates the degree in which items in the studied instrument remain true or consistent to the total instrument. Do the individual questions reflect the overall concept? The two common ways to show this are the split-half method or Cronbach's α.

Through the split-half method, instrument items are divided into two equal halves either by odd and even numbered items or the first and second halves. Correlation is then calculated to assess for consistency with a correlation coefficient of between 0.7 and 1.0 considered to indicate strong internal consistency [16].

The other common method is to calculate Cronbach's α, or item-total correlation, in which α is first calculated for the total instrument then after each subsequent removal of an item. If the Cronbach's α changes significantly after the removal of an item, that question should be re-evaluated and modified. A Cronbach's $\alpha > 0.70$ is considered acceptable.

Validity assesses the question: Does the instrument accurately measure what it intends to measure? For instance, if a questionnaire on OAB has an item on dyspareunia, this item would not accurately capture the effects of OAB and thus be invalid. Within the realm of validity, there are subgroups which describes various aspects.

Content validity evaluates how relevant or comprehensive the items in the instrument measure the concept. In other words, are the items in IIQ-7 relevant in describing OAB? Does the questionnaire capture all of the different aspects of OAB? There are different methods to measure this.

Content validity index (CVI) [23], the most widely reported approach [29], uses expert judges to rate the relevance of each item on the questionnaire on a four-point Likert scale with 0 meaning "nonrelevant" and 4 meaning "most relevant." Using three to ten expert judges, the individual CVI (I-CVI, relevancy of each item individually) or whole-scale CVI (S-CVI evaluates the instrument as a whole) can then be calculated.

For example, to calculate the S-CVI of the Incontinence Impact Questionnaire-Short Form (IIQ-7), Moore and colleagues [30] had six expert judges rate each item and determined that the $\frac{SCVI}{UA}$ was 0.88. Four items ("household chores, travel by car or bus more than 30 minutes away from home, emotional health, and feeling frustrated") each has I-CVI below 0.9.

Content validity ratio (CVR) [29] is another way to show content validity. Expert judges are asked to rate each item in the instrument on a three-point scale with 1 being "not necessary," 2 being "useful but not essential," and 3 as "essential." CVR is then calculated, and results can vary from −1 to 1, with higher scores indicating greater agreement between expert judges.

Face validity is considered the easiest way to assess validity, though it is also considered the weakest evidence as it does not provide objective analysis. It utilizes both expert and target population judges and assesses the degree to which an instrument *appears* to measure what it intended.

Construct validity evaluates how well the instrument measures the underlying theorem or construct. In other words, how well does the Nocturia Quality of Life (N-QOL) capture the construct of OAB? To prove this, one can see if different instruments yield similar results (convergent validity) or if different instruments yield appropriately different results (discriminant/divergent validity).

> *Convergent validity* assesses how a construct measured in different ways or with different instruments can give similar results [29]. For instance, the items relating to sleep quality on the N-QOL correlated strongly with the Pittsburgh Sleep Quality Index ($p < 0.01$), and the items relating to energy and social functioning correlated well with the SF-36 Health Survey ($p < 0.01$), indicating strong convergent validity [40].

> *Divergent/discriminant validity* is the assessment that the studied instrument can differentiate between different concepts. An instrument has discriminant validity if it has weak correlation with another instrument that was designed to measure a different concept, or if it is able to differentiate between different groups. For instance, discriminant validity was determined for the Prolapse Quality of Life Questionnaire (P-QOL) [30] by comparing the scores of symptomatic to asymptomatic women with POP. Using Student's *t*-test, they showed that each domain of the instrument was statistically different from each other ($p < 0.001$).

Criterion validity assess how well the studied instrument measures up to the standard, or criterion. If it is compared to the "gold standard," then concurrent criterion validity is being assessed [22]. The "gold standard" can be either objective tests (i.e., UDS, voiding diary, etc.) or other subjective instruments (i.e., other HRQL).

Responsiveness measures the instrument's ability to detect bidirectional treatment effects and changes to the patient's clinical status. Two commonly published variables are minimal clinically important difference (MCID) and cumulative distribution function (CDF).

Minimal Clinically Important Difference (MCID) or **Minimal Important Difference (MID)** According to Jaeschke et al. [31], MID is defined as "the smallest difference in score in the domain of interest which patients perceive as beneficial and which would mandate, in the absence of troublesome side effects and excessive cost, a change in the patient's management." Especially in clinical trials, MID provides comparative data to help distinguish truly beneficial treatments and to give real-life meaning to statistically significant data. The determination of the MID is an iterative process that typically uses two methodologies in combination: anchor based and distribution based [6].

Anchor-based approach utilizes an external tool, or "anchor," that can be an objective or subjective measurement. For example, in determining the MID for the ICIQ-UI SF, Sirls et al. [32] used the UDI, IIQ, PGI-I, and satisfaction as subjective anchors and incontinence episodes (IE) on the 7-day bladder diary as the objective anchor.

On the other hand, **distribution-based approach** is a statistical analysis of the scores, without including a patient's subjective experience based on the standard deviation.

Though an advantage of incorporating multiple methods is the accuracy of the result, it can also lead to a range of answers. Therefore, the iterative process includes compacting results, for example, when Sirls and colleagues triangulated results from the anchor- and distribution-based approaches to converge on the concluded MCID for the ICIQ-UI SF of -5 points at 12 months [32].

Cumulative Distribution Function (CDF). Another technique proposed by the FDA [7] that is more comprehensive and does not rely on a single value to estimate patient's responses over time is the CDF [6]. CDF graphs the percentage of patients (y axis) who scores at certain ranges on the studied instrument (x axis) to compare the effects of the treatment [33]. By trending the percentage of respondents who score a certain level in both the control and treatment groups, comparison can easily be made on the effects of treatment.

Linguistic and Cultural Validation

Researchers who wish to capture PRO data but do not have a validated one in a specific language may choose to develop a novel instrument or adapt a pre-existing one. With the latter option, if HRQL questionnaires are to be used in a country or a language different from its origin, it is important to appropriately translate and complete the validation process for the instrument in the new language. Once this process is completed, validation studies must be performed.

Grading System

Once analysis is completed, one can assess the overall quality of a questionnaire and determine the level of recommendation for usage. The International Consultation on Incontinence (ICI) established a grading system stated below [6].

Grade A "highly recommended": published evidence of the questionnaire being *valid, reliable, and responsive to change.*
A+: There is additional published evidence of content validity.
Grade B "recommended": published evidence of the questionnaire being *valid and reliable.*
B+: There is additional published evidence of content validity.

Grade C "potential": published evidence of *valid* or *reliable* or *responsive to change.*
C+: There is additional published evidence of content validity.

Factors to Consider for Research [6]

In reviewing the literature, there is an enormous amount of published PRO instruments for urinary, gynecological, sexual, and bowel dysfunction, so the need to develop a novel instrument is low. Therefore, it can be challenging to determine which instrument to use.

There are a few factors to consider beginning with determining the exact purpose of the instrument in your trial. What concept are you trying to capture – only OAB (OAB-V8) or urinary incontinence (IIQ)? Or do you wish to capture more than one concept, such as pelvic pain and urinary symptoms (UDI-6)?

Next, assess what type of PRO data you would like to gather. Are you looking to have the instrument screen for a disease or gather longitudinal information about the severity of the disease? Do you wish to capture quality-of-life data or satisfaction after treatment? As noted above, there are differences between these types, and validation studies are done with these specific goals in mind. Also assess if the instrument was validated for your intended study population and age and in the language of choice. An instrument validated for male urinary incontinence following a radical prostatectomy (Male Urogenital Distress Inventory, MUDI) should not be used to assess female urinary incontinence. If the instrument has not been translated and validated in the language of choice in the process described above, it cannot be accurately used.

Once those decisions are made, details such as the appropriate length of the instrument and frequency of administration should be evaluated. If assessing for clinical progression, consider the question of frequency: Should the instrument be administered every 2 months to capture a quick changing disease or will an annual survey suffice? This can impact the length of the instrument you choose. A four-question instrument may not be as burdensome to the patient as a 33-question survey; however, there may be a trade-off for quality or comprehensiveness of the data. Of note, many short forms of grade A instruments were developed to help with this issue and have equal grade A quality.

Below, we have compiled a list of published PRO instruments along with variables that will assist the reader in choosing the most appropriate instrument for their study design. It is organized by concepts with the various factors indicated for ease of use. Literature search was adapted from Abrams et al. [6] and performed using PubMed for validation work from January 2006 to July 2021. The following keywords used were "urinary incontinence," "urinary symptoms," "urgency," "lower urinary tract symptoms," "overactive bladder," "stress incontinence," "incontinence," "questionnaire," "epidemiology," "prostate," "prolapse," "fecal," "bowel," "anal," "quality of life," "sexual," "satisfaction," "symptom bother," "goal attainment," "screener," "internal consistency," "reliability," "responsiveness," "validity," "MCID," and "MID."

Conclusion

Understanding the abilities and limitations of PRO data along with the nuisances of psychometric measurements is key to conducting high-quality clinical research. We present a basic overview of these concepts in this chapter as it relates to urinary, gynecological, sexual, and bowel function and encourage further study of the field.

Cross-References

▶ Etiology, Diagnosis, and Management of Pelvic Organ Prolapse: Overview
▶ Pathophysiology and Clinical Evaluation of Chronic Pelvic Pain
▶ Pathophysiology and Diagnostic Evaluation of Stress Urinary Incontinence: Overview
▶ Pathophysiology, Diagnosis, and Treatment of Defecatory Dysfunction

References

1. Lim R, Liong ML, Leong WS, Yuen KH. Which outcome measures should be used in stress urinary incontinence trials? BJU Int. 2018;121(5):805–10.
2. Avery KN, Bosch JL, Gotoh M, Naughton M, Jackson S, Radley SC, et al. Questionnaires to assess urinary and anal incontinence: review and recommendations. J Urol. 2007;177(1):39–49.
3. Hewison A, McCaughan D, Watt I. An evaluative review of questionnaires recommended for the assessment of quality of life and symptom severity in women with urinary incontinence. J Clin Nurs. 2014;23 (21-22):2998–3011.
4. Nager CW, Kraus SR, Kenton K, Sirls L, Chai TC, Wai C, et al. Urodynamics, the supine empty bladder stress test, and incontinence severity. Neurourol Urodyn. 2010;29(7):1306–11.
5. Padmanabhan P, Nitti VW. Female stress urinary incontinence: how do patient and physician perspectives correlate in assessment of outcomes? Curr Opin Urol. 2006;16(4):212–8.
6. Abrams P, Cordozo L, Wagg A, Wein A. Incontinence. 6th ed; 2017.
7. U.S. Department of Health and Human Services FDA Center for Drug Evaluation and Research, U.S. Department of Health and Human Services FDA Center for Biologics Evaluation and Research, U.S. Department of Health and Human Services FDA Center for Devices and Radiological Health. Guidance for industry: patient-reported outcome measures: use in medical product development to support labeling claims: draft guidance. Health Qual Life Outcomes. 2006;4:79.
8. Brown JS, Bradley CS, Subak LL, Richter HE, Kraus SR, Brubaker L, et al. The sensitivity and specificity of a simple test to distinguish between urge and stress urinary incontinence. Ann Intern Med. 2006;144(10): 715–23.
9. Coyne KS, Zyczynski T, Margolis MK, Elinoff V, Roberts RG. Validation of an overactive bladder awareness tool for use in primary care settings. Adv Ther. 2005;22(4):381–94.
10. Homma Y, Yoshida M, Seki N, Yokoyama O, Kakizaki H, Gotoh M, et al. Symptom assessment tool for overactive bladder syndrome–overactive bladder symptom score. Urology. 2006;68(2):318–23.
11. Diokno AC, Brock BM, Brown MB, Herzog AR. Prevalence of urinary incontinence and other urological symptoms in the noninstitutionalized elderly. J Urol. 1986;136(5):1021–5.
12. Klovning A, Avery K, Sandvik H, Hunskaar S. Comparison of two questionnaires for assessing the severity of urinary incontinence: the ICIQ-UI SF versus the incontinence severity index. Neurourol Urodyn. 2009;28(5):411–5.
13. Donovan JL, Abrams P, Peters TJ, Kay HE, Reynard J, Chapple C, et al. The ICS-'BPH' Study: the

13. psychometric validity and reliability of the ICSmale questionnaire. Br J Urol. 1996;77(4):554–62.
14. Jackson S, Donovan J, Brookes S, Eckford S, Swithinbank L, Abrams P. The Bristol Female Lower Urinary Tract Symptoms questionnaire: development and psychometric testing. Br J Urol. 1996;77(6): 805–12.
15. Verghese T, Tryposkiadis K, Arifeen K, Middleton L, Latthe P. Minimal Clinically Important Difference for the International Consultation on Incontinence Questionnaire-Overactive bladder (ICIQ-OAB); 2017.
16. Lee YJ, Kim S, Kim S, Bai S. The significance and factors related to bladder outlet obstruction in pelvic floor dysfunction in preoperative urodynamic studies: a retrospective cohort study. Obstet Gynecol Sci. 2014;57:59–65.
17. Lemack GE, Zimmern PE. Predictability of urodynamic findings based on the Urogenital Distress Inventory-6 questionnaire. Urology. 1999;54(3):461–6.
18. Srikrishna S, Robinson D, Cardozo L. Validation of the Patient Global Impression of Improvement (PGI-I) for urogenital prolapse. Int Urogynecol J. 2010;21(5): 523–8.
19. Pleil AM, Coyne KS, Reese PR, Jumadilova Z, Rovner ES, Kelleher CJ. The validation of patient-rated global assessments of treatment benefit, satisfaction, and willingness to continue—the BSW. Elsevier; 2005.
20. Brubaker L, Khullar V, Piault E, Evans CJ, Bavendam T, Beach J, et al. Goal attainment scaling in patients with lower urinary tract symptoms: development and pilot testing of the Self-Assessment Goal Achievement (SAGA) questionnaire. Int Urogynecol J. 2011;22(8):937–46.
21. Brubaker L, Piault EC, Tully SE, Evans CJ, Bavendam T, Beach J, et al. Validation study of the Self-Assessment Goal Achievement (SAGA) questionnaire for lower urinary tract symptoms. Int J Clin Pract. 2013;67(4):342–50.
22. Boateng GO, Neilands TB, Frongillo EA, Melgar-Quiñonez HR, Young SL. Best practices for developing and validating scales for health, social, and behavioral research: a primer. Front Public Health. 2018;6:149.
23. Boparai JK, Singh S, Kathuria P. How to design and validate a questionnaire: a guide. Curr Clin Pharmacol. 2018;13(4):210–5.
24. Stokes T, Paty J. Developing and Validating Electronic Diaries. Amazon AWS. June 2003. chromeextension:// efaidnbmnnnibpcajpcglclefindmkaj/ https://alfresco-static-files.s3.amazonaws.com/alfresco_images/ pharma/2014/08/22/0e87fe25-0104-4b27-8446-b2dc49906d71/article-58534.pdf. Accessed August 2021.
25. Mukaka MM. A guide to appropriate use of correlation coefficient in medical research. Malawi Med J. 2012;24(3):69–71.
26. Flesch R. How to write plain English: let's start with the formula. University of Canterbury; 1979.
27. Health NIo. How to write easy-to-read health materials. Bethesda, MD: National Library of Medicine; 2013.
28. Weiss BD. Health literacy and patient safety: help patients understand. Manual for Clinicians: American Medical Association Foundation; 2007.
29. Zamanzadeh V, Ghahramanian A, Rassouli M, Abbaszadeh A, Alavi-Majd H, Nikanfar AR. Design and implementation content validity study: development of an instrument for measuring patient-centered communication. J Caring Sci. 2015;4(2):165–78.
30. Moore KN, Jensen L. Testing of the Incontinence Impact Questionnaire (IIQ-7) with men after radical prostatectomy. J Wound Ostomy Continence Nurs. 2000;27(6):304–12.
31. Jaeschke R, Singer J, Guyatt GH. Measurement of health status: ascertaining the minimal clinically important difference. Control Clin Trials. 1989;10(4): 407–15.
32. Sirls LT, Tennstedt S, Brubaker L, Kim HY, Nygaard I, Rahn DD, et al. The minimum important difference for the International Consultation on Incontinence Questionnaire-Urinary Incontinence Short Form in women with stress urinary incontinence. Neurourol Urodyn. 2015;34(2):183–7.
33. Wyrwich KW, Norquist JM, Lenderking WR, Acaster S. Methods for interpreting change over time in patient-reported outcome measures. Qual Life Res. 2013;22(3):475–83.

Part II

Diagnostic Evaluation

Clinical Evaluation of the Female Lower Urinary Tract and Pelvic Floor

7

Stephanie Gleicher and Natasha Ginzburg

Contents

Introduction	114
History	114
Focused Urologic History	114
General Medical History	115
Physical Exam	116
External Genitalia	116
Urethra	116
Pelvic Floor	117
Vaginal Vault	117
Cervix, Uterus, and Adnexa	118
Rectal Exam	118
Void Diary	118
Pad Test	118
Self-Reported Questionnaires	119
Urinalysis	121
Post-Void Residual	121
Dye Testing	122
Conclusion	122
References	122

Abstract

Perhaps the most important aspect of evaluation of female lower urinary tract issues is a thorough and well-focused history and physical examination. Accurately understanding patient symptoms requires a true grasp of the patient's perception of their problems, paired with a directed physical examination to link any anatomic findings with the patient's complaints.

S. Gleicher
Department of Urology, Vanderbilt University Medical Center, Nashville, TN, USA

N. Ginzburg (✉)
Department of Urology, SUNY Upstate Medical University, Syracuse, NY, USA
e-mail: Ginzburn@upstate.edu

© Springer Nature Switzerland AG 2023
F. E. Martins et al. (eds.), *Female Genitourinary and Pelvic Floor Reconstruction*,
https://doi.org/10.1007/978-3-031-19598-3_7

History taking should focus on the patient's symptoms including urinary, bowel, and pelvic floor symptoms as well as general health and medications. Physical exam can be focused on the female pelvic floor and should be performed with thoughtfulness to the sensitive nature of the exam as well as to the patient's specific concerns.

Adjunct testing as part of the initial history and physical exam may be helpful to further characterize the nature of the problem. Tests such as examination of urine, post-void residual measurements, voiding diaries, pad weights, and more specialized testing may be utilized for the appropriate patient and scenario.

Keywords

Pelvic floor · Prolapse · Incontinence · Overactive bladder

Introduction

A thorough history should be paired with a full clinical evaluation to accurately assess and diagnose disorders of the female pelvic floor. Studies have shown that patient history alone is not adequate and, at times, inaccurate in the diagnosis of various conditions [1, 2]. The initial clinical evaluation should be guided by patient complaints and might include a detailed history, comprehensive physical examination, voiding diaries, pad tests, self-reported questionnaires, urinalyses, post-void residuals (PVRs), and/or dye tests. After obtaining this information, additional testing or imaging may be recommended (i.e., urodynamics, ultrasounds, magnetic resonance imaging, etc.). Importantly, providers should have a systematic approach to diagnosis and evaluation of symptoms. This chapter provides a guide for the clinical evaluation of female urinary and pelvic floor disorders.

History

The goal of the history is to better understand and characterize the patient's lower urinary tract symptoms. It is also an opportunity to build rapport and trust with your patient, as many of their complaints are of a sensitive nature. For patients with multiple or related urologic complaints, we generally begin the conversation by asking, "What bothers you most?" Their subjective response guides further discussion.

Focused Urologic History

General Voiding Patterns

The history will begin by understanding current voiding patterns. It is important to classify the frequency of voids, void volumes, changes in voiding, urgency, and incontinence. Nighttime symptoms should be assessed. Women should be asked about the temporality of symptoms (i.e., day versus night, morning versus evening). Patients should be asked about incomplete emptying, straining to void, hesitancy, sensation of bladder fullness, and maneuvers to assist in emptying. It is important to address dysuria, history of urinary tract infections, dyspareunia, or pelvic pain. We should always ask about hematuria; if positive, inquire about smoking status, chemical exposures, and other risk factors [2]. It is important to determine the timing of symptom onset as well as progression of symptoms.

Incontinence

It is important to adequately characterize incontinence during history taking (i.e., leakage subtype – stress, urge, overflow, continuous, or mixed) based on when leakage occurs and sensation of bladder fullness. It is also important to assess the degree of bother. Providers need to quantify the leakage; this can be assessed by number of pads over 24 h. The onset of leakage should be obtained (acute versus chronic) and if the symptoms are worsening. Exacerbating factors should be discussed, including exposure to bladder irritants (i.e., carbonated, caffeinated, sugary beverages, acidic or spicy foods), bowel issues, or recent weight changes. Women should be asked about prior pelvic procedures, as well as pregnancy history (number of pregnancies, delivery type, and pelvic trauma). A thorough medication review should be performed to ensure no idiopathic contributions. Associated symptoms should be explored (i.e., hematuria, dysuria, recurrent urinary tract infections, pelvic pain, vaginal itching/burning); concerning symptoms, such as hematuria and recurrent infections, should be evaluated. Lastly, bowel health should be assessed.

Overactive Bladder

It is important to quantify urinary frequency, urgency, and nocturia among patients. Void volumes should be determined. If patients report primary nocturia, it is important to ask about sleep disorders, fluid retention, and/or snoring to assess for contributory medical conditions or etiologies of nocturnal polyuria. Subjects should be asked about diet to assess for bladder irritants (i.e., caffeine, soda, sugary drinks, alcohol, spicy foods, acidic foods, etc.). Women should be asked about prior interventions, including medications, physical therapy, or procedures. Again, associated symptoms should be explored, and concerning symptoms should be evaluated prior to discussion of treatments. Medical issues, including neurologic conditions, diabetes, and obesity, should be determined.

Prolapse

Patients are asked about sensation of, or pain associated with, tissue bulge in the vagina, as well as a urinary splinting or digital assistance with defecation. Studies have shown an 81% positive predictive value (PPV) and 76% negative predictive value (NPV) for prolapse when patients report bulge [3]. Prior pregnancies, trauma associated with childbirth, constipation, and prior pelvic surgeries should be determined. If the patient reports prolapse, the degree of bother should be assessed. Changes in voiding should also be determined (i.e., new-onset overactivity, straining to void, incomplete emptying, hematuria, recurrent urinary tract infections), and status of sexual activity should be documented.

Pelvic Pain

Subjects should be asked about the onset of pelvic pain, frequency of episodes, nature of pain, dysuria, dyspareunia, and an association with voiding. Women should be asked about hematuria and history of cystitis. If the patient reports

urinary tract infections, inquire about frequency, duration, association with sexual activity, or vaginal dryness/itching. It is important to ask about inciting events, exacerbating factors, and ameliorating techniques. Prior therapies should be discussed, as well as pelvic/abdominal surgeries. It is also important to inquire about bowel health, including constipation/diarrhea, tenesmus, etc.

Women should be asked about prior interventions (i.e., medications, physical therapy, behavioral changes, inserts, surgeries). Women should also be asked about their urologic history – childhood issues, recurrent urinary tract infections, kidney stones, bladder cancer, etc.

General Medical History

Providers should perform a global assessment of the patient. Many occult neurologic disorders may initially present with lower urinary tract symptoms (LUTS) [4]. The International Continence Society (ICS) established a consensus to correlate LUTS with neurologic conditions, such as multiple sclerosis, multiple system atrophy, spinal dysraphism, normal-pressure hydrocephalus, and Parkinson's disease [4]. This guide also outlines the next steps for providers if there is suspicion of neurologic issues. Similarly, underlying medical conditions (i.e., constipation, autoimmune disease, chronic heart failure, chronic obstructive pulmonary disease, chronic kidney disease, diabetes mellitus) may initially manifest as LUTS, and so providers must consider these during the clinical evaluation as well [5].

Prior surgeries (pelvic and abdominal) and a delivery history should be obtained. Women may be asked if they had a prior hysterectomy, pelvic radiation, mesh procedures, trauma, or other procedures that may impact urinary symptoms.

Medications

A comprehensive review of medications should be performed as these may contribute to symptomology. Various medications are known to impact voiding via altered sphincter control and detrusor function, as well as increased polyuria [6, 7]. Providers should consider the impact of antipsychotics, adrenergic agonists and antagonists, antidepressants, anticholinergics, and diuretics. Additionally, medications such as sodium-glucose cotransporter 2 (SGLT2) inhibitors may contribute to lower urinary symptoms due to the resultant glucosuria as part of the mechanism of action [8].

Ultimately, the history is tailored to the patient's symptoms. It is important to characterize the issues adequately, ensure no concerning symptoms are present that warrant workup, determine the degree of bother, and then proceed with physical exam. By the end of the initial conversation, providers should have a short list of possible etiologies for complaints and ideas for management. Further workup will better fine-tune the management options.

Physical Exam

After obtaining a complete history, providers should proceed with a comprehensive and systematic physical examination. A female pelvic exam for pelvic floor disorders encompasses the following general elements [9]:

- External genitalia
- Urethral meatus
- Urethra
- Bladder
- Vagina
- Cervix
- Uterus
- Adnexa
- Anus/perineum

External Genitalia

The preferred position for the female pelvic examination is lithotomy [2]. With regard to the external genitalia, providers should visually assess hair distribution, lesions, atrophy, or signs of estrogen deficiency [2]. Estrogen deficiency may manifest as receded labia or shiny, flat vulvar mucosa and a narrowed introitus [10]. Gentle palpation, often with a cotton swab, of the vulva should be performed to assess for tenderness that may be secondary to vulvodynia, vaginismus, or even

pelvic floor dysfunction [11, 12]. By gentle retraction, the clitoris and clitoral hood may be assessed for possible adhesions or pain. Retrospective studies have found that nearly 25% of women suffer from clitoral phimosis [13]. Providers may then assess glandular pathology, by gently palpating both the Skene's (periurethral) and Bartholin's (posterior) glands.

Urethra

The urethral meatus may appear prolapsed or with caruncle, also secondary to estrogen deficiency [2, 10]. Urethral caruncle appears as a fleshy mass, often on the inferior aspect of the meatus. It is soft and often easily reducible. Occasionally, the caruncle may become thrombosed, in which case it will appear more firm, well circumscribed, and often tender. A high index of suspicion should remain with any urethral mass for possible malignancy, and biopsy should be considered if clinically warranted. Urethral prolapse is similar in appearance but generally occurs circumferentially around the meatus.

The position of the meatus in relationship to midline should be assessed. Skene's gland cysts can appear as distal, fluctuant, rounded masses that displace the meatus off midline. Additionally, the size of the meatus can be inspected to ensure no meatal stenosis is present.

Urethral mobility, which is associated with stress urinary incontinence (SUI), can be assessed via the Q-tip test during Valsalva maneuver [2, 14, 15]. The urethral Q-tip test involves insertion of a well-lubricated Q-tip via meatus to the bladder neck and noting the angle of movement as the patient performs a Valsalva maneuver [2, 15, 16]. An angle greater than 30 degrees is associated with SUI [2, 15]. Additionally, a cough stress test may be performed where leakage is noted as the patient is asked to perform powerful coughs [14]. The bladder may be empty or full, but a positive response will diagnose SUI [14]. For women with an empty bladder (<100 mL) who have a positive cough test, this has been shown to have a 65–70% sensitivity and 67–76% specificity for intrinsic sphincter deficiency (ISD) [17].

Urethral palpation should be performed for tenderness, fluctuance, masses, and scarring [2]. In patients with a history of prior anti-incontinence surgery, palpation for mesh and inspection for hyper-suspension are important components of the examination.

Pelvic Floor

The pelvic floor musculature includes the levator ani complex (pubococcygeus, iliococcygeus, and coccygeus) and provides supportive and sphincteric function [18]. Functional pelvic floor dynamics allow for relaxation during voiding and defecation but contraction during stress maneuvers with feedback from abdominal pressure [18]. Palpation of the superficial and deep pelvic floor via the vagina may elicit tenderness, abnormalities in tonicity, incongruity with abdominal musculature, and fibromuscular banding [18, 19]. For patients with pelvic pain, a thorough examination of the pelvic floor muscles is critical to assess for pelvic floor hypertonicity as a source for the patient's symptoms.

Vaginal Vault

Lesions, masses, discharge, and tissue quality should be noted in the vault [2, 9]. In patients with prior vaginal surgery, scarring, mesh, and hyper-suspension may be seen. Inspection of the walls of the vagina is valuable to assess for any tissue abnormalities; excoriation from significant prolapse, vaginal wall cysts, or other lesions should be noted. If there is suspicion for fistula, pooling of urine or stool in the vaginal vault can be diagnostic.

A vaginal speculum should be used to assess vaginal prolapse, with attention paid to the anterior, apical, and posterior compartments as well as the genital hiatus and perineal body [2, 19]. Important to note, prolapse should be assessed in lithotomy position but may require the patient to stand. The goal is to elicit maximal prolapse/bulge that is subjectively experienced by the patient [20]. Various scales have been used to characterize vaginal prolapse, with the most widely used called the Pelvic Organ Prolapse Quantification (POP-Q) system [2, 19, 20]. The POP-Q scale utilizes the hymenal ring as a fixed reference point given its ease of identification. Defined points are assessed relative to the hymenal ring (defined as zero). If the anatomic position of these points is centimeters above or proximal to the hymen, a negative measure is assigned, while distal positions are assigned positive measures [19]. The lateral vaginal fornices should be inspected to assess for any paravaginal defects as well.

The first measurement is total vaginal length, "tvl," which represents the full vaginal depth with the vaginal canal in normal position [19]. This is measured with a half speculum retracting the posterior wall. The next measurements are apical defined points of the cervix, "C," and the posterior fornix, "D." Of note, "D" represents the level of uterosacral support and helps differentiate between compromised suspension and cervical elongation; when point "C" is significantly more positive than "D," cervical elongation should be suspected [19]. In women who have undergone hysterectomy, "C" represents the vaginal cuff, and "D" is not applicable [19]. A half speculum is used to retract the posterior vaginal wall, and the patient is prompted to perform a Valsalva maneuver, strong cough, or strain similar to a bowel movement. The distal edge of the cervix and the posterior fornix are then measured relative to the hymen; a cervix that is 2 cm beyond the hymen is scored "+2."

Similar technique is used to assess the anterior vaginal wall, with half speculum retracting the posterior vaginal wall. The defined points anteriorly are the fixed point 3 cm proximal to the hymen, "Aa," which delineates the urethrovesical junction, and the distal-most extent of the anterior wall, "Ba"; "Aa" ranges from −3 to +3, and Ba ranges from −3 to "tvl" [19].

The posterior vaginal wall requires half speculum retracting the anterior vaginal wall. Again, the patient is prompted to perform a Valsalva maneuver, strong cough, or strain similar to a bowel movement. The defined points posteriorly are the fixed point 3 cm proximal to the hymen, "Ap," and the distal extent of the posterior vaginal wall, "Bp." Similar to the anterior vaginal wall, "Ap" ranges from −3 to +3, and Bp ranges from −3 to "Tvl" [19].

With the patient performing a Valsalva maneuver, strong cough, or strain similar to a bowel movement, external measurements of the genital hiatus, "gh," and perineal body, "pb," are obtained. The "gh" represents the size of the vaginal opening and spans from the middle of the external urethral meatus to the posterior midline hymen. The "pb" represents the distance between the vagina and the anus and is measured from the posterior margin of the genital hiatus to the mid-anal opening [2, 19]. A widened gh and pb may be indicative of perturbed transverse perineal musculature support.

Figure 1, adapted from Bump et al., depicts these defined points [19].

Based on the scores, staging is assigned to characterize the severity of prolapse; stages range from 0 to IV (Table 1) based on the defined points for the anterior, apical, and posterior compartments [19].

Cervix, Uterus, and Adnexa

Bimanual exam may be performed to rule out pathology of the female internal genitalia [9]. Coexistent issues can occur in up to two thirds of women [21].

Rectal Exam

Female rectal exam may be useful in assessment of fecal impaction and rectocele [21]. By applying anterior pressure during the rectal exam, laxity of the posterior compartment may be identified [2]. Additionally, the bulbocavernosus reflex may be assessed. This tests sacral nerves 2–4 (S2–S4). By gently squeezing the clitoris or tugging a Foley catheter with balloon inflated at the bladder neck, the pelvic floor muscles contract, and a contraction of the anus is seen [2]. This reflex is important to test especially when there is question of neurologic integrity.

Void Diary

A voiding diary is a powerful tool for objectively assessing clinical symptoms [14, 22]. Also referred to as frequency/voiding charts, diaries generally capture information regarding time of void, void volume, incontinence episodes, urgency, and extent of leakage (Fig. 2) [22, 23]. Objective logs of urinary events help patients appreciate patterns, triggers, and the true nature of their issues versus subjective assessments of bother that are hindered by recall bias [14, 22]. Diaries also correlate associations or inciting triggers to urinary symptoms, which is helpful for patients. Diaries have varying durations, ranging from one to 7 days, but the current recommendation is 3 days. Shorter durations are not as reliable [23, 24]. When compared to diaries of longer durations, 3 days has been shown to have high reliability measures while also reducing patient burden [23, 25]. Numerous studies have reported significantly higher burden with diaries greater than 3 days which could lead to worse compliance with incomplete documentation [24, 25]. Voiding diary platforms have traditionally been hard copy, but numerous electronic versions have been developed to maximize compliance and convenience [26]. This option should be reconciled with a patient's level of comfort with computers and portable electronic devices.

Pad Test

Pad tests are another objective measure of urinary incontinence, yet they are not widely accepted as part of the standard evaluation of female urinary incontinence [2, 28]. The timing for pad tests ranges from 1 h to 24 h generally in clinical practice. The advantage of the 1-h pad test is that it is standardized and has been shown to have adequate test-retest reliability [21]. Patients empty their bladders and then consume 500 mL of fluid (preferably water; non-sodium rich) [29]. The subject then ambulates and performs stress maneuvers. If the patient feels that the leakage is representative of incontinence episodes, the pad is weighed [21, 29]. Severity has been defined as

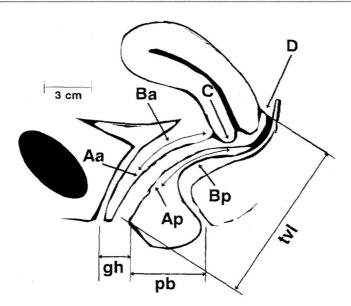

Fig. 1 Depiction of the Pelvic Organ Prolapse Quantification (POP-Q) Scale schematic with defined points delineated [19]; Tvl is total vaginal length in normal position without strain. Apex: C demarcates the cervix or cervical cuff, and D indicates the posterior fornix. Anterior wall: Aa is 3 cm proximal to hymen, and Ba is distal extent of anterior vagina. Posterior wall: Ap is 3 cm proximal to hymen, and Bp is distal extent of posterior vagina. Gh measures between the middle external urethral meatus and posterior midline of hymen; Pb measures from the posterior extent of genital hiatus to the anal opening

Table 1 Staging schematic for pelvic organ prolapse [2, 19]; Tvl is total vaginal length in normal position without strain. Apex: C demarcates the cervix or cervical cuff, and D indicates the posterior fornix. Anterior wall: Aa is 3 cm proximal to hymen, and Ba is distal extent of anterior vagina. Posterior wall: Ap is 3 cm proximal to hymen, and Bp is distal extent of posterior vagina

Stage 0	No prolapse in any compartment Aa, Ba, Ap, Bp at −3 cm and C or D ≤ (tvl −2) cm
Stage 1	Leading edge < −1 cm from hymen
Stage 2	Leading edge between −1 and +1 cm
Stage 3	Leading edge between +1 and <(tvl − 2) cm
Stage 4	Leading edge ≥ (tvl − 2) cm

"mild" (<11 g), "moderate" (11–50 g), and "severe" (>50 g) [29]. Importantly, vaginal discharge must be considered, and hydration status will impact results [29, 30]. The 24 h pad test is intended to better measure the severity of daily leakage based on normal activity (versus provocative maneuvers). Severity is considered "mild" if pad weight <20 g, "moderate" if pad weight 20–74 g, and "severe" if pad weight > 75 g [30].

Studies have shown that among women self-reporting incontinence, 97% will have a positive 1 h pad test (>1 g). However, the correlation between self-reported severity and pad weights is poor [31]. For this reason, pad tests remain underutilized as part of the clinical evaluation of incontinence [2, 21, 31].

Self-Reported Questionnaires

Self-reported questionnaires are an integral part of the clinical evaluation of urinary symptoms. Symptom perception can largely drive management decisions. Interestingly, studies have shown that providers underestimate the severity of perceived urinary symptoms 25–37% of the time [32]. Self-reported questionnaires or patient-reported outcome (PRO) tools undergo a rigorous design process prior to being utilized for clinical evaluation [33]. Designed by both physicians and patients, they have been studied extensively to confirm reliability, reproducibility, and validity

ICIQ-BLADDER DIARY (12/13) YOUR NAME: _____

Please complete this **3 day** bladder diary. Enter the following in each column against the time. You can change the specified times if you need to. In the time column, please write **BED** when you went to bed and **WOKE** when you woke up.

Drinks Write the amount you had to drink and the type of drink.

Urine output Enter the amount of urine you passed in millilitres (mls) in the urine output column, day and night. Any measuring jug will do. If you passed urine but couldn't measure it, put a tick in this column. If you leaked urine at any time write **LEAK** here.

Bladder sensation Write a description of how your bladder felt when you went to the toilet using these codes

  0 - If you had no sensation of needing to pass urine, but passed urine for "social reasons", for example, just before going out, or unsure where the next toilet is.

  1 - If you had a normal desire to pass urine and no urgency. *"Urgency" is different from normal bladder feelings and is the sudden compelling desire to pass urine which is difficult to defer, or a sudden feeling that you need to pass urine and if you don't you will have an accident.*

  2 - If you had urgency but it had passed away before you went to the toilet.

  3 - If you had urgency but managed to get to the toilet, still with urgency, but did not leak urine.

  4 - If you had urgency and could not get to the toilet in time so you leaked urine.

Pads If you put on or change a pad put a tick in the pads column.

Here is an example of how to complete the diary:

Time	Drinks		Urine output	Bladder sensation	Pads
	Amount	Type			
6am WOKE			350ml	2	
7am	300ml	tea			
8am			✓	2	
9am					
10am	cup	water	Leak	3	✓

DAY 1 DATE: _____/_____/_____

Time	Drinks		Urine output (mls)	Bladder sensation	Pads
	Amount	Type			
6am					
7am					
8am					
9am					
10am					
11am					
Midday					
1pm					
2pm					
3pm					
4pm					
5pm					
6pm					
7pm					
8pm					
9pm					
10pm					
11pm					
Midnight					
1am					
2am					
3am					
4am					
5am					

Fig. 2 Voiding diary, as adapted from the Incontinence Consultation on Incontinence Questionnaire Bladder Diary [27]. A three-day duration is adequate to reliably capture voiding habits

[33]. Each PRO attempts to characterize an outcome of interest, such as quality of life, screening for LUTS, symptom bother, urgency, and pelvic organ prolapse [33]. The ICS published a comprehensive list of validated PRO tools for the assessment of the various categories [33], and Kobashi

7 Clinical Evaluation of the Female Lower Urinary Tract and Pelvic Floor

et al. summarized them concisely [2]. Table 2 provides a snapshot of various questionnaires with ICS Grade A recommendation for women by category.

Urinalysis

Patients presenting with lower urinary tract symptoms should undergo urinalysis testing [2, 21, 22]. This is generally performed as a urine dipstick screening test and then further microscopy based on the results [34]. It is important to rule out infectious etiology of symptoms. Additionally, if the urine study demonstrates hematuria, a larger evaluation may be warranted to rule out malignant etiology. Other urine studies may show glucosuria or proteinuria, which imply possible medical etiology for symptoms [2].

Post-Void Residual

Subjects with incontinence should be evaluated for post-void residual (PVR). Patients with elevated PVRs who are being assessed for

Table 2 Summary of self-reported questionnaires by category for assessment in women with ICS Grade A recommendation. (Adapted from Staskin et al.'s guidelines [33])

Questionnaire	Outcome of interest
Health-Related Quality of Life (HRQOL)	
Bristol Female Lower Urinary Tract Symptoms Questionnaire (BFLUTS or ICIQ- FLUTS)	Lower urinary tract symptoms (LUTS), especially filling, voiding, incontinence
King's Health Questionnaire (ICIQ-LUTSqol)	Impact of LUTS on life restrictions and emotions
Overactive Bladder QoL Module (ICIQ-OABqol)	Impact of overactive bladder (OAB) on sleep, social interactions, anxiety, coping
Urinary Incontinence Questionnaire (ICIQ-UI)	Impact of urinary incontinence (UI) on QoL, as well as frequency and severity
Vaginal Symptom Questionnaire (ICIQ-VS)	Evaluation of vaginal symptoms and impact on QoL and sexual activity
Incontinence Impact Questionnaire (IIQ)	Impact of UI, primarily stress urinary incontinence (SUI), on QoL
Nocturia QoL Questionnaire (N-QoL or ICIQ-Nqol)	Impact of nocturia on QoL
Protection, Amount, Frequency, Adjustment, Body Image (PRAFAB)	Evaluate treatment effects for UI
Urinary Incontinence Severity Score (UISS)	Assess UI symptom severity and impact on everyday life
Screeners	
Bladder Self-assessment Questionnaire (BCSQ)	Screening tool for LUTS
Leicester Urinary Symptom Questionnaire (LUSQ)	Screening for storage LUTS
OAB Symptom Score (OAB-SS)	7-item assessment of symptom severity
OAB Awareness Tool (OAB-V8)	8-item assessment to identify OAB
Questionnaire for UI Diagnosis (QUID)	6-item assessment to diagnose stress versus urge UI
Symptom Bother	
Patient perception of Bladder condition (PPBC)	Assess perception of urinary issues
Urogenital Distress Inventory-6 (UDI-6)	Assess bother of LUTS
Urgency	
Indevus Urgency Severity Scale (IUSS)	Quantify urgency via voiding diaries
Pelvic Organ Prolapse QoL (POPQoL)	
Pelvic Floor Distress Inventory (PFDI)	Impact of pelvic floor disorders (i.e., POP, LUTS, colorectal-anal dysfunction) on QoL
Pelvic Floor Impact Questionnaire (PFIQ)	Impact of pelvic floor disorders on travel, social, emotional, and physical activity

interventions for urgency or stress urinary incontinence may be mismanaged. PVR can be measured with external bladder ultrasound or intermittent catheterization [2]. While catheterization is the gold standard for determination of PVR, studies have shown that bladder ultrasounds are cheap, less invasive, and quick, with sensitivity of 67% and specificity of 96% for volumes greater than or equal to 100 ml, making them a comparable option [35]. If patients are found to be retaining large volumes of urine, this will impact their lower urinary symptoms. Per the International Continence Society guidelines, normal emptying results in a PVR < 50 mL, and an elevated PVR is considered >300 mL [2, 21, 36]. Additionally, palpation of bladder fullness may represent elevated residuals.

Dye Testing

Based on clinical symptoms and history, a dye test may be helpful to rule out a vesicovaginal or ureterovaginal fistula [37]. This test involves simultaneous administration of oral phenazopyridine, which turns urine orange, and intravesical methylene blue, which turns urine blue, while the patient is wearing a tampon. If the tampon turns orange, a ureterovaginal fistula is suspected. If the tampon turns blue, a vesicovaginal fistula is diagnosed. Both colors may appear on the tampon implying two fistulous communications with the vagina [2, 37].

Conclusion

Various tools are available to provide a comprehensive clinical evaluation of the female pelvic floor and lower urinary tract symptoms. A combination of objective and subjective instruments can be utilized to best guide the next steps and management decisions. It is important that providers have a systematic approach for navigating the evaluation and diagnosis of various urinary and pelvic floor disorders. This chapter serves as a framework for optimizing clinical assessments.

References

1. Jensen JK, Nielsen FR Jr, Ostergard DR. The role of patient history in the diagnosis of urinary incontinence. Obstet Gynecol. 1994;83(5 Pt 2):904–10.
2. McDougal WS, et al. Campbell-Walsh urology. 10th ed. Elsevier Health Sciences; 2011. Review E-book
3. Tan JS, et al. Predictive value of prolapse symptoms: a large database study. Int Urogynecol J Pelvic Floor Dysfunct. 2005;16(3):203–9. discussion 209
4. Roy HA, et al. Assessment of patients with lower urinary tract symptoms where an undiagnosed neurological disease is suspected: a report from an International Continence Society consensus working group. Neurourol Urodyn. 2020;39(8):2535–43.
5. Yu C-J, Hsu C-C, Lee W-C, et al. Medical diseases affecting lower urinary tract function. Urological Science. 2013;24(2):41–45. https://doi.org/10.1016/j.urols.2013.04.004
6. Gormley EA, et al. Polypharmacy and its effect on urinary incontinence in a geriatric population. Br J Urol. 1993;71(3):265–9.
7. Tsakiris P, Oelke M, Michel MC. Drug-induced urinary incontinence. Drugs Aging. 2008;25(7):541–9.
8. Liu J, et al. Effects of SGLT2 inhibitors on UTIs and genital infections in type 2 diabetes mellitus: a systematic review and meta-analysis. Sci Rep. 2017;7(1):2824.
9. CMS.gov. 1997 Documentation Guidelines for Evaluation and Management Services. 1997 [cited 2021 Jul 25]. Available from: https://www.cms.gov/Outreach-and-Education/Medicare-Learning-Network-MLN/MLNEdWebGuide/Downloads/97Docguidelines.pdf
10. Mac Bride MB, Rhodes DJ, Shuster LT. Vulvovaginal atrophy. Mayo Clin Proc. 2010;85(1):87–94.
11. Bates CK, Carroll N, Potter J. The challenging pelvic examination. J Gen Intern Med. 2011;26(6):651–7.
12. O'Connell HE, et al. The anatomy of the distal vagina: towards unity. J Sex Med. 2008;5(8):1883–91.
13. Aerts L, et al. Retrospective study of the prevalence and risk factors of clitoral adhesions: women's health providers should routinely examine the glans clitoris. Sex Med. 2018;6(2):115–22.
14. Ghoniem G, et al. Evaluation and outcome measures in the treatment of female urinary stress incontinence: International Urogynecological Association (IUGA) guidelines for research and clinical practice. Int Urogynecol J Pelvic Floor Dysfunct. 2008;19(1):5–33.
15. Crystle CD, Charme LS, Copeland WE. Q-tip test in stress urinary incontinence. Obstet Gynecol. 1971;38(2):313–5.
16. Walters MD, Diaz K. Q-tip test: a study of continent and incontinent women. Obstet Gynecol. 1987;70(2):208–11.
17. Lobel RW, Sand PK. The empty supine stress test as a predictor of intrinsic urethral sphincter dysfunction. Obstet Gynecol. 1996;88(1):128–32.
18. Devreese A, et al. Clinical evaluation of pelvic floor muscle function in continent and incontinent women. Neurourol Urodyn. 2004;23(3):190–7.

19. Bump RC, et al. The standardization of terminology of female pelvic organ prolapse and pelvic floor dysfunction. Am J Obstet Gynecol. 1996;175(1):10–7.
20. Baden WF, Walker TA, Lindsey JH. The vaginal profile. Tex Med. 1968;64(5):56–8.
21. Walters MD, Karram MM. In: Walters MD, Karram MM, editors. Urogynecology and reconstructive pelvic surgery. 4th ed. Philadelphia: Elsevier/Saunders; 2015.
22. Abrams P, et al. Fourth International Consultation on Incontinence Recommendations of the International Scientific Committee: evaluation and treatment of urinary incontinence, pelvic organ prolapse, and fecal incontinence. Neurourol Urodyn. 2010;29(1):213–40.
23. Bright E, et al. Developing and validating the international consultation on incontinence questionnaire bladder diary. Eur Urol. 2014;66(2):294–300.
24. Yap TL, Cromwell DC, Emberton M. A systematic review of the reliability of frequency-volume charts in urological research and its implications for the optimum chart duration. BJU Int. 2007;99(1):9–16.
25. Ku JH, et al. Voiding diary for the evaluation of urinary incontinence and lower urinary tract symptoms: prospective assessment of patient compliance and burden. Neurourol Urodyn. 2004;23(4):331–5.
26. Rabin JM, McNett J, Badlani GH. A computerized voiding diary. J Reprod Med. 1996;41(11):801–6.
27. International Consultation on Incontinence Questionnaire Bladder Diary 2019 [cited 2021 Aug 9]. Available from: https://iciq.net/iciq-bladder-diary
28. Krhut J, et al. Pad weight testing in the evaluation of urinary incontinence. Neurourol Urodyn. 2014;33(5):507–10.
29. Klarskov P, Hald T. Reproducibility and reliability of urinary incontinence assessment with a 60 min test. Scand J Urol Nephrol. 1984;18(4):293–8.
30. O'Sullivan R, et al. Definition of mild, moderate and severe incontinence on the 24 hour pad test. BJOG. 2004;111(8):859–62.
31. Abdel-fattah M, Barrington JW, Youssef M. The standard 1-hour pad test: does it have any value in clinical practice? Eur Urol. 2004;46(3):377–80.
32. Rodríguez LV, et al. Discrepancy in patient and physician perception of patient's quality of life related to urinary symptoms. Urology. 2003;62(1):49–53.
33. Staskin D, et al. Initial assessment of urinary and faecal incontinence in adult male and female patients. In: Abrams P, Cardozo L, Khoury S, Wein A. eds. (2013) Incontinence: Proceedings of the Fifth International Consultation on Incontinence, February, 2012. Fifth. Health Publications Limited, pp. 361–428.
34. Simerville JA, Maxted WC, Pahira JJ. Urinalysis: a comprehensive review. Am Fam Physician. 2005;71(6):1153–62.
35. Goode PS, et al. Measurement of postvoid residual urine with portable transabdominal bladder ultrasound scanner and urethral catheterization. Int Urogynecol J Pelvic Floor Dysfunct. 2000;11(5):296–300.
36. Abrams P, et al. The standardisation of terminology of lower urinary tract function: report from the Standardisation Sub-committee of the International Continence Society. Neurourol Urodyn. 2002;21(2):167–78.
37. Raghavaiah NV. Double-dye test to diagnose various types of vaginal fistulas. J Urol. 1974;112(6):811–2.

Ultrasound Imaging of the Female Lower Urinary Tract and Pelvic Floor

8

Lewis Chan, Vincent Tse, and Tom Jarvis

Contents

Introduction	126
Pelvic Floor Ultrasound: Imaging Modalities	126
Use of Ultrasound as the Imaging Modality for Video Urodynamics	126
Dynamic Imaging	129
Pelvic Floor Ultrasound in the Evaluation of Sling and Mesh Complications	129
Sling Failure	129
Obstructive Sling	130
Sling Erosion	132
The Patient with Multiple Slings	132
Assessment of Pain	132
Pelvic Floor Ultrasound in the Assessment of Pelvic Organ Prolapse	134
Conclusion	136
Tips	136
Cross-References	137
References	137

Supplementary Information: The online version contains supplementary material available at https://doi.org/10.1007/978-3-031-19598-3_8.

L. Chan (✉) · V. Tse
Department of Urology, Concord Repatriation General Hospital and University of Sydney, Sydney, NSW, Australia
e-mail: lewis.chan@sydney.edu.au

T. Jarvis
Department of Urology, Prince of Wales Hospital and University of NSW, Randwick, NSW, Australia
e-mail: tomjarvis@ozdoctors.com

© Springer Nature Switzerland AG 2023
F. E. Martins et al. (eds.), *Female Genitourinary and Pelvic Floor Reconstruction*,
https://doi.org/10.1007/978-3-031-19598-3_8

Abstract

Urinary incontinence and pelvic organ prolapse are common conditions encountered in urologic/gynecologic practice. While transvaginal imaging is the technique of choice for imaging of the pelvic organs, there have been significant developments in the use of ultrasound in the assessment of pelvic floor disorders including 3D/4D ultrasound technologies. The dynamic nature of ultrasound imaging is ideally suited to imaging of the pelvic floor, which can be conducted by transabdominal, transvaginal, and transperineal approaches. This chapter discusses the role of pelvic floor ultrasound in the evaluation of the patient presenting with urinary incontinence, voiding dysfunction, pelvic organ prolapse, and mesh complications.

Keywords

Ultrasound · Pelvic floor · Translabial · Transperineal · Incontinence · Pelvic organ prolapse · Mesh · Sling · 3D ultrasound

Introduction

Assessment of the female patient with pelvic floor dysfunction is generally based on a through history, physical examination, and functional evaluation including urodynamics. Traditional imaging modalities such as urinary tract ultrasound and transvaginal ultrasound have established roles in general imaging survey of the urinary tract and genital tract, respectively. There is increasing utilization of ultrasound in the assessment of the female pelvic floor. The female pelvis can be imaged via transabdominal, transperineal, and transvaginal/introital approaches. While transvaginal imaging is the technique of choice for imaging of the pelvic organs, there have been significant developments in the use of ultrasound in the assessment of pelvic floor disorders including 3D/4D ultrasound in the assessment of pelvic organ prolapse over the past 15 years [1]. This chapter discusses the role of pelvic floor ultrasound imaging in the evaluation of female pelvic floor dysfunction, including urinary incontinence, voiding dysfunction, pelvic organ prolapse, and mesh complications.

Pelvic Floor Ultrasound: Imaging Modalities

Transabdominal ultrasound is often the initial modality of imaging in the assessment of patients with lower urinary tract symptoms. An ultrasound scan performed via the transabdominal route allows easy assessment of the bladder, post-void residual (PVR) urine measurements, identification of ureteric jets, and general survey of female pelvic organs. There is also a role in the assessment of upper urinary tract especially in cases of voiding dysfunction or suspected neurogenic bladder.

However, in the assessment of voiding dysfunction, urinary incontinence, and pelvic organ prolapse, transperineal or introital approaches (Fig. 1) allow for an easy, noninvasive method of imaging the three compartments of the pelvic floor. Furthermore, there is little distortion of anatomy and patient discomfort because the transducer is placed externally. The examination is relatively quick and easily performed at the bedside or clinic setting.

Transperineal imaging is often conducted with the patient in supine position (Fig. 1), but the standing position (Fig. 2) can be utilized and is useful for the assessment of incontinence and pelvic organ prolapse. Transperineal 2D ultrasound can be performed using standard grayscale ultrasound equipment and the curved array transducer (e.g., 2–5 MHz) used for transabdominal imaging (Tips 1). Introital ultrasound is performed using an endocavity transducer (e.g., 3–9 MHz) used for transvaginal imaging with the transducer placed at the introitus.

For most patients with voiding dysfunction, incontinence, and pelvic organ prolapse, 2D imaging is sufficient, but 3D imaging has an emerging role in the evaluation of prolapse and mesh complications.

Use of Ultrasound as the Imaging Modality for Video Urodynamics

Urodynamics are a commonly performed investigation in the evaluation of patients with bothersome urinary symptoms and incontinence and arguably remain the "gold standard" test. Traditionally video urodynamics have utilized fluoroscopic imaging. However, not all clinicians have access to radiological equipment, and there is the risk of radiation exposure to the patient and occupational exposure to the clinician, as well as the requirement to wear heavy protective garments.

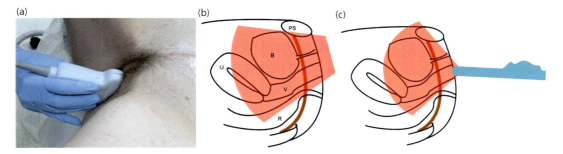

Fig. 1 Transducer placement for transperineal (translabial) (**a**, **b**) and introital (**c**) ultrasound

Fig. 2 Transducer placement for transperineal ultrasound with the patient standing (useful for demonstration of urethral hypermobility and pelvic organ prolapse)

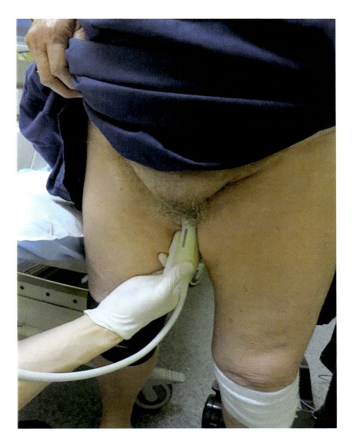

Furthermore, depending on the equipment, the patient may have to transfer on and off a fluoroscopy table. This poses difficulty for the elderly or patients with neurologic disease. Ultrasound imaging (abdominal and transperineal routes) provides an alternative imaging modality of the lower urinary tract during urodynamics (Fig. 3). Transperineal imaging, in particular, allows good visualization of the pelvic floor and arguably provides more information than contrast fluoroscopy in females for the assessment of urinary incontinence and pelvic organ prolapse as all three compartments of the pelvis can be demonstrated (Fig. 4). Ultrasound can also identify if there is mesh or sling present as these are easily visible on ultrasound imaging. A protocol for using ultrasound as an imaging modality during urodynamics is attached (Tips 2).

Fig. 3 Examination room setup for multi-channel urodynamics with ultrasound imaging

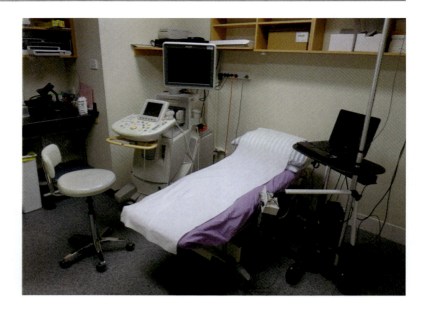

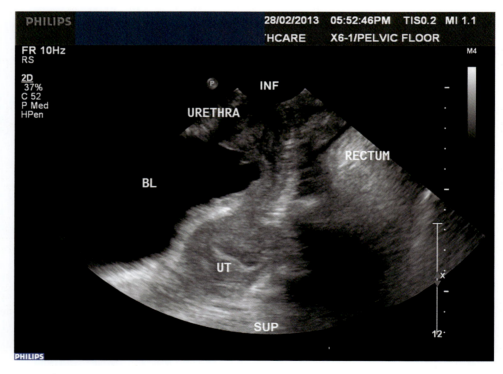

Fig. 4 Sagittal transperineal ultrasound image demonstrating the three compartments of the pelvis. B Bladder, U urethra, V vagina, R rectum, PS pubic symphysis, Inf- inferior/caudal, sup- superior/cranial

Dynamic Imaging

The ability of ultrasound to obtain real-time, dynamic imaging information is an important advantage of this modality of imaging in the assessment of the pelvic floor. This should be tailored to the clinical problem, hence the importance of clinician input in the performance of scans.

Dynamic assessment during transperineal ultrasound includes evaluation of the bladder neck and urethral mobility (see Video 1), pelvic organ prolapse during Valsalva and cough, as well as pelvic floor contractions. Some of these may be best performed with the patient in the standing position (Fig. 2). Dynamic imaging can be incorporated as part of video urodynamics.

Pelvic floor ultrasound can also be used as an adjunct for pelvic floor physiotherapy. This can be performed via transabdominal or more recently transperineal approaches and is usually performed with some urine in the bladder (e.g., about 1–200 mls) but not overfilled. Dynamic 2D imaging can detect pelvic floor contraction/"lift" (see Video 2). 3D/4D imaging may be utilized in guiding botulinum toxin injections to the pelvic floor in the treatment of chronic pelvic pain related to pelvic floor hyperactivity [2].

Pelvic Floor Ultrasound in the Evaluation of Sling and Mesh Complications

The mid-urethral synthetic sling (MUS) procedure has been a common treatment for female stress urinary incontinence with durable medium- to long-term outcomes. Multiple studies have demonstrated the efficacy of the MUS with a low morbidity [3]. However, a small number of patients will have complications following MUS including failure, obstructive voiding, sling erosion, or chronic pain [4, 5]. These issues are especially topical with the current controversy regarding the safety of synthetic mesh use in vaginal surgery for the treatment of pelvic organ prolapse and withdrawal of mesh products in many countries.

Apart from a thorough history and careful physical examination, the evaluation of a patient with potential sling complications includes functional assessment (such as urinary flow study, post-void residual urine measurement, and urodynamics), cystourethroscopy, and imaging. For complex patients, multiple investigative modalities may be necessary to fully evaluate the situation and formulate a management plan.

A synthetic mid-urethral sling is very echogenic and is easily visualized on ultrasound imaging compared to other imaging modalities such as CT scan and MRI where the mesh is generally difficult to visualize. The development of 3D and dynamic 3D (so-called 4D) ultrasound technologies allows the assessment of sling and pelvic structures in multiple imaging planes, similar to what can be achieved with MRI (Fig. 5). 3D ultrasound of the pelvic floor can be performed using the transperineal approach or introital approach (with intracavity 3D transducer). Ultrasound allows real-time dynamic imaging of the sling and other pelvic structures with better temporal resolution than single plane functional MRI and can contribute to functional as well as anatomic assessment of sling problems.

Sling Failure

There is imaging evidence to suggest that the synthetic mid-urethral sling provides posterior support to the urethra and, in particular, urethral compression during cough and Valsalva. This has been demonstrated on real-time imaging and suggests that this is a mechanism of action of these types of sling (Video 3) [6–8]. Ultrasound, therefore, has a role in the evaluation of the patient who has ongoing stress incontinence following placement of a mid-urethral sling. The various parameters reported in the literature include distance of sling to the urethra, sling to pubic symphysis, sling angle, and location of the sling relative to the mid-urethra or bladder neck [1, 9].

While the reported studies correlating these measurement parameters to clinical outcomes/success have been inconclusive [7, 10, 11], it is

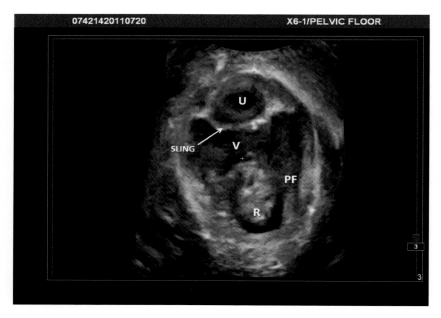

Fig. 5 Axial reconstruction of 3D volume in patient with stress incontinence cured by a trans-obturator synthetic sling. U urethra, V vagina, R rectum, PF pelvic floor muscle

important to realize that there can be multiple reasons for sling failure rather than just inadequate compression or poor positioning. For example, imaging findings such as an open bladder neck or proximal urethra may suggest the presence of intrinsic urethral sphincter deficiency (Fig. 6a, b).

The lack of dynamic compression on imaging may suggest either loosening of the sling (which may have occurred if the patient return to vigorous activity early postoperatively) or indeed technical failure with poor positioning of the sling at the time of the procedure. Longitudinal ultrasound studies of sling location have shown that there is no significant change in sling position over time [12].

Obstructive Sling

Patients with an obstructive mid-urethral sling may present with voiding dysfunction, an elevated post-void residual, worsening of overactive bladder symptoms, or pain; a high index of suspicion is warranted in such patients. While urodynamics remains the gold standard in evaluating obstruction in male patients, there is currently no consensus regarding the urodynamic parameters for the diagnosis of bladder outlet obstruction in females. As such, the diagnosis of sling obstruction is often a clinical decision based on de novo symptoms and signs following sling insertion. Ultrasound imaging, therefore, adds to the evaluation armamentarium for the patient with an obstructive sling and can provide information on sling location, bladder/urethral axis, and dynamics of sling motion during rest and on Valsalva. This can be demonstrated easily with the echogenicity of the synthetic sling but can also be seen in patients with pubovaginal fascial slings (Video 4). This is important especially given that some patients are Valsalva voiders. A common finding in patients with an obstructive sling is the angulation of the urethral axis (Fig. 7) especially if this is observed in the resting state [13]. Other sonographic findings reported in obstructive slings include a short distance between the sling and the urethra/pubic symphysis and abnormalities of sling configuration around the urethra [11, 13].

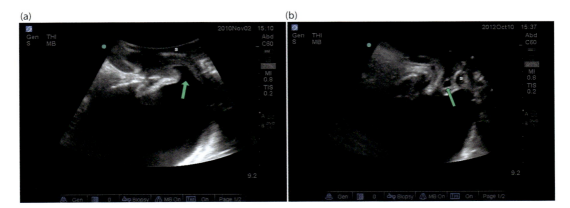

Fig. 6 (a) Failed mid-urethral sling. Transperineal ultrasound in a patient with persisting urinary incontinence following mid-urethral sling surgery. Note open bladder neck/proximal urethra due to intrinsic urethral sphincter deficiency (arrow). Mid-urethral sling (s). (b) Post injection of bulking agent. Transperineal ultrasound in the same patient (as **a**) following injection of bulking agent (Bulkamid®, hypoechoic area – arrow) demonstrating coaptation of the proximal urethra above the level of the sling

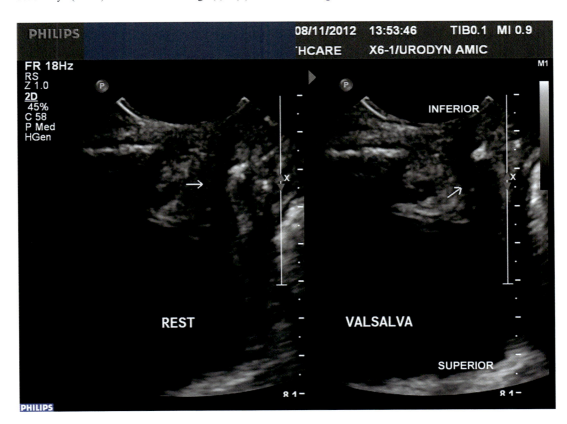

Fig. 7 Transperineal ultrasound images in a patient with voiding dysfunction post mid-urethral sling demonstrating angulation and kinking of the urethra by the sling (arrow) both at rest and during Valsalva (right image)

Sling Erosion

While sling exposure or extrusion into the vagina is easily assessed on clinical examination and erosion of the sling into the urethra is generally diagnosed on cystourethroscopy, these findings can also be demonstrated on ultrasound (Fig. 8) [14, 15]. Slings which have eroded into the urinary tract for a long period of time may become calcified and easily visible on ultrasound. Furthermore, information about the configuration of the arms of the sling outside the urethra and location of any bulking agents obtained on imaging, especially using 3D ultrasound volume reconstruction, may assist the surgeon in operative management (Fig. 9).

The Patient with Multiple Slings

Both 2D and 3D ultrasound can be useful in the assessment of the complex patient who has undergone several sling procedures or has persisting problems despite surgery for sling-related complications. In the patient who has persisting voiding dysfunction following sling division for obstruction, 3D ultrasound with multiplanar reconstruction can assess whether sufficient sling division has been achieved (Fig. 10a, b).

3D transperineal ultrasound is of particular value in the assessment of complex patients with multiple slings or other meshes in the anterior or apical compartment of the pelvis. 3D imaging can demonstrate the location of sling(s), while 2D imaging can demonstrate the dynamics of the slings with activity. This can be useful if division or excision of one or more slings is planned (Fig. 11).

Assessment of Pain

Pain following mesh procedures is often multifactorial and best managed in the context of

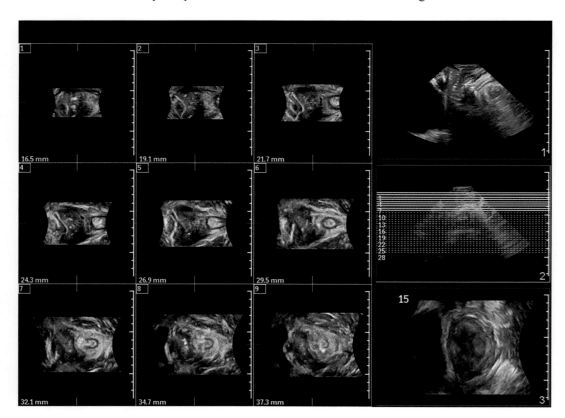

Fig. 8 Multiplanar reconstruction of 3D volume in patient with voiding dysfunction and two previous suburethral slings showing erosion of the first sling into urethral lumen (images 3-6)

8 Ultrasound Imaging of the Female Lower Urinary Tract and Pelvic Floor 133

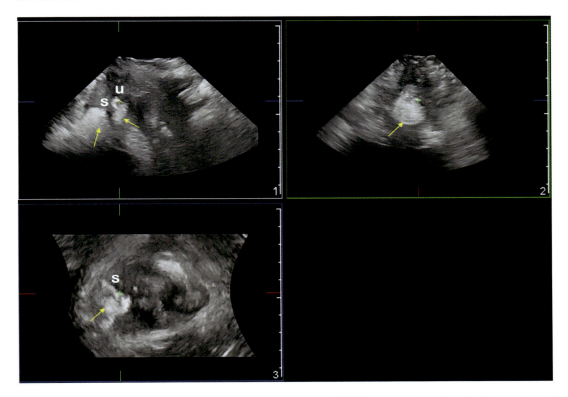

Fig. 9 Multiplanar reconstruction of 3D pelvic floor volume (Image 1 – sagittal, Image 2 – coronal, Image 3 – axial plane). Patient with recurrent urinary infections and voiding dysfunction following previous transobturator sling and bulking agent injection showing erosion of sling (s) into urethral lumen and echogenic bulking agent (arrow, Macroplastique® implant) anterior and posterior to the urethra (u)

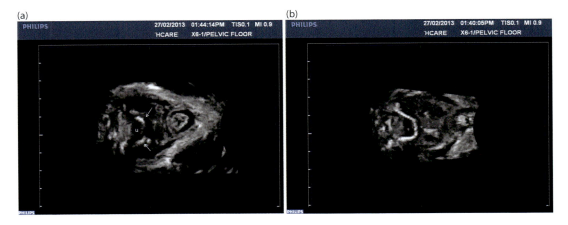

Fig 10 (**a**, **b**) Transperineal 3D ultrasound images in patient with persisting voiding dysfunction post sling division demonstrating insufficient division of the sling with a segment of sling continuity (**b**)

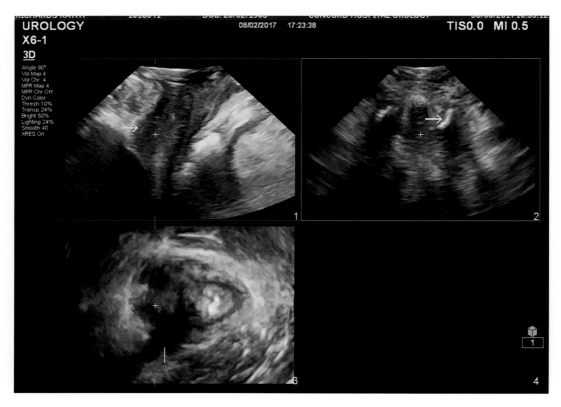

Fig. 11 Multiplanar reconstruction of 3D volume showing obstructive fascial sling (arrow, image1) and residual synthetic sling post division (arrow, image 2)

multidisciplinary team and multimodal approach. Imaging is of value in assessing the extent of mesh and the surrounding pelvic structures. 2D dynamic ultrasound can demonstrate the position of the mesh with movement, different postures, and activity. 3D ultrasound is of use in demonstrating mesh material and the relationship with pelvic organs. However, the retropubic or transobturator parts of the MUS may be difficult to visualize on ultrasound due to shadow artifact from adjacent bony structures. In the patient with suspected infected mesh material as the cause of pain, an MRI scan is of value in detecting inflammatory changes around the mesh (increased signal intensity on T2-weighted sequence). Transvaginal ultrasound can be used to correlate pain on examination with the presence or absence of mesh material at the site of pain (Video 5). This information may be valuable to assist the surgeon in planning the optimal surgical approach and providing informed consent as a number of such patients will eventually undergo excision of the mesh [14].

Pelvic Floor Ultrasound in the Assessment of Pelvic Organ Prolapse

Advances in 2D/3D ultrasound imaging has opened new opportunities for studying the functional anatomy of the pelvic floor. Pelvic organ prolapse (POP) can be imaged by transperineal (translabial) or introital approaches (Fig. 1). While POP is routinely assessed by clinical examination, 2D/3D pelvic floor ultrasound can clearly demonstrate to the pelvic floor surgeon which pelvic viscera are involved in the prolapse and the degree (stage) of prolapse (Fig. 12, Videos 6 and 7). The imaging findings can add to the

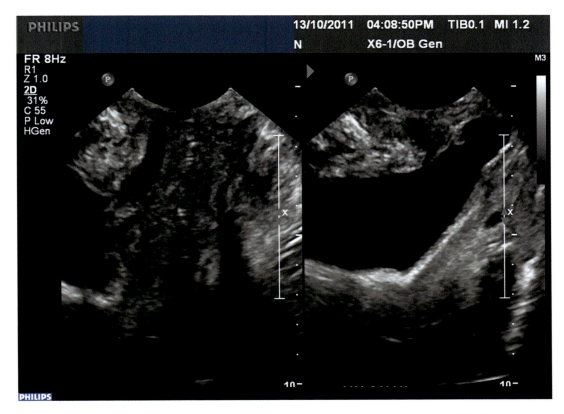

Fig. 12 Sagittal transperineal ultrasound images of patient with POP-Q stage 3 cystocele at rest (left) and on Valsalva (right). Note that the urethral axis tilts caudally almost 90 degrees during maximal Valsalva, and a large cystocele is seen protruding through the region of the introitus

clinical examination findings and assist the surgeon in deciding what type of reconstruction is most suitable for the patient. Occasionally, what is seen during physical examination may represent clinical understaging or false negatives of the actual prolapse present. This is due to levator co-activation which can prevent the maximal extent of the prolapse from presenting at the bedside. This phenomenon can often be seen on ultrasound and may be due to a generalized defensive reflex [16]. A protocol for ultrasound imaging of POP is attached (Tips 3).

One of the pathophysiological factors in POP is levator avulsion (LA), thought to be predominantly related to obstetric trauma [17, 18]. 3D imaging is of particular importance in the assessment of this entity as the levator ani muscle is well demonstrated in the axial plane (Fig. 5). Dietz et al. [19] have reported in uro-gynecological patient cohorts that the presence of LA is associated with a twofold increased risk of stage 2 or above POP (mainly cystocele and uterine prolapse). Furthermore, when LA is identified, it is often associated with paravaginal defects and may have implications regarding surgical reconstructive approach (Fig. 13). In patients undergoing native tissue cystocele repair, the presence of LA on pelvic floor ultrasound may be associated with an increased risk of treatment failure/recurrence [20]. Thus, the presence of LA, enterocele, rectocele, or entero-rectocele, and associated adnexal pathology on imaging may give the pelvic floor reconstructive surgeon further preoperative planning information in regard to surgical approaches. However, levator defects are not associated with urinary symptoms or voiding dysfunction [19].

3D pelvic floor ultrasound is also useful in understanding what happens when surgery fails,

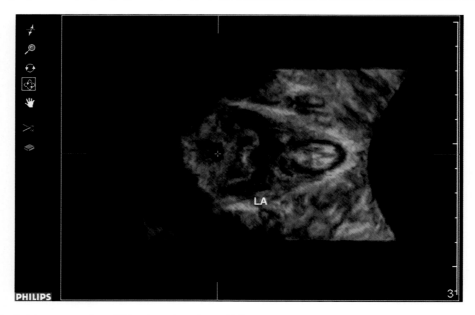

Fig. 13 Axial reconstruction of 3D volume in patient with levator tear (LA) and stage 1 rectocele

especially if there has been placement of synthetic meshes. Shek et al. demonstrated on 3D imaging that POP recurrence after anterior mesh reconstruction can occur dorsal to the mesh, implying dislodgement of the mesh arms [21].

If a patient presents with de novo dyspareunia after mesh repair, 3D ultrasound may also be useful in assessing the configuration and location of the mesh in addition to clinical vaginal examination. The mesh may appear crenulated and folded on ultrasound, corresponding to induration or firm bands palpable on clinical examination. Identification of such findings may reflect on the technical issues during mesh placement and assist in planning surgical correction/mesh removal.

Conclusion

2D and 3D pelvic floor ultrasound has an emerging role in the evaluation of patients with voiding dysfunction, pelvic organ prolapse, and complications following sling surgery. Imaging findings should be interpreted in the context of clinical presentation, physical examination, and urodynamic findings. 3D pelvic floor ultrasound can assist the clinician in the management of complex patients especially those who have multiple mid-urethral slings or mesh complications.

Tips

1. **A technique of transperineal 2D imaging**
    Indications
    Assessment of urinary incontinence, pelvic organ prolapse, and slings/mesh complications.
    Equipment
    Transperineal (translabial) 2D ultrasound can be performed using standard grayscale ultrasound equipment and the curved array transducer (e.g. 2–5 MHz) used for transabdominal imaging.
    Transducer placement
    The transducer is placed on the perineum in the sagittal plane (Fig. 1), and the image can be orientated according to the preference of the clinician. The key anatomic landmarks are the pubic symphysis, urethra, bladder, vagina, and rectum (Fig. 4).

Scanning position

Patient can be scanned in the supine or standing positions. It is important to avoid excessive pressure of the transducer against the perineum as this may cause discomfort and/or distort anatomy.

Movements of the transducer

The "rocking" maneuver allows the field of view to be adjusted covering the compartment of interest (anterior, middle, or posterior). It is important to adjust the depth-of-view setting to the region of interest.

2. **Imaging protocol for ultrasound urodynamics in the female patient**

   (a) Transabdominal imaging of bladder at beginning of filling phase to confirm catheter position if necessary

   (b) Bladder imaging at filling volume of 150 ml

   (c) Upper tract imaging (hydronephrosis/calculi) especially in neurogenic bladder patients

   (d) Repeat bladder imaging ± upper tract imaging at or near capacity (to identify reflux)

   (e) Dynamic translabial imaging (bladder neck/urethra/ POP) performed with patient standing after removal of filling catheter, at rest and on Valsalva/cough

   (f) Bladder neck descent/mobility measured relative to inferior aspect of pubic symphysis in mid sagittal plane

   (g) Assessment of pelvic floor contraction

   (h) Post-void residual measurement at the end of urodynamics

3. **Protocol for ultrasound imaging of POP**

   - Lighting should be dim in the examination room.
   - Female chaperone should be present during the examination.
   - Imaging can be performed in the setting of urodynamic testing or in the office with at least 200 ml of bladder volume.
   - Static images obtained first of the disposition of the pelvic viscera.
   - Dynamic images with the patient at rest and performing a Valsalva maneuver, noting bladder neck/urethra mobility and the presence of urodynamic stress incontinence or occult stress incontinence after reduction of the prolapse; also note the most dependent point of the prolapse for POP-Q assessment.

   - Avoid excessive pressure on the introitus with the transducer during the examination as it may cause discomfort and may obscure the severity of the prolapse.
   - Upper tract imaging (hydronephrosis/calculi) especially in higher stage prolapse or in a patient with unexplained deterioration in renal function.
   - Assessment of pelvic floor contraction.
   - Post-void residual measurement if done in conjunction with urodynamics.

Cross-References

▶ Clinical Evaluation of the Female Lower Urinary Tract and Pelvic Floor
▶ Endoscopic Evaluation
▶ Urodynamic Evaluation: Traditional, Video, and Ambulatory Approaches

Author's Contributions L. Chan – project development, data collection, manuscript writing
V. Tse – data collection, manuscript writing, editing
T. Jarvis – manuscript writing and editing
The authors have no potential conflicts of interest to disclose.

References

1. Shek KL, Dietz HP. Imaging of slings and meshes. Australas J Ultrasound Med. 2014;17(2):61–71.
2. Nesbitt-Hawes EM, Dietz HP, Abbott JA. Four-dimensional ultrasound guidance for pelvic floor botulinum toxin-A injection in chronic pelvic pain: a novel technique. Ultrasound Obstet Gynecol. 2018;51(3): 396–400.
3. Fusco F, Abdel-Fattah M, Chapple CR, Creta M, La Falce S, Waltregny D, et al. Updated systematic review and meta-analysis of the comparative data on colposuspensions, pubovaginal slings, and midurethral tapes in the surgical treatment of female stress urinary incontinence. Eur Urol. 2017;72(4):567–91.
4. Blaivas JG, Purohit RS, Benedon MS, Mekel G, Stern M, Billah M, et al. Safety considerations for synthetic sling surgery. Nat Rev Urol. 2015;12(9):481–509.

5. Brubaker L, Norton PA, Albo ME, Chai TC, Dandreo KJ, Lloyd KL, et al. Adverse events over two years after retropubic or transobturator midurethral sling surgery: findings from the Trial of Midurethral Slings (TOMUS) study. Am J Obstet Gynecol. 2011;205(5): 498 e1–6.

6. Shek KL, Chantarasorn V, Dietz HP. The urethral motion profile before and after suburethral sling placement. J Urol. 2010;183(4):1450–4.

7. Hegde A, Nogueiras M, Aguilar VC, Davila GW. Dynamic assessment of sling function on transperineal ultrasound: does it correlate with outcomes 1 year following surgery? Int Urogynecol J. 2017;28 (6):857–64.

8. Dietz HP, Wilson PD. The 'iris effect': how two-dimensional and three-dimensional ultrasound can help us understand anti-incontinence procedures. Ultrasound Obstet Gynecol. 2004;23(3):267–71.

9. Dietz HP. Pelvic floor ultrasound in incontinence: what's in it for the surgeon? Int Urogynecol J. 2011;22(9):1085–97.

10. Kociszewski J, Fabian G, Grothey S, Kuszka A, Zwierzchowska A, Majkusiak W, et al. Are complications of stress urinary incontinence surgery procedures associated with the position of the sling? Int J Urol. 2017;24(2):145–50.

11. Takacs P, Larson K, Scott L, Cunningham TD, DeShields SC, Abuhamad A. Transperineal sonography and urodynamic findings in women with lower urinary tract symptoms after sling placement. J Ultrasound Med. 2017;36(2):295–300.

12. Majkusiak W, Pomian A, Tomasik P, Horosz E, Zwierzchowska A, Kociszewski J, et al. Does the suburethral sling change its location? Int J Urol. 2017;24: 848–53.

13. Larson K, Scott L, Cunningham TD, Zhao Y, Abuhamad A, Takacs P. Two-dimensional and three-dimensional transperineal ultrasound findings in women with high-pressure voiding after midurethral sling placement. Female Pelvic Med Reconstr Surg. 2017;23(2):141–5.

14. Manonai J, Rostaminia G, Denson L, Shobeiri SA. Clinical and ultrasonographic study of patients presenting with transvaginal mesh complications. Neurourol Urodyn. 2016;35(3):407–11.

15. Staack A, Vitale J, Ragavendra N, Rodriguez LV. Translabial ultrasonography for evaluation of synthetic mesh in the vagina. Urology. 2014;83(1): 68–74.

16. Dietz HP. Why pelvic floor surgeons should utilize ultrasound imaging. Ultrasound Obstet Gynecol. 2006;28(5):629–34.

17. Dietz HP, Simpson JM. Levator trauma is associated with pelvic organ prolapse. BJOG. 2008;115(8):979–84.

18. Steensma AB, Konstantinovic ML, Burger CW, de Ridder D, Timmerman D, Deprest J. Prevalence of major levator abnormalities in symptomatic patients with an underactive pelvic floor contraction. Int Urogynecol J. 2010;21(7):861–7.

19. Dietz HP, Steensma AB. The prevalence of major abnormalities of the levator ani in urogynaecological patients. BJOG. 2006;113(2):225–30.

20. Dietz HP, Chantarasorn V, Shek KL. Levator avulsion is a risk factor for cystocele recurrence. Ultrasound Obstet Gynecol. 2010;36(1):76–80.

21. Shek KL, Dietz HP, Rane A, Balakrishnan S. Transobturator mesh for cystocele repair: a short- to medium-term follow-up using 3D/4D ultrasound. Ultrasound Obstet Gynecol. 2008;32(1):82–6.

Electrophysiologic Evaluation of the Pelvic Floor

9

Simon Podnar and David B. Vodušek

Contents

Clinical Introduction	140
Tests of Function: An Overview	141
Electromyography: An Overview	141
Pelvic Floor Muscle EMG: An Overview	142
The Motor Unit and the EMG	143
Motor Control and the EMG	143
The Concentric Needle EMG Electrode	144
Placement of Electrodes	144
EMG Findings in the Normal Muscle	144
EMG Findings Due to Muscle Denervation	145
EMG Findings Due to Muscle Reinnervation	145
EMG in Practice	147
EMG Changes After Vaginal Delivery: EMG in Idiopathic Incontinence	148
EMG in Women with Urinary Retention	148
EMG Changes in Primary Muscle Disease	149
Testing Conduction Across Nerves and Nervous Pathways: An Overview	149
Testing Motor Conduction in the Pelvic Area: An Overview	150
Testing Sensory Conduction in the Pelvic Area: An Overview	151

S. Podnar (✉)
Division of Neurology, University Medical Centre
Ljubljana, Ljubljana, Slovenia
e-mail: simon.podnar@kclj.si

D. B. Vodušek
Institute of Clinical Neurophysiology, Division of
Neurology, University Medical Centre Ljubljana,
Ljubljana, Slovenia

© Springer Nature Switzerland AG 2023
F. E. Martins et al. (eds.), *Female Genitourinary and Pelvic Floor Reconstruction*,
https://doi.org/10.1007/978-3-031-19598-3_9

Testing Reflexes in the Pelvic Area: An Overview	152
Testing Autonomic Reflexes in the Pelvic Area: An Overview	153
The Sympathetic Skin Response	153
Usefulness of Uroneurophysiology	153
Conclusion	154
References	154

Abstract

An urogynecological patient with a suspected neurogenic pelvic floor/pelvic organ dysfunction requires a basic neurological history and examination. Such patients may for various reasons be candidates for uroneurophysiological testing. Particularly (quantitative) concentric needle EMG and recording the clitorocavernosus/bulbocavernosus reflex is recommended as standard (and standardized) procedure in selected patients, particularly if they are candidates for invasive therapeutic procedures. The limitations of functional testing of the lower urinary tract innervation have to be acknowledged. In this chapter, all uroneurophsiological tests are described and commented.

Keywords

Pelvic floor EMG · Bulbocavernosus reflex · Pudendal somatosensory evoked potentials · Motor evoked potentials · Striated sphincter denervation

Clinical Introduction

This chapter aims at describing clinical neurophysiological (electrophysiological) tests of the pelvic floor and their clinical utility. It has to be understood that such testing needs to be placed in the context of the overall clinical picture of the patient, and particularly considering the neurological aspects. Therefore, we begin – same as the electrophysiological evaluation should begin – by considering the clinical information.

Electrophysiological evaluation is considered in selected patients with an ano-genito-urinary dysfunction (often called also "pelvic floor dysfunction") in whom a neurological origin of their dysfunction is suspected. In these patients a neurological examination should be performed first.

A neurological consult will be most fruitful if the neurologist is experienced in the field of uroneurology, which is to say with patients with neurogenic lower urinary tract, anorectal, and sexual dysfunction. The preference for such a consult is obvious, but may not be available everywhere. When the patient has to be seen by a physician without such experience, he/she should be acquainted with the neurocontrol of pelvic organs, the somatic and autonomic innervation of the body, and the pathophysiology of neurogenic autonomic dysfunctions.

As for the clinical "uro-neurological" assessment a pragmatic "minimum" is recommended.

The history should include an inquiry into neurologic symptoms (sensory, motor, autonomic, cognitive). Sensory phenomena (like paresthesiae) are the most sensitive indicators of nervous system involvement, as already damage to few sensory axons produces symptoms (for motor symptoms, the deficit has to be significantly larger to become noticed). All autonomic symptoms need to be explored (not only urinary, bowel, and sexual symptoms, but also orthostatic intolerance and alterations in sweating). Previous history of surgeries and trauma is important as these might have lesioned the innervation of pelvic organs.

A brief assessment of cognition is recommended. The overall motility, muscle tone and strength (particularly in lower limbs), myotatic reflexes, and the plantar response are to be examined. Checking for loss of fine touch and pain (pinprick) sensations is useful. While for the mentioned exam the patient would be wearing underwear, the neurologic exam of the lower sacral segments is obviously performed (discreetly) without underwear. Inspection of the lower back for nevus, hypertrichosis, or sinus, the feet for deformities, or muscle atrophy, and the anogenital area for morphological particularities might provide clues for the nature of the problem.

The motor and the sensory regional exams may reveal abnormalities not suspected by performing the general exam. The motor part of the examination of the anogenital region involves palpation of the levator ani and the anal sphincter for tone, voluntary contraction, and reflex contraction. The anal reflex (S2 to S4/5 segments) should be tested on both sides.

The finished clinical assessment will support (or not) the suspicion of a neurological cause of the dysfunction. It may qualify the suspicion with a hypothesis of the location and the nature of the neurological lesion.

The logical extensions of the clinical examination are functional tests, although in practice laboratory testing and imaging are often the first to be prescribed.

Normal function of pelvic organs requires intact central and peripheral neural control. Changes within relevant neural pathways (structural, ischemic, demyelinating) can cause LUT dysfunction. MRI of the brain, spinal cord, or pelvis can reveal these changes, but it has to be remembered that changes in morphology and function cannot be equated and often do not correlate well.

Tests of Function: An Overview

Function (motor, sensory, autonomic, cognitive) is assessed by history, followed by examination and methods developed to test individual function. Functional tests are direct extensions of the clinical examination. They can be divided into tests of the nervous system and muscle function, and tests of the pelvic organ function. The main tests of the nervous system and muscle function are quantitative sensory tests and clinical neurophysiological tests. The tests of pelvic organ function are urodynamics, anorectal functional tests, and genital function tests (not dealt with in this chapter).

Quantitative sensory tests have been advocated to add to the diagnosis of neuropathy in the anogenital region. Measuring the vibration perception threshold on the glans clitoris has been advocated for diagnosing sensory neuropathy [4]. Testing for clitoral and perineal thermal sensation may be informative about the presence of autonomic neuropathy, as autonomic fibers also are small diameter nerve fibers [35].

Recordings of bioelectrical activity from the nervous system and striated muscles have been found clinically useful in neuromuscular disorders. These tests are many and are grouped together into subcategories according to different criteria. It is practical to distinguish the recordings from muscle (electromyography) and the tests of nerve and nervous pathway function (conduction studies). Clinical neurophysiological tests applied in the diagnosis of pelvic organ dysfunction diagnostics have also been called "uroneurophysiological" [43].

In this chapter we explain the common and – at least to some extent – clinically useful uroneurophysiological tests without going into technical details, which can be found in longer texts aimed at clinical neurophysiologists [1]. As uroneurophysiology has developed from "general" clinical neurophysiology, the explanation of uroneurophysiological tests follows some general remarks on basic clinical neurophysiological tests.

Electromyography: An Overview

Depolarized (activated) striated muscle fibers generate electrical activity. This electrical activity can be recorded using the method called electromyography (EMG).

EMG can be recorded with different type of electrodes, broadly differentiated into intramuscular and "surface." While surface electrodes (usually plaques of varying size made of transducing rubber) record from a larger tissue volume, the intramuscular electrodes (made of metal) record only from the vicinity of the recording surfaces (the electrodes are wires or needles, with limited non-insulated areas that serve for recording). The surface electrodes record a more representative sample of the muscle of interest. But they are also less selective (in case the recording is from small muscles with other muscles lying in close proximity). Recordings are also easily contaminated by "artefacts." (Artifacts are everything that is not the EMG of the muscle of interest). Intramuscular electrodes are more selective, but also invasive [18].

In the (normal) relaxed muscle there is no electrical activity. This is true for most striated muscles apart from sphincters, where there is always – even during sleep – an ongoing firing of some motor units; this is the so-called tonic activity. The sphincters are truly "relaxed" only during voiding or defecation.

Muscle contraction is accompanied by electrical activity (derived from depolarization of muscle cells/fibers, not contraction itself). Thus, periods of muscle contraction are "marked," characterizing the pattern of activity/relaxation of a particular muscle within a particular time period. Such recordings are of interest in rehabilitation medicine and have been called kinesiologic EMG (assessing, for instance, the sequence of activity of leg muscles during walking). For kinesiological EMG, surface electrodes are used as a rule, since there is no need for "high fidelity" recording of the electrical muscle signal.

EMG recordings are furthermore used to diagnose muscle pathology, i.e., distinguish between normal, denervated, reinnervated, or myopathic muscle. For this purpose, needle electrodes are used in practice. In research, some progress is being made by sophisticated computer analysis of the EMG signal from surface recordings [13].

In diagnostics of muscle pathology the usefulness of EMG depends on its ability to detect the so-called (pathological) spontaneous activity and its ability to detect changes in motor unit potential changes.

In summary, EMG may thus be performed (as just described) for two quite distinct, although complementary, purposes. On the one hand, it can reveal the "behavior" (i.e., patterns of activity) of a particular muscle; on the other hand, it can be used to demonstrate whether a muscle is normal, myopathic, or denervated/reinnervated. Although the distinction in purpose is marked, this division is usually not specified and both types of investigation are just called "EMG," which can cause the occasional confusion.

Pelvic Floor Muscle EMG: An Overview

For anatomical, physiological, and practical reasons there are specificities of the pelvic floor and perineal EMG, but the techniques are intrinsically the same for all striated muscles.

Clinical EMG studies of the pelvic floor were sparse till the 1970s. Since then, EMG has been used increasingly in neurourology, urogynecology, and proctology research, and then more and more also as a routine diagnostic investigation.

Pelvic floor/sphincter EMG is also used in some urodynamic laboratories in assessment of lower urinary function. The "kinesiologic" type of EMG recording of the sphincter muscle is applied to demonstrate the (dis)coordination of striated sphincter and bladder contraction [39].

The behavior of the external anal sphincter is recorded by EMG in some laboratories in the assessment of anorectal dysfunction. The "kinesiological" type of pelvic floor EMG is also used as a "biofeedback" tool in pelvic floor physiotherapy. EMG recordings are furthermore used to diagnose pelvic floor/perineal muscles pathology (i.e., whether they are denervated or reinnervated) [24]. For this purpose, the same concentric needle electrodes are used as in general EMG, of different lengths – for the examination of muscles lying close to the skin (anal sphincter) or deep (pubococcygeus).

Apart from anatomical particularities, the sphincter muscles differ in the characteristics of motor units and their recruitment from the limb muscles [29]. Their motor units are smaller and are active throughout the micturition or defecation cycle, apart from the actual bladder and rectal emptying, when they relax.

The Motor Unit and the EMG

Fundamental to understanding the application of EMG methods is knowledge of the structure and function of the motor unit.

Striated muscles are innervated by alpha ("lower") motor neurons in the anterior horns of spinal cord. The motor neurons from the Onuf (striated sphincter) nucleus in the lower sacral segments have several specifics, but this is not crucial in the understanding of the motor unit concept. The axons of the sphincter motor neurons travel as part of the pudendal nerves to the muscle, where the motor axon tapers and branches into several axon terminals; each of them innervates one muscle cell, because of their shape usually called muscle fibers. Thus one lower motor neuron innervates many muscle fibers. The whole unit (one lower motor neuron plus all muscle fibers it innervates) constitute the motor unit. The additional characteristic of the muscle fibers constituting one motor unit is that they are mixed by muscle fibers from other motor units – scatterboard pattern.

EMG activity is generated by depolarization of muscle fibers. The activation of the motor neuron depolarizes all its muscle fibers simultaneously. As a consequence, the needle electrode in the vicinity of this motor unit will record all muscle fibers' action potentials at the same time, thus allowing for summation of individual muscle fiber action potentials into a motor unit potential (MUP). Depolarization of muscle fibers from other motor units will not appear synchronously with the previously mentioned motor unit and will constitute their motor unit potentials. Thus, activation of motor units is recorded as MUPs, each with a typical shape, and quantitative descriptors (e.g., amplitude and duration). Slight contraction will produce a few well-separated MUPs. By contrast, strong muscle contraction will make MUPs to merge into an "interference pattern" where individual MUPs are no longer discernible.

The contraction properties of a motor unit depend on the nature of its constituent muscle fibers. Muscle fibers can be classified according to their twitch tension, speed of contraction, and histochemical staining properties. The fatigue-resistant Type 1 fibers constitute motor units that fire for prolonged periods of time at lower firing frequencies, i.e., "tonically." Type 2 fibers make up motor units that fire briefly and rapidly in bursts, i.e., "phasically." Unfortunately, there is no clinical electrophysiological method that can estimate the proportion of motor units of different muscle fiber types. Nevertheless, in the pelvic floor and sphincters, the majority of muscle fibers are Type 1 (with some regional variation).

Motor Control and the EMG

Motor control of sphincter muscles (and pelvic floor muscles – pubococcygeus, etc.) can be assessed by the kinesiological EMG recording. The distinguishing feature of these muscles is the presence of continuous activity of motor units (even on "relaxation" of the subject), except during micturition or defecation. This "spontaneous" electrical activity in sphincters is due to tonic activity of motor units – and makes sense for the function of sphincter! During voluntary activation or reflex stimulation additional motor units are recruited.

The "behaviour" of muscles depends on the intactness of their motor control. Apart from the voluntary control exerted by the motor cortex, and the regional (sacral) reflexes, sphincter activity is reflexly coordinated with bladder activity. The responsible reflex center is in the pons (brainstem). Lesions of pathways between the pontine micturition center and Onuf's nucleus (the motor nucleus of striated sphincters in the lower sacral segments) cause loss of coordination between the motor command to the bladder and sphincter; instead of a decrease, there is an increase of urethral sphincter contraction during detrusor contraction. This is called detrusor–sphincter dyssinergia and can be demonstrated by simultaneous measurement of sphincter EMG and a pressure flow study (urodynamics) [39]; it can also be "seen" on video-urodynamics.

Poor relaxation and voluntary sphincter contractions during attempt to void (dysfunctional voiding) may mimic dyssinergia in uncooperative patients or in cases of learned abnormal behaviors such as in Hinman syndrome ("non-neurogenic neurogenic bladder") [11].

The Concentric Needle EMG Electrode

Modern EMG started with the introduction of the concentric needle electrode in 1929 [14], the design of which has endured ever since, almost unchanged. Nowadays a single-use disposable electrode is used. It consists of a central insulated platinum wire encased within a steel cannula and the tip ground to give an elliptical area of 580–150 µm. It records spike activity from about 20 muscle fibers. The number of motor unit potentials recorded depends both upon the local arrangement of muscle fibers within the motor unit and the level of contraction of the muscle.

Placement of Electrodes

The anal sphincter is easily located underneath the brownish corrugated skin surrounding the anal aperture, the insertion to be made cc. 1 cm from the aperture. The urethral sphincter in the female is reached with a needle insertion 0.5 cm laterally to the urethral orifice, not very deep beneath the mucosa. The bulbospongiosus muscle is reached by an insertion through the mucosa laterally of the vulva between the small and large labia. A short needle is preferable for examination of the sphincter and bulbospongiosus muscles. The levator ani (pubococcygeus muscle) is "located" by transrectal or transvaginal palpation and reached by a transcutaneous/transperineal insertion of a long needle electrode (Fig. 1.).

EMG Findings in the Normal Muscle

On needle insertion, whenever muscle tissue is penetrated, a burst of potentials indicates depolarization of the excitable membranes of muscle

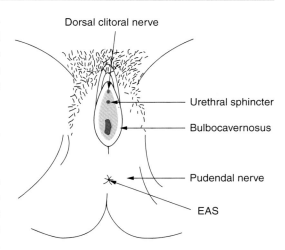

Fig. 1 Needle electrode insertions into pelvic floor and sphincter muscles and positions for electrical stimulation of peripheral nerves in the female perineum. Insertion into the subcutaneous external anal sphincter (EAS) muscle is at about 1 cm from the anal orifice, to a depth of 3–6 mm. For the bulbocavernosus muscle, the needle is inserted 2–3 cm in front of the anal orifice through the skin lateral to the labia majora. The female urethral sphincter is reached from the perineum 0.5 cm lateral to the urethral orifice. The puborectalis (part of levator ani) is inserted at a depth of 5 cm at the anal orifice, at an angle of about 30 degrees to the anal canal axis. The pubococcygeus (part of levator ani) muscle can be located by transrectal or transvaginal palpation and reached transcutaneously from the perineum or transvaginally. The dorsal clitoral nerves are stimulated with the cathode applied to the dorsal clitoris and the anode lateral to it. The pudendal nerves are stimulated posterolateral to the anal orifice by applying firm compression against the medial aspect of the ischial bones

fibers by the mechanical stimulus. This burst is called "insertion activity" and proves the presence of muscle (it is absent after the lesioned muscle fibroses). In the "relaxed subject" the electrode in the sphincter muscle (and most parts of the levator ani) will always – even during sleep – detect an ongoing firing of a few (small amplitude) motor unit potentials (MUPs) – tonic (motor unit) activity. The bulbospongiosus muscle has no tonic activity as it has no "sphincter function."

Reflex and voluntary activation recruits additional MUPs, many of which have somewhat larger amplitudes (but as a rule not above 2 mV). On strong voluntary contraction many MUPs appear, so that practically no "baseline" is seen on the screen anymore, just an "interference pattern" of MUPs.

Most of MUPs are of simple shape, up to 15% are polyphasic. The MUP duration is below 10 ms. The electrode position should be changed systematically in the examined muscle to "sample" the electrical activity in the muscle in a representative way. It is recommended that at least 20 motor unit potentials are sampled.

With computerized EMG machines the sampled MUPs are measured and the sample is statistically evaluated whether the parameters are within reference limits ("quantitative EMG") [30]. An experienced electromyographer can reach the same conclusion by "eyeballing" the electrical activity on the screen, and listening to the sound the various muscle electrical potentials produce. (The frequency content differs between the various examples of muscle electrical activity).

EMG Findings Due to Muscle Denervation

After a lesion of the motorneuron or its axon, all the muscle fibers of that motor unit become denervated. The motor unit is no longer depolarized by its motor neuron; if it is not reinnervated, the muscle fibers will slowly degenerate and finally fibrose.

If the whole motor nerve to the muscle is damaged, all muscle fibers are denervated. There will obviously be no more activation of that muscle. As a consequence, there is no activity ("electrical silence") even on attempted contraction for several days. Between 10 and 20 days after the injury, due to the denervation hypersensitivity of the muscle fibers, insertion activity becomes prolonged and then abnormal spontaneous activity in the form of short biphasic spikes ("fibrillation potentials") and biphasic potentials with prominent positive deflections ("positive sharp waves") appear [33]. In perineal muscles, complete denervation can be observed after traumatic lesions to the lumbosacral spine and damage to the cauda equina.

Most noxes will, however, cause only partial denervation. In partially denervated muscle, some MUPs remain and mingle eventually with abnormal spontaneous activity. As the MUPs in sphincter muscles are also short and mostly bi- or triphasic, and are firing spontaneously (tonical activity), it requires experience to recognize abnormal spontaneous activity in the presence of surviving motor units. The bulbospongiosus muscle, which has no tonic activity, is ideal to demonstrate fibrillation potentials and positive sharp waves after partial denervation in the lower sacral segments.

In long-standing partially denervated muscle, another type of abnormal insertion/spontaneous activity appears: the so-called repetitive discharges (Fig. 2). These are made up of repetitively firing (groups of) potentials. Hypersensitive muscle fibers become depolarized (by the mechanical stimulation of the electrode) and the depolarization spreads to neighboring fibers due to ephaptic transmission, and may become repetitive [33].

Interestingly, in the striated female urethral sphincter such discharges may occasionally be recorded without other indication of neuromuscular disease. When profuse, these discharges can point to the presence of Fowler syndrome [9].

EMG Findings Due to Muscle Reinnervation

After complete denervation, axonal reinnervation may occur. Muscle fibers become innervated, small MUPs appear; first short bi- and triphasic, soon becoming polyphasic, serrated, and of prolonged duration (Fig. 3). After partial denervation, there is a loss of motor units; some MUPs remain. Collateral reinnervation takes place: surviving motor axons will grow out to reinnervate the muscle fibers, which lost their nerve supply. Thus, a previously normal motor unit will obtain additional muscle fibers, becoming "bigger." The arrangement of its muscle fibers within the unit will also change and several muscle fibers belonging to the same motor unit come to be adjacent to one another [32].

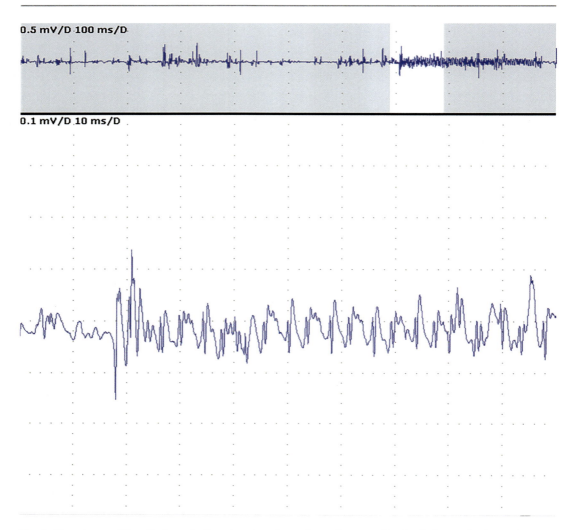

Fig. 2 Complex repetitive discharge in the external anal sphincter muscle of a 57-year-old female patient 1 year after a herpes zoster infection of the sacral segments. She was still suffering from pain in the anogenital area. Neurologically educated reader would note the similarity to the spike and wave epileptic discharges in the EEG. EMG furthermore showed a prevalence of prolonged polyphasic potentials and a delayed latency of the clitoro-anal reflex

Early in the process of reinnervation, the newly outgrown motor sprouts are thin and therefore conduct slowly so that the time taken for excitatory impulses to spread through the axonal tree is abnormally prolonged. This is reflected by prolongation of the waveform of the MUP, which also becomes polyphasic and gets small "late components." Neuromuscular transmission in these newly grown sprouts may also be insecure so that the MUP may show "instability": single muscle fibers' potentials pop in and out of the polyphasic MUP.

The axonal sprouts increase in diameter over time. Their conduction velocity increases. Thus, activation of all parts of the reinnervated bigger motor unit becomes more synchronous; as a consequence the MUP amplitude increases and the duration of the MUP shortens toward normal [32].

There are several conditions in which gross changes of reinnervation may be detected in

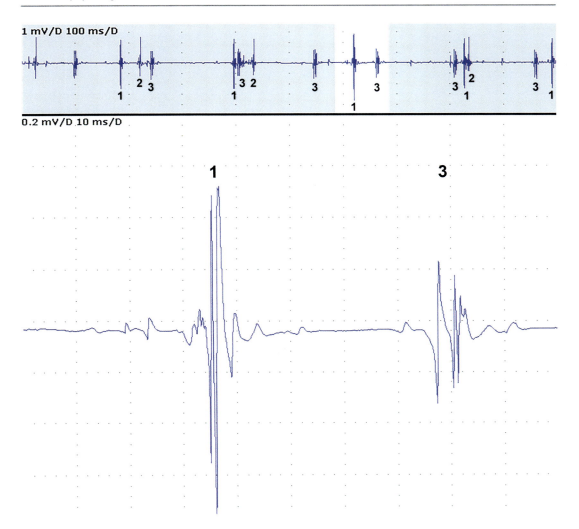

Fig. 3 Two polyphasic motor unit potentials (MUPs) of prolonged duration in the external anal sphincter muscle of a 62-year-old female patient 1 year after an acute onset of pain in the back radiating into both legs, with loss of sensation of bladder fullness and during defecation. An ischemic lesion of the conus was diagnosed. Large majority (80%) of MUPs in that muscle were of similar characteristics. In addition, reduction in the number of voluntarily and reflexly recruited MUPs have also been found

motor units of the pelvic floor: typically after pudendal nerve lesions, cauda equina lesions, in dysraphism and due to some neurodegenerative diseases (as Multiple system atrophy) [24].

EMG in Practice

The EMG exam in the neurophysiological laboratory is performed after an explanation of the procedure to the patient and a clinical appraisal of the clinical problem. The neurological examination focuses on lumbosacral segments and particularly on examination of sensation and reflexes in the anogenital region, which are seldom performed by the referring physicians.

A concentric needle is used for the recording of EMG without application of a local anesthetic, which is mostly unnecessary, and might interfere with the reflexes. As a rule, the exam would start with the anal sphincter. In patients with suspected lesions of sacral myotomes this is the most useful muscle to examine because it is easily accessible and has sufficient muscle bulk. If additional information on abnormal spontaneous activity is necessary, the bulbospongiosus muscles are examined; the tonic motor unit activity present in sphincters if abundant is interfering with the detection of fibrillation potentials and positive sharp waves. The striated urethral sphincter is examined in females with urinary retention (for the presence of repetitive discharges) [9]. The pelvic floor muscles (primarily the pubococcygeus) are examined if required by the clinical hypothesis.

The EMG exam starts with assessment of the "kinesiological" parameters: the activity of motor units during relaxation, during reflex stimulation and on voluntary contraction. In the striated sphincters (and in most insertions in the pelvic floor muscles) tonic activity is diminished after lesions in the sacral reflex arc, and increased in anxious patients. Brisk recruitment of motor units is observed during any patient activity (talking, coughing) and on reflex activation (pricking with a pin in the sacral area). Brisk recruitment should be obtained on voluntary contraction. The demonstration of voluntary and reflex recruitation of motor units in pelvic floor muscles and sphincters is proof of the integrity of respective neural pathways. Also, such recording demonstrates the amount of muscle activation during the particular maneuvers, i.e., the quantity of motor units recruitable reflexly and voluntarily. Because of limitations of the strength of reflex stimuli and the uncertainty of voluntary effort, the real number of (preserved) motor units is not always easy to estimate. The preservation of coordinated bladder-sphincter activity can only be assessed in the urodynamic laboratory [39].

Next, MUPs are evaluated by "eyeballing" (MUPs in tonic activity and on slight reflex and/or voluntary activation), or a quantitative EMG procedure using the algorithm in the EMG machine [30]. The EMG exam of one half of sphincter is as a rule followed by recording the clitoro-anal reflex (see below). The procedure is repeated in the other half of sphincter, and then possibly in other muscles as required to explore the pathology, or support the clinical hypothesis.

EMG Changes After Vaginal Delivery: EMG in Idiopathic Incontinence

Electrophysiological methods have played a major role in establishing the neuromuscular lesion due to vaginal delivery as a risk factor for incontinence and pelvic organ prolapse (in addition to histopathological findings) [10]. The finding of decreased intramuscular nerve density in the female urethral sphincter, which correlates with decreased muscular tissue, provides validation for the reported EMG abnormalities [23]. The abnormalities demonstrated in the anal sphincter have been suggested to be of pathogenetic significance and also for idiopathic fecal incontinence [38].

The development of imaging techniques has improved the diagnosis of postpartum structural (anatomical) damage to pelvic floor structures (including sphincters).

> The usefulness of EMG in individual patients with idiopathic incontinence is limited as its predictive value for treatment outcome has not been established. EMG of pelvic floor muscles in women after vaginal delivery and/or with undefined urinary incontinence should be restricted to the rare cases in whom a substantial pudendal nerve or sacral plexus involvement is suspected [44].

EMG in Women with Urinary Retention

Bladder denervation resulting in poor emptying (retention) would often be accompanied by denervation of pelvic floor muscles (as due to a cauda equina lesion), and thus the underlying pathology may be diagnosed by EMG (unfortunately only 3 weeks after the acute lesion). As the lesion may be occult and the dysfunction chronic, pathological MUP changes (due to reinnervation) will support the diagnosis of a previous lesion of motor neurons in the lower sacral segments [24]. In women with dysfunctional voiding, kinesiologic EMG recorded during an urodynamic assessment of voiding shows inappropriate (voluntary?) activation of sphincter motor units [6].

Some of young women in retention may, however, show profuse complex repetitive discharges on concentric needle EMG of the urethral sphincter and are finally diagnosed as Fowler's syndrome [40]. It has been hypothesized that the abnormal activity leads to sphincter contraction and – as a consequence – an inhibitory effect on the bladder. Isolated urinary retention in young women may rarely be due to multiple sclerosis and in this case no sphincter EMG abnormalities are expected.

EMG Changes in Primary Muscle Disease

So far, concentric needle EMG abnormalities reflecting neurogenic muscle lesions were discussed. EMG changes reflecting primary muscle disease are due to degeneration and loss of muscle fibers within motor units, not due to loss of whole motor units [32]. Reports of EMG features in pelvic floor muscles of patients with myopathy are scarce. Clinically, there seems to be little need for diagnostic sphincter EMG in patients with myopathy.

Testing Conduction Across Nerves and Nervous Pathways: An Overview

Electrophysiological conduction studies examine the capacity of a nerve (or nervous pathway) to transmit a test volley of depolarization elicited by a stimulus along its length (Fig. 4). Tests have been as a rule introduced for limb nerves (and their central connections) and only later modified for uroneurophysiology. Electrical stimulation of a motor (or mixed) nerve along its course will elicit a muscle response, which can be recorded by EMG (the response is called the compound muscle action potential or M wave) [8]. The

nerve roots carrying motor axons for particular muscles can be stimulated over the spinal column, thus testing the conduction over the whole length of the peripheral nerve.

The stimulation of the motor cortex area for particular muscle groups can be achieved from the scalp, thus testing the whole motor pathway (both central and peripheral). The EMG recorded muscle responses on stimulation over the spine and scalp are called motor evoked potentials (MEPs) [5].

Because the motor cortex and spinal nerve roots are distant from the electrodes placed on the surface, their depolarization requires high electrical current (causing pain). Magnetic stimulation achieves such depolarization painlessly and is thus the routine method to elicit muscle responses by spinal or scalp stimulation. Electrical stimulation is used, however, in intraoperative monitoring.

Both the time taken from the application of the stimulus to muscle activation (latency) and the amplitude of the muscle response are measured in limb nerves. The amplitude recorded by surface electrodes that detect from the whole muscle depends on the number of activated motor units and reflects the number of depolarized motor axons, whereas the motor latency (i.e., time to onset of response) and the motor conduction velocity along the nerve reflect the conduction speed of the fastest conducting motor axons [8].

The stimulating and recording pair of electrodes can be placed at some distance from each other on a peripheral nerve. On stimulation, the conducted depolarization of the nerve (called the compound nerve action potential or neurogram) is recorded. The amplitude of this response is related to the number of nerve axons being depolarized. If the stimulated nerve is purely sensory (a peripheral cutaneous nerve) the response is called the sensory neurogram (sensory nerve action potential – SNAP) [8].

On stimulation of sensory nerves or the innervated skin or mucosa the wave of depolarization travels along sensory pathways to the somatosensory cortex. It can be recorded from the spinal

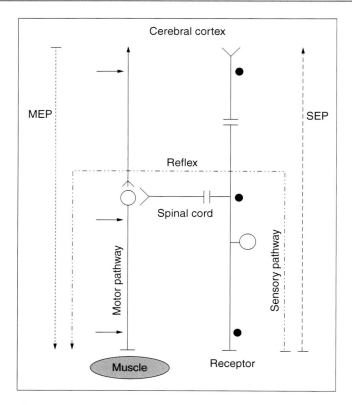

Fig. 4 Components of the somatic sensory and somatic motor systems and the electrophysiological tests that evaluate them. Arrows on the motor (left) side indicate different stimulation sites (from above) of the motor cortex, spinal roots, and peripheral nerves (terminal motor latency test). Small circles on the sensory (right) side indicate different recording sites (from below) from peripheral nerve (sensory nerve action potential, SNAP), spinal roots/cord, and somatosensory cortex. Note that for SNAP recording both distal stimulation and proximal recording or reverse could be employed. In addition, concentric needle electromyography (CNEMG) and single fiber electromyography (SFEMG) assess the lower motor neuron and muscle. Kinesiological EMG evaluates the integrity of upper motor neuron and neurocontrol reflex arcs. *MEP* motor evoked potential, *SEP* somatosensory evoked potential

cord and the brain by surface electrodes (and after averaging many repeated responses). The recorded potentials are called somatosensory evoked potentials (SEPs) [43].

As is appreciated clinically, certain stimuli will elicit particular reflex responses. The physiological stimulation can be replaced by electricity, and the clinical observation of the response by an EMG recording of the respective reflex muscle response. The commonly adopted technique for recording what is clinically called the bulbocavernosus reflex is to apply several repeated single electrical stimuli via surface electrodes to the dorsal clitoral nerve (on the clitoris) and record the consecutive reflex responses from the anal sphincter with a concentric needle EMG electrode. The obtained response has been also called the clitoro-anal reflex [25].

Testing Motor Conduction in the Pelvic Area: An Overview

Measurement of motor conduction velocity is routinely carried out to evaluate limb motor nerves. However, the pudendal nerve is not accessible to noninvasive stimulation at several anatomical points, but only distally. Thus, only the terminal motor latency of the sphincter muscle response (MEP or M wave) can be tested. On electrical stimulation perianally/perineally a M wave can be recorded from the anal sphincter muscle [45]. The more widely employed technique of obtaining the pudendal terminal motor latency relies on stimulation with a special "surface electrode assembly" fixed on a gloved index finger [15]. It consists of a bipolar stimulating electrode fixed to the tip of the gloved finger with the recording electrode pair placed 5 cm proximally on the base of the finger. The finger is inserted into the rectum or vagina and stimulation is performed close to the ischial spine. A "rounded" response is recorded from the surface electrodes at the base of the finger (which is claimed to be the M wave from the external anal sphincter) with a typical latency around 2 ms. This test is usually referred to as the "pudendal nerve terminal motor latency (PNTML) test" [36]. If a catheter-mounted electrode is used, responses from the urethral sphincter can also be obtained. In studies, as a rule, only latencies have been studied (as amplitudes of the M wave response have proved too variable). Research using this test indicated occult damage to the pudendal innervation vaginal delivery, being of pathogenetic importance for idiopathic stress urinary incontinence, fecal incontinence, and pelvic floor prolapse [37]. In many clinics this test was performed in isolation as the only clinical neurophysiological test to prove "pudendal neuropathy."

Most experts now doubt the clinical usefulness of the test: A lack of correlation to sphincter pressure measurements has been demonstrated [47], and the test was also not found to be useful in guiding therapy of fecal incontinence [36]. The American Gastroenterological Association statement indicated that "PNTMLT cannot be recommended for evaluation of patients with fecal incontinence" [3].

In summary, no truly reliable measurement of pelvic floor M waves' amplitude is available. The demonstrated presence of M waves on pudendal nerve stimulation, and MEPs on spinal nerve roots and the motor cortex stimulation can, however, prove the patency of the respective nervous pathways. A selective needle recording of a (sphincter or pelvic floor) muscle response (M wave) on appropriate electrical stimulation may be informative in selected patients with suspected "lower

motor neuron–type" lesions. A well-formed sphincter MEP with a normal latency in a patient with a functional disorder or a medicolegal case may on occasion be helpful.

The anal sphincter MEP has been introduced as an intraoperative monitoring technique in surgeries on the spinal column/spinal cord when the functions of pelvic organs are in danger of an iatrogenic lesion [34]. MEPs allow research on excitability of the motor cortex. It has been demonstrated that in comparison to the motor area for hand muscles, the anal sphincter motor cortex has less intracortical inhibition [16].

Testing Sensory Conduction in the Pelvic Area: An Overview

In the woman, the dorsal clitoral nerve is too short for measuring a sensory neurogram (sensory nerve action potential). However, on electrical stimulation of the clitoral nerve an electroencephalographic (EEG) response can be recorded over the scalp by surface electrodes after averaging many (typically 128) responses. The response is called the pudendal somatosensory evoked response (SEP) [43]. This SEP is of highest amplitude at the recording site Cz -2 cm: Fz (EEG terminology for placement of scalp electrodes), and is highly reproducible. The configuration of the pudendal SEP shows a main positive deflection at c. 40 ms (the P40) [42]. The later waves are interindividually variable.

Pudendal SEP are abnormal in patients with spinal cord lesions, cauda equina lesions, and peripheral nerve lesions [20]. While prolonged SEP latencies in patients with demyelinating lesions may be an early sign of such pathology, most patients with suspected neurogenic involvement of pelvic functions suffer from disorders inducing axonal lesions. Such lesions when mild are not easily detectable by conduction studies because in partial lesions the remaining axons conduct normally and produce a normal latency of the response. Thus, pudendal SEP were less sensitive than a clinical examination when investigating urogenital symptoms for detecting relevant neurological disease [7]. However, when a patient is complaining of loss of bladder or vaginal sensation it may be reassuring to be able to record a normal pudendal SEP. SEPs on clitoral stimulation were reported as a possibly valuable intraoperative monitoring method in patients with cauda equina or conus at risk of a surgical procedure [21].

Pudendal SEPs were used to study the mechanism of sacral neuromodulation [19].

Evoked cortical potentials can also be obtained on stimulation of the bladder urothelium [2], posterior urethra, the anal canal, the rectum, and sigmoid colon [17]. These cerebral potentials have also been shown to have a maximum amplitude over the midline (Cz −2 cm: Fz); but the responses are of a very low amplitude and of variable configuration; it was not possible to identify them in all control subjects. These tests have not been introduced into routine diagnostics.

Testing Reflexes in the Pelvic Area: An Overview

The anal and the bulbocavernosus reflex are elicited in clinical practice to assess the S2–S4 reflex arc. Electrophysiological correlates of these reflexes have been described and are more reliable than the clinically assessed response (e.g., observing or palpating the contraction), particularly in females [46]. Electrical [45], mechanical [31], or magnetic stimulation can be applied to elicit the reflex and the response is recorded as EMG from the target muscle. Apart from the clitoris and the perianal region also the bladder neck/proximal urethra can be stimulated using a catheter-mounted ring electrode and reflex responses obtained from perineal muscles.

Reflex responses can be recorded from any pelvic floor/perineal muscle and the stimuli can be applied at various parts of the anogenital area and pelvic organs; therefore the responses as a group have been referred to as "sacral reflexes." For particular reflex responses it has been suggested to use a compound term consisting of the part where the stimulus was applied and the muscle whose response was recorded (for instance the clitoro-anal reflex for what is traditionally known as the bulbocavernosus reflex) [25].

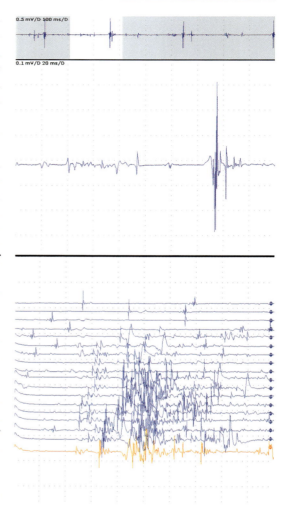

Fig. 5 Concentric needle EMG recordings in the left external anal sphincter of a 61-year-old woman with 6 months history of a subacute onset flaccid paraparesis with urinary incontinence and anorectal sensory loss. Three weeks before examination she had an uneventful embolization of arteriovenous malformation at the level of the third lumbar vertebra. Her urinary incontinence persists. Above high amplitude, long duration, polyphasic motor unit potential that is intermittently recruited (uppermost trace) on full voluntary activation is shown. Below a clitoro-anal reflex of prolonged latency obtained on strong electrical stimulation of the dorsal clitoral nerve is shown. As the stimulus strength was slowly increased (from top to bottom), the reflex first appeared and then stepwise increased in intensity and shortening in the latency

The typical reflex response obtained on electrical stimulation of the dorsal clitoral nerve has a latency between 30 ms and 45 ms in the anal sphincter (Fig. 5). The electrophysiological assessment of sacral reflexes is a more quantitative, sensitive, and reproducible way of assessing the S2–S4 reflex arcs than any of the clinical methods. Clitoro-cavernosus reflex testing is suggested as a complementary test to concentric needle EMG examination of pelvic floor muscles in patients with suspected peripheral nervous lesions [26]. A single electrical pulse is sufficient to elicit a normal reflex, and a reflex in a patient with a minor lesion. In more severe partial lesions a double stimulus will demonstrate the persisting patency of the reflex pathway. An absent reflex response on double stimulus of sufficient current strength indicates severe pathology, possibly the absence of continuity in the reflex arc. A prolonged reflex latency also indicates pathology involving the lower sacral reflex arc. However, a reflex with a normal latency does not exclude the possibility of a partial axonal lesion. A very short reflex latency is seen in tethered cord [12], the shorter latency being attributed to the low location of conus. Continuous intraoperative recording of sacral reflex responses on clitoris stimulation is feasible if double pulses or a train of stimuli are used and has become established in some neurosurgical centers focusing on lower spine surgery [34].

Testing Autonomic Reflexes in the Pelvic Area: An Overview

The uroneurophysiological methods discussed so far assess only the myelinated fibers, whereas it is the autonomic nervous system, and the parasympathetic component in particular, that is most relevant for sacral organ function. While it is true that lesions in the spinal canal (such as trauma, compression, etc.) usually involve both somatic and parasympathetic nerve fibers simultaneously (and thus uroneurophysiological test results may be extrapolated to the parasympathetic fibers), the lesions outside of the spinal canal (such as mesorectal excision of carcinoma or radical hysterectomy) may cause a pure autonomic lesion. Information on parasympathetic bladder innervation can, to some extent, be obtained by cystometry, but direct electrophysiological testing would be desirable.

In cases where a general involvement of autonomic fibers is suspected (as in diabetic polyneuropathy), cardiovascular autonomic innervation can be tested by measuring the respiratory variation of the R-R interval of the EKG signal. An indirect way to examine autonomic fibers (which are thin) is to assess thin sensory fiber function. As unmyelinated afferent fibers transmit temperature sensation and pain, unmyelinated fiber neuropathy can be identified by testing thermal sensitivity, available also as a quantitative sensory testing.

The "sympathetic skin response" (SSR) is the potential shift recorded with surface electrodes (from the skin of the palms, soles, and also from perineal skin) on "stressful stimulation" [22]. The SSR is a polysynaptic reflex with several afferent pathways, a complex central integrative mechanism, and a common sympathetic efferent limb (including postganglionic nonmyelinated C-fibers).

The Sympathetic Skin Response

The testing has to be performed in a warm quiet room with subdued light to allow for complete relaxation of the patient. The stimulus used in clinical practice is an electric pulse delivered to the upper or lower limb (to mixed nerves). The responses are easily habituated and have to be repeated (to ensure reproducibility of the response) at random with pauses of 2 min and above. The responses depend on a number of endogenous and exogenous factors including skin temperature, which should be at least above 28 °C. Particularly the absence of the SSR is accepted as a sign of pathology.

Diabetic cystopathy was associated with autonomic neuropathy as detected by SSR [41]. Information on the clinical usefulness of the test is still very limited.

Usefulness of Uroneurophysiology

An urogynecological patient with a suspected neurogenic pelvic floor/pelvic organ dysfunction requires a basic neurological history and examination. If the clinical suspicion of a neurological condition is strengthened, the patient is best referred to a neurologist.

Patients with LUT dysfunction and a suspected lesion of the peripheral innervation in the lower sacral segments may for various reasons be candidates for uroneurophysiological testing. Particularly (quantitative) concentric needle EMG and recording the clitoro-cavernosus/bulbocavernosus reflex is recommended as standard (and standardized) procedure in selected patients, particularly if they are candidates for invasive therapeutic procedures [28]. It has been demonstrated that both techniques are indeed complementary and have – performed in the same patient – a higher sensitivity than each test on its own (i.e., 96%) [26, 27].

The limitations of functional testing of the lower urinary tract innervation have to be acknowledged. Tests measuring conduction through somatic nervous pathways (motor, sensory, and reflex) are sensitive to demyelinative but not to axonal lesions, which predominate in clinical practice. The only available autonomic electrophysiological test – the sympathetic skin response – assesses the sympathetic, and not the more relevant parasympathetic pathways.

The relationship between a neurologic lesion/a neurophysiologic test abnormality and organ dysfunction is not straightforward – the tests assess nervous system function, not pelvic organ function.

Conclusion

Uroneurophysiological tests continue to be useful in selected patients suspected to have a neurogenic pelvic organ dysfunction due to involvement of the lower motor neurons and the reflex arcs of the second to fourth sacral segments including their nerve roots and peripheral nerves. They are less useful in diagnostics of lesions above the sacral spinal cord. Uroneurophysiological techniques are more and more included in the armamentarium of intraoperative techniques for identification and monitoring of nervous structures, and they remain useful for research.

References

1. Aminoff MJ. Aminoff's electrodiagnosis in clinical neurology. 6th ed. Saunders; 2012.
2. Badr G, Carlsson CA, Fall M, Friberg S, Lindström L, Ohlsson B. Cortical evoked potentials following stimulation of the urinary bladder in man. Electroencephalogr Clin Neurophysiol. 1982;54:494–8.
3. Barnett JL, Hasler WL, Camilleri M. American Gastroenterological Association medical position statement on anorectal testing techniques. American Gastroenterological Association. Gastroenterology. 1999;116:732–60.
4. Both S, Ter Kuile M, Enzlin P, Dekkers O, van Dijk M, Weijenborg P. Sexual response in women with type 1 diabetes mellitus: a controlled laboratory study measuring vaginal blood flow and subjective sexual arousal. Arch Sex Behav. 2015;44:1573–87.
5. Brostrom S. Motor evoked potentials from the pelvic floor. Neurourol Urodyn. 2003;22:620–37.
6. Deindl FM, Vodusek DB, Bischoff C, Hofmann R, Hartung R. Dysfunctional voiding in women: which muscles are responsible? Br J Urol. 1998;82:814–9.
7. Delodovici ML, Fowler CJ. Clinical value of the pudendal somatosensory evoked potential. Electroencephalogr Clin Neurophysiol. 1995;96:509–15.
8. Falck B. Neurography – motor and sensory nerve conduction studies. In: Staberg E, editor. Clinical neurophysiology of disorders of muscle and neuromuscular junction, including fatigue. 1st ed. Amsterdam: Elsevier; 2003. p. 269–321.
9. Fowler CJ, Christmas TJ, Chapple CR, Parkhouse HF, Kirby RS, Jacobs HS. Abnormal electromyographic activity of the urethral sphincter, voiding dysfunction, and polycystic ovaries: a new syndrome? Br Med J. 1988;297:1436–8.
10. Gilpin SA, Gosling JA, Smith AR, Warrell DW. The pathogenesis of genitourinary prolapse and stress incontinence of urine. A histological and histochemical study. Br J Obstet Gynaecol. 1989;96:15–23.
11. Groutz A, Blaivas JG, Pies C, Sassone AM. Learned voiding dysfunction (non-neurogenic, neurogenic bladder) among adults. Neurourol Urodyn. 2001;20:259–68.
12. Hanson P, Rigaux P, Gilliard C, Biset E. Sacral reflex latencies in tethered cord syndrome. Am J Phys Med Rehabil. 1993;72:39–43.
13. Holobar A, Farina D, Gazzoni M, Merletti R, Zazula D. Estimating motor unit discharge patterns from high-density surface electromyogram. Clin Neurophysiol. 2009;120:551–62.
14. Kazamel M, Warren PP. History of electromyography and nerve conduction studies: a tribute to the founding fathers. J Clin Neurosci. 2017;43:54–60.
15. Kiff ES, Swash M. Normal proximal and delayed distal conduction in the pudendal nerves of patients with idiopathic (neurogenic) faecal incontinence. J Neurol Neurosurg Psychiatry. 1984;47:820–3.

16. Lefaucheur JP. Excitability of the motor cortical representation of the external anal sphincter. Exp Brain Res. 2005;160:268–72.
17. Loening-Baucke V, Read NW, Yamada T. Further evaluation of the afferent nervous pathways from the rectum. Am J Phys. 1992;262:G927–33.
18. Mahajan ST, Fitzgerald MP, Kenton K, Shott S, Brubaker L. Concentric needle electrodes are superior to perineal surface-patch electrodes for electromyographic documentation of urethral sphincter relaxation during voiding. BJU Int. 2006;97:117–20.
19. Malaguti S, Spinelli M, Giardiello G, Lazzeri M, Van Den Hombergh U. Neurophysiological evidence may predict the outcome of sacral neuromodulation. J Urol. 2003;170:2323–6.
20. Niu X, Shao B, Ni P, Wang X, Chen X, Zhu B, et al. Bulbocavernosus reflex and pudendal nerve somatosensory-evoked potentials responses in female patients with nerve system diseases. J Clin Neurophysiol. 2010;27:207–11.
21. Ogiwara H, Morota N. Pudendal afferents mapping in posterior sacral rhizotomies. Neurosurgery. 2014;74: 171–5.
22. Opsomer RJ, Pesce F, Abi AA. Electrophysiologic testing of motor sympathetic pathways: normative data and clinical contribution in neurourological disorders. Neurourol Urodyn. 1993;12:336.
23. Pandit M, DeLancey JO, Ashton-Miller JA, Iyengar J, Blaivas M, Perucchini D. Quantification of intramuscular nerves within the female striated urogenital sphincter muscle. Obstet Gynecol. 2000;95:797–800.
24. Podnar S. Which patients need referral for anal sphincter electromyography? Muscle Nerve. 2006;33:278–82.
25. Podnar S. Nomenclature of the electrophysiologically tested sacral reflexes. Neurourol Urodyn. 2006;25:95–7.
26. Podnar S. Sphincter electromyography and the penilocavernosus reflex: are both necessary? Neurourol Urodyn. 2008;27:813–8.
27. Podnar S. Neurophysiologic studies of the sacral reflex in women with "non-neurogenic" sacral dysfunction. Neurourol Urodyn. 2011;30:1603–8.
28. Podnar S, Vodusek DB. Protocol for clinical neurophysiologic examination of the pelvic floor. Neurourol Urodyn. 2001;20:669–82.
29. Podnar S, Vodusek DB, Stalberg E. Standardization of anal sphincter electromyography: normative data. Clin Neurophysiol. 2000;111:2200–7.
30. Podnar S, Vodusek DB, Stalberg E. Comparison of quantitative techniques in anal sphincter electromyography. Muscle Nerve. 2002;25:83–92.
31. Podnar S, Vodusek DB, Trsinar B, Rodi Z. A method of uroneurophysiological investigation in children. Electroencephalogr Clin Neurophysiol. 1997;104: 389–92.
32. Rubin DI. Normal and abnormal voluntary activity. Handb Clin Neurol. 2019;160:281–301.
33. Rubin DI. Normal and abnormal spontaneous activity. Handb Clin Neurol. 2019;160:257–79.
34. Sala F, Squintani G, Tramontano V, Arcaro C, Faccioli F, Mazza C. Intraoperative neurophysiology in tethered cord surgery: techniques and results. Childs Nerv Syst. 2013;29:1611–24.
35. Santiago S, Ferrer T, Espinosa ML. Neurophysiological studies of thin myelinated (A delta) and unmyelinated (C) fibers: application to peripheral neuropathies. Neurophysiol Clin. 2000;30:27–42.
36. Saraidaridis JT, Molina G, Savit LR, Milch H, Mei T, Chin S, et al. Pudendal nerve terminal motor latency testing does not provide useful information in guiding therapy for fecal incontinence. Int J Color Dis. 2018;33:305–10.
37. Smith AR, Hosker GL, Warrell DW. The role of partial denervation of the pelvic floor in the aetiology of genitourinary prolapse and stress incontinence of urine. A neurophysiological study. Br J Obstet Gynaecol. 1989;96:24–8.
38. Snooks SJ, Swash M, Mathers SE, Henry MM. Effect of vaginal delivery on the pelvic floor: a 5-year follow-up. Br J Surg. 1990;77:1358–60.
39. Stoffel JT. Detrusor sphincter dyssynergia: a review of physiology, diagnosis, and treatment strategies. Transl Androl Urol. 2016;5:127–35.
40. Szymański JK, Słabuszewska-Jóźwiak A. Fowler's syndrome-the cause of urinary retention in young women, often forgotten, but significant and challenging to treat. Int J Environ Res Public Health. 2021;18(6):3310.
41. Ueda T, Yoshimura N, Yoshida O. Diabetic cystopathy: relationship to autonomic neuropathy detected by sympathetic skin response. J Urol. 1997;157:580–4.
42. Vodusek DB. Pudendal SEP and bulbocavernosus reflex in women. Electroencephalogr Clin Neurophysiol. 1990;77:134–6.
43. Vodusek DB. Evoked potential testing. Urol Clin North Am. 1996;23:427–46.
44. Vodusek DB. The role of electrophysiology in the evaluation of incontinence and prolapse. Curr Opin Obstet Gynecol. 2002;14:509–14.
45. Vodusek DB, Janko M, Lokar J. Direct and reflex responses in perineal muscles on electrical stimulation. J Neurol Neurosurg Psychiatry. 1983;46:67–71.
46. Wester C, FitzGerald MP, Brubaker L, Welgoss J, Benson JT. Validation of the clinical bulbocavernosus reflex. Neurourol Urodyn. 2003;22:589–91.
47. Wexner SD, Marchetti F, Salanga VD, Corredor C, Jagelman DG. Neurophysiologic assessment of the anal sphincters. Dis Colon Rectum. 1991;34: 606–12.

Urodynamic Evaluation: Traditional, Video, and Ambulatory Approaches

10

Miguel Miranda and Ricardo Pereira e Silva

Contents

Introduction	158
Urodynamics in the Female Setting	158
Bladder Diaries and Pad Testing	159
Voiding Diaries	159
Pad Testing	159
Uroflowmetry	159
Flow Patterns	160
PVR Assessment	162
Cystometry and Pressure-Flow Studies	162
Patient and Equipment Setup	162
End of the Study	165
Clinical Application	167
Videourodynamics	169
Filling Phase/Full at Rest	170
Voiding	170
Ambulatory Urodynamics	170
Equipment and the Study	171
Indications	171
Urethral Pressure Profile	171
Neurophysiology	173
Conclusion	174
References	174

M. Miranda
Urology Department, Centro Hospitalar Universitário
Lisboa Norte, Lisbon, Lisboa, Portugal

R. Pereira e Silva (✉)
Urology, Faculdade de Medicina, Universidade de Lisboa;
Centro Hospitalar Universitário Lisboa Norte, Lisbon,
Portugal

© Springer Nature Switzerland AG 2023
F. E. Martins et al. (eds.), *Female Genitourinary and Pelvic Floor Reconstruction*,
https://doi.org/10.1007/978-3-031-19598-3_10

Abstract

Urodynamic techniques allow for an objective assessment of the lower urinary tract system, with the aim of interpreting the different array of subjective symptoms and establishing a precise diagnosis. It compiles a wide variety of tests that range from less invasive and simpler ones, such as the bladder diary and the uroflowmetry, to others more complex and invasive, such as the filling cystometry, the pressure-flow study and videourodynamics. Anatomy and physiology of the female lower urinary tract have particular differences from the male counterpart which implies a distinct approach and interpretation. In women, the main complaints occur mostly during the filling phase of the micturition cycle and the physiological bladder outlet resistance is less pronounced. Therefore, urodynamics have an important role in the assessing the differential diagnosis of overactive bladder and the underlying mechanisms of urinary incontinence, predicting the outcomes of female urology surgery, and characterizing the phenotype of systemic neurological disorders. Nevertheless, standardization and clinical correlations are the still lacking, so effort should be made to report further data and develop less invasive and more accurate techniques.

Keywords

Urodynamics · Lower urinary tract · Neurogenic dysfunction · Cystometry · Pressure-flow studies · Urethral pressure profile

Introduction

Urodynamic studies (UDS) refer to a group of tests used to assess the lower urinary tract (LUT). These techniques aim to evaluate patient's storage and voiding phases together, reproducing the daily symptoms in order to allow for a more objective assessment and establish several measurable parameters. This data may be used to formulate a precise diagnosis and grade the severity of the complaints and eventually for an objective evaluation of treatment response.

These tests can be noninvasive, such as uroflowmetry and post-void residual volume (PVR) measurement, or invasive when requiring catheter, probes, or needle insertion (Table 1).

Urodynamic tests should be performed in the order to ask specific questions, such as the following: What is the diagnosis? How severe is the condition? What is the most appropriate treatment?

Table 1 Urodynamic techniques

Urodynamic techniques	
Noninvasive	Invasive
Micturition/time chart	Urethral pressure profile
Frequency/volume chart	Cystometry
Bladder diary	Pressure/flow study
Pad testing	Electromyography
Uroflowmetry +/− residual volume assessment	Videourodynamics
	Ambulatory urodynamics

Therefore, prior to urodynamics, a complete clinical history (including medical history and validated symptom and/or bother scores) and physical examination should be performed. A urinalysis to screen for infection or hematuria is also recommended before urodynamics.

Urodynamics in the Female Setting

The female urinary tract has anatomical differences from the male counterpart which have an impact on urodynamics. The female urethra is shorter, and the bladder neck is significantly weaker, partly due to the longitudinal disposition of the muscle fibers, opposite to the circular orientation in the male bladder neck. Furthermore, the absence of the prostate gland and smooth muscle fibers in prostatic urethra contributing to bladder outlet resistance makes the female continence mechanism more reliant on the integrity of the pelvic floor structures.

Taking into account the Poiseuille law (Fig. 1), the flow rate (Q) is significantly affected by the urethral length and caliber. Hence, the distinctions between the male and female anatomy will alone produce different urodynamic values, and the obtained results must always be interpreted in that context.

Key Points in Urodynamics
- Preceded by complete cynical history and physical examination.
- Performed in a standardized manner.

(continued)

Q	Flow rate
P	Pressure
r	Radius
η	Fluid viscosity
l	Length of tubing

$$Q = \frac{\pi \mathrm{Pr}^4}{8\eta l}$$

Fig. 1 Poiseuille law which determines the flow rate of a fluid in a tubing, according to the variables: (P) pressure gradient; (r) radius; (n) viscosity; (l) length

- Aim to ask specific questions and adapt the exam to each question.
- Consider anatomical differences.

Bladder Diaries and Pad Testing

Voiding Diaries

Voiding diaries are an initial, simple, and noninvasive tool to assess LUT symptoms and the impact on the quality of life. They portray the voiding pattern in a more objective manner, being an important complement to the clinical history. These questionnaires are classified according to the recorded information [1]:

- *Micturition time chart* – records the number of micturitions and during which time of the day and night it occurred, for at least 24 h.
- *Frequency volume chart* (*FVC*) – records the time and volume of each micturition, for at least 24 h.
- *Bladder diary* – records not only the time and volume but also the degree of urgency, use of pads, fluid intake, and episodes of incontinence.

Bladder diaries have an important role in discriminating increased frequency due to an overactive bladder (OAB) syndrome or reduced anatomical capacity from an increased production of urine due to high fluid intake. The number of episodes of incontinence and use of pads are also surrogate markers for assessing the impact on daily life.

Although definitions have changed little since their terminology standardization [2], continuous efforts have been made to design simpler and more user-friendly diaries that increase patient compliance [3]. Furthermore, translation and validation to different languages allowed a wider application of a standardized questionnaire in non-English-speaking patients [4, 5].

Pad Testing

Pad testing is a noninvasive urodynamic test which aims to detect and quantify urinary incontinence. It consists of measuring the change of weight of a pad used as a containment device to assess the presence and degree of urine loss. Pad tests can last a 1 h period or extend to 24–48 h. During this period the patient should perform different routine activities. Although ICS guidelines have been developed [6], standardization of this tool is still a challenge. This test can be more specifically used to assess incontinence surgery outcomes [7], vesicovaginal fistula repair outcomes [8], or the need for incontinence surgery during pelvic organ prolapse repair [9].

Uroflowmetry

Uroflowmetry is a first-line screening tool for the LUT assessment since it is a noninvasive, cheap, accessible, and very informative test. It is particularly useful to assess voiding symptoms and, together with the measurement of PVR, may help in the assessment of voiding dysfunction.

In women, it is particularly relevant when planning urinary stress incontinence surgery. An abnormally reduced flow with high PVR may suggest an underlying voiding dysfunction, which can be exacerbated with surgery and cause acute/chronic urinary retention or recurrent UTIs.

The female patient voids in the sitting position, to a recipient over a flowmeter that quantifies the urinary flow in milliliters per second (mL/s). The flowmeter produces a chart with the voiding time on the horizontal axis and the flow rate (Q) on the vertical axis.

The interpretation of the exam should encompass the shape of the curve as well as the absolute values:

- Maximum flow rate (Q_{max})
- Average flow rate (volume voided/flow time)
- Volume voided
- Voiding time
- Flow time
- Time to maximum flow
- PVR

Flow Patterns

Normal Flow

A normal flow curve has a "bell" shape, characterized by a rapid increase in the flow and peak (Q_{max}) reached within the first 5 s from the onset of voiding (Fig. 2).

Detrusor Overactivity

These patients have a normal flow curve but with a high amplitude due to the very high Q_{max} reached in the first 1–3 s. This is caused not only by the strong detrusor contraction but also by the rapid relaxation of the bladder neck and decreased outflow resistance.

Prolonged Flow

These flows typically include a delayed and low-amplitude Q_{max}, followed by a slow decrease in the flow rate. These curves are typical in patients with BOO (Q_{max} obtained normally in the first 10 s) and with DU (Q_{max} in the middle of the voiding time).

Intermittent Flow

An intermittent trace may be associated with a continuous or interrupted flow. In the first case, the voiding time is equal to the flow time, while in the second the voiding time is higher than the sum of the flow times of the different curves. The irregular trace may be caused by abdominal straining to compensate the BOO, neurological disorders that may cause a premature and involuntary rhabdosphincter contraction (detrusor

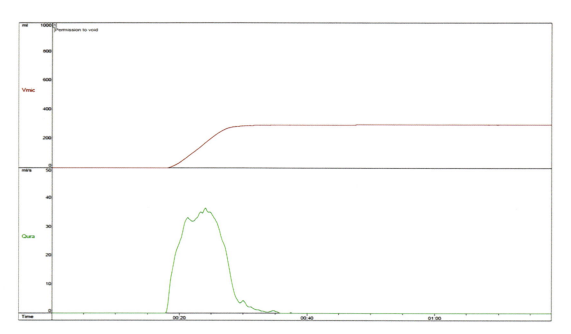

Fig. 2 Normal flow pattern in a woman

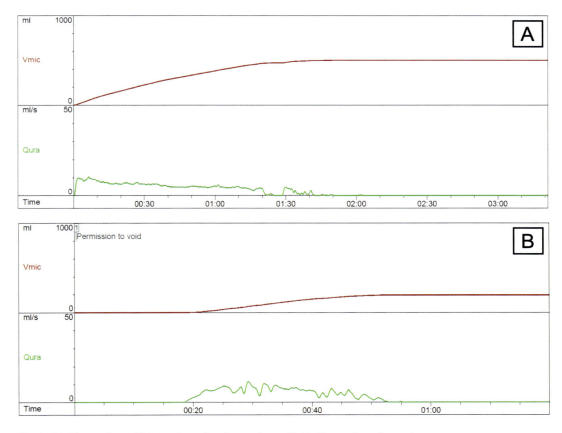

Fig. 3 (**a**) *Plateau* flow; (**b**) intermittent flow in a patient with bladder outflow obstruction

sphincter dyssynergia), fluctuations in detrusor contractility due to neurological problems or anxiety and pelvic floor contraction (Fig. 3). The interrupted flow at the end of the micturition is frequent in patients with BOO (terminal dribbling).

Plateau Flow

This trace shows a prolonged and constant flow rate, without a peak, which illustrates a diminished urethral caliber in the presence of a normally functioning detrusor. Irrespective of the detrusor contraction, the urethral stricture limits the Q_{max} to a steady level (Fig. 3).

The interpretation of the flow rates and shape of the curve should always take into consideration the patient's age and sex. A flow rate of at least 20 mL/s is generally considered to be normal for younger males, while this value physiologically decreases with age. In females, the flow rates are generally 5–10 mL/s higher. Nomograms have been designed throughout the years to allow for a better understanding of the whole range of normal function and dysfunction that may be seen during voiding in males and females. Siroky and Bristol nomograms are examples for the male population; however, there are few validated nomograms for females based on uroflowmetry data. The Solomon-Greenwell [10] and the Blaivas-Groutz [11] nomograms were developed and validated to assess the probability of BOO in women based on pressure-flow studies.

As previously illustrated by the Poiseuille law, the flow rate depends on both the pressure gradient (generated by the detrusor contraction) and the radius (represented by the urethral patency). One of the main limitations of uroflowmetry concerns the absence of pressure recording. As such, it doesn't allow to distinguish whether a low Q_{max} is associated with a prolonged flow time due to bladder outlet/urethral obstruction (high pressure) or detrusor underactivity (low pressure). Although the shape of the curve may suggest one of the former, there is significant overlap between traces that must usually be clarified using pressure-flow studies. Other confounding factors should be considered as they can lead to an artificial/misleading increase (abdominal stranding) or decrease of the flow rate (abnormal sphincter relaxation).

PVR Assessment

PVR is normally measured by ultrasound, rather than catheterization as it is less invasive. The PVR determination is essential since poor voiding efficiency, as demonstrated by high residual volume, may be asymptomatic in a significant number of patients [12–14]. Higher PVR might be related to chronic urinary retention and result in hydronephrosis, recurrent UTIs, and bladder stones. High PVR is also associated with an increased risk of acute urinary retention [15].

In women without significant LUTS, 95% had a PVR < 100 mL [16]. However, there is no clear consensus regarding the "normal" PVR value. The bladder voiding efficiency (BVE), which represents the proportion of the total bladder volume that is voided by the patient (BVE = voided volume/(voided volume + PVR) × 100), is another useful parameter to characterize and grade the severity of voiding dysfunction.

The intrinsic connection between the urinary and nervous systems outlines the importance and consequences of the patient's emotional status on the results. Therefore a comprehensive interpretation of the uroflowmetry should include not only technical aspects, such as a representative voiding volume (>150 mL) and the patient's preferred voiding position, but also situational and emotional factors. Hence, ensuring adequate privacy, clear explanation of the procedure itself and its goals (e.g., explanatory and concise leaflets), avoiding bladder overfilling, and postponing voiding are measures that help reduce anxiety and discomfort.

> **Key Points in Uroflowmetry**
> - Uroflowmetry is an excellent first-line LUT study.
> - Normal flow rates vary with age and sex.
> - The shape of the curve and the objective parameters should always be described together to assess the bladder and urethral function as well as investigate underlying voiding dysfunction.
> - PVR determination is useful for assessing the severity and risk of complications of voiding dysfunction.
> - The technical, situational, and emotional factors are essential to reduce artifacts and optimize the results in urodynamics.

Cystometry and Pressure-Flow Studies

Cystometry and pressure-flow studies are required in patients for whom noninvasive assessment does not allow for a clear functional diagnosis. These tests pretend to simulate the storage and voiding phases of the bladder cycle in order to objectively evaluate the LUT function.

Patient and Equipment Setup

The achievement of optimal results rely heavily on quality control, assured by following strict and standardized protocols according to international good practices [17] and on regular calibration of the equipment according to manufacturers.

The patient can be either standing or sitting during the exam, depending on the usual positioning during daily life. Bladder filling should be performed in the upright position, unless there is a clear and exceptional reason for the patient to be in supine position (e.g., neurogenic detrusor overactivity with severe urgency incontinence, impairing artificial filling even at a low rate).

The pressure measurement is performed with external pressure transducers positioned at the upper level of the pubic symphysis and with fluid-filled catheters. This method has proved to be the most accurate and reliable, although air-filled and microtip catheters may be used as alternatives. When using these catheters, however, one should keep in mind that the vast majority of the available studies concerning UDS, including nomograms, used water-filled systems, so differences in measurements may exist. The transurethral catheter should be as thin as possible (6–7F) and ideally comprise a double lumen system (for filling and pressure recording). The abdominal pressure should be measured in the rectal ampulla with thin (6F) catheters. It is recommended to fix the catheters with tape and avoid blocking the urethral meatus. In women the catheter can be fixed to the inner side of the labia.

Before starting the procedure, the atmospheric pressure should be set to zero and the fluid-filled lines be flushed to avoid artifacts caused by air bubbles.

An infusion pump is responsible for filling the bladder at a defined rate. The filling rate should be representative of the physiological bladder filling. Thus the recommended flow should be in the range of 20–30 mL/s (¼ of the estimated body weight) or eventually higher in the specific cases where the patient's regular voided volumes are acquainted.

The data collected from the transducers and the flowmeter are centralized in a computer station and illustrated in a continuous pressure-flow chart.

A standard urodynamic study usually encompasses at least *three phases*:

Free Uroflowmetry and PVR Determination

Filling Cystometry

This procedure intends to reproduce the storage phase and begins when the infusion pump is switched on (Table 2). The bladder is artificially filled with atmosphere temperature saline fluid. The intravesical (P_{ves}) and intra-abdominal (P_{abd}) pressures are continuously measured. The detrusor pressure (P_{det}) is then mathematically calculated as the difference between those two variables ($P_{det} = P_{ves} - P_{abd}$) and displayed by the software as an additional pressure line. At rest, the P_{ves} and P_{abd} are typically the same; up to 5 cm, H_2O may be accepted as a minor, clinically nonsignificant difference. If the subtraction reveals a higher value, exclusion of kinks and leaks or repositioning of the catheters should be performed. Asking the patient to cough at the beginning and throughout the test ensures a trustworthy recording of the pressure as both the P_{ves} and the P_{abd} should spike in the same range with the P_{det} being close to zero. Any significant rise or fall of the P_{det} should prompt an inspection to rule out catheter displacement. The filling phase ends when the patient experiences a strong desire to void.

Bladder Sensation

During the filling phase, the patient should report three sensation parameters:

- *First sensation of filling (FSF)* – the first perception of stored urine
- *First desire to void (FDV)* – the first sensation at which the patient may go to the toilet if desirable
- *Normal desire to void (NDV)* – a comfortable sensation for which the patient would go to the toilet in a daily life setting
- *Strong desire to void (SDV)* – strong sensation of bladder repletion for which the patient would not postpone voiding, although not associated with urgency, pain, or fear of leakage

Table 2 Summary of filling cystometry assessment

Filling cystometry				
Replicated phase	Quantified parameters	Objective assessment	Subjective assessment	Replicated LUTS
Storage	Pdet Pves Pabd Urinary volume Leaked volume ALPP	Bladder compliance Bladder capacity Detrusor involuntary activity Leakage (spontaneous or due to provocative maneuvers)	Bladder sensation: FSF FDV SDV	Urgency Incontinence

Other sensations such as urgency, with or without leak, fear of leakage, or pain should also be reported.

The bladder sensation can be divided in:

- *Normal*
- *Reduced* – decreased sensation, described by a late FSF and FDV
- *Absent* – when the patient reports no bladder sensation for a normal bladder capacity in the general population (e.g., 500 mL)
- *Increased* – manifested by an early onset the FSF, for volumes normally below 100 mL, which restrict bladder capacity due to strong desire to void

Bladder Compliance

Compliance is defined as the property of the bladder to accommodate large volumes of urine without a significant increase in the P_{det}, due to its elastic properties. It is measured in mL/cm H_2O and is measured by the $\Delta volume/\Delta P_{det}$.

A normal bladder compliance is >40 mL/cm H_2O. Values below this threshold can be caused by tuberculosis, radiotherapy, neurologic conditions (multiple sclerosis or spinal cord injury), or chronic bladder outlet obstruction [18]. A high filling rate can artificially suggest low compliance.

Bladder Capacity

- Cystometric capacity – depicts the bladder volume at the end of the filling phase, when the patient has normal desire and before starting the voiding phase.
- Maximum cystometric capacity – is the volume at which the patient has strong desire to void and can no longer postpone micturition. In women this value should normally be around 500 mL [19].
- Maximum anesthetic capacity – represents the maximum volume that the bladder can be filled under general or spinal anesthesia.

Detrusor Activity

In this phase detrusor can be classified as normal or overactive. *Normal detrusor* should be relaxed during all the filling phase so that the bladder can accommodate increasing urine volumes without significant changes in pressure. This prevents urinary incontinence and allows the urine to be transferred from the ureters to the bladder following a pressure gradient due to ureteral peristalsis. Any detrusor contraction during storage is considered detrusor involuntary activity. *Detrusor overactivity* (DO) can be spontaneous or provoked by several maneuvers such as changing position, coughing, Valsalva, fast filling, or running water. Most commonly DO is idiopathic in nature and no underlying disorder is found. In some cases DO is a symptom of neurological disorders such as cerebrovascular diseases, multiple sclerosis, or spinal cord injury, being therefore termed neurogenic DO. The detrusor contraction description should include the volume at which it occurred, its duration, its rise in amplitude, and whether it was followed by leakage. DO is usually defined by a phasic and transient increase in P_{det}, which can be then associated with urgency and incontinence (Fig. 4).

Urethral Function

The urethra plays a pivotal role in maintaining continence due to the urethral smooth muscle contraction and the mucosal coaptation related to the submucosal high vascular plexus which create a watertight seal [20].

In the presence of an incompetent urethral closure mechanism, leakage may occur in the absence of a detrusor contraction. The rise of the intravesical pressure will overcome the urethral pressure and lead to incontinence. This can be tested by asking the patient to cough or perform the Valsalva maneuver which will generate a transient increase of the P_{ves}. If the urethral function is normal, no leakage should be recorded by the flowmeter. The urethral and bladder neck function can be objectively evaluated by the abdominal leak point pressure (ALPP), which refers to the lowest P_{ves} at which the leakage occurs during an intentional increase in the abdominal pressure, without a detrusor contraction. It is named cough leak point pressure (CLPP) or Valsalva leak point pressure (VLPP) according to the applied provocative maneuver. The ALPP correlates with the severity of the stress incontinence, and a value <60 cm H_2O is highly suggestive of intrinsic sphincter deficiency (ISD). On the other hand, women with urinary stress incontinence due to urethral hypermobility tend to have ALPP >90 cm H_2O [21, 22]. Despite the importance of

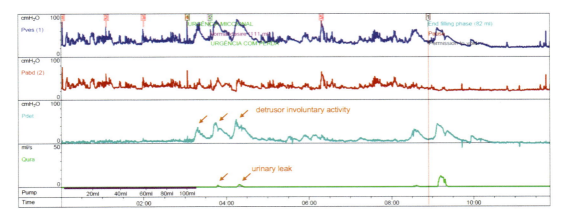

Fig. 4 Detrusor overactivity portrayed by sudden and transient rises in P_{det} which correspond to detrusor involuntary activity with associated urinary leakage

establishing cutoffs and objectively quantifying the severity of stress incontinence before treatment, these parameters have a low reproducibility and are yet to be standardized and validated (Table 2).

Pressure-Flow Study

Pressure-flow studies simulate the voiding phase of the micturition cycle (Table 3). It starts with "permission to void" and ends either when the patient finishes the micturition and/or the flow rate is null and/or the detrusor pressure returns to the baseline. The main goal is to assess the (1) bladder outflow function and the (2) detrusor contraction. It is of utmost importance to respect the patient's privacy during this part of the exam.

In the normal setting, the voiding phase starts with an isometric contraction of the detrusor, where the P_{det} rises against a closed sphincter without modification of the intravesical volume (Fig. 5). When the parasympathetic nerve impulse instructs the sphincter to relax, the flow rate (Q) gradually increases until reaching a maximum flow (Q_{max}). The P_{det} at the Q_{max} is recorded ($P_{det}Q_{max}$) and commonly follows the maximum pressure as there is a physiological delay between the pressure and flow curves.

Detrusor Activity

- Normal – normal voiding is achieved when the detrusor contractility produces a normal flow rate and allows complete emptying of the bladder. However, the urinary flow rate and the capacity of emptying the bladder are not only dependent on the detrusor contraction but also on bladder outlet resistance. Thus, the ICS recommends to assess detrusor activity and urethral resistance based on pressure-flow plot nomograms rather than rigid cutoffs.
- Underactive – this happens when detrusor contraction is of low amplitude or prolonged in time, thus causing an incomplete emptying or a lengthened voiding (Fig. 6).
- Acontractile – when no change in P_{det} is recorded due to absence of detrusor contraction.

Urethral Function

During voiding in women, the physiological relaxation of the urethra and pelvic floor will allow to generate flow without a significant increase in the intravesical pressure. However, in some cases there may be bladder outlet obstruction, either due to mechanical causes, such as urethral strictures, or due to bladder neck/pelvic floor overactivity. The latter can be caused by detrusor sphincter dyssynergia, dysfunctional voiding, or non-relaxing urethral sphincter obstruction.

End of the Study

Before ending the study, patients should be asked to cough in order to assess the quality of the pressure recording and subtraction between the P_{ves} and

Table 3 Summary of pressure-flow study assessment

Pressure-flow study				
Replicated phase	Quantified parameters	Objective interpretation	Subjective interpretation	Replicated LUTS
Voiding	Pdet Pves Pabd Voided volume Voiding and flow time Flow rate (Q) Qmax and Qaverage PdetQmax Time to Qmax	Detrusor activity Urethral function PVR		Weak stream Hesitancy Intermittency Straining Feeling of incomplete voiding

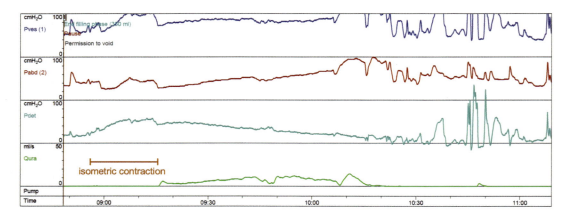

Fig. 5 Excessively prolonged isometric contraction phase in a patient with a delayed opening of the bladder neck during voiding

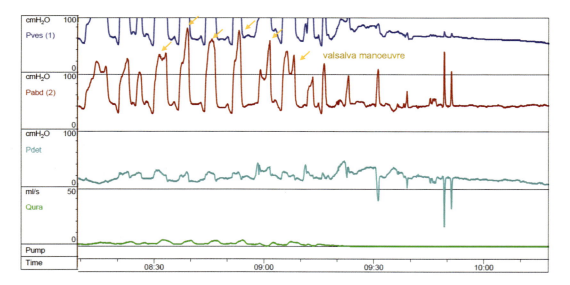

Fig. 6 Patient with severe underactive detrusor. The weak urinary flow ($Q_{max} < 5$ mL/s) is mainly due to the increased abdominal pressure from Valsalva maneuvers. The P_{det} intermittent rises are artifactual subtraction defects

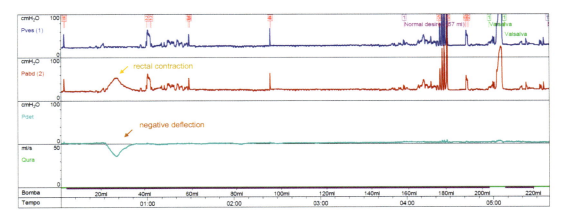

Fig. 7 Rectal activity produces an artificial negative deflection since the contraction in the rectal ampulla is not transmitted to the bladder

P_{abd}. This is particularly useful to exclude dampening artifacts which happen when there is any error in the pressure transmission either caused by air bubbles in the system, misplacement of the transducer, or kinking of the catheter (for instance, due to abdominal straining during voiding) (Fig. 7).

The PVR is measured at the end of the procedure as part of the complete assessment of pressure-flow studies. Care must be taken when interpreting this value, since a high PVR may be caused by obstruction due to the vesical catheter, overfilling of the bladder, or inhibition due to absence of adequate privacy conditions.

Clinical Application

Urodynamic role is vast and includes [23]:

- Assessment on the etiology of LUTS
- Prediction of the possible impact of the LUT dysfunction on the upper urinary tract
- Treatment selection and prediction of outcomes and side effects of the selected treatment
- Better understanding of the physiopathology behind refractory LUT dysfunction

Unlike men where the main indications for urodynamics are related to bladder outlet obstruction, the main lower urinary tract disorders and complaints in women fall in the specter of bladder filling disorders, which typically present with urgency, frequency, nocturia, and incontinence. In the female setting, urodynamics has an important role in assessing incontinence, the bladder sensation, the detrusor activity during filling and voiding, the sphincter, and the pelvic floor function.

OAB is a syndrome with several phenotypes and complex underlying mechanisms suggesting a more comprehensive and patient-tailored approach [24]. However, the ICS concluded that neither the severity of symptoms nor the specific mechanism of action of the OAB is helpful in treatment selection or predict response to treatment [25]. Therefore, current guidelines do not recommend UDS as a routine in patients with uncomplicated OAB symptoms [26].

Urinary incontinence (UI) is a particularly common and bothersome symptom with severe impact on the quality of life and represents one of main indications for urodynamic assessment. The prevalence increases with age as there is a tendency for the bladder to become more overactive. Therefore, urgency UI (UUI) is more prevalent in older ages, being twice more common in patients over 60 years old than the ones below 40 [27]. On the other hand, stress UI (SUI) is more prevalent in the middle age with a peak incidence between 45 and 59 years [28]. In a significant proportion of cases, both types of incontinence can be present (mixed UI, MUI).

The role of urodynamics prior to incontinence surgery has been subject of debate. UDS in this setting could have added value in the differential diagnosis of SUI and UUI, therefore being able to select the best patients who would benefit from surgical treatments [29]. Furthermore, it is useful in revealing patients at higher risk of treatment failure or complication by identifying poor outcome factors, such as intrinsic sphincter deficiency, detrusor overactivity, and voiding dysfunction [30]. However, preoperative DO in women with MUI was not associated with treatment failure after incontinence surgery due to postoperative UUI [31]. A randomized clinical trial (RCT) showed that for uncomplicated SUI, an office evaluation with positive result on provocative stress test, normal PVR, exclusion of UTI, and urethral mobility on Q-tip test was non-inferior to UDS in the preoperative evaluation [32]. These findings have been further supported by another RCT where treatment based on urodynamic findings was not inferior mid urethral sling operation after clinical assessment [33].

Pelvic organ prolapse (POP) is particularly common in women with LUTS and incontinence [34]. Before POP correction, urinary symptoms may be attributed to the prolapse itself or be perceived as "normal" by the patients. However, LUT dysfunction can be simultaneously present and be uncovered after surgery in the form of storage symptoms due to underlying DO or urinary retention due to detrusor underactivity. Furthermore, de novo SUI was found in a significant number of patients after POP surgical treatment [35, 36]. This raises the question whether preemptive diagnosis of SUI could allow for combined prolapse and SUI surgery. While UDS have no predictive value on POP correction outcomes, it may help better patient counselling, hence improved decision-making and overall management [37]. Current guidelines do not include UDS as part of POP diagnostic workup, however, recommend filling cystometry and pressure-flow studies in patients proposed for SUI surgery with concurrent anterior or apical prolapse [38].

Patients with diseases of the nervous system are more keen to develop LUT dysfunction. The neurogenic LUT dysfunction is associated with an increased risk of chronic renal disease, bladder stones, and UTI, namely, sepsis [39]. Considering the potential complications, a correct and timely diagnosis is of utmost importance. However, the diagnosis solely based on the clinical history and physical examination is often challenging. Although some patterns of neurogenic bladders can be recognized depending on the lesion location (Table 4), it is common to find a mismatch between neurologic signs and urodynamic findings. For instance, frontal lobe tumors may cause DO and UI, while in rarer cases also urinary retention [40]. Similar findings were reported in 19 poststroke patients, where 37% showed DO, 21% detrusor underactivity, and 5% detrusor sphincter dyssynergia [41]. Furthermore, systemic disorders, such as multiple sclerosis or Parkinson's disease, can present with multiple site lesions and a vast array of bladder dysfunction symptoms

Table 4 Patterns of neurogenic dysfunction

Above the brainstem	Detrusor overactivity and involuntary bladder contractions:
	Urinary frequency
	Urgency
	Urgency urinary incontinence
	Low risk of developing high-pressure neurogenic bladders
Brainstem/pontine and suprasacral spinal cord	Detrusor overactivity Detrusor sphincter dyssynergia Bladder hyposensitivity High risk of high voiding pressures, vesicoureteral reflux, and renal damage
Below sacral spinal cord (peripheral nerve and cauda equina)	Different patterns depending on the injured pathway:
	Complete lesion: acontractile detrusor and bladder hyposensitivity
	Pelvic nerve lesion: underactive detrusor and hypertonic externa urinary sphincter, causing urinary retention
	Pudendal nerve lesion: spastic bladder with detrusor overactivity and an incompetent urethra, causing incontinence

[42]. Therefore, an objective and comprehensive assessment of the LUT through urodynamics is of pivotal importance in aiding in the diagnosis and guiding a patient-tailored treatment.

DO is a common urodynamic finding in multiple neurological disorders and an important cause of UI which can per se lead to embarrassment, social isolation, depression, dermatitis, and skin ulcers. When DO is followed by high pressures, there is an increased risk of upper urinary tract lesion. Detrusor leak point pressure (DLPP) is a marker used to identify patients at high risk for upper urinary tract injury. It is defined by the ICS as the lowest detrusor pressure at which urine leakage occurs in the absence of either a detrusor contraction or increased abdominal pressure [43]. DLPP is measured during a filling cystometry, and a cutoff of >40 cm H_2O has been used to predict long-term upper urinary tract deterioration [44]. However, this value has shown to have low sensitivity and in some studies low reliability, maybe due to the lack of standardization [45, 46]. Furthermore, neurogenic patients can have high DLPP and simultaneous SUI and low ALPP due to ISD. Currently DLPP should not be used alone to make a decision on invasive therapies, such as argumentative cystoplasty [43].

Detrusor sphincter dyssynergia occurs when there is a loss of coordination between detrusor and the external striated sphincter contraction, resulting in an attempt to expel the urine against a closed sphincter. The inadequate voiding may lead to long-term bladder wall thickening and consequential diminished bladder compliance, high voiding pressures, vesicoureteral reflux, hydronephrosis, and kidney failure. It is typically associated to neurological injury in the pontine micturition center and suprasacral spinal cord which coordinates the detrusor and sphincter activity. The most common causes are spinal cord injury, multiple sclerosis, acute transverse myelitis, and myelomeningocele [47]. In multiple sclerosis, detrusor sphincter dyssynergia is more frequent in cervical lesions [48], and it correlates with cervical plaque formation and increased cerebrospinal fluid myelin basic protein [49]. After spinal cord injury, spinal shock may develop causing autonomic dysfunction, namely, the loss of the neurological reflex and bladder contractility. Therefore, during this period, there is an acontractile detrusor and complete urinary retention. Spinal shock typically lasts 6–12 weeks, and UDS should be delayed until 3–4 months after the trauma in order to wait for the reestablishment of the reflex activity and allow for an unbiased interpretation of the LUT function.

It is impractical to perform a filling cystogram and pressure-flow study in all patients, and benefits must be weighted against the inherent risks [50]:

- Invasive test causing physical discomfort and embarrassment to the patient [51]
- Low but non-negligible risk of UTI which can be as high as 4% in neurogenic lower urinary tract disturbance [52]
- Urinary retention after the urodynamic investigation
- Transient discomfort, dysuria, or hematuria following the exam

Key Points in Cystometry and Pressure-Flow Studies
- Indicated for study and management of complex or equivocal cases.
- For a trustworthy and accurate test, it is essential to regular calibration and good practices compliance.
- Cystometry and pressure-flow studies are the gold standard for diagnosing detrusor overactivity.
- Pressure-flow studies are particularly useful to clarify equivocal dysfunctional voiding, especially when to differentiate bladder outlet obstruction from detrusor underactivity.
- Invasive tests that comprise risks which must be weighted against its benefits.

Videourodynamics

Videourodynamics (VUD) refers to the combination of cystometry and pressure-flow studies with fluoroscopic imaging and radiographic contrast. The exam should not be routinely performed, due to the radiation exposure, availability, and costs. Instead it is indicated for patients where anatomical disorders may play a significant role in the underlying filling or voiding disorder.

The sequential outline of the upper and lower urinary tract as the contrast flows during the different phases of micturition cycle allows for an anatomical assessment together with the recording of the following:

Filling Phase/Full at Rest

The filling of the bladder with contrast media will depict its shape and contour which may show the presence of bladder diverticula, fistulae, or vesicoureteral reflux at rest (Fig. 8). During the filling phase, the patient may be asked to cough or strain in order to visualize the bladder base descent and bladder neck competence. Bladder neck opening during this phase can be secondary to detrusor involuntary activity or to intrinsic incompetence.

Voiding

In physiological conditions, voiding begins with bladder base descent followed by an appropriate bladder neck opening. Failure to open may be due to bladder neck fibrosis, benign prostatic hyperplasia, detrusor underactivity with insufficient increase of P_{det}, or detrusor-bladder neck dyssynergia. VUD is also useful for detailing the site of obstruction, such as posterior urethral valves.

As the urinary stream flows, the P_{det} rises, and the contrast media is progressively emptied from the bladder. During this phase the caliber and shape of the urethra are assessed as well as the presence of vesicoureteral reflux during voiding. The presence of contrast media at the end of voiding can also be measured as PVR.

For more complex cases, such as neurogenic bladders and when more measurements are deemed important, this test can be combined with simultaneous electromyography and intraurethral pressure assessment for assessing sphincter activity and urethral pressure, respectively.

Indications for VUD in women:

- Recurrent stress incontinence – before invasive treatment
- Bladder outlet dysfunction – differential diagnosis between bladder neck dysfunction, urethral stricture, cystocele, or poor relaxation of the pelvic floor [53–55]
- Lower urinary tract dysfunction in patients with neurological conditions or congenital malformations
- Patients with known or suspected vesicoureteric reflux or with upper urinary tract deterioration possibly related to the lower urinary tract
- Severe lower urinary tract dysfunction as demonstrated by very high PVR or bladder diverticula

> **Key Points in Videourodynamics**
> - Allows for combined anatomical and functional assessment of the lower and upper urinary tract
> - Indicated only for specific and complex cases

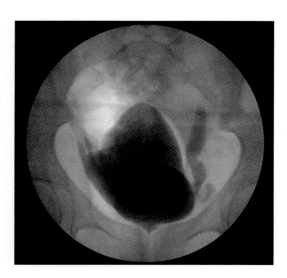

Fig. 8 Vesicoureteral reflux during the filling phasing

Ambulatory Urodynamics

Ambulatory urodynamics (AUDS) was introduced in the 1980s and relies on the same principles of conventional urodynamics using, however, a physiological-filling cystometry in an outpatient setting. In AUDS the filling fluid is urine at body temperature and at kidney production rate, instead of artificial filling with ambient-temperature saline. Despite having a slower filling rate, it has the advantage of allowing the patient to perform his or her daily activities, therefore rendering a more natural assessment of the micturition cycle.

Equipment and the Study

Patient setup and catheter positioning are similar to cystometry and pressure/flow studies. In some cases, these catheters can be air-charged instead of water-filled and have wireless connection through Bluetooth. Care must be taken to ensure the catheters are securely fixed and have adequate length to avoid displacement during movement. At the beginning of the test, the patient is asked to cough, and periodic coughs should be repeated thereafter to check adequate subtraction of the pressures. The patient carries a portable device that is connected to the vesical and rectal catheters, which perform the normal readings. The data is later downloaded for processing. At least three different cycles in different situations should be recorded:

1. At rest
2. Deambulation
3. Performing incontinence provocative maneuvers

During the physiological filling, the patient is instructed to record the bladder sensation, urgency and leakage episodes, time and amount of volume intake, performance of provocative maneuvers, and voluntary voids. The latter should be recorded using a flowmeter to assess the flow rate. Urinary leakage can be reported by the patient's diary system or by an alarm pad that detects urine through changing in the resistance of an electric circuit.

Indications

AUDS should be performed when traditional urodynamics are not sensitive enough to reproduce the symptoms [56]. Standard cystometry fails to detect DO in up to 50% of the cases [57], and AUDS has shown increased detection rates of DO [58]. This is attributed to several caveats/ pitfalls in conventional cystometry, namely, the unfamiliar environment, motionless position, and artificial filling rate.

AUDS also plays a role in diagnosing urinary incontinence that is not demonstrated in conventional urodynamics as it allows recording of leakage during everyday activities. Furthermore it may outperform traditional tests in determining whether the main cause of incontinence is DO or sphincter weakness.

Future applications for AUDS include treatment response assessment and optimization of sacral neuromodulation as investigators found a correlation between sacral neuromodulation patient-reported outcomes and AUDS findings [59, 60].

However, technical issues, which can be as high as 25% [61], have deemed this test to be challenging and to have variable reproducibility. With movement and in an uncontrolled scenario, the catheters can be easily displaced hindering precise measurement (Fig. 9). Patient cooperation is also of major importance. The technology and devices used to measure urinary leak and intravesical volumes have yet to be improved.

Overall, and despite its advantages over conventional urodynamics, AUDS is a time-consuming exam and requires significant expertise for its interpretation, therefore being only recommended in a specific setting of patients.

> **Key Points in Ambulatory Urodynamics**
> - Second-line diagnostic tool when traditional urodynamics fails to explain symptoms.
> - Is time-consuming and requires specialized equipment and training.
> - Patient cooperation and standardization are mandatory for reliable recordings and reproducible results.

Urethral Pressure Profile

Urinary continence is achieved by a complex interaction between pelvic structures, namely, the striated urogenital sphincter, the pelvic floor muscles, and the urethral smooth muscle and the highly vascularized submucosa. As long as the urethral

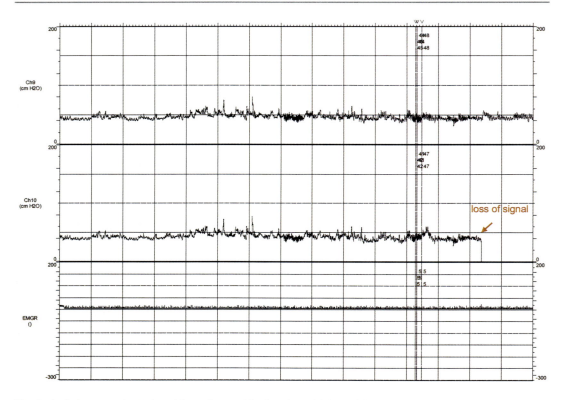

Fig. 9 Ambulatory urodynamics without abnormal findings but with loss of signal due to catheter displacement

closure pressure is superior to the intravesical pressure, continence is maintained. During certain activities, such as coughing or Valsalva maneuvers, a transient increase in the abdominal pressure is transmitted to the bladder and the urethra. In case the pressure transmission is 100%, both the bladder and urethral closure pressures increase in the same proportion, thus preventing any urinary leak. On the other hand, whether there is an inefficient transmission pressure or there is an insufficient sphincter deficiency, the bladder pressure will surpass the urethral closure pressure and cause urinary leakage [20].

Urethral pressure profile (UPP) is a test that records the urethral intraluminal pressure along its length. There are several methods to measure the urethral pressure, the Brown and Wickham technique being the most commonly used. This method requires insertion of a 4 to 10Ch catheter into the bladder which is slowly removed at a constant speed. The catheter has side holes that flush water at a steady rate. The urethral pressure corresponds to the pressure needed to overcome the urethral wall and perfuse the catheter. Other devices include balloon catheter profilometry, catheter tip transducers, and air-charged catheters. UPP records the following:

- *Maximum urethral pressure (MUP)* – the maximum measured pressure
- *Maximum urethral closure pressure (MUCP)* – (MUP, P_{ves})
- *Functional profile length* – the length of the urethra along which the urethral pressure exceeds the bladder pressure
- *Pressure transmission ratio* – the change in percentage of the incremental intravesical pressure compared to the urethral pressure (Fig. 10)

In females the MUP varies with age. Mean MUP values for women between 25 and 44 years normally range between 75 and 90 cm H_2O. With aging there is a significant decline after menopause that can reach up to 50% [62]. This process is multifactorial and thought to be due to loss of striated muscle fibers and nerve injury [20].

$$PTR\ (\%) = \frac{\triangle P_{ura}}{\triangle P_{ves}}\ X\ 100$$

Fig. 10 Pressure transmission ratio (PTR) equation, where ΔP_{ura} is the difference between urethral pressure at stress and at rest and ΔP_{ves} is the difference between intravesical pressure at stress and at rest

A functional and competent sphincter mechanism will be relaxed and permit unobstructed urinary flow during voiding and efficiently close during filling to avoid incontinence. This way, UPP should be performed either at:

- *Rest* – UPP at rest is targeted to characterize storage LUTS, namely, incontinence. Continent women show a greater baseline MUP and greater increase in MUP during filling [63]. Furthermore, MUCP correlates with the severity of SUI [64]. A low MUCP is associated with a poor urethral function due to ISD, which is considered one of the main mechanisms involved in stress incontinence [65]. These parameters may help identify patients in which the main cause of incontinence is ISD, rather than urethral hypermobility and which will have less benefit from urethral support surgery such as urethral slings [66].
- *Stress* – UPP performed simultaneous with maneuvers that increase abdominal pressure can further simulate and quantify parameters in patients with SUI. VLPP inversely correlates with the severity of SUI. VLPPs lower than 60 cm H_2O are associated with a shorter urethral functional length and lower sphincter activity. In SUI there is an inadequate pressure transmission that causes an insufficient increase in the urethral closure pressure to prevent urine leakage. A low PTR can be a surrogate marker for urethral hypermobility and has shown correlation with the Q-tip angle [67]. The association between the PTR and the grade of SUI has been reinforced by the findings of an increase of PTR in patients submitted to midurethral surgery and resolution of SUI [68].
- *Voiding* – UPP during voiding is useful to study obstructive symptoms, to define the severity of obstruction by measuring the

urethral pressure and to determine the site of obstruction. In adult young women, Fowler's syndrome, also called high-tone non-relaxing sphincter, is characterized by idiopathic voiding dysfunction with or without urinary retention and is thought to be caused by external urethral sphincter spasms (Fig. 11). It is typically associated with high MUCP (>100 cm H_2O), large bladder capacity, and normal bladder filling [69].

> **Key Points in Urethral Pressure Profile**
> - Useful for portraying urethral function.
> - Parameters tend to correlate with severity of SUI and predict response to treatment.
> - Low specificity and lack of standardization prevent its application in routine practice.

Neurophysiology

Neurophysiological studies are mainly used in research for a better and comprehensive understanding of the urinary tract function. These tests are most commonly applied in patients with neurological conditions. The micturition cycle runs through a complex interaction between neurological circuits, including somatic nerves running through the pudendal nerve, parasympathetic nerves emerging from sacral routes, and sympathetic nerves coming from the hypogastric nerves. Neurophysiological urodynamic investigations help detect defects in nerve conduction and consequent abnormal muscle contraction which causes either voiding dysfunction or storage disorders.

- **Electromyography** – through the application of needles or surface electrodes, it is possible to assess the muscle or electrical activity in response to nerve stimulation, namely, the pelvic floor striated musculature and urinary sphincters. Some of its indications include:
  - Diagnosis and study: Fowler's syndrome; detrusor sphincter dyssynergia and cauda

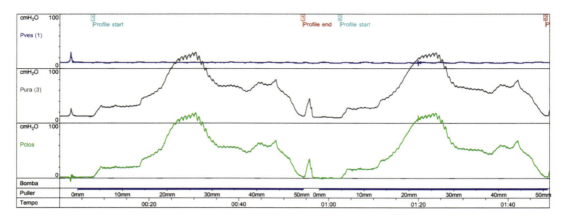

Fig. 11 Patient with Fowler's syndrome and high MUCP (>100 cm H$_2$O)

- equina syndrome with bladder sacral nerve compression
- Treatment: physiotherapy and biofeedback muscle training
- **Nerve conduction latency studies** - determines the time from the moment of peripheral nerve stimulation and muscle contraction. The aforementioned correlation of neuropathy in older women with incontinence can be objectified with electrophysiology studies. Pudendal nerve terminal motor latency is significantly increased in patients with incontinence when compared to controls [70].

Key Points in Neurophysiology
- Most added value in neurogenic patients
- Limited clinical usage

Conclusion

The lower urinary tract is a complex system with close interaction between neurological circuits, voluntary and involuntary musculature, and pelvic organs. Any damage or malfunction in one of these components can lead to either storage or voiding dysfunction. Urodynamics is a valuable tool to assess in an objective fashion the lower urinary tract symptoms, which helps to diagnose the underlying disorder exclude complications of the upper tract and guide treatment choice. As each urodynamic test has its indications, advantages, risks, and costs, the clinician must have a comprehensive knowledge of their benefits in order to choose the appropriate test and accurately interpret the results. With the development of new technologies, the tests have become more sophisticated, less invasive, and more precise.

In the future, goals should be focused on standardizing the procedures and reporting of the results, finding and strengthening correlations between urodynamic parameters and treatment indications, as well as investing on development of less invasive and more accurate technology.

References

1. Abrams P, Cardozo L, Fall M, Griffiths D, Rosier P, Ulmsten U, et al. The standardisation of terminology of lower urinary tract function: report from the Standardisation Sub-committee of the International Continence Society. Neurourol Urodyn. 2002;21: 167–78.
2. Bright E, Cotterill N, Drake M, Abrams P. Developing and validating the International Consultation on Incontinence Questionnaire bladder diary. Eur Urol. 2014;66:294–300.
3. de la Blanca R, Medina Polo J, Arrébola Pajares A, Hernández Arroyo M, Peña Vallejo E, Teigell Tobar J, Alonso Isa M, Garcia Gómez B, Romero Otero J, Rodriguez Antolin A, SP. Design and preliminary validation of a simpler version of the bladder diary for the evaluation of lower tract urinary symptoms. In: International Continence Society 51st Annual Meeting. Melbourne 14–17 October. Abstract #293. International Continence Society 51st Annual Meeting. Melbourne. 14–17 October, Hospital Universitario 12 de Octubre; n.d.

4. Pereira E Silva R, Lopes F, Fernandes M, Polido J, Ponte C, Esteves A, et al. Translation and validation of the Portuguese version of the International Consultation on Incontinence Questionnaire (ICIQ) Bladder Diary. Int Urogynecol J. 2022.

5. Tayebi S, Salehi-Pourmehr H, Hajebrahimi S, Hashim H. Translation and validation of the Persian ICIQ bladder diary. Int Urogynecol J. 2021;32:3287–91.

6. Krhut J, Zachoval R, Smith PP, Rosier PFWM, Valanský L, Martan A, et al. Pad weight testing in the evaluation of urinary incontinence. Neurourol Urodyn. 2014;33:507–10.

7. Bezerra CA, Bruschini H, Cody DJ. Traditional suburethral sling operations for urinary incontinence in women. Cochrane Database Syst Rev. 2005: CD001754.

8. Pope R, Ganesh P, Wilkinson J. Pubococcygeal sling versus refixation of the pubocervical fascia in vesicovaginal fistula repair: a retrospective review. Obstet Gynecol Int. 2018;2018:6396387.

9. Chang T-C, Hsiao S-M, Chen C-H, Wu W-Y, Lin H-H. Utilizing preoperative 20-minute pad testing with vaginal gauze packing for indicating concomitant midurethral sling during cystocele repair. Eur J Obstet Gynecol Reprod Biol. 2014;172:127–30.

10. Lindsay J, Solomon E, Nadeem M, Pakzad M, Hamid R, Ockrim J, et al. Treatment validation of the Solomon-Greenwell nomogram for female bladder outlet obstruction. Neurourol Urodyn. 2020;39:1371–7.

11. Mytilekas K-V, Oeconomou A, Sokolakis I, Kalaitzi M, Mouzakitis G, Nakopoulou E, et al. Defining voiding dysfunction in women: bladder outflow obstruction versus detrusor underactivity. Int Neurourol J. 2021;25:244–51.

12. Haylen BT, Lee J, Logan V, Husselbee S, Zhou J, Law M. Immediate postvoid residual volumes in women with symptoms of pelvic floor dysfunction. Obstet Gynecol. 2008;111:1305–12.

13. Lukacz ES, DuHamel E, Menefee SA, Luber KM. Elevated postvoid residual in women with pelvic floor disorders: prevalence and associated risk factors. Int Urogynecol J Pelvic Floor Dysfunct. 2007;18:397–400.

14. Milleman M, Langenstroer P, Guralnick ML. Post-void residual urine volume in women with overactive bladder symptoms. J Urol. 2004;172:1911–4.

15. Emberton M. Definition of at-risk patients: dynamic variables. BJU Int. 2006;97(Suppl 2):12–5. discussion 21–2.

16. Gehrich A, Stany MP, Fischer JR, Buller J, Zahn CM. Establishing a mean postvoid residual volume in asymptomatic perimenopausal and postmenopausal women. Obstet Gynecol. 2007;110:827–32.

17. Rosier PFWM, Schaefer W, Lose G, Goldman HB, Guralnick M, Eustice S, et al. International Continence Society Good Urodynamic Practices and Terms 2016: urodynamics, uroflowmetry, cystometry, and pressure-flow study. Neurourol Urodyn. 2017;36:1243–60.

18. Arunachalam D, Heit M. Low bladder compliance in women: a clinical overview. Female Pelvic Med Reconstr Surg. 2020;26:263–9.

19. D'Ancona CAL, Gomes MJ, Rosier PFWM. ICS teaching module: cystometry (basic module). Neurourol Urodyn. 2017;36:1673–6.

20. Ashton-Miller JA, DeLancey JOL. Functional anatomy of the female pelvic floor. Ann N Y Acad Sci. 2007;1101:266–96.

21. Kalejaiye O, Vij M, Drake MJ. Classification of stress urinary incontinence. World J Urol. 2015;33:1215–20.

22. Bump RC, Elser DM, Theofrastous JP, McClish DK. Valsalva leak point pressures in women with genuine stress incontinence- reproducibility, effect of catheter caliber, and correlations with other measures of urethral resistance.pdf. Am J Obstet Gynecol. 1995;173:551–7.

23. Padilla-Fernández B, Ramírez-Castillo GM, Hernández-Hernández D, Castro-Díaz DM. Urodynamics before stress urinary incontinence surgery in modern functional urology. Eur Urol Focus. 2019;5:319–21.

24. Peyronnet B, Mironska E, Chapple C, Cardozo L, Oelke M, Dmochowski R, et al. A comprehensive review of overactive bladder pathophysiology: on the way to tailored treatment. Eur Urol. 2019;75:988–1000.

25. Rosier PFWM, Kuo H-C, De Gennaro M, Gammie A, Finazzi Agro E, Kakizaki H, et al. International Consultation on Incontinence 2016; executive summary: urodynamic testing. Neurourol Urodyn. 2019;38:545–52.

26. Harding CK, Lapitan MC, Arlandis S, Bø K, Costantini E, Groen J, et al. EAU guidelines on management of non-neurogenic female lower urinary tract symptoms (LUTS). In: European Association of Urology Guidelines. 2021 edition. European Association of Urology Guidelines Office; 2021. [Internet]. Available at. https://uroweb.org/wp-content/uploads/EAU-Guidelines-on-Non-Neurogenic-Female-LUTS-2021.pdf

27. Irwin DE, Milsom I, Hunskaar S, Reilly K, Kopp Z, Herschorn S, et al. Population-based survey of urinary incontinence, overactive bladder, and other lower urinary tract symptoms in five countries: results of the EPIC study. Eur Urol. 2006;50:1306–14. discussion 1314–5.

28. Irwin DE, Kopp ZS, Agatep B, Milsom I, Abrams P. Worldwide prevalence estimates of lower urinary tract symptoms, overactive bladder, urinary incontinence and bladder outlet obstruction. BJU Int. 2011;108:1132–8.

29. Nager CW, Brubaker L, Daneshgari F, Litman HJ, Dandreo KJ, Sirls L, et al. Design of the Value of Urodynamic Evaluation (ValUE) trial: a non-inferiority randomized trial of preoperative urodynamic investigations. Contemp Clin Trials. 2009;30:531–9.

30. Fletcher SG, Lemack GE. Clarifying the role of urodynamics in the preoperative evaluation of stress urinary incontinence. ScientificWorldJournal. 2008;8: 1259–68.

31. Nager CW, Sirls L, Litman HJ, Richter H, Nygaard I, Chai T, et al. Baseline urodynamic predictors of

31. treatment failure 1 year after mid urethral sling surgery. J Urol. 2011;186:597–603.
32. Nager CW, Brubaker L, Litman HJ, Zyczynski HM, Varner RE, Amundsen C, et al. A randomized trial of urodynamic testing before stress-incontinence surgery. N Engl J Med. 2012;366:1987–97.
33. van Leijsen SAL, Kluivers KB, Mol BWJ, Hout J't, Milani AL, Roovers J-PWR, et al. Value of urodynamics before stress urinary incontinence surgery: a randomized controlled trial. Obstet Gynecol. 2013;121:999.
34. Lowder JL, Frankman EA, Ghetti C, Burrows LJ, Krohn MA, Moalli P, et al. Lower urinary tract symptoms in women with pelvic organ prolapse. Int Urogynecol J. 2010;21:665–72.
35. Brubaker L, Cundiff GW, Fine P, Nygaard I, Richter HE, Visco AG, et al. Abdominal sacrocolpopexy with Burch colposuspension to reduce urinary stress incontinence. N Engl J Med. 2006;354:1557–66.
36. Wei JT, Nygaard I, Richter HE, Nager CW, Barber MD, Kenton K, et al. A midurethral sling to reduce incontinence after vaginal prolapse repair. N Engl J Med. 2012;366:2358–67.
37. Serati M, Giarenis I, Meschia M, Cardozo L. Role of urodynamics before prolapse surgery. Int Urogynecol J. 2015;26:165–8.
38. NICE guidance – urinary incontinence and pelvic organ prolapse in women: management: © NICE (2019) urinary incontinence and pelvic organ prolapse in women: management. BJU Int. 2019(123):777–803.
39. Ginsberg D. The epidemiology and pathophysiology of neurogenic bladder. Am J Manag Care. 2013;19:s191–6.
40. Fowler CJ. Neurological disorders of micturition and their treatment. Brain. 1999;122(Pt 7):1213–31.
41. Gelber DA, Good DC, Laven LJ, Verhulst SJ. Causes of urinary incontinence after acute hemispheric stroke. Stroke. 1993;24:378–82.
42. Koprowski C, Friel B, Kim C, Radadia KD, Farber N, Tunuguntla H, et al. Urodynamic evaluation of adult neurogenic lower urinary tract dysfunction: a review. Am J Urol Res. 2017;2(2):029–37.
43. Tarcan T, Demirkesen O, Plata M, Castro-Diaz D. ICS teaching module: detrusor leak point pressures in patients with relevant neurological abnormalities. Neurourol Urodyn. 2017;36:259–62.
44. McGuire EJ. Urodynamics of the neurogenic bladder. Urol Clin North Am. 2010;37:507–16.
45. Combs AJ, Horowitz M. A new technique for assessing detrusor leak point pressure in patients with spina bifida. J Urol. 1996;156:757–60.
46. Tarcan T, Tinay I, Sekerci CA, Alpay H, SimSek F. Is 40 cm H2O detrusor leak point pressure (DLPP) cut-off really reliable for upper urinary tract (UUT) protection in children with myelodysplasia? J Urol. 2009;181:312.
47. Castro-Diaz D, Taracena Lafuente JM. Detrusor-sphincter dyssynergia. Int J Clin Pract Suppl. 2006;60:17–21.
48. Araki I, Matsui M, Ozawa K, Takeda M, Kuno S. Relationship of bladder dysfunction to lesion site in multiple sclerosis. J Urol. 2003;169:1384–7.

49. Litwiller SE, Frohman EM, Zimmern PE. Multiple sclerosis and the urologist. J Urol. 1999;161:743–57.
50. Klingler HC, Madersbacher S, Djavan B, Schatzl G, Marberger M, Schmidbauer CP. Morbidity of the evaluation of the lower urinary tract with transurethral multichannel pressure-flow studies. J Urol. 1998;159:191–4.
51. Suskind AM, Clemens JQ, Kaufman SR, Stoffel JT, Oldendorf A, Malaeb BS, et al. Patient perceptions of physical and emotional discomfort related to urodynamic testing: a questionnaire-based study in men and women with and without neurologic conditions. Urology. 2015;85:547–51.
52. Takami N, Mukai S, Nomi M, Yanagiuchi A, Sengoku A, Maeda K, et al. Retrospective observational study of risk factors for febrile infectious complications after urodynamic studies in patients with suspected neurogenic lower urinary tract disturbance. Urol Int. 2022;106:722–729
53. Ong HL, Lee C-L, Kuo H-C. Female bladder neck dysfunction-a video-urodynamic diagnosis among women with voiding dysfunction. Low Urin Tract Symptoms. 2020;12:278–84.
54. Peng C-H, Chen S-F, Kuo H-C. Videourodynamic analysis of the urethral sphincter overactivity and the poor relaxing pelvic floor muscles in women with voiding dysfunction. Neurourol Urodyn. 2017;36:2169–75.
55. Hsiao S-M, Lin H-H, Kuo H-C. Videourodynamic studies of women with voiding dysfunction. Sci Rep. 2017;7:6845.
56. Abelson B, Majerus S, Sun D, Gill BC, Versi E, Damaser MS. Ambulatory urodynamic monitoring: state of the art and future directions. Nat Rev Urol. 2019;16:291–301.
57. Radley SC, Rosario DJ, Chapple CR, Farkas AG. Conventional and ambulatory urodynamic findings in women with symptoms suggestive of bladder overactivity. J Urol. 2001;166:2253–8.
58. Digesu GA, Gargasole C, Hendricken C, Gore M, Kocjancic E, Khullar V, et al. ICS teaching module: ambulatory urodynamic monitoring. Neurourol Urodyn. 2017;36:364–7.
59. Kocher NJ, Damaser MS, Gill BC. Advances in ambulatory urodynamics. Curr Urol Rep. 2020;21:41.
60. Drossaerts J, Rademakers KLJ, Rahnama'i SM, Marcelissen T, Van Kerrebroeck P, van Koeveringe G. The value of ambulatory urodynamics in the evaluation of treatment effect of sacral neuromodulation. Urol Int. 2019;102:299–305.
61. Pannek J, Pieper P. Clinical usefulness of ambulatory urodynamics in the diagnosis and treatment of lower urinary tract dysfunction. Scand J Urol Nephrol. 2008;42:428–32.
62. Pipitone F, Sadeghi Z, DeLancey JOL. Urethral function and failure: a review of current knowledge of urethral closure mechanisms, how they vary, and how they are affected by life events. Neurourol Urodyn. 2021;40:1869–79.
63. Geynisman-Tan J, Mou T, Mueller MG, Kenton K. How does the urethra respond to bladder filling in

continent and incontinent women? Female Pelvic Med Reconstr Surg. 2021.

64. Dompeyre P, Pizzoferrato A-C, Le Normand L, Bader G, Fauconnier A. Valsalva urethral profile (VUP): a urodynamic measure to assess stress urinary incontinence in women. Neurourol Urodyn. 2020;39:1515–22.

65. DeLancey JOL, Trowbridge ER, Miller JM, Morgan DM, Guire K, Fenner DE, et al. Stress urinary incontinence: relative importance of urethral support and urethral closure pressure. J Urol. 2008;179:2286–90. discussion 2290.

66. Lo T-S, Ng KL, Lin Y-H, Hsieh W-C, Kao CC, Tan YL. Impact of intrinsic sphincter deficiency on mid-urethral sling outcomes. Int Urogynecol J. 2021.

67. Wu C-J, Ting W-H, Lin H-H, Hsiao S-M. Clinical and urodynamic predictors of the Q-tip test in women with lower urinary tract symptoms. Int Neurourol J. 2020;24:52–8.

68. Hsiao S-M, Sheu B-C, Lin H-H. Sequential assessment of urodynamic findings before and after transobturator tape procedure for female urodynamic stress incontinence. Int Urogynecol J Pelvic Floor Dysfunct. 2008;19:627–32.

69. Biers SM, Harding C, Belal M, Thiruchelvam N, Hamid R, Sahai A, et al. British Association of Urological Surgeons (BAUS) consensus document: management of female voiding dysfunction. BJU Int. 2022;129:151–9.

70. Snooks SJ, Badenoch DF, Tiptaft RC, Swash M. Perineal nerve damage in genuine stress urinary incontinence. An electrophysiological study. Br J Urol. 1985;57:422–6.

Endoscopic Evaluation

11

Francisco E. Martins, Natalia Martins, Liliya Tryfonyuk, and José Bernal Riquelme

Contents

Introduction	180
Historical Perspective	180
Types of Endoscopes and Equipment	181
Rigid Cystourethroscopy	181
Flexible Cystourethroscopy	183
Personnel and Preparation	184
Technique	184
Indications	185
Contraindications	185
Complications	185
Normal Endoscopic Findings	185
Pathologic Urethral Findings	186
Pathologic Bladder Findings	186

F. E. Martins (✉)
Department of Urology, Reconstructive Urology Unit,
School of Medicine, Hospital Santa Maria, CHULN,
University of Lisbon, Lisbon, Portugal

N. Martins
Urology Division, Armed Forces Hospital, Lisbon,
Portugal

L. Tryfonyuk
Urology Division, Rivne Regional Hospital, Rivne,
Ukraine

J. B. Riquelme
Urology Division, Hospital Sotero Del Rio, Santiago,
Chile

© Springer Nature Switzerland AG 2023
F. E. Martins et al. (eds.), *Female Genitourinary and Pelvic Floor Reconstruction*,
https://doi.org/10.1007/978-3-031-19598-3_11

Conclusions	193
Cross-References	193
References	193

Abstract

Cystoscopy is a basic urologic skill necessary for the endoscopic evaluation of the lower urinary tract, specifically the urethra and bladder. It is one of the most important diagnostic tools used by urologists to evaluate the lower urinary tract. It is relatively simple and can be performed under local anesthesia as an office procedure in numerous cases, or in the operating room under general anesthesia. There are essentially two types of cystoscopies: rigid (used for both diagnostic and therapeutic purposes) and flexible (mostly used for diagnostic purposes). It is a very useful means of diagnosis for numerous urologic conditions, and it also has a therapeutic role when needed. Indications for cystoscopy may range from major health-threatening conditions such as bladder cancer or severe hematuria to milder, bothersome conditions such as micturition problems, bladder stones, recurrent lower urinary tract infections, and bladder pain syndrome. This is a simple procedure that every urologist should be able to perform as part of their clinical routine practice, either for diagnostic or therapeutic purposes.

Keywords

Cystoscopy · Cystourethroscopy · Endoscopic evaluation · Flexible cystoscopy · Lower urinary tract

Introduction

Endoscopy of the lower urinary tract (cystourethroscopy), specifically the urethra and bladder, is one of the most common procedures performed by urologists. It allows for direct visualization of the urethra, urethral sphincter, bladder, and ureteral orifices in the female. There are both flexible and rigid cystoscopes and a variety of tools that can be

incorporated during cystoscopy, depending on the situation. Cystoscopy is mostly a diagnostic procedure, but there are a limited number of therapeutic procedures that can also be performed. There are various indications to perform a cystoscopy. It can be performed as a simple office procedure or as a procedure in the operating room with the patient under general anesthesia. This chapter describes the indications, contraindications of cystoscopy, necessary equipment, potential complications, and the role of the interprofessional team in managing patients with problems of the lower urinary tract.

The goals of this chapter are (1) to describe the technique of cystourethroscopy, (2) to discuss the indications for cystourethroscopy, (3) to outline its complications, and (4) to elucidate the importance of adequate effort coordination among health care professionals to optimize the delivery of care for patients undergoing cystourethroscopy.

Historical Perspective

In 1805, Philip Bozzini (1773–1809), a young German army surgeon, developed the first endoscopic instrument that was the ancestor of the modern endoscope that would allow him to investigate the cavities of the human body, including the possibility of locating bullets in his army patients. Although not highly successful due to its size and rudimentary candlelight illumination, this invention sparked enormous interest and improvements by future urologists for the evaluation of the female lower urinary tract, including urethra and bladder [1]. However, the procedure involved a cumbersome device with poor illumination provided by a candle reflected through a funnel in the urethral limiting visibility. Additionally, to achieve a better view, the operator inevitably burnt himself if the stand had to be tilted to improve the view. In the nineteenth century, refinements to this crude instrument included a surrounding cannula followed by a lens system to provide magnification of the field and better view. Nonetheless, the greatest drawback of these early endoscopes was poor illumination, despite efforts to get around this obstacle using reflective mirrors and, finally, an incandescent light source. Even after all these improvements, visualization remained deficient without bladder distension. Therefore, cystoscopy was simply a complement to the established practice of urethral dilatation and bimanual palpation of the bladder.

In 1894, Kelly, a genitourinary surgeon at Johns Hopkins Hospital, changed the role of cystoscopy with the introduction of a technique that allowed simultaneous adequate distension of the bladder. Although not innovative, the Kelly cystoscope, essentially a hollow tube without a lens, was introduced with an obturator, with the patient in the knee-chest position. With the patient in this position, a negative intra-abdominal pressure was created allowing air to distend the bladder when the cystoscope was introduced. A head mirror used by the physician would reflect an electric light and illuminate the bladder (Fig. 1) [2]. Due to its simplicity and good view, this technique rapidly became accessible to all physicians. Also, in the late 1800s, Maximilian Nitze devoted most of his life to the development of endoscopes with new properties and applications [3].

The twentieth century provided the stage for several innovations in cystoscopy. In 1954, Hopkins and Kopany introduced a fiberoptic telescope followed later by a rod lens system. These innovations dramatically improved light transmission and resolution. Further developments in lens and light technology led to significant refinements [4]. In 1966, Karl Storz introduced a system of transmitting cold light from an external source through noncoherent fibers to provide excellent illumination, ending up with a revolutionary improved instrument of smaller diameter and better image [5].

The flexible endoscope is the most recent development in cystoscopy. The advantages of the flexible cystoscope are the flexibility of the fiberoptic lens system allowing the cystoscope to bend and thus to increase the range of the view field and patient tolerance.

Types of Endoscopes and Equipment

Urological cystourethroscopes can be divided into two types: rigid and flexible endoscopes. Rigid endoscopes use the Hopkins rod-lens optical system. Light is transmitted to illuminate the target to be seen by the examiner's eye. The Hopkins rod-lens system has the advantage of yielding better optical definition when compared with the fiberoptic bundles used in flexible cystoscopes. However, the advent of flexible digital cystoscopes has narrowed this gap. Visualization is also superior in the rigid cystoscope due to the greater irrigant flow rate. Rigid cystoscopes also have larger working channels, which allow the simultaneous use of a wider variety of instruments. The advantage of the flexible cystoscopes is that they are smaller in size providing superior patient comfort. This is the main reason why they are used for routine flexible cystourethroscopy in the office setting. Another advantage of the flexible endoscope is its easy passage with a patient in the supine position, unlike the rigid cystoscope that requires the patient to be in the frog-leg or lithotomy position. Another excellent advantage is the mobility of the tip of the flexible cystoscope, which allows for easier inspection of the bladder. With a rigid cystoscope, it is necessary to use multiple lenses with varying degrees of angle to achieve proper inspection of the entire bladder.

Rigid Cystourethroscopy

Rigid cystoscopes are produced in sets that consist of an optical lens, bridge, sheath, and obturator (Fig. 2). The optical lenses come with different tip angles that range from 0 to 120 degrees to allow optimal visualization of the lower urinary tract. Zero-degree or 12° lens are ideal for urethroscopy (straight view urethral visualization), whereas cystoscopy (bladder visualization) usually requires a 12°, 30° (forward-oblique view), or a 70° (lateral view) lens. The most common lens degrees used during a typical rigid cystourethroscopy include the 30-degree lens and the 70-degree lens. The 30° lens is more commonly used for therapeutic purposes. The 70° lens is

Fig. 1 Air cystoscopy: the history of an endoscopic technique from the late nineteenth century. (Schultheiss, BJU International (1999); 83: 571–577. Wiley Online Library (reproduced with permission))

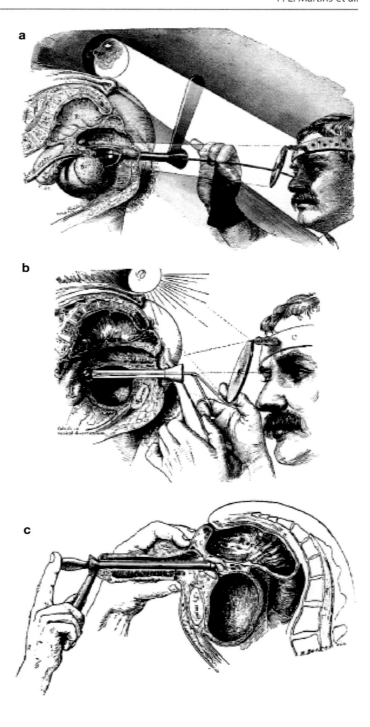

more useful to inspect the anterior, inferolateral walls, dome, and bladder neck. These different angles allow visualization of the entire bladder walls.

The cystourethroscope employs a bridge that connects the optical lens to the sheath. Basically, there are three types of bridges: (1) diagnostic bridge that has no working channel; (2) bridge

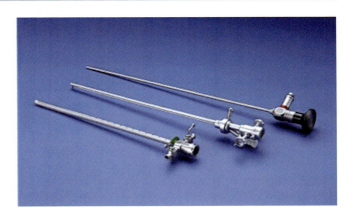

Fig. 2 Olympus rigid cystoscope. Existing rigid cystoscopes, regardless of size, are composed of three main parts: external sheath with obturator, intermediate piece (bridge), and telescope (optical system). Courtesy of Olympus Corporation. Copyright Olympus Corporation

having 1 or 2 working channels used for therapeutic purposes; and (3) the Albarran bridge, a specialized model that contains a lever that deflects wires or catheters that pass through the working channel to facilitate entrance into the ureteric orifice.

The cystourethroscopy sheaths are expressed in French (Fr) and come in a variety of sizes. The Fr measurement system refers to the external circumference in millimeters. One Fr equals one-third of a millimeter. Sheaths can range in size from 15/17 Fr to 25 Fr. Smaller sheaths are ideal for diagnostic cystoscopy and cause less trauma. Larger sheaths are used for therapeutic procedures as they allow more irrigant flow and larger working channels for instruments. Each sheath has an obturator that blunts the distal end of the sheath for passage into the bladder without visual assistance. Blind endoscope passage is generally only recommended to be performed in a female.

Flexible Cystourethroscopy

Unlike the rigid model, the flexible cystourethroscope combines the optical systems and irrigation-working channel in a single unit (Fig. 3). They range between 16 and 17 Fr. The optical system consists of two bundles of optic fibers, one single image-bearing fiberoptic bundle for illumination (noncoherent optical fibers) and two light-bearing fiberoptic bundles for image (coherent optical fibers). The fiber flexibility allows incorporation of a distal tip-deflecting mechanism, controlled by a lever at the eyepiece that deflect the tip 270° in a single plane making complete maneuverability possible [6]. The irrigation and instruments must pass through the same working channel. The amount of irrigation is significantly decreased with the instrument passing through the channel. The slower flow of the irrigant through this narrower caliber scope may significantly decrease clear visualization compared to a rigid scope. A working channel is present to allow passage of guidewires, needles, and forceps. These flexible materials do not resist high temperatures in an autoclave. Therefore, decontamination is recommended to clean flexible scopes instead of sterilization. Gentle handling is critical to good visualization and material longevity.

Both Karl Storz and Olympus produce fiberoptic and digital models. Digital scopes are now available in high definition (1920 × 1080 pixels) and standard definition (720 × 480 pixels). These scopes do not require focusing or white balancing. Studies have been performed to compare the resolution, contrast evaluation, depth of field, color representation, and the illumination of fiberoptic, standard, and high-definition flexible cystoscopes. All the parameters studied showed overall improvement, except illumination that was much better in the fiberoptic models compared to digital [7]. In a randomized study performed in 2009 comparing optics, performance, and durability of fiberoptic and standard-definition digital scopes, Okhunov et al. reported a

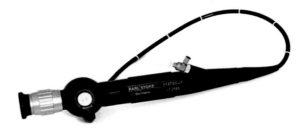

Fig. 3 Storz 11272CU1 flexible cystoscope (Courtesy of Karl Storz Endoscopy, Culver City, CA) We acknowledge copyright and ownership to Copyright KARL STORZ SE & Co. KG, Tuttlingen, Germany

trend of surgeon optical ranking in favor of digital scopes, and no difference in durability between models [8].

Irrigant material depends on the situation, but sterile water or normal saline is most commonly used. Nonionic irrigants (water, glycine, and sorbitol) are required when using monopolar electrocautery. Isotonic irrigating fluids (normal saline/lactated ringers) can be used when using bipolar electrocautery instruments. Sterile water should be used when bladder samples are collected for cytologic evaluation.

Personnel and Preparation

The personnel required for endoscopic evaluation of the lower urinary tract depends on the setting it is being performed, that is as an office or operating room procedure. A simple office cystourethroscopy requires minimal personnel, as it does not involve anesthesia. It is helpful to have a nurse as an assistant, especially when these procedures need to be performed more easily with an extra pair of hands. An ideal example is to perform a cystoscopy to remove an indwelling ureteral stent. This would allow the surgeon to operate the cystoscope while having his/her assistant operate the flexible grasper. However, when performing endoscopic evaluation in the operating room, an anesthesia staff, scrub, and circulating nurses are needed for assistance.

Informed consent should be obtained before the procedure, as this is an invasive procedure and prone to iatrogenic injury. A urinalysis and urine culture should be performed before the procedure. However, many centers do not consider this as mandatory. Most best practice policy statements on antimicrobial prophylaxis do not recommend antibiotic administration for routine diagnostic cystoscopy in the absence of patient-related risk factors such as (1) advanced age, (2) diabetes mellitus, (3) other immunodeficiency states, (4) chronic steroid use, (5) poor nutritional status, (6) colonized endogenous or exogenous material, (7) prolonged coexistent infection, and (8) chronic circulatory deficiency status. Either a fluoroquinolone or a trimethoprim-sulfamethoxazole can be recommended as prophylaxis lasting less than 24 h for therapeutic procedures. Two-antibiotic combination alternatives may include an aminoglycoside with or without ampicillin, a first- or second-generation cephalosporin, or amoxicillin/clavulanate [9]. Otherwise, antibiotic prophylaxis should be administered according to local practice standards.

Technique

First, the patient's external genitalia should be inspected for any lesions or anatomic abnormalities. The cystourethroscope should be assembled correctly and connected to sterile irrigant fluid at around 90 cm above the patient's pelvis.

In female patients, rigid cystourethroscopy insertion can be performed using a sheath obturator. The scope will need to be directed anteriorly as it is advanced into the bladder. A flexible scope can be inserted similarly as a Foley catheter, with active deflection being used as needed. Prior to the procedure, the skin should be scrubbed with an antiseptic agent such as aqueous-based iodopovidone-containing products such as Betadine are safe on all skin surfaces and are most commonly used for preparation [9]. Alcohol-based solutions can be damaging to mucus membranes and, therefore, should not be recommended for use on the genitalia.

If a halogen light source is used, a white balance of the lighting system should be performed. The urethral meatus and channel should be lubricated with an anesthetic gel and followed by gentle insertion and passage of the cystourethroscope. Inspection of the urethra and bladder should be meticulously performed, including identification of both ureteral orifices and followed by inspection of the lateral, posterior, anterior walls, and bladder dome and neck. A 70° lens or a flexible endoscope is required for this inspection.

Indications

There are several indications for office-based cystourethroscopy. Office cystoscopy is performed mostly for diagnostic purposes. Endoscopic evaluation of the female lower urinary tract is not performed routinely as it is not indicated in the diagnostic workup of a patient with lower urinary tract symptoms alone.

The most common indication for cystourethroscopy is hematuria, either gross (macroscopic or frank hematuria) or microscopic (nonvisible, diagnosed by dipstick urinalysis). Other formal indications are persistent obstructive or irritative lower urinary tract symptoms (LUTS), these same symptoms in the context of prior vesicourethral or vaginal surgery, suspicion of urethral stricture, a history of a difficult placement of a midurethral sling, and the presence of certain urological symptoms strongly associated with specific pathology, such as pneumaturia and/or fecaluria suggesting colovesical fistula. Persistent, continuous urine leakage suggesting vesicovaginal fistula, or more rarely an ectopic ureter opening in the vagina and bypassing the urinary sphincter. Postvoid dribbling or recurrent urethral discharge in the female may be indicative of a urethral diverticulum, and its opening may be visible at urethroscopy. Some authors perform cystourethroscopy routinely after vaginal mesh surgery to ensure that the urethra or bladder has not been inadvertently injured. Another important indication for cystourethroscopy is routine surveillance of bladder cancer.

In summary, formal indications for cystourethroscopy include: (1) hematuria (gross and microscopic), (2) persistent lower urinary tract symptoms (obstructive and irritative), (3) history of previous vaginal surgery, (4) history of pelvic trauma, (5) suspicion of fistula, presence of foreign body in the lower urinary tract, (6) presence of abnormal imaging of bladder, and (7) surveillance of bladder malignancy.

Contraindications

Contraindications to cystoscopy are relatively easy to list. Any evidence of acute urinary tract infection should contraindicate the procedure as it can put the patient at risk for developing sepsis from a urinary infectious source. For this reason, it should be recommended to obtain a urinalysis 5–7 days before any scheduled cystoscopy procedure. If a UTI is identified, the patient should be treated appropriately before the procedure. A contraindication for flexible cystoscopy in the office setting would be any intolerance to pain or discomfort with the procedure. In this case, the procedure should be rescheduled to the operating room (OR) under sedation. A urethral stricture can be a relative contraindication depending on the stricture severity, eventually making cystoscopy impossible, as the scope will not be able to pass through the stenotic urethral segment.

Complications

Complications of cystoscopy are generally insignificant and inconsequential such as urinary tract infection, hematuria, irritative voiding symptoms, and injury to the bladder or urethra. The development of an iatrogenic urethral stricture is a known possibility of instrumentation.

Normal Endoscopic Findings

In normal conditions, the urethral mucosa has a pink color and smooth surface with a longitudinal ridge, called the urethral crest. The urethrovesical junction (UVJ) is usually round or inverted horseshoe-shaped and completely coapted until the irrigating fluid expands the urethral lumen and the UVJ. The UVJ has minimal mobility and closes quickly on Valsalva maneuver.

Normally, the bladder mucosa has a smooth surface with a pale pink to glistening whitish hue. A translucent mucosa allows easy visualization of the submucosa vasculature. The dome thickens and obtains a granular texture as it transitions to the trigone. The trigone has a roughly triangular shape with the inferior apex pointing toward the UVJ and the ureteral orifices as the superior apices. The interureteric ridge is a visible elevation that forms in the trigone between the ureteral orifices at the bottom of the field of vision. Although some variations are possible, the ureteral orifices generally have a circular or slit-like appearance. With efflux of urine, the slit opens, and the mound retracts towards the intramural portion of the ureter.

When distended, the bladder assumes a roughly spherical shape, but numerous mucosal folds are apparent in the empty or partially filled state (Fig. 4). The uterus and cervix can be seen indenting the posterior and superior walls of the bladder, which usually creates posterolateral pouches where the bladder blankets the uterus into the paravaginal spaces. At times, manual pressure on the lower abdomen is needed to visualize the bladder dome properly.

Pathologic Urethral Findings

Congenital urethral anomalies are rare. However, urethral duplication has been reported, and typically, the most anterior lumen drains the true bladder. Because the false urethra has a blind end with the possibility of urine pooling and entrapment, resection of the abnormal duplicate urethral channel may be necessary. Urethral stones and strictures are other relatively common findings (Fig. 5). Fronds and polyps, found most commonly in the proximal urethra or at the UVJ, have been associated with chronic inflammation. Urethral diverticulum may appear as ostia on the lateral or posterior surface of the urethra, eventually discharging an exudate upon milking of the ventral aspect of the urethra. They can be generally described as a periurethral cystic structure adjacent to the urethra. Foreign material, such as exposed synthetic mesh used for anti-incontinence midurethral sling placement can be detected.

The urethral hypermobility, typical of stress incontinence assessed by urodynamic study, causes the UVJ to open and descend in response to cough and Valsalva maneuver, with the patient not being able to close the UVJ to hold and squeeze instructions. Furthermore, urethroscopy may typically show a rigid, fixed urethra with poor coaptation (Fig. 6). In severe ISD cases, the UVJ may not respond to commands and the lumen is visualized in its full length from external meatus to UVJ.

Pathologic Bladder Findings

Pathologic conditions involving the bladder can be grouped as mucosal lesions or structural variations. The former group is either inflammatory or neoplastic in nature, although their concurrent existence is common. Cystoscopy should be

Fig. 4 Endoscopic view of normal bladder

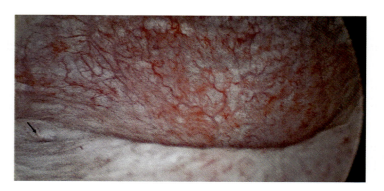

Fig. 5 Bladder stones

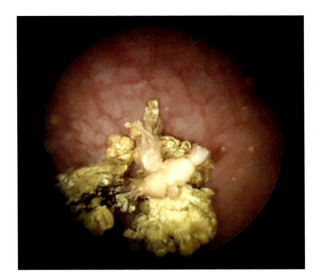

Fig. 6 Endoscopic view of rigid fixed urethra with poor coaptation

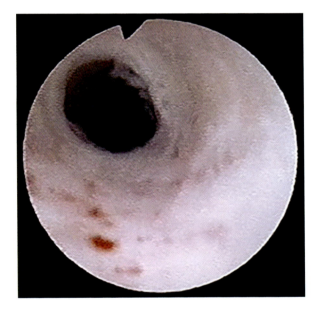

avoided in the presence of active acute infectious cystitis. However, if performed inadvertently, it may show different findings. In its mildest form, bacterial cystitis can be unremarkable, with a few pink macules or papules. In more severe cases, mucosal edema and hypervascularity are evident, including submucosal hypovascular pattern and marked vascular dilatation. In hemorrhagic cystitis, such as following heavy irradiation, these changes may be associated with gross hematuria and irritative voiding symptoms.

Hematuria is one of the most common indications for cystoscopy. This symptom can occur alone or in combination with irritative voiding. Several conditions may be the cause, such as chronic inflammatory conditions including hemorrhagic cystitis following administration of chemotherapeutic drugs (e.g., cyclophosphamide), radiation cystitis, tuberculous cystitis, schistosomiasis cystitis, interstitial cystitis, chronic use of anticoagulants, and other less common forms of cystitis, such as inflammatory

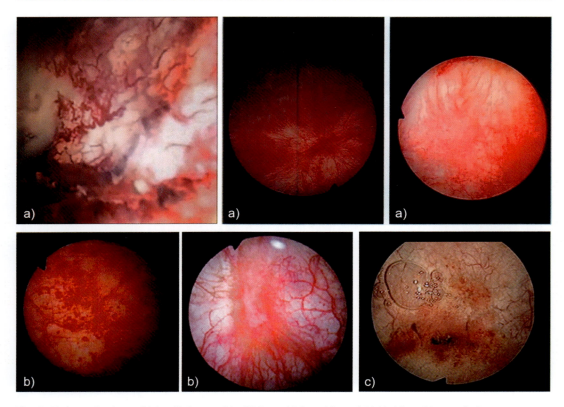

Fig. 7 Endoscopic views of (**a**) radiation cystitis, (**b**) interstitial cystitis, and (**c**) bladder schistosomiasis

polyps, cystitis cystica, cystitis glandularis, eosinophilic cystitis, emphysematous cystitis, and bladder stones (Fig. 7). Endometriosis of the urinary tract is relatively rare, accounting for less than 1% of all cases of endometriosis, the bladder being the most affected organ (Fig. 8). Bladder stones may result from urinary stasis due to bladder outlet obstruction or the presence of a foreign body, or coalescence of an inflammatory exudate, which functions as a lithogenic nidus. They can become attached to exposed mesh, any synthetic material, or nonabsorbable sutures used in prior surgery. Bladder cancer is a common cause of hematuria, macroscopic or microscopic, monosymptomatic or not. It is twice as common in men than in women and may be of different histopathologic types. Transitional cell carcinoma is the most common type followed by squamous cell carcinoma and adenocarcinoma.

Structural variations or congenital anomalies of the bladder and ureters may be anatomical or functional. Additional ureteral orifices are rare anatomic anomalies that reflect anomalies of the renal collecting system. They often enter the bladder wall at a slightly superior level to the trigone and in proximity to the other ureteral orifice. Ureteroceles develop in the distal, intravesical ureteral segment as laxity of the ureteral lumen, and herniate into the bladder cavity during efflux of urine.

Trabeculations of the inner surface of the bladder represent hypertrophied detrusor musculature. These trabeculations result from detrusor hyperactivity and functional or anatomic outlet obstruction. A bladder diverticulum may develop when high intravesical pressure produces enlargement

Fig. 8 Bladder endometriosis

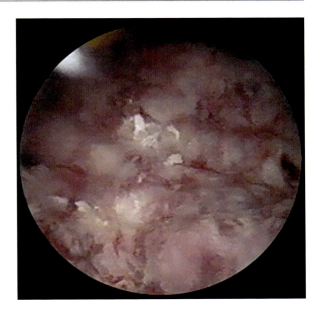

Fig. 9 Bladder diverticulum

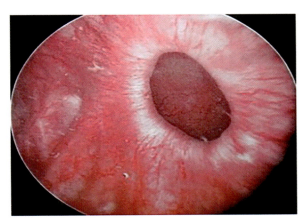

and outpouching of the intervening sacculation or herniation of the bladder wall (Fig. 9). Bladder diverticula may be acquired or congenital. Both the neck diameter and size of the diverticulum may vary significantly. It has been reported that bladder diverticula may lodge malignant neoplasms in up to 10% [10].

Leukoplakia of the bladder is a rare condition. It is characterized by squamous metaplasia of the transitional epithelium and keratinization. Addition of keratin deposition appears as a white flaky substance floating in the bladder. Leukoplakia may occur in other organs that are covered by squamous cell epithelium and is considered a premalignant condition. However, cytogenetic studies of bladder leukoplakia are consistent with a benign lesion, and no treatment is required.

Urinary tract fistulae represent an abnormal, extra-anatomic communication between the urinary tract urothelium and other mucosal-lined structure or organ, or the skin surface. Potentially, a fistula can form between any segment of the urinary tract, such as kidney, ureters, bladder, and urethra, and virtually any other body cavity.

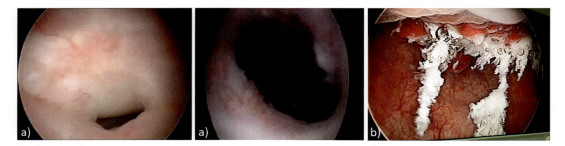

Fig. 10 Endoscopic views of bladder fistulation: (**a**) vesicovaginal fistula and (**b**) vesicoenteric fistula with exuberant inflammatory reaction associated

Cystoscopy is mandatory in the diagnostic workup of urinary tract fistulae.

In the industrialized world, the most common etiology (75%) of vesicovaginal fistula (VVF) is incidental, unrecognized injury to the bladder at the time of gynecologic surgery, usually abdominal hysterectomy (Fig. 10) [11, 12]. The diagnostic workup and treatment are described elsewhere in this textbook. However, in this setting, a thorough vaginal examination and a methylene dye test should always be part of the diagnosis. Vesicovaginal fistulae may also result from vaginal hysterectomies, urological procedures, vaginal synthetic mesh procedures, radiotherapy, cancer, obstetric trauma, and prolonged unattended labor. Early in its development, immature fistulae may have a less well-defined area of localized bullous edema without an apparent ostium. Well-developed fistulae show smoother margins with ostia of varying sizes (few millimeters to several centimeters). It is not uncommon to initially miss the exact fistula tract in a small VVF. Even methylene blue dye test may be misleading in cases of very small fistulae. The surgeon should attempt to pass a guidewire endoscopically through the fistula tract. Visualization of the guidewire in the vaginal cavity would confirm the diagnosis and the exact location of the VVF on both the vesical and vaginal sides. Sometimes, there may exist more than one collateral fistula tract. In patients with prior history of pelvic cancer or irradiation, a biopsy of the fistula is mandatory to exclude tumor recurrence. Post-hysterectomy fistulae are usually found in the bladder base above the interureteric ridge and at the level of the vaginal cuff.

Vesicoenteric fistula is an abnormal communication between the intestine and the bladder. The etiology varies, including diverticular disease (by far the most common, 65–79%), cancer (second in frequency, accounting to 10–20%), chronic intestinal inflammatory diseases, irradiation, injuries, and foreign bodies [13–15]. These fistulae uniformly have a surrounding inflammatory reaction with erythema, edema, and congestion. Although cystoscopy is accepted to have the highest yield in identifying a potential lesion, the findings may be nonspecific and may hinder its identification in 54–65% of cases [15–17]. Colonoscopy is not particularly valuable in detecting these fistulae. The detection rate can vary from as low as 8.5% and up to 55% [16–19]. However, as 10–15% of vesicoenteric fistulae result from malignancy, endoscopic examination of the colon should be an integral part of the diagnostic evaluation of these fistulae.

Chronic pelvic/bladder pain syndrome/interstitial cystitis has been characterized by the triad of pelvic/bladder pain, urinary frequency, and urgency. This syndrome is defined as a chronic health problem associated with bladder pain, bladder pressure, and sometimes with concurrent pelvic pain. The pain may be perceived to be originating from the bladder and vary in severity from mild discomfort to severe, incapacitating pain. This condition is part of a spectrum of diseases known as painful bladder syndrome, which includes interstitial cystitis.

Primary diagnostic tests should include urine analysis and culture, testing for sexually transmitted infections, and urine cytology in patients

Fig. 11 Endoscopic view of a patient's bladder with painful bladder syndrome

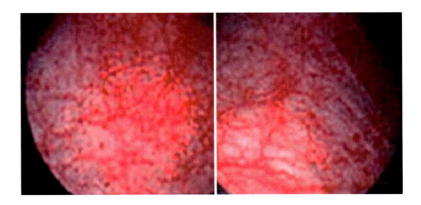

considered to be at high risk of urothelial malignancy. Pelvic imaging usually yields limited information and should be performed only if an alternative diagnosis is strongly suspected. Cystoscopy is essential to exclude other pathology and to aid accurate phenotyping of bladder painful syndrome (Fig. 11). Cystoscopy can evaluate bladder capacity and identify the presence of Hunner lesions and/or glomerulations for which targeted treatment could be recommended. Patients can be classified using the International Society for the Study of BPS criteria (ESSIC) based on cystoscopic and histological findings [20]. For this, patients are required to undergo cystoscopy with hydrodistension and biopsy, with hydrodistension often acting as a therapeutic as well as diagnostic intervention. The technical protocol of cystoscopy and hydrodistension is associated with significant variation and lack of consensus. The National Institute of Diabetes and Digestive and Kidney Diseases (NIDDK) recommended cystoscopy and hydrodistension to be performed under sedation. Despite variations in technical details regarding filling pressure, duration of hydrodistension, and number of cycles of distension, all the existent guidelines agree that cystoscopy and hydrodistension should be performed under anesthesia [21–24]. However, in a study by Cole EE et al, hydrodistension could not identify any statistically significant differences in post-distension objective findings or therapeutic benefits according to categorization of patients' presenting symptoms [25]. On the contrary, Lamale LM et al, observed a strong correlation between pain and cystoscopic findings with hydrodistension [26]. Nonetheless, and all in all, cystoscopy with hydrodistension under anesthesia provides a simple, safe, and important role in differential diagnosis, including some beneficial therapeutic efficacy in painful bladder syndrome/interstitial cystitis and, therefore, should be included in the routine diagnostic evaluation of these conditions [27].

Initially called ulcers, Hunner lesions correspond to an inflammatory process with rupture through the mucosa and submucosa when the bladder is distended. Hunner lesions are tiny vessels radiating from a central scar, which is covered by coagulum. When bladder distention causes their rupture, petechial hemorrhage occurs in a waterfall manner. Hunner lesions are uncommon, being present in only 10–15% of patients with interstitial cystitis/bladder pain syndrome. Glomerulations have been long described and constitute a separate entity, and they are characterized as small submucosal petechiae that become evident upon bladder distension [28]. However, these lesions were not considered pathognomonic for interstitial cystitis, as they may be present in other bladder pathologies and even in otherwise healthy women [29, 30].

Cystoscopy is considered a safe and well-tolerated procedure with only anecdotal report of bladder rupture, bladder necrosis, and acute pyelonephritis [31].

Malignant bladder lesions are common, being rated as the second most common cancer in the genitourinary tract (Fig. 12) [32]. They are the 11th most commonly diagnosed cancer and the 14th leading cause of death by cancer

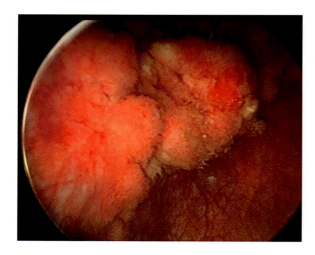

Fig. 12 Exuberant exophytic bladder neoplasm

worldwide [33]. The estimated number of new cases and deaths in 2008 were 382,700 and 150,300, respectively [34]. Known risk factors for bladder cancer include tobacco use, *Schistosoma haematobium* infection, occupational exposure to aromatic amines and polycyclic aromatic hydrocarbons, dietary patterns, environmental pollution, and genetic predisposition. While smoking is the predominant etiologic factor of bladder cancer in the industrialized world, infection with *S. haematobium* is the major cause of the disease in most parts of Africa and the Middle East where the parasite is endemic [35, 36].

These lesions should be investigated with transurethral cold-cup biopsies or resection for histopathologic characterization. Urinary cytology and other urinary markers are helpful but not sensitive enough to avoid the need for tissue histopathology. Therefore, the diagnosis and initial staging of bladder cancer are made by cystoscopy and transurethral resection. Superficial, low-grade lesions usually consist of single or several papillary lesions, while high-grade tumors are larger and sessile, sometimes with necrotic areas. Carcinoma in situ (CIS) may have a characteristic red, velvety appearance resembling areas of inflammation with mucosal irregularity.

Use of fluorescent cystoscopy with blue light can enhance the detection rate of bladder cancer lesions by approximately 20% [37]. These blue-light techniques are thought to improve tumor detection rate, help to improve tumor resection, and thereby reduce residual tumor and recurrence [38]. With the introduction of photosensitizing drugs such as 5-aminolevulinic acid (5-ALA) and its derivate hexylaminolevulinate (HAL, Hexvix®, Photocure ASA, Oslo, Norway), bladder cancer cells accumulate avidly these hematoporphyrin derivatives and are shown as glowing red, as cancer cells emit red fluorescence while benign cells appear blue green, which helps to identify the borders of the tumors more accurately (Fig. 13) [38]. Blue-light cystoscopy (BLC) appears to be beneficial in all initial transurethral resections of bladder tumors in decreasing the rate of residual tumor, and of particular benefit in the diagnosis of CIS [38]. Nonetheless, the updated European guidelines recommend the use of BLC in patients who are suspected of harboring a high-grade tumor, for example, for biopsy guidance in patients with positive cytology or with history of high-grade tumor. Especially when centers already have experience and expertise and the right equipment is available, BLC could support diagnosis in certain cases. Prospective, randomized future studies could add to the discussion of the benefit of BLC, especially the impact BLC can have on progression and survival and overall costs for health care in patients with NMIBC [39].

Approximately 90% of bladder cancers are transitional cell carcinomas. They may be grouped as superficial (papillary, exophytic appearance) or less

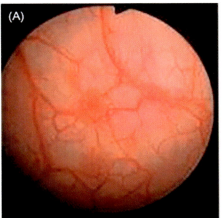 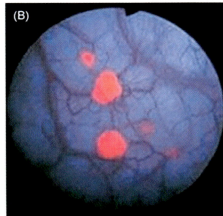

Fig. 13 Blue-light cystoscopy of papillary lesions

commonly invasive (sessile or ulcerated). Adenocarcinomas account for <2% of all bladder cancers, sometimes being preceded by chronic cystitis and metaplasia. They usually arise along the bladder base, while those related to the urachus arise at the bladder dome. Squamous cell carcinomas are often associated with chronic infection, bladder lithiasis, chronic indwelling catheters, or *Schistosoma haematobium* infection. These tumors are often solid, nodular, and invasive at the time of diagnosis.

Metastatic lesions have been reported, including deposits from melanoma, breast adenocarcinoma, and several other origins, often resulting in macroscopic hematuria. Locally advanced cancers, particularly from the colon and rectum, cervix, and uterus can directly invade the bladder wall, disrupt the bladder mucosa, and cause an abnormal cystoscopic aspect and the resulting hematuria.

Conclusions

Cystourethroscopy is one of the most common and important diagnostic tools used by urologists and a key procedure for the diagnostic evaluation, and treatment when needed, of bladder conditions. In female patients, it allows for direct visualization of the urethra, bladder, and ureteral orifices. It is relatively simple and can be performed as a simple office procedure or in the operating room with the patient under general anesthesia.

Cross-References

▶ Endoscopic Evaluation

References

1. Gunning JE, Rosenzweig BA. Evolution of endoscopic surgery. In: White RA, Klein SR, editors. Endoscopic surgery. St. Louis: Mosby; 1991.
2. Kelly HA. The direct examination of the female bladder with elevated pelvis: the catheterization of the ureters under direct inspection, with and without elevation of the pelvis. Am J Obstet Dis Women Child. 1894;25:1.
3. Shah J. Endoscopy through the ages. BJU Int. 2002;89: 645–52.
4. Hopkins HH, Kopany NS. A flexible fiberscope, using static scanning. Nature. 1954;179:30.
5. Yassin MS, Henderson JM, Keely FX. Endoscopy. In: Cardozo L, Staskin D, editors. Textbook of female urology and urogynecology. Boca Raton: CRC Press, Taylor & Francis Group; 2017.
6. Kouri T, Fogazzi G, Gant V, et al. European urinalysis guidelines. Scand J Clin Lab Invest. 2000;60(Supplement 231):1–96.
7. Quayle SS, Ames CD, Lieber D, Yan Y, Landman J. Comparison of optical resolution with digital and standard fiberoptic cystoscopes in an in vitro model. Urology. 2005 Sep;66(3):489–93.
8. Okhunov Z, Hruby GW, Mirabile G, Marruffo F, Lehman DS, Benson MC, Gupta M, Landman J.

Prospective comparison of flexible fiberoptic and digital cystoscopes. Urology. 2009 Aug;74(2):427–30.

9. Wolf JS, Bennett CJ, Dmochowski RR, Hollenbeck BK, Pearle MS, Schaeffer AJ. Urologic surgery antimicrobial prophylaxis best practice policy panel. Best practice policy statement on urologic surgery antimicrobial prophylaxis. J Urol. 2008 Apr;179(4):1379–90.

10. Melekos MD, Asbach HW, Barbalias GA. Vesical diverticula: etiology, diagnosis tumorgenesis and treatment. Analysis of 74 cases. Urology. 1987;30:453–7.

11. Hadley HR. Vesicovaginal fistula. Curr Urol Rep. 2002;3:401–7. https://doi.org/10.1007/s11934-002-0085-5.

12. Gerber GS, Schoenberg HW. Female urinary tract fistulas. J Urol. 1993;149(2):229–96.

13. Mileski WJ, Joehl RJ, Rege RV, Nahrwold DL. One-stage resection and anastomosis in the management of colovesical fistula. Am J Surg. 1987;153(1):75–9.

14. Pollard SG, Macfarlane R, Greatorex R. Colovesical fistula. Ann R Coll Surg Engl. 1987;69(4):163–5.

15. Daniels IR, Bekdash B, Scott HJ, Marks CG, Donaldson DR. Diagnostic lessons learnt from a series of enterovesical fistulae. Color Dis. 2002;4(6):459–62.

16. Melchior S, Cudovic D, Jones J, Thomas C, Gillitzer R, Thüroff J. Diagnosis and surgical management of colovesical fistulas due to sigmoid diverticulitis. J Urol. 2009;182(3):978–82.

17. Solkar MH, Forshaw MJ, Sankararajah D, Stewart M, Parker MC. Colovesical fistula—is a surgical approach always justified? Color Dis. 2005;7(5):467–71.

18. Kwon EO, Armenakas NA, Scharf SC, Panagopoulos G, Fracchia JA. The poppy seed test for colovesical fistula: big bang, little bucks! J Urol. 2008;179(4):1425–7.

19. Kavanagh D, Neary P, Dodd JD, Sheahan KM, O'Donoghue D, Hyland JMP. Diagnosis and treatment of enterovesical fistulae. Color Dis. 2005;7(3):286–91.

20. Van de Merwe J, Nordling J, Bouchelouche P, et al. Diagnostic criteria, classification and nomenclature for painful bladder syndrome/interstitial cystitis: an ESSIC proposal. Eur Urol. 2008;53(1):60–7. https://doi.org/10.1016/j.eururo.2007.09.019.

21. Engeler DS, Baranowski AP, Dinis-Oliveira P, Elneil S, Hughes J, Messelink EJ, van Ophoven A, Williams AC, European Association of Urology. The 2013 EAU guidelines on chronic pelvic pain: is management of chronic pelvic pain a habit, a philosophy, or a science? 10 years of development. Eur Urol. 2013 Sept;64(3):431–9.

22. Homma Y, Ueda T, Ito T, Takei M, Tomoe H. Japanese guideline for diagnosis and treatment of interstitial cystitis. Int J Urol. 2009 Jan;16(1):4–16.

23. Hanno P, Lin A, Nordling J, Nyberg L, van Ophoven A, Ueda T, Wein A. Bladder Pain Syndrome Committee of the International Consultation on Incontinence Bladder Pain Syndrome Committee of the International Consultation on Incontinence. Neurourol Urodyn. 2010;29(1):191–8.

24. Hanno PM, Erickson D, Moldwin R, Faraday MM, American Urological Association. Diagnosis and treatment of interstitial cystitis/bladder pain syndrome: AUA guideline amendment. J Urol. 2015 May;193(5):1545–53.

25. Cole EE, Scarpero HM, Dmochowski RR. Are patient symptoms predictive of the diagnostic and/or therapeutic value of hydrodistention? Neurourol Urodyn. 2005;24(7):638–42.

26. Lamale LM, Lutgendorf SK, Hoffman AN, Kreder KJ. Symptoms and cystoscopic findings in patients with untreated interstitial cystitis. Urology. 2006 Feb;67(2):242–5.

27. Aihara K, Hirayama A, Tanaka N, Fujimoto K, Yoshida K, Hirao Y. Hydrodistension under local anesthesia for patients with suspected painful bladder syndrome/interstitial cystitis: safety, diagnostic potential and therapeutic efficacy. Int J Urol. 2009 Dec;16(12):947–52.

28. Hand JR. Interstitial cystitis; report of 223 cases (204 women and 19 men). J Urol. 1949 Feb;61(2):291–310.

29. Walsh A. Interstitial cystitis. In: Harrison JH, Gittes RF, Perlmutter AD, editors. Campbell's urology. 4th ed. Philadelphia: W. B. Saunders; 1978. p. 693.

30. Waxman JA, Sulak PJ, Kuehl TJ. Cystoscopic findings consistent with interstitial cystitis in normal women undergoing tubal ligation. J Urol. 1998 Nov;160(5):1663–7.

31. Grossklaus DJ, Franke JJ. Vesical necrosis after hydrodistension of the urinary bladder in a patient with interstitial cystitis. BJU Int. 2000 July;86(1):140–1.

32. American Cancer Society. Cancer facts & figures 2007. Atlanta: American Cancer Society; 2007. http://www.cancer.org/downloads/STT/CAFF2007PWsecured.pdf

33. Chavan S, Bray F, Lortet-Tieulent J, Goodman M, Jemal A. International variations in bladder cancer incidence and mortality. Eur Urol. 2014;66:59–73.

34. Ferlay J, Shin HR, Bray F, Forman D, Mathers C, Parkin DM. GLOBOCAN 2008 v2.0, cancer incidence and mortality worldwide: IARC Cancer Base No. 10. [Internet]. International Agency for Research on Cancer website http://globocan.iarc.fr

35. Burger M, Catto JWF, Dalbagni G, et al. Epidemiology and risk factors of urothelial bladder cancer. Eur Urol. 2013;63:234–41.

36. Parkin DM. The global health burden of infection-associated cancers in the year 2002. Int J Cancer. 2006;118:3030–44.

37. Jocham D, Witjes F, Wagner S, et al. Improved detection and treatment of bladder cancer using hexaminolevulinate imaging: a new prospective, phase III multicenter study. J Urol 2005; 174(3):862–866.; discussion 866.

38. Elfering PO, Witjes JA. Blue-light cystoscopy in the evaluation of non-muscle-invasive bladder cancer. Ther Adv Urol. 2014;6(1):25–33.

39. Jichlinski P, Jacqmin D. Photodynamic diagnosis in non-muscle invasive bladder cancer. Eur Urol Suppl. 2008;7:529–35.

Part III
Bladder Storage and Emptying Disorders

Idiopathic Urinary Retention in the Female

12

Abdulghani Khogeer, Lysanne Campeau, and Mélanie Aubé-Peterkin

Contents

Introduction	198
Etiology and Physiology of Urinary Retention	199
Idiopathic Urinary Retention-Related Syndrome	199
Fowler's Syndrome	199
Dysfunctional Voiding	200
Primary Bladder Neck Obstruction	200
Idiopathic Detrusor Underactivity	200
Chronic Intestinal Pseudo-Obstruction	201
Pathophysiology of Urinary Retention	201
Diagnosis and Management	201
Diagnostic Workup	201
History and Physical Exam	201
Investigations	202
Management	202
Bladder Drainage	203
Oral Pharmacotherapy	203
Surgical Therapy	203
Conclusion	204

A. Khogeer
Department of Surgery, Faculty of Medicine, Rabigh, King
Abdulaziz University, Jeddah, Saudi Arabia
e-mail: Abdulghani.khogeer@mail.mcgill.ca

L. Campeau
Department of Urology, Jewish General Hospital,
Montreal, QC, Canada
e-mail: Lysanne.campeau@mcgill.ca

M. Aubé-Peterkin (✉)
Department of Surgery/Urology, McGill University Health
Center and Lachine Hospital, Montreal, QC, Canada
e-mail: Melanie.aube-peterkin@mcgill.ca

© Springer Nature Switzerland AG 2023
F. E. Martins et al. (eds.), *Female Genitourinary and Pelvic Floor Reconstruction*,
https://doi.org/10.1007/978-3-031-19598-3_17

Cross-References 204

References 204

Abstract

Urinary retention is characterized by the inability to voluntary void urine despite persistent effort. It is a multifactorial condition with several anatomical and functional etiologies. Female urinary retention is a rare and poorly understood entity when compared to the synonymous condition commonly encountered in men. Urinary retention in females can be classified as anatomical or functional. Idiopathic female urinary retention is a diagnosis of exclusion with a spectrum in the severity of the condition ranging from difficult voiding to complete retention. The diagnosis is based on a detailed history, physical examination, and appropriate workup including urodynamics and psychoneurological analysis aiming to eliminate all possible differential diagnoses. Understanding the pathophysiology of urinary retention is the key element to providing an appropriate management strategy. Treatment depends on the severity of the condition and patient's general status while taking in consideration the different patient phenotypes and related conditions. The management may range from watchful waiting and post-void residual surveillance to bladder drainage either by clean intermittent self-catheterization or indwelling catheter insertion. No oral medication yet has shown effectiveness in restoring normal micturition. Perineal and pelvic physiotherapy with biofeedback could improve symptoms in select patients. Surgical intervention may be a suitable option in select or refractory cases either by posterior tibial or sacral nerve stimulation.

Keywords

Urinary retention · Idiopathic urinary retention · Chronic urinary retention · Female urinary retention · Bladder outlet obstruction · Detrusor underactivity · Fowler's syndrome

Introduction

Urinary retention describes the acute or chronic inability to voluntarily pass urine over an adequate amount of time. The exact incidence of female urinary retention is unknown, but it is a rare condition occurring in up to seven cases per 100,000 population per year according to some studies. Urinary retention predominantly affects men with a male-to-female ratio of 13: 1 and is most commonly related to prostatic enlargement [1]. It can be classified as acute/transient urinary retention (AUR) or chronic/persistent urinary retention (CUR). Urinary retention has multiple presentations ranging from complete retention to incomplete or insufficient voiding with an elevated post-void residual (PVR) and may be symptomatic or asymptomatic. According to the International Continence Society (ICS), AUR presents as painful, palpable, or percussable bladder with inability to pass any urine when the bladder is full. CUR is defined as a nonpainful bladder with chronic high PVR [2]. However, there is no absolute definition of CUR or accepted standardized criteria regarding bladder volume or defined quantitative PVR which is associated with urinary retention in women. The lack of a standardized definition is a limitation for uniform reporting of this condition in medical literature. According to the American Urological Association (AUA), CUR can be defined as an elevated PVR above 300 mL that has persisted for at least six months and is documented on two or more separate occasions [3]. This cutoff PVR measurement (>300 ml) is frequently used in certain studies and represents the minimal amount of urine associated with a palpable urinary bladder on physical examination [4]. CUR is a clinical sign and is not considered as a formal diagnosis and may have various manifestations in different populations [5]. To date, there is a lack of dedicated studies comparing female and male urinary retention. Female urinary retention is a commonly misunderstood urologic condition that risks being mismanaged as many urologists focus on urethral and anatomical causes of retention. Idiopathic urinary retention (IUR) refers to any form of urinary retention without any identifiable underlying cause. Truly IUR in women is a rare condition to diagnose, especially when eliminating patients with anatomical or functional obstruction including all possible neurological abnormalities. This condition is likely a manifestation of underactive bladder, a diagnosis challenging to ascertain. In the past, women with urinary retention were often judged to be affected by a psychological disorder [6]. Currently, thanks to many diagnostic tools, psychological urinary retention is considered to be a diagnosis of exclusion.

Etiology and Physiology of Urinary Retention

Anatomical and functional causes of female urinary retention are detailed in Table 1. Anatomical origin can be related to any cause of bladder outlet obstruction (BOO), for example, prolapse of pelvic organs, giant uterine fibroids, urethral diverticula, urethral caruncle, urethral stricture, ectopic obstructing ureterocele, or as a result of stress urinary incontinence surgeries [7]. Iatrogenic injuries caused by urologic, gynecologic, or colorectal surgical interventions may in turn cause BOO. On the other hand, functional urinary retention is relevant to either bladder dysfunction or bladder outlet dysfunction. Bladder dysfunction may refer to detrusor underactivity or detrusor atony. Bladder outlet dysfunction can be categorized into two main subgroups: primary bladder neck obstruction and dysfunctional voiding. Uniquely, some patients may present with a failure in sphincteric relaxation called Fowler's

syndrome. The most common cause of outlet obstruction in females has not been clearly determined. However, urethral causes in women are rare, while detrusor muscle failure is considered as a prevalent cause of female retention in most series [1, 8]. The term nonobstructive urinary retention (NOUR) can be defined as the inability to empty the bladder with no anatomical or functional interference to the urine flow. It can occur as a result of a neurological condition, or it can be idiopathic. If no underlying cause is found, the problem is referred to as an idiopathic retention of urine [9]. IUR is a heterogenous condition with divergent pathophysiological mechanisms resulting in a failure to void and is a diagnosis of exclusion. Investigating any possible underlying cause of urinary retention is essential to reveal any reversible cause as well any possible comorbid conditions including functional and neuropsychological disorders, opiate consumption, chronic pain syndrome, chronic intestinal pseudo-obstruction, etc. [10–13].

In rare scenarios, severe and long-term psychosocial disturbances may impact normal voiding function. This likely results from subconscious central nervous system inhibition of detrusor activity by many complex pathways from the brain to the sacrum [14].

Idiopathic Urinary Retention-Related Syndrome

Fowler's Syndrome
Fowler's syndrome (FS) is a rare disorder affecting younger women in which the urethral sphincter fails to relax to allow urine to pass normally [15, 16]. It is a clinical diagnosis based on a multidisciplinary evaluation of the patient. Dr. Clare Fowler in 1985 described a

Table 1 Etiology of female urinary retention

Bladder dysfunction	Bladder outlet obstruction	Bladder outlet dysfunction
Aging Neurological diseases Inflammatory disorders Chronic disease: Diabetes mellitus Medications (e.g., opiates, anticholinergics) Acute or chronic pain Urinary tract infection	Pelvic organ prolapse Postoperative: Stress urinary incontinence Urethral/meatal stenosis Urethral diverticulum/caruncle Gynecological causes Stones Ureterocele Foreign body Malignancies	Primary bladder neck obstruction Dysfunctional voiding Sphincter-detrusor dyssynergia Fowler's syndrome

characteristic failure of external urethral sphincter (EUS) relaxation on electromyography (EMG) along with unexplained high-volume painless urinary retention [17]. This syndrome affects mostly young post-menarche women from the second to third decades of age. It is not uncommon to find a triggering event like a surgical history or a precipitating acute illness, and there is an association with polycystic ovarian syndrome. The principal clinical finding shows painless high-volume urinary retention usually greater than one liter [18]. There are no identified structural or neurological etiologies responsible for the urinary retention in these cases [19]. Workup includes several tests: urethral sphincteric EMG (high EUS with complex repetitive discharges and decelerating bursts), urethral profilometry (increased maximal urethral closure pressure), and transvaginal ultrasound (increased sphincter volume). Video-urodynamic studies show an increased bladder capacity with low sensation and reduced or absent detrusor contraction and urinary flow with visible opening in the bladder neck associated with narrowing at the mid-urethra with or without dilatation of the proximal urethra [20]. Treatment options are based on bladder drainage and sacral nerve modulation (SNM). Currently, SNM is the only effective treatment able to restore normal micturition in patients with FS [21].

Dysfunctional Voiding

Also named "Hinman's syndrome," dysfunctional voiding is likely the most commonly described disorder of both non-neurologic and nonanatomical cause of voiding disorder in females [22–24]. It is believed to occur due to an acquired maladaptive habit which is characterized by an intermittent flow rate resulting from involuntary contractions of the EUS and/or pelvic floor muscles during voiding in an anatomically and neurologically intact patient [25]. This disorder is present in up to 2% of patients referred for urodynamic assessment [2]. It is hypothesized that this learned attitude or behavior is caused by a response to various conditions such as trauma, inflammation, organ infection (urethra, bladder, vagina), or a remote incident during childhood or adult life [4, 26]. It is associated with larger incidence of psychological disorder than in the general population and is of much higher incidence in sexual abuse patients [27, 28]. The diagnosis can be established using video-urodynamics and sphincter EMG (augmented activity during voiding) [29]. Urodynamics may reveal high-pressure and low-flow voiding with normal bladder sensation and capacity. Fluoroscopy may show narrowing at the level of the EUS with proximal urethral ballooning [26, 29]. Initial management usually includes cognitive therapy and timed voiding. Physiotherapy with pelvic and perineal floor muscle relaxation may restore normal micturition [2].

Primary Bladder Neck Obstruction

Primary bladder neck obstruction is described as the failure of bladder neck relaxation resulting in impaired urine flow [30]. This syndrome can be found in 9% to 16% of urodynamic studies done for urinary retention [31]. The cause may be related to primary smooth muscle hypertrophy or due to augmented sensitivity of the bladder neck to sympathetic stimulation [32–34]. Urodynamic studies show normal bladder capacity and sensation with a high-pressure and low-flow voiding with increased PVR. The EMG activity is usually normal. Voiding fluoroscopy shows no opening of the bladder neck. Regarding management, watchful waiting may be advised in the absence of upper or lower urinary tract impairment. Alpha-blockers could significantly improve patient symptoms and correct urodynamic parameters in 67% of patients [35]. In case of failure of medical therapy, surgical treatment by transurethral incision of bladder neck could be discussed. Incisions can be made at 5 o'clock and/or 7 o'clock [36]. Patients should be informed about the benefits and risks of bladder neck incision, notably failure, urethral stricture, and urinary incontinence.

Idiopathic Detrusor Underactivity

Idiopathic detrusor underactivity is most commonly observed in elderly individuals. Etiology is likely due to underlying afferent neuromyogenic dysfunction resulting in abnormal central nervous control of lower urinary tract function with failure of detrusor contraction [21, 37]. Idiopathic detrusor underactivity is a rare pathology without an identifiable cause. In urodynamic studies, the EMG is normal. The typical urodynamic finding is a low-pressure and low-flow voiding. Currently, there are no available effective treatments, and bladder drainage with or without timed voiding is the mainstay management option. This entity is discussed in detail in ▶ Chap. 13, "Overview of Diagnosis and Pharmacological Treatment of Overactive and Underactive Bladder Disorders".

Chronic Intestinal Pseudo-Obstruction

This is a rare condition that is associated with chronic bowel obstruction symptoms and no identifiable structural cause. Chronic intestinal pseudo-obstruction is associated with 10%–69% of cases of detrusor muscle failure with lower urinary tract dysfunction [38–40]. The underlying mechanism is not known and is probably related to visceral myopathic or neuropathic processes affecting the intestines. Patients often can void by Valsalva maneuver and pelvic floor relaxation. Urodynamic studies may show increased bladder capacity, reduced sensation, and low-pressure low-flow voiding with high PVR measurements. The EMG is normal and the treatment consists of bladder drainage and Valsalva voiding.

Pathophysiology of Urinary Retention

Insufficient emptying or complete retention is related to any form of disorder affecting the detrusor strength and/or duration of contraction or any increase in outlet resistance. Retention may also be related to an impaired detrusor-sphincteric coordination [41, 42]. The act of micturition runs through a very complex pathway. The lower urinary tract consists of the urethra and urinary bladder which plays the role of an expanding reservoir for urine. The continence mechanism is composed of both internal and external urethral sphincters which inhibit urine loss on filling phase. A variety of neurological control pathways (sympathetic, parasympathetic, and somatic) are associated with several reflexes (afferent and efferent) which are mediated by numerous central and peripheral neurotransmitters that are dedicated to both storage and voiding phases. These lower motor nerves are under the regulation of higher motor function in the brain. The storage phase of micturition is mainly mediated through stimulation of β_3-adrenergic receptors (sympathetic control), the α-adrenergic receptors of the internal urethral sphincter (sympathetic control), and the external urethral sphincter (somatic control). As previously mentioned, there are two mechanisms of urinary retention: bladder outlet dysfunction/obstruction and detrusor impairment, and these conditions can coincide.

Diagnosis and Management

Diagnostic Workup

History and Physical Exam

The aim of the workup is to identify the presence of urinary retention and its underlying causes. The evaluation of any woman presenting with urinary retention should always begin with a full history and physical examination. A thorough history plays a very important role in the investigation of urinary retention. The symptoms of urinary retention are variable and include abdominal pain or discomfort, storage symptoms such as frequency and urgency, voiding symptoms such as decreased stream and straining to void, and sensation of incomplete emptying associated with or without urinary incontinence. The timing of onset of symptoms may help elucidate the appropriate diagnosis. The physician must screen for the presence of recurrent urinary tract infections (UTI) and gross hematuria. Assessment of fluid intake and voiding patterns with a voiding diary provide additional information. Bowel dysfunction and sexual issues must be assessed while taking history. Validated questionnaires are helpful and important tools to evaluate future symptomatic changes throughout follow-up. Past medical and surgical conditions and any medications should be queried to exclude any secondary or iatrogenic causes of urinary retention. If workup reveals no organic etiology, psychological investigation may be warranted to rule out the presence of a psychological component to the urinary retention.

During physical examination, abdominal exam may reveal a palpable bladder. Complete pelvic, vaginal, and rectal exams should be performed. Presence of a pelvic mass, pelvic organ prolapse, or tight and/or tender pelvic floor muscles may help elucidate etiology of retention. A digital rectal exam may exclude fecal impaction or changes in sphincter tone. A full neurological exam is recommended. Ancillary exams include uroflowmetry with measuring of PVR with either a bladder scanner or via catheterization. A minimum of two readings are recommended to reduce the risk of false-positives results (e.g., excessive fluid intake, inadequate time to complete voiding, or stress). There is no absolute cutoff PVR value that confers a diagnosis of CUR. In current literature, "acceptable" PVRs range between 100 mL and 500 mL, and a cutoff value of 300 mL is frequently used in literature [3, 4, 43, 44]. Voiding efficiency can be assessed by taking into account the voided volume. Some authors promote not to designate a fixed numerical PVR value to diagnose urinary retention and to rather base the diagnosis on signs, symptoms, and clinical judgement [45].

Investigations

Urinalysis and culture are recommended to exclude microscopic hematuria and UTI. Evaluation should include abdominal imaging to rule out hydronephrosis, hydroureter, bladder stones, or a pelvic mass. Renal function should be assessed with serum creatinine and calculated clearance. Magnetic resonance imaging (MRI) of the spine can be done to rule out any suspected underlying neurological etiology.

Urodynamic testing is very useful in the evaluation of urinary retention and the gold standard to identify the functional cause of BOO, with video-urodynamics if available. The suggested revised criteria for female BOO are a maximum flow rate (Qmax) of 12 mL/s or less, combined with a voiding pressure (PdetQmax) of 25 cm H20 or more [31, 46]. The Solomon-Greenwell nomogram was recently validated as a female BOO index (BOOIf). It is calculated using the formula BOOIf = PdetQmax – 2.2*Qmax. A BOOIf <0 provides a < 10% probability of obstruction; a BOOIf >5 is likely obstructed (50%); and if BOOIf >18, obstruction is almost certain (>90%) [47].

Urodynamic studies can record detrusor muscle activity during filling and voiding phases, urinary bladder capacity, and sensation which add to their diagnostic value. Urethral profilometry or sphincter EMG evaluates sphincter activity and may rule out a persistently elevated urethral sphincter tone. Nevertheless, urinary retention may occur in the absence of any notable findings. The use of simultaneous fluoroscopy with video-urodynamics is helpful to identify the level of obstruction, if present, by imaging the bladder neck and the urethra while noting the presence of a continuous detrusor contraction with a concomitant reduced or delayed flow rate [48]. Regarding detrusor activity, one must note that the absence of a detrusor contraction does not always signify that the detrusor is unable to contract, only that the contraction was not recorded throughout the study. The International Continence Society (ICS) describes primary detrusor muscle underactivity as "a contraction of reduced strength and/or duration, resulting in prolonged bladder emptying and/or failure to achieve complete bladder emptying within a normal time span" [4, 49, 50].

Urethro-cystoscopy is an invasive but effective procedure notably used to diagnose the site of BOO in women (after urodynamic testing) and can also provide a therapeutic role (e.g., urethral dilation in the presence of a urethral stricture). Cystoscopy should also be performed as part of the workup for hematuria if present.

It is well understood that CUR may eventually cause deterioration of upper urinary tract function with a risk of severe and irreversible complications that may progress to end-stage renal failure if not treated. Indeed, CUR may present as an incidental finding in asymptomatic patients, and many patients with untreated CUR do not suffer any morbidity from their condition.

Management

Management is based on addressing the possible etiological cause of the retention and providing adequate intervention and follow-up. Acute retention or chronic retention causing renal impairment should immediately be treated by relieving the obstruction [51]. In the latter case, observation for post-obstructive diuresis should be performed.

Conservative management is preferred in patients with secondary dysfunctional voiding related to sexual abuse, history of depression or anxiety, or other identified psychosocial causes as many similar cases might resolve with physical therapy, cognitive therapy, or both. Patients with secondary retention triggered by an acute or organic event may recover after removal or treatment of the inciting cause. For example, retention occurring after mid-urethral sling placement can be treated with sling incision; significant pelvic organ prolapse with BOO is best treated by surgical repair or conservatively via pessary placement. Opioid analgesics or drugs with anticholinergic effects should be avoided as these may worsen the condition. Pelvic floor physical therapy with biofeedback is a useful treatment modality for patients suffering from dysfunctional voiding [52].

Patients with IUR englobe many pathological phenotypes (pelvic floor muscle disorder, detrusor underactivity) that render treatment in some situations quite challenging. Therefore, identifying these subtypes clinically may enable the tailoring of treatment. Not all patients with IUR necessarily require treatment, and for some, intervention may place them at risk for complications (e.g., urethral dilation without evidence of stricture may in itself cause urethral stricture).

Bladder Drainage
In settings of complete or symptomatic retention, treatment starts with bladder drainage via either an indwelling urethral or suprapubic catheter or intermittent self-catheterization (ISC). Conversely, in patients with partial retention, PVR surveillance with timed voiding may be justified. ISC is an appropriate first option for dexterous women with urinary retention and is successful in most patients. ISC may improve or restore function of the decompensated bladder and allow patients to resume spontaneous voiding. There exists no standard of care regarding the ideal ISC interval and suitable catheter type or size to be used; however, care should be tailored according to an individualized bladder management plan. Insertion of indwelling catheter may be necessary in patients unable or unwilling to perform ISC. Unfortunately, bladder drainage is associated with poor patient tolerance and compliance. Indwelling catheterization and ISC can increase the risk of UTI, urethral injury, and decreased quality of life [53]. Open communication with the patient is necessary to ensure adequate compliance despite these risks.

Oral Pharmacotherapy
The role of oral treatment in women with NOUR is not well defined. Alpha-blockers may improve in cases of outlet obstruction caused by primary bladder neck obstruction. Conversely, alpha-blockers provide marginal or no benefit in female with NOUR [54]. The use of sildenafil citrate for the increase of nitric oxide-mediating muscle relaxation has shown no significant advantage over placebo regarding Qmax, PVR, standardized symptom scores, and voiding diary parameters [55]. Furthermore, cholinergic treatments have been shown to be ineffective [56].

Surgical Therapy
Surgical management should be considered when noninvasive treatment regimens have failed. Sacral neuromodulation (SNM) could effectively restore spontaneous voiding in a proportion of patients and is authorized by the FDA for the management of NOUR in patients with reduced bladder contractility. However, the mechanism of action is not well understood. SNM is thought to have a double peripheral and central nervous system effect on lower urinary tract function by restoring the afferent transmissions to the brain which affect and modulate sacral afferents, spinal cord reflexes, and brain centers [57]. The intention is to release the detrusor muscle from presumed inhibition that emanates from the pathologic sphincter afferent activity [16]. The efficacy of SNM has been confirmed in a meta-analysis regarding NOUR with a mean PVR decrease of 236 mL [58]. Long-term studies have also demonstrated its efficacy in the treatment of IUR in women [59, 60]. However, not all female with IUR respond to SNM, highlighting the importance of recognizing the causal and prognostic factors responsible for different types of urinary

retention, and concomitant physical and cognitive therapy may still be warranted. As previously mentioned, SNM has allowed some women with Fowler's syndrome to recover their ability to void.

Alternatively, less invasive treatment options in patients with NOUR are transcutaneous electrical nerve stimulation (TENS) and percutaneous tibial nerve stimulation (PTNS). These treatments may show beneficial effects on various objective and subjective parameters of bladder function and, therefore, may merit a trial before opting for the more invasive SNM [61]. Intra-sphincteric injection of botulinum toxin type A is used to treat detrusor-sphincter dyssynergia but has not shown efficacy in dysfunctional voiding. Nonetheless, some trials have recognized short-term success with very limited literature on dysfunctional voiding cases [62, 63]. Alternatively, injection of botulinum toxin type A within the pelvic floor muscles can be an effective management for various pelvic floor disorders, but its applicability to treat IUR in women remains uncertain. However, this technique requires further investigation and a greater understanding of its mechanism of action in order to enhance its use in the future [64, 65]. Lastly and as discussed earlier, transurethral bladder neck incision is feasible and can be performed on patients suspected with a primary bladder neck obstruction. However, this approach is associated with a low risk (3%) of stress urinary incontinence and bladder neck stenosis [66].

Conclusion

Idiopathic urinary retention in female is a rare and poorly understood condition that has an important impact on patients' quality of life. Urinary retention in women must be carefully evaluated to identify etiology and rule out any reversible causes. However, an underlying etiology can be difficult to identify. Understanding the pathophysiology of urinary retention is a key element to providing adequate management. Full clinical, radiological, and urodynamic workup is warranted and will guide appropriate selection of either conservative or more invasive management options. The use of video-urodynamics has majorly contributed to establishing proper diagnosis and management of female urinary retention. Adequate management may mitigate the risk of developing long-term complications, notably upper tract deterioration. A multidisciplinary approach among urologists, physiotherapists, and mental health-care professionals may be required in complex or refractory cases, especially if past psychosocial factors have been identified. Future research in IUR is needed. Effectively, facing the rarity and limited cohort of patients, it is challenging to build strong clinical trials.

Cross-References

▶ Behavioral Modification and Conservative Management of Overactive Bladder and Underactive Bladder Disorders
▶ Bladder Dysfunction and Pelvic Pain: The Role of Sacral, Tibial, and Pudendal Neuromodulation
▶ Overview of Diagnosis and Pharmacological Treatment of Overactive and Underactive Bladder Disorders
▶ Voiding Dysfunction After Female Pelvic Surgery

References

1. Klarskov P, Andersen J, Asmussen C, Brenoe J, Jensen SK, Jensen IL, et al. Acute urinary retention in women: a prospective study of 18 consecutive cases. Scand J Urol Nephrol. 1987;21:29–31.
2. Haylen BT, et al. An International Urogynecological Association (IUGA)/International Continence Society (ICS) joint report on the terminology for female pelvic floor dysfunction. Neurourol Urodyn. 2010;29:4–20.
3. AUA Non-Neurogenic Chronic Urinary Retention Consensus Definition, Management Strategies, and Future Opportunities. https://www.auanet.org//guide lines/guidelines/chronic-urinary-retention
4. Abrams P, Cardozo L, Fall M, et al. The standardisation of terminology of lower urinary tract function: report from the Standardisation Sub-committee of the International Continence Society. Neurourol Urodyn. 2002;21:167–78.
5. Asimakopoulos AD, De NC, Kocjancic E, Tubaro A, Rosier PF, Finazzi-Agro E. Measurement of post-void residual urine. Neurourol Urodyn. 2016;35:55.
6. Knox SJ. Psychogenic urinary retention after parturition, resulting in hydronephrosis. BMJ. 1960;2:1422–4.

7. Montague DK, Jones LR. Psychogenic urinary retention. Urology. 1979;13:30–5.
8. Ahmad I, Krishna NS, Small DR, Conn IG. Aetiology and management of acute female urinary retention. Br J Med Surg Urol. 2009;2:27–33.
9. Wein AJ, Barrett DM. Voiding function and dysfunction. Yearbook Medical Publishers; 1988. p. 326–7.
10. Fox M, Jarvis GJ, Henry L. Idiopathic chronic urinary retention in the female. Br J Urol. 1976;147:797.
11. Hoeritzauer I, Stone J, Fowler C, Elneil-Coker S, Carson A, Panicker J. Fowler's syndrome of urinary retention: a retrospective study of comorbidity. Neurourol Urodyn. 2016;35(5):601–3.
12. Groutz A, Blaivas JG. Non-neurogenic female voiding dysfunction. Curr Opin Urol. 2002;12:311–6.
13. Van Koeveringe GA, Vahabi B, Andersson KE, KirschnerHerrmans R, Oelke M. Detrusor underactivity: a place for new approaches to a common bladder dysfunction. Neurourol Urodyn. 2011;30:723–8.
14. Abdel Raheem A, Madersbacher H. Voiding dysfunction in women: how to manage it correctly. Arab J Urol. 2013;11:319–30.
15. Krane RJ, Siroky MB. Psychogenic voiding dysfunction in the adult female. In: Raz S, editor. Female urology. Philadelphia: WB Saunders; 1983. p. 337–43.
16. NICE interventional procedure consultation document, June 2015 Sacral nerve stimulation for idiopathic chronic non-obstructive urinary retention.
17. Wiseman O, Kitchen N, Fowler C. Long term results of sacral neuromodulation for woman with urinary retention. BJU Int. 2004;94(3):335–7.
18. Fowler CJ, Kirby RS, Harrison MJ. Decelerating burst and complex repetitive discharges in the striated muscle of the urethral sphincter, associated with urinary retention in women. J Neurol Neurosurg Psychiatry. 1985;48:1004–9.
19. Swinn MJ, Wiseman OJ, Lowe E, Fowler CJ. The cause and natural history of isolated urinary retention in young women. J Urol. 2002;167:151–6.
20. Kavia RB, Datta SN, Dasgupta R, Elneil S, Fowler CJ. Urinary retention in women: its causes and management. BJU Int. 2006;97:281–7.
21. DasGupta R, Fowler CJ. Urodynamic study of women in urinary retention treated with sacral neuromodulation. J Urol. 2004;171:1161–4.
22. Osman N, Chapple C. Fowler's syndrome–a cause of unexplained urinary retention in young women. Nat Rev Urol. 2014;11:87–98. https://doi.org/10.1038/nrurol.2013.277.
23. Hinman F, Baumann FW. Vesical and ureteral damage from voiding dysfunction in boys without neurologic or obstructive disease. J Urol. 1973;109:727–32.
24. Allen TD, Bright TC 3rd. Urodynamic patterns in children with dysfunctional voiding problems. J Urol. 1978;119:247–9.
25. Carlson KV, Fiske J, Nitti VW. Value of routine evaluation of the voiding phase when performing urodynamic testing in women with lower urinary tract symptoms. J Urol. 2000;164:1614–8.
26. Groutz A, Blaivas JG, Pies C, Sassone AM. Learned voiding dysfunction (non-neurogenic, neurogenic bladder) among adults. Neurourol Urodyn. 2001;20:259–68.
27. Carlson KV, Rome S, Nitti VW. Dysfunctional voiding in women. J Urol. 2001;165:143–7.
28. Fan YH, Lin AT, Wu HM, Hong CJ, Chen KK. Psychological profile of female patients with dysfunctional voiding. Urology. 2008;71:625–9.
29. Pannek J, Einig EM, Einig W. Clinical management of bladder dysfunction caused by sexual abuse. Urol Int. 2009;82:420–5.
30. Brucker BM, et al. Urodynamic differences between dysfunctional voiding and primary bladder neck obstruction in women. Urology. 2012;80:55–60.
31. Diokno AC, Hollander JB, Bennett CJ. Bladder neck obstruction in women: a real entity. J Urol. 1984;132:294–8.
32. Nitti VW, Tu LM, Gitlin J. Diagnosing bladder outlet obstruction in women. J Urol. 1999;161(5):1535–40.
33. Leadbetter GW Jr, Leadbetter WF. Diagnosis and treatment of congenital bladder-neck obstruction in children. N Engl J Med. 1959;260:633–7.
34. Crowe R, et al. An increase of neuropeptide Y but not nitric oxide synthase-immunoreactive nerves in the bladder neck from male patients with bladder neck dyssynergia. J Urol. 1995;154:1231–6.
35. Hickling D, Aponte M, Nitti V. Evaluation and management of outlet obstruction in women without anatomical abnormalities on physical exam or cystoscopy. Curr Urol Rep. 2012;13:356–62.
36. Kessler TM, Studer UE, Burkhard FC. The effect of terazosin on functional bladder outlet obstruction in women: a pilot study. J Urol. 2006;176:1487–92.
37. Jin X-B, Qu H-W, Liu B, Wang J, Zhang Y-d. Modified trans urethral incision for primary bladder neck obstruction in women: a method to improve voiding function without urinary incontinence. Urology. 2012;79(2):310–3.
38. Tyagi P, Smith P, Kuchel G, et al. Pathophysiology and animal modeling of underactive bladder. Int Urol Nephrol. 2014;46:S11–21.
39. Mousa H, Hyman PE, Cocjin J, Flores AF, Di Lorenzo C. Long-term outcome of congenital intestinal pseudo-obstruction. Dig Dis Sci. 2002;47:2298–305.
40. Lapointe SP, Rivet C, Goulet O, Fekete CN, Lortat-Jacob S. Urological manifestations associated with chronic intestinal pseudo- obstructions in children. J Urol. 2002;168:1768–70.
41. Vargas JH, Sachs P, Ament ME. Chronic intestinal pseudo obstruction syndrome in pediatrics. Results of a national survey by members of the North American Society of Pediatric Gastroenterology and Nutrition. J Pediatr Gastroenterol Nutr. 1988;7(3):323–32. PMID: 3290417.
42. Wein A, Barret D. Voiding function and dysfunction. Chicago Year Book Medical; 1988. p. 371.
43. Brucker BM, Nitti VW. Evaluation of urinary retention in women: pelvic floor dysfunction or primary bladder

neck obstruction. Curr Bladder Dysfunct Rep. 2012;7: 222–9.

44. Kaplan SA, Wein AJ, Staskin DR, et al. Urinary retention and post void residual urine in men: separating truth from tradition. J Urol. 2008;180:47.

45. Gallien P, Reymann JM, Amarenco G, et al. Placebo controlled, randomised, double blind study of the effects of botulinum a toxin on detrusor sphincter dyssynergia in multiple sclerosis patients. J Neurol Neurosurg Psychiatry. 2005;76:1670.

46. Thomas AW, Cannon A, Bartlett E, et al. The natural history of lower urinary tract dysfunction in men: the influence of detrusor underactivity on the outcome after transurethral resection of the prostate with a minimum 10-year urodynamic follow-up. BJU Int. 2004;93:745.

47. Defreitas GA, Zimmern PE, Lemack GE, Shariat SF. Refining diagnosis of anatomic female bladder outlet obstruction: comparison of pressure flow study parameters in clinically obstructed women with those of normal controls. Urology. 2004;64:675–9.

48. Solomon E, Yasmin H, Duffy M, Rashid T, Akinluyi E, Greenwell TJ. Developing and validating a new nomogram for diagnosing bladder outlet obstruction in women. Neurourol Urodyn. 2018;37(1):368–78. https://doi.org/10.1002/nau.23307. Epub 2017 Jun 30. PMID: 28666055

49. Blaivas JG, Groutz A. Bladder outlet obstruction nomogram for women with lower urinary tract symptomatology. Neurourol Urodyn. 2000;19:553–64.

50. Osman NI, Chapple CR, Abrams P, et al. Detrusor underactivity and the underactive bladder: a new clinical entity. A review of current terminology, definitions, epidemiology, aetiology, and diagnosis. Eur Urol. 2014;65:389.

51. Miyazato M, Yoshimura N, Chancellor MB. The other bladder syndrome: underactive bladder. Rev Urol. 2013;15:11.

52. Voorham Van der Zalm P, Pelger R, Stiggelbout A, Elzeveveir H, Nijeholt GAL. Effects of magnetic stimulation in the treatment of pelvic floor dysfunction. BJU Int. 2006;97:1035–8.

53. Xu D, Qu C, Meng H, Ren J, Zhu Y, Min Z, et al. Dysfunctional voiding confirmed by transdermal perineal electromyography, and its effective treatment with baclofen in women with lower urinary tract symptoms: a randomized double-blind placebo controlled crossover trial. BJU Int. 2007;100(3):588–92.

54. Wilde MH, McMahon JM, Tang W, et al. Self-care management questionnaire for long-term indwelling urinary catheter users. Neurourol Urodyn. 2016;35:492.

55. Costantini E, Lazzeri M, Bini V, et al. Open label, longitudinal study of tamsulosin for functional bladder outlet obstruction in women. Urol Int. 2009;83:311.

56. Datta SN, Kavia RB, Gonzales G, Fowler CJ. Results of double blind placebo controlled crossover study of sildenafil citrate(Viagra) in women suffering from obstructed voiding or retention associated with the primary disorder of sphincter relaxation (Fowler's syndrome). Eur Urol. 2007;51:489–95.

57. Wein AJ, Malloy TR, Shaffer F, Roeger DM. The effects of bethanechol chloride on urodynamic parameters in normal women and in women with significant residual urine volumes. J Urol. 1980;124:397.

58. Ernstein AJ, Peters KM. Expanding indications for neuromodulation. Urol Clin North Am. 2005;32(1): 59–63.

59. Gross C, Habli M, Lindsell C, South M. Sacral neuromodulation for nonobstructive urinary retention: a meta-analysis. Female Pelvic Med Reconstr Surg. 2010;16(4):249–53.

60. Dasgupta R, Wiseman OJ, Kitchen N, Fowler CJ. Long term results of sacral neuromodulation for women with urinary retention. BJU Int. 2004;94(3):335–7.

61. Van Kerrebroeck PE, van Voskuilen AC, Heesakkers JP, et al. Results of sacral neuromodulation therapy for urinary voiding dysfunction: outcomes of a prospective, worldwide clinical study. J Urol. 2007;178(5): 2029–34.

62. Coolen RL, et al. Transcutaneous electrical nerve stimulation and percutaneous tibial nerve stimulation to treat idiopathic nonobstructive urinary retention: a systematic review. Eur Urol Focus. 2020;7(5):1184–94.

63. Jiang YH, Wang CC, Kuo HC. On a botulinum toxin a urethral sphincter injection as treatment for non-neurogenic voiding dysfunction: a randomized, double-blind, placebo-controlled study. Sci Rep. 2016;6:38905.

64. Panicker JN, Seth JH, Khan S, et al. Open label study evaluating outpatient urethral sphincter injections of on a botulinum toxin A to treat women with urinary retention due to a primary disorder of sphincter relaxation (Fowler's syndrome). BJU Int. 2016;117(5): 809–13.

65. Malde S, Apostilidis A, Selai C, et al. Botulinum toxin A for refractory OAB and idiopathic urinary retention: can phenotyping improve outcome for patients: ICI-RS. Neurourol Urodyn. 2019;2019:1–9.

66. Peng CH, Kuo HC. Transurethral incision of bladder neck in treatment of bladder neck obstruction in women. Urology. 2005;65:275–8.

Overview of Diagnosis and Pharmacological Treatment of Overactive and Underactive Bladder Disorders

13

S. Saad, N. Osman, O. A. Alsulaiman, and C. R. Chapple

Contents

Introduction	208
Definitions	208
Epidemiology	209
Bladder Neurophysiology	209
Etiopathogenesis of OAB and UAB	210
Diagnosis	211
History	211
Examination	211
Investigations	213
Management	215
Overactive Bladder	215
Underactive Bladder	217
Conclusion	218
References	218

Abstract

In this chapter, we focus on the underlying pathophysiology, diagnosis, and pharmacological management of over- and underactive bladder. Overactive bladder syndrome (OAB) is a symptom complex defined by ICS as "urinary urgency, usually accompanied by frequency and nocturia, with or without urgency urinary incontinence, in the absence of urinary tract infection (UTI) or other obvious pathology." Urgency is the pivotal symptom of OAB. Underactive bladder (UAB) is a syndrome "characterized by a slow urinary stream, hesitancy, and straining to void, with or without a feeling of incomplete bladder emptying sometimes with storage symptoms." The medical treatment of choice of OAB is anticholinergics. Where anticholinergics are contraindicated or ineffective, the β3 agonist mirabegron can be offered. Patients failing oral

S. Saad · N. Osman · O. A. Alsulaiman ·
C. R. Chapple (✉)
Department of Urology, Sheffield Teaching Hospitals NHS Foundation Trust, Sheffield, UK
e-mail: c.r.chapple@shef.ac.uk

© Springer Nature Switzerland AG 2023
F. E. Martins et al. (eds.), *Female Genitourinary and Pelvic Floor Reconstruction*,
https://doi.org/10.1007/978-3-031-19598-3_12

medical therapy can be offered intravesical injections of botulinum toxin A, but the effect is temporary, and regular injections are needed. In specialized centers, sacral neuromodulation or posterior tibial nerve stimulation can be offered. No effective pharmacotherapy exists for underactive bladder. Electrical stimulation has been used in some cases with varying success. OAB and UAB represent a diagnostic challenge due to varied presentation and overlapping symptoms. The exact mechanisms behind OAB and UAB are poorly understood. Treatment is tailored to the patient's symptoms with options more established for OAB than UAB, the latter being defined recently. Further research is required to better understand these disorders.

Keywords

Overactive bladder · Underactive bladder · Pharmacotherapy · Anticholinergics · Intravesical botox · Neuromodulation

Introduction

Lower urinary tract symptoms (LUTS) encompass storage symptoms (frequency, urgency, urgency incontinence, and nocturia), voiding symptoms (hesitancy, intermittency, slow stream, splitting/spraying, straining, terminal dribble), and post-voiding symptoms (sensation of incomplete bladder emptying, double voiding, post-void incontinence, and post-micturition urgency). LUTS arise due to a failure of storage and/or failure of emptying [1]. It is well recognized that individual LUTS do not always correlate with specific underlying pathophysiology which gave rise to the aphorism that the "bladder is an unreliable witness" [2] .Moreover, the primary role of the bladder in pathophysiology is now well recognized, in contrast to previous thinking which focused on the prostate. In this chapter we review the terminology, symptoms, pathophysiology, and urodynamic findings of storage and voiding bladder dysfunction as well as their management.

Definitions

The International Continence Society (ICS) has standardized the terminology of LUTS [3]. *Urinary incontinence* has been described as an involuntary leakage of urine. If this is preceded or accompanied by a sense of urgency, it is termed *urgency urinary incontinence (UUI)*. *Urgency* is the "sudden and compelling desire to void which is difficult to defer" [4]. This differs from *urge* which is the normal physiological sensation to void as the bladder approaches fullness.

Overactive bladder syndrome (OAB) is a symptom complex defined by the ICS as "urinary urgency, usually accompanied by frequency and nocturia, with or without urgency urinary incontinence, in the absence of urinary tract infection (UTI) or other obvious pathology" [3, 5]. Urgency is the pivotal symptom of OAB. OAB may be classed as "wet" or "dry" depending on the presence or absence of urgency incontinence respectively. Detrusor overactivity (DO) is a urodynamic observation characterized by involuntary contractions of the detrusor muscle during the filling phase. Detrusor overactivity is present in 40% of dry women with overactive bladder and 60% of those with incontinence. The contrasting figures for men who are dry and wet are 60% and 90%, respectively [6].

The number of voids leading to wakening from sleep is defined as *nocturia*. Each void must be preceded and followed by sleep [4].

Underactive bladder represents the symptom associated with detrusor underactivity. It is more complex to define than overactive bladder as there is no pathognomonic clinical symptom that correlates well with any underlying abnormality in the detrusor muscle (c.f. urgency) [7]. *Detrusor underactivity* (DUA) has been defined by the ICS as "a contraction of reduced strength and/or duration, resulting in prolonged bladder emptying within a normal time span measured by urodynamics" [3, 5]. *Acontractile detrusor* is defined as "one that cannot contract during urodynamic studies" [3].

The symptoms of UAB are diverse and overlap with other conditions like bladder outlet obstruction (BOO) and OAB. A recent consensus definition proposed by Chapple et al. in 2018 defines UAB as a syndrome "characterized by a slow urinary stream, hesitancy, and straining to void, with or without a feeling of incomplete bladder emptying sometimes with storage symptoms" (note: underactive bladder occurs in association with diverse pathophysiologies, and based on current knowledge, there is no single distinguishing symptom. Storage symptoms are varied and may be highly prevalent, including nocturia, increased daytime frequency, reduced sensation of filling, and incontinence. Underlying mechanisms of storage symptoms are diverse and are often related to a significant PVR urine volume) [8].

Epidemiology

Multiple population-based studies demonstrate OAB to be highly prevalent and increasing in prevalence with age. The overall prevalence of OAB is 10.8% males and 12.2% females as per the European Prospective Investigation into Cancer and Nutrition (EPIC) study, rising to 13.1% and 14.6%, respectively, in those aged 40 and above [9]. 44.5% of females and 28% of males experienced incontinence, and over half of these patients had bothersome symptoms [4].

Given the significant overlap of symptoms, there is no reliable epidemiological data estimating the prevalence of UAB. Clinical studies demonstrate 9–28% of men younger than 50 years of age and 48% older than 70 years of age undergoing UDS to be affected by DU. 12–45% of women undergoing UDS have DUA. DUA is more prevalent in the elderly who are institutionalized [7].

Bladder Neurophysiology

Normal functioning of the bladder relies on a complex interplay between the autonomic, central, and somatic nervous system as well as neurohormonal modulation. Although the human bladder does not have Pacinian corpuscles found in the bladder of other mammals, stretch and fullness are sensed via the afferent nerve fibers (mechanoreceptor A-delta), myofibroblasts, and urothelium which act together as an integrated stretch receptor organ, interconnected by interstitial cells [10, 11]. There are two main afferent nerve fibers, the myelinated A-delta fibers and unmyelinated C fibers that carry sensory information. In addition, the extent of bladder wall distension is influenced by the non-neuronal release of neurotransmitters from the urothelium, namely, agents like nitrous oxide (NO), adenosine triphosphate (ATP), and acetyl choline (ACh). Impulses passing from the bladder terminate in the dorsal horn of the lumbosacral spinal cord and reach the limbic system of the brain via the pelvic, pudendal, and hypogastric nerves. They terminate in the dorsal horn of the lumbosacral spinal cord at levels T11–L2 and S2–S4 [12]. From there, the afferent nerves ascend via the lateral or dorsal funiculus to terminate in the periaqueductal gray (PAG) matter, among other areas, to convey sensory information to the pontine micturition center (PMC) which then initiates micturition [12]. The afferent Aδ fibers, found in the detrusor smooth muscle layer, are the primary mediators of bladder fullness [13–15], whereas C fibers in the urothelium and lamina propria only activate in response to extreme stretch, temperature changes, or chemical irritation, as well as pathological situations [10]. In addition to the afferent nerves, the role of the urothelium, lamina propria, and myofibroblasts in bladder control has been recently highlighted [11]. The urothelial cells can cause reflex bladder contractions or local vascular changes by exciting local nerves via direct release of mediators like ATP, NO, ACh, neurokinin A, and nerve growth factor (NGF) [16]. The urothelium also expresses various receptors like nicotinic, muscarinic, adrenergic, tachykinin, bradykinin, and transient receptor potential vanilloid receptors (e.g., TRPV1, TRPV2, and TRPV4) which respond to afferent nerve signaling [10]. The suburothelial fibroblasts (interstitial cells) also have a role in relaying information between the detrusor and urothelium [17], as well as communicating with afferent nerves and responding to urothelial release of ATP [10].

The efferent control of the bladder involves the autonomic and somatic (sphincteric) nervous pathways. The autonomic nerve fibers are sympathetic (adrenergic) and parasympathetic (cholinergic). The sympathetic nerves originate in the thoracolumbar spinal cord at T11–L2 level and synapse in the bladder and urethra via the hypogastric and pelvic plexuses [12]. The postganglionic sympathetic neurons release noradrenaline which relaxes the smooth muscle in the body of the bladder via the β3-adrenoceptors and contracts the smooth muscle at the bladder neck via the a1α-adrenoceptors [10]. The parasympathetic nerves originate from the sacral segments of the spinal cord (S2–S4) and travel via the pelvic nerve to synapse in the pelvic plexus or autonomic ganglia in the detrusor [12]. They cause bladder contraction via the release of ACh which stimulates M3 muscarinic receptors in the bladder wall [10].

The somatic efferent fibers originate in Onuf's nucleus in the ventral horn of the spinal cord (S2–S4). They cause contraction of the external sphincter striated muscle via ACh release by the pudendal nerve.

When the bladder is in the storage phase, the "guarding reflex" causes detrusor relaxation and contraction of the urethral sphincter to prevent bladder emptying as the bladder fills. Once the bladder volume reaches a certain threshold, afferent fibers passing through the PAG area remove the tonic inhibition of the PMC exerted by the higher centers in the limbic system to initiate voiding by relaxing the external urethral sphincter and contracting the detrusor [10] (Figs. 1 and 2).

Etiopathogenesis of OAB and UAB

Although the pathophysiology of DO is poorly understood, three hypotheses have been proposed. The myogenic hypothesis proposed initially by Brading suggests increased excitability of the detrusor myocytes with an increased tendency to spread across the bladder leading to a coordinated detrusor contraction [18]. Drake et al.

proposed a modular arrangement of the detrusor muscle with each module controlled by a myovesical plexus made of intramural ganglia and myofibroblasts [19]. When these modules increase in excitability, their micromotions synchronize and lead to detrusor contraction causing urgency, among other symptoms of the OAB symptom complex [10].

The neurogenic hypothesis implicates loss of descending inhibitory pathways from the higher centers in causing DO [12]. Damage to spinal axons has been suggested to cause a greater role of unmyelinated C fibers in the reflex arc, increasing detrusor excitability [4].

These hypotheses attempt to explain the motor component of OAB seen with detrusor overactivity. The integrative hypothesis attempts to explain the cardinal symptom of OAB, urgency, which is a sensory symptom. This hypothesis considers the urothelium and the underlying suburothelial layer to be a closely communicating integrated functional unit which responds to local mechanical and chemical stimuli by increasing afferent activity of adjacent nerves [10]. This increased afferent activity can lead to perception of urgency and detrusor contractions. The urothelium expresses various receptors like P2X, nicotinic, muscarinic, and TRPV1 which can increase afferent activity in response to different chemical stimuli like ATP, ACh, and NO [4, 10]. Other mechanisms of increased afferent activity may include sensitization of one organ by local inflammatory damage leading to increased excitability in another [10]. This was demonstrated in a study which showed irritable bowel syndrome to occur concurrently in 33.3% of patients with OAB [20]. This can be explained by the similar and closely integrated innervation of the bladder and rectum.

The mechanisms underlying DUA are broadly classified into (a) **myogenic** which involve processes that change the structure and function of detrusor muscle and (b) **neurogenic** which involve the afferent, efferent, and central neural pathways that control micturition. The major etiological factors and pathogenetic factors are summarized in (Figs. 3 and 4).

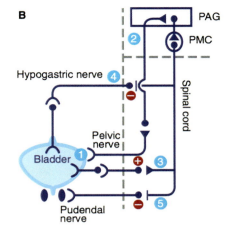

Fig. 1 Reflex control of the bladder. (**a**) Storage reflexes. (1) Minimal distension leads to low-level afferent firing in pelvic nerve. (2) Activation of sympathetic activity in hypogastric nerve. (3) Contraction of bladder outlet and inhibition of detrusor contraction. (4) Activation of sympathetic activity in pudendal nerve leads to contraction of the external urethral sphincter. (**b**) Voiding reflexes. (1) Increased distension leads to intense afferent firing in the pelvic nerve. (2) Activation of the spinobulbospinal reflex pathway involving the PAG and PMC. (3) Stimulation of parasympathetic activity to bladder and urethral smooth muscle. (4) Inhibition of sympathetic activity in hypogastric nerve leading to relaxation of bladder outlet and detrusor contraction. (5) Inhibition of sympathetic activity in pudendal nerve leads to relaxation of the external urethral sphincter. PAG, periaqueductal gray; PMC, pontine micturition center; PSC, pontine storage center. (Reproduced with permission from Professor Chapple [10])

Diagnosis

History

Assessment of patients with OAB/UAB starts with a detailed urological and medical history. The cardinal symptom in OAB is urgency. Patients usually describe how long they can hold their urine before they leak. They may also plan their daily activities based on proximity to toilet facilities. OAB can also present in conjunction with bladder outflow obstruction, especially in the elderly males. It is essential to take a dietary history especially caffeine intake. A frequency volume chart maintained over 3 days is especially useful to get an objective idea of symptoms. In keeping with recommendations of the European Association of Urology (EAU), a standardized questionnaire such as OAB-q or ICIQ-OAB should be used to assess the impact of OAB on patient's quality of life (QoL).

There are no pathognomonic symptoms of UAB, and the symptoms are diverse and overlap with those seen in OAB and bladder outlet obstruction (BOO). While UAB is a voiding disorder, often there are associated storage symptoms due to elevated post-voiding residuals in some cases. The patients may complain of a weak stream with hesitancy, intermittency, and straining. Some may complain of increased frequency, whereas others may report infrequent voiding and a reduced urge to void. They may also report a feeling of incomplete bladder emptying after voiding. A careful drug history should be taken to identify any drugs that reduce bladder contractility.

Examination

Examination should include the abdomen, external genitalia, and prostate followed by a full neurological exam. Any neurological deficits should be explored further and assessed with relevant investigations to rule out any neurological cause for urological symptoms.

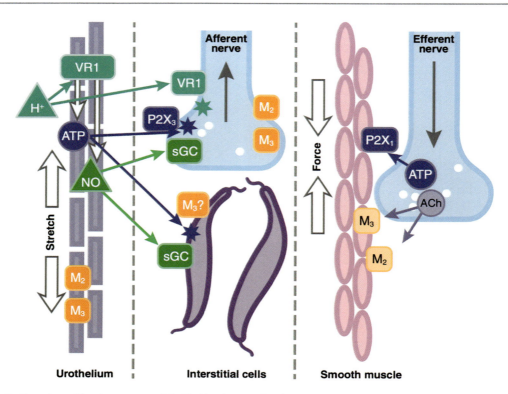

Fig. 2 Overview of the ultrastructure of the bladder showing the urothelium, interstitial space, and detrusor smooth muscle. On the left, neurotransmitters from the urothelium are transmitted via the interstitial cells to the bladder afferents. On the right, faulty efferent signaling causes involuntary detrusor activity. ACh, acetylcholine; NO, nitric oxide; P2X3, purinergic receptor; sGC, soluble guanylyl cyclase; VR1, vanilloid receptor 1. (Reproduced with permission from Professor Chapple [10])

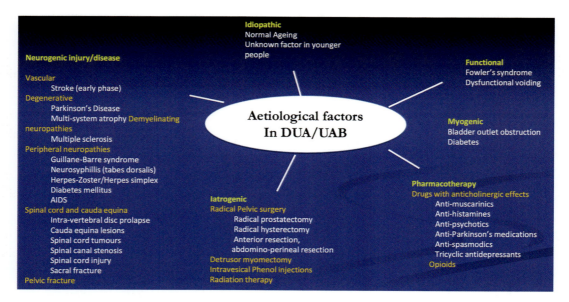

Fig. 3 Etiological factors in underactive bladder. DUA: Detrusor underactivity; UAB: Underactive bladder. (Reproduced with permission from Professor Chapple)

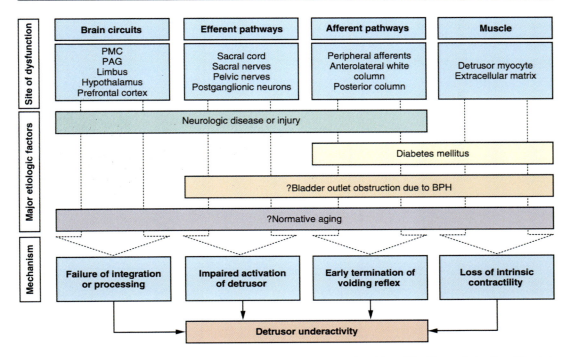

Fig. 4 Etiology and pathogenesis of Detrusor Underactivity (DUA). (Reproduced from [7] with permission from Elsevier)

Investigations

Investigations should start with urinalysis to exclude urinary tract infection, hematuria, proteinuria, or glycosuria. This should be followed by a flow rate and measurement of post-void residual volume (PVR), especially in patients complaining of voiding difficulties. A frequency volume chart or bladder diary helps to quantify the symptoms as well as demonstrating the individual's voiding pattern. It also shows if a patient has 24 h polyuria, which is defined as passage of more than 2.8 L urine per 24 h [4], or nocturnal polyuria, which is passage of more than one-third of urine during the night over the age of 40 years (a lesser proportion may equate with nocturnal polyuria in younger age groups). Nocturnal polyuria usually results from increased urine production at nighttime due to sleep apnea which results in the production of atrial natriuretic peptide, increased fluid retention in daytime, or increased imbibition of fluid at nighttime [4]. To calculate nocturnal urine production, the last void before going to bed is excluded, and all voids since then and the first void on waking are included [4].

Patients who do not respond to behavioral modifications and pharmacological management proceed to urodynamics. The important questions to ask during the filling phase are the first filling sensation, initial desire to void, normal desire to void, and a desperate desire to void [4]. In a patient with OAB, these sensations occur at lesser filling volumes than a normal individual. Although the normal bladder capacity is variable, a range of 400–500 ml is considered normal [4]. Poor detrusor compliance shows up as an upward slope on the urodynamic trace and is caused by an increase of more than 10 cm H20 above 400 ml of filling [4]. Presence of urgency and urgency incontinence should be noted if present. Involuntary detrusor contractions may coincide with urgency. Provocation maneuvers such as running a tap or asking patient to rub their hands together or bounce up and down on toes can be used to provoke detrusor overactivity [4]. Approximately 69% of men and 44% of women with OAB-dry and 90% of men and 58% of women with OAB-wet symptoms demonstrate detrusor overactivity [4].

Since UAB lacks a pathognomonic symptom, the only diagnostic modality available is an invasive urodynamics test. Most methods of measuring detrusor voiding function assess only the strength of contraction rather than sustainability or speed of contraction.

An important relationship to consider is the relationship between the post-voiding residual and the functional bladder capacity, the so-called voiding efficiency. Voiding efficiency = residual/residual + voided volume. A voiding efficiency greater than 40% is considered to be abnormal and represents a trend to a significant degree of incomplete bladder emptying.

Assessing Detrusor Contraction Strength

The two parameters commonly used to estimate detrusor contraction strength are the maximal urinary flow rate or Qmax and detrusor pressure at maximal urinary flow rate or Pdet@Qmax. The threshold values for both these parameters are set at the lower limits of the normal range, which, for men, is derived from a historical series of men undergoing bladder outflow surgery [21, 22]. This approach to measuring detrusor contraction strength has a few limitations. The bladder output relation or BOR was introduced by Griffiths in 1972 and depicts the relation between bladder pressure and uroflow. It measures the bladder function independent of the urethra and posits that the higher the bladder pressure, the lower the flow and vice versa [23]. If the urine flow is stopped, the detrusor pressure will rise to reach its highest possible value (isovolumetric contraction), and on resuming urinary flow, the pressure will decrease. By this relation, Pdet@Qmax measures the lowest detrusor pressure at the maximal urinary flow [24]. Secondly, bladder outlet resistance variability is not considered. So, if the Pdet is low, a low Qmax can be attributed to an increased outflow resistance and vice versa [7]. Thirdly, this cannot be applied to women as they have considerably different voiding dynamics. Women void with a lower detrusor pressure and pelvic floor relaxation with or without augmentation by abdominal straining [40].

To accurately assess contraction strength by measuring isovolumetric pressure, methods were developed based on post hoc mathematical analysis or mechanical/voluntary interruption to urinary flow during UDS, but they are complicated and impractical for routine clinical use [7].

An alternative method was proposed by Schafer (1995) to estimate isovolumetric contraction strength by modifying his pressure-flow nomogram. He superimposed the BOR as a simplified straight line on his nomogram and projected the point representing Pdet@Qmax back to the y-axis (Pdet) to obtain the isovolumetric pressure (Fig. 5) [7]. The projected isovolumetric pressure (PIP) can be calculated using the formula.

$$PIP = PDet@QMax + KQMax$$

K is a fixed constant representing the angle of the BOR [25], and its value is taken as 5cmH20/ml/sec in men with BPH and 1 cm H20/ml/sec in older women [26] (Fig. 5).

The detrusor coefficient (Deco) is obtained by dividing the PIP by 100. A value less than one signifies a weak contraction.

$$PIP = PDet@QMax + 5 \, QMax/100$$

The bladder contractility index (BCI) is also calculated using the same formula and has three ratings: (a) strong >150, (b) normal 100–130, and (c) weak <100 [27].

The Schäfer nomograms cannot be applied to female patients as they overestimate detrusor contractility in these patients [42]. Tan et al. proposed a modification of the calculation for PIP by taking the value of K as 1 cm H20 for older women [42]. The equation they proposed was.

$$PIP_1 = PDet@QMax + QMax$$

They derived this calculation from retrospectively analyzing urodynamic data in 100 elderly females aged 53 or above suffering from urge incontinence and randomized to either a trial of oxybutynin or placebo. Based on their calculations for this group, they classed contractions

Fig. 5 Determination of projected isovolumetric curve by plotting Pdet@Qmax on Schäfer's contractility nomogram and projecting it back to y-axis. (Reproduced from [7] with permission from Elsevier)

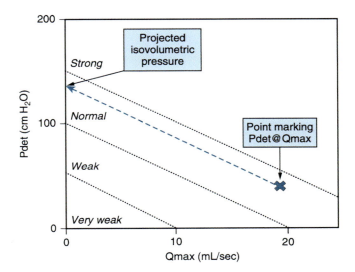

with PIP$_1$ less than 30 cm H20 as weak, between 30 and 75 cm H20 as typical for this group, and greater than 75 cm H20 as unusually strong. There are a few limitations to this study. It cannot be applied to younger women. These values cannot be considered normal bladder pressure values as the patient group was symptomatic.

The advantages of using these calculations are their simplicity, and the measurements are easy to obtain. However, they may not be applicable to other groups, e.g., men with post-prostatectomy incontinence and younger women. Also, they are less reliable than occlusion tests.

Occlusion tests can be used to directly measure isovolumetric pressure by mechanically obstructing the flow of urine. These can be classified into (1) voluntary stop test where the urine flow is interrupted after it has begun and (2) continuous occlusion test where urine outflow is blocked before and during the course of the voiding contraction. In their comparison of different stop test methods in female patients, Tan et al. concluded that the continuous stop test is the more reliable and preferred method of measuring detrusor contraction strength [41]. The voluntary stop test can underestimate contraction strength, whereas there's a need to repeat the voiding phase in the continuous occlusion test. Although these tests provide a real-time indication of isovolumetric strength and a good test-retest reliability without any calculations, they are painful, impractical, and impossible in some patients.

Management

Overactive Bladder

Conservative

The first-line management of OAB includes lifestyle modifications like reducing excessive fluid and caffeine intake. Additionally, fluid intake should be spaced throughout the day rather than concentrated at particular times. A significant fluid intake can also occur with increased consumption of fruits and vegetables. Patients should also be told to time their voids at certain parts of the day and leave longer periods between each void to train their bladder. A bladder diary is helpful in these cases.

Pharmacological

Pharmacological management is reserved for patients who fail to respond to lifestyle and behavioral modification.

Anticholinergics

These are first-line medications to manage OAB symptoms. They are antimuscarinic, and the traditional view is that they inhibit nonvoluntary detrusor contractions by inhibition of parasympathetic (efferent) activity principally by acting on the M3 receptor [28]. Other muscarinic receptors (M2, M4, and M5) exist in the bladder, but their role is less defined. Muscarinic receptors are also present in the urothelium and sensory nerves, and inhibition of these receptors may also explain the effect of these agents on OAB symptoms. As muscarinic receptors are present in other parts of the body, e.g., M1 in the CNS, M1 and M3 in salivary glands, M2 in the heart, M3 and M5 in the eyes, and M2 and M3 in the gastrointestinal system, these drugs can have side effects corresponding to their receptor selectivity. These include dry mouth, constipation, cognitive impairment, and dry eyes [4]. This class of medications is contraindicated in closed-angle glaucoma and urinary retention.

B3 Agonists

The bladder also contains B-adrenergic receptors (b-1, b-2, and b-3) which, on stimulation, can lead to detrusor relaxation via increased cyclic AMP levels [4]. This action is mainly mediated by the b3 receptor in humans. Mirabegron is a b-3 agonist which relaxes the detrusor by specifically binding to this receptor. Recent phase 3 trials have demonstrated its safety with a dose of 50 mg proving the most efficacious [4]. This drug can be used with most beta blockers (except metoprolol for reasons due to metabolism via the same hepatic pathway) and is relatively free of side effects which are comparable to placebo. There is a contraindication to its use in patients with uncontrolled hypertension but otherwise has been shown to not significantly raise the blood pressure in other patients.

Botulinum Toxin

The bacterium *Clostridium botulinum* produces botulinum toxin A(BTX) which can be injected into the bladder of patients who fail to respond to pharmacotherapy. BTX is a bacterial extract, and the various available BTX compounds differ in their constituents and efficacy. The only licensed BTX is onabotulinum toxin A (Botox). BTX acts by decreasing the release of all neurotransmitters onto the post-nerve terminals which prevents

nerve impulses from crossing the synaptic junction. BTX modulates the efferent neural pathway by disrupting the SNARE (soluble N-ethylmaleimide-sensitive factor attachment protein receptor) complex which leads to a highly specific neuromuscular blockade of ACh release at somatic and autonomic nerve terminals [4]. There is growing evidence that the mechanism of action of BTX might be more complex since urgency and painful bladder are sensory symptoms and other neurotransmitters like ATP, substance P, etc. may be involved [4].

Of the seven serotypes of BTX (A–G), BTX-A is the most commonly used, and a dose of 100 U has been shown to sufficiently reduce symptoms and improve quality of life (QoL) [29]. The patients must be counselled on the need to perform intermittent self-catheterization (ISC) if they develop voiding difficulty (which is more common with increasing age and occurs in up to 10% of patients with idiopathic OAB, albeit in younger age groups an incidence of less than 5% is the norm). Adverse events like impaired vision, dry mouth, and muscular weakness are rare and increase with increased doses of the toxin [4]. BTX can be safely injected into the bladder as an outpatient procedure using flexible cystoscopy.

Sacral Neuromodulation

Sacral neuromodulation, developed by Tanagho and Schmidt 40 years ago [30], presents another treatment modality for patients suffering from severe OAB symptoms especially with incontinence. Although the mechanism of action is not fully understood, it is believed to modulate spinal cord reflexes and higher centers as opposed to directly stimulating the bladder efferents to the detrusor [4]. A minimally invasive two-stage approach is utilized to insert the neuromodulator [31]. In the first stage, a tined lead is inserted into a foramen depending on the best sensory response from S2, S3, and S4. The lead is tunnelled into the skin via a gluteal skin incision, and once the wound has healed, it is connected to an external stimulator to test the response. A successful response is defined as a $> 50\%$ improvement in symptoms as judged by the bladder diary variables [4]. Once successful, the external stimulator is removed, and a neuromodulator is inserted internally through the gluteal skin incision made previously. Five-year success rates of 56–68% have been reported [32]. Problems may include battery failure, loss of efficacy, lead migration, and infection [4].

PTNS

Percutaneous tibial nerve stimulation (PTNS) is a form of neuromodulation that involves the use of a fine needle inserted just above the ankle. The resulting feedback loop projects to the S2–4 junction of the sacral plexus via the posterior tibial nerve and provides neuromodulation to the pelvic floor [4]. In a randomized study, patients on PTNS reported a subjective cure rate of 79.5% as compared to 58.4% for patients on tolterodine [33]. Reported adverse effects include headache, swelling, worsening of symptoms, leg cramps, and pain [4].

Underactive Bladder

Conservative Management

Initial management options of UAB include behavioral interventions like scheduled voiding to increase the frequency of voids especially in patients with impaired bladder sensation. Double voiding is another technique used by patients to effectively empty their bladder. Patients can also strain to empty their bladder using the Valsalva or Crede maneuver, but this should be used only in a small subset of patients (e.g., DUA with incompetent sphincter), or they risk damage to the urinary tract due to high vesical pressures [7].

Pelvic floor physiotherapy and biofeedback can be used to help patients with impaired relaxation of the pelvic floor and external urethral sphincter which can cause urinary retention and reflexively inhibit detrusor contractility [7]. Indeed, this therapy has shown good results in children and adults with impaired voiding [34, 35].

Catheterization is another option to ensure adequate drainage of the bladder. ISC is the preferred method over an indwelling/suprapubic catheter as it is associated with less infection rates [7]. It does require a patient to have good manual dexterity. In patients who are unable or unwilling to perform ISC, an indwelling urethral catheter should be avoided in the long term, and a suprapubic catheter would be the better option [7].

Pharmacotherapies

No effective pharmacotherapy for UAB exists at present. Medications have been aimed at increasing extra-vesical pressure/bladder contractility and decreasing outlet resistance but to no avail. There is a need to elucidate the mechanisms that lead to detrusor underactivity which can serve as pharmacological targets in the future, but at present, there are no potential candidate drugs in clinical trials [7].

Electrical Stimulation

Various forms of electrical stimulation have been used with varying success in specific cases of UAB. Brindley et al. [36, 37] developed a device for patients with complete spinal cord injury to stimulate the anterior sacral roots using an implantable receiver, an external transmitter, and stimulation wires. This method requires a patient with an intact neural efferent pathway and a bladder capable of contracting. As the relaxation time of the striated sphincter is shorter than that of the detrusor muscle, voiding occurs in spurts [38].

Sacral neuromodulation is another option that has been successfully used in a select group of patients with nonobstructive retention and DUA. Van Kerrebroeck et al. reported the results of a prospective, randomized, multicenter study where they investigated 31 patients who underwent sacral neuromodulation for urinary retention. At the end of a 5-year follow-up, they reported a decrease in mean number of daily catheterizations from 5.3 ± 2.8 to 1.9 ± 2.8, with a success rate of 58%. Similarly, there was a decrease in the mean volume of per catheterization from 379.9 ± 183.8 mL to 109.2 ± 184.3 mL, with a success rate of 71% [32].

Intravesical electrotherapy (IVE) involves application of current through the bladder wall by filling the bladder with saline and passing a current through an electrode at the catheter tip. A neutral electrode is applied to an area of normally sensitive skin to close the circuit [7]. IVE has been shown in animal studies to activate afferent mechanoreceptors in the bladder wall which causes a central reflex activation of the detrusor [7]. IVE has shown encouraging results in children with Gladh et al. demonstrating return-to-normal voiding in 83% of children with neurogenic and idiopathic DUA [39]. IVE is quite time- and resource-intensive requiring ten daily 60 min sessions followed by home treatment, at least thrice a week until bladder function normalizes.

Surgical Options

Intrasphincteric Botulinum Toxin

Botulinum neurotoxin A (BoNT-A) can be injected into the urethral sphincter to reduce outlet resistance and overcome reflex inhibition of detrusor contraction, although its action is short-lived, and it is not licensed for use outside of clinical trials [7].

Reconstructive Surgery

There have been reports of various reconstructive surgical procedures for UAB such as latissimus dorsi detrusor myoplasty (LDDM), rectus abdominis detrusor myoplasty, and reduction cystoplasty. All these procedures are considered experimental.

Conclusion

OAB and UAB are challenging to diagnose due to a varied presentation and shared symptomatology. The exact mechanisms behind OAB and UAB are poorly understood. Treatment is tailored to the patient's symptoms with options more established for OAB than UAB, the latter being defined recently. Further research is needed to better understand these disorders which would help develop effective therapeutic agents to treat patients suffering from OAB and UAB.

References

1. Chapple CR. Lower urinary tract symptoms revisited. Eur Urol. 2009;56(1):21–3.
2. Bates CP, Whiteside CG, Turner-Warwick R. Synchronous cine-pressure-flow-cysto-urethrography with special reference to stress and urge incontinence. Br J Urol. 1970;42(6):714–23.
3. Abrams P, et al. The standardisation of terminology of lower urinary tract function: report from the standardisation sub-committee of the international continence society. Neurourol Urodyn. 2002;21(2):167–78.
4. Chapple CR, Mangera A. Urgency incontinence and overactive bladder. In: Oxford textbook of urological surgery. Oxford: Oxford University Press; 2017. p. 282–8.
5. Haylen BT, et al. An International Urogynecological Association (IUGA)/International Continence Society (ICS) joint report on the terminology for female pelvic floor dysfunction. Neurourol Urodyn. 2010;29(1):4–20.
6. Hashim H, Abrams P. Is the bladder a reliable witness for predicting detrusor overactivity? J Urol. 2006;175(1):191–4.
7. Chapple CR, Osman NI. The underactive detrusor. In: Partin AW, Peters CA, Kavoussi LR, Dmochowski RR, Wein AJ, editors. Campbell-Walsh-Wein urology. Elsevier; 2020. p. 2650–63.
8. Chapple CR, et al. Terminology report from the International Continence Society (ICS) working group on Underactive Bladder (UAB). Neurourol Urodyn. 2018;37(8):2928–31.
9. Irwin DE, et al. Population-based survey of urinary incontinence, overactive bladder, and other lower urinary tract symptoms in five countries: results of the EPIC study. Eur Urol. 2006;50(6):1306–14. discussion 1314–5
10. Chapple C. Chapter 2: pathophysiology of neurogenic detrusor overactivity and the symptom complex of "overactive bladder". Neurourol Urodyn. 2014;33(Suppl 3):S6–13.
11. Wiseman OJ, Fowler CJ, Landon DN. The role of the human bladder lamina propria myofibroblast. BJU Int. 2003;91(1):89–93.
12. Daly D, Chapple CR. Anatomy, neurophysiology and pharmacological control mechanisms of the bladder. In: Oxford textbook of urological surgery. Oxford: Oxford University Press; 2017. p. 215–29.
13. Morrison J. The activation of bladder wall afferent nerves. Exp Physiol. 1999;84(1):131–6.
14. Michel MC, Chapple CR. Basic mechanisms of urgency: roles and benefits of pharmacotherapy. World J Urol. 2009;27(6):705–9.
15. Banakhar MA, Al-Shaiji TF, Hassouna MM. Pathophysiology of overactive bladder. Int Urogynecol J. 2012;23(8):975–82.
16. Birder LA, de Groat WC. Mechanisms of disease: involvement of the urothelium in bladder dysfunction. Nat Clin Pract Urol. 2007;4(1):46–54.
17. Davidson RA, McCloskey KD. Morphology and localization of interstitial cells in the guinea pig bladder: structural relationships with smooth muscle and neurons. J Urol. 2005;173(4):1385–90.
18. Brading AF. A myogenic basis for the overactive bladder. Urology. 1997;50(6):57–67.

19. Drake MJ, Mills IW, Gillespie JI. Model of peripheral autonomous modules and a myovesical plexus in normal and overactive bladder function. Lancet. 2001;358 (9279):401–3.
20. Matsumoto S, et al. Relationship between overactive bladder and irritable bowel syndrome: a large-scale internet survey in Japan using the overactive bladder symptom score and Rome III criteria. BJU Int. 2013;111(4):647–52.
21. Abrams PH, Griffiths DJ. The assessment of prostatic obstruction from urodynamic measurements and from residual urine. Br J Urol. 1979;51(2):129–34.
22. Schäfer W. Editorial comment. Neurourol Urodyn. 1989;8(5):499–503.
23. Nitti VW. Pressure flow urodynamic studies: the gold standard for diagnosing bladder outlet obstruction. Rev Urol. 2005;7:S14–21.
24. Osman NI, et al. Detrusor underactivity and the underactive bladder: a new clinical entity? A review of current terminology, definitions, epidemiology, aetiology, and diagnosis. Eur Urol. 2014;65(2):389–98.
25. Schafer W. Analysis of bladder-outlet function with the linearized passive urethral resistance relation, linPURR, and a disease-specific approach for grading obstruction: from complex to simple. World J Urol. 1995;13(1):47–58.
26. Griffiths D. Detrusor contractility–order out of chaos. Scand J Urol Nephrol Suppl. 2004;215:93–100.
27. Abrams P. Bladder outlet obstruction index, bladder contractility index and bladder voiding efficiency: three simple indices to define bladder voiding function. BJU Int. 1999;84(1):14–5.
28. Hegde SS, Eglen RM. Muscarinic receptor subtypes modulating smooth muscle contractility in the urinary bladder. Life Sci. 1999;64(6–7):419–28.
29. Dmochowski R, et al. Efficacy and safety of onabotulinumtoxinA for idiopathic overactive bladder: a double-blind, placebo controlled, randomized, dose ranging trial. J Urol. 2010;184(6):2416–22.
30. Tanagho EA, Schmidt RA. Bladder pacemaker: scientific basis and clinical future. Urology. 1982;20(6):614–9.
31. Spinelli M, et al. New sacral neuromodulation lead for percutaneous implantation using local anesthesia:

description and first experience. J Urol. 2003;170(5): 1905–7.
32. van Kerrebroeck PE, et al. Results of sacral neuromodulation therapy for urinary voiding dysfunction: outcomes of a prospective, worldwide clinical study. J Urol. 2007;178(5):2029–34.
33. Peters KM, et al. Randomized trial of percutaneous tibial nerve stimulation versus extended-release tolterodine: results from the overactive bladder innovative therapy trial. J Urol. 2009;182(3):1055–61.
34. de Jong TP, et al. Effect of biofeedback training on paradoxical pelvic floor movement in children with dysfunctional voiding. Urology. 2007;70(4):790–3.
35. Minardi D, et al. The role of uroflowmetry biofeedback and biofeedback training of the pelvic floor muscles in the treatment of recurrent urinary tract infections in women with dysfunctional voiding: a randomized controlled prospective study. Urology. 2010;75(6):1299–304.
36. Brindley GS, Polkey CE, Rushton DN. Sacral anterior root stimulators for bladder control in paraplegia. Paraplegia. 1982;20(6):365–81.
37. Brindley GS, et al. Sacral anterior root stimulators for bladder control in paraplegia: the first 50 cases. J Neurol Neurosurg Psychiatry. 1986;49(10):1104–14.
38. Sauerwein D. Surgical treatment of spastic bladder paralysis in paraplegic patients: sacral deafferentiation with implantation of a sacral anterior root stimulator. Urologe A. 1990;29:196–203.
39. Gladh G, Mattsson S, Lindstrom S. Intravesical electrical stimulation in the treatment of micturition dysfunction in children. Neurourol Urodyn. 2003;22(3): 233–42.
40. Nitti VW, Tu LM, Gitlin J. Diagnosing bladder outlet obstruction in women. J Urol. 1999;161(5):1535–40.
41. Tan TL, Bergmann MA, Griffiths D, Resnick NM. Which stop test is best? Measuring detrusor contractility in older females. J Urol. 2003;169(3):1023–7. https://doi.org/10.1097/01.ju.0000043810.43273.d7.
42. Tan TL, Bergmann MA, Griffiths D, Resnick NM. Stop test or pressure-flow study? Measuring detrusor contractility in older females. Neurourol Urodyn. 2004;23 (3):184–9. https://doi.org/10.1002/nau.20020.

Behavioral Modification and Conservative Management of Overactive Bladder and Underactive Bladder Disorders

14

Alain P. Bourcier and Jean A. Juras

Contents

Overactive Bladder 221
Lifestyle Interventions 223
Behavioral Therapy 228
Complementary and Alternative Medicine 231
Pelvic Floor Muscle Training 232
Urgency Inhibition and Suppression Techniques 233
Biofeedback Therapy 234
Electrical Stimulation 239
Electrical Stimulation: At Home 241
Percutaneous Tibial Nerve Stimulation (PTNS) 242
Self-Rehabilitation at Home 245
Conclusion 246

Underactive Bladder 246
Conservative Management 247
Conclusion 248

References 248

Keywords

Overactive bladder · Pelvic floor muscles training · Lifestyle modifications · Biofeedback · Intermittent catheterization

A. P. Bourcier (✉)
Centre d'Imagerie Médicale Cardinet, International Committee of Postpartum Management, Paris, France

J. A. Juras
Centre d'Imagerie Médicale Cardinet, Paris, France

© Springer Nature Switzerland AG 2023
F. E. Martins et al. (eds.), *Female Genitourinary and Pelvic Floor Reconstruction*,
https://doi.org/10.1007/978-3-031-19598-3_13

Overactive Bladder

Overactive bladder (OAB), a common lower urinary tract dysfunction, is defined by the International Continence Society as a syndrome characterized by urinary urgency, with or without urgency incontinence, usually with frequency and nocturia [1, 2]. OAB can be classified as OAB wet (with incontinence) or OAB dry (without incontinence). A prerequisite for the diagnosis is the absence of urinary tract infection or other detectable underlying disease.

OAB is a symptom-based diagnosis. This is distinct from the urodynamic diagnosis of detrusor overactivity (DO). DO is defined as a urodynamic observation characterized by involuntary detrusor contractions during the filling phase that may be spontaneous or provoked (Figs. 1 and 2). DO is subdivided into idiopathic detrusor overactivity (IDO) and neurogenic detrusor overactivity (NDO). However, patients with OAB do not always present with DO.

OAB is highly prevalent in the female population, and it represents a significant public health burden. Individuals with OAB report a significant impairment to overall quality of life [3]. Women with symptoms of OAB have reported that OAB interfered with daily activities, including staying at home, decreased physical activities, and weight gain because of an inability to exercise [4]. Many authors have described the associations between psychological conditions and OAB. Kinsey et al. recently systematically reviewed the psychological impact of OAB [5]. In this analysis, results from 32 papers reveal that the most widely studied associations are depression and anxiety. However, their results also suggest that OAB significantly affects self-esteem, sexuality, and relationships.

Individuals with symptoms of OAB often delay seeking treatment or even discussing their symptoms with healthcare providers. Increased symptom severity or bother appears to be a driving force for patients to seek treatment [6].

Conservative management is a type of medical treatment defined by the avoidance of invasive measures such as surgery or other invasive

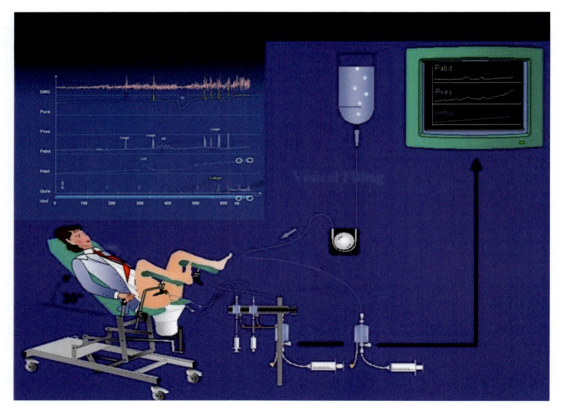

Fig. 1 OAB with detrusor overactivity. This multichannel trace shows multiple involuntary phasic contractions occurring at maximum filling capacity. Note that the provocative tests (running water and coughs) induced detrusor overactivity. Pves: intravesical pressure; Pura: intraurethral pressure; Pabd: abdominal pressure; Pdet: detrusor pressure (calculated by subtracting Pves from Pura)

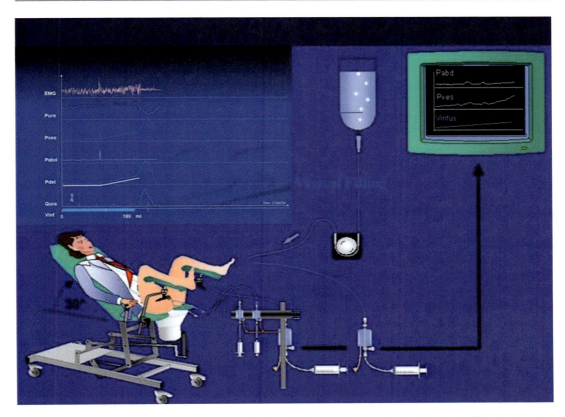

Fig. 2 The detrusor overactivity (DO) starts early after the bladder is filled with 150 ml and immediately leads to a complete loss of stored urine. In that case, the very high pressure of detrusor contractions may be indicative of a neurological etiology rather than idiopathic. Neurogenic detrusor overactivity is frequently observed in patients with conditions such as multiple sclerosis and spinal cord injury. In this example, there is a phasic DO, which rapidly leads to leakage (OAB/wet): leakage occurs with a relaxation of the EMG of the PFMs. This trace also shows a bladder-reduced compliance. Pves: intravesical pressure; Pura: intraurethral pressure; Pabd: abdominal pressure; Pdet: detrusor pressure calculated by subtracting Pve from Pura

procedures, usually with the intent to preserve function or body parts. Conservative management is an approach, utilizing nonsurgical treatment options, such as physical therapy, medication, and other therapies. The first-line treatments of OAB are lifestyle interventions, behavioral modifications, pelvic floor muscle training (PFMT), biofeedback therapy (BT), and electrical stimulation (ES). A conservative approach is often justified, especially if symptoms are only mild or easily manageable.

Behavioral modification is a group of therapies used to modify OAB symptoms by changing the bladder habits or by teaching new skills: bladder retraining, timed voiding, prompted voiding, fluid management, and elimination of bladder irritants [7–10] with the aim of educating the patient about her condition and providing the patient with strategies to reduce symptoms. In some countries, lifestyle modifications, bladder training, and scheduled voiding regimes are encompassed by the term "behavioral therapy," defined as an approach that seeks to alter the individuals' actions or their environment in order to improve bladder control.

Lifestyle Interventions

Changing a patient's behavior, environment, or lifestyle can mitigate or reduce symptoms like urinary incontinence, urgency, frequency, and nocturia. The interventions include lifestyle changes: cessation of smoking, weight reduction, elimination of dietary bladder irritants, adequate fluid intake, bowel regulation, smoking habits, and adaptation of physical stressors [8–10]. Patients seeking care for lower urinary tract symptoms (LUTS) are frequently instructed to modify daily behaviors to reduce symptoms. Diet, fluid intake, and caffeine, alcohol, and tobacco use may have effects on LUTS [11]. It is important to communicate to the patient that treatment demands patience and motivation, otherwise long-term improvements will not be achieved.

Smoking

Smoking irritates the bladder and can make symptoms worse. Smoking can cause frequent urination (caused by nicotine-induced bladder contractility). Smoking increases the risk of developing all forms of urinary incontinence, especially stress urinary incontinence, mainly due to violent and frequent prolonged coughing increasing downward pressure on the pelvic floor, causing repeated stretch injury to the pudendal and pelvic nerves. In addition, tobacco may have anti-estrogenic hormonal effects, which may influence collagen synthesis. There may also be an association between nicotine and increased detrusor contractions (nicotine-induced bladder contractility and some other toxins that can be bladder irritants). Smoking habits indicate that smoking can cause symptoms of urgency incontinence and urgency and frequency [8, 12]. Nuotio and coworkers [13] showed a correlation between smoking and urinary urgency in a population-based survey of 1059 women and men aged 60–89 years. Smokers were more likely to report incontinence than nonsmokers. Kawara and associates [14] have studied the correlation between smoking habit and lower urinary tract symptoms in women and showed that the prevalence of urgency and urgency UI correlated with age and smoking habits, and both current and ex-smokers show an increased prevalence compared with nonsmokers, especially younger women. In their final remarks, the authors wrote that the prevalence of LUTS, including OAB and UUI, increases with age. Furthermore, a smoking habit

exacerbates LUTS symptoms, especially among young women [14]. Based on this study, the authors recommend smoking cessation, which can be an effective way to reduce the urgency symptom over time. The cessation of smoking might reversely decrease the prevalence of urgency and UUI, but not daytime frequency and nocturia. Tähtinen RM and colleagues [15] estimate the relation of smoking status and smoking intensity with bladder symptoms by sending 3000 questionnaires mailed to women (aged 18–79 years). They concluded that urgency and frequency are approximately three times more common among current than never smokers. Nocturia and SUI are not associated with smoking. These results suggest an additional rationale for smoking cessation in women seeking medical attention for bladder symptoms and highlight the diversity between such symptoms [15].

Obesity

Obesity is an independent risk factor for the prevalence of urinary incontinence (UI). The precise mechanisms explaining the relationship among obesity, overweight, and OAB are not well understood. Some authors report that excess body weight increases intra-abdominal pressure, which in turn increases bladder pressure and intravesical pressure, leading to excessive activity of the urinary bladder. Several authors have investigated the relationship between obesity – assessed only by body mass index (BMI) – and OAB symptoms [16–20]. Most of these studies have shown high BMI to be a risk factor for UI in women. Maintaining normal weight through adulthood may be an important factor in the prevention of UI. Weight reduction should be recommended as part of the conservative management and behavior modification for obese women with UI [8, 21].

Metabolic factors may play a role in the development of OAB, UI, and other lower urinary tract symptoms. Massive weight loss significantly decreases UI in morbidly obese women. Lai and associates [22] described the relationship between metabolic factors and LUTS, OAB, and UI in a study with 920 participants. Central obesity (per 10 cm larger waist) was associated with higher odds of UI in both sexes, OAB in females, as well as frequency and nocturia. They concluded that central and general obesity were key metabolic factors associated with UI in both males and females and with OAB in females but not in males [22].

Auwad et al. [23] assessed the effect of moderate weight loss in obese women with urodynamically proven UI using the International Consultation on Incontinence recommended outcome measures. Sixty-four incontinent women were offered a weight reduction program with a low-calorie diet and exercise and a target loss of 5–10%. An anti-obesity drug (Orlistat) was offered to those who failed to achieve their target. Forty-two (65%) achieved the target weight loss and had significant reduction in BMI and girth. Weight loss was associated with significant reduction in pad test loss (median difference, 19 g; 95% confidence interval, 13–28 g; $p < 0.001$). The authors concluded that there was a reduction in OAB symptoms objectively confirmed following the 12-week program for the reduction of abdominal fat.

The objective of the study of Hagovska and colleagues [24] was to reduce symptoms of OAB through a three-month exercise program in young overweight women with OAB. The sample consisted of 70 women (mean age 26.7 ± 4.8 years), 36 being treated and 34 in the control group. They used a body composition analyzer with the assessment of skeletal muscle mass (kg), body fat mass (kg), body fat percentage (%), visceral fat area (cm^2/level), and the waist/hip circumference index. The intervention was a program for the reduction of abdominal fat with aerobic training, strengthening of the abdominal muscles, and stretching. They concluded that body composition analysis confirmed a reduction of BMI, body weight, body fat percentage, visceral abdominal fat, the WHR index, and waist circumference in the other parameters. A reduction in OAB symptoms was also objectively confirmed following the exercise program.

Impact of Food and Dietary Habits

First-line treatment for OAB is behavioral and dietary modifications because they have minimal side effects and high potential benefits. There is increasing evidence that diet may have a significant role in the development of lower urinary tract symptoms. Also good dietary habits and good nutrition are important in the management of LUTS. While high fluid intake is known to affect lower urinary tract function, the effects of other fluids than caffeine may have a direct impact on LUTS. Among these, alcohol, carbonated drinks, and artificial sweeteners are less well understood, and studies are sometimes contradictory [11]. Given the available evidence, lifestyle interventions and fluid modification may have an important role in the primary prevention of LUTS. However, more research is needed to determine the precise role of caffeine, carbonated drinks, and alcohol in the pathogenesis and management of these symptoms [25].

High fruit and vegetable consumption was negatively associated with nocturia. High intake of tea and dietary sodium showed a positive association with nocturia. Several foods have also been directly linked to changes in diuresis rate. At present, there is limited evidence to suggest that certain foods may contribute to the pathogenesis of nocturia.

Overall, there is evidence to suggest that certain foods, electrolytes, and specific compounds may contribute to the pathogenesis of nocturia, but there remains poor overall evidence with regard to specific conclusions and largely insufficient evidence to establish causality. High dietary intake of fruits and vegetables showed a negative association with nocturia, whereas high intake of tea showed a positive association with nocturia in observational studies [25–27].

Fluid Intake

Whether fluid intake should be restricted in UI patients is another issue. Patients with OAB symptoms may subscribe to either restrictive or excessive fluid intake behaviors. It is important to teach the patient that adequate fluid intake is necessary to eliminate irritants from the bladder and prevent UI [8, 20, 28]. Adequate fluid intake is very important for older adults, who already have a decrease in their total body weight and are at increased risk for dehydration. Although drinking less liquid does result in less urine in the bladder, the smaller amount of urine may be more highly concentrated and irritating to the bladder mucosa. In addition, inadequate fluid intake is a risk factor for constipation.

Swithinbank and associates [29] performed a four-week randomized, prospective, crossover study to determine the effect of caffeine restriction and of increasing and decreasing fluid intake on urinary symptoms. Sixty-nine women with a mean age of 54.8 years completed the study, including 39 with SUI and 30 with IDO. This study shows that a decrease in fluid intake improves some of these symptoms in patients with SUI and IDO.

Hashim and Abrams assessed how the symptoms of OAB and quality of life in 24 adults were affected by decreasing or increasing fluid input. There was a significant reduction in frequency, urgency, and nocturia when patients decreased their fluid input by 25%, but no effect on their UI. They concluded that fluid manipulation is a cheap, noninvasive, and easy way to help reduce the symptoms of OAB [30].

Zimmern et al. explored [31] whether instruction in fluid management resulted in changes in fluid intake and incontinence over a 10-week study period in women with urgency UI. Patients in both groups received general fluid management instructions, while in the drug + behavior arm, those with excessive urine output (>2.1 L/day) had additional individualized instruction during each of four study visits to learn behavioral strategies. They conluded that general fluid instructions can contribute to the reduction in UUI symptoms for women taking anticholinergic medications, but additional individualized instructions along with other behavioral therapies did little to further improve the outcome.

Caffeine

Caffeine is a xanthine derivative, a natural diuretic, and a bladder irritant. It acts similarly to thiazide diuretics. Caffeine is a central nervous system stimulant that reaches peak blood concentrations within 30–60 min after ingestion and has an average half-life of 4–6 hours [21].

Caffeine can cause a significant rise in detrusor pressure, leading to urinary urgency and frequency after caffeine ingestion. Caffeine has an excitatory effect on the detrusor muscles. Patients with symptoms of frequency and urgency often complain that their symptoms are exacerbated by tea or coffee [28].

Bryant and coworkers [32] conducted a prospective randomized trial of persons with symptoms of urgency, frequency, and urgency UI who routinely ingested 100 mg or more of caffeine per day. Both groups were taught bladder training, but the intervention group was also instructed to reduce caffeine intake to less than 100 mg/day. Patients should be advised about the possible adverse effects caffeine may have on the detrusor muscle and the possible benefits of reduction of caffeine intake [21]. They also should be instructed to switch to caffeine-free beverages and foods or to eliminate them and see if urinary urgency and frequency decrease. If they wish to continue to consume caffeine, patients with incontinence and OAB should ingest no more than 100 mg/day in order to decrease urgency and frequency.

Lohsiriwat and colleagues evaluated the effect of caffeine at the dose of 4.5 mg/kg on bladder function in OAB adults. They showed that caffeine at 4.5 mg/kg caused diuresis and decreased the threshold of sensation at filling phase, with an increase in flow rate and voided volume. They recommended that individuals should avoid or be cautious in consuming caffeine containing foodstuffs [33].

The goal of the study of Gleason et al. [34] was to characterize associations between caffeine consumption and severity of UI in US women who participated in the 2005–2006 and 2007–2008 National Health and Nutrition Examination Survey (NHANES), a cross-sectional, nationally representative survey. They stated that caffeine intake of ≥204 mg/day was associated with any UI but not with moderate/severe UI in US women.

Caffeine may also affect bladder function via central micturition centers, and in their study, Young-Sam and associates [35] suggested that caffeine facilitates bladder instability through enhancing neuronal activation in the central micturition centers. In addition to caffeine serving as a bladder irritant, caffeine is a weak diuretic, increases urine output, and contributes to urinary frequency.

Bladder Irritants

Certain foods and drinks have been associated with worsening symptoms of urinary frequency, urgency, urgency incontinence, or bladder pain. Some people find that certain foods or beverages seem to make their OAB symptoms worse and try to reduce the amount or eliminate them. The most common are (Table 1):

Anecdotal evidence suggests that elimination of dietary factors such as artificial sweeteners (aspartame) and certain foods (e.g., highly spiced foods, citrus juices, tomato-based products) may promote urinary incontinence [21, 36].

Alcohol is a diuretic, which means it promotes water loss through urine. It does this by inhibiting the production of a hormone called vasopressin, which plays a large role in the regulation of water excretion. Drinking alcohol inhibits the body's release of the hormone vasopressin. When we drink alcohol, the excess urine production can lead to dehydration and urine that is more concentrated. Alcoholic beverages generally contain a lot of sugar, which can also cause irritation in the bladder. If a patient suffers from any kind of bladder control issue, it is a good idea to watch her alcohol intake. Beer, white wine, champagne, spirits, and other alcoholic beverages can act as a bladder stimulant and ultimately lead to OAB. Hence, reducing alcohol consumption can help reduce any irritation of the bladder that could exacerbate any urgency or frequency symptoms [21].

Table 1 Patient Education Tool: List of Bladder Irritants

Acidic foods: Lemons, limes, oranges, grapefruit, and tomatoes and tomato products (like tomato sauce or salsa) are among the chief reported offenders
Acidic fruit juices, such as orange or grapefruit juice, can alter the pH of urine and exacerbate OAB symptoms
Highly spiced foods: Some people say chilies or wasabi wreaks havoc on their bladder
Artificial sweeteners in beverages and foods: Aspartame, saccharin, and others
Chocolate: Contains caffeine
Salty foods: Potato chips, salted nuts, and other salty foods can cause the body to retain water, which eventually goes to the bladder

People with OAB symptoms may also benefit from avoiding alcohol because of its diuretic properties.

The aim of the study of Robinson et al. [25] was to appraise the available evidence on the effect of caffeine, alcohol, and carbonated drinks on LUTS. They searched literature using the terms "fluid intake," "caffeine," "alcohol," "carbonated" and "urinary incontinence," "detrusor overactivity," "overactive bladder," and "OAB." They stated that in addition to fluid intake, there is some evidence to support the role of caffeine, alcohol, and carbonated beverages in the pathogenesis of OAB and LUTS. They concluded that lifestyle interventions and fluid modification may have an important role in the primary prevention of LUTS. However, more research is needed to determine the precise role of the bladder irritants.

Nutriments

Studies suggest that low intake levels of certain micronutrients may be associated with increased risk of OAB onset, the most significant association being with vitamin D. Vitamin D and its metabolites are steroid hormones and have many important functions. Cumulative studies have shown that vitamin D may be associated with LUTS, but the findings have been inconsistent. Different studies have found that low vitamin D levels are linked to OAB.

In the study of Dallosso and associates [37], results suggested that low intake levels of certain micronutrients may be associated with increased risk of OAB onset, the most significant association being with vitamin D. Vitamin D and its metabolites are steroid hormones and have many important functions. Low vitamin D status is involved in the pathogenesis of several chronic diseases. Muscle wasting is a symptom of osteomalacia, the clinical condition resulting from vitamin D deficiency in adults, and muscle atrophy has been described histopathologically in type II fibers. The potential role of vitamin D in the function of the detrusor muscle needs to be considered. Because it is produced phytochemically in the skin by exposure to ultraviolet light, the level of dietary intake is not usually very important. Apart from the elderly and other at-risk groups, there is no recommended level of vitamin D intake in the United Kingdom. Vitamin D supplements and improved calcium intake may improve urinary and psychological symptoms and quality of life among patients with OAB. Assessment for vitamin D status in patients with OAB may be warranted. This study [34] also provided some evidence that lower intake levels of the B vitamins niacin and B_6 may be associated with OAB onset. Bread and chicken are sizeable sources of niacin in the diet. Lower intake levels of both of these food groups showed an association with onset of OAB in another analysis [38, 39].

The literature also reports associations with folate and vitamin B_{12}; this suggests that the B_6 association with homocysteine may be because the three vitamins share the same food sources [40]. Potassium is very widespread in the diet, and a low intake is rare, sometimes occurring in people with bizarre or extremely low energy intakes.

Potassium depletion in the body never results solely from an inadequate intake and is always associated with abnormal losses from the body. The largest sources in the diet are fruit and vegetables (30%) and refined grains (21%) [41]: High intakes of vegetables and breads were associated with a reduced risk of OAB onset. A high potassium intake is generally considered an indicator of a "good quality diet," mainly because of its association with high fruit and vegetable content. The associated reduced risk of OAB onset could therefore be related to some aspect of a "healthy diet." [21].

Maserejian et al. [42] tested the hypothesis that carotenoid, vitamin C, zinc, and calcium intakes are associated with LUTS and UI in women during an observational, cross-sectional, population-based epidemiologic study of 2060 women (age 30–79 years). They observed that high-dose intakes of vitamin C and calcium were positively associated with urinary storage or incontinence, whereas vitamin C and β-cryptoxanthin from foods and beverages were inversely associated with voiding symptoms. Results indicate that micronutrient intakes may contribute to LUTS in dose-dependent and symptom-specific ways.

In conclusion for this first part, women with OAB can implement lifestyle modifications to control their OAB symptoms, such as losing weight, regulating fluid intake, and avoiding caffeine.

Behavioral Therapy

Bladder Training, Frequency Volume Charts

Behavioral therapy for OAB was first reported by Jeffcoate and Francis in the 1960s, when they advocated the practice of voiding "by the clock" for urgency UI [43]. Bladder training (sometimes called "bladder drill," "bladder retraining," or "bladder re-education") is a type of behavioral therapy that can help by minimizing the frequent urge to urinate. It involves a program of patient education along with a scheduled voiding regimen with gradually progressive voiding intervals. Other pioneers recommend this approach in the management of "urgency incontinence," "involuntary bladder contraction," and "instable bladder," which is now entitled OAB [44–46].

Despite the similarity in the basic framework, treatment protocols often differ, particularly with respect to where the intervention is delivered (such as outpatient, inpatient, and home environments). Bladder training instruction is usually provided directly by healthcare providers, although pamphlets, educational materials, or information and communication technology occasionally used [47]. Treatment frequently consists of bladder re-training by "bladder drill," to relearn the cortical inhibition of detrusor contractions. This may be time-consuming and frustrating, and correct diagnosis is necessary to ensure maximum patient compliance with treatment. Behavioral modification improves central control of bladder function, avoiding the mortality and morbidity of surgery, and the side effects of drug treatment. However, this type of treatment requires high levels of motivation and encouragement and suffers from high relapse rates.

Frequency volume charts provide an objective measure of bladder function, which is essential to support the treatment of urological problems.

A frequency volume chart is a simple, easy-to-use, noninvasive tool that is useful in the assessment of patients with LUTS. The frequency volume chart is the systematic registration of voiding habits by patients in their own environment for a specified period of time.

Using charts to record the times urine is passed and the volumes voided over a period of time gives an objective measure of bladder performance [8, 21]. The charts are usually completed by patients after they have been taught how to do so by a health professional. They provide valuable information which must be recorded on the chart and will be determined by the assessor based on the capabilities of the patient, who must be able to safely void into a container and measure and record the volume of fluid. The first advance came when the 24 h period was divided into daytime when the patient is awake and nighttime when asleep. Later modifications included asking the patient to document fluid intake (type and volume), the volumes of urine voided, the number of episodes of urgency, incontinence, and the use of incontinence aids such as pads. A 1–3-day chart is commonly used in clinical practice, and evidence has shown that this is as useful as those charts kept for longer periods [8, 21].

It is useful but needs to provide data with a complete bladder diary which records the times of micturition and voided volumes, episodes of incontinence, pad use, other information such as the degree of urgency, degree of incontinence, and fluid intake and type.

Charts or diaries should be completed for a minimum of 3 days [48]. The use of these charts encourage women to complete the diaries and to inform them concerning variations in their usual activities. The frequency/volume chart provides the best tool for following the result of treatment in patients with the urge syndrome.

Although recommended by many urologists, frequency volume charts are not widely used. This is more likely to be due to doctors not giving patient charts. When a chart is returned, one should collate the information for each day to identify the following: *daytime frequency*, the number of voids recorded during waking hours, including the last void before sleep and the first void after rising in the morning; and *nocturia*, the number of voids recorded during a night's sleep, where each void was preceded and followed by sleep. Bladder diary must be used to determine the maximum voided volume (the largest volume of urine voided during a single micturition). Comparing the results with what is considered normal bladder function may indicate areas of dysfunction and may be used to confirm a diagnosis.

It is important to remember that it is difficult to define a "normal" or healthy bladder function as normal parameters depending on age and gender, as well as many other internal and external factors such as fluid intake and type [49]. Despite their simplicity, frequency volume charts are useful, and their use should be encouraged, both in primary care and specialist practice.

Habit Training and Scheduled Voiding Regimens

Habit training is a toileting schedule that is matched to the patient's voiding pattern. Using the patient's voiding chart, a toileting schedule is assigned to fit a time interval that is shorter than the patient's normal voiding pattern and precedes the time period when incontinent episodes are expected. Thus, the voiding interval may be lengthened or shortened throughout the day, depending on the patient's voiding pattern with the goal to preempt UI. Habit training is usually implemented by caregivers, but patients may also be encouraged to suppress the urge to void until the assigned time. Habit training has been used primarily in institutional settings with cognitively and/or physically impaired adults. It is potentially useful for adults without cognitive or physical impairment, who have a consistent pattern of UI.

Timed voiding is a fixed voiding schedule that remains unchanged over the course of treatment. The goal of timed voiding is to prevent UI by providing regular opportunities for bladder emptying prior to exceeding bladder capacity. Timed voiding has been recommended for patients who cannot participate in independent toileting. It has been primarily used in institutional settings as a passive toileting assistance program where a caregiver takes the patient to void every 2–4 hours including at night. It is used to teach people with or without cognitive impairment to initiate their own toilet through requests for help and positive reinforcement from caregivers when they do so. Although it has been used primarily in institutionalized settings with cognitively and physically impaired older adults, prompted voiding has applicability for use with homebound older adults.

A frequently used treatment regimen [50] can be broken into the following components [8]:

- Exclude pathology.
- Explain the condition to the patient.
- Explain the treatment and its rationale to the patient.
- Instruct the patient to void at set times during the day, for instance, every 2 hours. The patient must not void between these times; she must wait or be incontinent.
- Increase voiding interval by increments after the initial goal is achieved, then repeat the process.
- The patient should have a normal fluid intake.
- The patient should keep her own input and output chart. The increasing volumes of urinary output at increasing intervals act as a reinforcement reward.
- The patient should receive praise and encouragement on reaching her daily targets.

Prompted voiding is a toileting program appropriate for older adults with all types of UI and individuals who may have impaired cognitive function. Fink and colleagues [51] determined the efficacy and safety of treatments for nursing home residents (1161 patients) with UI in a systematic review conducted for randomized controlled trials published from 1985 through 2008. Compared with usual care, prompted voiding alone or prompted voiding plus exercise reduced daytime incontinence and increased appropriate toileting. In nursing home residents with UI, prompted voiding alone and prompted voiding with exercise were associated with modest short-term improvement in daytime UI. Results do not clearly support an independent effect of exercise in improving UI. They concluded that these trials should include measures of UI, patient quality of life, and cost outcomes.

In a recent study, Martin-Losada and coworkers [52] assessed the efficacy of a prompted voiding program for restoring urinary continence at discharge in hospitalized older adults who presented with reversible UI on admission to a functional recovery unit. The study included 221 participants aged 65 and over with a history of reversible UI in the previous year that were on a prompted voiding program throughout their hospitalization period. The primary outcomes were UI assessed at discharge and at 1 month, 3 months, and 6 months after discharge. Their conclusion was that prompted voiding program can reverse UI or decrease the frequency and amount of urine loss in hospitalized older adults. Prompted voiding will enhance the health, functional ability, and quality of life of older adults with UI, resulting in the reduction of associated healthcare costs and the risk of developing complications.

The purposes of a narrative literature review of Reisch [53] described the rationale and theory for behavioral training techniques for OAB. Most outcomes are favorable, but there is inadequate evidence to support any specific training protocol. They stated that behavioral treatment for OAB is well supported by solid theoretical rationales, but evidence for the treatment is equivocal and leaves practitioners with many unanswered questions.

In conclusion for this second part, behavioral therapy, including bladder training and frequency volume charts, improves central control of bladder function, requires high levels of motivation and encouragement, and suffers from high relapse rates. It is noteworthy that bladder training needs to be performed for at least 6 weeks in order to achieve a satisfactory benefit. This part of the conservative treatment appears to be equal or superior to drug treatment and may have greater long-term benefits. There are numerous areas for future studies. There is a need for comparison between bladder retraining and other physical interventions.

Complementary and Alternative Medicine

There is a growing popularity of the use of complementary and alternative medicine (CAM) to treat illness and promote well-being. It is important for health professionals to understand how patients use CAM in addition to and/or as a substitute for allopathic care. CAM refers to a series of medical and health-care practices and products that are not considered part of conventional medicine.

The National Center for Complementary and Integrative Health has grouped CAM into five domains: dietary modifications and nutraceuticals (herbal products, dietary supplements); biofeedback therapy and yoga; body-based approaches, massage; energy therapies; and acupuncture and naturopathy [54–56]. Besides lifestyle changes, CAM can also be used to relieve UI symptoms, but there is limited information on the specific use of CAM among women with UI. In an international study, it was found that 42% of women with UI use CAM [57]. Another study that aimed to identify the use of CAM by women with UI was identified; this study reported that 33% of women with UI used CAM, with the most common therapy being prayer [58].

Yoga, a series of exercises originated in ancient India, can regulate the physical and mental function spontaneously. It is reported that yoga can modulate pelvic floor muscle tone, which contributes to LUTS relief [59]. A study showed that yoga could improve the symptoms of UUI and enhance the quality of life [60]. In a randomized, controlled trial, 19 women with SUI, UUI, or MUI were allocated to yoga therapy or control group. After 6-week therapy, women in yoga therapy group presented a more significant decrease in daily episode of UI than their counterparts in the control group (1.8 vs. 0.3) [61]. In terms of specific yoga postures, frog pose, fish pose, locust pose, plank pose, and seated twist may be beneficial for UI [59].

Acupuncture, as an effective therapy, has gained acceptance in urologists over the past decades [62]. It is described as one of the "complementary and alternative medicine/therapies,"

showing promising efficacy in the treatment of many conditions and resulting in fewer adverse effects compared with some conventional medical treatments. Equally, acupuncture stimulation of the sacral vertebra has a suppressive action on patient with OAB resulting in stress and urge incontinence. Acupuncture has been used to treat urinary incontinence since ancient times in China [63]. Acupuncture works by stimulating points with needles. In traditional Chinese medicine theory, acupuncture is thought to regulate qi circulation. For OAB, needling at points on the kidney or bladder meridians could reinforce qi and promote the recovery of bladder function [64]. A systematic review protocol detailed the proposed methods for evaluating the effectiveness and safety of acupuncture for OAB [65]. RCTs in English or Chinese have been included without restriction of publication type. Participants of any race or gender with a diagnosis of OAB were included. The conclusions drawn from this review will benefit patients and clinicians seeking effective and minimally invasive methods for treating OAB. The authors declared that this study might have some limitations. Specifically, different forms of acupuncture therapies and qualities of methodology may cause significant heterogeneity.

Electroacupuncture has also been used for treatment in patients with OAB. Electroacupuncture is a typical treatment that is effective at suppressing excessive contractions and activities of the detrusor muscle, improving bladder compliance, maintaining normal urination. However, the efficacy and safety of electroacupuncture are still controversial. Baliao acupoints, especially Zhongliao, are the main targets of acupuncture for dysuria and can improve urination symptoms. The Sanyinjiao acupoint is also commonly used. Of note, the tibial nerve is located deeply behind the Sanyinjiao [66]. Consequently, electrical stimulation can transmit the nerve impulse to the sacral segment through the posterior tibial nerve, which produces a regulatory effect [66, 67].

The purpose of the study of Aenouk et al. [68] was to catalog the most recent available literature regarding the use of conservative measures in the treatment of pelvic floor disorders. The literature was reviewed for articles published on physical, complementary, and alternative treatments for pelvic floor disorders over the past 5 years. Review of pelvic floor muscle physiotherapy (PFMT) and biofeedback (BF) shows a benefit for patients suffering from bladder dysfunction (incontinence, overactive bladder), bowel dysfunction (constipation, fecal incontinence), pelvic organ prolapse, and sexual dysfunction (pelvic pain). Combination of PFMT and BF has shown improved results compared to PFMT alone, and some studies find that electrical stimulation can augment the benefit of BF and PFMT. Additionally, acupuncture and cognitive behavioral therapy have been shown to be an effective treatment for pelvic floor disorders, particularly with respect to pelvic pain [68].

Pelvic Floor Muscle Training

Conservative treatment of women with UI, specifically pelvic floor muscle training (PFMT) and bladder retraining, is recognized as an effective therapy [69, 70]. Therapy is usually based on improving PFM function (in particular, the ability to sustain a contraction) and then using the improved muscle function in a bladder retraining program. The rationale for use of PFMT in OAB and UUI is that contraction of the muscles can reflexively or voluntarily inhibit contraction of the detrusor muscle. PFMT is defined as any program of repeated voluntary pelvic floor muscle contractions taught by a healthcare professional. The core consists of different groups of muscles, including respiratory diaphragm at the apex of the abdomen, the abdominal muscles (transversus abdominis) in the front, the lumbar paraspinal muscles in the back, and the pelvic floor muscles at the base. Strengthening the core can reduce urinary incontinence by restoring support to the pelvic organs and helping to control against leakage.

PFMT should pay attention to these other groups and specifically the obturator internus, the hip external rotators, and the glutei muscles. It is important to recognize the specific triggers that induce urgency or incontinence, and prior to

exposure to a trigger or at the time of the perceived urgency, rhythmic pulsing of the PFMs can either preempt the abnormal bladder contraction before it occurs or diminish the bladder contraction after it begins.

Reflex inhibition of a detrusor contraction may be possible by producing a voluntary contraction of the striated muscles of the pelvic floor and activating the perineo-detrusor inhibitory reflex, as described by Mahony and colleagues [71]. PFM exercises are also used for the treatment of OAB. The rationale behind the use of PFMT to treat urge incontinence is the observation that electrical stimulation of the pelvic floor inhibits detrusor contractions. The aims of this approach are to inhibit detrusor muscle contraction by voluntary contraction of the PFMs when the patient has the urge to void and to counteract the fall in urethral pressure or urethral relaxation that occurs with an involuntary detrusor contraction. It has been suggested that reflex inhibition of detrusor contractions may accompany repeated voluntary PFM contraction or maximum contractions. A study by Shafik [72] demonstrated that striated urethral sphincter contraction effected the inhibition of vesical contraction and suppression of the desire to void, an action suggested to be mediated through the "voluntary urinary inhibition reflex." Twenty-eight patients with OAB and 17 healthy volunteers were enrolled in the study. The results of this study encourage the treatment of overactive bladder with PFM contractions.

Burgio [73] focused on programs that include PFMT as a component in treatment for women or men. When it became evident that voluntary pelvic floor muscle contraction can be used to control bladder function, PFMT was also integrated into the treatment of urge incontinence and OAB as part of a broader behavioral urge suppression strategy. It can be combined with all other treatment modalities and holds potential for the prevention of bladder symptoms.

The study of Voroham and associates [74] aimed to determine the efficacy of 9 weeks of biofeedback-assisted PFMT on OAB symptoms and to detect changes in EMG activity of individual PFM with the MAPLe. They concluded that EMG BAPFMT is effective in significantly reducing symptoms and complaints of OAB and increases quality of life for patients.

Dumoulin and colleagues [75] assessed the effects of PFMT for women with UI in comparison to no treatment, placebo or sham treatments, or other inactive control treatments and summarized the findings of relevant economic evaluations. They used randomized or quasi-randomized controlled trials in women with SUI, UUI, or MUI (based on symptoms, signs, or urodynamics). One arm of the trial included PFMT. Another arm was a no treatment, placebo, sham, or other inactive control treatment arm. The review included 31 trials (10 of which were new for this update) involving 1817 women from 14 countries. Based on the data available, the authors can be confident that PFMT can cure or improve symptoms of SUI and all other types of UI. The findings of the review suggest that PFMT could be included in first-line conservative management programs for women with UI. The long-term effectiveness and cost-effectiveness of PFMT needs to be researched further.

Bo et al. [76] evaluated the effect of PFMT on OAB symptoms in women and assessed the influence of PFMT on PFM function, satisfaction with treatment, side effects, adherence, and the quality of exercise reporting. There was considerable heterogeneity of PFMT protocols, outcome measures, and follow-up periods. PFMT provided a significant reduction of OAB symptoms in five studies with a reduction in urinary frequency ($n = 1$) and urgency urinary incontinence ($n = 4$). The authors stated that PFMT might reduce OAB symptoms; however, due to many limitations of the published studies, it is not possible to clearly determine the effect of PFMT on OAB symptoms and PFM function.

Clearly, the necessary knowledge and skills were imparted to enable women to perform PFMT and bladder training at levels that resulted in significant differences in pelvic floor contraction strength and lengthened inter-void interval. The greater efficiency of instruction when provided to groups rather than individually warrants further study to document cost-effectiveness outcomes.

Urgency Inhibition and Suppression Techniques

In the management of OAB symptoms, patients can be taught to control urgency by performing general relaxation techniques, including slow deep breathing exercises to relax the bladder, decrease the intensity of the urgency, and allow the patient to delay voiding. Distraction techniques in which patients get involved in tasks that involve mental concentration could also be proposed. Wyman et al. suggested some techniques including checkbook balancing, using self-motivational statements, such as "I can wait," "I can take control," and "I will conquer this." [77] When urgency comes, urge suppression technique is usually done by concentrating on squeezing the pelvic floor muscles quickly and tightly several times (Fig. 3). This way of squeezing the pelvic floor muscles signals the bladder to relax. If the patient is able to isolate and perform a PFM contraction, they can be taught to suppress urgency by performing either a 10-s PFM contraction or five or six rapid and intense PFM contractions [72]. These contractions appear to induce their effects by preventing internal sphincter relaxation produced by the micturition reflex, which then results in detrusor relaxation [72].

Although strong PFM contractions will be more effective than weak contractions in suppressing urgency, simply making the patient aware of the importance of a well-timed PFM contraction is likely to provide benefit. A well-timed, volitional anal sphincter contraction (reflecting pelvic floor muscles) is able to suppress fully developed detrusor contractions, prevent the occurrence of further contractions, and hence suppress urgency [78]. Patients are also taught to avoid rushing to the bathroom, which may increase abdominal pressure and trigger bladder contractions. Instead, they are instructed to walk at a normal pace to the bathroom and pausing, if needed, to contract their PFMs. Reacting to the first sense of urgency by running to the bathroom needs to be substituted with urgency inhibition techniques [21].

A prospective experimental study was conducted between 2015 and 2019 by Pal et al.

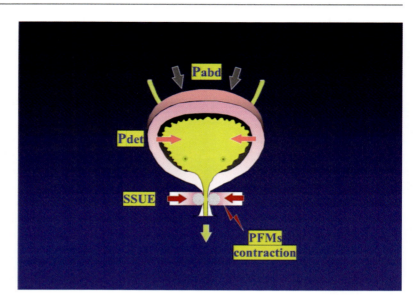

Fig. 3 PFMs strength and power are important in the control of urgency incontinence. Patients are taught "urgency strategies" to prevent loss of urine. The goal is to challenge the urgency by using PFMs to inhibit the involuntary detrusor contraction. This is accomplished by rapidly contracting them and taking a deep breath. Pabd: abdominal pressure; Pdet: detrusor pressure; Pves: intravesical pressure; SSUE: external striated urethral sphincter; PFMs: pelvic floor muscles

[79] Women complaining of OAB were enrolled. The women were asked to perform the urge suppression technique whenever urgency occurred. Ninety-one women ultimately completed the study. Frequency and nocturia were reduced. Seventy-six women had improvement of their urgency sensation ($P < 0.001$), whereas urgency urinary incontinence reduction was statistically not significant ($P > 0.05$). The authors concluded that urge suppression and modified fluid consumption are good adjunct in female OAB management.

Biofeedback Therapy

Biofeedback therapy (BT) can be defined as the use of monitoring equipment to measure internal physiologic events, or various body conditions of which the person is usually unaware, to develop conscious control of body processes. Biofeedback uses instruments to detect, measure, and amplify internal physiologic responses to provide the patient with feedback concerning those responses [80].

A major reason for the high interest is that the patient is actively involved in the treatment. The instruments include sensors (EMG, pressure sensors) for detecting and measuring the activity of anal or urinary sphincters and PFMs, and techniques also have been developed to measure activity of the detrusor muscle for treatment of UI called cystometric BT but is not yet popularized. During cystometry, bladder pressure readings are available to the patients and may provide a mechanism for feedback that allows them to acquire better control. Cystometric biofeedback was used to teach the patient on how to recognize and inhibit detrusor contractions. The original technique for BF of idiopathic detrusor instability was described by Cardozo and colleagues [81, 82].

For BT to be useful, several conditions must be met. There must be a readily detectable and measurable response (e.g., bladder pressure, PFM activity), and there must be a perceptible cue (e.g., the sensation of urgency) that indicates to the patient when control should be performed. In the application of BT to the treatment of UI, the concepts of neurophysiology of voiding and learning and conditioning are combined to accomplish the clinical objective of voluntary control of bladder function [83]. Simultaneous measurement of abdominal activity should be done with all BT techniques. Intra-abdominal pressure can be measured easily using an internal rectal balloon or surface electrodes. Electromyographic activity of the rectus abdominis muscles can be determined by surface electrodes. The abdominal muscle activity is displayed via two active electrodes placed 3 cm apart just below the umbilicus. A ground electrode is placed on the iliac crest [84, 85].

Biofeedback equipment has become sophisticated, and there are two basic types designed to suit the setting in which biofeedback is implemented: the outpatient clinic (Fig. 4), where the patient is trained using a comprehensive clinic system, and the individual's home (Fig. 5), where a smaller unit is used, generally on a more frequent basis. Abdominal muscle activity should be monitored simultaneously with PFMs so that patients can learn to contract the PFMs selectively. These measurements can be accomplished through a two- channel system.

Another approach to biofeedback for UI [84, 85] combines bladder pressure and PFMs in a procedure that provides simultaneous visual feedback of bladder, external anal sphincter, and intra-abdominal pressures. Using two-channel biofeedback (one with surface electrodes and one using an internal rectal balloon), patients are taught to contract and relax the PFMs selectively without increasing bladder pressure or intra-abdominal pressure.

The initial step in treatment is to help the patient identify the PFMs. It is important to test contractility and to know how the patient contracts the PFMs when instructed to squeeze these muscles. Very often, the contraction is performed incorrectly (Fig. 6). Instead of lifting up with the muscles, the patient is observed to be bearing down, which is counterproductive because it increases intra-abdominal pressure and therefore bladder pressure [84, 85].

Other investigators have found that a sizeable minority of women with SUI seeking medical care are unable to initially contract their pelvic floor muscles correctly. When asked to "squeeze as if trying to stop the flow of urine," about a third of women initially contract the gluteal, hip adductors, or abdominal muscles, rather than the levator ani muscles [86–88]. This response has been referred to as a "reversed perineal command" [84, 85, 89] or a "paradoxical perineal command." The frequency of such incorrect contraction is about 30% in women after childbirth, and it decreases to about 10% in women in the perimenopausal period. These women contract the gluteal, hip adductor, or abdominal muscles or are bearing down [90]. The vast majority are sportswomen who have had the constant abdominal muscle

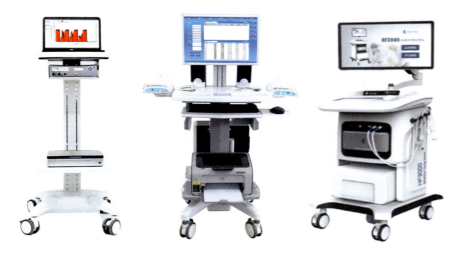

Fig. 4 Stationary devices with a wide range of electrical parameters, multichannel systems, used to provide electrical stimulation (ES) in the office or clinic under the control of a health care professional. It is also possible to connect the home care unit utilized by the patient at home to a stationary equipment

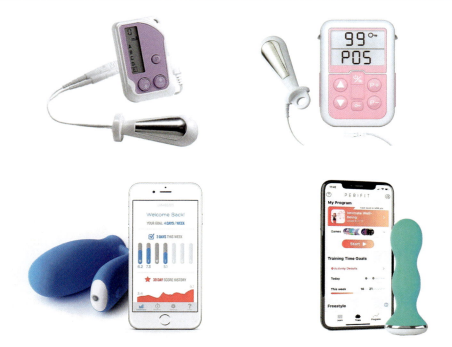

Fig. 5 Home biofeedback devices use a unit with a vaginal or anal electrode. Home-based biofeedback comprises 20 min self-training sessions twice per day, in which a self-inserted probe is used to provide visual feedback via a handheld monitoring device of vaginal or anal probe (top). Sensors connected to smartphones are available (bottom)

recruitment involved in their physical activities [91, 92]. Bump and colleagues [93] reported that 50% of women were unable to perform a voluntary PPFM contraction after brief verbal instruction, and as many as 25% mistakenly performed a Valsalva maneuver.

This type of improper PFM activity needs to be identified and eliminated as soon as possible. It seems clear that patients who bear down in this way must be identified before being asked to practice Kegel exercises at home, or the efforts will be futile. In addition, such maneuvers might increase vaginal wall descent or worsen UI by increasing intra-abdominal pressure. Except for the group of patients who are unable to perform a proper voluntary pelvic floor contraction, it seems very rare to perform a voluntary pelvic floor contraction without a co-contraction of the abdominal muscles. We suggest that it is not possible to maximally contract the PFMs without co-contraction of transverse abdominal muscle (transversus abdominis). Contraction of this muscle can be observed as a pulling in of the abdominal wall with no movement of the pelvis. During the initial biofeedback session, it is also common to observe patients perform pelvic muscle contractions accompanied by contraction of synergistic muscles such as adductors (pressing the knees) or gluteal muscles (squeezing the buttocks). This natural substitution of the stronger muscles for the weakened or minimally perceived motor response can also have negative consequences [91, 92].

An instrumentation system allows multiple measurements and modalities to be displayed on a monitor and stored in a computer database (Fig. 4). Patients should be able to recognize that the proper muscles are being used appropriately. Therapy is first concentrated on the inhibition of the antagonist muscles and decreasing the activity of surrounding muscles while increasing the response of the agonists. When the substituting muscles contract, their afferents can mask low-intensity sensory signals that may be

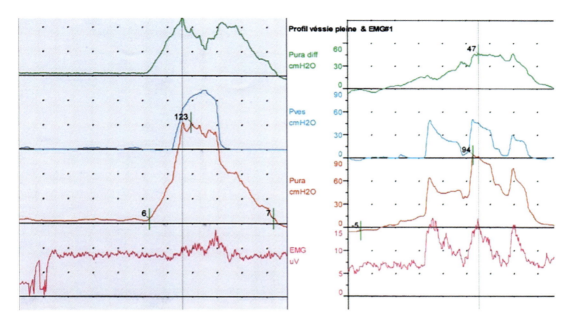

Fig. 6 Recording of electromyographic surface activity of PFMS, urethral pressure, and vesical pressure during a hold maneuver. The graphs demonstrate abnormal voluntary perineal contractions. Left, paradoxical perineal command: instead of lifting up the anus and vagina in drawing up, the patient is bearing down or pushing, which is counterproductive. From bottom to top, four tracings: surface EMG of PFMs activity (bottom); urethral pressure (second); vesical pressure (third); differential pressure (top). Right, co-contraction of abdominal muscles. Some patients use antagonist muscles when contracting the PFMs. From bottom to top, four tracings: surface EMG of PFMs activity (bottom); urethral pressure (second); vesical pressure (third); differential pressure (top)

generated by the weakened PFMs. This faulty maneuver perpetuates the substitution pattern and delays the development of increased awareness of the isolated PFMs. When the patient is instructed to relax the abdominal or surrounding muscles (adductors/gluteal), substitution of the interfering muscles may be detected by the biofeedback equipment (Fig. 7). An abdominal substitution pattern used when attempting to "hold back" leads to a false maneuver of pushing down, which causes a rise in intra-abdominal pressure. To minimize inappropriate tensing, it is helpful to train patients to keep these muscles relaxed when trying to prevent urine loss. For this purpose, patients are instructed to breathe evenly and to relax abdominal muscles. During the training sessions, the patient is also asked to place one hand on her lower abdomen to palpate the faulty abdominal contraction.

The evolution of women's professional activities and stressful environments represent high-risk factors for pelvic floor dysfunction. We may assume a certain relationship between pelvic floor support and intra-abdominal pressure. In our practice [84, 91, 92], we use office equipment that allows patients to different positions as they learn to use the PFMs to prevent urgency incontinence. We help them change their reactions by establishing targets and assisting them to develop new habits and modify their physical activities. It is optimal for patients to be standing when they performed these exercises (Fig. 7).

Summary of the Scientific Evidence for Biofeedback Therapy

Stein and colleagues evaluated the long-term effectiveness of transvaginal or transrectal EMG biofeedback in 28 patients with stress and urgency UI [94]. Sixty percent of the patients had detrusor overactivity, as demonstrated by urodynamics. Biofeedback successfully treated five of 14 patients (36%) with SUI and nine of

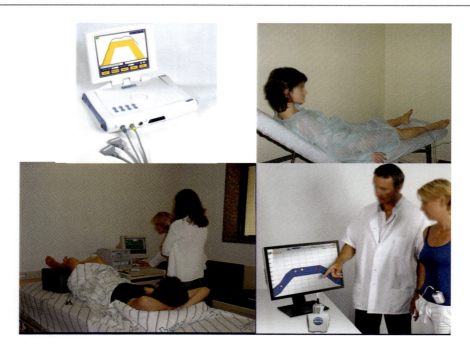

Fig. 7 The initial step in behavioral therapy (BT) is to help the patient identify the PFMs. At the end of this first stage, the use of new skills during exercises in standing position represents the applied BT. (Top left): Recordings of PFMs during a hold maneuver showing that the patient can sustain the contraction for more than 5 seconds without using the abdominal muscles. (Top right and bottom left): The patient is comfortably installed with relaxation of the lower part of the body before she attempts to contract properly the PFMs. To minimize inappropriate tensing, it is helpful to train patients to keep these muscles relaxed in breathing evenly and asked to place one hand on their lower abdomen. (Bottom right): A short vaginal probe or two sensor electrodes without wire used for a PFMT program in standing position. The patient contracts the PFMs at different periods and is asked to move

21 (43%) with UUI. The treatment response was durable throughout follow-up, from 3 to 36 months, in all of the responding patients. The authors concluded that biofeedback is a moderately effective treatment for SUI and UUI and should be offered to patients as a treatment option.

Wyman and colleagues [95] compared the efficacy of bladder training, PFMs with biofeedback-assisted instruction and combination therapy in women with genuine SUI and in those with detrusor overactivity. This was a large randomized clinical trial with three treatment groups. Women with incontinence (145 with SUI and 59 with urgency incontinence) received a 12-week intervention program, including six weekly office visits and six weekly mail or telephone contacts. The combination therapy group had significantly fewer incontinent episodes, better quality of life, and greater treatment satisfaction immediately after the therapy. They concluded that combination therapy had the greatest immediate efficacy in the management of female UI.

Burgio and associates [96] examined the role of BT in a multicomponent behavioral training program for urgency incontinence in community-dwelling older women ($n = 222$, age 55–92 years). Patients were randomly assigned to receive 8 weeks (4 visits) of biofeedback-assisted behavioral training ($n = 73$), 8 weeks (4 visits) of behavioral training without biofeedback or 8 weeks of self-administered behavioral treatment using a self-help booklet. They concluded that BF to teach PFM control, verbal feedback based, and a self-help booklet in a first-line behavioral training program all achieved comparable improvements in urge incontinence in community-dwelling older women.

A total of 124 patients entered the study of Liaw and Kuo [97], but only 68 (55%) completed the program. Among these patients, 52 (76%) had symptomatic improvement. After PFMT, the maximum flow rate and voided volume all increased in both genders and in patients with OAB as well as those with voiding dysfunction. The results of this study demonstrated that with a proper training program, 77% of patients with OAB and voiding dysfunction can achieve improvement in symptoms using biofeedback PFMT. The severity of frequency urgency symptoms can be reduced, and voided volume and Qmax can be increased.

Electrical Stimulation

Electrical Stimulation: Office Therapy

Electrical stimulation (ES) is used as a resource for UI treatment and can be offered in the outpatient clinic by an adequately trained nurse or physical therapist. Electrical currents are applied therapeutically to stimulate muscle contraction, usually through activation of nerves that supply muscles. ES was first used in the management of UI in 1952, when Bors [98] described the influence of ES on the pudendal nerves, and in 1963, when Caldwell and coworkers [99] developed electrodes that were permanently implanted into the pelvic floor and controlled by radiofrequency. Godec and associates [100] first described the use of non-implanted stimulators specifically for bladder inhibition. ES is an effective treatment of OAB. The technique uses natural pathways and micturition reflexes, and its efficacy relies on a preserved reflex arc, with complete or partial integrity of the PFM innervation [101].

The rationale behind the use of ES for patients with OAB or urgency UI is based on studies that observed bladder muscle inhibition following direct pudendal nerve stimulation. Appropriate ES may restore the inhibition effect. The mechanism of ES for urgency incontinence is a reflex inhibition of detrusor contraction. Bladder inhibition is accomplished through three mechanisms: activation of afferent fibers within the pudendal nerve by activation of the hypogastric nerve at low intravesical pressure corresponding to the filling phase, direct inhibition of the pelvic nerve within the sacral cord at high intravesical pressure, and supraspinal inhibition of the detrusor reflex [102, 103]. It is thought that PFM stimulation leads to reflex contraction of the striated paraurethral and periurethral muscles with simultaneous reflex inhibition of the detrusor muscle. In principle, defective control of the urinary bladder, resulting in urgency incontinence, is caused by a central nervous dysfunction that affects central inhibitory control of the micturition reflex. Appropriate ES may restore the inhibition effect [103].

Threshold intensity varies inversely with fiber diameter. Any pulse configuration can provide nerve activation, and many stimulation waveforms have been used to cause neural excitation [102, 104]. The sacral afferent nerves, particularly the autonomic nerves of the pelvic organs, are poorly myelinated (A) or unmyelinated (C) fibers, which conduct current at a slow rate of 5–20 Hz. Thus, in the treatment of OAB wet and OAB dry, low frequency stimulation is applied to the pudendal nerve afferents through probes. The different parameters for ES include biphasic capacitively coupled pulses, monophasic square pulses, biphasic square pulses, and monophasic capacitively coupled spike pulses. Pulse durations range from 0.08 ms up to 100 ms, but the most common used pulse duration is 0.2 ms. In both forms of ES, the frequencies are chosen based on the clinical diagnosis. To minimize electrochemical reactions at the electrode-mucosa interface, biphasic or alternating pulses are recommended [104].

It is thought that pelvic floor muscle stimulation leads to reflex contraction of the striated paraurethral and periurethral muscles with simultaneous reflex inhibition of the detrusor muscle. Different types of ES include office therapy and the home treatment program [105, 106]. Outpatient therapy is also called the outpatient program or in-clinic treatment (Fig. 4). With this approach, a stationary device with a wide range of electrical parameters is used in the office or clinic under the control of the therapist. The system can be modified to suit the needs of each patient.

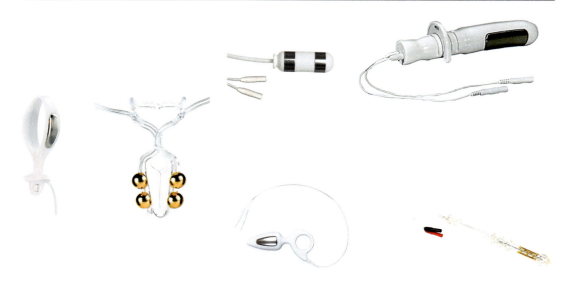

Fig. 8 Many probes are available with special conditions affecting the choice. The use of probes depends on the size and the shape of the vagina. Standard electrostimulation probes and biofeedback of muscle activity in current practice (top right). Probes designed specifically for patients with a wide vaginal hiatus (middle left). It is also possible to utilize anal probes in certain conditions (bottom right)

Many probes exist for ES as well as BT (Fig. 8). The currently available probes must be anatomically shaped in order to give good contact and to provide an efficient response to the electrical stimulus without discomfort or pain. We have selected those that could be proposed to our patients all over the world. There are a standard two-ring vaginal probe, an intra-anal probe, and a two-channel vaginal and anal insertion probe. Special conditions that affect the choice of probe include the following: vaginal size (depth of 4–12 cm), shape (e.g., atresia or gaping vagina), vaginal angle (10–45°), quality of the levator ani (thin or thick fibers), and type and degree of vaginal wall descent. Accurate assessment of individual anatomic differences allows the therapist to select the appropriate electrodes to obtain the most effective results. Some stimulators have controls to adjust frequency, duty cycle, and timing. The stimulus and intensity of the current are also adjustable, and all of these systems allow easy graduation in the intensity of contraction.

The main contraindications to ES are as follows: demand heart pacemakers; pregnancy, if the risk of pregnancy exists; post void residual greater than 100 mL; obstruction of the urethra, fixed and radiated urethra; bleeding; urinary tract infection or vaginal discharge; complete peripheral denervation of the PFMs; and severe genital prolapse with complete eversion of the vagina [107, 108].

Many patients will not accept treatment with vaginal or anal probes because of ethical and religious beliefs. These concerns must be taken into account before this therapy is advocated. This issue is especially relevant when home treatment is being considered, because some patients will not agree to insert the device themselves, and some will refuse this type of treatment altogether. Functional, anatomic, and attitudinal barriers are more common in frail elderly people. Cognitively or functionally impaired subjects require a participating caregiver. In the elderly, home care treatment could be performed by a nurse or a physical therapist. Different pelvic stimulators accommodate a variety of needs and vaginal sizes. One model relaxes the detrusor; another is designed to treat mixed UI; the third model treats double (urinary and fecal) incontinence. All require custom fitting by a women's health specialist.

Summary of the Scientific Evidence for Office Therapy

Brubaker indicated that there is also strong evidence that ES affects striated muscle [109]. The therapy can cause hypertrophy of skeletal muscle fibers, possibly by the recruitment of faster-conducting motor units, which would not normally be recruited during voluntary efforts. There is good evidence that the use of vaginal electrical stimulators can reduce the occurrence of symptoms of overactive bladder in about half of the patients treated. The use of non-implanted devices is effective and well tolerated and should precede the use of implanted devices. A direct comparison with other effective methods of treatment for overactive bladder is warranted.

Yamanishi et al. [110] evaluated the usefulness of ES for UI due to detrusor overactivity in a randomized, double-blind manner on 68 patients (29 men, 39 women, 70.0 ± 11.2 years). OAB was urodynamically defined as involuntary detrusor contractions of more than 15 cm H2O during the filling phase. Ten-hertz square waves of 1-ms pulse duration were used. A vaginal electrode was used in women, and stimulation was given for 15 min twice daily for 4 weeks. Of the 17 patients in the active group, 13 remained cured or improved for an average of 8.4 months after completion of the 4-week treatment. They concluded that ES was useful in treating urinary incontinence due to detrusor overactivity.

Amaro and coworkers [111] compared effective and sham intravaginal ES in treating mixed urinary incontinence in 40 women randomly distributed, in a double-blind study, into two groups: group G1 ($n = 20$), effective ES, and group G2 ($n = 20$), sham ES, with follow-up at 1 month. The pretreatment urodynamic study showed no statistical difference in urodynamic parameters between the groups. There was no statistically significant difference between the groups. They concluded that significant improvement was provided by effective and sham electrostimulation, questioning the effectiveness of electrostimulation as a monotherapy.

Firinci et al. [112] carried out a study on the efficacy of single and combined use of BF and ES added to bladder training on incontinence-related quality of life (QoL) and clinical parameters in women with idiopathic OAB. Seventy women were randomized into four groups as follows: Group 1 received BT alone ($n = 18$), Group 2 received BT + BF ($n = 17$), Group 3 received BT + ES ($n = 18$), and Group 4 received BT + BF + ES ($n = 17$). They concluded that in the first-line conservative treatment of women with idiopathic OAB, (i) adding BF and/or ES to BT increases treatment effectiveness, (ii) clinical efficiency is greater when the combination includes ES, and (iii) BT + BF + ES (triple combination) is the most effective treatment option in reducing nocturia and improving quality of life.

Yildiz and associates [113] studied the efficacy of intravaginal ES added to bladder training on incontinence-related quality of life and clinical parameters in women with idiopathic OAB. Sixty-two women with idiopathic OAB were randomized into two groups: Group 1 received bladder training alone (n:31), and Group 2 received bladder training + intravaginal electrical stimulation ($n = 31$). IVES was performed for 20 min 3 days a week over a course of 8 weeks for a total of 24 sessions. A statistically significant improvement was found in all parameters for all groups at the end of the treatment. Incontinence severity, frequency of voiding, nocturia, incontinence episodes, number of pads, symptom severity, and quality of life were significantly improved in Group 2 compared to those in Group 1 ($p < 0.05$). The authors concluded that BT + IVES were more effective than BT alone on both incontinence-related quality of life and clinical parameters in women with OAB.

Electrical Stimulation: At Home

Transcutaneous Electrical Nerve Stimulation

Transcutaneous electrical nerve stimulation (TENS) is a simple, noninvasive analgesic technique that is used extensively in health-care settings by physiotherapists, nurses, and midwifes. It has been demonstrated that TENS is of significant benefit in the management of vulvar and sexual pain (vulvodynia), and it can also have a relevant role in the treatment of pelvic floor dysfunction where we have the development of hypertonic muscles. TENS can also be used to strengthen pelvic muscles in the management of hypotonic pelvic floor dysfunction. TENS can be effective alone or combined with other therapies in the treatment of urinary incontinence, but there is no consensus on the electrical parameters to be used. The feasibility and effectiveness of sacral TENS (S-TENS) have been demonstrated in the treatment of fecal incontinence, primarily assessing patient continence scores. TENS is carried out with surface electrodes and, therefore, provides a noninvasive alternative to other stimulation modalities [114]. Transcutaneous tibial nerve stimulation (TTNS) is a specific form of TENS used in the treatment of OAB. The terms TTNS and TENS are used interchangeably.

Portable, disposable, and home self-applied transcutaneous electrical nerve stimulation device is effective for reducing OAB symptoms (Fig. 9). TENS consists of sessions of 30 min once a week for 12 weeks using biphasic square waves at a 20 Hz frequency with 200 cycles per second. Areas of stimulation are the dermatomes of S2 and S3 and the thigh area. Stimulation frequency is 20–50 Hz, and the pulse width is 200 μs. Stimulation is carried out daily during 2–6 weeks.

Percutaneous Tibial Nerve Stimulation (PTNS)

Percutaneous tibial nerve stimulation or posterior tibial nerve stimulation (PTNS) is a minimally invasive neuromodulation procedure. In the PTNS, the posterior tibial nerve is stimulated. The posterior tibial nerve is a distal branch of the sciatic nerve that originates in the pelvis (L5–S3 spinal roots) and descends toward the lower extremities, which are the same roots that innervate the parasympathetic pathway of the bladder (S2–S4). This nerve closely relates to pelvic nerves for bladder and perineal floor; therefore, a retrograde stimulation of S3 roots and of sacral spinal cord can be obtained [115].

This technique involves one-sided stimulation of the posterior tibial nerve, 5 cm above the medial malleolus of the ankle (Fig. 10). Stimulation can be carried out transcutaneously with a surface electrode or percutaneously by placing a

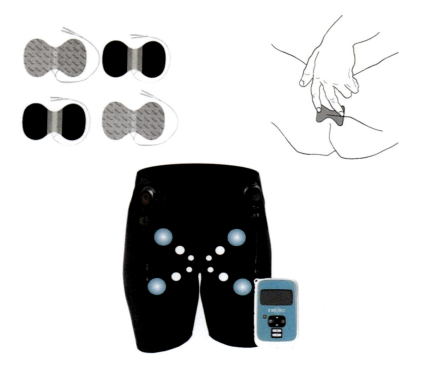

Fig. 9 Electrical stimulation (ES) of nerves activates sensory fibers that cause inhibition of bladder voiding via a reflex mechanism in the spinal cord. A stimulator sends electrical impulses by placing intra-cavitary probes, surface electrodes on the skin, either on the perineum (top right) or to the lower back (top left). These devices are compact, designed for home use. They have different programs for stress, urgency, and mixed incontinence. Another type is a non-invasive multipath technology, which recruits and engages the PFMs painlessly, stimulated by the electrodes which sit at the front and the back of a shorts (bottom)

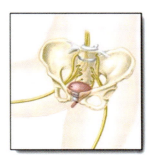

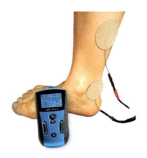 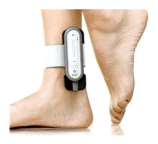 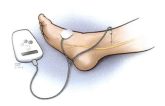

Fig. 10 Electrical stimulation (ES) can be carried out with a surface electrode, or percutaneously by placing a needle through the skin of the lower leg. The signal is conducted retrogradely through nerve fibers originating from L4 to S3 (top). The electrode is connected to an electrical stimulator (pulse generator) outside the body (bottom, middle). In PTNS, the stimulator sends pulses to the electrode (bottom right), which stimulates the tibial nerve with specific parameters. Standardized stimulation parameters will be applied: 1020 Hz frequency; pulse width of 200 μs; and duration of 30 min/weekly

needle through the skin. The signal is retrogradely conducted through nerve fibers originating from L4 to S3. The evidence shows that this procedure is effective in reducing urinary and bowel symptoms, and there are no major safety concerns, so it can be offered routinely as a treatment option for people with an overactive bladder and/or urge fecal incontinence. This is a simple, noninvasive, well-tolerated technique considered as a conservative and effective therapy for patients with UUI and OAB [109, 115]. Stimulation can be achieved via a percutaneous needle electrode (by inserting a 34-gauge needle 4–5 cephalad to the medial malleolus) or a transcutaneous surface electrode (stimulation is given via two 50 mm × 50 mm electrode pads, placed posterior and superior to the medial malleolus) [115–117].

The electrical current used for PTNS is a continuous square waveform with a duration of 200 Us, a frequency of 200 Hz and continuous stimulation at a pulse width of 200 μs, and a frequency of 10 Hz. The intensity of the current is determined by the highest level tolerated by the patient. The stimulation sessions last for 30 min. TENS seems to be as good as PTNS in terms of symptom improvement and may be an option for those patients who find needle insertion unacceptable [118].

Summary of the Scientific Evidence for TENS and PTNS

Ugurlucan and associates [119] compared the effects of transvaginal ES and PTNS in a randomized controlled trial. The study demonstrated that there was no statistically significant difference between the two groups in objective measurements. Quality-of-life assessments showed improvements in both groups but only a significant difference in the social limitations domain between ES and posterior nerve stimulation (ES significantly better than PTNS).

Zhu et al. [120] looked for randomized controlled trials that studied ES in OB treatment with subject headings and keywords using literature searches and manual retrieval. Ten randomized controlled trials involving 719 patients were included. The therapeutic effect of ES combined with other therapies for increasing the maximum bladder capacity was better compared with other therapies alone. No significant difference was noted between ES alone and other therapies alone. Based on current evidence, ES has certain effects on OAB. ES is safe, efficacious, and worthy of clinical use.

Another randomized controlled trial compared PTNS and ES with PFMT in 60 women with OAB with 30 participants allocated to each arm [121]. When the two groups were compared after treatment, women treated with PTNS showed statistically significant improvement compared with those treated with ES and PFMT as well as improvement in quality-of-life assessment.

Iyer and associates [122] retrospectively reviewed 183 patients with refractory OAB over a 9-year period who received 30-min sessions of PTNS for 12 weeks. There was a statistically significant improvement in urinary frequency, nocturia, and urgency incontinence episodes in the PTNS group, with the effect seen by week 10 of treatment; 61.5% of participants self-reported >50% improvement in symptoms with the number of PTNS sessions increasing the odds of subjective success.

Furtado-Albanezi and coworkers [123] randomized 40 women with nocturia into two groups of weekly transcutaneous electrical nerve stimulation (TENS) sessions compared with PFMT and behavioral therapy for a 12-week treatment period. Both treatments resulted in an improvement in the quality of sleep with a reduction in the number of awakenings to urinate (45% in both groups reduced by 1).

Vandoninck and associates [124] evaluated urodynamic changes after PTNS for the treatment of OAB with the aim of finding urodynamic-based predictive factors. Ninety patients underwent 12 PTNS sessions. The objective success rate was 56% (leakages/24 hours). They concluded that

PTNS could not abolish DO. PTNS increased cystometric capacity and delayed the onset of DO. Cystometry seemed useful to select good candidates: Patients without DO or with late DO onset proved to be the best candidates for PTNS.

In a nonsystematic review by De Wall and Heesakkers [125], they presented a summary of the history and theories on the pathophysiology behind neuromodulation, the clinical results, and latest developments in PTNS. They stated that PTNS seems not to be cost-effective as a primary treatment compared to antimuscarinics, but PTNS minimally invasive and not costly, it is time-consuming.

Peters and coworkers [126] compared the device Urgent PC vs Sham Effectiveness in Treatment of Overactive Bladder Symptoms was a multicenter, double-blind, randomized, controlled trial comparing the efficacy of PTNS to sham through 12 weeks of therapy. This multicenter, double-blind, randomized, sham-controlled trial provides level I evidence that PTNS therapy is safe and effective in treating overactive bladder symptoms. The compelling efficacy of PTNS demonstrated in this trial is consistent with other recently published reports and supports the use of peripheral neuromodulation therapy for OAB.

Burton et al. [127] evaluated the effectiveness of PTNS in treating OAB symptoms by systematic review of the literature up to April 2011 (Medline, EMBASE, Google Scholar). The studies report variable initial success rates (37–82%) for treating OAB symptoms with PTNS. The authors concluded that there is evidence of significant improvement in OAB symptoms using PTNS, which is comparable to the effect of antimuscarinics but with a better side effect profile. In order to recommend PTNS as a practical treatment option, long-term data and health economic analysis are needed.

Martin-Garcia et al. [128] compared the effectiveness of TTNS to PTNS in sustaining symptom improvement over a 6-month period in women with idiopathic OAB who had responded to an initial 12-week course of PTNS. Twenty-four women diagnosed with idiopathic OAB successfully treated with PTNS were included in this study. Participants were assessed at 6 weeks, 3 months, and 6 months after completing the initial course of PTNS. Urinary frequency, episodes of urinary urgency and episodes of UUI did not change significantly between baseline and 6 months in either group. TTNS is effective in the maintenance of symptom improvement in women with OAB who had positively responded to a course of 12 weekly PTNS sessions.

A randomized controlled clinical trial conducted by Padilha and colleagues [129] included 99 women, randomly allocated into three groups: TTNS, parasacral TES, and placebo. The current used for the TENS will be a symmetrical balanced biphasic pulsed current, for 12 sessions, twice a week, for 20 min. The parasacral TES will be used as an option for positioning the electrodes alternatively to the tibial nerve region in special populations, such as amputees or people with severe lower limb sensory impairment.

Ramirez-Garcia and associates [130] compared the efficacy of TTNS with PTNS regarding patient-reported outcome measures, specifically quality-of-life improvement and patient's treatment benefit, on symptoms associated with OAB. Sixty-eight adult patients (67.6% women) were included in the intention to treat analysis. The scores of the OAB-q-SF scales showed no statistically significant differences between the two groups. A significant improvement of quality of life was observed in both TTNS and PTNS groups. These findings along with TTNS ease of application and less invasiveness may lead to an increased indication of this technique for OAB.

The study of Bacchi Ambrosano Giarreta et al. [131] verified whether the addition of vaginal electrical stimulation to transcutaneous tibial nerve electrical stimulation is more beneficial than transcutaneous tibial nerve electrical stimulation alone for women with OAB. A total of 106 women aged >18 years with OAB or mixed UI with prevalent OAB symptoms were randomly divided into two groups, Group 1, TTNS ($n = 52$); Group 2, TTNS + VS ($n = 54$). After treatment, a reduction in urinary frequency of 1.5 micturitions was observed in Group 2, which was not clinically relevant despite being statistically significant. They concluded that the addition of VS to TTNS

for the treatment of OAB was not more effective than TTNS as a single therapy.

The above studies presented show that the main side effect from the percutaneous approach is pain at the needle insertion site. Inflammation and pain at the insertion site of the implantable device resulted in device removal. The use of PTNS in isolation in patients with OAB does seem to provide improvement in symptoms; however, the evidence from combination studies with PTNS and an antimuscarinic demonstrates that the two together provide greater symptom improvement. TTNS showed similar results to PTNS. Overall, the evidence shows that PTNS results in short- and long-term OAB symptom improvement. It could be argued that side effects with this treatment are more tolerable than those seen with antimuscarinics such as dry mouth and constipation.

Self-Rehabilitation at Home

The pandemic caused by coronavirus disease (COVID-19) increased the awareness and efforts to provide care from a distance using information technologies. Telehealth or telemedicine intends to facilitate effective delivery of health services such as physical therapy.

Da Mata and associates [132] reviewed the recent literature about the practice and effectiveness of the rehabilitation of the female pelvic floor dysfunction via telehealth, and four studies were included. They concluded that telehealth promoted a significant improvement in urinary symptoms, PFM function, and quality of life, but more studies are needed to draw more conclusions.

Based on this concept, we proposed a new therapeutic strategy called "auto-rééducation à domicile" (self-rehabilitation at home) in 2019. The literature has shown that home PFMT provides equal benefit to outpatient PFMT in reducing urinary symptoms when the patients attend some outpatient sessions to monitor their exercises during their treatment [133].

Therefore, before starting a PFMT program, one must ensure that the patients are able to perform a correct PFM contraction [86, 88, 89].

In order to avoid improper voluntary PFMs, which will not improve the patient's symptoms, we assess the PFMs function during her first visit. The physical examination consists of inspection at rest and inspection during effort with a digital palpation, assessing the PFM strength and endurance, identifying any prolapse, overweight, core muscles, and postural abnormalities. After this examination, we propose a specific exercise program with different sequences to practice daily for 15 min following a strict protocol. We also provide our patients with a leaflet sent by email giving information on the "management of your overactive bladder." This brochure includes different items: What is an overactive bladder? What are the symptoms? Lifestyle measures and urgency strategy. We asked the patient to have a second visit between 2 and 3 weeks to evaluate the improvement and to measure the degree of patient's satisfaction. If she is cured or greatly improved, we recommend to keep on practicing PFMs and follow the previous instructions written in the leaflet. In case of minor improvement, we prescribe a home-based neuromuscular electrical stimulation or home-based biofeedback device during 4 weeks. At the end of this period, we check for the third and last time the results of the combined therapy. Until now we have treated 290 patients and we are in the process to, we expect to publish the findings at the end of 2022.

Conclusion

Clinicians should be able to provide their patients with information regarding conservative treatment options for OAB. If caregivers do not have the time or interest in managing pharmacotherapy, they may refer to a specialist for medication management. Currently, there are several options for treatment with first-line therapies including behavioral modification and pelvic floor physical therapy. Although adjunctive therapies are useful because they may actively involve the patient in treatment, a combination of behavioral and pharmacologic approaches to the OAB syndrome offers the greatest chance of success.

Underactive Bladder

Underactive bladder (UAB) is a voiding disorder that generates disabling LUTS, defined by the ICS as a symptom complex characterized by a slow urinary stream, hesitancy, and straining to void, with or without the feeling of incomplete bladder emptying, sometimes with storage symptoms. It has received less attention than the condition of OAB.

Causes of UAB include neurogenic, myogenic, aging, and medication side effects (Table 2) [134]. The prevalence of UAB in different patient groups suggests that multiple etiologies are implicated. It can be observed in many neurologic conditions and myogenic failure. Diabetic cystopathy is the most important and inevitable disease developing from UAB and can occur early in the disease course. Careful neurologic and urodynamic examinations are necessary for the diagnosis of UAB.

Detrusor underactivity reflects the urodynamic observation of UAB and is due to a contraction of reduced strength and/or duration resulting in prolonged bladder emptying and/or a failure to achieve complete bladder emptying within a normal time span. Low detrusor pressure or short detrusor contraction time results in prolonged bladder emptying measured by urodynamics (detrusor hypocontractility) [135–137].

Symptoms such as retention and high post void residual urine in women are more likely due to detrusor underactivity, in regard to the low incidence of bladder outlet obstruction (BOO) in women (2.7–8%) [138].

The long-term effects of UAB may lead to significant complications. Urine left behind in

Table 2 Main causes of underactive bladder

Diabetes mellitus (diabetic cystopathy)
Bladder outlet obstruction
Aging
Neurologic disorders (multiple sclerosis, Parkinson's disease)
Acute cerebrovascular accidents
Injury to the spinal cord, cauda equina, and pelvic plexus
Herniated disc, lesions of the pudendal nerve

the bladder can lead to urinary tract infections, which, if become chronic, can lead to kidney damage and blood infections [139].

Conservative Management

Proper management focuses on the prevention of upper urinary tract damage, avoidance of over-distension, and reduction of residual urine (Table 3). Incomplete bladder emptying is a serious risk factor for urinary tract infection. Scheduled voiding and intermittent self-catheterization are the typical conservative treatment options. Methods to improve the voiding process are therefore practiced. UAB treatment requires increased detrusor pressure or decreased bladder outlet pressure.

Many health-care professionals are not familiar with UAB, specifically general practitioners, physical therapists, and nurse practitioners commonly seeing patients with disorders or symptoms related to pelvic floor muscle dysfunction. On the other hand, urologists usually treat patients with UAB, and most treatments focus on techniques to promote and assist bladder emptying such as intermittent self-catheterization and indwelling catheters [136].

There are no proven standard treatment options for UAB. However, proposed UAB treatments, include behavioral therapy, pharmacological, clean intermittent catheterization (CIC) strategies, and neuromodulation [140, 141].

The common techniques used are:

- *Timed voiding and prompt voiding: A fixed time interval toileting assistance program, a behavioral therapy used mainly in nursing homes.*

Table 3 The goals for bladder management include

Protecting upper urinary tracts
Achieving regular bladder emptying, avoiding stasis and bladder overdistension
Preventing and treating complications, UTIs, and stones
Maintaining continence and avoiding frequency and urgency

Prompt voiding is induced by a caregiver, while timed voiding is regulated by the patients themselves to empty the bladder before UI occurs at the scheduled time [142–144]. The goal is for the patient to follow a planned schedule that is shorter than the patient's normal voiding pattern and is timed prior to a possible UI episode. A family or a professional caregiver may ask the patient at regular time intervals (2 hours during the daytime and 4 hours at night) regarding the need to void and thereby provide assistance with the visit to the toilet. It is most successful with residents who are mobile or able to follow simple instructions.

- *Bladder expression: Various maneuvers aimed at increasing intravesical pressure in order to facilitate bladder emptying.*

There are various techniques such as abdominal straining, Valsalva's maneuver, and Crede's maneuver. The downward movement of the lower abdomen by suprapubic compression (Credé) or by abdominal straining (Valsalva) leads to an increase in intravesical pressure and generally also causes a reflex sphincter contraction [145]. The high pressures created during these procedures are hazardous for the urinary tract [146]. Potential complications of the Credé and Valsalva maneuvers include high bladder pressure, abdominal bruising with the Credé method, hernia, and hemorrhoids [147].

- *Bladder reflex triggering: Various maneuvers performed by the patient or the therapist in order to elicit reflex detrusor contraction by exteroceptive stimuli.*

Stimulation of the sacral or lumbar dermatomes can elicit a reflex detrusor contraction [144]. This comprises various maneuvers performed by the patient or the therapist to elicit reflex bladder emptying by exteroceptive stimuli [148]. The most commonly used maneuvers are tapping the suprapubic area, pulling the pubic hair, stroking the skin of the thigh or sole of the foot, and digital rectal stimulation. The patient should find the best individual trigger zone and points.

- *Intermittent self-catheterization (ISC) or clean intermittent catheterization (CIC)*

  This is a technique whereby the patient is taught to empty the bladder by passing a catheter into the bladder to drain out urine, which is then immediately removed and discarded. The procedure is taught to the patient by a specialist continence nurse or urotherapist. There are a wide variety of materials used and techniques applied for CIC. Several complications with CIC/ISC have been described: UTIs, urethral bleeding, urethritis, urethral stricture, and bladder stones [149]. CIC alone or in combination with another bladder-emptying method is the most frequently used method of bladder emptying [149, 150].

- *Electrical stimulation (ES): Sacral neuromodulation can be offered to selected cases, but it is an invasive procedure. Less invasive alternatives are TENS and PTNS.*

  These methods of ES might be effective and safe for treating neurogenic LUTS [151]. Coolen et al. [152] assessed the efficacy of TENS and PTNS for treating idiopathic nonobstructive urinary retention. A total of 3307 records were screened, and 8 studies met the inclusion criteria. The authors reported that the efficacy of TENS and PTNS in the treatment of idiopathic nonobstructive urinary retention is limited and should be verified in larger randomized studies before application in clinical practice. Intravesical electro-stimulation can increase bladder capacity and improve bladder compliance and bladder filling sensation. In patients with neurogenic detrusor underactivity, intravesical electro-stimulation (IVES) may also improve voiding and reduce residual volume. Few studies have reported that intravesical electrical stimulation may have direct effect on the bladder, especially on the detrusor muscle, and such approach may be more effective for relieving urinary retention or neurogenic bladder dysfunction [153]. IVES could be a promising treatment for bladder dysfunction in clinical practice.

Conclusion

UAB is an unmet medical condition, which has received less attention than the condition of OAB. Current treatments are the use of prescription medications, physiotherapy, and the use of intermittent self-catheterizations to drain the bladder. These treatments may not represent a cure, but instead they reduce the consequences of the disorder, limiting the damage done by UAB on the bladder and kidneys. There is currently no standard protocol for the treatment of UAB that allows an effective prevention of possible complications commonly associated to this condition or that promote a considerable improvement in the quality of life of patients [151, 154, 155].

References

1. Abrams P, Cardozo L, Fall M, et al. The standardisation of terminology of lower urinary tract function: report from the Standardisation Sub-Committee of the International Continence Society. Neurourol Urodyn. 2002;21:167–78.
2. Haylen BT, de Ridder D, Freeman RM, et al. An International Urogynecological Association (IUGA)/International Continence Society (ICS) joint report on the terminology for female pelvic floor dysfunction. Neurourol Urodyn. 2010;29:4–20.
3. Coyne KS, Wein A, Nicholson S, et al. Comorbidities and personal burden of urgency urinary incontinence: a systematic review. Int J Clin Pract. 2013;67(10): 1015–33.
4. Dmochowski RR, Newman DK. Impact of overactive bladder on women in the United States: results of a national survey. Curr Med Res Opin. 2007;23(1): 65–76.
5. Kinsey D, Pretorius S, Glover L, et al. The psychological impact of overactive bladder: a systematic review. J Health Psychol. 2016;21(1):69–81.
6. Reynolds WS, Fowke J, Dmochowski R. The burden of overactive bladder on US public health. Curr Bladder Dysfunct Rep. 2016;11(1):8–13.
7. Srikrishna S, Robinson D, Cardozo L, et al. Management of overactive bladder syndrome. Postgrad Med J. 2007;83(981):481–6.
8. Bourcier AP. Behavioral modification and conservative management of overactive bladder cht 19. In: Female urology. E-Book. 2008.
9. Gormley EA, Lightner DJ, Burgio KL, et al. Diagnosis and treatment of overactive bladder (non-neurogenic) in adults: AUA/SUFU guideline. J Urol. 2012;188:2455.

10. Lightner DJ, Gomelsky A, Souter L, et al. Diagnosis and treatment of overactive bladder (non-neurogenic) in adults: AUA/SUFU guideline amendment. J Urol. 2019;202:558.

11. Bradley CS, Erickson BA, Messersmith EE. Evidence for the impact of diet, fluid intake, caffeine, alcohol and tobacco on lower urinary tract symptoms: a systematic review. J Urol. 2017;198(5):1010–20.

12. Hannestad YS, Rortveit G, Daltveit AK, et al. Are smoking and other lifestyle factors associated with female urinary incontinence? The Norwegian EPINCONT study. BJOG. 2003;110:247–54.

13. Nutio M, Jylha M, Luukkaala M, Tammela TLJ. Health problems associated with lower urinary tract symptoms in older women. Scand J Prim Health Care. 2005;23:209–14.

14. Kawahara T, Ito H, Yao M, Uemura H. Impact of smoking habit on overactive bladder symptoms and incontinence in women. Int J Urol. 2020;27(12):1078–86.

15. Tähtinen RM, Auvinen A, Cartwright R, et al. Smoking and bladder symptoms in women. Obstet Gynecol. 2011;118(3):643–8.

16. Hunskaar S. A systematic review of overweight and obesity as risk factors and targets for clinical intervention for urinary incontinence in women. Neurourol Urodyn. 2008;27(8):749–57.

17. Hakki U, Orhan Ünal Z. Metabolic syndrome in female patients with overactive bladder. Urology. 2012;79:72–5.

18. Bunn F, Kirby M, Pinkney E, L., et al. Is there a link between overactive bladder and the metabolic syndrome in women? A systematic review of observational studies. Int J Clin Pract. 2015;69(2):199–217.

19. Hagovska M, Svihra J, Bukova A. The relationship between overweight and overactive bladder symptoms. Obes Facts. 2020;13:297–306.

20. Baytaroglu C, Sevgili E. Association of metabolic syndrome components and overactive bladder in women. Cureus. 2021;13(4):e14765.

21. Newman DK. Lifestyle interventions, chapter 27. In: Bourcier AP, Mc Guire EJ, Abrams P, editors. Pelvic floor disorders. Philadelphia: Elsevier Saunders; 2004. p. 269–76.

22. Lai HH, Helmut ME, Smith AR, et al. Relationship between central obesity, general obesity, overactive bladder syndrome and urinary incontinence among male and female patients seeking care for their lower urinary tract symptoms. Urology. 2019;123:34–43.

23. Auwad W, Steggles P, Bombieri L, et al. Moderate weight loss in obese women with urinary incontinence: a prospective longitudinal study. Int J Urogynecol. 2008;19:1251–9.

24. Hagovska M, Švihra J, Alena Buková A, et al. Effect of an exercise programme for reducing abdominal fat on overactive bladder symptoms in young overweight women. Int Urogynecol J. 2020;31:895–902.

25. Robinson D, Hanna-Mitchel A, Rantell A, et al. Are we justified in suggesting change to caffeine, alcohol, and carbonated drink intake in lower urinary tract disease? Report from the ICI-RS 2015. Neurourol Urodyn. 2017;36(4):876–81.

26. Tomohiro M, Nakamura Y, Yasuda T, et al. Effect of restricted salt intake on nocturia. Eur Urol Suppl. 2017;16(3):e698. 10.1016. https://doi.org/10.1016/S1569-9056(17)30463-3

27. Matsuo T, Miyata Y, Sakai H. Daily salt intake is an independent risk factor for pollakiuria and nocturia. Int J Urol. 2017;24(5):384–9. https://doi.org/10.1111/iju.13321.

28. Wyman JF, Burgio KL, Newman DK. Practical aspects of lifestyle modifications and behavioural interventions in the treatment of overactive bladder and urgency urinary incontinence. Int J Clin Pract. 2009;63(8):1177–91.

29. Swithinbank L, Hashim H, Abrams P. The effect of fluid intake on urinary symptoms in women. J Urol. 2005;174(1):187–9.

30. Hashim H, Abrams P. How should patients with an overactive bladder manipulate their fluid intake? BJU Int. 2008;102(1):62–6.

31. Zimmern P, Litman HJ, Mueller E, et al. Effect of fluid management on fluid intake and urge incontinence in a trial for overactive bladder in women. BJU Int. 2010;105(12):1680–5.

32. Bryant CM, Dowell CJ, Fairbrother G. A randomised trial of the effects of caffeine upon frequency, urgency and urge incontinence (Abstract number 96). Neurourol Urodyn. 2000;19(4):501–2.

33. Lohsiriwat S, Hirunsai M, Chaiyaprasithi B. Effect of caffeine on bladder function in patients with overactive bladder symptoms. Urol Ann. 2011;3(1):14–8.

34. Gleason JL, Richter HE, Redden DT, et al. Caffeine and urinary incontinence in US women. Int Urogynecol J. 2013;24(2):295–302.

35. Young-Sam C, Il-Gyu K, Sung-Eun K, et al. Caffeine enhances micturition through neuronal activation in micturition centers. Mol Med Rep. 2014;10:2931–6.

36. Newman DK. Managing and treating urinary incontinence. Baltimore: Health Professions Press; 2002.

37. Dallosso HM, McGrother CW, Matthews RJ, et al. Nutrient composition of the diet and the development of overac-tive bladder: a longitudinal study in women. Neurourol Urodyn. 2004;23:204–10.

38. Gregory J, Foster K, Tyler H. The dietary and nutritional survey of British adults. London: HMSO; 1990.

39. Dallosso HM, McGrother CW, Matthews RJ, et al. The association of diet and other lifestyle factors with overactive bladder and stress incontinence: a longitudinal study in women. BJU Int. 2003;92:69–77.

40. De Bree A, Verschuren WMM, Blom HJ, et al. Association between B vitamin intake and plasma homocysteine concentration in the general Dutch population aged 20 65 y. Am J Clin Nutr. 2001;73:1027–33.

41. Lin P, Aickin M, Champagne C. Food group sources of nutrients in the dietary patterns of the DASH-Sodium trial. J Am Diet Assoc. 2003;103:488–96.

42. Maserejian NM, Giovannuci EL, Mc KT, et al. Intakes of vitamins and minerals in relation to urinary incontinence, voiding, and storage symptoms in women: a cross-sectional analysis from the Boston Area Community Health Survey. Eur Urol. 2011;59(6):1039–47.

43. Jeffcoate TN, Francis WJ. Urgency incontinence in the female. Am J Obstet Gynecol. 1966;94:604–8.

44. Jarvis GJ. Bladder retraining, chapter 32. In: Bourcier AP, Mc Guire EJ, Abrams P, editors. Pelvic floor disorders. Philadelphia: Elsevier Saunders; 2004. p. 311–3.

45. Jarvis GJ. The management of urinary incontinence due to primary vesical sensory urgency by bladder drill. Br J Urol. 1982;54(4):374–6.

46. Fantl JA, Hurt WG, Dunn LJ. Detrusor instability syndrome: the use of bladder retraining drills with and without anticholinergics. Am J Obstet Gynecol. 1981;140(8):885–90.

47. Fantl JA, Newman DK, Colling J, et al. Urinary incontinence in adults: acute and chronic management. Clinical practice guideline, no. 2. Rockville: Department of Health and Human Services. Public Health Service, Agency for Health Care Policy and Research; 1996.

48. NICE Clinical Guidelines. The management of urinary incontinence in women. National Collaborating Centre for Women's and Children's Health (UK); 2013. No. 171.

49. Lukacz ES. A healthy bladder: a consensus statement. Int J Clin Pract. 2011;65(10):1026–36.

50. Jarvis GJ. Bladder retraining, chapter 32. In: Bourcier AP, McGuire EJ, Abrams P, editors. Pelvic floor disorders. Philadelphia: Elsevier Saunders; 2004. p. 311–3.

51. Fink HA, Taylor BC, Tacklind JW, et al. Treatment interventions in nursing home residents with urinary incontinence: a systematic review of randomized trials. Mayo Clin Proc. 2008;83(12):1332–43.

52. Martin-Losada L, Parro-Moreno AI, Serrano-Gallardo MP, et al. Efficacy of prompted voiding for reversing urinary incontinence in older adults hospitalized in a functional recovery unit: study protocol. Adv Nurs. 2021;77(8):3542–52.

53. Reisch R. Interventions for overactive bladder: review of pelvic floor muscle. J Women's Health Phys Ther. 2020;44(1):19–25.

54. Lowe FC, Patel T. Complementary and alternative medicine in urology: what we need to know in 2008. BJU Int. 2008;102(4):422–4.

55. Jackson CB, Taubenberger SP, Botheho E, et al. Complementary and alternative therapies for urinary symptoms: use in a diverse population sample qualitative study. Urol Nurs. 2012;32(3):149–57.

56. Pang R, Chang R, Zhou XY et al. Complementary and alternative medicine treatment for urinary incontinence. synopsis in the management of urinary incontinence. 2017. https://doi.org/10.5772/66705.

57. Fitzgerald MP, Link CL, Litman HJ, Travison TG, et al. Beyond the lower urinary tract: the association of urologic and sexual symptoms with common illnesses. Eur Urol. 2007;52(2):407–15.

58. Öz Ö, Altay B. Relationships among use of complementary and alternative interventions, urinary incontinence, quality of life, and self-esteem in women with urinary incontinence. J Wound Ostomy Continence Nurs. 2018;45(2):174–8.

59. Ripoll E, Mahowald D. Hatha Yoga therapy management of urologic disorders. World J Urol. 2002;20(5): 306–9.

60. Tenfelde S, Janusek LW. Yoga: a biobehavioral approach to reduce symptom distress in women with urge urinary incontinence. J Altern Complement Med. 2014;20(10):737–42.

61. Huang AJ, Jenny HE, Chesney MA, et al. A group-based yoga therapy intervention for urinary incontinence in women: a pilot randomized trial. Female Pelvic Med Reconstr Surg. 2014;20(3):147–54.

62. Tempest H, Reynard J, Bryant RJ, et al. Acupuncture in urological practice-a survey of urologists in England. Complement Ther Med. 2011;19(1):27–3.

63. Zhang L, Yang Y, Liu HL, et al. Urinary incontinence in ancient Chinese Medical literature. J Tradit Chin Med Lit. 2013;2:54–6.

64. Wang Y, Zhishun L, Peng W, et al. Acupuncture for stress urinary incontinence in adults. Cochrane Database Syst Rev. 2013;7:CD009408.

65. Mo Q, Wang Y, Ye Y, et al. Acupuncture for adults with overactive bladder: a systematic review protocol. BMJ Open. 2015;5:e006756.

66. Shen J, Luo R, Zhang L, et al. Using electro-acupuncture with optimized acupoint positioning to predict the efficacy of sacral neuromodulation of refractory overactive bladder. Medicine. 2019;98(45):e17795.

67. Yu XZ, Wang JQ. Twenty-four cases of overactive bladder treated with acupuncture. Shangdong J Tradit Chin Med. 2011;30:245–6.

68. Aenouk A, De E, Rehfuss A, et al. Physical, complementary, and alternative medicine in the treatment of pelvic floor disorders. Curr Urol Rep. 2017;18(6):47.

69. Wilson PD, Bo K, Hay-Smith J, et al. Conservative management in women. In: Abrams P, Cardozo L, Khoury S, Wein A, editors. International consultation incontinence. 2nd ed. Plymouth: Plymbridge Distributors; 2002.

70. Herbert JH. Pelvic floor muscle exercises, chapter 28. In: Bourcier AP, McGuire EJ, Abrams P, editors. Pelvic floor disorders. Philadelphia: Elsevier-Saunders; 2004. p. 277–80.

71. Mahony DT, Laferte RO, Blais DJ. Incontinence of urine due to instability of micturition reflexes: part I. Detrusor reflex instability. Urology. 1980;15:229–39.

72. Shafik A, Shafik IA. Overactive bladder inhibition in response to pelvic floor muscle exercises. World J Urol. 2003;20(6):374–7.

73. Burgio KL. Update on behavioral and physical therapies for incontinence and overactive bladder: the role of pelvic floor muscle training. Curr Urol Rep. 2013;14(5):457–64.
74. Voorham JC, De Wachter S, Van den Bos TWL, et al. The effect of EMG biofeedback assisted pelvic floor muscle therapy on symptoms of the overactive bladder syndrome in women: a randomized controlled trial. Neurourol Urodyn. 2017;36(7):1796–803.
75. Dumoulin C, Cacciani LP, Hay-Smith EJC. Pelvic floor muscle training versus no treatment, or inactive control treatments, for urinary incontinence in women. Cochrane Database Syst Rev. 2018;10(10):CD005654.
76. Bo K, Ferndandes ACNL, Duarte TB, et al. Is pelvic floor muscle training effective for symptoms of overactive bladder in women? A systematic review. Physiotherapy. 2020;106:65–76.
77. Wyman JF, Fantl JA. Bladder training in ambulatory care management of urinary incontinence. Urol Nurs. 1991;11:11–7.
78. Burgio KL, Locher JL, Goode PS, et al. Behavioral vs drug treatment for urge urinary incontinence in older women: a randomized controlled trial. JAMA. 1998;280:1995–2000.
79. Pal M, Chowdhury RR, Bandyopadhyay S. Urge suppression and modified fluid consumption in the management of female overactive bladder symptoms. Urol Ann. 2021;13(3):263–7.
80. Olson RP. Definitions of biofeedback. In: Schwartz MS, editor. Bio-feedback: a practitioner's guide. New York: Guilford Press; 1987. p. 33–7.
81. Cardozo LD, Stanton SL, Hafner J. Biofeedback in the treatment of detrusor instability. Br J Urol. 1978;50(Suppl 5A):250–4.
82. Cardozo LD. Biofeedback in overactive bladder. Br J Urol. 2000;85(Suppl 3):24–8.
83. O'Donnell PD. Biofeedback therapy. In: Raz S, editor. Female urology. Philadelphia: WB Saunders; 1996. p. 253–62.
84. Bourcier AP. Pelvic floor rehabilitation. In: Raz S, editor. Female urology. Philadelphia: WB Saunders; 1996. p. 263–81.
85. Bourcier AP, Burgio KL. Biofeedback therapy. In: Bourcier AP, McGuire EJ, Abrams P, editors. Pelvic floor disorders. Philadelphia: Elsevier-Saunders; 2004. p. 297–311.
86. Bø K, Larsen S, Oseid S, et al. Knowledge about and ability to correct pelvic floor muscle exercises in women with urinary stress incontinence. Neurourol Urodyn. 1988;7:261–2.
87. Hay-Smith EJ, Herderschee R, Dumoulin C, Herbison GP. Comparisons of approaches to pelvic floor muscle training for urinary incontinence in women. Cochrane Database Syst Rev. 2011;(12):CD009508.
88. Henderson JW, Wang S, Egger MJ, et al. Can women correctly contract their pelvic floor muscles without formal instruction? Female Pelvic Med Reconstr Surg. 2013;19(1):8–12.
89. Bourcier AP, Bonde B, Haab F. Functional assessment of pelvic floor muscles. In: Appell RA, Bourcier AP, La Torre F, editors. Pelvic floor dysfunction: investigations and conservative treatment. Rome: Casa Editrice Scientifica Internazionale; 1999. p. 97–106.
90. Kim S, Wong V, Moore KH. Why are some women with pelvic floor dysfunction unable to contract their pelvic floor muscles? Aust N Z J Obstet Gynaecol. 2013;53(6):574–9.
91. Bourcier AP, Juras A, Haab F. Physical activities, sports and female pelvic floor: update management. Lead Opin Gynäkol Geburtshilfe. 2020;2:27–33.
92. Bourcier AP, Haab F, Juras JA. Physical activities, sports and female pleivc floor: from causes to management: a review. Acta Sci Med Sci. 2020;4(6):55–65.
93. Bump RC, Hurt G, Fantl A, Wyman J. Assessment of Kegel muscle exercise performance after brief verbal instruction. Am J Obstet Gynecol. 1991;165:332–29.
94. Stein M, Discippio W, Davia M. Biofeedback for the treatment of stress and urge incontinence. J Urol. 1995;153:641–3.
95. Wyman JF, Fantl JA, McClish DK. Comparative efficacy of behavioural interventions in the management of female urinary incontinence. Continence Program for Women Research Group. Am J Obstet Gynecol. 1998;1998(179):999–1007.
96. Burgio KL, Goode PS, Locher JL, et al. Behavioral training with and without biofeedback in the treatment of urge incontinence in older women: a randomized controlled trial. JAMA. 2002;288:2293–9.
97. Liaw YM, Kuo HC. Biofeedback pelvic floor muscle training for voiding dysfunction and overactive bladder. Incont Pelvic Floor Dysfunct. 2007;1:13–5.
98. Bors E. Effect of electrical stimulation of the pudendal nerves on the vesical neck: its significance for the function of cord bladders. J Urol. 1952;167:925.
99. Caldwell KPS, Cook PJ, Flack FC, et al. Stress incontinence in females: report on 31 cases of treated electrical implants. J Obstet Gynaecol Br Commonw. 1968;75:777.
100. Godec C, Cass AS, Ayala G. Bladder inhibition with functional, electrical stimulation. Urology. 1975;6:663–6.
101. Lindstrom S, Fall M, Carlsson CA, et al. The neurophysiological basis of bladder inhibition in response to intravaginal electrical stimulation. J Urol. 1983;129:405.
102. Fall M, Lindstrom SHG. Inhibition of overactive bladder by functional electrical stimulation. In: Appell RA, Bourcier AP, La Torre F, editors. Pelvic floor dysfunction: investigations and conservative treatment. Rome: Casa Editrice Scientifica Internazionale; 1999. p. 267–72.
103. Vodusek DB, Light JK, Libby JM. Detrusor inhibition induced by stimulation of pudendal nerve afferents. Neurourol Urodyn. 1986;5:381–9.
104. Plevnik S, Janez J, Vrtacnick P, et al. Short-term electrical stimulation: home treatment for urinary incontinence. World J Urol. 1986;4:24–6.

105. Bourcier AP. Office therapy and home care perineal stimulation. Urodynam Neurourodynam Continence. 1992;2:83–5.

106. Bourcier AP, Juras JC. Electrical stimulation: home treatment versus office therapy. Eighty-ninth Annual Meeting of American Urological Association, San Francisco, May 14–19, 1994. J Urol. 1994;151:1171.

107. Bourcier AP, Mamberti-Dias A, Susset J. Functional electrical stimulation in uro-gynecology. In: Appell RA, Bourcier AP, La Torre F, editors. Pelvic floor dysfunction: investigations and conservative treatment. Rome: Casa Editrice Scientifica Internazionale; 1999. p. 259–66.

108. Bourcier AP, Park TAE. Electrical stimulation. In: Bourcier AP, McGuire EJ, Abrams P, editors. Pelvic floor disorders. Philadelphia: Elsevier-Saunders; 2004. p. 281–91.

109. Brubaker L. Electrical stimulation in overactive bladder. Urology. 2000;55(5 Suppl 1):17–23.

110. Yamanishi T, Yasuda K, Sakakibara R, et al. Randomized, double-blind study of electrical stimulation for urinary incontinence due to detrusor overactivity. Urology. 2000;55(3):353–7.

111. Amaro JL, Gameiro MO, Padovani CR. Intravaginal electrical stimulation: a randomized, double-blind study on the treatment of mixed urinary incontinence. Acta Obstet Gynecol Scand. 2006;85(5):619–22.

112. Firinci S, Yildiz N, Alkan H, et al. Which combination is most effective in women with idiopathic overactive bladder, including bladder training, biofeedback, and electrical stimulation? A prospective randomized controlled trial. Neurourol Urodyn. 2020;39(8): 2498–508.

113. Yildiz N, Alkan H, Sarsan A. Efficacy of intravaginal electrical stimulation added to bladder training in women with idiopathic overactive bladder: a prospective randomized controlled trial. Int Braz J Urol. 2021;47(6):1150–9.

114. Slovak M, Chapple CR, Barker AT. Non-invasive transcutaneous electrical stimulation in the treatment of overactive bladder. Asian J Urol. 2015;2:92–101.

115. Giani I. Tibial nerve stimulation. In: Electrical stimulation for pelvic floor disorders. Cham: Springer; 2014. p. 119–28.

116. Gaziev G, Topazio L, Iacovelli V, et al. Percutaneous tibial nerve stimulation (PTNS) efficacy in the treatment of lower urinary tract dysfunctions: a systematic review. BMC Urol. 2013;13:61.

117. Ramirez-Garcia I, Blanco-Ratto L, Kauffman S, et al. Efficacy of transcutaneous stimulation of the posterior tibial nerve compared to percutaneous stimulation in idiopathic overactive bladder syndrome: randomized control trial. Neurourol Urodyn. 2019;38:261–8.

118. Bhide AA, Tailor V, Fernando R, et al. Posterior tibial nerve stimulation for overactive bladder—techniques and efficacy. Int Urogynecol J. 2020;31(5):865–70.

119. Ugurlucan FG, Onal M, Aslan E, et al. Comparison of the effects of electrical stimulation and posterior tibial nerve stimulation in the treatment of overactive bladder syndrome. Gynecol Obstet Investig. 2013;75(1):46–52.

120. Zhu T, Feng XJ, Zhou Y, Wu JX. Therapeutic effects of electrical stimulation on overactive bladder: a meta-analysis. Springerplus. 2016;5(1):2032.

121. Scaldazza CV, Morosetti C, Giampieretti R, Lorenzetti R. Percutaneous tibial nerve stimulation versus electrical stimulation with pelvic floor muscle training for overactive bladder syndrome in women: results of a randomized controlled study. Int Braz J Urol. 2017;43(1):121–6.

122. Iyer S, Laus K, Rugino A, et al. Subjective and objective responses to PTNS and predictors for success: a retrospective cohort study of percutaneous tibial nerve stimulation for overactive bladder. Int Urogynecol J. 2019;30(8):1253–9.

123. Furtado-Albanezi D, Jürgensen SP, Avila MA, et al. Effects of two nonpharmacological treatments on the sleep quality of women with nocturia: a randomized controlled clinical trial. Int Urogynecol J. 2019;30(2): 279–86.

124. Vandoninck V, van Balken MR, Finazzi AE. Percutaneous tibial nerve stimulation in the treatment of overactive bladder: urodynamic data. Neurourol Urodyn. 2003;22(3):227–32.

125. De Wall LL, Heesakkers JPFA. Effectiveness of percutaneous tibial nerve stimulation in the treatment of overactive bladder syndrome. Res Rep Urol. 2017;9: 145–57.

126. Peters KM, Carrico DJ, Perez-Marrero RA, et al. Randomized trial of percutaneous tibial nerve stimulation versus Sham efficacy in the treatment of overactive bladdersyndrome: results from the SUmiT trial. J Urol. 2010;183:1438–43.

127. Burton C, Sajja A, Latthe PM. Effectiveness of percutaneous posterior tibial nerve stimulation for overactive bladder: a systematic review and meta-analysis. Neurourol Urodyn. 2012;31(8):1206–16.

128. Martin-Garcia M, Crampton J. A single-blind, randomized controlled trial to evaluate the effectiveness of transcutaneous tibial nerve stimulation in Overactive Bladder symptoms in women responders to percutaneous tibial nerve stimulation. Physiotherapy. 2019;105(4):469–75.

129. Padilha JF, Avila MA, Seidel EJ, et al. Different electrode positioning for transcutaneous electrical nerve stimulation in the treatment of urgency in women: a study protocol for a randomized controlled clinical trial. Trials. 2020;21:166.

130. Ramirez-Garcia I, Kauffmann S, Blanco-Ratto L, et al. Patient-reported outcomes in the setting of a randomized control trial on the efficacy of transcutaneous stimulation of the posterior tibial nerve compared to percutaneous stimulation in idiopathic overactive bladder syndrome. Neurourol Urodyn. 2021;40(1):295–302.

131. Bacchi Ambrosano Giarreta F, Milhem Haddad J, de Carvalho S, Fusco HC, et al. Is the addition of vaginal electrical stimulation to transcutaneous tibial nerve

electrical stimulation more effective for overactive bladder treatment? A randomized controlled trial. Actas Urol Esp (Engl Ed). 2021;45(1):64–72.

132. da Mata KRU, Costa RCM, Carbone ÉDSM, et al. Telehealth in the rehabilitation of female pelvic floor dysfunction: a systematic literature review. Int Urogynecol J. 2021;32(2):249–59.

133. Fitz FF, Gimenez MM, de Azevedo FL, et al. Pelvic floor muscle training for female stress urinary incontinence: a randomised control trial comparing home and outpatient training. Int Urogynecol J. 2020;31(5): 989–98.

134. Chapple CR, Osman NI, Birder L, et al. Terminology report from the ICS, Working Group on Underactive Bladder. Neurourol Urodyn. 2018; 37(8):2928–2931. https://doi.org/10.1002/nau.23701

135. D'Ancona C, Haylen B, Oelke M, et al. The International Continence Society (ICS) report on the terminology for adult male lower urinary tract and pelvic floor symptoms and dysfunction. Neurourol Urodyn. 2019;38(2):433–77.

136. Miyazato M, Yoshimura N, Chancellor MB. The other bladder syndrome: underactive bladder. Rev Urol. 2013;15(1):11–22.

137. Aldamanhori R, Osman NI, Chapple CR. Underactive bladder: pathophysiology and clinical significance. Asian J Urol. 2018;5(1):17–21.

138. Carr LK, Webster GD. Bladder outlet obstruction in women. Urol Clin North Am. 1996;23:385–91.

139. Chancellor MB, Bartolone SN, Lamb LE, et al. Underactive bladder; review of progress and impact from the International CURE-UAB Initiative. Int Neurourol J. 2020;24(1):3–11.

140. Osman NI, Chapple CR, Abrams P, et al. Detrusor underactivity and the underactive bladder: a new clinical entity? A review of current terminology, definitions, epidemiology, aetiology, and diagnosis. Eur Urol. 2014;65(2):389–98.

141. Cho KJ, Kim JC. Management of urinary incontinence with underactive bladder: a review. Int Neurourol J. 2020;24(2):111–7.

142. Ouslander JG, Schnelle JF, Uman G, et al. Predictors of successful prompted voiding among incontinent nursing home residents. J Am Med Assoc. 1995;273(17):1366–70.

143. Eustice S, Roe B, Paterson J. Prompted voiding for the management of urinary incontinence in adults. Cochrane Database Syst Rev. 2000:CD002113.

144. Ostaszkiewicz J, Johnston L, Roe B. Habit retraining for the management of urinary incontinence in adults. Cochrane Database Syst Rev. 2004: CD002801.

145. Barbalias GA, Klauber GT, Blaivas JG. Critical evaluation of the Crede maneuver: a urodynamic study of 207 patients. J Urol. 1983;130:720.

146. Wyndaele JJ, Mandersbacher H, Radziszewski P, et al. Neurologic urinary incontinence. Neurourol Urodyn. 2010;29:159.

147. Chang SM, Hou CL, Dong DQ, Zhang H. Urologic status of 74 spinal cord injury patients from the 1976 Tangshan earthquake, and managed for over 20 years using the Credé maneuver. Spinal Cord. 2000;38(9): 552–4.

148. Gazewski JB, Schurch B, Hamid R, et al. An International Continence Society (ICS) report on the terminology for adult neurogenic lower urinary tract dysfunction (ANLUTD). Neurourol Urodyn. 2017 Nov 17. https://doi.org/10.1002/nau.23397.

149. Madersbacher H, Wyndaele JJ, Igawa Y, et al. A conservative management in neuropathic urinary incontinence. In: Abrams P, Khoury S, Wein A, editors. Incontinence. 2nd ed. Plymouth: Health Publication Ltd; 2002. p. 697–754.

150. Hansen RB, Biering-Sørensen F, Kristensen JK. Bladder emptying over a period of 10–45 years after a traumatic spinal cord injury. Spinal Cord. 2004;42(11):631–7.

151. Yamany T, Elia M, Lee JJ, Singla AK. Female underactive bladder – current status and management. Indian J Urol. 2019;35(1):18–24.

152. Coolen RL, Jeroen JG, Scheepe JT. Transcutaneous electrical nerve stimulation and percutaneous tibial nerve stimulation to treat idiopathic nonobstructive urinary retention: a systematic review. Eur Urol Focus. 2021;7(5):1184–94.

153. Cao T, Xie B, Yang S, et al. Low-frequency intravesical electrical stimulation for the treatment of acute urinary retention: a promising therapeutic approach. Front Med. 2021;8:572846. https://doi.org/10.3389/fmed.2021.572846.

154. Bayrak Ö, Dmochowski RR. Underactive bladder: a review of the current treatment concepts. Turk J Urol. 2019;45(6):401–9.

155. Santos-Pereira M, Charrua A. Understanding underactive bladder: a review of the contemporary literature. Porto Biomed J. 2020;5(4):e070.

Bladder Dysfunction and Pelvic Pain: The Role of Sacral, Tibial, and Pudendal Neuromodulation

15

Ly Hoang Roberts, Annah Vollstedt, Jason Gilleran, and Kenneth M. Peters

Contents

Introduction	256
Sacral Plexus	257
Surgical Technique	258
Percutaneous Nerve Evaluation (PNE)	260
Complications	261
Programming	261
Indications	264
Overactive Bladder (OAB)	264
Urinary Retention	265
Chronic Pelvic Pain	265
Pudendal Nerve	265
Surgical Technique	266
Complications	267
Indications	268
Tibial Nerve	268
Surgical Technique	269
Complications	269
Indications	269
Conclusion	270
Cross-References	270
References	270

L. Hoang Roberts (✉) · J. Gilleran · K. M. Peters
William Beaumont School of Medicine, Beaumont
Hospital, Oakland University, Royal Oak, MI, USA
e-mail: Ly.Hoang@beaumont.org;
Jason.Gilleran@beaumont.edu;
kenneth.peters@beaumont.edu

A. Vollstedt
Department of Urology, University of Iowa Hospitals and
Clinics, Iowa City, IA, USA

© Springer Nature Switzerland AG 2023
F. E. Martins et al. (eds.), *Female Genitourinary and Pelvic Floor Reconstruction*,
https://doi.org/10.1007/978-3-031-19598-3_15

Abstract

Neural damage or nociceptive stimuli may cause detrusor or pelvic floor dysfunction and pain. With any disruption in the complex neural system of the lower urinary tract, there is a risk of uninhibited voiding reflex leading to urgency, frequency, or incontinence. Chronic urethral obstruction or peripheral vascular disease can also lead to detrusor ischemia with resulting smooth muscle cell and neuronal damage. The regeneration of nerves can result in bladder instability and hence, urgency and frequency. With pelvic floor dysfunction, visceral stimuli from either infection, trauma, surgery, or chronic straining can be a noxious trigger resulting in pain, so that over time, hyperalgesia can occur. Lesser understood predisposing factors include chronic illnesses such as depression, anxiety, pain, irritable bowel syndrome, and fibromyalgia.

Neuromodulation uses the complex pelvic and bladder neuroanatomy to treat lower urinary tract symptoms and pelvic floor dysfunction. The history of neuromodulation, or the use of electrical stimulation to modulate or modify a function, has roots back to Roman times when Scribonius used shock from contact with a torpedo fish to treat gout pain. Since then, in-depth study of the neural system has advanced medicine so that the first implantable stimulator was developed in 1967 for spinal pain. Neuromodulation for bladder dysfunction was first postulated in 1895 by Langley and Anderson, but the focus on the pelvic nerve with its opposing concomitant effects of external urethral sphincter and detrusor contraction limited its success. Further work with animal models led to the understanding of the sacral nerve roots such that Tanagho and Schmidt were able to develop the first electrode to be safely implanted at S3. Evolution of this concept has now included research in understanding the role of the pudendal nerve in modulating both bladder and pelvic muscles.

In this chapter, we will concentrate on the three specific nerves (sacral, tibial, and pudendal) that have been used as targets for neuromodulation in urology. For each neural target, we will describe the relevant anatomy, surgical technique, possible complications, and relevant data on the efficacy in treating overactive bladder, underactive bladder, and pelvic floor dysfunction.

Keywords

Bladder dysfunction · Overactive bladder · Underactive bladder · Pelvic floor

dysfunction · Pelvic pain · Lower urinary tract dysfunction · Neuromodulation · Sacral nerve · Tibial nerve · Pudendal nerve

Introduction

The urinary bladder has two functions: storage and emptying. Both functions are regulated by a complex communication between the brain, spinal cord, and peripheral nervous systems. Bladder storage, or continence, is a result of the inhibition of detrusor muscle contraction via the lumbar sympathetic system and activation of the external urethral sphincter via the somatic system. Bladder emptying, or voluntary voiding, is initiated by a neural reflex that involves afferent neurons within the bladder to send signals through the sacral spinal cord to the pontine micturition center (PMC) and to the bladder efferent parasympathetic neurons [1]. As a result, the external urethral sphincter relaxes, and the detrusor muscle contracts via the parasympathetic system. Storage and voiding rely on the interactions of the central nervous system (CNS), made up of the brain and the spinal cord, and the peripheral nervous system (PNS), made up of the afferent (sensory) and efferent (motor) neurons [1].

The neuroanatomy of the pelvis is complex, as it includes both visceral (i.e., bladder, rectum, reproductive organs) and somatic structures (i.e., bony pelvis, ligaments, and muscles). The visceral organs are innervated by visceral afferents which run parallel with the sympathetic system, via the superior and inferior hypogastric plexus from T10 to L2, and the parasympathetic system, via the inferior hypogastric plexus from the pelvic splanchnic nerves (S2–S4). As they travel caudally, these nerves give rise to various plexuses including the rectal, vesical (bladder), ovarian, testicular, deferential plexus (vas deferens, epididymis, seminal vesicle, prostate), cavernous (penis and clitoris), and uterovaginal (uterus, vagina). The primary nerve that provides both motor and sensory capabilities to the somatic structures is the pudendal nerve (S2–S4) [2]. This innervates the main supporting structures of the pelvic floor, the levator ani muscles, which consists of the pubococcygeus, puborectalis, and iliococcygeus. Other supporting structures include the perineal membrane and body [3]. In addition, other regional muscles provide afferent signals to the lumbar or sacral plexus when nociceptive input is encountered.

Pathology occurs when neural damage or nociceptive stimuli result in detrusor or pelvic floor dysfunction and pain. With any disruption in the complex neural system, there is a risk of uninhibited voiding reflex leading to urgency, frequency, or incontinence seen in upper motor neuron lesions or hypotonicity in lower motor neuron lesions [4]. Chronic urethral obstruction or peripheral vascular disease can also lead to detrusor ischemia with resulting smooth muscle cell and neuronal damage [5–7]. The regeneration of nerves can result in bladder instability and, hence, urgency and frequency [7]. With pelvic floor dysfunction, visceral stimuli from either infection, trauma, surgery, or chronic straining can be a noxious trigger resulting in pain, so that over time, hyperalgesia can occur [8]. Lesser understood predisposing factors include chronic illnesses such as depression, anxiety, pain, irritable bowel syndrome, and fibromyalgia [9].

Neuromodulation uses the complex pelvic and bladder neuroanatomy to treat lower urinary tract symptoms and pelvic floor dysfunction. The history of neuromodulation, or the use of electrical stimulation to modulate or modify a function, has roots back to Roman times when Scribonius used shock from contact with a torpedo fish to treat gout pain [10, 11]. Since then, in-depth study of the neural system has advanced medicine so that the first implantable stimulator was developed in 1967 for spinal pain [12]. Neuromodulation for bladder dysfunction was first postulated in 1895 by Langley and Anderson [13], but the focus on the pelvic nerve with its opposing concomitant effects of external urethral sphincter and detrusor contraction limited its success. Further work with animal models led to the understanding of the sacral nerve roots such that Tanagho and Schmidt were able to develop the first electrode to be safely implanted at S3 [14]. Evolution of this concept has now included research in understanding the role of the pudendal nerve in modulating both bladder and pelvic muscles. Though the exact mechanism of action of neuromodulation is unclear, it is hypothesized that electrical stimulation

of the afferent nerves in the spinal roots leads to the modulation of continence and voiding neural pathways in the central nervous system by inhibiting sensory processing in the spinal cord [15]. This same mechanism has been used to interrupt pain at the spinal cord with great success [8].

In this chapter, we will concentrate on the three specific nerves (sacral, tibial, and pudendal) that have been used as targets for neuromodulation in urology. For each neural target, we will describe the relevant anatomy, surgical technique, possible complications, and relevant data on the efficacy in treating overactive bladder, underactive bladder, and pelvic floor dysfunction.

Sacral Plexus

The sacral plexus is formed by the nerve roots of lumbar spinal nerves L4 and L5 and the anterior divisions of the sacral spinal nerves S1, S2, S3, and S4 and is located on the surface of the posterior pelvic wall, anterior to the piriformis muscle (Fig. 1).

The sacrum is composed of five modified vertebrae which are fused together. It is a triangular bone mass extending from the inferior vertebral column and containing the sacral and coccygeal nerves. At each vertebral level, paired spinal nerves leave the spinal cord via the intervertebral foramina of the vertebral column. Each nerve then divides into anterior and posterior nerve fibers. The sacral plexus begins as the anterior fibers of the spinal nerves S1, S2, S3, and S4. They are joined by the fourth and fifth lumbar roots, which combine to form the lumbosacral trunk. This descends into the pelvis to meet the sacral roots as they emerge from the spinal cord.

The anterior rami of the S1–S4 spinal roots (and the lumbosacral trunk) divide into several cords. These cords combine to form the five major peripheral nerves of the sacral plexus. These nerves descend the posterior pelvic wall and have two main courses: (1) exit the pelvis via the greater sciatic foramen to enter to the gluteal region that includes the sciatic nerve which branches above the popliteal fossa to become the common peroneal and tibial nerve which innervates the lower limb, and (2) remain in the pelvis to innervate the pelvic floor muscles, organs, and perineum [17].

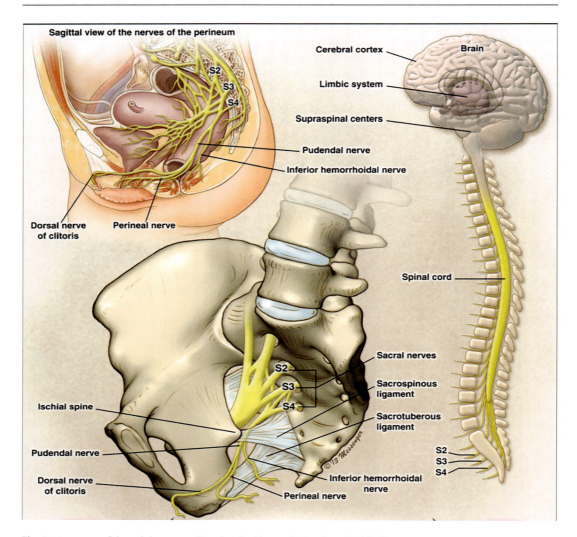

Fig. 1 Anatomy of the pelvic nerves. (Reprinted with permission from Ref. [16])

The five major nerve branches of the sacral plexus branches are the superior gluteal nerve (L4, L5, S1), inferior gluteal nerve (L5, S1, S2), sciatic nerve (L4, L5, S1, S2, S3), posterior femoral cutaneous nerve of the thigh (S1, S2, S3), and pudendal nerve (S2, S3, S4). In addition to the five major branches, there are also several small nerve branches, including the nerves that innervate the piriformis muscles, obturator internus, and quadratus femoris [17].

The S3 foramen is the targeted foramen for placement of the lead for sacral neuromodulation, as the S3 nerve has the most control over bladder function but minimal effect on the leg and the foot. The S3 foramen can be seen fluoroscopically, but knowledge of the anatomical landmarks is critical for proper lead placement. The location of the S3 foramen is approximated by measuring 9 cm cephalad to the coccyx and 1–2 cm lateral to the midline on either side [18].

Surgical Technique

Staged Sacral Neuromodulation (SNM). In 1982 Tanagho and colleagues developed the first spiral electrode that can be placed with minimal nerve damage [14]. The technique was then described in 1997 by Janknegt and colleagues [19]; the two-staged SNM includes the implantation of the permanent lead for a trial period (stage 1) and then of the implantable pulse generator (IPG) (stage 2).

The patient is positioned prone with moderate sedation, and local anesthesia is used to infiltrate the skin. Using fluoroscopic guidance, the anterior-posterior (AP) view is used to make a transverse mark (A) across the inferior aspect of the sacroiliac joint which is palpable approximately 9 cm cephalad to the coccyx. Next, longitudinal lines (B) are marked 1–2 cm from the midline at the medial edge of the sacral foramen bilaterally. The point of intersection indicates the location of the S3 foramen (Fig. 2). Beginning 2 cm cephalad from this point at a 30–60° angle from the skin, a needle can be advanced into the S3 foramen. Lateral fluoroscopic views can help show the S3 foramen midway between the base of the sacrum and the coccyx with a distinct sciatic notch. The S3 nerve can be found best medially and superiorly in the foramen, with the entrance of the needle at 90° to the sacrum because of sacral curvature. Confirmation is done using both motor with or without a sensory response. Stimulating the S3 nerve should provide contraction of the pelvic floor resulting in a visible "bellow" of the pelvic muscles with or without toe flexion. If sensory response is captured, a tapping sensation in the vaginal, rectal, or scrotal region is most common. If other motor responses are seen (Table 1), the lead may be in S2 or S4, and the needle should be adjusted appropriately based on motor and fluoroscopic findings. Because of anesthesia, confirmation based on motor responses

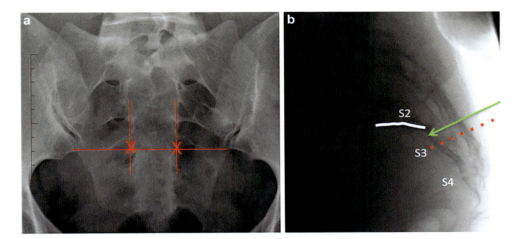

Fig. 2 Radiographic images with key landmarks for lead placement in sacral neuromodulation. (**a**) With AP views, horizontal line marked at the inferior edge of the sacroiliac joints. Two vertical lines marked at the medial aspects of the sacral foramen. The intersection marks the S3 foramen. (**b**) With lateral views, the S3 foramen is identified at sciatic notch. (Reprinted with permission from Axonics)

Table 1 Appropriate S3 motor responses are bellows and/or plantar flexion. Comparison of the different motor and sensory responses of each S2–S4 [22]

Nerve	Motor response	Sensory response
S2	Leg or hip rotation, plantar flexion of entire foot, contraction of calf, contraction of superficial pelvic floor	At genital area and leg
S3	Contraction of levator ani resulting in bellows or "anal wink," plantar flexion of big toe	At rectum, perineum, scrotum or vagina
S4	Contraction of posterior levator ani, no lower extremity response	At rectum only

alone are sufficient as sensory data does not impact clinical outcomes [20, 21]. The goal should be to obtain a motor response under low current (<2 mA) to preserve battery life.

Once the best position is found, a guidewire is passed through the foramen needle lumen at a similar depth and then removing the needle. The introducer sheath is placed over the guidewire using Seldinger technique such that the radio-opaque marker is midway between anterior and posterior edges of the sacrum. The internal metal trocar is removed leaving the sheath in place, and the quadripolar lead is placed with the curve pointing lateral so that the lead follows the natural plane of the nerve root. If the sheath is placed too deep, it can create a false passage, and the lead will have minimal contact with the nerve.

The lead is referred to as quadripolar because it has four electrodes, numbered 0–3 from deep to superficial. Proximal to the four electrodes are the tines, which decrease the risk of lead migration. The lead should be deployed so that the anterior edge of the sacrum straddles electrode 3, but this varies based on motor response testing on each electrode. Using a hook electrode, motor responses and thresholds can be checked on each electrode, and the current needed to activate a motor response on each can be recorded for future reference to aid in programming. Ideally, a motor response is seen on each electrode at 2 mA or less. A site is chosen on the ipsilateral buttock for a future IPG, a 1 cm transverse incision is made, and subcutaneous pocket is created. Marking this area with the patient siting in pre-op is ideal to be certain the IPG sits in a comfortable area. Once the lead is deployed, the proximal end is tunneled to this and then connected to a percutaneous extension lead that is tunneled to the contralateral buttock to reduce infection of the permanent lead. Bipolar programs are created based on the best motor response at the lowest thresholds, and the device is activated in the post-op area and the power increased until a sensory response is noted. A trial period of 7–14 days is given, in which the patient records a voiding diary and bladder symptoms. If the patient reports >50% improvement in overall symptoms, they can proceed to second-stage implant.

The second-stage implant is also done under IV sedation and local anesthesia. The previous 1 cm transverse incision is carefully opened, and the permanent lead and extension lead are externalized, the permanent lead freed and the extension lead removed from the skin surface outward. The incision is extended, and a subcutaneous pocket is created to accommodate the implantable pulse generator. The IPG is connected to the permanent lead and placed in the pre-made subcutaneous pocket.

Percutaneous Nerve Evaluation (PNE)

This office procedure is performed by placing a monopolar lead in the S3 foramen under local anesthesia in the office with or without fluoroscopic guidance. Appropriate motor response along with perineal sensory activation indicates proper positioning. A temporary dressing is used to immobilize the lead to the skin, and stimulation is delivered from an external device. If the patient reports >50% symptom improvement within 3–7 days, the monopolar temporary lead is removed; afterward the patient can be scheduled for a single-stage permanent quadripolar lead, and IPG is then placed in the operating room [23]. Advantages include avoiding multiple trips to the OR with anesthesia with the associated risks and costs. However, PNE reliability on clinical outcome, especially with the ease of lead migration based on its design, is often inferior to the staged permanent lead. Bosch et al. reported that 28% of patients had a discrepancy in PNE results compared to when the permanent lead was placed, suggesting that the PNE did not help with final clinical response [24]. In a prospective randomized trial of PNE vs two-staged SNM, a total of 24% ($n = 10/40$) of patients failed therapy, though more ($n = 7$) significantly seen in the PNE cohort vs the two-stage group ($n = 2$). Logistic regression analysis supported this as it correlated failure with PNE [25]. Therefore, if a patient fails to respond to a PNE, they should be offered a staged trial with the permanent lead.

Complications

Complications for SNM include lead migration, pain at IPG site, loss of efficacy, infection, revision and explanation, or battery failures [26–28]. Intraoperative bleeding is rare and is typically successfully treated with manual pressure and electrocautery [29]. After stage 1, Hijaz et al. reported an explantation rate due to infection rate of 8% ($n = 4/50$) and revisions secondary to frayed subcutaneous extension wire ($n = 6$), marginal response ($n = 13$), lead infection ($n = 3$), and improper localization of stimulus ($n = 1$) [27]. After stage 2, the Sacral Nerve Stimulation Study Group reported a revision rate of 33% with the most common reason being pain at subcutaneous pocket site (15.3%) and lead migration (8.4%). Other complications included infection (6.1%), transient electric shock (5.5%), and pain at lead site (5.4%) [26]. However, more contemporary studies report a lead migration rate of 0.6–2.1% with the introduction of the tined lead, infection rate of 2–12% that can be reduced with 5 days of perioperative antibiotics, and 10% of pocket site discomfort after the positioning of the IPG on the buttock instead of the anterior abdomen [25, 27, 30].

Programming

One advantage to the SNM is its ability to create different programs of stimulation with varying parameters such as frequency, amplitude, pulse width, and cycling. In brief, each electrode on the quadripolar lead has an anode (+ pole) and a cathode(− pole) so that the movement of the electron from the − pole to the + pole results in electrical stimulation of the nerve in between the electrodes. Based on Ohm's law ($V = IR$), amplitude, v, is defined as the difference in maximum and minimum voltage (V) or current (I) or, in other words, how much electrical current is stimulating the nerve. Because the IPG produces a pulsed waveform, the frequency (Hz, i.e., how fast the nerve is being stimulated) and the pulse width (μs, i.e., pulse duration can determine how wide the area of stimulation is) can be adjusted.

Cycling (s) is a feature which allows intermittent stimulation to reduce battery charge or the theoretical risk of overstimulating the nerve. Default setting for frequency is 14 Hz with a range of 2.1–130 Hz, pulse width 210 μs with a range of 60–250 μs, and cycling ranges from 0.1 s to 24 h [31].

Impedance (Ω, R), or resistance, can be tested so that it should typically be between 400 and 1500 Ω; however, those between 1500 and 4000 Ω can be within normal limits and clinically insignificant as tissue encapsulation can increase resistance. Clinically significant impedances are <50 Ω which suggests a short circuit and >4000 Ω which suggest an open circuit [32]. A short circuit can be due to water between the connection and a fused wire, whereas an open circuit is due to broken wires. Impedance issues can lead to depletion of pulse generator battery life if not recognized. Programs are varying configurations of + or − at the four available electrodes or with the case as the cathode (+ pole). At our institution, programming is done intraoperatively during the first stage with the lowest motor threshold recorded at each electrode. Based on this, programs are tested and set at the end of the case. Each device has default programs, but if customized programs are to be set, the electrode with the lowest minimal threshold should be set as the cathode(−), and the electrode that creates the ideal electric field should be the anode (+). For instance, if the most proximal electrode (0) showed some S2 stimulation, having the electric field targeted closer to the anterior sacrum would be advisable. Using two electrodes creates a targeted elliptical bipolar electric field, whereas, if the case is made to be the anode (+), this creates a larger, radial monopolar field [31]. Of note, program 1+/2− has been reported as the most commonly preferred program by patients [33].

A dedicated staff with knowledgeable programming skills is paramount to managing a neuromodulation practice since troubleshooting the SNM is an artform [32]. Reprogramming should only be done for adverse events or loss of efficacy, but routine device interrogation should be done to confirm lead integrity and battery life.

Patients with subsensory stimulation but still benefitting from stimulation should not have their programs changed as this is to be expected [33]. The goal of reprogramming any parameters should be a comfortable sensation in the pelvic area, achieved at the lowest minimal threshold. If a program is changed, patients should monitor symptoms for at least 2 weeks on those settings before attempting another program. There are published literatures on reprogramming algorithms, including an AUA update series. Below, we briefly list how to trouble shoot common programming scenarios, adapted from our work on the AUA Update Series: *Programming of Sacral Neuromodulation Devices: What the Practicing Clinician Should Know.*

1. *Loss of efficacy*: Loss of efficacy over time can occur in 3–38% of patients [32]. Medical conditions such as UTI or constipation or changes in dietary behaviors can be culprits, so that prompt investigation and treatment should be done before programming changes. Other causes include inadvertent powering off the device, impedance changes, or lead migration. Below is a systematic algorithm to check for all causes.
   - **Interrogate the device**. It is important to note the current program electrodes, amplitude, impedance, battery life, and location of sensation. Comparing this to intraoperative measurements of each electrode can help assess if electric field has been optimized. Abnormal values such as for impedance can indicate specific issues. If parameters are normal, continue below.
   - **Reprogram**. Most reprogramming occurs in the first year of implantation and decreases over time (2.15 sessions in year 1 vs. 0.7 in year 2) [34], with only a minority (17%) requiring ≥ 3 attempts [35]. However, if needed, a new program can be used by comparing programs to intraoperative measurements for optimization. For instance, if intraoperative measurements show that electrode 0 had a minimum threshold of 1.5 V, 1 at 1 V, 2 at 0.7 V, and 3 at 0.5 V, programs which utilize electrodes

2 or 3 (ex// 3−, 2+ or 3−, case +) are ideal because of concepts presented above. Choose the program with the lowest minimal threshold. If no programs can be found with a threshold <2 V, proceed with the following step.
   - **Increase pulse width in increments of 100 μs with maximum of 450 μs** [32]. Increasing the pulse width, or pulse duration, can increase the area of stimulation and recruit more nerve fibers. Therefore, this can be adjusted to amplify a signal or dampen it, depending on the desired effects. Using a program with the lowest minimal threshold or one best corresponding with intraoperative measurements, increase the pulse width in increments of 100 μs until appropriate sensation is felt. Once sensation is felt, amplitude can also be decreased to maximize battery life. If appropriate sensations cannot be achieved, proceed with the following step.
   - **Increase frequency in increments of 10 Hz with max of 130 Hz** [32]. Increasing frequency can strengthen the signal, though too high of a frequency can theoretically cause muscle fatigue to important structures like the urethral sphincter [31, 36]. Like above, adjust the frequency in increments of 10 Hz until appropriate sensation is felt. If maximum frequency is reached without appropriate sensation, proceed with the following step.
   - **Obtain AP and lateral sacral X-ray**. Lead migration can occur in 1.6–2.1% of patients ranging from 3 weeks to 8 months post-implantation [30, 37]. Therefore, if reprogramming fails, lead migration should be ruled out. Obtain an AP and lateral sacral X-ray, and compare to all prior films, including intraoperative ones. If migration is shown, lead revision is recommended.

2. *Impedance issues* [27]: As discussed above, abnormal impedances can signify lead compromise or increasing scarring around the lead. However, before final diagnosis, it is important to rule out a false-positive result by rechecking impedance at a higher power level

or increased pulse width. If impedance remains <50 or >4000, then consider the following [32]:

- **Short Circuit**. Common clinical signs of this is a decrease in efficacy with concomitant shocking sensation at the IPG site [27]. If this is the case, proceed with the following.
  - **Reprogram**. A short (impedance <50) occurs between to bipolar electrodes. If the patient is on this electrode combination, change the program to a different combination where a short does not exist based on device interrogation and set ideal stimulation parameters. A benefit of a quadripolar electrode is that multiple electrode combinations exist that can allow the provider to bypass the short and continuing therapy without revision. If reprogramming does not result in symptom improvement, remove and replace the lead. The original IPG can be used if it has adequate battery life remaining.
- **Open Circuit**. This can occur if there is a break in the lead resulting in current leak. During device interrogation, the impedance is tested between the CASE and the electrode. If the impedance is >4000, that particular electrode cannot be used for any program. Thus, reprogram using other electrode combinations. If reprogramming does not lead to a good clinical response, remove and replace the lead.

3. *Pain at IPG*: Pain at the IPG site is common (15.3%) [26], with causes such as infection, waistline irritation, IPG malrotation, short circuit, sensitivity to monopolar stimulation, erosion, neuropathy, and seroma [27].
   - **Examine the pocket and lead insertion sites**. If the sites are erythematous with discharge, have fluctuance, or have visible lead extruding from incision, this may suggest infection, seroma, or erosion, respectively. Also assess for the waistline and the relative position of the IPG to this as friction can cause irritation over time. IPG malrotation, or "torsion" can also cause pain, and this

can be confirmed on a sacral or pelvic X-ray. All of the above would require intraoperative revisions. If none of the above, proceed with the following.

- **Turn off stimulator**. If the discomfort is from the stimulation, turning off the stimulation should resolve the pain within a few minutes. If this occurs, interrogating the device may discover a short circuit (see *Impedance Issues*). If this is not the case and the patient was on a monopolar program, consider switching to a bipolar stimulation.
- **Assess level of discomfort**. Determine the strength and nature of the pain, as well as the patient's bother factor. If not very bothersome, reassure the patient that this will not harm the tissue [27]. If bothersome, proceed to the OR.
- **Intraoperative revisions**. Depending on the underlying issue, extent of revisions can range from repositioning the IPG in a deeper pocket for more subcutaneous fat cushioning, drainage of seroma, complete lead revision, or explantation. If infection is noted, the lead and IPG should be removed and can be replaced in future, once infection has resolved.

4. *Pain down leg/transient shock*: S2 nerve root stimulation, typically from a high electrode (2 or 3) or irritation from the lead itself, can cause pain down the leg [32]. A transient shock, on the other hand, can be due to both nerve irritation or impedance issues (see *Impedance Issues*).
   - **Turn off stimulator**. If the discomfort is from the stimulation, turning off the stimulation should resolve the pain, though the patient assess this for 2–3 weeks. If the pain is persistent, this may be from sciatica, or lead irritation. If pain resolves, proceed to the following step.
   - **Reprogram**. Narrow the electric field to the distal electrodes (ex// 0− or 1−), or lower the pulse width. If reprogramming does not improve, proceed to the following step.
   - **Intraoperative revision**. If pain persists, this may be secondary to lead migration so

that lead revision may be required. Lead placement can be attempted on the contralateral side to avoid irritation of the same nerve.

5. *Fever/pain at incision sites*: Infection after stage I or II has been estimated to be 2–12% [38–41], usually prevented with 5 days of antibiotics postimplantation. If this occurs, authors recommend complete explantation since salvage surgery has been shown to also eventually lead to explant of device [27].

Indications

Since 1997, SNM has been FDA-approved for urinary urgency and later in 1999, for frequency, urinary urge incontinence, fecal incontinence, and nonobstructive urinary retention. Per the AUA/SUFU guidelines, it can be offered as a third-line therapy after failure of conservative measures and medical therapy [42, 43]. Though no exclusion criteria have been clearly defined, those with cognitive deficits which may interfere with managing the device may not be the right candidate for this. With the advent of the MRI compatible leads, patients who may need future imaging are not excluded.

Overactive Bladder (OAB)

Multiple studies over the years have shown SNM to be an effective treatment for OAB [41]. Hassouna et al. performed the first prospective multicenter RCT comparing SNM ($n = 25$) to the control ($n = 26$) and reported improvements in the experimental arm for urinary frequency on voiding diary (16.9 ± 9.7–$9.3 \pm 5.1, p < 0.0001$), volume per void (118 ± 74–226 ± 124 ml), urgency (rank 2.2 ± 0.6–1.6 ± 0.9, $p = 0.01$), quality of life (physical health 77 vs. 48, $p < 0.0001$), and maximum bladder capacity (253 ± 93–325 ± 185 ml, $p = 0.008$) at 6 months. The control cohort had no changes from baseline, but 15 patients chose to cross over when given the option at 6 months. Stimulation was then turned off with patients reporting the return of baseline symptoms, with

all patients (37/51) requesting a reactivation of the stimulation therapy [41]. Similarly, both van Kerrebroeck et al. [40] and Siegel et al. [26] reported success rates (i.e., >50% improvement) of 68% and 59%, respectively, in their multicenter prospective trials. Schmidt et al. had a 76% success rate with 47% of which achieving complete dryness. Results were sustained at 18 months [44]. Retrospective studies by Al-Zahrani [45], Sutherland [46], and Latini [47] report higher sustained success rates of 85%, 69%, and 90%, respectively. The risk for revision is relatively high of 30% [42]. Risk factors for needing revision include a history of trauma, decrease in BMI, being enrolled in pain clinic, or history of adverse events related to the SNM implantation [48].

Technology and surgical technique have improved over the years, and contemporary studies report improved clinical outcomes with reduced complications. The INSITE trial [49], a prospective, multicenter, randomized controlled trial, compares the Interstim™ SNM to standard medical therapy. With a cohort of 340 participant enrolled, there were 1-, 2-, 3-, and 5-year success rates of 82%, 79%, 76%, and 67%, respectively, for OAB symptoms, where success was defined as >50% improvement in symptoms. For those with urinary incontinence, there was an average reduction of 1.7 ± 2.1 leaks/day compared to baseline ($p < 0.0001$) with 38% achieving complete dryness at 5 years. Regarding urinary frequency, of the 57% of patients who had an improvement in symptoms, there was an average reduction of 4.4 ± 4.4 voids/day from baseline ($p < 0.0001$). Eighty-four percent of participants also reported "improved" or "greatly improved" quality of life on the ICIQ-OABqol. Interestingly, sexual function scores were better on the FLUTSsex questionnaires among the female cohort. The INSITE trial reported an overall rate of 22.4% of complications which ranged from undesirable change in stimulation (22%), site pain (15%), and inefficacy (13%), though incidence of lead migration at 3 years was noted to be 4% with the majority occurring between 12 and 24 months [50]. This is in comparison to the ARTISAN-SNM [51] trial which is a 2-year single-arm, prospective, multicenter trial which evaluates clinical outcomes of patients who has OAB and treated with Axonic® sacral neuromodulation. With a total of 121 participants, success rates at 1 and 2 years were 89% and 88%, respectively. Urinary incontinence episodes decreased from an average baseline of 5.6 ± 0.3 to 1.0 ± 0.2 episodes/day ($p < 0.0001$), with 37% achieving complete continence. Urinary frequency decreased from 11.6 ± 0.3 to 8.5 ± 0.2 voids/day ($p < 0.0001$). Fecal incontinence was also evaluated using the Cleveland Clinic Florida- Fecal Incontinence Score (CCF-FIS) which saw a reduction from 9.3 ± 0.5 at baseline to 3.7 ± 0.5 at 2 years ($p < 0.001$). Authors reported device-related adverse events in 16% of participants and 12% procedure-related adverse events with the most common also being uncomfortable change in stimulation (9%). Site pain was reported in two participants (1.7%), lead migration in 1 (<1%), inefficacy in 1 (<1%), and infection in 1 (<1%). Twelve participants obtained MRI after SNM without any adverse events reported.

Urinary Retention

Since 1999, SNM has been FDA-approved for nonobstructive urinary retention due to overwhelming data on its efficacy. In 2015, it was approved by the UK National Institute for Health and Care Excellence (NICE, 2015). In a retrospective multicenter study, Carderelli et al. reported improved PVR (321 ± 153.5–87.2 ± 96.9 ml, $p < 0.001$) and frequency of daily self-catheterization (3.8 ± 1.4–1.3 ± 1.3, $p < 0.001$) at a median of 11 months for urinary retention patients who underwent SNM [52]. Similarly, Jones et al. published that in 177 patients with idiopathic urinary retention, the mean volume per catheterization and mean frequency of daily catheterizations were reduced significantly ($p < 0.001$) enough that 69% were able to stop catheter usage at 6 months. Inactivation of the SNM correlated with an elevation of the post-void residual. Effects were sustained at 18 months [53]. A meta-analysis of 14 studies with 751 patients came to the same conclusion: the mean difference in PVR and voided volume were 236 and 344 ml, respectively,

favoring SNM [54]. Even complex patients such as those with Fowler's syndrome have been shown to respond well to SNM and can be given another option besides lifelong self catheterization [38, 55].

Chronic Pelvic Pain

Although SNM is not FDA-approved for pelvic pain, several small case studies have reported success in managing this challenging condition. In 2001, Siegel et al. reported an average decrease of pain from 9.7 to 4.4 at a median of 19 months for ten patients who underwent SNM for chronic pelvic pain [56]. In a larger study of 64 patients with OAB, UR, or pelvic pain, Aboseif reported that the pelvic pain cohort ($n = 41$) had a mean pain score decrease from 5.8 to 3.7 at a mean follow-up of 24 months after undergoing SNM [57]. In 2004, Peters and colleagues performed SNM in 21 patients with refractory interstitial cystitis (IC)/bladder pain syndrome. At a mean of 15.4 months, 20 reported moderate or marked improvement in pain with an average decrease of 36% in narcotics use [58]. Data from Zabihi et al. supported this as they report the pain score improved by 40% ($p = 0.04$) in the 23/30 patients who had permanent implantation at the sacral nerve [59]. Feler et al. reported a case series of four patients who suffered from vulvodynia, epididymo-orchitis, and IC who were all successfully treated with SNM [60]. In 2011, Martellucci et al. reported a significant decrease in mean visual analog pain score from 8.2 to 1.9 at 6 months and 1.8 at 36 months in 17 patients who developed chronic pelvic pain after pelvic surgery [61]. This remains an active area of research.

Pudendal Nerve

As discussed, the pudendal nerve is made up of contributions from the ventral (anterior), rami of nerves from the S2, S3, and S4 sacral nerve roots. Arising from the sacral plexus, the pudendal provides visceral and somatic (motor and sensory) innervation to most of pelvic muscles and viscera.

The pudendal nerve traverses the ventral surface of the piriformis muscle within the greater sciatic foramen. From the piriformis muscle, the pudendal nerve courses behind the sacrospinous ligament and the overlying coccygeus muscle, just medial to the ischial spine [62]. Given the proximity to the ischial spine, this bony landmark is clinically relevant to palpate the pudendal nerve on a transvaginal or transrectal exam. It then reenters the pelvis through the lesser sciatic foramen and enters Alcock's canal, which is located on the lateral wall of the ischioanal fossa. Alcock's canal is formed by the splitting of the obturator internus muscle fascia. Approximately one-third of the length of the pudendal nerve is contained within Alcock's canal [62].

The pudendal nerve has three branches: inferior rectal nerve, dorsal nerve to the penis/clitoris, and perineal nerve. The inferior rectal nerve innervates the external anal sphincter, anal canal, and the perianal skin. The perineal nerve branches and supplies the ischiocavernosus, bulbocavernosus, the superficial transverse perineal muscles, external urethral sphincter, and skin of the labia.

Stimulation of the pudendal nerve modulates the bladder afferent reflex that works through the sacral interneurons that then activate storage through the pudendal nerve.

Since the pudendal nerve innervates the bladder, external urethral and anal sphincters, and pelvic floor muscles, direct stimulation of the pudendal nerve can have a wider range of effects compared to sacral stimulation [62]. Studies have shown that pudendal stimulation leads to a greater improvement in urinary urgency, frequency, and bowel function, compared to sacral stimulation [63].

Damage to the pudendal nerve can result in neuralgia with the diagnostic criteria of (a) pain in the territory of the pudendal nerve, (b) pain predominantly while sitting, (c) pain that does not wake the patient at night, (d) pain without objective sensory impairment, and (e) pain relieved by pudendal nerve block [64]. The most common etiology for pudendal neuralgia is vaginal childbirth [65], though other reasons include pelvic trauma, entrapment between the sacrotuberous and sacrococcygeal ligaments [66], compression at Alcock's canal [67], infection [68, 69], surgical trauma, and chronic irritation from a bicycles [70] or equestrian saddle [71].

Surgical Technique

Multiple techniques for localizing the pudendal nerve have been published [72–74]. Below, the Peters technique is described. Like SNM, the procedure is done with the patient prone under IV sedation and with local anesthetic. Perirectal EMG needles are placed at the 3 and 9 o'clock positions of the anal sphincter for intraoperative electromyography (EMG) monitoring. By starting medial to the marked ischial tuberosity and traveling laterally toward the ischial spine with the foramen needle, the pudendal nerve can be found traversing the ischiorectal space. On AP views, the needle should head toward the superolateral edge of the obturator foramen toward the ischial spine. On lateral views, the ischial spine can be seen as a notch anterior to the lower the sacrum. Continuous stimulation of the foramen needle with 5 mA and 5 Hz will help localize the nerve. An anal wink and positive compound muscle action potential (CMAP) confirm pudendal stimulation. Once found, the same technique of placing the bidirectional guidewire and introducer sheath as SNM is done, with the exception that the inner metal introducer is continuously stimulated during placement. Next, a 41 cm quadripolar lead is placed and each electrode tested for the lowest motor threshold, as this length lead is necessary to reach the potential IPG site at the upper buttock. Additionally, given that the lead can move several mm while sitting or lying down, testing should be done with manual pressure on the buttocks pushing cranially and then anteriorly to simulate these positions, respectively. The lead is then tunneled toward the subcutaneous pocket which is at the same location on the upper buttock as the SNM. The rest of the steps are similar to SNM (see Fig. 3).

The Spinelli technique utilizes two anatomical landmarks – the greater trochanter and pubic rami – with Bock adding a finger transrectally to guide the needle. The STAR method by Heinze

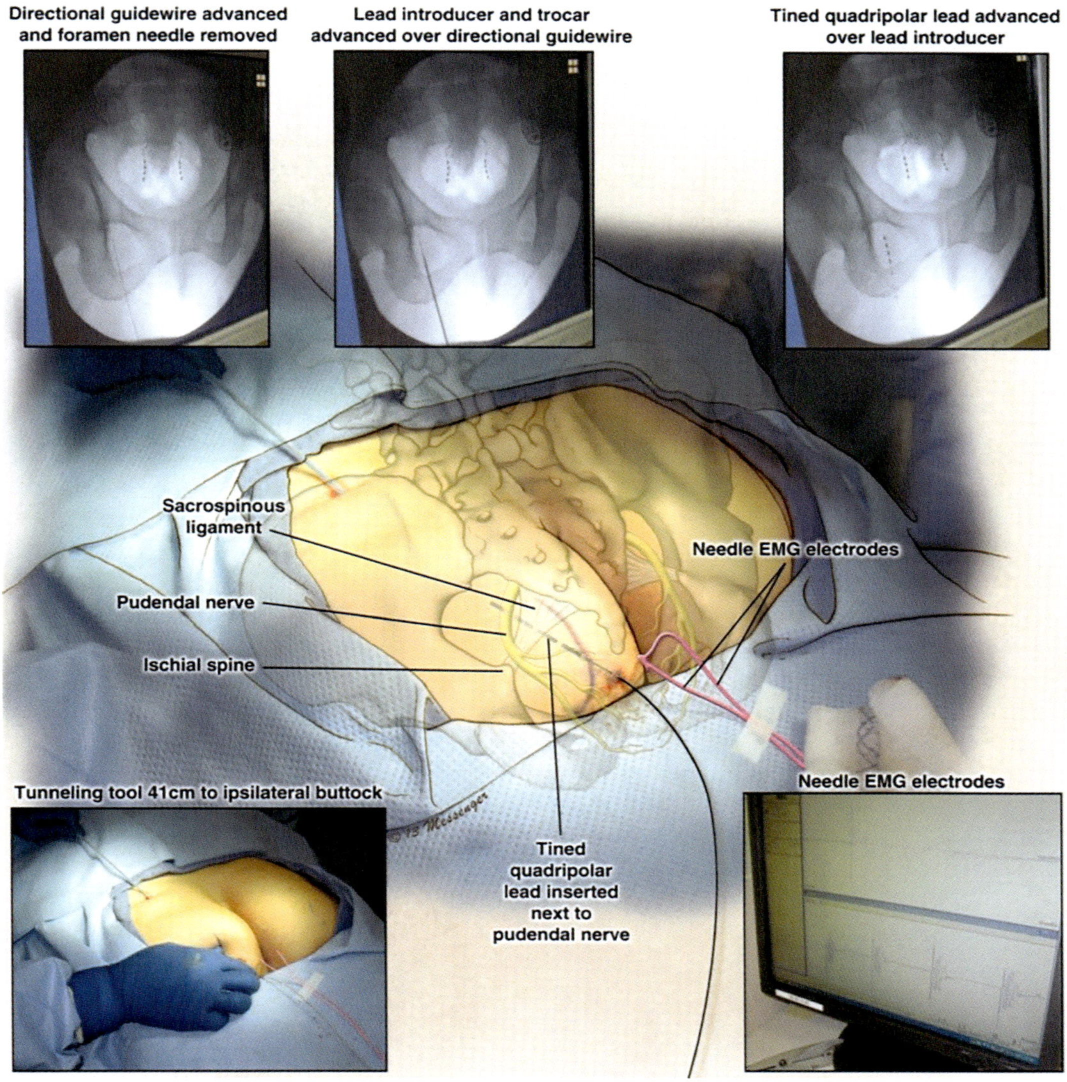

15 Bladder Dysfunction and Pelvic Pain: The Role of Sacral, Tibial, and Pudendal Neuromodulation

Fig. 3 The Peters technique for pudendal neuromodulation. (Reprinted with permission from Ref. [16])

triangulates the pudendal nerve using a series of steps. First, one draws a horizontal line on the skin surface across the acetabulum and a vertical line across the center of the ischial tuberosity to find the ischial spine at the intersection. Next, a parallel line is made from the ischial tuberosity to the anal rim. Lastly, using the anal rim as the third corner, one can locate the pudendal nerve in the center of the triangle.

Recent work in using 3D technology to better localize the pudendal nerve shows promise [75].

Other access techniques have been explored such as the laparoscopic approach [76], but this has not been widely adopted as there is greater inherent risk and cost [77].

Complications

Complications of PNM include lead migration (15.3%) [78] and loss of efficacy [79]. The higher rate of lead migration compared to SNM may be due to the lack of an anchoring tissue for PNM compared to the sacral periosteum for SNM. Other complications include local irritation at insertion site during sitting or aberrant lower leg stimulation. Further research is needed to completely capture risks of PNM.

Indications

Pudendal neuromodulation (PNM) has not been FDA-approved for OAB, urinary retention, or pelvic floor dysfunction. However, research interest began in 2005 when a randomized control trial was published comparing SNM to pudendal neuromodulation for patients with LUTS. Patients were randomized in a blinded fashion to receive neuromodulation at the sacral or pudendal nerve initially for 7 days and then were crossed over to the other location for 7 days. While blinded, 79% of the patients found reported the pudendal lead to be better than the sacral lead, and this corresponded to a 63% reduction of symptoms with the pudendal stimulation compared to 46% for the sacral ($p = 0.02$) [63].. Using the transgluteal approach on 15 patients with neurogenic urge incontinence, Spinelli reported an increase of maximum cystometric capacity on urodynamics of 153 ± 50–331 ± 111 ml, a reduction of daily incontinent episodes (7 ± 3.3–2.6 ± 3.3, $p < 0.02$) with 8 achieving complete continence, and 8 reported bowel improvements [73]. In a prospective study of 84 patients treated with pudendal neuromodulation for OAB or bladder pain, 71% reported >50% improvement of symptoms. Of note, 44 patients were refractory to SNM. For underactive bladder, animal models show that pudendal stimulation increases voiding efficiency by 40–50% [80] and increases bladder capacity [81], but no clinical trials in humans have been done to date.

Pudendal neuralgia is a severe pain condition that is difficult to diagnose and treat. Treatment often includes medical therapy, pelvic floor physical therapy, nerve blocks, pudendal nerve entrapment surgery, or neuromodulation. In 2014, Peters et al. conducted a pilot study of 19 patients with pudendal neuralgia and found that 3 patients had complete relief of pain, 3 almost complete, 10 significant/remarkable, and 3 small/slight. At a mean of 2.95 years, only five patients had their devices explanted secondary to symptom resolution ($n = 1$), loss of efficacy ($n = 3$), and patient stopped using the devise ($n = 1$) [79]. In a pilot study of 13 patients with pudendal neuralgia who failed prior therapies, Hoang Roberts et al. [78] reported a success rate of 76.9% and a cure rate of 46.1% after the trial period using Stimwave® to modulate the pudendal nerve. After permanent implant and long-term follow-up, 5/9 patients reported >50% pain improvement.

Tibial Nerve

Understanding of the anatomy of the tibial nerve is important in order to understand needle placement for percutaneous tibial nerve stimulation. The tibial nerve is a mixed sensory and motor nerve that arises from L4, L5, S1, S2, and S3 spinal nerve roots. The tibial nerve is a branch of the sciatic nerve. At the apex of the popliteal fossa, the sciatic nerve divides into the common peroneal nerves and the tibial nerve before proceeding down the leg, as tibial nerve then passes posteriorly and inferiorly to the medial malleolus through the tarsal tunnel. Here, it gives rise to the branches that provide cutaneous innervation to the heel. It then terminates into sensory branches that innervate the sole of the foot.

The peripheral nerves involved in sensory and motor control of the bladder, and pelvic floor also arises from L4 to S3 [82, 83]. Thus, it is thought that the neuromodulation of the tibial nerve modulates the lower urinary tract via the shared tracts [84]. Researchers have hypothesized that stimulation of the afferent nerve fibers of the tibial nerve remodels the detrusor inhibition reflex. Others have demonstrated that neuromodulation of the tibial nerve may work centrally through direct modulation of the pontine micturition center [85].

Neuromodulation is thought to work by changing afferent signaling. Stimulating a distal nerve such as the tibial may lead to more afferent signals, through more nerve roots reaching the spinal cord and brain, and this could potentially lead to a more robust clinical response [63]. The tibial nerve, with its five afferent nerve roots, is a new, exciting target for implantable, chronic stimulation.

Surgical Technique

The percutaneous tibial nerve stimulation (PTNS) procedure is performed in the clinic without any IV or local anesthesia. Patient is placed in a sitting position with the target ankle elevated. A grounding pad is placed on the ipsilateral foot and a 34 gauge needle is percutaneously inserted approximately three fingerbreadths above the medial malleolus for a depth of 3 cm. Stimulation is then increased at incremental amplitudes until plantar flexion or toe fanning is seen. Tingling of the bottom of the feet can be experienced. Each session lasts 30 min and induction treatment is one session every week for 12 weeks. If OAB symptoms improve at the end of induction, maintenance therapy can begin with one session every month (see Fig. 4).

Complications

Given that PTNS is minimally invasive, very few complications have been reported and are usually self-limited, such as minor discomfort at needle site. From the SUmiT trial, no complications were reported [86].

Indications

PTNS was first described in 1983 by Nakamura et al. [87] and FDA-approved in 2000 for OAB [88] and recommended as a third-line therapy along with SNM and intra-detrusor Botox® injections for OAB. Though retrospective studies demonstrated the efficacy of PTNS for OAB, this procedure was not widely considered until 2010 when the SUmiT trial, a multicenter double-blinded RCT, proved its efficacy and safety [86]. Authors randomized 220 patients to either 12 weeks of PTNS or sham therapy [86]. Authors randomized 220 patients to either 12 weeks of PTNS or sham therapy. At 13 weeks, 54.5% of patients in the experimental arm reported moderately or markedly improved responses compared to 20.9% of the sham ($p < 0.001$). Urinary frequency, nocturia, urgency, and episodes of urge incontinence were all significantly improved. Long-term follow-up of 50 responders from the SUmiT trial showed that 77% continued to have significant improvement at a median of 36 months if given 1 PTNS treatment/month as maintenance therapy. Compared to antimuscarinics, PTNS also performed well, according to the Overactive Bladder Innovative Therapy Trial (OrBIT). Patients

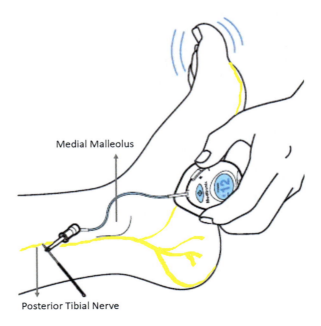

Fig. 4 PTNS technique. Needle is placed approximately three fingerbreadths cranial from medial malleolus at the posterior tibial nerve. (Adapted from Medtronic with permission)

($n = 100$) with OAB were randomized to PTNS or tolterodine for 12 weeks after which the PTNS cohort was given the option to continue with treatment for a total of 12 months. At 12 weeks, 79.5% of the PTNS group had significant improvement from baseline compared to only 54.8% in the tolterodine cohort ($p = 0.01$). Out of the 35 patients who initially responded to PTNS, 33 chose to continue for 12 months, and treatment improvements were sustained in 94% at 6 months and 96% at 12 months [89]. PNM has limited research in the setting of urinary retention and chronic pelvic pain and is currently not FDA-approved for these conditions.

Conclusion

Technological advances in medicine have made the modulation of complex neural networks feasible and safe. The treatment of OAB, non-obstructive retention, and pelvic pain via neuromodulation of the sacral, pudendal, and tibial nerves has provided significant clinical relief, especially in patients refractory to traditional therapies. The future of neuromodulation holds many possibilities to extend its use in managing other complex conditions.

Cross-References

▸ Behavioral Modification and Conservative Management of Overactive Bladder and Underactive Bladder Disorders
▸ Overview of Diagnosis and Pharmacological Treatment of Overactive and Underactive Bladder Disorders

References

1. Leng WW, Chancellor MB. How sacral nerve stimulation neuromodulation works. Urol Clin. 2005;32(1): 11–8.
2. Gorniak G, King PM. The peripheral neuroanatomy of the pelvic floor. J Women's Health Phys Therapy. 2016;40(1):3–14.
3. Corton MM. Anatomy of pelvic floor dysfunction. Obstet Gynecol Clin. 2009;36(3):401–19.
4. Bartley J, Gilleran J, Peters K. Neuromodulation for overactive bladder. Nat Rev Urol. 2013;10(9):513–21. https://doi.org/10.1038/nrurol.2013.143.
5. Schröder A, Chichester P, Kogan BA, et al. Effect of chronic bladder outlet obstruction on blood flow of the rabbit bladder. J Urol. 2001;165(2):640–6.
6. Sibley G. Developments in our understanding of detrusor instability. Br J Urol. 1997;80:54–61.
7. Mills IW. The pathophysiology of detrusor instability and the role of bladder ischaemia in its aetiology. Oxford, UK: University of Oxford; 1999.
8. Tahseen S. Role of sacral neuromodulation in modern urogynaecology practice: a review of recent literature. Int Urogynecol J. 2018;29(8):1081–91. https://doi.org/10.1007/s00192-017-3546-6.
9. Steers WD. Pathophysiology of overactive bladder and urge urinary incontinence. Rev Urol. 2002;4(Suppl 4):S7.
10. Stillings D. A survey of the history of electrical stimulation for pain to 1900. Med Instrum. 1975;9(6):255–9
11. Gildenberg PL. History of electrical neuromodulation for chronic pain. Pain Med. 2006;7(Suppl 1):S7–S13. https://doi.org/10.1111/j.1526-4637.2006.00118.x.
12. Sweet W, Wepsic J. Treatment of chronic pain by stimulation of fibers of primary afferent neuron. Trans Am Neurol Assoc. 1968;93:103–7.
13. Langley J, Anderson H. The innervation of the pelvic and adjoining viscera. IV. The internal generative organs. J Physiol. 1895;19:122–30.
14. Tanagho EA, Schmidt RA. Bladder pacemaker: scientific basis and clinical future. Urology. 1982;20(6):614–9.
15. Yoshimura N, Chancellor MB. Chapter 60. Pathophysiology and pharmacology of the bladder and urethra. In: Wein AJ, et al., editors. Campbell-Walsh urology. 10th ed. Philadelphia: Elsevier; 2012. p. 1786–833.
16. Peters KM. Pudendal neuromodulation for sexual dysfunction. J Sex Med. 2013;10(4):908–11. https://doi.org/10.1111/jsm.12138.
17. The Sacral Plexus. Updated April 21 2020. https://teachmeanatomy.info/lower-limb/nerves/sacral-plexus/. Accessed 26 July 2021.
18. Sandip Vasavada RR. Chapter 10. Electrical stimulation and neuromodulation in storage and emptying failure. In: Wein AJ, Kavoussi LR, Novick AC, editors. Campbell-Walsh urology. 10th ed. Philadelphia: Elsevier; 2012. p. 2026–46.
19. Janknegt RA, Weil EH, Eerdmans PH. Improving neuromodulation technique for refractory voiding dysfunctions: two-stage implant. Urology. 1997;49(3):358–62. https://doi.org/10.1016/S0090-4295(96)00506-7.
20. Peters KM, Killinger KA, Boura JA. Is sensory testing during lead placement crucial for achieving positive outcomes after sacral neuromodulation? Neurourol Urodyn. 2011;30(8):1489–92. https://doi.org/10.1002/nau.21122.
21. Cohen BL, Tunuguntla HS, Gousse A. Predictors of success for first stage neuromodulation: motor versus sensory response. J Urol. 2006;175(6):2178–80.

Discussion 2180–1. https://doi.org/10.1016/s0022-5347(06)00315-6.

22. Vignes J, De Seze M, Dobremez E, Joseph P, Guerin J. Sacral neuromodulation in lower urinary tract dysfunction. Adv Tech Stand Neurosurg. 2005;30:177–224.

23. Fulton M, Peters KM. Neuromodulation for voiding dysfunction and fecal incontinence: a urology perspective. Urol Clin North Am. 2012;39(3):405–12. https://doi.org/10.1016/j.ucl.2012.05.008.

24. Bosch JL, Groen J. Sacral nerve neuromodulation in the treatment of patients with refractory motor urge incontinence: long-term results of a prospective longitudinal study. J Urol. 2000;163(4):1219–22.

25. Everaert K, Kerckhaert W, Caluwaerts H, et al. A prospective randomized trial comparing the 1-stage with the 2-stage implantation of a pulse generator in patients with pelvic floor dysfunction selected for sacral nerve stimulation. Eur Urol. 2004;45(5):649–54.

26. Siegel SW, Catanzaro F, Dijkema HE, et al. Long-term results of a multicenter study on sacral nerve stimulation for treatment of urinary urge incontinence, urgency-frequency, and retention. Urology. 2000;56(6):87–91.

27. Hijaz A, Vasavada S. Complications and troubleshooting of sacral neuromodulation therapy. Urol Clin. 2005;32(1):65–9.

28. Blandon RE, Gebhart JB, Lightner DJ, Klingele CJ. Re-operation rates after permanent sacral nerve stimulation for refractory voiding dysfunction in women. BJU Int. 2008;101(9):1119–23.

29. Carmel ME, Vasavada SP, Goldman HB. Troubleshooting sacral neuromodulation issues. Curr Urol Rep. 2012;13(5):363–9. https://doi.org/10.1007/s11934-012-0268-7.

30. Deng DY, Gulati M, Rutman M, Raz S, Rodríguez LV. Failure of sacral nerve stimulation due to migration of tined lead. J Urol. 2006;175(6):2182–5.

31. Knowles CH, de Wachter S, Engelberg S, et al. The science behind programming algorithms for sacral neuromodulation. Color Dis. 2021;23(3):592–602.

32. Powell C. Troubleshooting interstim sacral neuromodulation generators to recover function. Curr Urol Rep. 2018;19(10):1–9.

33. Lehur PA, Sørensen M, Dudding TC, et al. Programming algorithms for sacral neuromodulation: clinical practice and evidence – recommendations for day-to-day practice. Neuromodulation. 2020;23(8):1121–9.

34. Cameron AP, Anger JT, Madison R, Saigal CS, Clemens JQ, Urologic Diseases in America Project. Battery explantation after sacral neuromodulation in the Medicare population. Neurourol Urodyn. 2013;32(3):238–41.

35. Amundsen CL, Komesu YM, Chermansky C, et al. Two-year outcomes of sacral neuromodulation versus onabotulinumtoxinA for refractory urgency urinary incontinence: a randomized trial. Eur Urol. 2018;74(1):66–73.

36. Thüroff JW, Bazeed MA, Schmidt RA, Wiggin DM, Tanagho EA. Functional pattern of sacral root stimulation in dogs I. Micturition. J Urol. 1982;127(5):1031–3.

37. Marcelissen TA, Leong RK, de Bie RA, van Kerrebroeck PE, de Wachter SG. Long-term results of sacral neuromodulation with the tined lead procedure. J Urol. 2010;184(5):1997–2000.

38. Dasgupta R, Wiseman OJ, Kitchen N, Fowler CJ. Long-term results of sacral neuromodulation for women with urinary retention. BJU Int. 2004;94(3):335–7.

39. Everaert K, De Ridder D, Baert L, Oosterlinck W, Wyndaele J. Patient satisfaction and complications following sacral nerve stimulation for urinary retention, urge incontinence and perineal pain: a multicenter evaluation. Int Urogynecol J. 2000;11(4):231–6.

40. van Kerrebroeck PE, van Voskuilen AC, Heesakkers JP, et al. Results of sacral neuromodulation therapy for urinary voiding dysfunction: outcomes of a prospective, worldwide clinical study. J Urol. 2007;178(5):2029–34.

41. Hassouna MM, Siegel SW, Lycklama Ànÿeholt A, et al. Sacral neuromodulation in the treatment of urgency-frequency symptoms: a multicenter study on efficacy and safety. J Urol. 2000;163(6):1849–54.

42. Gormley EA, Lightner DJ, Faraday M, Vasavada SP, American Urological Association, Society of Urodynamics, Female Pelvic Medicine. Diagnosis and treatment of overactive bladder (non-neurogenic) in adults: AUA/SUFU guideline amendment. J Urol. 2015;193(5):1572–80. https://doi.org/10.1016/j.juro.2015.01.087.

43. Lightner DJ, Gomelsky A, Souter L, Vasavada SP. Diagnosis and treatment of overactive bladder (non-neurogenic) in adults: AUA/SUFU guideline amendment 2019. J Urol. 2019;202(3):558–63. https://doi.org/10.1097/JU.0000000000000309.

44. Schmidt RA, Jonas U, Oleson KA, et al. Sacral nerve stimulation for treatment of refractory urinary urge incontinence. J Urol. 1999;162(2):352–7.

45. Al-Zahrani AA, Elzayat EA, Gajewski JB. Long-term outcome and surgical interventions after sacral neuromodulation implant for lower urinary tract symptoms: 14-year experience at 1 center. J Urol. 2011;185(3):981–6.

46. Sutherland SE, Lavers A, Carlson A, Holtz C, Kesha J, Siegel SW. Sacral nerve stimulation for voiding dysfunction: one institution's 11-year experience. Neurourol Urodyn. 2007;26(1):19–28.

47. Latini JM, Alipour M, Kreder KJ Jr. Efficacy of sacral neuromodulation for symptomatic treatment of refractory urinary urge incontinence. Urology. 2006;67(3):550–3.

48. White WM, Pickens RB, Dobmeyer-Dittrich C, Klein FA. Incidence and predictors of complications with sacral neuromodulation. J Urol. 2008;179(4S):487.

49. Siegel S, Noblett K, Mangel J, et al. Five-year followup results of a prospective, multicenter study of patients

with overactive bladder treated with sacral neuromodulation. J Urol. 2018;199(1):229–36.

50. Siegel S, Noblett K, Mangel J, et al. Three-year follow-up results of a prospective, multicenter study in overactive bladder subjects treated with sacral neuromodulation. Urology. 2016;94:57–63.

51. Pezzella A, McCrery R, Lane F, et al. Two-year outcomes of the ARTISAN-SNM study for the treatment of urinary urgency incontinence using the Axonics rechargeable sacral neuromodulation system. Neurourol Urodyn. 2021;40(2):714–21. https://doi.org/10.1002/nau.24615.

52. Cardarelli S, D'Elia C, Cerruto MA, et al. Efficacy of sacral neuromodulation on urological diseases: a multicentric research project. Urologia. 2012;79(2):90–6. https://doi.org/10.5301/ru.2012.9278.

53. Jonas U, Fowler C, Chancellor M, et al. Efficacy of sacral nerve stimulation for urinary retention: results 18 months after implantation. J Urol. 2001;165(1):15–9.

54. Gross C, Habli M, Lindsell C, South M. Sacral neuromodulation for nonobstructive urinary retention: a meta-analysis. Female Pelvic Med Reconstr Surg. 2010;16(4):249–53.

55. Kessler TM, Fowler CJ. Sacral neuromodulation for urinary retention. Nat Clin Pract Urol. 2008;5(12):657–66. https://doi.org/10.1038/ncpuro1251.

56. Siegel S, Paszkiewicz E, Kirkpatrick C, Hinkel B, Oleson K. Sacral nerve stimulation in patients with chronic intractable pelvic pain. J Urol. 2001;166(5):1742–5.

57. Aboseif S, Tamaddon K, Chalfin S, Freedman S, Kaptein J. Sacral neuromodulation as an effective treatment for refractory pelvic floor dysfunction. Urology. 2002;60(1):52–6. https://doi.org/10.1016/s0090-4295(02)01630-8.

58. Peters K, Konstandt D. Sacral neuromodulation decreases narcotic requirements in refractory interstitial cystitis. BJU Int. 2004;93(6):777–9.

59. Zabihi N, Mourtzinos A, Maher MG, Raz S, Rodríguez LV. Short-term results of bilateral S2–S4 sacral neuromodulation for the treatment of refractory interstitial cystitis, painful baldder syndrome, and chronic pelvic pain. Int Urogynecol J. 2008;19(4):553–7.

60. Feler CA, Whitworth LA, Fernandez J. Sacral neuromodulation for chronic pain conditions. Anesthesiol Clin North Am. 2003;21(4):785–95.

61. Martellucci J, Naldini G, Del Popolo G, Carriero A. Sacral nerve modulation in the treatment of chronic pain after pelvic surgery. Color Dis. 2012;14(4):502–7.

62. Jason GIlleran NG. Chapter 7. Pudendal neuromodulation. In: Gilleran JP, Alpert SA, editors. Adult and pediatric neuromodulation. Cham: Springer; 2018. p. 89–104.

63. Peters KM, Feber KM, Bennett RC. Sacral versus pudendal nerve stimulation for voiding dysfunction: a prospective, single-blinded, randomized, crossover trial. Neurourol Urodyn. 2005;24(7):643–7. https://doi.org/10.1002/nau.20174.

64. Labat J-J, Riant T, Robert R, Amarenco G, Lefaucheur J-P, Rigaud J. Diagnostic criteria for pudendal neuralgia by pudendal nerve entrapment (Nantes criteria). Neurourol Urodyn. 2008;27:306–10.

65. Snooks S, Henry M, Swash M. Faecal incontinence due to external anal sphincter division in childbirth is associated with damage to the innervation of the pelvic floor musculature: a double pathology. Br J Obstet Gynaecol. 1985;92(8):824–8.

66. Pisani R, Stubinski R, Datti R. Entrapment neuropathy of the internal pudendal nerve: report of two cases. Scand J Urol Nephrol. 1997;31(4):407–10.

67. Tognetti F, Poppi M, Gaist G, Servadei F. Pudendal neuralgia due to solitary neurofibroma: case report. J Neurosurg. 1982;56(5):732–3.

68. Howard EJ. Postherpetic pudendal neuralgia. JAMA. 1985;253(15):2196.

69. Layzer RB, Conant MA. Neuralgia in recurrent herpes simplex. Arch Neurol. 1974;31(4):233–7.

70. Silbert P, Dunne J, Edis R, Stewart-Wynne E. Bicycling induced pudendal nerve pressure neuropathy. Clin Exp Neurol. 1991;28:191–6.

71. Abdi S, Shanouda P, Patel N, Saini B, Bharat Y, Calvillo O. A novel technique for pudendal nerve block. Pain Physician. 2004;7(3):319–22.

72. Bock S, Folie P, Wolff K, Marti L, Engeler DS, Hetzer FH. First experiences with pudendal nerve stimulation in fecal incontinence: a technical report. Tech Coloproctol. 2010;14(1):41–4. https://doi.org/10.1007/s10151-009-0554-7.

73. Spinelli M, Malaguti S, Giardiello G, Lazzeri M, Tarantola J, Van Den Hombergh U. A new minimally invasive procedure for pudendal nerve stimulation to treat neurogenic bladder: description of the method and preliminary data. Neurourol Urodyn. 2005;24(4):305–9. https://doi.org/10.1002/nau.20118.

74. Heinze K, Hoermann R, Fritsch H, Dermietzel R, van Ophoven A. Comparative pilot study of implantation techniques for pudendal neuromodulation: technical and clinical outcome in first 20 patients with chronic pelvic pain. World J Urol. 2015;33(2):289–94. https://doi.org/10.1007/s00345-014-1304-7.

75. Gu Y, Lv T, Jiang C, Lv J. Neuromodulation of the pudendal nerve assisted by 3D printed: a new method of neuromodulation for lower urinary tract dysfunction. Front Neurosci. 2021;15:619672. https://doi.org/10.3389/fnins.2021.619672.

76. Possover M. A novel implantation technique for pudendal nerve stimulation for treatment of overactive bladder and urgency incontinence. J Minim Invasive Gynecol. 2014;21(5):888–92.

77. Li AL, Marques R, Oliveira A, Veloso L, Girão MJ, Lemos N. Laparoscopic implantation of electrodes for bilateral neuromodulation of the pudendal nerves and S3 nerve roots for treating pelvic pain and voiding dysfunction. Int Urogynecol J. 2018;29(7):1061–4.

78. Hoang Roberts L, Vollstedt A, Volin J, McCartney T, Peters KM. Initial experience using a novel nerve stimulator for the management of pudendal neuralgia. Neurourol Urodyn. 2021; https://doi.org/10.1002/nau.24735.

79. Peters KM, Killinger KA, Jaeger C, Chen C. Pilot study exploring chronic pudendal neuromodulation as a treatment option for pain associated with pudendal neuralgia. Low Urin Tract Symptoms. 2015;7(3):138–42. https://doi.org/10.1111/luts.12066.

80. Chen SC, Lai CH, Fan WJ, Peng CW. Pudendal neuromodulation improves voiding efficiency in diabetic rats. Neurourol Urodyn. 2013;32(3):293–300.

81. Hokanson JA, Langdale CL, Sridhar A, Grill WM. Stimulation of the sensory pudendal nerve increases bladder capacity in the rat. Am J Physiol Renal Physiol. 2018;314(4):F543–50.

82. Mcguire EJ, Shi-chun Z, Horwinski ER, Lytton B. Treatment of motor and sensory detrusor instability by electrical stimulation. J Urol. 1983;129(1):78–9. https://doi.org/10.1016/S0022-5347(17)51928-X.

83. Nguyen LN, Chowdhury ML, Gilleran JP. Outcomes for intermittent neuromodulation as a treatment for overactive bladder. Curr Bladder Dysfunct Rep. 2017;12(1):66–73. https://doi.org/10.1007/s11884-017-0411-x.

84. Wolff GF, Krlin RM. Posterior tibial nerve stimulation. In: Gilleran JP, Alpert SA, editors. Adult and pediatric neuromodulation. Cham: Springer; 2018.

85. Tai C, Shen B, Chen M, Wang J, Roppolo JR, de Groat WC. Prolonged poststimulation inhibition of bladder activity induced by tibial nerve stimulation in cats. Am J Physiol Renal Physiol. 2011;300(2):F385–92. https://doi.org/10.1152/ajprenal.00526.2010.

86. Peters KM, Carrico DJ, Perez-Marrero RA, et al. Randomized trial of percutaneous tibial nerve stimulation versus sham efficacy in the treatment of overactive bladder syndrome: results from the SUmiT trial. J Urol. 2010;183(4):1438–43. https://doi.org/10.1016/j.juro.2009.12.036.

87. Nakamura M, Sakurai T, Tsujimoto Y, Tada Y. Transcutaneous electrical stimulation for the control of frequency and urge incontinence. Hinyokika Kiyo. 1983;29(9):1053–9.

88. Peters KM, Carrico DJ, MacDiarmid SA, et al. Sustained therapeutic effects of percutaneous tibial nerve stimulation: 24-month results of the STEP study. Neurourol Urodyn. 2013;32(1):24–9.

89. Peters KM, MacDiarmid SA, Wooldridge LS, et al. Randomized trial of percutaneous tibial nerve stimulation versus extended-release tolterodine: results from the overactive bladder innovative therapy trial. J Urol. 2009;182(3):1055–61.

Voiding Dysfunction After Female Pelvic Surgery

16

Shirin Razdan and Angelo E. Gousse

Contents

Introduction	276
Surgical Anatomy of the Pelvic Nervous System	276
Surgical Anatomy of the Pelvic Floor	277
Pathophysiology of Voiding Dysfunction After Pelvic Surgery	278
Evaluation of Voiding Dysfunction	278
History and Physical Exam	278
Urinalysis	279
Postvoid Residual (PVR)	279
The Role of Urodynamics	280
The Role of Cystoscopy	284
Voiding Dysfunction After Radical Hysterectomy	285
Voiding Dysfunction After Surgery for Stress Urinary Incontinence	286
Voiding Dysfunction and Pelvic Organ Prolapse Surgery	288
Anterior Prolapse	290
Apical Prolapse	292
Posterior Prolapse	293
Voiding Dysfunction After Endometriosis Surgery	293
Voiding Dysfunction After Colorectal Surgery	295
Conclusion	295
References	296

S. Razdan
Department of Urology, Icahn School of Medicine at Mount Sinai Hospital, New York, NY, USA

A. E. Gousse (✉)
Department of Urology, Larkin Hospital Palm Springs Teaching Hospital, Miami, FL, USA

Abstract

Pelvic surgery can result in voiding dysfunction. Neuropathic inadvertent iatrogenic trauma to the pelvic plexus occurs most often after radical gynecological and colorectal surgeries. In benign conditions, transvaginal and abdominal retropubic surgery performed for

© Springer Nature Switzerland AG 2023
F. E. Martins et al. (eds.), *Female Genitourinary and Pelvic Floor Reconstruction*,
https://doi.org/10.1007/978-3-031-19598-3_16

pelvic organ prolapse and urinary incontinence lead to voiding dysfunction because of anatomic changes and overcorrections. In the latter categories, bladder outlet obstruction remains the most prevalent cause of voiding dysfunction, rather than neuropathy. Long-standing bladder outlet obstruction can lead to overactive bladder or even myopathic detrusor failure. Surgery for pelvic organ prolapse can lead to outcomes in voiding behaviors with urinary retention, overactive bladder, and stress urinary incontinence.

In this chapter, we describe the surgical anatomy of the pelvic nervous system and the pelvic floor and discuss the pathophysiology and evaluation of voiding dysfunction after pelvic surgery, including surgery for stress urinary incontinence, pelvic organ prolapse, endometriosis, hysterectomy, and colorectal surgery.

Keywords

Voiding dysfunction · Pelvic organ prolapse · Stress urinary incontinence · Midurethral sling · Pubovaginal sling · Radical hysterectomy

Introduction

Pelvic surgery either performed abdominally or transvaginally can result in voiding dysfunction. Neuropathic inadvertent iatrogenic trauma to the pelvic plexus occurs most often after radical, gynecological, and colorectal surgeries. In benign conditions, transvaginal and abdominal retropubic surgery performed for pelvic organ prolapse and urinary incontinence lead to voiding dysfunction because of anatomic changes and overcorrections. In the latter categories, bladder outlet obstruction remains the most prevalent cause of voiding dysfunction, rather than neuropathy. It is noteworthy that long-standing bladder outlet obstruction can lead to overactive bladder or even myopathic detrusor failure. Surgery for pelvic organ prolapse can lead to outcomes in voiding behaviors with urinary retention,

overactive bladder, and stress urinary incontinence all reported in the literature.

Surgical Anatomy of the Pelvic Nervous System

The bladder receives innervation from the pelvic plexus (i.e., input from the S2 to S4 spinal cord segments), which is situated on the lateral aspect of the rectum. The portion of the pelvic plexus that specifically supplies the bladder is also called the vesical plexus.

Sympathetic preganglionic pathways that arise from the T11–L2 spinal segments pass to the sympathetic chain ganglia and then to prevertebral ganglia in the superior hypogastric and pelvic plexus and also to short adrenergic neurons in the bladder and urethra [1]. Sympathetic postganglionic nerves that release norepinephrine provide an excitatory input to smooth muscle of the urethra and bladder base, an inhibitory input to smooth muscle in the body of the bladder, and an inhibitory and facilitatory input to vesical parasympathetic ganglia [2]. The sympathetic nerve supply to the detrusor muscle and urethral muscle is overall sparse, with alpha adrenergic receptors concentrated in the bladder base and proximal urethra, whereas β-adrenergic receptors are most prominent in the bladder body [3, 4].

The primary supply to the detrusor is by parasympathetic nerves that are uniformly and diffusely distributed throughout the detrusor. In women, numerous parasympathetic nerves, identical to those innervating the detrusor, supply the bladder neck and urethral muscle. The superior hypogastric plexus is a fenestrated network of fibers anterior to the lower abdominal aorta. The hypogastric nerves exit bilaterally at the inferior poles of the superior hypogastric plexus that lie at the level of the sacral promontory. The network of nerve structures is located between the endopelvic fascia and the peritoneum. The hypogastric nerves unite the superior hypogastric plexus and the inferior hypogastric plexus (or pelvic plexus) bilaterally. The inferior hypogastric plexus has connections with the sacral roots from S2-S4 [5]. The superior hypogastric plexus and hypogastric nerves are mainly sympathetic, the pelvic splanchnic nerves are mainly parasympathetic, and the inferior hypogastric plexus contains both types of fibers.

Somatic efferent pathways to the external urethral sphincter are carried in the pudendal nerve from anterior horn cells in the third and fourth sacral segments of the human spinal cord [1]. Afferent axons in the pelvic, hypogastric, pudendal, and levator ani nerves transmit information from the lower urinary tract and pelvic floor to second-order neurons in the lumbosacral spinal cord [6, 7].

Disruption anywhere along the spinal cord and peripheral nerves can influence bladder function and sphincter control. While suprapontine lesions result in overactive bladder with synergic sphincters, suprasacral lesions typically result in detrusor sphincter dyssynergia. More pertinent to the pelvic surgeon is peripheral nerve injury which results in a triad of underactive detrusor, bladder neck incompetence, and fixed striated sphincter tone.

Neuropathic injury can also cause pelvic organ prolapse. The pudendal nerve supplies the urethral and anal sphincters and perineal muscles. The nerves to the levator muscles, which originate from S3 to S5 nerve roots, innervate the main musculature of the pelvic floor. Pelvic floor nerve injury can occur during vaginal delivery or surgery and predispose women to disruption in support of the pelvic viscera.

Surgical Anatomy of the Pelvic Floor

A mastery of the surgical anatomy of the pelvic floor is vital to understanding the pathophysiology and treatment options for pelvic organ prolapse and stress urinary incontinence that will be discussed later in this chapter.

The pubovesical ligaments help support the urethra and bladder neck but may also play a role in relaxation of the bladder neck during micturition. The anterior vagina provides support to the urethra through its lateral attachments to the pubococcygeus and arcus tendineus fascia pelvis.

DeLancey described different levels of pelvic organ support. Level I is represented by the cardinal ligaments and uterosacral ligaments providing support to the uterus, cervix, and upper vagina. Level II support runs from the paravaginal attachments to the arcus tendineus fascia pelvis and to the arcus tendineus rectovaginalis. Anterior vaginal wall prolapse results from loss of level II support. Level III support is created by the distal vaginal attachments to the levator muscles laterally, anteriorly to the urethra, and posteriorly to the perineal body. Level III support provides foundation to the urethra, and disruption leads to urethral hypermobility and stress urinary incontinence [8].

DeLancey also hypothesized that healthy women have a "suburethral hammock" attached laterally that supports the urethra and maintains urinary continence. However, in women with stress urinary incontinence, there is a deficiency of this supporting layer that is evidenced by hypermobility of the bladder neck and urethra. It was theorized that descent of these structures inferiorly allowed for unequal pressure transmission and subsequent stress urinary incontinence. Therefore a pubovaginal sling placed at the bladder neck can eliminate stress incontinence by providing a strong layer of tissue that provides dynamic compression of the urethra during times of increased intra-abdominal pressure [9]. Another theory postulated that the midurethra is the mediator of urinary continence. The pubococcygeus muscles insert at the level of the midurethra just outside the vaginal epithelial wall and play a vital role in the midurethral continence mechanism. Westby et al. (1982) and Asmussen and Ulmsten (1983) demonstrated that maximum urethral closure pressure (MUCP) occurs at the midurethra in continent women, and this phenomenon is most likely caused by the combined contribution of anatomic structures in this location [10, 11]. Thus, the midurethral sling was created to further augment any potential deficit in this area that may contribute to stress urinary incontinence.

Pelvic organ support strongly depends on the interaction between the levator ani muscles and the endopelvic fascia. Once the pelvic organs are unsupported by the levator muscles, the entire support for the pelvic organs has to be provided by the ligaments of the endopelvic fascia. After a period of time, these ligaments tend to fail and prolapse ensues. Injury or stretching of these ligaments can occur during vaginal delivery, hysterectomy, chronic straining, or with normal aging [12].

Petros and Ulmsten proposed a unifying concept called the integral theory, which postulated that adequate function of the pubourethral ligaments, suburethral vaginal hammock, and pubococcygeus muscles was the most important factor for preservation of urinary continence in women. Injury to any of these three components from surgery, parturition, aging, or hormonal deprivation could lead to impaired midurethral function and subsequent stress urinary incontinence [13].

Pathophysiology of Voiding Dysfunction After Pelvic Surgery

Voiding dysfunction after pelvic surgery may be caused by anatomic or functional disturbances of the lower urinary tract. A concept popularized by Dr. Alan Wei, voiding dysfunction may be divided into two broad categories: failure to store and failure to empty.

Failure to store may be caused by detrusor overactivity, which may result from denervation supersensitivity after pelvic dissection or from surgery-induced bladder outlet obstruction (e.g., after a tight suburethral slingplasty). Bladder outlet obstruction may be the most common factor in the development of postoperative voiding dysfunction [14]. Some have proposed that parasympathetic denervation supersensitivity develops as a result of bladder outlet obstruction, while others have postulated that denervation hypersensitivity may develop from the surgical dissection alone in the absence of bladder outlet obstruction [15–17]. Other studies suggested that bladder outlet obstruction might result in changes in cholinergic and purinergic signaling.

Failure to empty: Bladder outlet obstruction after suburethral sling surgery is most often related to increased tension resulting in urethral compression [14, 18]. Retropubic and transvaginal needle suspensions stabilize lateral periurethral tissues, with obstruction relating to hyperelevation of the bladder neck and kinking of the proximal urethra. Pubovaginal slings provide suburethral support to augment urethral coaptation during periods of increased intra-abdominal pressure. Obstruction after midurethral sling placement has been attributed to compression from excessive tension or sling misplacement or migration [19]. While some patients may present with urinary urgency, frequency, urge incontinence, or pelvic pain, others develop complete failure to void requiring an indwelling catheter or intermittent catheterization.

Voiding dysfunction after nonurologic pelvic surgery, particularly after cancer surgery, is often due to damage to the hypogastric and pelvic plexuses and can have a myriad presentation, including detrusor instability or even frank urinary retention [20].

Evaluation of Voiding Dysfunction

A detailed knowledge of the preoperative voiding history is of paramount importance in the assessment and evaluation of postsurgical voiding dysfunction. The presence and extent of preoperative storage and voiding symptoms are important for comparison with de novo or persistent symptoms after incontinence surgery. Important factors include preoperative emptying status and PVR volume. These assessments are important for those with elevated PVR volumes after slingplasty. If preoperative voiding parameters and emptying are normal, incomplete emptying or retention after surgery increases the suspicion for postoperative bladder outlet obstruction or iatrogenic traumatic neuropathy. At that point, a postoperative evaluation becomes mandatory.

History and Physical Exam

Postoperative evaluation demands a comparative thorough history that includes assessment of storage symptoms such as frequency, dysuria, urgency, and urge incontinence and voiding symptoms such as hesitancy, incomplete emptying, straining, positional voiding, and complete urinary retention before and after surgery. The physical examination evaluates anatomical evidence of a hypersuspended urethra and bladder neck, degree of urethral mobility, and kinks underneath the urethra. Furthermore, the presence of stress urinary incontinence (SUI), worsening or new-onset pelvic organ prolapse, and erosion of mesh or allografts in the vaginal canal or within the lumen of the urethra should be noted. At times, the mesh cannot be seen but can be palpated underneath bleeding friable granulation tissue. New onset and unexplained vaginal bleeding should always be carefully evaluated after female pelvic surgery, as it can be a sign of foreign body extrusion through the vaginal wall. In postmenopausal women with a uterus, the differential diagnosis of unexplained vaginal bleeding postpelvic surgery should also include endometrial hyperplasia or carcinoma, with appropriate gynecologic referral.

The findings on physical examination may vary from normal anatomy to a clearly hypersuspended urethra. Midurethral slings do not typically result in overcorrection of the urethrovesical angle unless the surgeon is too aggressive in tensioning of the sling or places it incorrectly underneath the urethra. To prevent overtensioning, many surgeons place a "spacer" underneath the urethra while the sling is being deployed and adjusted. (Fig. 1). A 13 Hegar can be used as a spacer (Fig. 2). Inexperienced surgeons are more likely to use excessive tension when adjusting the sling, resulting in outlet obstruction (Fig. 3).

Bladder neck slings, however, can pull or scar the urethra against the pubic bone and result in a negative urethrovesical angle. Anterior compartment prolapse may create a fulcrum or point of obstruction and should be excluded in the evaluation of voiding dysfunction after sling surgery. Urethral or vaginal erosion of the sling, SUI, and persistent urethral hypermobility also should be considered [21].

Urinalysis

A urinalysis can provide the surgeon with very valuable information when evaluating voiding dysfunction after pelvic surgery. While a completely clear urine analysis is very encouraging, it does not necessarily eliminate the possibility of complications after pelvic surgery. It is possible to have overactive bladder symptoms, an elevated postvoid residual, or even frank urinary retention with a normal urinalysis. However, it is rare to have a normal urinalysis in the face of urethral erosion. Pyuria and microscopic hematuria, with or without a positive nitrite on urine dipstick, signals a urinary tract infection. The clinician should have a low threshold to obtain a urine culture after pelvic surgery when the urinalysis is abnormal. Elevated postvoid residual volumes can result in urinary tract infections (UTIs). Of note, UTIs can mimic overactive bladder symptoms. Therefore, it is recommended to obtain a urinalysis in all patients after female pelvic surgery with voiding dysfunction to better characterize the possible etiology of symptoms.

Postvoid Residual (PVR)

The assessment of the urinary bladder's ability to empty (postvoid residual) post female pelvic surgery cannot be emphasized enough. The postvoid residual can be measured using bladder scan ultrasonography or postvoid urethral catheterization. The postvoid residual remains at the cornerstone of every postoperative initial evaluation given the ease of determination and clinical significance.

Documentation of adequate bladder emptying is important, as it often will change patient management. An elevated PVR can be related to bladder underactivity, lack of adequate bladder contractility, or bladder outlet anatomic obstruction. Note that functional bladder obstruction is rare post pelvic surgery but may exist secondary to levator spasm or pseudodyssynergia. By far, anatomic fixed bladder outlet obstruction is most commonly seen. A preoperative PVR is valuable and should be obtained prior to undergoing female

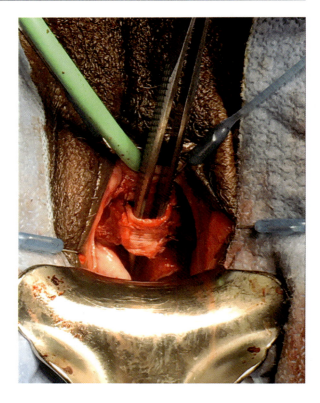

Fig. 1 Spacing an autologous pubovaginal rectus sling to prevent postoperative voiding dysfunction. Overtensioning of a pubovaginal sling predisposes to urinary retention

pelvic surgery. At times, preexisting causes for bladder emptying exist and must be assessed and explained prior to surgery. The change in PVR from preoperative value to postoperative value is one of the most important clinical information available to the clinician when evaluating voiding dysfunction after female pelvic surgery.

Preoperatively, increased PVR volumes due to loss of detrusor contractility or bladder outlet obstruction, or both, can place a patient at greater risk for postoperative voiding dysfunction. Postoperatively, the PVR volume should be documented, although an elevated PVR cannot differentiate bladder outlet obstruction from impaired detrusor contractility. In these complicated cases, when indicated, multichannel urodynamics is most useful.

The Role of Urodynamics

Although commonly performed by most clinicians, the evidence-based value of urodynamic study (UDS) in the evaluation of voiding dysfunction after incontinence surgery remains controversial [22]. Urodynamic studies may provide information on detrusor overactivity or impaired compliance in patients in urinary retention or increased PVR capacity (Fig. 4). They may also confirm the diagnosis of bladder outlet obstruction as demonstrated by high pressure with low flow [23] (Fig. 5). Many studies indicate that that the presence of an adequate detrusor contraction has no association with successful voiding after transvaginal urethrolysis and sling takedown [24–26]. As such, UDS findings must be analyzed in context when managing voiding dysfunction after pelvic and redo surgery.

When counseling a patient with voiding dysfunction after pelvic surgery, prior to resorting to UDS evaluation, a full clinical impression of the type of dysfunction must be ascertained. In other words, a determination of the predominant symptom must be made –whether storage or voiding. Bladder outlet obstruction can often be suspected on physical exam without need for adjunctive

Fig. 2 Spacing a midurethral synthetic sling with a #13 Hegar spacer diminishes postoperative urination retention associated with overt tensioning

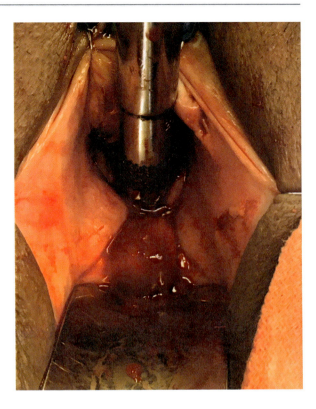

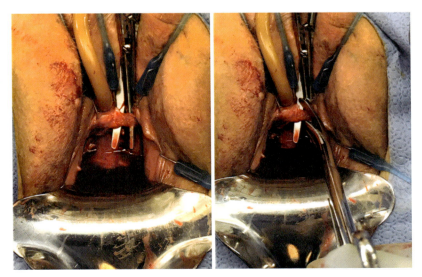

Fig. 3 A synthetic suburethral sling placed too tight and too distal which leads to postoperative urinary retention. Note mesh between blades of the Metzenbaum scissors

UDS. For more complex voiding pathologies, UDS can be used to tease out the nuances of detrusor and urethral function. Video urodynamics (VUDS) can also be considered for direct visualization of bladder emptying, urethral anatomy, and sphincter relaxation. In general, the clinical suspicion for postoperative bladder outlet obstruction related to a hypersuspended and compressed bladder outlet is of greater importance than the urodynamic findings. When there is

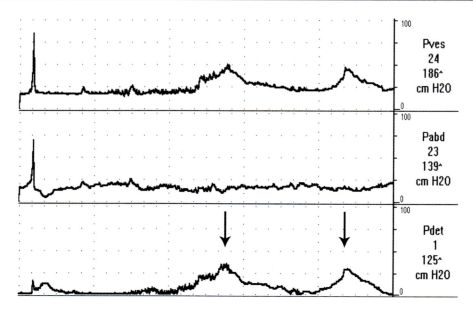

Fig. 4 Detrusor overactivity noted during multichannel urodynamics after postsling urinary retention

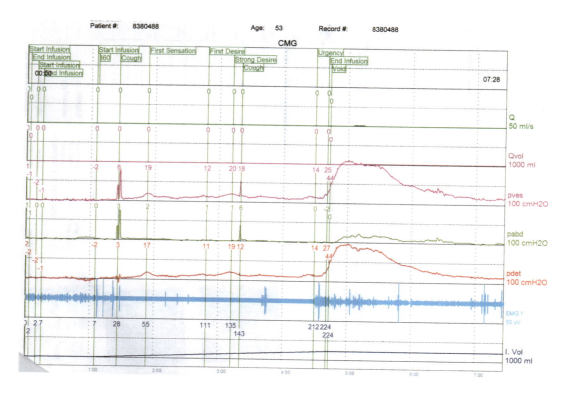

Fig. 5 High pressure and low flow consistent with bladder outlet obstruction after a synthetic suburethral sling

clear evidence of a temporal relationship for voiding dysfunction after female pelvic surgery, a urodynamic study, in itself, should never dissuade a surgeon from performing a sling takedown and urethrolysis in a symptomatic patient.

Miller et al. performed a study to determine which urodynamic parameters can best predict postoperative voiding dysfunction following pubovaginal sling surgery. The records of 98 consecutive women who had undergone pubovaginal sling surgery with allograft fascia lata between July 1998 and July 2000 were reviewed. Urodynamic and follow-up data were sufficient for evaluation of 73 patients. Average time to return of efficient voiding was 3.92 days (median 3). Of 21 women who voided without a detrusor contraction, urinary retention developed in 4 (23%) versus 0 of 48 who voided with detrusor contraction (p = 0.007). Urinary retention was defined as the need to perform even occasional self-catheterization. All four women with urinary retention had a detrusor pressure of less than 12 cm H_2O (0 in 3, 4 in 1). None of the women with a detrusor pressure of greater than 12 cm H_2O had urinary retention (p = 0.047). The presence of Valsalva voiding in women without a detrusor contraction did not affect the incidence of urinary retention (11.1%) compared to those who did not demonstrate Valsalva voiding (5.1%) (p = 0.603). Peak flow rate, detrusor instability on preoperative urodynamics, and postvoid residual urine volume were not associated with postoperative urinary retention. Finally, postvoid residual urine volume predicted delayed return to normal voiding (p = 0.001). There were no other urodynamic parameters that were significantly associated with urinary retention, delayed return to normal voiding, or postoperative urgency symptoms including peak flow rate, capacity, or compliance. The authors concluded that women who void without or with a weak detrusor contraction on urodynamics are most likely to have urinary retention postoperatively. The authors concluded that preoperative urodynamic evaluation may be used to counsel women regarding the risk of urinary retention following the pubovaginal sling procedure [27].

Other authors have also explored the utility of preoperative UDS in predicting functional outcomes after midurethral sling surgery. Duckett et al. found resolution of OAB symptoms in 51% of women who underwent MUS; the persistence of OAB symptoms was predicted by a significant decrease (20.0 to 14.0 mL/s) in the maximum flow rate after the MUS (P = 0.027) and a significant increase in the detrusor pressure at maximum flow after the MUS (P = 0.04) [28]. Panayi et al. determined that elevated preoperative opening detrusor pressure predicted persistence of DO after MUS surgery in women with preoperative mixed urinary incontinence [29].

Liang et al. investigated the contributing factors of persistent detrusor overactivity (DO) in women with advanced pelvic organ prolapse (POP) after transvaginal mesh (TVM) repair. The authors retrospectively evaluated consecutive patients with DO and advanced POP who had undergone TVM in a tertiary hospital between 2010 and 2014. All patients received evaluations, including a structured urogynecological questionnaire, pelvic examination using the POP-Quantification System, scores of the Urogenital Distress Inventory and Incontinence Impact Questionnaire, and urodynamic testing before transvaginal mesh repair and 6 months after surgery. Of 326 patients with POP who underwent vaginal mesh repair, 63 with preoperative DO were included. Urinary urgency was present in 27 (42.9%), and urgency incontinence was present in 26 (41.3%) patients. Nineteen (30.2%) patients had persistent DO after surgery. Patients with persistent DO had lower preoperative maximal flow rate, higher preoperative detrusor pressure at maximum flow, higher postoperative residual urine volume, and higher rates of concomitant sacrospinous ligament suspension compared to those without DO. Twenty percent of women with advanced POP had DO, and most of these cases resolved after prolapse repair. For women with lower preoperative mean flow rate and concomitant sacrospinous ligament suspension, the authors concluded that preoperative counseling should consist of a discussion about persistent DO and relevant urinary symptoms following transvaginal mesh repair [30].

The Role of Cystoscopy

All patients with persistent storage symptoms after sling surgery should undergo cystoscopy to rule out urethral erosion and bladder perforation from sutures, the suture passer, or sling material (Figs. 6–7). Cystourethroscopy may also show a hypersuspended midurethra or bladder neck

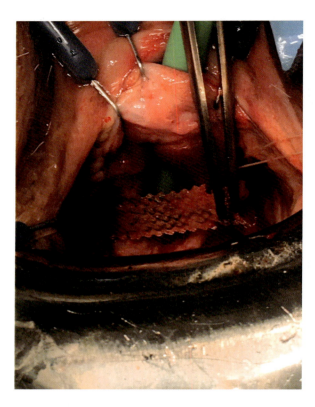

Fig. 6 Patient with urinary retention post midurethral sling surgery. Early synthetic mesh suburethral erosion with exposure of the urethral Foley

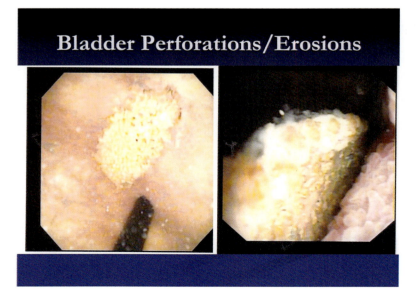

Fig. 7 Mesh erosion near the bladder neck associated with urinary retention, recurrent UTI, and calcified synthetic mesh in the urinary bladder

(indicating excessive sling tension), scarring, deviation of the urethra, sling misplacement, sling migration, fistula formation, and calcified eroded synthetic sling material in the urethra or the urinary bladder. Vaginoscopy also can be performed to exclude vaginal extrusion of a sling. Any time a patient reports gross hematuria or persistent vaginal bleeding, if there is presence of microscopic hematuria on urinalysis, or recurrent UTIs, a cystoscopy and vaginoscopy must be performed.

Voiding Dysfunction After Radical Hysterectomy

Voiding dysfunction is relatively common after radical hysterectomy, with a reported rate of 52–85%, with prolonged Foley catheter required in as many as 42% of patients [31, 32]. It is more common with radical hysterectomy than subtotal hysterectomy for benign disease [33]. Loss of bladder filling sensation is the suggested pathophysiologic mechanism of urinary retention after hysterectomy, suggested to be due to deafferentiation of bladder wall and bladder neck [34]. Decreased visceral sensation of the bladder or bladder neck is associated with neurogenic disease [35]. Functionally, these patients have absent filling sensation on cystometry, together with partial or complete sensory denervation of the bladder, resulting in increased bladder capacity and secondary urinary retention. Compared with subtotal hysterectomy, total or radical hysterectomy has been associated with a more prominent decrease in voiding frequency and increased bladder capacity [33]. Partial or complete deafferentiation, together with a concomitant factor (e.g., preexisting pelvic floor dysfunction, histrionic personality, and medications) may result in urinary retention [36].

Both early and late voiding dysfunction have been reported after radical hysterectomy. During the initial phase, a significant reduction of bladder compliance and maximum urethral closure pressure at 3–6 months postoperatively have been noted [37, 38]. PVR volumes tend to increase at 2 and 6 weeks after surgery. At uroflowmetry, the mean flow rate and the maximal flow rate showed a reduction at 2 weeks, 6 weeks, and 3 months after surgery [37]. This may be attributed to impaired parasympathetic motor innervation, as a result of pelvic nerve or pelvic plexus injury, in maintaining detrusor contractility. Studies have shown that transvaginal hysterectomy is more likely to result in voiding dysfunction than transabdominal laparoscopic hysterectomy. This ultimately results in longer hospital stay and increased risk of postoperative UTI [39].

Long-term bladder function after hysterectomy is marked by significant reduction of bladder compliance, increase of residual urine volume, increase of first voiding desire, and reduction of the maximum cystometric capacity [40–42]. Reduced bladder compliance, detrusor overactivity, and urinary incontinence may disappear within 6 to 12 months but may also persist for a longer period of time. Somatic as well as autonomic demyelination with or without denervation might be responsible for changes in urethrovesical function [37, 43, 44].

There is a subset of women who report improved voiding symptoms after hysterectomy. These are typically women with preexisting overactive bladder symptoms, stress urinary incontinence, and nocturia [45, 46]. This improvement may result from the postoperative changes in the urodynamics and mobility of the bladder neck, with investigators suggesting that these effects may be attributed to the anchoring of the vaginal cuff to the cardinal-uterosacral ligament complex during hysterectomy [47].

Nerve-sparing radical hysterectomy has been described as a means to decrease the incidence of early and late bladder dysfunction, with minimally invasive approaches facilitating greater nerve preservation [42, 48, 49].

When counseling women about the long-term effects of hysterectomy on voiding symptoms, it is important to describe that early postoperative voiding dysfunction (requiring prolonged catheterization of at least a month) is more likely to result in high postvoid residual volumes and abdominal straining on micturition at least 2 years after the index surgery, although this is unlikely to affect quality of life [50].

Another concern with vaginal hysterectomy is the risk of iatrogenic pelvic organ prolapse (POP) or stress urinary incontinence (SUI). The odds ratio of POP and SUI after vaginal hysterectomy has been reported to be 4.9 and 6.3, respectively, irrespective of the reason for hysterectomy (i.e., for treatment of POP vs. other gynecologic diagnoses) [51]. Surgery for pelvic organ prolapse is also increased after prior hysterectomy [52]. That being said, hysterectomy is also within the treatment paradigm of apical prolapse, as will be discussed later in this chapter. This further corroborates the previously mentioned nuance in neural and structural contributors to urinary continence and pelvic organ support that are in balance and counterbalance after pelvic surgery.

Voiding Dysfunction After Surgery for Stress Urinary Incontinence

Anti-incontinence procedures are designed to correct SUI by restoring support to the urethrovesical junction and, in cases of intrinsic sphincter dysfunction, by improving coaptation of the urethra. Persistent voiding dysfunction from postoperative urethral hypersuspension is a known complication after female anti-incontinence surgery. It has been reported to occur in 2.5% to 24% of patients [53]. In a large series of 503 patients comparing the Burch colposuspension with Stamey endoscopic needle suspension, voiding dysfunction was found to be the most common complication (12.1%) [54]. In most patients, postoperative voiding dysfunction is caused by obstruction from the incontinence procedure itself [14, 55].

Bladder outlet obstruction occurs in 5% to 20% of patients after a Marshall-Marchetti-Krantz procedure, in 4% to 7% after a Burch colposuspension, in 5% to 7% after a needle suspension, and in 4% to 10% after pubovaginal sling operations [56–58]. Burch colposuspension has also been associated with pelvic floor dysfunction concerning for bowel dysfunction (e.g., incomplete emptying of bowel, gas and stool incontinence, etc.) [59]. Although midurethral slings are placed without tension, studies have shown that they may still be associated with voiding

dysfunction in 4.9% to 10% of patients [53, 60]. Preoperative UDS has not been found to be predictive of voiding dysfunction after Burch colposuspension or pubovaginal sling placement [61]. Other predictors of obstructive voiding symptoms after transobturator sling surgery include older age, narrow vaginal canals, preoperative overactive bladder symptoms, and prior pelvic organ prolapse surgery [62].

Yang et al. described the risk factors for development of de novo urinary urgency and urgency incontinence after autologous pubovaginal sling. From 2013 to 2016, they reviewed the results of 347 patients who underwent autologous pubovaginal sling. The authors described de novo urinary urgency/urge incontinence as treatment (medication, botulinum toxin injection, and sacral neuromodulation) for urgency postoperatively that was not required before surgery [63]. A total of 109 patients underwent rectus fascia pubovaginal sling. Of this cohort, 23 (21.1%) patients were treated for de novo urgency/urge incontinence, 18 (78.2%) with anticholinergic, 4 (17.3%) with botulinum toxin injection, and 2 (8.69%) with sacral neuromodulation. The only risk factor predictive of de novo urinary urgency was prior pelvic organ prolapse surgery [63]. There is not an insignificant need for postoperative clean intermittent catheterization in women who undergo pubovaginal sling placement for SUI. Risk factors for this include preoperative PVR > 100 mL or Qmax < or = 20 mL/s [64].

Autologous pubovaginal sling represents an important technique in the arsenal of female pelvic reconstructive urologists, as it is a versatile sling that can be utilized even in the face of prior midurethral sling failure [65]. Milose et al. reviewed the charts of 66 women who underwent autologous pubovaginal sling with rectus fascia after one or more failed synthetic midurethral sling from 2007 to 2012. They found that at a mean of 14.5 months after autologous pubovaginal sling, 46 (69.7%) patients reported cure of stress urinary incontinence. Of these patients, 25 (37.9%) had complete cure with no stress or urgency incontinence, 17 had cure of stress urinary incontinence but had persistent urgency incontinence, and 4 had cure of stress urinary incontinence but experienced do novo urgency incontinence [65]. Patients with pure stress urinary incontinence were significantly more likely to be cured of all incontinence (62.5%) than those women with preoperative mixed incontinence (30.0%) (p = 0.006) [65].

In women with prior failed MUS surgery or with mesh-related complications, autologous pubovaginal sling can be a successful alternative. McCoy et al. evaluated 46 patients who underwent autologous fascial pubovaginal sling following removal of transvaginal synthetic mesh in a simultaneous or staged fashion. All 46 patients had received at least one prior mesh sling for incontinence and 8 (17%) had received prior transvaginal polypropylene mesh for pelvic organ prolapse repair. With a mean follow-up of 16 months, 22% of patients required a mean of 1.8 subsequent interventions an average of 6.5 months after autologous sling placement with no difference in median quality of life at final follow-up. At last follow-up, 42 of 46 patients (91%) and 35 of 46 (76%) had achieved objective and subjective success, respectively. There was no difference in subjective success between patients treated with a staged mesh removal versus a concomitant removal (69% vs 80%, p = 0.48) [65].

Virseda-Chamorro et al. determined that women with a preoperative rectocele and detrusor overactivity are at a greater risk to develop postoperative detrusor overactivity after pelvic organ prolapse surgery and should be counseled of this potential sequela [66]. Gamble et al. determined that women with preoperative mixed urinary incontinence, older age, nocturia, greater maximum cystometric capacity, and bladder neck slings (vs. retropubic MUS and transobturator MUS) were at increased risk of persistent DO after transvaginal sling surgery [67].

There is a unique subset of mesh-related complications that must also be discussed with patients preoperatively. Recurrent infections, mesh extrusion, or perforation has been studied extensively in the literature. Punjani et al. found that postoperative urinary retention and hospital presentation for UTI symptoms are associated with an increased risk of reoperation for MUS

complications. These patients should be followed and investigated for mesh complications when appropriate. Funk et al. found an overall low 9-year risk of sling revision or removal (3.7%). This risk, however, was elevated among women who had a concomitant anterior or apical prolapse procedure, and those between ages 18 and 29 [68].

Rates of midurethral sling (MUS) failure are reported at 5–20% [69]. Zimmern et al. performed a secondary analysis of the SISTEr and ToMUS trials of women who underwent primary treatment of stress urinary incontinence with recurrence of stress incontinence [70]. The investigators found that 5-year retreatment-free survival rates (and standard errors) were 87% (3%), 96% (2%), 97% (1%), and 99% (0.7%) for Burch, autologous fascial sling, transobturator MUS, and retropubic MUS groups, respectively (p < 0.0001) [70]. The overall retreatment rate was 6% at 5 years, with most women electing either transurethral bulking agents or autologous pubovaginal sling.

When comparing outcomes of colposuspension, midurethral slings, and pubovaginal slings for treatment of stress urinary incontinence, a recent systematic review and meta-analysis found MUS to be superior to Burch colposuspension in ensuring durable responses with both higher overall and objective cure rates [71]. Pubovaginal sling was equivalent in outcomes to MUS in their analysis. When comparing retropubic and transobturator midurethral slings, the former was significantly more likely to cause postoperative urinary tract infections and voiding dysfunction [71].

Risk factors for urinary retention after MUS surgery include old age, concomitant surgery, vaginal vault prolapse, poorly performed intraoperative cough test, low preoperative urinary flow rate, and low detrusor contractility [72, 73]. While most women will pass a voiding trial on their first attempt after MUS surgery, those who fail are at increased risk of postoperative urinary tract infection or developing long-term impaired bladder emptying after passing a subsequent voiding trial [74]. Although it is often transient and self-limiting, chronic postmidurethral sling voiding dysfunction may lead to irreversible changes affecting detrusor function. Initial management includes intermittent catheterization, and addressing circumstantial factors interfering with normal voiding, such as pain [75].

For urinary retention after synthetic midurethral sling surgery, conventional teaching is sling incision should be performed after a month, as voiding dysfunction is not likely to spontaneously improve [76, 77]. However, the rate of recurrent SUI after sling incision has been reported to be as high as 60%, and patients should be counseled about this fact [78, 79]. There have been reports of sling mobilization to relieve outlet obstruction and improve voiding symptoms, although the data in this sphere is sparse at best. [79, 80] This is different for autologous pubovaginal slings, where intermittent self-catheterization can stretch the sling and relieve outlet obstruction up to three months after index surgery. If persistent obstructive voiding exists at that point, sling incision can be performed with reasonable outcomes [81, 82]. The current literature supports CIC, sling incision, and sling mobilization, as well as urethrolysis, as viable options for treatment of de novo obstructive voiding after MUS placement and pubovaginal sling placement [83].

In surgery for retention after slingplasty, a midline incision over the sling should be attempted initially. If the sling cannot be identified or bladder neck mobility is not restored, formal transvaginal urethrolysis should be performed [14]. Suprameatal dissection may be helpful in lysing scarred fibrous attachments between the urethra and pubis. Retropubic urethrolysis is reserved for patients with voiding dysfunction after retropubic suspension and for initial transvaginal urethrolysis failures. Resuspension of the urethra may be considered if the patient has concomitant SUI. Patients with persistent obstruction or voiding dysfunction after initial urethrolysis should undergo a workup similar to that for primary voiding dysfunction after anti-incontinence surgery and may be considered for aggressive repeat urethrolysis if obstruction is diagnosed. This approach may prevent chronic bladder dysfunction [84].

Oliver and Raz described their technique and outcomes of suprameatal urethrolysis with Martius flap (SMUM) for those women with refractory bladder outlet obstruction (BOO) after SUI surgery [85]. After a median follow-up of 10.8 months (range 3.1–20.1), the procedure was successful in nine patients (82%). Postoperative median PVR was 29 ml (range 0–425) and median change in PVR was a 280 ml (range 29–1050) decrease ($p < 0.01$). Among the seven patients who required catheterization preoperatively, five patients (71%) recovered volitional voiding. Two patients (18%) continued to require indwelling or intermittent catheterization and underwent additional surgery for BOO. SUI recurred in one patient (9%). The authors concluded that SMUM is successful in improving or relieving refractory BOO in this challenging patient population. After transvaginal urethrolysis, the authors believe that Martius flap interposition is critical to preventing recurrent fixation of the urethra to the pubic bone and thus achieving improved voiding [85] (Figs. 8, 9, and 10).

Voiding Dysfunction and Pelvic Organ Prolapse Surgery

Pelvic organ prolapse (POP) refers to the downward descent of pelvic organs, which may result in symptoms of pelvic pressure or pain, vaginal "bulge," urinary retention, urinary urgency, splinting on defecation, or other dysfunctional bowel or bladder habits. POP occurs due to loss of vaginal support of the pelvic structures and is most commonly due to conditions that cause increase in abdominal or pelvic pressure that subsequently transmits to pelvic contents: obesity, advancing age, and vaginal delivery. Compromise in any of the vaginal levels of support as previously discussed in this chapter is the leading mechanism of pelvic organ descent.

POP can be characterized using various quantification systems, but the most commonly accepted system is the Pelvic Organ Prolapse Quantification (POPQ) system, which was first created in 1993 and subsequently updated in 2002 [86]. Six defined points in the vagina are identified: points Aa and Ba for the anterior vagina, Ap and Bp for the posterior vagina, and C and D for the cervix/vault. Point D is not used in

Fig. 8 Fibrofatty Martius flap being prepared to cover suprameatal dissected space

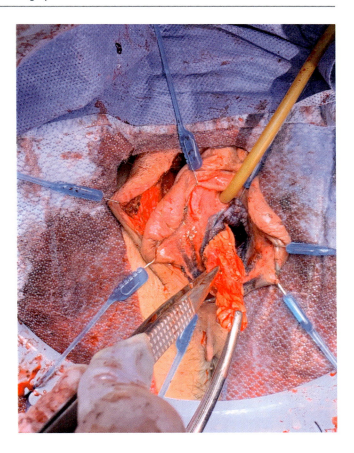

women who previously had a hysterectomy. The patient is asked to strain, ideally when in the standing position, to elicit the POP to its maximum extent. The location of the defined points is then gauged relative to the hymenal ring and recorded on a grid [86]. Staging pelvic organ prolapse then relies on identifying the lowest extent of any part of the six defined points.

There are four stages of POP. Stage 0 refers to no prolapse. Stage I prolapse is when the most distal extent of prolapse is greater than 1 cm proximal to the hymen. Stage II prolapse is when distal extent of prolapse is between 1 cm proximal to 1 cm distal to the hymen. Stage III prolapse occurs when the distal extent of prolapse is greater than 1 cm distal to the hymen but not complete vaginal eversion. Stage IV prolapse is when the distal extent of prolapse is 2 cm less than the total vaginal length or complete vaginal eversion. Studies have shown that most POP does not become symptomatic until at least reaching the hymenal ring (Stage II prolapse) [87].

Loss of vaginal or uterine support in women visit can be seen in up to 43% to 90% of patients [88, 89]. It is now clear that stage I prolapse of the anterior and posterior vaginal wall are so common that they are likely to be part of the normal spectrum in healthy women. In a multicenter observational study of 1004 patients seeking routine gynecologic care, only 24% of patients had no prolapse. The prevalence of stages I, II, and III prolapse was 38%, 35%, and 2%, respectively [87]. Thus, some loss of uterovaginal support is present in the majority of the adult female population and surgical treatment should not automatically be offered for these women without concomitant symptoms.

Overall, outcomes from surgery for pelvic organ prolapse are durable, although with rates of de novo bladder overactivity reported at 12%

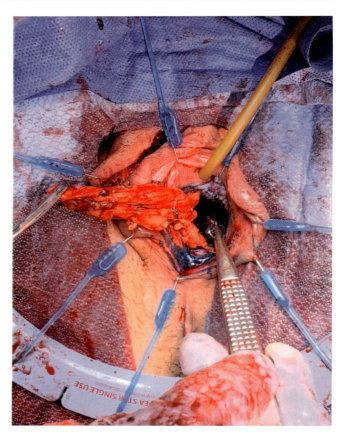

Fig. 9 Fibrofatty Martius flap being developed to be placed in suprameatal space

and de novo voiding dysfunction (including SUI) at 9% [90]. Most patients with advanced pelvic organ prolapse and elevated PVR volumes demonstrate normalization of the PVR volumes after surgical correction of the pelvic organ prolapse [91]. Predicting which patients with POP will develop de novo SUI after prolapse repair is challenging. A recent literature review, however, found that trial of an ambulatory pessary accurately predicted persistent urgency and frequency as well as occult SUI in 20% of patients. This, when combined with preoperative UDS, can provide the clinician with a better understanding of a patient's unique voiding signature [92]. Theofrastous and coworkers reported improvement in the length of postoperative bladder catheterization in postmenopausal women undergoing pelvic organ prolapse repair with preoperative estrogen replacement [93].

When reviewing the different surgeries for prolapse and their resultant effects on voiding function, we will organize the discussion into compartments: anterior, apical, and posterior. Anterior compartment prolapse typically refers to prolapse of the bladder (cystocele). Apical prolapse is usually the uterus or vaginal cuff post-hysterectomy. It can also, rarely, describe enteroceles. Posterior prolapse is typically prolapse of the rectum (rectocele). While organ-specific terminology is often used to describe the prolapse, it is prudent to use the more generic compartment to describe type of prolapse as on physical exam alone it is impossible to truly determine which organ is prolapsing.

Anterior Prolapse

Solitary anterior compartment prolapse without concomitant apical prolapse is rare. However, in the clinical scenario where this were to occur, anterior colporrhaphy, a native tissue repair, is

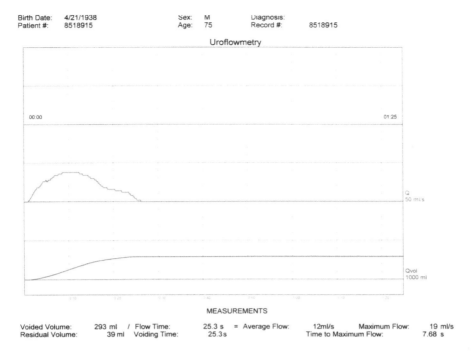

Fig. 10 Adequate and a normal flow curve is often reassuring after a period of postpelvic surgery voiding dysfunction

the most commonly performed surgical treatment. Outcomes of this procedure are durable, and suture material used (rapid absorbable multifilament suture compared to slowly absorbable monofilament suture) has not been shown to affect recurrence rate [94].

For women with concomitant SUI and cystocele, anterior colporrhaphy can be performed along with sling placement. Ahmed et al. compared whether transvaginal mesh was more effective than a transobturator midurethral sling with anterior colporrhaphy at treating comorbid SUI at the time of cystocele repair. The authors found that the mesh group tended to have better objective, subjective, and anatomical outcomes than the group with native tissue repair and midurethral sling, although these differences did not reach statistical significance. The combined treatment group also had more short-term voiding dysfunction at 3 months that resolved by 1 year [95]. While the authors concluded that there is no significant difference in outcomes with combined approach versus 4-armed subvesical vaginal mesh, the utilization of mesh for prolapse repair has fallen out of favor and is, in fact, associated with a serious warning by the FDA for significant postoperative complications. In fact, other studies have shown that prosthetic device use for repair of prolapse results in significantly more complications, such as vaginal erosion, bleeding, infection, pain, or urethral and bladder perforation [96].

There is scant literature describing voiding dysfunction after anterior colporrhaphy. Lakeman et al. performed UDS on 17 women postoperative day 1 after anterior colporrhaphy and found no significant evidence of bladder outlet obstruction. Overall, detrusor pressure and maximum flow rate remained equivalent preoperatively and postoperatively [97]. In our experience, for women with symptomatic cystoceles or other anterior compartment prolapse, native tissue repair represents the safest and most durable treatment option. Attendant SUI can be addressed with a midurethral sling with minimal additional complication risk or voiding dysfunction.

Apical Prolapse

There are multiple surgical treatment options for the repair of apical compartment prolapse. These therapies can be performed transabdominally or transvaginally depending on patient factors such as prior surgeries and surgeon preference and comfort. Uterine descent is the most common cause of apical prolapse, and there is significant debate regarding utility of hysteropexy or vault suspension post hysterectomy as the therapy of choice for this form of apical prolapse. Schulten et al. performed a study on women with stage II uterine prolapse comparing sacrospinous hysteropexy to vaginal hysterectomy with uterosacral ligament suspension and found a greater risk of recurrent apical prolapse in the hysterectomy with uterosacral ligament suspension group at 5 years [98]. The patients undergoing sacrospinous hysteropexy also had greater subjective improvement in symptoms. This group identified specific risk factors for recurrence of prolapse after both procedures and found body mass index, smoking, and POP-Q point Ba were statistically significant risk factors for their composite outcome of failure (prolapse beyond the hymen, bothersome bulge symptoms, repeated surgery, or pessary use for recurrent prolapse) in the period of 5 years after surgery [99]. Of note, the authors also showed that vaginal hysterectomy was a risk factor for posterior compartment recurrence when compared with sacrospinous hysteropexy.

A randomized controlled trial out of the Netherlands compared sacrospinous hysteropexy with vaginal hysterectomy and uterosacral ligament suspension and found that sacrospinous hysteropexy was noninferior to hysterectomy with ligament suspension for preventing recurrence apical prolapse at 12 months [100]. This group also found no difference in sexual function postoperatively after the two procedures [101]. Similarly, a randomized clinical trial comparing uterosacral ligament suspension with sacrospinous ligament suspension with or without perioperative behavioral therapy found no significant difference in surgical or anatomic failure with either surgical technique [102]. A recent systematic review and meta-analysis comparing sacrospinous ligament suspension and uterosacral ligament suspension for apical prolapse found no significant difference in efficacy and complication rates for patients. However, sacrospinous ligament suspension seems to have lower complication rates of vaginal granulation tissue and urethral injury. It is also associated with shorter operative time and thus greater surgeon preference [103].

When examining the risk of de novo or recurrent voiding symptoms after apical prolapse surgery, Cespedes reported outcomes of treating total vault prolapse with concomitant stress urinary incontinence using bilateral sacrospinous ligament fixation through an anterior vaginal approach in 28 patients. All patients had grade 3 or 4 vault prolapse, and all patients had associated enteroceles, cystoceles, and/or rectoceles. At a mean follow-up of 17 months (range 5 to 35 months), SUI had been cured in all patients; however, two patients continued to have mild urge incontinence requiring less than one pad per day. One patient had elevated PVR volumes requiring intermittent catheterization for 2 months [104]. The technique of bilateral sacrospinous ligament fixation was also described more recently by Solomon et al., with almost 37% of all patients requiring short-term Foley catheterization postprocedure [105].

There are defined risk factors for voiding dysfunction after extensive vaginal reconstructive surgery with or without mesh for pelvic organ prolapse. According to Lo et al. patients with diabetes mellitus, concurrent midurethral sling insertion, preoperative detrusor pressure at maximal flow <10 cm H_2O, and postvoid residual volume ≥ 200 ml in patients with advanced pelvic organ prolapse (stage III or IV) were more likely to experience voiding dysfunction postoperatively [106]. Sacrocolpopexy is a commonly performed surgical treatment for apical prolapse, performed via an abdominal approach. Now performed primarily minimally invasively, sacrocolpopexy is often compared to transvaginal repairs in terms of safety and outcomes. Haraki et al. found that sacrocolpopexy resulted in fewer episodes of postoperative acute urinary retention, urinary tract infections, and ED visits for voiding difficulty [107]. Minimally invasive sacrocolpopexy was also associated with fewer 30-day readmissions

[108]. On the contrary, Eto et al. found no significant differences between vaginal uterosacral ligament suspension, sacrospinous ligament fixation, and robotic sacrocolpopexy in terms of transient voiding dysfunction postapical prolapse repair. Concomitant anti-incontinence procedure, however, was associated with increased risk of postoperative voiding dysfunction [109].

Postoperative urinary retention has been reported in 13–32% of patients that undergo pelvic organ prolapse (POP) repair. Yune et al. compared rates of urinary retention between transvaginal and robotic transabdominal approaches and identified risk factors for postoperative urinary retention following POP repair. Out of 484 patients reviewed, 333 underwent POP repair with a transvaginal approach, and 151 underwent robotic-assisted sacrocolpopexy. Postoperative urinary retention was identified in 128 (26.4%) patients, where 113 underwent transvaginal high uterosacral ligament suspension and 15 underwent robotic-assisted sacrocolpopexy. The odds ratio (OR) of postoperative urinary retention following transvaginal high uterosacral ligament suspension was 3.26 (CI 1.72–6.18; P < 0.001) compared to robotic-assisted sacrocolpopexy. Older age was also a risk factor for postoperative urinary retention (OR 1.03, CI 1.01–1.05; P = 0.012). While parity, preoperative PVR, and rates of concomitant transvaginal anterior/posterior repair were significantly higher in patients that developed postoperative urinary retention on univariate analysis, these factors did not demonstrate significance on multivariate analysis. [110] Postoperative pain has also been found to be a significant predictor of urinary retention after vaginal reconstructive procedures [111]. When comparing laparoscopic and robotic approach to sacrocolpopexy, Turner et al. did not find any significant predictors of postoperative urinary retention [112].

Posterior Prolapse

Posterior vaginal wall prolapse almost universally refers to rectocele repair. The most commonly performed surgical repair is a plication given its ease of performance and durability. Urinary incontinence is not usually associated with posterior wall prolapse or repair of such prolapse, as the most common symptoms associated with the defect are related to defecation. A systematic review showed that surgery in the posterior vaginal compartment typically has a high rate of success for anatomical outcomes, obstructed defecation, and bulge symptoms, although these improvements may not be durable in the long term. Additionally, to ensure maximized outcomes, a native-tissue transvaginal rectocele repair should be preferentially performed [113].

Voiding Dysfunction After Endometriosis Surgery

As previously discussed, dissection close to the autonomic nerve plexuses of the sacral spinal cord can risk damage to both pre- and postganglionic nerves responsible for synergic voiding. While the focus of this chapter has been on voiding dysfunction after gynecologic surgery, colorectal surgery and deep pelvic surgery for endometriosis have also been associated with significant effect on postoperative voiding parameters.

There is an entire body of literature examining voiding function after colorectal surgery for endometriosis. Dubernard et al. found that the most common pelvic locations for endometriosis deposits were involving the intestine, specifically colorectum, with a smaller component involving the rectovaginal septum. In their study looking at 86 women who underwent laparoscopic surgery for deep pelvic endometriosis, almost all patients reported significant urinary complications, consisting of hesitancy (p = 0.02), strain to start (p = 0.04), stopping flow (p = 0.01), incomplete emptying (p = 0.008), and reduced stream (p = 0.02) [114]. De novo hesitancy (p = 0.02), stopping flow (p = 0.02), and incomplete emptying (p = 0.004) occurred more frequently after colorectal resection than after resection of other locations [114]. The authors found that urinary complications mainly occurred after segmental colorectal endometriosis resection combined with bilateral uterosacral ligament resection.

This suggests that while anatomic preservation of autonomic plexuses contributes greatly to our patients' ability to engage in normal micturition, there is a not insignificant contribution of pelvic fascial support that should also be preserved.

Two recent systematic reviews and meta-analyses sought to describe outcomes after colorectal surgery for endometriosis. Bendifallah et al. specifically assessed the impact type of surgery for colorectal endometriosis – rectal shaving, discoid resection, or segmental colorectal resection – had on surgical outcomes. Of 168 articles that were eligible, 60 were included in the qualitative analysis, and 9 described voiding dysfunction <30 days after surgery. Disc excision was associated with more voiding dysfunction <30 days than rectal shaving (OR = 12.9; 95% CI, 1.40–119.34; p = 0.02; and I2 = 0%) [115]. No difference was found in the occurrence of voiding dysfunction <30 days between segmental resection and rectal shaving (OR = 3.05; 95% CI, 0.55–16.87; p = 0.20; and I2 = 0%) or between segmental colorectal and discoid resections (OR = 0.99; 95% CI, 0.54–1.85; p = 0.99; and I2 = 71%) [115]. Vesale et al. performed a similar review, finding 201 articles suitable for eligibility, with 51 reviewed systematically, and 13 included in the meta-analysis. Rectal shaving was statistically less associated with postoperative voiding dysfunction than segmental colorectal resection (Odds ratio [OR] 0.34; 95% confidence intervals [CI], 0.18–0.63; I2 = 0%; and p < 0.001) or discoid excision (OR 0.22; 95% CI, 0.09–0.51; I2 = 0%; and p < 0.001) [116]. No significant difference was noted when comparing discoid excision and segmental colorectal resection. Likewise, rectal shaving was associated with a lower risk of self-catheterization >1 month than segmental colorectal resection (OR 0.3; 95% CI, 0.14–0.66; I2 = 0%; and p = 0.003) [116]. The researchers concluded that colorectal surgery for endometriosis has a significant impact on urinary function regardless of technique. However, rectal shaving causes less postoperative voiding dysfunction than discoid excision or segmental resection.

Investigators from Switzerland evaluated the prognostic factors for developing voiding dysfunction after surgery for deep infiltrating endometriosis (DIE). They studied 198 women with endometriosis of the posterior compartment who underwent surgery and a postoperative bladder scan. They found that 41% of the patients initially experienced voiding dysfunction (defined as >100 mL postvoid residual urine volume at second bladder scan) [117]. Among those with a need for self-catheterization after discharge (n = 17), voiding dysfunction lasted for a median of 41 days before a return to residual urine volume of <100 mL. The preoperative presence of DIE nodules in the ENZIAN compartment B was associated with postoperative voiding dysfunction (p = 0.001). The hazard ratio for elevated residual urine volume was highest when the disease stage was B3 (hazard ratio 6.43; CI, 2.3–18.2; and p < 0.001), describing a nodule diameter of >3 cm in lateral distension [117].

Spagnolo et al. performed urodynamic evaluation and anorectal manometry on women who underwent bowel shaving for bulky posterior DIE. Intestinal and urinary function was evaluated in patients with bulky posterior DIE (>30 mm in largest diameter) using urodynamic and anorectal manometry. Results of urodynamic studies and anorectal manometry were similar before and after nerve-sparing surgical excision of the posterior DIE nodule, suggesting that nerve-sparing does not influence the motility or sensory capacity of the bladder and rectosigmoid colon [118]. This is in contradistinction to a study by Bonneau et al., who performed a review of the literature between 1995 and 2012 and found that in women undergoing surgery for DIE, nerve-sparing did result in improvement in urodynamic parameters and incidence of voiding dysfunction [119]. The authors also found that in women with colorectal endometriosis, about half of all the patients had abnormal preoperative urodynamic test results. DIE surgery is associated with a risk of urinary dysfunction mainly corresponding to de novo voiding dysfunction in 1.4% to 29.2% of cases with a mean value of 4.8% [119]. Risk factors of postoperative voiding dysfunction are the need for partial colpectomy, parametrectomy, and patients requiring colo-anal anastomosis. For patients with urinary tract endometriosis, the incidence of preoperative voiding dysfunction is comprised between 24.4% and 79.2% with a rate of postoperative voiding dysfunction ranging from 0% to 16.9% with a mean value of 11.1% [119].

Other predictors of voiding dysfunction after endometriosis surgery include need for parametrectomy at the time of surgery [120]. Concomitant resection of the uterus, uterosacral ligaments, and vagina along with the parametrium also significantly increases the incidence of postoperative voiding dysfunction [120]. Once again, the role of the uterosacral ligaments has been described in ensuring adequate normal voiding parameters post endometrial surgery. The anatomic basis has already been previously discussed, with these ligaments serving as scaffolding for the female pelvic structures, but additionally studies have found that the inferior hypogastric plexus sits just cephalad to the proximal portion of the uterosacral ligaments, and thus may inadvertently get damaged by resection of these structures either unilateral- or bilaterally [121].

Voiding Dysfunction After Colorectal Surgery

The most commonly studied colorectal procedures resulting in postoperative voiding dysfunction are low anterior resection (LAR) and abdominoperineal resection (APR). A cross-sectional Danish study examining urinary voiding patterns and quality of life postsurgical treatment for colorectal cancer found voiding (p < 0.0001) and incontinence scores (p < 0.0001) were significantly higher after treatment for rectal cancer than after colon cancer. In the rectal cancer group, abdominoperineal excision was found to be a significant risk factor for both voiding (p < 0.0001) and incontinence (p = 0.011), while radiotherapy only impaired continence (p = 0.014) [122]. When comparing men and women who underwent APR for rectal cancer, Ledebo et al. reported that 36% of the men and 57% of the women were incontinent postoperatively, compared to 15% and 37% of the men and women in the "normal" reference group [123]. This suggests that while women at baseline are more likely to experience urinary incontinence, they should still be counseled that they are at increased risk of experiencing de novo voiding dysfunction after APR than their male counterparts.

Risk factors for de novo voiding dysfunction after APR include tumors situated between 4 and 8 cm from the anal verge and lymphadenectomy that includes more than ten nodes. These tumor and surgical characteristics are more likely to result in autonomic nerve damage [124]. A seminal study describing the urodynamic parameters after APR found a significant decrease in effective bladder capacity and increases in first sensation to void and residual urine postoperatively [125]. Expected peak and average urinary flow rates can also be expected to decrease significantly post-APR. On the contrary, researchers found no significant changes in urethral sphincter electromyography [125]. These findings as a whole suggest that damage to parasympathetic nerves (sacral plexus) results in an atonic bladder with diminished contractile ability, often necessitating intermittent catheterization after APR.

Low anterior resection, typically preferred for treatment of proximal rectal cancers, has fewer data describing significant postoperative voiding dysfunction. While APR is more likely to result in postoperative micturition difficulty, performing a concomitant lateral pelvic lymph node dissection (LPLD) at the time of LAR has been shown to result in an increased need for medication for voiding difficulty postoperatively [126]. In fact, LPLD was the single most important factor predicting urinary dysfunction post LAR [126]. A "low anterior resection" syndrome has also been described but predominantly involves defecatory dysfunction with occasional voiding symptoms [127, 128]. For those experiencing significant urinary symptoms, both posterior and tibial nerve stimulation have been reported to result in meaningful symptom relief [129].

Conclusion

Female bladder outlet obstruction after pelvic surgery is a multifaceted and dynamic topic. Short-term and long-term bladder dysfunction remains a common side effect after radical hysterectomy, with bladder atony reported in as many as 42% of patients. Bladder outlet obstruction can occur after a Marshall-Marchetti-Krantz procedure, Burch colposuspension, midurethral sling, and pubovaginal sling procedure. Urethral erosion may occasionally manifest with obstructive or irritative voiding symptoms. Most patients with advanced pelvic organ prolapse and elevated post void residual volumes had normalization of residual volumes after surgical correction of the pelvic organ prolapse. Postoperative stress incontinence may occur in 10% of patients when the bladder neck and urethra are not adequately supported. Evaluation of voiding dysfunction after female pelvic surgery should take into account risk factors for obstructive voiding, operative details, as well as clinical data such as cystoscopic, postvoid residual, PVR, and urodynamic findings. Treatment of postpelvic surgery voiding dysfunction includes the gamut of watchful waiting and clean intermittent catheterization to sling incision or removal, urethrolysis, recurrent prolapse repair, or even more complex repair with Martius flap incorporation. Colorectal surgery is also associated with postoperative voiding dysfunction, most likely due to autonomic nerve damage, and is characterized by an atonic bladder with fixed external urethral sphincter tone.

References

1. de Groat WC, Yoshimura N. Anatomy and physiology of the lower urinary tract. Handb Clin Neurol. 2015;130:61.
2. Anderson KE. Pharmacology of lower urinary tract smooth muscles and penile erectile tissues. Pharmacol Rev. 1993;45:253.
3. Andersson KE, Arner A. Urinary bladder contraction and relaxation: physiology and pathophysiology. Physiol Rev. 2004;84:935.
4. Gosling J. The structure of the bladder and urethra in relation to function. Urol Clin North Am. 1979;6:31.
5. Havenga K, DeRuiter MC, Enker WE, et al. Anatomical basis of autonomic nerve-preserving total mesorectal excision for rectal cancer. Br J Surg. 1996;83:384.
6. De Groat WC. Spinal cord projections and neuropeptides in visceral afferent neurons. Prog Brain Res. 1986;67:165.
7. de Groat WC, Griffiths D, Yoshimura N. Neural control of the lower urinary tract. Compr Physiol. 2015;5:327.

8. DeLancey JO. Functional anatomy of the female lower urinary tract and pelvic floor. Ciba Found Symp. 1990;151:57.
9. DeLancey JO. Structural support of the urethra as it relates to stress urinary incontinence: the hammock hypothesis. Am J Obstet Gynecol. 1994;170:1713.
10. Westby M, Asmussen M, Ulmsten U. Location of maximum intraurethral pressure related to urogenital diaphragm in the female subject as studied by simultaneous urethrocystometry and voiding urethrocystography. Am J Obstet Gynecol. 1982;144:408.
11. Asmussen M, Ulmsten U. On the physiology of continence and pathophysiology of stress incontinence in the female. Contrib Gynecol Obstet. 1983;10:32.
12. DeLancey JO. The hidden epidemic of pelvic floor dysfunction: achievable goals for improved prevention and treatment. Am J Obstet Gynecol. 2005;192:1488.
13. Petros PE, Ulmsten U. I.: an integral theory of female urinary incontinence. Experimental and clinical considerations. Acta Obstet Gynecol Scand Suppl. 1990;153:7.
14. Gomelsky A, Nitti VW, Dmochowski RR. Management of obstructive voiding dysfunction after incontinence surgery: lessons learned. Urology. 2003;62:391.
15. Harrison SC, Hunnam GR, Farman P, et al. Bladder instability and denervation in patients with bladder outflow obstruction. Br J Urol. 1987;60:519.
16. Speakman MJ, Brading AF, Gilpin CJ, et al. Bladder outflow obstruction–a cause of denervation supersensitivity. J Urol. 1987;138:1461.
17. Cardozo LD, Stanton SL, Williams JE. Detrusor instability following surgery for genuine stress incontinence. Br J Urol. 1979;51:204.
18. Patel BN, Kobashi KC, Staskin D. Iatrogenic obstruction after sling surgery. Nat Rev Urol. 2012;9:429.
19. Tse V, Chan L. Outlet obstruction after sling surgery. BJU Int. 2011;108(Suppl 2):24.
20. Cheung F, Sandhu JS. Voiding dysfunction after non-urologic pelvic surgery. Curr Urol Rep. 2018;19:75.
21. Tran H, Rutman M. Female outlet obstruction after anti-incontinence surgery. Urology. 2018;112:1.
22. Murray S, Lemack GE. Defining the role of urodynamics in predicting voiding dysfunction after anti-incontinence surgery: a work in progress. Curr Opin Urol. 2010;20:285.
23. Sweeney DD, Leng WW. Treatment of postoperative voiding dysfunction following incontinence surgery. Curr Urol Rep. 2005;6:365.
24. McGuire EJ, Letson W, Wang S. Transvaginal urethrolysis after obstructive urethral suspension procedures. J Urol. 1989;142:1037.
25. Nitti VW, Raz S. Obstruction following anti-incontinence procedures: diagnosis and treatment with transvaginal urethrolysis. J Urol. 1994;152:93.
26. Cross CA, Cespedes RD, English SF, et al. Transvaginal urethrolysis for urethral obstruction after anti-incontinence surgery. J Urol. 1998;159:1199.

27. Miller EA, Amundsen CL, Toh KL, et al. Preoperative urodynamic evaluation may predict voiding dysfunction in women undergoing pubovaginal sling. J Urol. 2003;169:2234.

28. Duckett JR, Basu M. The predictive value of preoperative pressure-flow studies in the resolution of detrusor overactivity and overactive bladder after tension-free vaginal tape insertion. BJU Int. 2007;99:1439.

29. Panayi DC, Duckett J, Digesu GA, et al. Pre-operative opening detrusor pressure is predictive of detrusor overactivity following TVT in patients with pre-operative mixed urinary incontinence. Neurourol Urodyn. 2009;28:82.

30. Liang CC, Hsieh WC, Lin YH, et al. Predictors of persistent detrusor overactivity in women with pelvic organ prolapse following transvaginal mesh repair. J Obstet Gynaecol Res. 2016;42:427.

31. Artman LE, Hoskins WJ, Bibro MC, et al. Radical hysterectomy and pelvic lymphadenectomy for stage IB carcinoma of the cervix: 21 years experience. Gynecol Oncol. 1987;28:8.

32. Mundy AR. An anatomical explanation for bladder dysfunction following rectal and uterine surgery. Br J Urol. 1982;54:501.

33. Roovers JP, van der Bom JG, Huub van der Vaart C, et al. Does mode of hysterectomy influence micturition and defecation? Acta Obstet Gynecol Scand. 2001;80:945.

34. Everaert K, De Muynck M, Rimbaut S, et al. Urinary retention after hysterectomy for benign disease: extended diagnostic evaluation and treatment with sacral nerve stimulation. BJU Int. 2003;91:497.

35. Wyndaele JJ. Is abnormal electrosensitivity in the lower urinary tract a sign of neuropathy? Br J Urol. 1993;72:575.

36. Weber AM, Walters MD, Schover LR, et al. Functional outcomes and satisfaction after abdominal hysterectomy. Am J Obstet Gynecol. 1999;181:530.

37. Chuang TY, Yu KJ, Penn IW, et al. Neurourological changes before and after radical hysterectomy in patients with cervical cancer. Acta Obstet Gynecol Scand. 2003;82:954.

38. Lin LY, Wu JH, Yang CW, et al. Impact of radical hysterectomy for cervical cancer on urodynamic findings. Int Urogynecol J Pelvic Floor Dysfunct. 2004;15:418.

39. Ghezzi F, Cromi A, Uccella S, et al. Immediate Foley removal after laparoscopic and vaginal hysterectomy: determinants of postoperative urinary retention. J Minim Invasive Gynecol. 2007;14:706.

40. Scotti RJ, Bergman A, Bhatia NN, et al. Urodynamic changes in urethrovesical function after radical hysterectomy. Obstet Gynecol. 1986;68:111.

41. Benedetti-Panici P, Zullo MA, Plotti F, et al. Long-term bladder function in patients with locally advanced cervical carcinoma treated with neoadjuvant chemotherapy and type 3-4 radical hysterectomy. Cancer. 2004;100:2110.

42. Laterza RM, Sievert KD, de Ridder D, et al. Bladder function after radical hysterectomy for cervical cancer. Neurourol Urodyn. 2015;34:309.

43. Chen GD, Lin LY, Wang PH, et al. Urinary tract dysfunction after radical hysterectomy for cervical cancer. Gynecol Oncol. 2002;85:292.

44. Axelsen SM, Petersen LK. Urogynaecological dysfunction after radical hysterectomy. Eur J Surg Oncol. 2006;32:445.

45. Long CY, Hsu SC, Wu TP, et al. Effect of laparoscopic hysterectomy on bladder neck and urinary symptoms. Aust N Z J Obstet Gynaecol. 2003;43:65.

46. Virtanen H, Mäkinen J, Tenho T, et al. Effects of abdominal hysterectomy on urinary and sexual symptoms. Br J Urol. 1993;72:868.

47. Long CY, Jang MY, Chen SC, et al. Changes in vesicourethral function following laparoscopic hysterectomy versus abdominal hysterectomy. Aust N Z J Obstet Gynaecol. 2002;42:259.

48. Possover M, Stöber S, Plaul K, et al. Identification and preservation of the motoric innervation of the bladder in radical hysterectomy type III. Gynecol Oncol. 2000;79:154.

49. Puntambekar SP, Patil A, Joshi SN, et al. Preservation of autonomic nerves in laparoscopic total radical hysterectomy. J Laparoendosc Adv Surg Tech A. 2010;20:813.

50. Manchana T, Prasartsakulchai C, Santingamkun A. Long-term lower urinary tract dysfunction after radical hysterectomy in patients with early postoperative voiding dysfunction. Int Urogynecol J. 2010;21:95.

51. Forsgren C, Lundholm C, Johansson AL, et al. Vaginal hysterectomy and risk of pelvic organ prolapse and stress urinary incontinence surgery. Int Urogynecol J. 2012;23:43.

52. Huang HK, Ding DC. Pelvic organ prolapse surgery following hysterectomy with benign indication: a national cohort study in Taiwan. Int Urogynecol J. 2018;29:1669.

53. Dörflinger A, Monga A. Voiding dysfunction. Curr Opin Obstet Gynecol. 2001;13:507.

54. Wang A. C.: Burch colposuspension vs. Stamey bladder neck suspension. A comparison of complications with special emphasis on detrusor instability and voiding dysfunction. J Reprod Med. 1996;41:529.

55. Klutke JJ, Klutke CG, Bergman J, et al. Bladder neck suspension for stress urinary incontinence: how does it work? Neurourol Urodyn. 1999;18:623.

56. Zimmern PE, Hadley HR, Leach GE, et al. Female urethral obstruction after Marshall-Marchetti-Krantz operation. J Urol. 1987;138:517.

57. Conrad DH, Pacquee S, Saar TD, et al. Long-term patient-reported outcomes after laparoscopic Burch colposuspension. Aust N Z J Obstet Gynaecol. 2019;59:850.

58. Holschneider CH, Solh S, Lebherz TB, et al. The modified Pereyra procedure in recurrent stress urinary incontinence: a 15-year review. Obstet Gynecol. 1994;83:573.

59. Kjølhede P, Wahlström J, Wingren G. Pelvic floor dysfunction after Burch colposuspension–a comprehensive study. Part II Acta Obstet Gynecol Scand. 2005;84:902.

60. Karram MM, Segal JL, Vassallo BJ, et al. Complications and untoward effects of the tension-free vaginal tape procedure. Obstet Gynecol. 2003;101:929.

61. Lemack GE, Krauss S, Litman H, et al. Normal preoperative urodynamic testing does not predict voiding dysfunction after Burch colposuspension versus pubovaginal sling. J Urol. 2008;180:2076.

62. Romics M, Keszthelyi V, Brodszky V, et al. Narrow vagina as a predictor of obstructive voiding dysfunction after Transobturator sling surgery. Urol Int. 2021;105:1092.

63. Yang PS, Delpe S, Kowalik CG, et al. Risk factor of De novo urgency and urge incontinence after autologous fascia Pubovaginal sling. Res Rep Urol. 2021;13:591.

64. Mitsui T, Tanaka H, Moriya K, et al. Clinical and urodynamic outcomes of pubovaginal sling procedure with autologous rectus fascia for stress urinary incontinence. Int J Urol. 2007;14:1076.

65. Milose JC, Sharp KM, He C, et al. Success of autologous pubovaginal sling after failed synthetic mid urethral sling. J Urol. 2015;193:916.

66. Virseda-Chamorro M, Salinas-Casado J, Tapia-Herrero AM, et al. Effect of pelvic organ prolapse repair on detrusor overactivity in women following incontinence surgery: a multivariate analysis. Neurourol Urodyn. 2017;36:2083.

67. Gamble TL, Botros SM, Beaumont JL, et al. Predictors of persistent detrusor overactivity after transvaginal sling procedures. Am J Obstet Gynecol. 2008;199:696.e1.

68. Jonsson Funk M, Siddiqui NY, Pate V, et al. Sling revision/removal for mesh erosion and urinary retention: long-term risk and predictors. Am J Obstet Gynecol. 2013;208:73.e1.

69. Fong ED, Nitti VW. Review article: mid-urethral synthetic slings for female stress urinary incontinence. BJU Int. 2010;106:596.

70. Zimmern PE, Gormley EA, Stoddard AM, et al. Management of recurrent stress urinary incontinence after Burch and sling procedures. Neurourol Urodyn. 2016;35:344.

71. Fusco F, Abdel-Fattah M, Chapple CR, et al. Updated systematic review and meta-analysis of the comparative data on Colposuspensions, Pubovaginal slings, and Midurethral tapes in the surgical treatment of female stress urinary incontinence. Eur Urol. 2017;72:567.

72. Takacs P, Medina CA. Tension-free vaginal tape: poor intraoperative cough test as a predictor of postoperative urinary retention. Int Urogynecol J Pelvic Floor Dysfunct. 2007;18:1445.

73. Hong B, Park S, Kim HS, et al. Factors predictive of urinary retention after a tension-free vaginal tape procedure for female stress urinary incontinence. J Urol. 2003;170:852.

74. Ripperda CM, Kowalski JT, Chaudhry ZQ, et al. Predictors of early postoperative voiding dysfunction and other complications following a midurethral sling. Am J Obstet Gynecol. 2016;215:656.e1.

75. Bazi T, Kerkhof MH, Takahashi SI, et al. Management of post-midurethral sling voiding dysfunction. International Urogynecological association research and development committee opinion. Int Urogynecol J. 2018;29:23.

76. Malacarne DR, Nitti VW. Post-sling urinary retention in women. Curr Urol Rep. 2016;17:83.

77. Croak AJ, Schulte V, Peron S, et al. Transvaginal tape lysis for urinary obstruction after tension-free vaginal tape placement. J Urol. 2003;169:2238.

78. Viereck V, Rautenberg O, Kociszewski J, et al. Mid-urethral sling incision: indications and outcomes. Int Urogynecol J. 2013;24:645.

79. Moksnes LR, Svenningsen R, Schiøtz HA, et al. Sling mobilization in the management of urinary retention after mid-urethral sling surgery. Neurourol Urodyn. 2017;36:1091.

80. Rautenberg, O., Kociszewski, J., Welter, J. et al.: Ultrasound and early tape mobilization–a practical solution for treating postoperative voiding dysfunction. Neurourol Urodyn, 33: 1147, 2014.

81. Nitti VW, Carlson KV, Blaivas JG, et al. Early results of pubovaginal sling lysis by midline sling incision. Urology. 2002;59:47.

82. Thiel DD, Pettit PD, McClellan WT, et al. Long-term urinary continence rates after simple sling incision for relief of urinary retention following fascia lata pubovaginal slings. J Urol. 2005;174:1878.

83. Celik H, Harmanlı O. Evaluation and management of voiding dysfunction after midurethral sling procedures. J Turk Ger Gynecol Assoc. 2012;13:123.

84. Leng WW, Davies BJ, Tarin T, et al. Delayed treatment of bladder outlet obstruction after sling surgery: association with irreversible bladder dysfunction. J Urol. 2004;172:1379.

85. Oliver JL, Raz S. Suprameatal urethrolysis with Martius flap for refractory bladder outflow obstruction following stress incontinence surgery in females. Neurourol Urodyn. 2018;37:449.

86. Madhu C, Swift S, Moloney-Geany S, et al. How to use the pelvic organ prolapse quantification (POP-Q) system? Neurourol Urodyn. 2018;37:S39.

87. Swift S, Woodman P, O'Boyle A, et al. Pelvic organ support study (POSST): the distribution, clinical definition, and epidemiologic condition of pelvic organ support defects. Am J Obstet Gynecol. 2005;192:795.

88. Durnea CM, Khashan AS, Kenny LC, et al. Prevalence, etiology and risk factors of pelvic organ prolapse in premenopausal primiparous women. Int Urogynecol J. 2014;25:1463.

89. Samuelsson EC, Victor FT, Tibblin G, et al. Signs of genital prolapse in a Swedish population of women 20 to 59 years of age and possible related factors. Am J Obstet Gynecol. 1999;180:299.

90. Maher, C., Feiner, B., Baessler, K. et al.: Surgical management of pelvic organ prolapse in women. Cochrane Database Syst Rev: Cd004014, 2013.

91. Fitzgerald MP, Kulkarni N, Fenner D. Postoperative resolution of urinary retention in patients with advanced pelvic organ prolapse. Am J Obstet Gynecol. 2000;183:1361.
92. Chen A, McIntyre B, De EJB. Management of Postoperative Lower Urinary Tract Symptoms (LUTS) after pelvic organ prolapse (POP) repair. Curr Urol Rep. 2018;19:74.
93. Theofrastous JP, Addison WA, Timmons M. C.: voiding function following prolapse surgery. Impact of estrogen replacement. J Reprod Med. 1996;41:881.
94. Valtersson E, Husby KR, Elmelund M, et al. Evaluation of suture material used in anterior colporrhaphy and the risk of recurrence. Int Urogynecol J. 2020;31:2011.
95. Ahmed AA, Abdellatif AH, El-Helaly HA, et al. Concomitant transobturator tape and anterior colporrhaphy versus transobturator subvesical mesh for cystocele-associated stress urinary incontinence. Int Urogynecol J. 2020;31:1633.
96. Balzarro M, Rubilotta E, Porcaro AB, et al. Long-term follow-up of anterior vaginal repair: a comparison among colporrhaphy, colporrhaphy with reinforcement by xenograft, and mesh. Neurourol Urodyn. 2018;37:278.
97. Lakeman MM, Hakvoort RA, Van de Weijer EP, et al. Anterior colporrhaphy does not induce bladder outlet obstruction. Int Urogynecol J. 2012;23:723.
98. Schulten SFM, Detollenaere RJ, Stekelenburg J, et al. Sacrospinous hysteropexy versus vaginal hysterectomy with uterosacral ligament suspension in women with uterine prolapse stage 2 or higher: observational follow-up of a multicentre randomised trial. BMJ. 2019;366:l5149.
99. Schulten SF, Detollenaere RJ, IntHout J, et al. Risk factors for pelvic organ prolapse recurrence after sacrospinous hysteropexy or vaginal hysterectomy with uterosacral ligament suspension. Am J Obstet Gynecol. 2022;227:252.e1.
100. Detollenaere RJ, den Boon J, Stekelenburg J, et al. Sacrospinous hysteropexy versus vaginal hysterectomy with suspension of the uterosacral ligaments in women with uterine prolapse stage 2 or higher: multicentre randomised non-inferiority trial. BMJ. 2015;351:h3717.
101. Detollenaere RJ, Kreuwel IA, Dijkstra JR, et al. The impact of sacrospinous Hysteropexy and vaginal hysterectomy with suspension of the uterosacral ligaments on sexual function in women with uterine prolapse: a secondary analysis of a randomized comparative study. J Sex Med. 2016;13:213.
102. Jelovsek JE, Barber MD, Brubaker L, et al. Effect of uterosacral ligament suspension vs sacrospinous ligament fixation with or without perioperative behavioral therapy for pelvic organ vaginal prolapse on surgical outcomes and prolapse symptoms at 5 years in the OPTIMAL randomized clinical trial. JAMA. 2018;319:1554.
103. Chen Y, Peng L, Zhang J, et al. Sacrospinous ligament fixation vs uterosacral ligaments suspension for pelvic organ prolapse: a systematic review and meta-analysis. Urology. 2022;166:133.
104. Cespedes RD. Anterior approach bilateral sacrospinous ligament fixation for vaginal vault prolapse. Urology. 2000;56:70.
105. Solomon ER, St Marie P, Jones KA, et al. Anterior bilateral sacrospinous ligament fixation: a safe route for apical repair. Female Pelvic Med Reconstr Surg. 2020;26:e33.
106. Lo TS, Shailaja N, Hsieh WC, et al. Predictors of voiding dysfunction following extensive vaginal pelvic reconstructive surgery. Int Urogynecol J. 2017;28:575.
107. El Haraki AS, Burns J, Crafton CL, et al. Voiding function after sacrocolpopexy versus native tissue transvaginal repair for apical pelvic organ prolapse in an ERAS era: a retrospective cohort study. Int Urogynecol J. 2021;1
108. Berger AA, Tan-Kim J, Menefee SA. Readmission and emergency department visits after minimally invasive sacrocolpopexy and vaginal apical pelvic organ prolapse surgery. Am J Obstet Gynecol. 2021;225:552.e1.
109. Eto C, Ford AT, Smith M, et al. Retrospective cohort study on the perioperative risk factors for transient voiding dysfunction after apical prolapse repair. Female Pelvic Med Reconstr Surg. 2019;25:167.
110. Yune JJ, Cheng JW, Wagner H, et al. Postoperative urinary retention after pelvic organ prolapse repair: vaginal versus robotic transabdominal approach. Neurourol Urodyn. 2018;37:1794.
111. Yadav M, Patel K, Turrentine MA, et al. Postoperative pain and urinary retention after vaginal reconstructive surgery. Female Pelvic Med Reconstr Surg. 2021;27:e497.
112. Turner LC, Kantartzis K, Shepherd JP. Predictors of postoperative acute urinary retention in women undergoing minimally invasive sacral colpopexy. Female Pelvic Med Reconstr Surg. 2015;21:39.
113. Grimes CL, Schimpf MO, Wieslander CK, et al. Surgical interventions for posterior compartment prolapse and obstructed defecation symptoms: a systematic review with clinical practice recommendations. Int Urogynecol J. 2019;30:1433.
114. Dubernard G, Rouzier R, David-Montefiore E, et al. Urinary complications after surgery for posterior deep infiltrating endometriosis are related to the extent of dissection and to uterosacral ligaments resection. J Minim Invasive Gynecol. 2008;15:235.
115. Bendifallah S, Puchar A, Vesale E, et al. Surgical outcomes after colorectal surgery for endometriosis: a systematic review and meta-analysis. J Minim Invasive Gynecol. 2021;28:453.
116. Vesale E, Roman H, Moawad G, et al. Voiding dysfunction after colorectal surgery for endometriosis: a systematic review and meta-analysis. J Minim Invasive Gynecol. 2020;27:1490.

117. Imboden S, Bollinger Y, Härmä K, et al. Predictive factors for voiding dysfunction after surgery for deep infiltrating endometriosis. J Minim Invasive Gynecol. 2021;28:1544.
118. Spagnolo E, Zannoni L, Raimondo D, et al. Urodynamic evaluation and anorectal manometry pre- and post-operative bowel shaving surgical procedure for posterior deep infiltrating endometriosis: a pilot study. J Minim Invasive Gynecol. 2014;21:1080.
119. Bonneau C, Zilberman S, Ballester M, et al. Incidence of pre- and postoperative urinary dysfunction associated with deep infiltrating endometriosis: relevance of urodynamic tests and therapeutic implications. Minerva Ginecol. 2013;65:385.
120. Benoit L, Dabi Y, Bazot M, et al. Parametrial endometriosis: a predictive and prognostic factor for voiding dysfunction and complications. Eur J Obstet Gynecol Reprod Biol. 2022;276:236.
121. Deffieux X, Raibaut P, Hubeaux K, et al. Voiding dysfunction after surgical resection of deeply infiltrating endometriosis: pathophysiology and management. Gynecol Obstet Fertil. 2007;35(Suppl 1):S8.
122. Kristensen MH, Elfeki H, Sinimäki S, et al. Urinary dysfunction after colorectal cancer treatment and impact on quality of life-a national cross-sectional study in males. Color Dis. 2021;23:394.
123. Ledebo A, Bock D, Prytz M, et al. Urogenital function 3 years after abdominoperineal excision for rectal cancer. Color Dis. 2018;20:O123.
124. Burgos FJ, Romero J, Fernandez E, et al. Risk factors for developing voiding dysfunction after abdominoperineal resection for adenocarcinoma of the rectum. Dis Colon Rectum. 1988;31:682.
125. Chang PL, Fan HA. Urodynamic studies before and/or after abdominoperineal resection of the rectum for carcinoma. J Urol. 1983;130:948.
126. Matsuoka H, Masaki T, Sugiyama M, et al. Impact of lateral pelvic lymph node dissection on evacuatory and urinary functions following low anterior resection for advanced rectal carcinoma. Langenbeck's Arch Surg. 2005;390:517.
127. Bulfone G, Del Negro F, Del Medico E, et al. Rehabilitation strategies for low anterior resection syndrome. A systematic review, vol. 56. Ann Ist Super Sanita; 2020. p. 38.
128. Keane C, Wells C, O'Grady G, et al. Defining low anterior resection syndrome: a systematic review of the literature. Color Dis. 2017;19:713.
129. Altomare DF, Picciariello A, Ferrara C, et al. Short-term outcome of percutaneous tibial nerve stimulation for low anterior resection syndrome: results of a pilot study. Color Dis. 2017;19:851.

Bladder Augmentation and Urinary Diversion

17

Henriette Veiby Holm

Contents

Introduction 302

Indications and Options for Bladder Augmentation and Urinary Diversion 303
Indications and Patient Selection 303
Options 304

Preoperative Investigations 304

Bladder Augmentation 306
Surgical Technique 306
Postoperative Care, Outcome, and Complications 307

Continent Catheterizable Channel and Combinations 309
Mitrofanoff CCC 309
Transversely Tubularized Bowel Segments (TTBS): Yang-Monti Channel
and Modifications 310
Continent Cutaneous/Catheterizable Ileocecocystoplasty (CCIC) 312
Hemi-Kock CCC and Cystoplasty 314

Supravesical Urinary Diversion 315
Continent Cutaneous Urinary Diversion 315
Incontinent Urinary Diversion 317

Pregnancy 318

Cross-References 320

References 320

Abstract

Bladder augmentation and urinary diversion are surgical options for patients with bladder storage and emptying disorders, when

conservative measures have failed. Surgical treatment can be required for the preservation of renal function, for incontinence, or for a combination of both. However, it can also be required to regain quality of life in patients with intractable bladder dysfunction without the immediate risk of renal deterioration or severe incontinence. Patients include those with neurogenic lower urinary tract

H. V. Holm (✉)
Section of Reconstructive Urology and Neurourology,
Department of Urology, Oslo University Hospital
Rikshospitalet, Oslo, Norway

© Springer Nature Switzerland AG 2023
F. E. Martins et al. (eds.), *Female Genitourinary and Pelvic Floor Reconstruction*,
https://doi.org/10.1007/978-3-031-19598-3_18

dysfunction (NLUTD) and those with severe idiopathic or iatrogenic (non-neurogenic) lower urinary tract dysfunction (LUTD).

For patients with a bladder emptying disorder but good reservoir function of low pressure, a continent catheterizable channel (CCC) can be an option. In the opposite scenario, in patients with only a storage disorder due to bladder dysfunction such as severe detrusor overactivity or poor compliance, neurogenic or non-neurogenic, a bladder augmentation may be indicated. In the case of concomitant bladder storage and emptying disorder, a combination of augmentation cystoplasty and a continent catheterizable channel is possible, if the patient is suited, and otherwise a supravesical continent or incontinent supravesical urinary diversion may be indicated. Urinary diversion may be a last resort for patients with devastated outlet after iatrogenic injury.

Long-term consequences of bladder augmentation and urinary diversion include recurrent urinary tract infections, bladder/reservoir stones, metabolic disturbance, strictures, and perforation. Nevertheless, these reconstructive options may give appropriately selected patients the opportunity for improved urinary storage capacity, continence, and preservation of renal function, as well as an improved quality of life.

Keywords

Bladder augmentation · Cystoplasty · Urinary diversion · Urinary conduit · Urinary reservoir · Continent catheterizable channel · Cystoenterocutaneostomy · Yang-Monti · Mitrofanoff · Hemi-Kock · Bricker · Devastated bladder outlet

---

Introduction

Bladder augmentation and urinary diversion include many surgical options to treat several conditions and types of patients with bladder storage and emptying disorders. These options are usually only applied after conservative measures have failed. Surgical treatment can be required for the preservation of renal function, for incontinence, or for a combination of both. However, it can also be required to regain quality of life in patients with intractable bladder dysfunction without the immediate risk of renal deterioration or severe incontinence. Patients include those with neurogenic lower urinary tract dysfunction (NLUTD) and those with severe idiopathic or iatrogenic (non-neurogenic) lower urinary tract dysfunction (LUTD). Urinary diversion may be a last resort for patients with devastated outlets after iatrogenic injury.

Bladder storage requires accommodation of increasing volumes of urine without increase of intravesical pressure (normal compliance), absence of involuntary bladder contractions (detrusor overactivity, DO), and competent outlet that remains closed during filling and increases with intra-abdominal pressure. Failure of these functions may result in incontinence, frequency, pain, and potentially upper tract deterioration. Detrusor compliance is defined as the change in detrusor volume divided by the change in detrusor pressure ($\Delta V/\Delta P$) during the urodynamic filling phase [1]. Poor (reduced) compliance often occurs with long-standing obstruction, neurogenic and non-neurogenic, or postradiation. Poor compliance is associated with reduced capacity, elevated intravesical pressures, and vesicoureteral reflux. Increased intravesical pressure due to poor compliance or DO is a risk factor for upper urinary tract deterioration and renal damage.

Bladder emptying requires the simultaneous contraction of the detrusor and relaxation of the outlet. Dyssynergy of the two, commonly seen in neurological patients, or the failure of either, will cause a bladder emptying disorder. Detrusor sphincter dyssynergia is another cause of elevated intravesical pressures that can be detrimental to renal function.

For patients with a bladder emptying disorder (and a bladder with a good reservoir function) but inability to perform urethral clean intermittent self-catheterization (CISC), a continent catheterizable channel (CCC) with an abdominal stoma can be an option. Storage disorders due to reduced bladder compliance, reduced capacity, or severe DO can be treated with augmentation cystoplasty. In the case of concomitant bladder storage *and* emptying disorders, a combination of augmentation cystoplasty and a CCC is possible, if the patient is suited. In other cases, a supravesical urinary diversion may be indicated. Permanent catheter drainage, like a suprapubic cystostomy, may be the right solution for selected patients.

Surgical treatment of severe LUTD warrants careful investigations of the lower urinary tract function and dysfunction, the upper urinary tract function, as well as the patient's general and cognitive condition, to make the right treatment decision for each patient.

In this chapter, we review the indications for and different methods of bladder augmentation and urinary diversion. Urinary diversion following cystectomy for bladder cancer specifically is not covered in this book, neither are congenital abnormalities and the pediatric population. Some historic perspectives will be mentioned but not in detail.

Indications and Options for Bladder Augmentation and Urinary Diversion

Indications and Patient Selection

Augmentation cystoplasty effectively improves bladder compliance, capacity, and incontinence in patients with refractory detrusor overactivity (DO), impaired compliance, or reduced capacity secondary to, e.g., radiation therapy. Inability to perform urethral clean intermittent self-catheterization (CISC) may be alleviated by a continent catheterizable channel (CCC) with an abdominal stoma. In severe cases of bladder dysfunction or devastated outlet, a supravesical urinary diversion should be considered. Individualized treatment selection is crucial for a successful outcome for each patient.

Patients include those with neurogenic lower urinary tract dysfunction (NLUTD) and those with severe idiopathic, iatrogenic, or post-traumatic lower urinary tract dysfunction (LUTD). The EAU and AUA/SUFU Guidelines briefly mention bladder augmentation and urinary diversion in the chapters *Neuro-urology/NLUTD*, respectively, but hardly, if at all, in the chapters *Non-neurogenic Female LUTS/Incontinence/Overactive Bladder*, respectively [2, 3]. However, this option should not be overlooked in the non-neurogenic population with severe LUTD.

Congenital abnormalities including bladder exstrophy and epispadias are usually but not always treated in childhood. Nevertheless, these patients may need revisions or new reconstructive solutions as adults. (The pediatric patient population is not covered especially in this book, but some surgical options are similar to other patient groups.)

Neurogenic causes for lower urinary tract dysfunction include spinal cord injury (SCI), multiple sclerosis (MS), spina bifida, Parkinson's disease, etc. In neurogenic patients, preservation of kidney function is just as important as restoring quality of life and continence, as severe NLUTD may be detrimental for the upper urinary tract. Individuals with suprasacral SCI, adult spina bifida, and MS are at the highest risk for elevated intravesical pressures and upper tract deterioration [4].

Idiopathic LUTD include severe detrusor overactivity, sensory urgency, and chronic cystitis including interstitial cystitis, tuberculous cystitis, and schistosomiasis. Iatrogenic causes include any pelvic cancer treatment, surgical and/or radiotherapy, as well as surgery for benign conditions such as sling procedures for incontinence and hysterectomy. The latter group may consist of patients with severe incontinence, radiation cystitis, and fistulas [5]. Trauma may also cause long-lasting LUTD of varying degrees depending on the initial trauma and primary treatment.

While all of the above may be indications for bladder augmentation or urinary diversion, contraindications must be carefully considered. These include patient factors such as age, comorbidities, obesity, previous treatments (especially abdominopelvic surgery and radiotherapy), concomitant lower or upper urinary tract disorders, and/or a so-called devastated bladder outlet. Other factors to be considered include bowel disease (Mb. Crohn, ulcerative colitis, short bowel syndrome, and congenital anomalies), cognitive function, psychiatric illness (e.g., Münchausen syndrome), and manual dexterity.

The exact extent of the lower urinary tract disorder has to be diagnosed, and any concomitant LUTD needs to be identified prior to surgery. Upper urinary tract function or abnormalities may affect the treatment choice and outcome. Pre-existing renal insufficiency may be exacerbated due to electrolyte abnormalities caused by absorption by the bowel mucosa when incorporated into the urinary tract, especially in bladder augmentation and continent reservoirs, where urine is exposed to the mucosa for a long period of time.

Additionally, when choosing continent solutions like bladder augmentation, continent catheterizable channel, and urinary reservoir, patient and caregivers need to understand and handle clean intermittent catheterization at timely intervals.

Hence, complete lower urinary tract investigation and assessment of upper tract function should be performed, as well as careful consideration of the patients' manual dexterity and cognitive function. When the preoperative investigations are completed and the problems identified, one needs to carefully assess which options are available for each patient. Solutions will be different for patients with bladder storage disorders, bladder emptying disorders, or both.

To summarize, in many cases of LUTD of benign (neurogenic or non-neurogenic) etiology in need of reconstructive surgical treatment, the bladder can be preserved and augmented. However, in some cases a supravesical urinary diversion is the most appropriate option for the patient. Moreover, in some cases the LUTD is so severe that the bladder and outlet need to be abandoned and a supravesical urinary diversion will be the only choice [5]. When the available and appropriate options are clear, they need to be discussed with the patient. The final decision depends on the preference and experience of the surgeon responsible for the patient.

Options

There are many reconstructive options for patients with bladder storage and emptying disorders. The different reconstructive solutions will be discussed in more detail in the following paragraphs. The options can be classified as the following (Table 1):

i) Bladder augmentation (BA) aka augmentation cystoplasty (AC), enterocystoplasty
ii) Continent catheterizable channel (CCC) keeping native urinary bladder as reservoir
iii) Supravesical urinary diversion (continent/reservoir or incontinent/conduit)

A combination of bladder augmentation and CCC can be performed if indicated, also sometimes in conjunction with a continence procedure in case of outlet insufficiency.

Preoperative Investigations

Surgical treatment of severe LUTD warrants careful investigations of the exact lower urinary tract dysfunction, the upper urinary tract function, as well as the patient's general and cognitive condition to make the right treatment decision for each patient.

Functional investigations including urodynamic studies are indispensable to evaluate the native urinary bladder capacity and compliance, as well as the urethral function. Urodynamic studies include those of noninvasive and invasive nature, from bladder diaries and pad weighing, free uroflowmetry, cystometry and pressure-flow studies, as well as voiding cystourethrography in some cases.

In case of outlet insufficiency, obstruction, or devastated outlet, a combined procedure may be planned concomitantly as a CCC and/or AC. Patients who have had previous urinary diversion or a permanent suprapubic tube should practice bladder filling/cycling to show whether they have adequate bladder capacity, and their ability to store urine should be evaluated.

A voiding cystography is useful in some cases depending on background, to detect or exclude vesicoureteral reflux and to characterize any voiding dysfunction, such as detrusor sphincter dyssynergia or dysfunctional voiding.

Table 1 Bladder augmentation and urinary diversion options

Reconstructive option	Variants	LUTD indication	
Bladder augmentation	• Gastrocystoplasty • Ileocystoplasty • Cecocystoplasty • Colocystoplasty (sigmoid) • Ureterocystoplasty • Autoaugmentation	Bladder storage	Detrusor overactivity Reduced compliance Reduced capacity
Continent catheterizable channel (CCC)	• Mitrofanoff • Yang-Monti • Modifications: - Double Monti - Spiral Monti	Bladder emptying	Detrusor sphincter dyssynergia Inability to perform CISC Devastated outlet
Combination of bladder augmentation and CCC	• Hemi-Kock continent stoma with augmentation cystoplasty • Ileocecocystoplasty	Bladder storage and emptying	Combination of any of the above
Supravesical urinary diversion	• Continent cutaneous diversion (many variants, e.g., Kock, Mainz, Indiana, Lundiana) • Orthotopic (e.g., Studer, Mayo) • Incontinent cutaneous diversion (e.g., Bricker ileal conduit, ureterostomy)	Severe bladder storage and/or emptying disorder	Patient not suitable for abovementioned options

Cystourethroscopy is mandatory to rule out any additional abnormalities, such as bladder stones, erosion of foreign material, bladder cancer, etc.

Renal insufficiency is a relative contraindication to bladder augmentation and continent supravesical urinary diversion. Assessment of renal function and imaging studies of the upper urinary tract is a mandatory part of the preoperative investigation of patients with severe LUTD. Depending on underlying cause (neurogenic vs. non-neurogenic), renal function can be assessed by creatinine, cystatin C, or a radionuclide glomerular filtration rate measurement. Intravenous pyelography, CT urography, or a radionuclide scan will detect any upper tract obstruction or any other upper tract malformation or dysfunction.

Bladder augmentation leads to a high risk of being unable to void spontaneously; hence the patient or their caregiver needs to be aware, able and willing to perform clean intermittent self-catheterization (CISC). Inability or reluctance/unwillingness to catheterize is therefore a contraindication to bladder augmentation. In case of difficulty with CISC, a catheterizable continent channel (CCC) should be planned for as a

concomitant procedure. Patients with poor dexterity due to paralysis of upper extremities or any other reason are not good candidates for bladder augmentation or a CCC and should rather be considered for an incontinent urinary diversion.

Bowel function assessment is important to detect any contraindication to the procedure being planned (inflammatory bowel disease, diverticulitis, gastric ulcer, short bowel syndrome, radiation therapy) or to plan for concomitant procedures (e.g., a colostomy in case of neurogenic bowel dysfunction). Some authors warn of chronic diarrhea and fecal incontinence if removing the ileocecal valve, especially in the neurogenic population; however, it seems those concerns are unsubstantiated [6]. When choosing which part of bowel to use for augmentation or continent, urinary reservoir assessment of any existing renal impairment and metabolic acidosis, as well as liver failure, should be included. For example, the utilization of ileum and colon can worsen acidosis, and increased absorption of ammonia by the intestine incorporated into the urinary tract can be detrimental to patients with liver failure.

Bladder Augmentation

Bladder augmentation has several synonyms: commonly referred to as augmentation cystoplasty, clam enterocystoplasty, etc., and often specifying the tissue used for augmentation, e.g., ileocystoplasty. The main indication is reconstruction of a dysfunctional bladder when all conservative management has failed, to create a compliant and large-capacity urinary storage unit. It is an effective treatment of reduced bladder compliance and/or capacity and incontinence due to bladder dysfunction. This may protect the upper urinary tract from high intravesical pressures and may provide urinary continence. The EAU Guidelines state that augmentation cystoplasty should be offered to patients with urinary incontinence who have failed all other treatment options; however, indications include many more diagnoses. Some indications have better reported outcomes, i.e., neurogenic or non-neurogenic overactive bladder (92%), than others have, i.e., inflammatory disorders including radiation cystitis (55%) [7]. The use of bladder augmentation in the treatment of interstitial cystitis (IC) and bladder pain syndrome is controversial. However, good results have been reported in classical IC patients with Hunner's lesions and small bladder capacity.

Tizzoni and Foggi were the first to describe augmentation ileocystoplasty in dogs (1888), shortly followed by von Mikulicz describing cystoplasty in humans (1889). Lemoine reported the use of colocystoplasty using sigmoid colon in humans in 1912. Intestinal segments for bladder augmentation gained popularity in the 1950s. The successful introduction of clean intermittent self-catheterization (CISC) by Lapides in 1971 reduced the indications for augmentation cystoplasty in patients with neurogenic bladders [8]. However, it also contributed significantly to the wide acceptance of the procedure by the 1980s and allowed augmentation cystoplasty to be offered to patients with NLUTD who were previously not candidates for this procedure (e.g., SCI patients).

Augmentation with almost any part of the gastrointestinal tract (gastrocystoplasty, ileocystoplasty, cecocystoplasty, colocystoplasty) and other tissues (ureter, gallbladder, fascia, and peritoneum) has been described. Synthetic materials have not yet been successful but are still being investigated [7, 9]. Augmentation with a detubularized patch of ileum is the most commonly used technique nowadays [7], but no single segment represents the perfect substitution, as each has its own complications. The gastrointestinal segment used should be based on the patient's past medical history, the intraoperative findings, and the surgeon's experience.

(Latissimus dorsi detrusor myoplasty was invented for the ease of spontaneous voiding without the need for CISC as a potential treatment for the acontractile bladder and was first reported by Stenzl in 1997, with reported success rates of 70–80% and mild–moderate complications [10, 11]. It has only been used for patients with bladder acontractility, not as an augmentation procedure, and will therefore not be discussed further.)

Surgical Technique

Augmentation cystoplasty is traditionally performed via laparotomy (lower midline or transverse/Pfannenstiel incision), bivalving the bladder coronally (left to right) or sagitally (ventral to dorsal) down to the level of the ureteric orifices and then anastomosing a detubularized segment of bowel onto the bivalved bladder. Extraperitoneal (with only a small fenestration for the harvesting of bowel) and laparoscopic (including robot-assisted) approaches have been described [12]. More important than the approach to the bladder and the direction of the cystotomy is the achievement of the widest possible opening, preventing an hourglass configuration of the enterocystoplasty. The "star modification" is achieved by both sagittal and coronal incision to divide each half of the bladder into two parts [13].

The most commonly used bowel segment is the ileum. It is taken 15–40 cm proximal to the Ileocecal valve to reduce the risk of metabolic acidosis and vitamin B deficiency. The 20–40 cm long segment is detubularized (antimesenteric, often asymmetrically) and usually folded in a U-shaped manner before it is anastomosed to the cystotomy starting posteriorly. The bowel may also be folded into an S or W shape [14, 15].

A suprapubic tube is left in place through the native bladder wall for 3 weeks postoperatively or until the patient is comfortable with starting/resuming CISC. Some surgeons prefer to do a cystogram at the time of removal of the suprapubic tube.

The most common alternative to ileum is the sigmoid colon, although a higher risk of UTI and larger amount of mucus production have been reported [7, 16]. Theoretically, there is a higher long-term risk of malignancy. A segment of 15–20 cm is detubularized and often folded in a U or S shape to give a more effective configuration and adequate bladder capacity. If indicated ureters can be reimplanted into the tenia. Seromuscular colocystoplasty lined with urothelium has been described as an option, in an effort to avoid some of the abovementioned morbidity associated with the use of the sigmoid colon [7, 16].

The cecum can be used in its original shape but is also usually detubularized. It is most commonly used in conjunction with the terminal ileum as an ileocecocystoplasty. The ileum can then be used for reimplantation of ureters (however, not tunneled) if indicated, or it can be used as a continent catheterizable channel (CCC) through the abdominal wall. The appendix can also be utilized as a CCC. This is elaborated in further detail below.

Other possibilities include the use of the stomach (gastrocystoplasty) or a preexisting massively dilated ureter (ureterocystoplasty), the latter mostly utilized in children with megureters and a nonfunctioning kidney. The use of stomach has the advantages that it does not lead to metabolic acidosis, the stomach produces less mucus than other gastrointestinal tract segments, ureters can easily be reimplanted into it, it is rarely included in fields of radiation, it readily decreases bladder pressures, and it has been associated with less stone formation.

Autoaugmentation, i.e., seromyotomy or detrusor myomectomy, is an option for bladders with poor compliance and detrusor overactivity but with normal or modestly reduced bladder capacity. In this procedure, a part of the detrusor is resected off the urothelium, creating a low-pressure bladder diverticulum. The cranial part of the remainder of the detrusor can be hitched to the respective psoas muscles bilaterally. The advantages include a low rate of long-term adverse effects, and it does not preclude further interventions.

Treatment of any sphincter/bladder outlet insufficiency should be considered and if indicated performed simultaneously as augmentation cystoplasty, with either bladder neck closure or a continence procedure, for example, an autologous (fascial) sling, urethrovesical or bladder neck suspension, or an artificial urinary sphincter. A continent catheterizable channel (CCC) can be created to permit bladder emptying and may be indicated in patients with functional or anatomical limitations preventing urethral CISC, including wheelchair dependence and neurologic conditions with reduced upper extremity dexterity. Reimplantation of ureters may also be indicated. These procedures are done before the augmentation cystoplasty, which then will be the last part of the operation.

Postoperative Care, Outcome, and Complications

Routine follow-up after bladder augmentation includes metabolic assessment and evaluation of vitamin B12 deficiency. The latter usually occurs only after 3–5 years after augmentation. Cystoscopic surveillance for tumors in the native bladder or interpolated bowel can be initiated 10 years following enterocystoplasty [14]. The EAU Guidelines state that patients with enterocystoplasty need lifelong surveillance; however, controversy persists over this issue [2, 7]. Long-term follow-up would be indicated to discover any metabolic disturbance (3.4%), renal function deterioration, diverticularization, stone formation (6–52%), and malignancy (4%). Other long-term complications include mucus retention (12.5%), bacteriuria (60%), urinary tract infections (UTI) (8–49%), bowel dysfunction (15%), and spontaneous perforation (1.9–3%) [2, 7, 17].

All gastrointestinal segments produce mucus, which can block spontaneous voiding or catheters, and mucus accumulation is associated with recurrent UTI and stone formation. Hence, daily bladder irrigation of mucus is recommended to decrease the incidence of long-term bladder stone formation and UTI. Clinical experience shows that this is not necessary in all patients, but some authors recommend irrigation with >120–240 mL sterile salt water daily, especially in patients prone to UTI and stones [18, 19]. So-called muco-regulatory drugs, including N-acetylcysteine, aspirin, and ranitidine, have been described to reduce the amount of mucus secretion and urine viscosity [20, 21]; however, their effectiveness could not be confirmed in a randomized, controlled trial [22].

In case of chronic or recurrent UTI, cystoscopy should be performed to look for mucus and stones. CISC through an abdominal CCC increases the risk of mucus accumulation and incomplete bladder emptying and hence UTI and stone formation. The presence of urea-splitting bacteria increases the risk of stone formation and should be treated with antibiotics, even in the absence of UTI symptoms.

Metabolic acidosis is a common complication and can lead to nausea, reduced appetite, and fatigue. If long-standing, metabolic acidosis can lead to demineralization, osteoporosis, and increased fracture risk, although this is rare. Metabolic acidosis can develop in patients with augmented bladders because of the longer-lasting exposure of urine to bowel mucosa. The colon and ileum secrete sodium and bicarbonate and reabsorb ammonia, ammonium, hydrogen ions, and chloride when exposed to urine. The longer the length of bowel used, the higher the risk of metabolic disturbances. In these patients, the renal reserve function can be an important factor because the kidneys need to excrete these reabsorbed molecules and water twice [15]. Many patients are able to compensate the acidosis, but some patients will need treatment with bicarbonate, and they should be monitored closely.

Intestinal dysfunction resulting from the resection of bowel segments is related to the function of the removed and the remaining bowel, not necessarily the length of bowel resected. The terminal ileum is the primary area for absorption of bile acids and vitamin B12. Hence, removal of the terminal ileum can interfere with normal enterohepatic circulation of bile acids, diminishing their absorption, and may cause diarrhea, due to an excessive amount of bile acids reaching the colon, as well as vitamin B12 deficiency. Resection of the ileocecal valve may aggravate this [15].

Spontaneous perforation of the augmented bladder can occur at any time. Perforation is associated with substance abuse, noncompliance with CISC, and the need for assistants to perform and monitor CISC [17]. Episodic overdistension causing bowel ischemia is thought to increase the risk. Diagnosis should be swift, as a delay may cause sepsis and death. Shoulder pain may be a sign of urine irritating the diaphragm. Especially spinal cord-injured patients may be difficult to diagnose correctly, as they may not present with classical symptoms of acute abdomen. A perforation may be missed on CT or cystogram if not done carefully. The bladder should be filled slowly to capacity and then again after the bladder is drained. Standard treatment is surgical repair, but a small perforation may close spontaneously with bladder drainage. Antibiotics and close observation is mandatory.

The incidence of tumors in the augmented bladder are reported to be similar to comparable patient groups (2.5–4%) [17]. However, the diagnosis of tumors may be delayed as hematuria, and frequency is common in this patient group. This may be an argument for routine cystoscopy; however, the random timing of a routine cystoscopy may be too late, as few present with localized disease if only examined routinely and not ad hoc [23]. Hence, new or sudden onset of symptoms should prompt investigations without delay. Tumors have most commonly been reported in the entero-urinary anastomosis [24].

Special considerations and complications for pregnant patients with bladder augmentation are handled at the end of this chapter.

Long-term outcome is reported to be good (53–92%), depending on the underlying disorder, including continence rates up to 100% [7]. As mentioned, patients undergoing augmentation cystoplasty have a high risk of having to perform clean intermittent self-catheterization (10–75%). Long-term success and high rate of CISC are reported more commonly in the neurogenic patient population than the non-neurogenic population [7].

Failure of the cystoplasty to resolve the underlying disorder has been reported in 5–42% of patients. A few patients undergoing bladder augmentation will present with small capacity, poor compliance, recurrent perforation, or persistent incontinence, often due to peristaltic contractions of the intestinal segment despite intraoperative detubularization. These can be treated with anticholinergics, beta3-agonist, botulinum toxin A injections, or augmentation of the augmented bladder [2, 25]. Bladder augmentation revision without additional bowel harvest can be done for certain suboptimal cystoplasty configurations [26]. Conversion to supravesical urinary diversion would be a last resort.

To conclude, we quote the EAU Guidelines: "The long-term scientific evidence shows that bladder augmentation is a highly successful procedure that stabilizes renal function and prevents anatomical deterioration; however, lifelong follow-up is essential in this patient group given the significant morbidity associated with this procedure."

Continent Catheterizable Channel and Combinations

In 1910 Makass published a German article titled: "Treatment of bladder exstrophy, by changing the isolated cecum into urinary bladder and the appendix into urethra" [27]. In 1922, Voelcker described the method in a general surgery textbook, also noting that it was continent and that the patients have to catheterize themselves through the appendix [28]. Mitrofanoff published the use of appendix as a continent vesicostomy for bladder catheterization in 1980 [29]. Since then a variety of techniques and tissue segments have been described for creating a continent catheterizable channel (CCC) to the bladder, including cecum, small bowel, stomach, ureter,

and bladder. Currently the two popular options remain the appendix and Yang-Monti transverse ileal tube, the latter with modifications like "the double Monti" and the "spiral Monti" [6]. Nevertheless, what is today referred to as "the Mitrofanoff principle" is based on the implantation of a supple tube within a submucosal tunnel with firm muscular backing of the detrusor for the continence (valve) mechanism. Filling of the bladder leads to coaptation of the channel, hence providing continence. The goal of the procedure is to achieve a stoma that is continent while it is also easy to catheterize. It should also have an appropriate caliber for mucus drainage and endoscopic manipulation, and it should be easy to perform.

The urinary reservoir can for some patients be their native bladder, for others an augmentation cystoplasty is also indicated, as described above. For the latter patient group, the Mitrofanoff or Yang-Monti CCC can, for example, be combined with an ileocystoplasty. Alternatively, the combination of a CCC and bladder augmentation could be created with a continent ileocecal cystoplasty or a hemi-Kock continent stoma with AC [6, 23].

Some of the most popular surgical techniques in current practice and their outcomes are described briefly below. No perfect solution exists; each has associated complications and relatively high revision rates (15–70%) [23]. For example, Husmann recently reported high stomal complication rates, with 21/30 (70%) for the Yang-Monti, 27/66 (41%) for the Mitrofanoff, and 13/63 (21%) for the ileocecocystoplasty CCC patients. BMI was a significant risk factor (50% of the patients), but even with a normal BMI, the revision rates were 53%, 26%, and 15%, respectively [18].

Mitrofanoff CCC

The particular advantage of the appendix is that it has a small lumen and its wall is relatively thick and robust; thus it forms a reasonably reliable guide for the intermittent passage of the catheter into the lumen of the urinary reservoir. Through a lower midline or Pfannenstiel incision, the bladder and ileocecal junction and appendix are

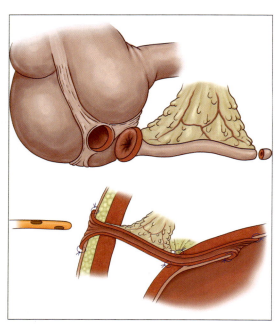

Fig. 1 Mitrofanoff continent catheterizable channel. (Illustration by Yohaksson Arias)

accessible. The appendix is identified and disconnected from the cecum with a cuff, while preserving its mesentery and blood supply (Fig. 1) [14, 15, 30]. If the appendix is short, some tubularized cecal wall can be incorporated as an extension of the appendix. After passing a Ch 14 catheter down the isolated appendix to check its patency and caliber, the distal end is tunneled submucosally for 3–4 cm into the bladder to achieve the continence mechanism. There are several methods for achieving this, e.g., the Ghoneim interserosal tunnel implantation without opening the bladder except for the small cystotomy where the appendix enters [31].

Stomas are usually placed in the umbilicus or in the right lower abdominal quadrant but should be individualized based on manual dexterity and anatomic considerations. The proximal end of the appendix (or tubularized cecum) is spatulated and secured to a wide-based V- or U-shaped skin flap at the apex of the spatulation. A catheter is left in the bladder via the stoma for 3 weeks before CISC is commenced. The catheter balloon should not be filled, as any drag on it may harm the continence mechanism; rather the catheter should be sutured to the skin of the abdomen.

Long-term outcome is reported to be good in children, but the appendix may often prove to be too small (short and narrow) for use in adults, especially in obese patients or patients who prefer their stoma in the umbilicus. Surgical revisions are fairly common (39–61%), from minor endoscopic or suprafascial procedures to complete channel revision, for difficult catheterization and/or incontinence [23]. Appendiceal perforation, necrosis, and stricture have also been reported [14, 30].

Transversely Tubularized Bowel Segments (TTBS): Yang-Monti Channel and Modifications

When an appendix of suitable dimensions is not available, a segment of ileum can be used for a CCC, tailored either by a longitudinal caliber-reducing resection, by invagination, or preferably by transverse tabularization. The transverse tabularization of a short segment of ileum has become known as the Monti principle, but it was originally described by Yang in 1993 (Fig. 2) [32, 33]. Several modifications are described, and collectively they are known as *transversely tubularized bowel segments*, TTBS [34]. Transverse reconfiguration of the bowel segment allows catheterization to occur parallel to the mucosal folds (valvulae conniventes), rather than perpendicularly, as in the case of tapered bowel segments, thereby decreasing the incidence of catheterization difficulties [34, 35].

A 2.5 cm (or longer if indicated) ileal segment is isolated, detubularized through a longitudinal incision halfway on the anterior side, and then transversally re-tubularized with running absorbable suture, obtaining a tube with short and long branches separated by the mesentery (Fig. 2). This method gives a tube length/lumen ratio of 4:1; hence, a 2.5-cm-long bowel segment creates a tube of 9–10 cm length with a caliber of Ch 16–18. The length and caliber of the tube can be adjusted individually; the longer the segment harvested, the wider the tube constructed. The

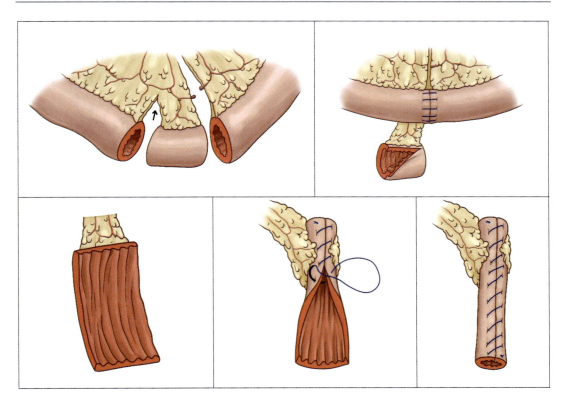

Fig. 2 Yang-Monti continent catheterizable channel. (Illustration by Yohaksson Arias)

long branch is implanted into the bladder and therefore must be at least 3- to 4-cm-long to secure adequate continence, since it is the submucosal zone that is responsible for the continence. The total length of the tube should be as short as possible to facilitate ease of catheterization [32].

If a longer tube is required, a "double-Monti" can be constructed (Fig. 3) [15]. Two adjacent 2.5 cm ileal segments are isolated and detubularized, and the two identical flaps are attached by the short branches. The resulting flap is tubularized, and a tube of two long branches separated by two insertions of mesentery is obtained. A longer channel can also be obtained by using a 3 to 4 cm segment of ileum and partially dividing it halfway close to the mesenteric border. This method was described by Casale in 1999 and is popularly called "spiral Monti" (Fig. 4) [36]. Chapple's modification involves a Z-plasty of the initial incision of the bowel segment, like Casale's, with a slightly different tabularizing method [15]. Both the latter versions have the advantage of avoiding the anastomosis between the two segments, also avoiding any difficulty with CISC potentially caused by the anastomosis.

For all of the above methods of creating a CCC, key technical points include construction of the shortest channel possible to facilitate ease of catheterization, avoid kinking, and, if possible, to fix the bladder to the undersurface of the abdominal wall [14]. If a combined procedure of CCC and bladder augmentation is done, the CCC should be implanted into the bladder, rather than the intestinal segment.

The same considerations regarding stomal placement as described above with the Mitrofanoff procedure apply. The stoma can be constructed using skin flaps (with V, VQZ, or VQ techniques) or resection of a circular skin fragment slightly wider in diameter than the tube [30]. In women, the stoma can be constructed in

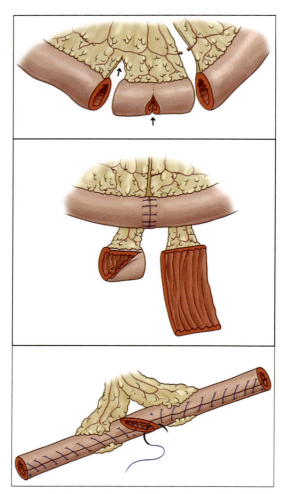

Fig. 3 Double-Monti continent catheterizable channel. (Illustration by Yohaksson Arias)

an orthotopic, vulvar position [33]. A catheter is left in the bladder via the CCC for 3 weeks before CISC is commenced. The catheter balloon should not be filled, as any drag on it may harm the continence mechanism; rather the catheter should be sutured to the skin of the abdomen.

Long-term results of TTBS are reported to be excellent, with continence rates of 91–98%. However, revision should be expected due to catheterization difficulty or incontinence (19–60%) [30, 35]. Overall complication rates of at least 20–30% with the need of revision surgery can be expected [23, 30]. Stomal stenosis at the skin level is reported to be the most common long-term problem (10–61%) [14, 23]. A longer extravesical segment of a CCC can lead to catheterization problems such as false passage and diverticuli, especially near the detrusor hiatus. Hence, minimizing extravesical portion of the channel decreases subfascial complications [35]. Fistulas between the CCC and the bladder, as well as stomal incontinence, are reported to be relatively rare (3–9%) [14, 34, 35]. The latter may be due to a short intramural tunnel or elevated bladder/reservoir pressure.

Continent Cutaneous/Catheterizable Ileocecocystoplasty (CCIC)

The two major reconstructive techniques for creation of a CCC include the *flap valve* (i.e., Mitrofanoff, Monti) and the *nipple valve* (i.e., invaginated ileum, ileocecal valve). The ileocecal valve is a natural nipple valve that can be incorporated into a continent cutaneous urinary reservoir (supravesical urinary diversion, e.g., Indiana, Lundiana techniques, described below) or into a continent cutaneous catheterizable ileocecocystoplasty onto the native bladder [6, 37]. Sarosdy described the continent cutaneous ileocecocystoplasty (CCIC) in 1992 as a way to augment the native bladder and creating a CCC using only one bowel segment (Fig. 5) [37]. The ileocecal valve itself functions as the continence mechanism, while the ileal limb is made smaller in caliber usually by tapering and occasionally by intussuscepting (invagination) [6].

The following three benefits of combining the CCC and augmentation in one with the CCIC have been argued [6]: (1) the use of a relatively short and single bowel resection with one mesentery pedicle. (2) The length and caliber of the channel is easier to modify with the tapered ileum to the adult population, especially in case of obesity. (3) There is no need to create a detrusor tunnel, which is beneficial in neurogenic patients with thick-walled bladders with inflamed mucosa.

It can either be done through a midline laparotomy or by a combined laparoscopic procedure (for the bowel mobilization) and a Pfannenstiel incision (for the reconstruction) [6]. About 10 cm

17 Bladder Augmentation and Urinary Diversion

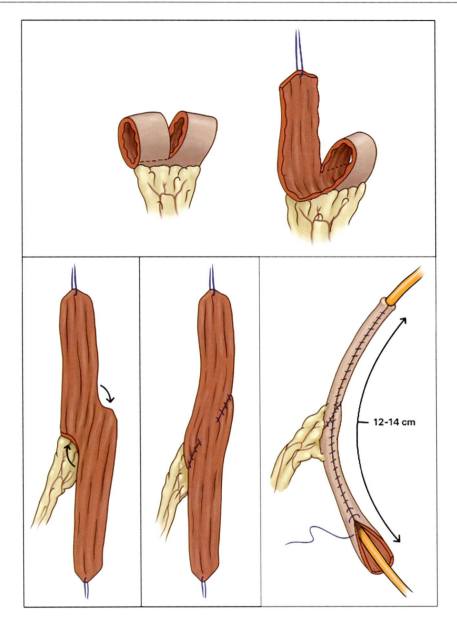

Fig. 4 The construction of a spiral Monti modified continent catheterizable channel. (Illustration by Yohaksson Arias)

of ileum and 10–20 cm of cecum is needed for the reconstruction. The cecum is detubularized between the tenia antimesenterically and appendectomy is performed. The ileum is tapered with a single pass of a GIA-100 stapler. It is important to avoid overlapping stapler lines to minimize catheterization problems. The continence mechanism is reinforced at the ileocecal valve with interrupted sutures. The detubularized cecal segment is then anastomosed to the bivalved bladder, and the efferent limb of the ileal segment can be brought out as a CCC (Fig. 5).

Long-term outcome is reported to be good, with excellent continence rates (>95%) and low revision rates due to stomal stenosis (3–9%) and catheterization problems (13–20%) which is

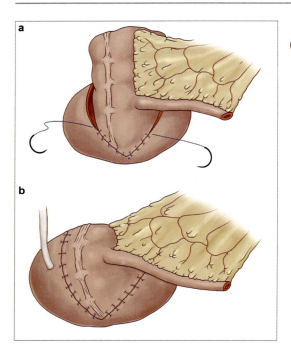

Fig. 5 Continent cutaneous catheterizable ileocecocystoplasty (CCIC). (**a**) The construction of a continent cutaneous catheterizable ileocecocystoplasty. (**b**) With suprapubic tube through bladder wall, to be left in situ for three weeks postoperatively until CISC is commenced

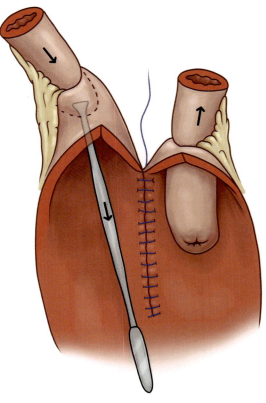

Fig. 6 Kock reservoir illustrating the construction of the efferent and afferent limbs. (Illustration by Yohaksson Arias)

relatively rare compared to the flap valves like Mitrofanoff or Monti [6, 23, 38, 39]. Regarding other complications, renal deterioration, vitamin B12 deficiency, and fecal incontinence are reported to be very rare [6]. Bowel function may actually improve in neurogenic patients who have previously had issues with constipation [6].

Hemi-Kock CCC and Cystoplasty

The flap valve (Mitrofanoff, Yang-Monti) and ileocecal (nipple) valve CCC techniques mentioned above have been widely reported. The hemi-Kock system, comprising a detubularized ileal segment with a stapled ileoileal intussusception, is a form of *nipple valve*. This method, originally described in 1988 by Skinner's group, has not been widely reported [6, 40]. Levy and Elliott attribute the lack of adoption to poor technical reproducibility and long-term durability and a propensity for dessusception of the continence mechanism [6]. However, Herschorn et al. recently reported good long-term results in terms of revision-free rates of <10% [23].

Kock et al. first described the use of an intussuscepted ileal nipple valve as a continence mechanism in 1982 (Fig. 6) [41]. For a hemi-Kock CCC with cystoplasty, a 35–55 cm segment of ileum is isolated, including 15 cm for catheterizable limb and valve and 20–40 cm for the bladder augmentation. The latter is detubularized and reconfigured in a U shape. The efferent limb is intussuscepted. Herschorn et al. have described several modifications leading to more successful outcome [23]. These include removal of the peritoneum on the mesentery to reduce the bulk of the intussusception and a small mesenteric window at the point of maximal stretch to maintain good vascularity, as well as tapering and reinforcement of the catheterizable

17 Bladder Augmentation and Urinary Diversion

limb (with three staple lines and imbricating sutures) to prevent valve eversion and facilitate catheterization.

Herschorn et al. reported success in 90% and failures in 10%, with complete continence without stomal leakage in 58% of 109 patients. Intervention during follow-up was required in 64%, mostly endoscopic bladder stone evacuation. Valve revision was done in 13% (9.4% after abovementioned modifications), parastomal hernia repair in 6.4%, stoma revision in 5.5%, and stoma incision in 6.4% [23].

Supravesical Urinary Diversion

Continent Cutaneous Urinary Diversion

Continent urinary diversions can be divided into ureterosigmoidostomy, continent cutaneous urinary diversion (CCUD, aka heterotopic), and orthotopic bladder reconstruction (aka neobladder). The first attempt on urinary diversion was done by ureterosigmoidostomy as early as 1852, but this technique is largely abandoned nowadays due to long-term complications including malignancy. Orthotopic bladder is anastomosed to the native urethra and is associated with a relatively high rate of urinary incontinence when utilized in women, as well as hypercontinence (i.e., with the need for CISC). This technique relies on a well-functioning rhabdosphincter for continence and is rarely used in patients with bladder dysfunction of benign etiology. Orthotopic diversion is therefore not discussed in this chapter, but a recent review by Zlatev et al. can be recommended for interested readers [42]. This chapter will focus on continent cutaneous urinary diversions (CCUD).

The first description of a catheterizable reservoir for urinary diversion was by Verhoogen in 1908, who reported early results after creation of a cecal reservoir, achieving the possibility of catheterization but not continence [43]. Continence and catheterization were first reported in 1949 by Gilchrist and Merricks. The modern era of CCUD started with the Kock continent ileostomy (aka Kock pouch) in 1975, later modified by

Skinner's group [41]. This technique involves a 70–80 cm segment of ileum, utilizing the central 50 cm for the creation of the reservoir and the two ends for valves with antireflux and continence mechanisms, respectively. The proximal/oral end of the segment (afferent limb) is anastomosed to the ureters, and the distal/aboral end (efferent limb) provides the CCC (Fig. 6). Improved functional outcomes and reduced complications were reported in the 1980s, with the use of detubularized bowel for the reservoir and flap valve (plication, intussusception) between the CCC and the reservoir to provide continence [43]. The Mainz group reintroduced the use of the appendix as the outlet, which offers the advantages of being "ready-made" and requiring a smaller portion of bowel. However, the appendix may not always be available or of adequate caliber.

In 1993, Bissada et al. highlighted the goals of continent cutaneous urinary diversions, principles that still hold true today [44]:

- Construction of an adequate volume, low-pressure reservoir with high compliance
- Reliable continence mechanism
- Prevention of intestinal ureteric reflux or stenosis
- Simplicity in construction
- Avoidance of use of synthetic material
- Avoidance of the use of excessive lengths of bowel
- Ease of catheterization
- Avoidance of need for revision
- Good cosmetic appearance

The reservoir (aka pouch) is constructed of detubularized bowel, usually with either ileum, right colon, or ileocecal segment [43]. Transverse colon can be utilized in case of pelvic irradiation and radiated bowel [45, 46]. The various bowel segments have different characteristics, regarding electrolyte and fluid exchange, mucus production, and muscular activity, as mentioned in the bladder augmentation paragraph.

There have been many modifications both regarding the creation of continence mechanisms and antireflux strategies. However, the necessity of preventing reflux in continent urinary reservoirs has been debated [45, 47, 48]. Those who advocate a direct refluxing anastomosis suggest that a tendency toward increased risk of stricture formation outweigh the potential benefits of reflux prevention [48]. However, in contemporary reports, anastomotic strictures have not been a frequent complication, with an incidence of, e.g., 2–4%, an incidence comparable to those of direct techniques [47]. Reflux prevention also reduces bacteriuria of the upper urinary tract [47]. Anti-reflux techniques include submucosal tunnels (described by Leadbetter 1951, Hohenfellner 1958, Goodwin 1959, Le Duc 1987), interserosal tunnels (Abol-Enein 1994), nipple valves (Ricard 1909, Kock 1982), as well as the chimney technique (Studer 1988).

Continence mechanisms are principally the same as described in the CCC paragraph, with a flap valve or a nipple valve, usually utilizing appendix, ileum, or the ileocecal valve [43, 52].

In total, there are a wide range of different combinations for the creation of a CCUD, regarding choice of bowel for the reservoir, the continence mechanism, and the ureter implantation technique. The choices are up to the surgeon responsible for each individual patient and usually depend somewhat on each center's tradition and expertise. A few techniques in contemporary use are described briefly in the following section. Acronyms or eponyms identify many of these techniques and their combinations (Table 2).

i. *The Mainz pouch I*: The continent cutaneous ileocecal reservoir (Mainz-pouch, "Mixed Augmentation Ileum 'n Zecum") was established in 1983 using 10–15 cm of cecum and ascending colon and two adjacent

ileal loops of equal length [50]. Originally, the continence mechanism was created using an additional ileal segment, which was intussuscepted, pulled through the ileocecal valve, and fixed by metal staples. Since 1990, the submucosally embedded in situ appendix stoma is used when possible for construction of the continent outlet. The bowel-flap tube was introduced another 5 years later serving as an alternative procedure especially in patients in whom the appendix is not available. In this technique, a small caliber conduit is created from large bowel wall at the lower pole of the cecum and tunneled in situ under the mucosa. The ureters were primarily implanted in an antirefluxing technique within a submucosal tunnel into the cecum (as described by Goodwin). The serosa-lined extramural tunnel (described by Abol Enein) is an alternative, beneficial technique when the ureters are dilated preoperatively [53, 54]. (The Mainz III pouch is quite different, originally described with the use of transverse colon and refluxing ureterointestinal anastomoses, beneficial in irradiated patients [46].)

Outcome reports are good with continence rates of up to 93%. Complications include stomal stenosis in 15–24% (intussuscepted ileal nipple vs. appendix), reservoir stones in 5.6–11%, and ureteroenteric stricture rate of 5–6.5% [53].

ii. *The Indiana pouch* (Fig. 7): In 1987, Rowland and colleagues reported the first use of the ileocecal valve as a dependable continence mechanism [55]. The Indiana pouch involves a right colon reservoir with the tapered terminal ileum functioning as the CCC and a

Table 2 Continent urinary reservoir options

Acronym/eponym	Bowel segment	Continence mechanism
Kock [41]	Ileum	Nipple valve
Mansoura [49]	Ileum	Tapered ileal segment or appendix
Mainz I [50]	Ileocecal	Intussuscepted ileal nipple or appendix or bowel-flap (cecum)
Mainz III [46]	Transverse colon	Tapered colon
Indiana [43, 51]	Right colon	Tapered ileal segment or appendix
Lundiana [43, 51]	Right colon	Tapered ileal segment or appendix

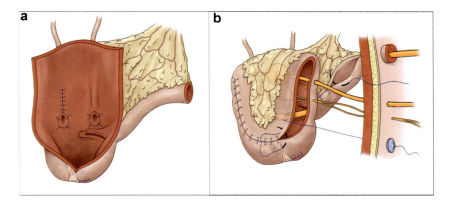

Fig. 7 The construction of an Indiana pouch. (Illustration by Yohaksson Arias)

reinforced ileocecal valve providing continence. The ileal segment is tapered over a Ch 16 catheter using a GIA stapler, and imbricating sutures are placed at the ileocecal valve. The isolated right colon segment is detubularized by incising along the tenia coli and then folded into a U configuration, and the back wall of the pouch is closed with a running, absorbable suture. Ureteroenteric anastomoses are created in a direct, end-to-side, freely refluxing manner.

Reported continence rates are up to 93–97% and reoperation rates 17% [43].

iii. *The Lundiana pouch*: The Lundiana is a modification of the Indiana pouch, also involving the right colon as pouch, tapered ileum as outlet, and reinforced ileocecal valve as continence mechanism [51]. The ureters are implanted into the colon by antireflux technique (according to Le Duc). The right colon is detubularized, opened along the anterior tenia coli down to the level of the ileocecal valve, and from there the incision is extended transversely to the base of the valve. The ileal segment is tapered over a Ch 12 catheter up to the junction using a GIA stapler. The staple line closes the transverse cecal wall incision, tapers the valve on the catheter, and tethers the narrowed ileocecal valve to the cecal wall [51]. The Lundiana method creates a uniform conduit and a narrowed and tethered ileocecal valve. The complexity is considered moderate, and the use of stapling technique makes the procedure standardized. The continence mechanism involves a combination of passive resistance and a flap valve.

The Lundiana technique has reported continence rate of 91% but also a relatively high revision rate, as 54% are reoperated at least once, due to ureteroenteric stricture (15%), pouch stone (14%), revision of outlet due to incontinence or catheterization difficulties (8%), stoma stenosis (8%), and pouch perforation (5%), etc. [51].

Incontinent Urinary Diversion

Cutaneous Ureterostomy

Cutaneous ureterostomy, anastomosing ureters directly to the abdominal wall, is p.t. performed only when bowel segments are unavailable for urinary tract reconstruction, e.g., in patients with bowel disease or in case of serious comorbidity. Stomal stenosis with subsequent skin problems, recurrent urinary tract infections, and compromise of renal function are frequent complications and limit the use of this technique [56].

Ureteroileal Conduit

The ureteroileal conduit was described in 1950 by Bricker as a means of a conduit between ureters and the skin after pelvic evisceration and published in 1950. This solution has no storage (reservoir/bladder) function [57]. Until that time, simple cutaneous ureterostomy had been utilized in these scenarios but were often complicated, as mentioned above.

The ureteroileal conduit is the gold-standard urinary diversion technique against which all others are measured today [58]. The original Bricker method is a short transperitoneal ileal conduit. Turner-Warwick developed an extra-peritoneal conduit (EPIC) procedure using a longer segment [15]. The transperitoneal conduit should be long enough to reach from its ureteroenteric anastomosis on the posterior abdominal wall to the stoma site on the anterior abdominal wall, but it needs to be as short as possible to prevent redundant intraperitoneal loops that may hinder free drainage.

The conduit is constructed either via a laparot-omy or laparoscopically, with or without robotic assistance. Approximately 15–20 cm ileal segment is isolated 15–20 cm from the ileocecal junction. It has to be long enough to reach the stoma site tension-free without disturbing the vascular arcade. When isolating and mobilizing the ureters, it is important to handle them with great care. The left ureter is usually pulled through a window created in the mesentery dorsal to the sigmoid colon. The conduit should be oriented iso-peristaltically, anastomosing the ureters to the proximal end of the conduit loop. The ileal segment should drain the urine freely; thus, anti-refluxing implantation is not necessary. This may minimize the incidence of ureteroenteric stenosis. Nevertheless, there are several methods for ureter implantation. Bricker originally used the method described by Nesbit in 1948, with separate end-to-side anastomoses. Wallace described two methods of conjoined end-to-end anastomoses (type 1 and type 2) in 1967 [15]. The Wallace type 1 involves an iso-peristaltic side-by-side anastomosis of the two ureters, while the Wallace type 2 involves an anti-peristaltic end-to-end anastomosis of the spatulated ureters, before the ureters are anasto-mosed to the end of the conduit. There are several modifications of these ureteroenteric anastomoses [15, 58]. No matter which technique is used, the same surgical principles apply, including mainte-nance of an adequate distal ureteral blood supply, a tension-free anastomosis, and avoidance of ure-teral kinking or twisting.

The quality of life of a patient with a ureteroileal conduit is dependent on achieving a leak-proof adhesion of the urine collecting bag attached around the stoma. To achieve this goal, it is neces-sary to select an appropriate stoma site with an undistorted surrounding surface as well as the cre-ation of a projecting, circumferentially everted, stoma cuff through the abdominal wall without narrowing nor risking a parastomal hernia (Fig. 8).

The ileal conduit can be used for a range of different indications, including malignant and benign, neurogenic, and non-neurogenic. There are only relative contraindications to the procedure, such as impaired cognition and impaired manual dexterity, although these challenges can be over-come by assistance. The same considerations regarding stomal placement as described above with the CCC procedures apply and should be carefully decided in collaboration with the ostomy therapist before surgery is commenced. The long-term management of the stoma requires stoma bags and anti-adhesive spray and occasionally stoma paste, stoma rings, and barrier cream. Follow-up by an ostomy therapist is essential.

Long-term complications include those involv-ing the stoma (parastomal hernia, stenosis, bleed-ing), UTI, renal and pouch stones, and renal failure. Metabolic complications can be of signif-icant consequence; hence regular follow-up is needed [58, 59].

Patients may struggle with the psychological impact of living with a stoma and should be appropriately counselled before surgery [58]. However, urinary diversion improves health-related and disease-specific quality of life in patients with disabling LUTD refractory to conservative treatments [60].

Pregnancy

Pregnancies with reconstructed urinary tracts were first reported in 1967 [61]. In published literature, the majority of pregnant patients with urinary diversion had an exstrophy-epispadias complex as underlying indication (42%), followed by neuro-genic bladder dysfunction (24%) [61].

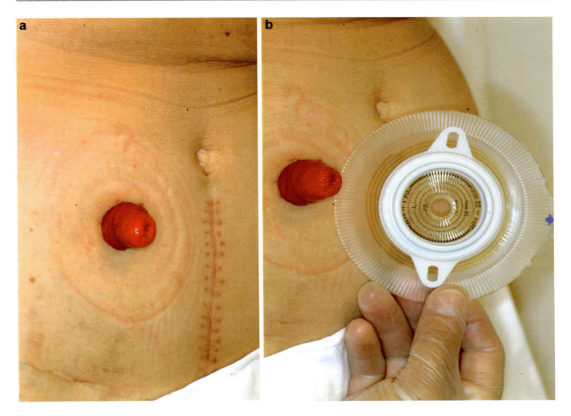

Fig. 8 (**a**) Bricker urostomy: The nipple of the ileal conduit. (**b**) The ostomy plate should be changed daily

Pregnancy after augmentation cystoplasty, ileal conduit urinary diversion, and ureterosigmoidostomy may be complicated by premature birth (16–20%), urinary tract infections (15–39%), CISC difficulty (30%), urinary obstruction (11–13%), deterioration in renal function, and intestinal obstruction (10%) [16, 61–63]. De novo urinary incontinence (8.5%) during pregnancy occurs mainly in patients with cystoplasty and is usually transient [61]. Premature labor is reported in 8% and preeclampsia in 3% [61]. Hence, recommendations for follow-up include routine monthly urine culture and treatment of bacteriuria to avoid its complications, even if asymptomatic. Antibiotic long-term prophylaxis is recommended only in cases of recurrent symptomatic infections. Detection of preeclampsia by measuring serum uric acid is more reliable than identifying proteinuria on urine dipsticks. If performing amniocentesis it is important to be careful of the augmented bladder's blood supply. Renal function should be carefully monitored with monthly serum creatinine levels, and if indicated a renal ultrasound can rule out hydronephrosis and obstruction. A temporary nephrostomy may be indicated, but conservative management is often possible.

A CCC or the efferent limb of a continent reservoir will be stretched during pregnancy, potentially causing tortuosity and CISC difficulties toward the end of the pregnancy and the first few weeks after delivery [61]. CISC difficulty is reported in 50% of pregnant women with a CCC and more commonly in patients with the stoma in the right iliac fossa compared to the umbilical site [63]. A permanent catheter in the CCC may alleviate this problem, and within a few weeks after pregnancy, CISC is usually possible to resume.

Delivery by caesarean section appears to have been the preferred delivery mode, but there is no empirical data to support this choice in all cases [61, 63]. Bey et al. recently reported in a systematic review that the etiology of any neurological disorder or the type of urological reconstruction did not appear to influence decision-making regarding delivery mode; however, underlying exstrophy-epispadias complex did, according to Huck et al. [61, 63]. Patients who have undergone augmentation cystoplasty alone or supravesical urinary diversion can deliver vaginally. Previously, caesarean section was recommended in those who had undergone bladder neck procedures or placement of artificial sphincters (AUS) to avoid disruption of the continence mechanism [16, 62]. However, vaginal delivery is reported to be safe in women who have undergone complex urological reconstruction, with few exceptions [63]. There has only been report of one patient whose AUS was damaged during instrumental (forceps) extraction [63], while the majority have been uncomplicated [61]. Complications were more frequent during caesarean section than vaginal delivery, and the rates of postpartum incontinence were similar in both groups and transient in most [63].

The most complex pathology regarding pregnancy and delivery is bladder exstrophy. Associated breech or transverse fetal position (50%), high incidence of genital prolapse (8%), and several previous surgeries including reconstructed genitalia may justify planned caesarean section in these patients [63]. This group also has an increased risk of miscarriage (35%) [61].

In any case, a caesarean section should preferably be a nonemergency procedure in the presence of a urologic surgeon, as it requires specific precautions. Adhesions between the bladder reconstruction and anterior surface of the uterus can make the procedure more challenging [16, 62]. A midline and high uterine incision is preferable to avoid injury in patients with bladder augmentation and/or CCC, while a Pfannenstiel incision is to be recommended in patients with continent cutaneous reservoirs [61]. Any injury to the bladder, CCC, reservoir, or the blood supply of reconstructed urinary tract should be identified and repaired, followed by catheter drainage for at least 10 days postoperatively.

Cross-References

▶ Indications and Use of Bowel in Female Lower Urinary Tract Reconstruction: Overview
▶ Options for Surgical Reconstruction of the Heavily Irradiated Pelvis

References

1. Abrams P, Cardozo L, Fall M, Griffiths D, Rosier P, Ulmsten U, et al. The standardisation of terminology of lower urinary tract function: report from the Standardisation Sub-committee of the International Continence Society. Neurourol Urodyn. 2002;21(2): 167–78. https://doi.org/10.1002/nau.10052.
2. Blok B, Castro-Diaz D, Del Popolo G, Groen J, Hamid R, Karsenty G, et al. EAU guidelines on neuro-urology. 2022. https://uroweb.org/guidelines/neuro-urology. Accessed June 1, 2022.
3. Ginsberg DA, Boone TB, Cameron AP, Gousse A, Kaufman MR, Keays E, et al. The AUA/SUFU guideline on adult neurogenic lower urinary tract dysfunction: treatment and follow-up. J Urol. 2021;206(5):1106–13. https://doi.org/10.1097/JU.0000000000002239.
4. Vince RA Jr, Klausner AP. Surveillance strategies for neurogenic lower urinary tract dysfunction. Urol Clin North Am. 2017;44(3):367–75. https://doi.org/10.1016/j.ucl.2017.04.004.
5. Martins FE, Holm HV, Lumen N. Devastated bladder outlet in pelvic cancer survivors: issues on surgical reconstruction and quality of life. J Clin Med. 2021;10(21):14920. https://doi.org/10.3390/jcm10214920.
6. Levy ME, Elliott SP. Reconstructive techniques for creation of catheterizable channels: tunneled and nipple valve channels. Transl Androl Urol. 2016;5(1): 136–44. https://doi.org/10.3978/j.issn.2223-4683.2016.01.04.
7. Biers SM, Venn SN, Greenwell TJ. The past, present and future of augmentation cystoplasty. BJU Int. 2012;109(9):1280–93. https://doi.org/10.1111/j.1464-410X.2011.10650.x.
8. Lapides J, Diokno AC, Silber SJ, Lowe BS. Clean, intermittent self-catheterization in the treatment of urinary tract disease. Trans Am Assoc Genitourin Surg. 1971;63:92–6.
9. Affas S, Schafer FM, Algarrahi K, Cristofaro V, Sullivan MP, Yang X, et al. Augmentation cystoplasty of diseased porcine bladders with bi-layer silk fibroin grafts. Tissue Eng Part A. 2019;25(11–12):855–66. https://doi.org/10.1089/ten.TEA.2018.0113.
10. Stenzl A, Ninkovic M, Willeit J, Hess M, Feichtinger H, Schwabegger A, et al. Free neurovascular transfer of latissimus dorsi muscle to the bladder. I. Experimental studies. J Urol. 1997;157 (3):1103–8.

11. van Koeveringe G, Rademakers K, Stenzl A. Latissimus dorsi detrusor myoplasty to restore voiding in patients with an acontractile bladder – fact or fiction? Curr Urol Rep. 2013;14(5):426–34. https://doi.org/10.1007/s11934-013-0349-2.

12. Grilo N, Chartier-Kastler E, Grande P, Crettenand F, Parra J, Phe V. Robot-assisted supratrigonal cystectomy and augmentation cystoplasty with totally intracorporeal reconstruction in neurourological patients: technique description and preliminary results. Eur Urol. 2021;79(6):858–65. https://doi.org/10.1016/j.eururo.2020.08.005.

13. Keating MA, Ludlow JK, Rich MA. Enterocystoplasty: the star modification. J Urol. 1996;155(5):1723–5. https://doi.org/10.1016/s0022-5347(01)66182-2.

14. Smith JA Jr, Howards SS, Preminger GM. Hinman's atlas of urologic surgery. 3rd ed. Philadelphia: Elsevier Saunders; 2012.

15. Turner-Warwick R, Chapple C. Perspectives of urinary diversion and cystoplasty. In: Functional reconstruction of the urinary tract and gynaeco-urology. Hoboken: Blackwell Science; 2002. p. 679–819.

16. Niknejad KG, Atala A. Bladder augmentation techniques in women. Int Urogynecol J Pelvic Floor Dysfunct. 2000;11(3):156–69. https://doi.org/10.1007/s001920070043.

17. Husmann DA. Mortality following augmentation cystoplasty: a transitional urologist's viewpoint. J Pediatr Urol. 2017;13(4):358–64. https://doi.org/10.1016/j.jpurol.2017.05.008.

18. Husmann DA. Lessons learned from the management of adults who have undergone augmentation for spina bifida and bladder exstrophy: incidence and management of the non-lethal complications of bladder augmentation. Int J Urol. 2018;25(2):94–101. https://doi.org/10.1111/iju.13417.

19. Peycelon M, Szymanski KM, Francesca Monn M, Salama AK, Risk H, Cain MP, et al. Adherence with bladder irrigation following augmentation. J Pediatr Urol. 2020;16(1):33.e1–8. https://doi.org/10.1016/j.jpurol.2019.10.029.

20. George VK, Gee JM, Wortley MI, Stott M, Gaches CG, Ashken MH. The effect of ranitidine on urine mucus concentration in patients with enterocystoplasty. Br J Urol. 1992;70(1):30–2. https://doi.org/10.1111/j.1464-410x.1992.tb15659.x.

21. Gillon G, Mundy AR. The dissolution of urinary mucus after cystoplasty. Br J Urol. 1989;63(4):372–4. https://doi.org/10.1111/j.1464-410x.1989.tb05220.x.

22. N'Dow J, Robson CN, Matthews JN, Neal DE, Pearson JP. Reducing mucus production after urinary reconstruction: a prospective randomized trial. J Urol. 2001;165(5):1433–40.

23. Herschorn S, Locke J, Vigil H. Hemi-Kock continent stoma with augmentation cystoplasty: modifications and outcomes. Urology. 2021; https://doi.org/10.1016/j.urology.2021.10.004.

24. Biardeau X, Chartier-Kastler E, Roupret M, Phe V. Risk of malignancy after augmentation cystoplasty: a systematic review. Neurourol Urodyn. 2016;35(6):675–82. https://doi.org/10.1002/nau.22775.

25. Sabiote L, Llorens E, Quiroz Y, Sierra L, Palou J, Bujons A. Is onabotulinum toxin-a combined injection in the bowel patch and the bladder remnant a safe alternative to bladder re-augmentation? Urology. 2021;157:227–32. https://doi.org/10.1016/j.urology.2021.03.035.

26. Pariser JJ, Elliott SP. Opportunities for augmentation cystoplasty revision without additional bowel harvest: "hourglass" deformity or non-detubularized augment. Can Urol Assoc J. 2019;13(5):E140–E4. https://doi.org/10.5489/cuaj.5548.

27. Makass M. Zur Behandlung der Blasenectopie. Umwandlung des ausgeschalteten Coecum zur Blase und der Appendix zur Urethra. Zentralblatt für Chirurgie (no. 33); 1910.

28. de Jong T, Schroeder RPJ. History of appendicovesicostomy, clean intermittent catheterisation and appendicostomy, who were the inventors? J Pediatr Urol. 2021;17(4):594–5. https://doi.org/10.1016/j.jpurol.2021.06.018.

29. Mitrofanoff P. Trans-appendicular continent cystostomy in the management of the neurogenic bladder. Chir Pediatr. 1980;21(4):297–305.

30. Farrugia MK, Malone PS. Educational article: the Mitrofanoff procedure. J Pediatr Urol. 2010;6(4):330–7. https://doi.org/10.1016/j.jpurol.2010.01.015.

31. Ghoneim MA, Shehab-El-Din AB, Ashamallah AK, Gaballah MA. Evolution of the rectal bladder as a method for urinary diversion. J Urol. 1981;126(6):737–40.

32. Yang WH. Yang needle tunneling technique in creating antireflux and continent mechanisms. J Urol. 1993;150(3):830–4. https://doi.org/10.1016/s0022-5347(17)35625-2.

33. Monti PR, Lara RC, Dutra MA, de Carvalho JR. New techniques for construction of efferent conduits based on the Mitrofanoff principle. Urology. 1997;49(1):112–5. https://doi.org/10.1016/S0090-4295(96)00503-1.

34. Monti PR, de Carvalho JR, Arap S. The Monti procedure: applications and complications. Urology. 2000;55(5):616–21. https://doi.org/10.1016/s0090-4295(99)00587-7.

35. Leslie JA, Cain MP, Kaefer M, Meldrum KK, Dussinger AM, Rink RC, et al. A comparison of the Monti and Casale (spiral Monti) procedures. J Urol. 2007;178(4 Pt 2):1623–7.; discussion 7. https://doi.org/10.1016/j.juro.2007.03.168.

36. Casale AJ. A long continent ileovesicostomy using a single piece of bowel. J Urol. 1999;162(5):1743–5.

37. Sarosdy MF. Continent urinary diversion using cutaneous ileocecocystoplasty. Urology. 1992;40(2):102–6. https://doi.org/10.1016/0090-4295(92)90503-o.

38. Redshaw JD, Elliott SP, Rosenstein DI, Erickson BA, Presson AP, Conti SL, et al. Procedures needed to

maintain functionality of adult continent catheterizable channels: a comparison of continent cutaneous ileal cecocystoplasty with tunneled catheterizable channels. J Urol. 2014;192(3):821–6. https://doi.org/10.1016/j.juro.2014.03.088.

39. Cheng PJ, Keihani S, Roth JD, Pariser JJ, Elliott SP, Bose S, et al. Contemporary multicenter outcomes of continent cutaneous ileocecocystoplasty in the adult population over a 10-year period: a Neurogenic Bladder Research Group study. Neurourol Urodyn. 2020;39 (6):1771–80. https://doi.org/10.1002/nau.24420.

40. Weinberg AC, Boyd SD, Lieskovsky G, Ahlering TE, Skinner DG. The hemi-Kock augmentation ileocystoplasty: a low pressure anti-refluxing system. J Urol. 1988;140(6):1380–4. https://doi.org/10.1016/s0022-5347(17)42050-7.

41. Kock NG, Nilson AE, Nilsson LO, Norlen LJ, Philipson BM. Urinary diversion via a continent ileal reservoir: clinical results in 12 patients. J Urol. 1982;128(3):469–75. https://doi.org/10.1016/s0022-5347(17)53001-3.

42. Zlatev DV, Skinner EC. Orthotopic urinary diversion for women. Urol Clin North Am. 2018;45(1):49–54. https://doi.org/10.1016/j.ucl.2017.09.005.

43. Pearce SM, Daneshmand S. Continent cutaneous diversion. Urol Clin North Am. 2018;45(1):55–65. https://doi.org/10.1016/j.ucl.2017.09.004.

44. Bissada NK, Marshall IY, Kaczmarek A. Continent urinary diversion and bladder substitution. J S C Med Assoc. 1993;89(9):435–8.

45. Bailey S, Kamel MH, Eltahawy EA, Bissada NK. Review of continent urinary diversion in contemporary urology. Surgeon. 2012;10(1):33–5. https://doi.org/10.1016/j.surge.2011.09.003.

46. Leissner J, Fisch M, Hohenfellner R. Colonic pouch (Mainz-pouch III) for continent urinary diversion. BJU Int. 2006;97(2):417–30. https://doi.org/10.1111/j.1464-410X.2006.06052.x.

47. Ghoneim MA. Editorial comment. J Urol. 2002;168(3):1016–7. https://doi.org/10.1016/S0022-5347(01)69444-8.

48. Hohenfellner R, Black P, Leissner J, Allhoff EP. Refluxing ureterointestinal anastomosis for continent cutaneous urinary diversion. J Urol. 2002;168(3):1013–6. Discussion 1016–7. https://doi.org/10.1097/01.ju.0000025142.28876.be.

49. Abol-Enein H, Salem M, Mesbah A, Abdel-Latif M, Kamal M, Shabaan A, et al. Continent cutaneous ileal pouch using the serous lined extramural valves. The Mansoura experience in more than 100 patients. J Urol. 2004;172(2):588–91. https://doi.org/10.1097/01.ju.0000129437.33688.4d.

50. Thuroff JW, Alken P, Riedmiller H, Engelmann U, Jacobi GH, Hohenfellner R. The Mainz pouch (mixed augmentation ileum and cecum) for bladder augmentation and continent diversion. J Urol. 1986;136(1):17–26. https://doi.org/10.1016/s0022-5347(17)44714-8.

51. Liedberg F, Gudjonsson S, Xu A, Bendahl PO, Davidsson T, Mansson W. Long-term third-party assessment of results after continent cutaneous diversion with Lundiana pouch. BJU Int. 2017;120 (4):530–6. https://doi.org/10.1111/bju.13863.

52. Wiesner C, Stein R, Pahernik S, Hahn K, Melchior SW, Thuroff JW. Long-term followup of the intussuscepted ileal nipple and the in situ, submucosally embedded appendix as continence mechanisms of continent urinary diversion with the cutaneous ileocecal pouch (Mainz pouch I). J Urol. 2006;176(1):155–9. Discussion 159–60. https://doi.org/10.1016/S0022-5347(06)00571-4.

53. Wiesner C, Bonfig R, Stein R, Gerharz EW, Pahernik S, Riedmiller H, et al. Continent cutaneous urinary diversion: long-term follow-up of more than 800 patients with ileocecal reservoirs. World J Urol. 2006;24(3):315–8. https://doi.org/10.1007/s00345-006-0078-y.

54. Wiesner C, Pahernik S, Stein R, Hahn K, Franzaring L, Melchior SW, et al. Long-term follow-up of submucosal tunnel and serosa-lined extramural tunnel ureter implantation in ileocaecal continent cutaneous urinary diversion (Mainz pouch I). BJU Int. 2007;100(3):633–7. https://doi.org/10.1111/j.1464-410X.2007.06991.x.

55. Rowland RG, Mitchell ME, Bihrle R, Kahnoski RJ, Piser JE. Indiana continent urinary reservoir. J Urol. 1987;137(6):1136–9. https://doi.org/10.1016/s0022-5347(17)44428-4.

56. Turner-Warwick R, Chapple C. Functional reconstruction of the urinary tract and gynaeco-urology. Hoboken: Blackwell Science; 2002.

57. Bricker EM. Bladder substitution after pelvic evisceration. Surg Clin North Am. 1950;30(5):1511–21. https://doi.org/10.1016/s0039-6109(16)33147-4.

58. Tanna RJ, Powell J, Mambu LA. Ileal conduit. Treasure Island: StatPearls; 2022.

59. Bakke A, Jensen KM, Jonsson O, Jonsson E, Mansson W, Paananen I, et al. The rationale behind recommendations for follow-up after urinary diversion: an evidence-based approach. Scand J Urol Nephrol. 2007;41(4):261–9. https://doi.org/10.1080/00365590600991284.

60. Schultz A, Boye B, Jonsson O, Thind P, Mansson W. Urostomy and health-related quality of life in patients with lower urinary tract dysfunction. Scand J Urol. 2015;49(1):2–7. https://doi.org/10.3109/21681805.2013.876095.

61. Huck N, Schweizerhof S, Stein R, Honeck P. Pregnancy following urinary tract reconstruction using bowel segments: a review of published literature. World J Urol. 2020;38(2):335–42. https://doi.org/10.1007/s00345-019-02781-z.

62. Hautmann RE, Volkmer BG. Pregnancy and urinary diversion. Urol Clin North Am. 2007;34(1):71–88. https://doi.org/10.1016/j.ucl.2006.10.001.

63. Bey E, Perrouin-Verbe B, Reiss B, Lefort M, Le Normand L, Perrouin-Verbe MA. Outcomes of pregnancy and delivery in women with continent lower urinary tract reconstruction: systematic review of the literature. Int Urogynecol J. 2021;32(7):1707–17. https://doi.org/10.1007/s00192-021-04856-1.

Pathophysiology and Diagnostic Evaluation of Stress Urinary Incontinence: Overview

18

Helal Syed and Matthias Hofer

Contents

Introduction	324
Epidemiology of Stress Urinary Incontinence	324
Terminology	324
Prevalence and Risk Factors	324
Pathophysiology	326
Normal Physiology and Continence	326
Abnormal Physiology	327
Diagnostic Evaluation	327
History	328
Physical Exam	329
Ancillary Studies	330
Conclusion	331
Cross-References	332
References	332

Abstract

Stress urinary incontinence is a common urological condition that affects all demographics of females but is more prevalent with increasing age. It is a condition that affects quality of life-socially, mentally, and physically-but also has a monetary cost associated with its evaluation and management as well as the loss of productivity with costs into the billions of dollars. We discuss the epidemiology and risk factors for SUI in females and provide an overview of the normal continence mechanisms in females as well as the pathophysiologic changes that contribute to SUI followed by the diagnostic evaluation for SUI.

Keywords

Bladder · Voiding · Stress urinary incontinence · Voiding physiology

H. Syed
Division of Urology, Department of Surgery, Children's Hospital Los Angeles | University of Southern California Keck School of Medicine, Los Angeles, CA, USA

M. Hofer (✉)
Urology San Antonio, San Antonio, TX, USA
e-mail: matthias.hofer@urologysa.com

© Springer Nature Switzerland AG 2023
F. E. Martins et al. (eds.), *Female Genitourinary and Pelvic Floor Reconstruction*,
https://doi.org/10.1007/978-3-031-19598-3_19

Introduction

Urinary incontinence (UI) is a common urological condition affecting both men and women, young and old, across all demographics, and regions across the world. UI can be broken down into stress urinary incontinence (SUI), urgency urinary incontinence (UUI), or mixed urinary incontinence (MUI). MUI can be further denoted as stress or urgency predominant based on the most bothersome symptom(s) for the patient. While it is not generally thought of as life-threatening, it substantially affects the quality of life of not only those afflicted but their family members and network as well. In addition, for those patients who are employed, it can lead to loss of productivity, missed worked, and wages and income. The direct and indirect costs of UI can be staggering. In the United States, over $12 billion are spent annually in the care of female stress urinary incontinence [1]. In 2007, the national cost of UUI was $65.9 billion, with projected costs of $82.6 billion in 2020 [2]. While the mechanisms of UUI are similar for both genders, in SUI, there are anatomic differences contributing to the gender specific presentation of the condition. The purpose of this chapter is to provide an overview of (1) the epidemiology of SUI in females, (2) the normal continence mechanisms in females, (3) the pathophysiologic changes that contribute to SUI, (4) risk factors for SUI, and (5) the diagnostic evaluation for SUI.

Epidemiology of Stress Urinary Incontinence

Terminology

Urinary incontinence (UI) is a broad term that encompasses all types of urinary incontinence. Generally, UI is broken down into three main subtypes: stress urinary incontinence (SUI), urgency urinary incontinence (UUI), and mixed urinary incontinence (MUI). MUI is when a patient has symptoms or signs of both stress and urgency urinary incontinence. MUI can be further broken down into MUI urgency predominant or

MUI stress predominant based on the patient's symptoms and signs. While there are additional and rather rare additional forms of incontinence defined by the International Continence Society (ICS) Glossary such as coital incontinence. These are associated with SUI, MUI, or UUI in the vast majority of patients and can be thought of being a subtype one of the three main types [3].

Additionally, when discussing UI, it is important to differentiate between signs and symptoms. A **symptom** is a complaint that the patient experiences. A **sign** is an observation that the clinician makes. This distinction is important as patients may experience symptoms of UI but not have signs and vice versa. This specifically is important to recognize during the evaluation of UI: for example, a patient may have **symptoms** that appear to be consistent with SUI but upon careful examination actually have **signs** rather consistent with UUI. According to the ICS, the **symptom** of SUI is defined as "complaint of involuntary loss of urine on effort or physical exertion including sporting activities, or on sneezing or coughing." The **sign** of SUI per ICS is defined as "observation of involuntary leakage from the urethral orifice synchronous with effort or physical exertion, or on sneezing or coughing" [4].

Prevalence and Risk Factors

The prevalence of UI has been reported around 50% of females with a prevalence of SUI particularly in 46% of all women [5, 6]. This number has been consistent since 2005 [7]. Below we will be discussing the demographic factors conferring risk and those which are protective of developing UI (Table 1).

Table 1 Risk factors for stress urinary incontinence

Age
Pregnancy
Race

Comorbid conditions:
   Smoking
   Obesity
   Diabetes
   Pelvic organ prolapse

Age

Age has been consistently positively associated with UI with an increased prevalence of UI in older women compared to their younger counterparts. For example, in the 2017–2018 period, approximately 34% of females between the ages of 20–39 years had SUI compared with 51% of those aged between 40 and 59 years and 53% in those greater than 60 years of age. Again, this has been steady since 2005 (Fig. 1) [7]. While the exact mechanism is unknown, it is thought to be due to "wear and tear" of the pelvic anatomy along with loss of a decrease of muscle mass and changes in the connective tissue composition [8–11].

Pregnancy

Pregnancy has been known to be associated with incontinence as well. A longitudinal cohort study that investigated the extent of persistent UI found that after 12 years after giving birth, 38% of females had persistent UI. In fact, in those females who had reported UI at 3 months after giving birth, approximately 76% continued to have UI at the 12-year mark [12]. Some of the risk factors associated with persistent UI were vaginal delivery, older age, greater parity, and other comorbid conditions such as obesity and smoking, which have independently been associated with SUI as well [12, 13]. Using data from the National Health and Nutrition Examination Survey from 2005 to 2018, pregnancy was associated with SUI with higher odds of having SUI with a vaginal delivery than with a cesarean delivery. However, both delivery types were noted to have higher odds of SUI than those who were nulliparous [7]. When comparing cesarean delivery to vaginal delivery, it was reported that the risk of long-term SUI was twofold higher in those who had vaginal delivery. Interestingly, there was no difference in the risk of SUI between spontaneous vaginal delivery and vaginal delivery with instrumentation (forceps, vacuum assisted) [14]. Furthermore, the greater number of children and duration of labor greater than 24 h were associated with UI. However, age at first and last childbirth, episiotomy, and birth weight over 4 kg of a child were not associated with UI [15]. It is thought that in addition to the changes related to increasing weight and size related to the growing uterus and fetus, biochemical and hormonal changes may lead to reduced strength and support of the pelvic floor musculature [13].

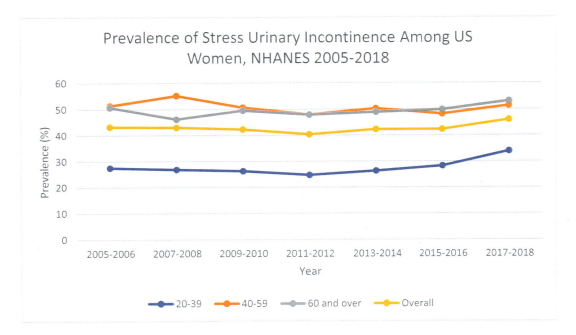

Fig. 1 SUI Trends in US Women. (Adapted from Abufaraj [7])

Race

Multiple studies have demonstrated that Caucasian females have a higher likelihood of experiencing SUI and Black females with the lowest risk. Hispanic and Asian females appear to have the same risk as Caucasian females [7, 16]. These differences are not explained by lifestyle and health-related factors, but studies have demonstrated differences in the pelvic floor musculature and support between White and African American females to include smaller levator ani muscle in White females and increased urethral closure pressure in Black females [16].

Comorbid Conditions

There are several comorbid conditions that have been associated with SUI to include smoking, obesity, diabetes, depression, and pelvic organ prolapse. Smoking status, obesity, and pelvic organ prolapse will be briefly discussed.

Smoking Status

There is some controversy regarding whether smoking is associated with SUI as studies have conflicting results [7, 15, 17]. Generally, smoking, specifically tobacco, is thought to contribute to degradation of tissues via vasoconstrictive effects of nicotine as well as direct endothelial damage of blood vessels from metabolites of tobacco leading to decreased tissue oxygenation [18]. Additionally, smoking causes an imbalance in the ratio between proteolytic enzymes and inhibitors which affects tissue quality as well as wound healing. While smoking cessation improved tissue oxygenation and the microenvironment after 4 weeks, there is permanent damage especially in regard to wound healing [19].

Obesity

Multiple studies have indicated obesity as a risk factor for SUI [7, 17, 20, 21]. In fact, these studies have demonstrated that increasing bodyweight even if not obese increases the risk for SUI. It is a modifiable risk factor, and thus, reduction in weight whether by surgical or non-surgical means has a beneficial effect on UI in these patients.

POP

Pelvic organ prolapse has been associated with stress urinary incontinence. On one hand, prolapse may cause urethral kinking leading to overflow incontinence due to a full bladder. On the other hand, prolapse of pelvic organs is a sign of loss of pelvic organ support to include the loss of support structures that maintain proper urethral orientation. In one study, up to 63% of patients who had POP also had concomitant urinary incontinence [15].

Pathophysiology

Normal Physiology and Continence

Continence is maintained by combination of sphincteric function as well as proper bladder compliance. This requires a combination of the proper neural control of the bladder and sphincter musculatures as well as the proper musculofascial elements of those structures. While neural control is thought to play a larger role in UUI than in SUI, pelvic surgery and trauma can damage the lumbosacral spinal cord and pelvic nerves which can impair sphincter function leading to incontinence.

Neural Control

Storage of urine is mediated by sympathetic function of the autonomic nervous system by way of the hypogastric nerve. The bladder essentially is under tonic control to allow for filling and storage. Simultaneously, spinal reflex arcs promote bladder neck closure via afferent signaling from the bladder which pass through the interneurons in the spinal cord to the efferent signaling to the bladder neck and the internal or smooth urethral sphincter. This is under sympathetic control as well. During this time, the pelvic nerves, which supply the parasympathetics to the bladder, are tonically inhibited. Additionally, Onuf's nucleus in the sacral spinal cord provides somatic motor neurons via the pudendal nerve to the external or striated urethral sphincter (also known as a the rhabdosphincter) resulting in tonic resistance to help maintain continence. During voiding, the pontine micturition center in the brainstem sends a signal that releases the parasympathetic neurons from their tonic inhibition and allows for bladder contraction with coordinated suppression of the sympathetic neurons and thus coordinated relaxation of the sphincters.

Musculofascial Control

There are two aspects to the musculofascial control of urine. The first is the location of the bladder which affects the anatomic position of the sphincter. This is particularly important for females who can have a more mobile pelvic floor compared to males which can affect the bladder neck position and function resulting in continence. The second aspect are the sphincteric mechanisms. The internal or smooth urethral sphincter is a continuation of the bladder neck muscle fibers and is not under volitional control. The external sphincter or rhabdosphincter is composed of concentric layers of type I (slow-twitch) skeletal muscles which allow for the tonic contraction of the muscle, thus maintaining urethral closure and continence.

Abnormal Physiology

Historically, three types of SUI have been described. Type 1 SUI occurred when there was a loss of the normal posterior urethrovesical angle and support of bladder neck. This would lead to increased pressure transmission of the forces experienced by the bladder to the urethra, therefore overpowering the distal urethral sphincter mechanism causing incontinence. Type 2 SUI was type 1 SUI with the addition of urethral hypermobility that would lead to further pressure transmittance [22, 23]. Several authors reported on these findings, and their contributions were collated into the pressure transmission.

An additional type of SUI, SUI type 3, also known as intrinsic sphincteric deficiency (ISD), is when there is weakness of the urethra specifically in the ability to coapt the walls of the urethra. The dysfunctional urethra is fixed and can be due to neural or structural issues. Classically, patients with ISD were described as having a "pipestem" urethra. ISD, while it can be the etiology for SUI on its own, can also be found concomitantly with other abnormal physiology such as urethral hypermobility. ISD is diagnosed through urodynamic testing when the maximal urethral closure pressure (MUCP) is less than 20 cm H_2O or a Valsalva leak point pressure (VLPP) of less than 60 cm H_2O [23, 24].

In addition to the above explanations, DeLancey et al. proposed the "hammock hypothesis" [25]. The hypothesis stated that the surrounding support structures of the urethra from the anterior vaginal wall extending laterally create a hammock for the urethra and that during periods of increased intra-abdominal pressure, those structures compress the urethra along with distal urethral sphincteric mechanisms, all of which contribute to continence.

The integral theory states that there is a point or zone of maximal continence that is located mid-urethra at the pubourethral ligaments. During bladder storage and times of increased intra-abdominal pressure when continence needs to be maintained, the pelvic floor adapts actively and passively to pull of the pubourethral ligaments to effectively close the urethra. When there is laxity of the ligament deviation of the forces, it leads to incontinence [26].

SUI on Prolapse Reduction (Occult or Latent SUI)

Related to the loss of pelvic support is the idea of occult stress urinary incontinence. This type of SUI is usually discovered after correction of anterior POP. It is thought the POP causes kinking of the urethra creating continence (this continence can be strong enough to actually create obstruction as well). By correcting the POP, this "continence" mechanism is removed, thus unmasking underlying SUI. Thus, at the time of evaluation of SUI, it is important to look for SUI in the presence of POP and also after reduction of POP (e.g., with a pessary).

Diagnostic Evaluation

Just as any encounter, a thorough history and physical examination is mandatory in the evaluation and management of SUI.

History

History of Present Illness

Components of a good history of present illness will elucidate when the symptoms started in association with any events. Often, incontinence will be associated after major events such as trauma, surgery, and pregnancy. The **onset** may be abrupt or gradual. It is also important to document if there has been **progression** of symptoms and how so. For example, there may be increasing frequency or increases in the amount of loss of urine during incontinent episodes. **Aggravating** factors are important to note and commonly will be activities that increase intra-abdominal pressure such as coughing, sneezing, laughing, changing positions, or engaging in physical activity such as running or weightlifting (specifically once that involve the use of the pelvic floor muscles such as deadlifts or squats). Alleviating factors are important to note as well but oftentimes will involve cessation of the offending activity.

When inquiring about incontinent episodes, it is important to ask if there is complete loss of urine and whether the patient is aware of the leakage. Additionally, most if not all patients will admit that they have resorted to wearing underwear liners or pads or in more severe cases adult diapers, and thus, it is prudent to document the quantity used and how moist these articles are. Finally, it is important to note the degree of bother of the symptoms. Occasionally, patients will have signs and/or symptoms of SUI but are not bothered by it and hence will not opt for management.

Past Medical History

It is crucial to take note of any comorbid conditions especially those that are known to affect the neurologic and vascular system such as hypertension and diabetes. Poorly controlled diabetes may lead to damage of the nerves supplying the bladder, and what was initially thought to be stress urinary incontinence is actually overflow incontinence secondary to poor emptying of the bladder. In addition, conditions that may affect the patient's surgical candidacy should also be documented such as cardiovascular or peripheral vascular diseases. Pertinent to females is obstetric history. While pregnancy is known to be a risk factor, the details surrounding the pregnancy are important as well. Patient age at each pregnancy should be noted as well as type of delivery and the use of aids such as vacuum devices or forceps and whether an episiotomy was performed.

Past Surgical History

A thorough surgical history is imperative to help identify possible etiologies for incontinence but also to help in surgical planning as well. Intra-abdominal and pelvic surgeries are generally asked about, but it is also important to elicit any history of orthopedic surgeries as well, especially those that involve the hips and lower extremities as those can affect positioning of the patient in lithotomy position. Explicitly asking patients the type of approach used (i.e., open vs. laparoscopic) as well as if there were any complications during any abdominopelvic surgery is important as patients will often not divulge that information readily. If patient is not able to elucidate and there is concern that the previous surgery may have been more complex, then it may be prudent to reach out to the operating surgeon to gather details. Of note, it is also important to inquire about any cardiac procedures as well, as patients often may not think of a cardiac stent or pacer placement as part of their past surgical history, which may affect their ability to undergo an incontinence procedure.

Medications, Family History, Social History, and Review of Systems

While there are no specific medications that cause stress urinary incontinence it is important to have a complete list especially for surgical planning purposes. For example, a patient may have concomitant overactive bladder and take medications for it. After SUI surgery, these same medications may put the patient into urinary retention. Additionally, it is important to take note of anticoagulants and antiplatelet agents as inadvertent continuing of those medications into surgery may cause excessive bleeding and possibly complications such as hematoma formation.

Other components of a history and physical examination such as family history, social history, and review of systems are important to record for completeness. Specifically, in regard to social history, documentation of smoking history is important as smoking is not only a risk factor for SUI as mentioned previously, but for patients who do undergo SUI surgery, it is associated with wound complications due to poor and delayed wound healing. When asking about review of systems (ROS), it is important to ask about other lower urinary tract symptoms as well such as dysuria, hematuria, urgency, frequency, feelings of incomplete bladder emptying, and nocturia. Additionally, feelings of vaginal bulging and any splinting maneuvers during voiding or defecation should be inquired about as well. The ROS should also ask about bowel habits and may include questions about diet and liquid intake as well. Gynecologic ROS should inquire about vaginal dryness, dyspareunia, or any pelvic pain.

Physical Exam

General

In the evaluation of SUI, most clinicians will perform a focused physical exam with attention given to the genital and in females, the vaginal exam. However, there are several key findings that clinicians should gather. BMI or an equivalent measure should be obtained as obesity has been demonstrated to be a risk factor for SUI, as mentioned previously. On abdominal exam, it is important to note any surgical scars as prior abdominopelvic surgeries can be a cause for SUI. In the day and age of minimally invasive surgery with small or few scars, often patients may forget to mention that they had abdominal surgery. Neurologic exam is important as well, as certain neurologic conditions will have a preferred pattern of expression. For example, in patients with Parkinson's disease, evidence of the Parkinsonian tremors and shuffled gait may lead to

sphincter bradykinesia and thus failure of the guarding reflex with subsequent SUI during moments of increased intra-abdominal pressure such as during changes of position.

Vaginal

A complete vaginal exam cannot be understated in the evaluation of UI in the female. Depending on the clinic setup, it can be done in conjunction with a cystoscopy if that is also being performed. Given the comprising nature of this specific portion of the exam, ensuring patient comfort is key. Ideally, the patient is in a medical gown with appropriate draping (can be done with a large towel or drawsheet) to ensure modesty. The room should have a comfortable temperature as well. Good lighting either with a lighted speculum or a spotlight should be available. During the exam, the provider should maintain good communication with the patient regarding the next steps. Oftentimes, it is beneficial to explain to the patient the steps that will be performed so that the patient is not taken by surprise. The patient should be in lithotomy position with the legs in stirrups to have adequate exposure. The sequencing of steps should be methodical to avoid any unnecessary movement. A lighted half speculum should be used if available.

The first thing to do is to inspect the vaginal canal looking for scarring, vaginal atrophy, or any other lesions such as urethral caruncles. Next, the anterior, posterior, and apical compartments should be examined for pelvic organ prolapse. This is accomplished by first examining each compartment with the half speculum with the patient first relaxed and then with the patient bearing down or doing a Valsalva maneuver. This will help determine the extent of descent of the compartment. The POPQ tool is an objective way to quantify any pelvic organ prolapse that may be present.

After POPQ measurements are completed, provocative maneuvers should be performed to evaluate for leakage of urine. This is usually done with the half speculum applied to the posterior compartment to visualize the urethra and anterior compartment. However, if the patient has any degree of pelvic organ prolapse, the prolapse should be reduced while performing the provocative maneuvers. The patient is asked to cough, and leakage of urine is evaluated. Additionally, urethral hypermobility should also be evaluated. Classically, a well-moistened cotton tip applicator is placed into the urethra, and the patient is asked to cough or bear down, and the degree of movement of the applicator is observed and recorded. Greater than 30 degrees confirms this finding. However, this can be an uncomfortable test, and many providers will just visualize how much the urethra moves without the applicator. Sometimes incontinence is not observed with the patient in lithotomy position, and the patient can be asked to stand up and cough over an absorbent pad or a towel, and incontinence is visualized.

The bimanual exam is performed to evaluate for any pelvic floor tightness and tenderness. Tenderness at the lateral vaginal walls can be indicative of injury to the arcus tendineus or the cardinal ligaments, which provide support to the vaginal walls and help maintain normal anatomical configuration. Additionally, the pelvic floor tone is measured with one or two fingers in the vaginal vault, and the patient is asked to squeeze or perform a Kegel exercise.

Ancillary Studies

Voiding Diary

Often patients are not able to recall specifics on their voiding habits. A voiding diary is a log of 1–3 days in length and sometimes even longer especially in the pediatric population, of when a patient voids, how much they have voided, and associated symptoms to include incontinence and whether it is associated with urgency and/or a cough, sneeze, straining, etc. This can help especially identify if there is a pattern or not with the voids. For example, a patient may only have daytime frequency and incontinence but no nighttime incontinence and vice versa. Some of these patterns may be associated with the use of certain medication such as diuretics.

In addition to the outputs recorded, liquid intake is also recorded—how much, what type, and when—during this time period. These data taken together help quantify whether there is appropriate input and output of fluids and if there may be an underlying condition as well.

Pad Weight

Some patients will go through several liners a day, but they will change at the faintest sign of moisture, while others will go through a couple of adult diapers that happen to be completely soaked. This can lead to ambiguity on the degree of incontinence, and thus, some providers will use pad weight as an objective measure. However, there is controversy regarding the optimal method of evaluating pad weights. There is a 1-h, 24-h, and even a 48-h pad weight test. The 1-h test can be done in office but may not be reproducible or reflect actual "real-life" scenarios, and the 48-h test collects more data but may be cumbersome to patients. The 6th edition of the ICS International Consultation on Incontinence concluded that a "24-h test correlates well with symptoms of incontinence" and that "a test lasting longer than 24 h has little advantage" (ICS ICI 6th edition, 2017). However, in their consensus statements, they write that the "pad test is an **optional** investigative tool in the routine evaluation of UI" and the "pad test is a useful outcome measure in clinical trials and research studies." They suggest that as standards, 1 g of weight gain in the 20 min to 1 h in office test with fixed bladder volume and more than 1.3 g/24 h for the 24-h ambulatory test as positive tests [27].

Urinalysis

Labs are generally not necessary in the workup of stress urinary incontinence. The exception to this is urinalysis. Sometimes UI is caused by infection especially in a patient that does not have typical cystitis symptoms such as dysuria, urgency, or frequency. Urinalysis can provide evidence of infection. Depending on whether microscopy was performed on the sample, evidence of nitrite, leukocyte, and esterase should prompt further investigation of the urinalysis prior to further investigation and management of stress urinary incontinence. It is important to obtain a proper sample that is not contaminated which result in a false-positive urinalysis. Additionally, sometimes a urinalysis will demonstrate microscopic hematuria, necessitating a different but important workup to rule out malignancy.

Post-Void Residual

A post-void residual (PVR) measures the amount of urine that remains in the bladder immediately after voiding. It is most often an in-office procedure performed with a bladder scanner device but can be performed with an ultrasound machine as well. A PVR is a required part of the evaluation for SUI to ensure that the patient is emptying appropriately and to ensure that the patient's incontinence is not simply overflow incontinence that is observed when intra-abdominal pressures are increased. Furthermore, SUI treatments increase the outlet pressure and can potentially lead to increased PVRs in patients which may lead to detrimental bladder function and in worser cases lead to obstructive uropathy with subsequent kidney injury. Generally speaking, most urologists would agree that a PVR of less than 100 cc is considered normal. PVRs can be performed along with noninvasive uroflowmetry in the same procedure to determine a flowrate, but in females, it is not necessary as the caliber of the female urethra is quite large. Flow-rate values concerning obstruction (typically rates below 15 ml/s in females) are usually associated with POP and/or dysfunctional voiding and can be further evaluated as necessary (▶ Chap. 12, "Idiopathic Urinary Retention in the Female").

UDS

Urodynamic testing (UDS) is performed to answer a specific question. It is not required as part of the initial evaluation of a patient with stress urinary incontinence as it is timely and costly and is invasive which can be stressful for patients. Additionally, given its invasive nature, it can lead to urinary tract infection. In simple terms, UDS involves the use of two pressure-transducing catheters, one placed into the bladder and one placed into the vagina or rectum to measure bladder and abdominal pressures, respectively, at various times during bladder filling and emptying. The pressure data is coupled with flow data, and the information is visualized on various graphs. In isolated SUI, it is not required but it may be helpful in patients who have concomitant POP, prior incontinence surgeries, MUI, and inability to diagnose based on history and physical examination (i.e., inability to demonstrate SUI during physical exam).

Cystoscopy

Similar to UDS, cystoscopy is not required as part of the initial evaluation of SUI. Oftentimes, it is performed in patients who have had a prior incontinence procedure to help evaluate and visualize the anatomy. This is especially pertinent in females who have had a prior urethral sling procedure to ensure that there is no erosion of the prior sling into the urethra especially if there is consideration to place another sling. It is usually performed in the office setting with the patient in stirrups and can be performed with a flexible cystoscopy or a rigid cystoscope (with both a 30-degree and a 70-degree lens). If performing a cystoscopy, ofttimes providers will do the pelvic exam and a PVR in the same setting.

Conclusion

Stress urinary incontinence is a common urological condition that affects all demographics of females but is more prevalent with increasing age. In addition to age, risk factors include pregnancy, BMI, and comorbid conditions. It is a condition that affects quality of life, socially, mentally, and physically but also has a monetary cost associated with its evaluation and management as well as the loss of productivity with costs into the billions of dollars. Evaluation for SUI includes a thorough history and physical examination with focus on the pelvic and vaginal exam. This helps in confirming pathophysiologic findings such as urethral hypermobility and/or a fixed urethral sphincter as well as laxity of support structures. Ancillary studies help to rule out other confounding diagnoses. Once the evaluation is complete, providers can than proceed to having a thorough discussion with patients regarding optimal treatment.

Cross-References

▶ Idiopathic Urinary Retention in the Female

References

1. Chong EC, Khan AA, Anger JT. The financial burden of stress urinary incontinence among women in the United States. Curr Urol Rep. 2011;12(5):358–62.
2. Coyne KS, Wein A, Nicholson S, Kvasz M, Chen C-I, Milsom I. Economic burden of urgency urinary incontinence in the United States: a systematic review. J Manag Care Pharm. 2014;20(2):130–40.
3. Lau H-H, Huang W-C, Su T-H. Urinary leakage during sexual intercourse among women with incontinence: incidence and risk factors. PLoS One. 2017;12(5): e0177075.
4. D'Ancona C, Haylen B, Oelke M, Abranches-Monteiro L, Arnold E, Goldman H, et al. The International Continence Society (ICS) report on the terminology for adult male lower urinary tract and pelvic floor symptoms and dysfunction. Neurourol Urodyn. 2019;38(2):433–77.
5. Markland AD, Richter HE, Fwu C-W, Eggers P, Kusek JW. Prevalence and trends of urinary incontinence in adults in the United States, 2001 to 2008. J Urol. 2011;186(2):589–93.
6. Dooley Y, Kenton K, Cao G, Luke A, Durazo-Arvizu-R, Kramer H, et al. Urinary incontinence prevalence: results from the National Health and Nutrition Examination Survey. J Urol. 2008;179(2):656–61.
7. Abufaraj M, Xu T, Cao C, Siyam A, Isleem U, Massad A, et al. Prevalence and trends in urinary incontinence among women in the United States, 2005–2018. Am J Obstet Gynecol. 2021;225(2):166. e1–166.e12.
8. Mannella P, Palla G, Bellini M, Simoncini T. The female pelvic floor through midlife and aging. Maturitas. 2013 Dec;76(3):230–4.
9. Falconer C, Blomgren B, Johansson O, Ulmsten U, Malmström A, Westergren-Thorsson G, et al. Different organization of collagen fibrils in stress-incontinent women of fertile age. Acta Obstet Gynecol Scand. 1998 Dec;77(1):87–94.
10. Goepel C. Differential elastin and tenascin immunolabeling in the uterosacral ligaments in post-menopausal women with and without pelvic organ prolapse. Acta Histochem. 2008 Dec;110(3):204–9.
11. Chen BH, Wen Y, Li H, Polan ML. Collagen metabolism and turnover in women with stress urinary incontinence and pelvic prolapse. Int Urogynecol J. 2002;13(2):80–7.
12. MacArthur C, Wilson D, Herbison P, Lancashire RJ, Hagen S, Toozs-Hobson P, et al. Urinary incontinence persisting after childbirth: extent, delivery history, and effects in a 12-year longitudinal cohort study. BJOG Int J Obstet Gynaecol. 2016;123(6):1022–9.
13. Sangsawang B. Risk factors for the development of stress urinary incontinence during pregnancy in primigravidae: a review of the literature. Eur J Obstet Gynecol Reprod Biol. 2014;178:27–34.
14. Tähtinen RM, Cartwright R, Tsui JF, Aaltonen RL, Aoki Y, Cárdenas JL, et al. Long-term impact of mode of delivery on stress urinary incontinence and urgency urinary incontinence: a systematic review and meta-analysis. Eur Urol. 2016;70(1):148–58.
15. Kılıç M. Incidence and risk factors of urinary incontinence in women visiting Family Health Centers. Springerplus. 2016;5(1):1331.
16. Townsend MK, Curhan GC, Resnick NM, Grodstein F. The incidence of urinary incontinence across Asian, black, and white women in the United States. Am J Obstet Gynecol. 2010;202(4):378.e1–7.
17. Richter HE, Burgio KL, Brubaker L, Moalli PA, Markland AD, Mallet V, et al. Factors associated with incontinence frequency in a surgical cohort of stress incontinent women. Am J Obstet Gynecol. 2005;193 (6):2088–93.
18. Silverstein P. Smoking and wound healing. Am J Med. 1992;93(1):S22–4.
19. Sørensen LT. Wound healing and infection in surgery. Ann Surg. 2012;255(6):1069–79.
20. Troko J, Bach F, Toozs-Hobson P. Predicting urinary incontinence in women in later life: a systematic review. Maturitas. 2016;94:110–6.
21. Townsend MK, Curhan GC, Resnick NM, Grodstein F. BMI, waist circumference, and incident urinary incontinence in older women. Obesity. 2008;16(4): 881–6.
22. McGuire EJ, Lytton B, Pepe V, Kohorn EI. Stress urinary incontinence. Obstet Gynecol. 1976;47(3): 255–64.
23. Parrillo LM, Ramchandani P, Smith AL. Can intrinsic sphincter deficiency be diagnosed by urodynamics? Urol Clin N Am. 2014;41(3):375–81.
24. McGuire EJ, Lytton B, Kohorn EI, Pepe V. The value of urodynamic testing in stress urinary incontinence. J Urol. 1980;124(2):256–8.
25. DeLancey JOL. Structural support of the urethra as it relates to stress urinary incontinence: the hammock hypothesis. Am J Obstet Gynecol. 1994;170(6):1713–23.
26. Petros PEP, Woodman PJ. The integral theory of continence. Int Urogynecol J. 2007;19(1):35–40.
27. Amarenco G, Doumouchtsis SK, Derpapas A, Fernando R, Sekido N, Shobeiri SA, et al. In: Abrams P, Cardoso L, Wagg A, Wein A, editors. Incontinence 6th edition. 6th ed. Bristol; 2017. p. 739–44.

Pudendal Nerve Entrapment Syndrome: Clinical Aspects and Laparoscopic Management

19

Renaud Bollens, Fabienne Absil, and Fouad Aoun

Contents

Introduction	334
Anatomy	334
Differential Diagnosis (Fig. 4)	336
Epidemiology	337
Pathophysiology	338
Compression	338
Stretching	338
Etiology (Fig. 5)	338
External Factors	338
Local Condition	339
Myofascial Syndrome (Fig. 6)	340
Trigger Factors	341
Clinical Aspects	342
Neurological Aspects	343
Arterial Aspects	345
Venous Aspects	345
Associated Pathology	346
Diagnosis	346
Patient History	346
Clinical Exam of a Pudendal Pathology	346
Complementary Exams	348

R. Bollens (✉)
Urology, Centre Hospitalier de Wallonie Picarde, Tournai, Belgium

Urology Department, Catholic University of North of France, Lille, France

F. Absil
Gynaecology, Epicura Hospital, Ath, Belgium

F. Aoun
Urology, Hôtel Dieu de France, Université Saint Joseph, Beyrouth, Lebanon

© Springer Nature Switzerland AG 2023
F. E. Martins et al. (eds.), *Female Genitourinary and Pelvic Floor Reconstruction*,
https://doi.org/10.1007/978-3-031-19598-3_20

Nantes Criteria	350
Treatment	350
Conservative Treatment	350
Laparoscopic Pudendal Decompression	353
Conclusion	357
Cross-References	357
References	357

Abstract

Since the description by the Nantes team in France many studies have analyzed pudendal neuralgia in the context of chronic pelvic pain syndrome. Although the pain mechanism has been extensively studied, the functional disturbances associated are still considered simple local sensitization problems due to the initial pain.

The initial surgical technique has been improved over time to allow a more complete distal dissection. The feedback of our patients has taught us the relationship between pudendal entrapment and many other functional syndromes. The improvement of several different problems reported by our patients has opened the window to a completely new approach to functional pelviperineal syndromes. From the principles of pudendal neuralgia, we have developed the concept of pudendal neuropathy and more recently the concepts of arterial and venous pudendal pathology. We have also developed a new theory explaining the pathophysiology of the origin of these syndromes to propose a new logical therapeutic approach. This theory can explain the efficiency of all treatments proposed to help the patients. The treatment must first target decompression of the nerve; hence surgery must be advocated as first-line treatment and not only in desperate cases.

Keywords

Pudendal nerve · Etiology · Pathophysiology · Laparoscopy · Treatment · Functional · Symptoms · Entrapment · Syndrome

Introduction

Our experience with treatment of pudendal entrapment started in 2014 when we watched a live laparoscopic surgical demonstration performed by Professor Tibet Erdogu in Barcelona [1, 2]. Since then, we have followed more than 1000 patients and operated on more than 400. The feedback from our patients has provided us with a new understanding of these pathologies in clinical terms, but also the understanding of the pathophysiology and the origin of the symptoms. In the beginning, we focused on the pain problem related to this pathology [3–5]. However, we rapidly realized that a part of the problem was also a functional one in many cases. Although the nerve entrapment is the main problem for most of the patients, it became evident that pathology of the pudendal artery, but also the pudendal vein, can be associated with some complaints of the patient. From the concept of *pudendal neuralgia*, we have developed the concept of *pudendal neuropathy*, which also encompasses the functional problems associated with the neurologic component. We have also developed the concept of pudendal arteriopathy and more recently the concept of pudendal venous pathology.

Anatomy

The pudendal nerve arises at the S2, S3, and S4 roots (Figs. 1 and 2). It runs between the pyriformis muscle and the sacrospinous ligament, and it is located near the sciatic nerve roots. The sciatic nerve exits the pelvis through the great sciatic notch before the sciatic spine. The pudendal nerve travels under the sciatic spine and the fibrotic part

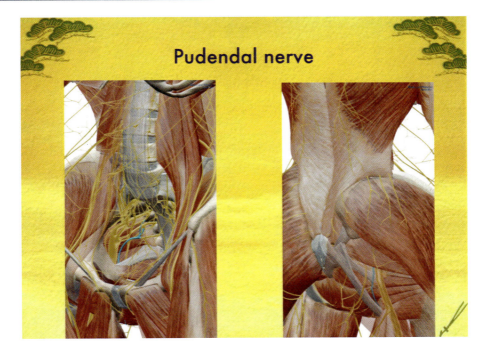

Fig. 1 Anatomy of the pudendal nerve

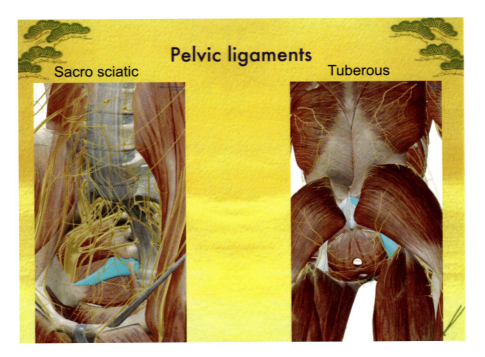

Fig. 2 Anatomy of the pudendal nerve

of the sacrosciatic ligament, to leave the pelvis through the small sciatic notch (Fig. 2). At that level, the rectal branch leaves the main pudendal trunk (Fig. 3) and passes through the tuberous ligament. After the sciatic spine, the pudendal nerve enters Alcock's canal (duplication of the internal obturator muscle aponeurosis). The main trunk is divided in, or just after, Alcock's canal into three main branches: the anterior, the median, and the posterior (Fig. 3). The territory of the innervation is extended from the coccyx to the pubis including the clitoris (or glans penis), the small and the large labia (or the scrotum), the urethra, the vestibulum of the vagina, the perianal area, and the anal canal [6]. The pudendal nerve contains sympathetic fibers, sensory fibers, and motor fibers (for the anal and urinary sphincters) [7, 8]. The pudendal artery follows the pudendal nerve and gives the blood supply for the pudendal nerve and the proximal part of the sciatic nerve. Some anatomical variations exist, and an accessory pudendal artery can run along the endopelvic fascia to join the prostatic dorsal plexus in males [9].

The venous system is certainly the most complex as the potential number of anatomical variations and anastomoses is very high. The most important to remember, to understand the clinical aspect, is that the internal pudendal vein drains the corpus cavernosum and the inferior rectal veins [10, 11].

Differential Diagnosis (Fig. 4)

The pudendal nerve is not the only nerve of the perineum. The perineum is also innervated by the iliohypogastric nerve (pubic area), the ilioinguinal nerve (inguinal area and anterior part of the labia majora), the genitofemoral nerve (inguinal area), the cluneal nerve (posterior part of the labia

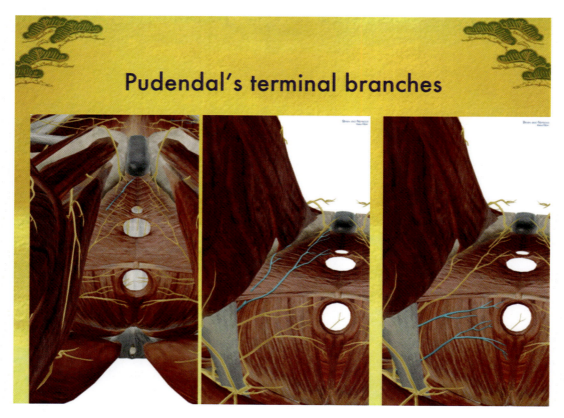

Fig. 3 Terminal branches of the pudendal nerve

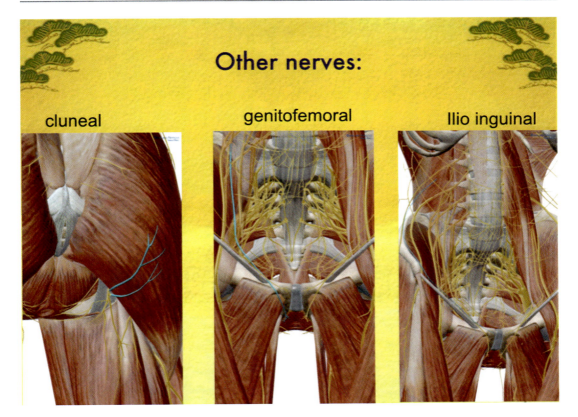

Fig. 4 Other perineal nerves

majora and posterior part of the perineum), and impar ganglia (perianal area) [12]. The clitoris and the glans, the vaginal vestibulum, the urethra, and the anal canal are specifically innervated by the pudendal nerve. The pudendal nerve is a sympathetic, motor, and sensory nerve, while the other nerves are mainly sensory.

Epidemiology

The real incidence of pudendal entrapment is uncertain due to the difficulty in defining a precise clinical condition. The Italian association for pudendal neuralgia has 5000 patients for 40 million inhabitants, which only includes patients with a pain syndrome. However, many patients may have functional symptoms without pain. When we consider the functional aspects of this pathology, from our point of view, we estimate the incidence to be around 15% of the adult population [13].

This pathology is not yet taught in medical school programs, which explains the mean delay of 5 years between the debut of symptoms and the correct diagnosis. In our outpatient clinics, some patients have more than 30 years of medical wandering. This lack of knowledge also explains why many patients have already consulted many different specialists involved with perineal problems, urologists, gynecologists, proctologists, dermatologists, and/or psychiatrists. For the same reason, a significant number of patients have had surgery for the wrong reason to try to help them (hysterectomy, colectomy, promontofixation, cystectomy, suburethral sling, radical prostatectomy, transurethral prostate resection, etc.). The clinical result after these surgeries may be limited and very short. The patients usually have a relapse after 1 week (duration of the effect of general anesthesia).

The incidence is accepted to be higher in women than in men (9:1 ratio). However, the difference between women and men is probably overestimated because many specific male problems are not yet recognized as pudendal pathology. Nevertheless, the incidence is certainly higher for women due to the specific obstetrical risk. The symptoms seem to appear mainly after 35 years. We have observed another group of patients with symptoms arising at adolescence or in young adulthood. The younger patients usually have specific risk factors. The most common is a congenital shorter lower limb and in rare cases hypersensitivity to compression of the fine nervous fibers [14]. This pathology is related to abnormal functioning of sodium channels [15].

Pathophysiology

Basically the mechanisms to create a neurological lesion are simple. The most common is compression. Stretching can also occur, particularly in women.

Compression

Many physicians believe compression is due to a fibrosis in Alcock's canal, but in reality, the compression is more commonly proximal. In this area, the nerve can be compressed on the sacrosciatic ligament by another element. The compression can be external, for example, seen in sports using a saddle or simply by a chair in professions in a seated position. The pudendal elements can also be compressed by the pyriformis muscle itself [16]. This muscle can develop a chronic contraction in case of postural problem. A symmetric anterior pelvic rotation can increase the pressure on the pudendal nerve simply due to a modification of the relative position between the piriformis muscle and the pudendal elements. The rectal branch can be selectively compressed in the passage through the tuberous ligament,

causing a selective anorectal symptom. The authors have seen a patient who had a perineal resection of the rectal branch and still had anal pain. Laparoscopic decompression was performed without rectal branch dissection (supposedly, it had already been resected). However, due to the persistence of the symptoms, a second laparoscopic exploration of the rectal branches was performed, and the stump of the rectal branches was found still compressed in the tuberous passage. After the release of the nerve stump segment, the pain disappeared.

Stretching

Theoretically, stretching of the nerve can result from sport activities associated with the practice of leg splitting (e.g., karate, classic dance). In the authors' experience, no such case has been seen yet. Most commonly, several women have been observed presenting with a descending perineum syndrome associated with pudendal nerve entrapment symptoms, particularly with an anorectal condition. In the descending perineum syndrome, the rectal branch is particularly exposed to traction because the main trunk is fixed in Alcock's canal.

Etiology (Fig. 5)

The origin of this problem is not related to a single underlying cause. In fact, several risk factors can be defined. When patients combine any number of these risk factors, they may develop symptoms.

External Factors

The types of sports at the highest risk are bicycling and horse riding due to the use of a saddle. A saddle creates a direct pressure through the perineum on to the pudendal structures. The second most common sport is jogging. This group of patients can develop pudendal compression from the pyriformis muscle when they have an uncompensated postural problem.

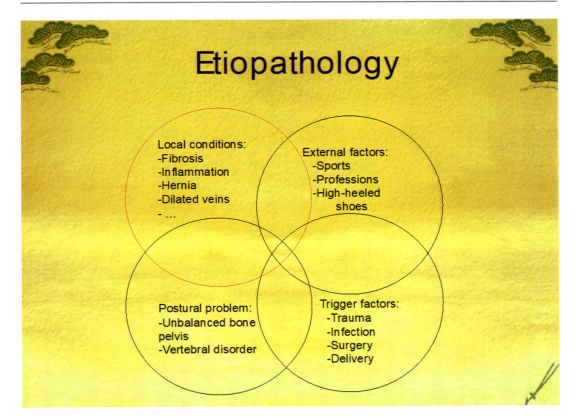

Fig. 5 Etiology of pudendal nerve entrapment

Professions in a seated position, like informaticians, secretaries, teachers, drivers, etc., are at risk. After the increased periods of time spent teleworking from home during the Covid pandemic, a significant number of patients have presented with pudendal symptoms. They have moved from an ergonomic office chair to the kitchen chair to work. This change of the professional environment may explain this observation. The use of high-heeled shoes increases the symmetric anterior rotation of the bony pelvis and the pressure of the pyriformis muscle on the pudendal elements. It also represents a risk factor for the women who wear them daily.

Local Condition

During surgery some specific conditions can be observed, including fatty hernias under the edge of the sacrosciatic ligament and in other cases significant fibrosis of the ligament at the level of the sciatic spine. If the ligament itself is not a dynamic element of compression, this fibrosis increases the counter resistance when the pyriformis muscle is contracted. If the ligament is more elastic, the muscle contraction will not be as efficient in compressing the pudendal element. The pudendal vein can be extremely dilated in some cases. It is difficult to know if this venous dilatation can compress the nerve significantly. It may be a consequence rather than the origin of the problem.

Some specific situations are associated with local inflammation, urinary fistulation with urinoma, or endometriosis. The uterosacral ligament is commonly involved by the endometriotic lesions. The sacrosciatic ligaments are localized a few centimeters apart from the uterosacral ligament. This proximity explains the common association between endometriosis and pudendal nerve symptoms. Strange symptoms reported by some patients with endometriosis may be caused by pudendal neuropathy. If association of both problems is suspected, resection of the endometriotic lesion should be completed by pudendal surgical decompression.

Myofascial Syndrome (Fig. 6)

Muscle contraction, particularly of the pyriformis muscle, is central to the etiology of pudendal compression. The contracted muscle can create a pressure on the pudendal nerve and at the same time on the sciatic nerve roots.

Localized Pelviperineal Muscle Contraction

In most cases, the clinical examination reveals a muscle contracture of the pelvis and the perineum [17]. The transverse muscle of the perineum, the internal obturator muscle, and the levator muscle but also the muscles around the hip can be contracted. The origin of the contraction can be different from patient to patient. Pain seems to be the trigger factor in many cases. Some patients describe a light trauma like a shock to the coccyx, and a few days after this initial event, they develop a typical pudendal nerve symptom. In case of pain, the body reacts with a muscle contraction around the painful place to try to immobilize the area. Like in a case of shoulder dislocation, it is easy to reduce in the first hours; however, it becomes possible only under anesthesia on the day after. Finally, a light event can create a painful situation. The pain induces a reflex muscle contracture of the perineum including the pyriformis muscle. The contracted pyriformis increases the pressure on the pudendal nerve. When the pudendal neuralgia begins, the patient develops a vicious circle: the pain induces muscle contracture, and the muscle contracture induces pain (due to the pudendal neuralgia). This theory can explain many individual underlying events, like a delivery, a urinary tract infection, sexual abuse, etc.

Postural Disorder and Global Myofascial Syndrome

Asymmetry of the length of the legs is a risk factor to develop pudendal nerve entrapment, but the incidence of a congenital asymmetry is much lower than the incidence of this disease [18]. Systematic scanometry of patients' legs showed that the length was symmetric in most of the patients. There is a predominance of the right-sided pathology in our patient group. Initially, it was assumed

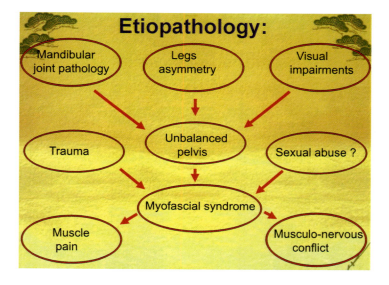

Fig. 6 Etiopathology of the pudendal nerve entrapment

to be due to a bias in the manner the patient was examined. Apparently, this proved to be the case, as being right-handed, we likely pushed harder on the right side than on the left. However, changing our examination technique (right hand to exam the right side and left hand for the left side) did not affect this predominance.

Our research found a significant incidence of functional unbalanced pelvis. It means that there is a natural tendency to adopt an asymmetric position when standing up: the right knee is slightly flexed when we are right-handed and the opposite if we are left-handed. This asymmetric position creates a false shorter leg that is not visible when we do a scanometry of the legs ("soldier standing to attention" position on X-ray). When the patient has an unbalanced bone pelvis position related to a functional problem or a real shorter leg, she can develop a global myofascial syndrome. Many muscles can be contracted and hence the origin of chronic pain. The fascia lata muscle can exert tension on the knee and create chronic pain in the external chamber of the knee. On the other extremity, this muscle may cause trochanteritis. In the buttock, the contracted pyriformis muscle pushes on the sciatic roots and pudendal nerve and can cause a painful spot in the buttock. The patient potentially presents with a paravertebral muscle contraction from the lower back to the cervical area. This muscle contraction is the trigger of chronic back pain and may explain the origin of Maigne's syndrome that is sometimes observed in this patient population [19]. This syndrome results from compression of a sensory nerve originating at the level of the last thoracic and the first lumbar vertebrae. It manifests as neurologic pain in the upper part of sacroiliac joint, the iliac crest, and the inguinal area, particularly in the epididymis in men. In our experience, the correction of posture can solve the pudendal nerve problem and chronic back pain.

Trigger Factors

Many patients report a specific event at the origin of their problem. The patient history may identify various small preexisting symptoms. This specific event could be identified as a trigger event rather than the real origin of the pudendal pathology. A pelvic inflammatory condition such as urethritis, prostatitis, or a simple cystitis have been reported by the patients. It is difficult to know the exact mechanism causing the pudendal symptoms, but it is most likely multifactorial: the inflammatory process, the pain, and the reflex muscle contraction.

A surgical procedure can also be a trigger event. Some procedures are performed in the vicinity of the pudendal nerve, but others do not seem to be close enough to explain a direct injury of the pudendal structures. The list of surgeries reported by patients to be the trigger event includes sub-urethral sling, vaginal hysterectomy, anorectal perineal amputation, transurethral prostate resection, transurethral bladder resection, ureteroscopy, etc. The common denominator of these is the lithotomy position used during the procedure. Most experts do not understand the problem fully, but the relation between the two events is established without the proof of real causation. An intense sport activity can trigger the symptoms, especially when the intensity of the effort is unusually high. Off-road bicycling, intense road bicycling, bodybuilding, long jogging, and intensive gardening (equivalent to intensive squat exercise) have been reported. A long travel in a seated position has also been reported as the debut of the pathology.

In our experience, few women report delivery as the origin of the symptoms. The potential trauma of labor or delivery is evident [20]. In most cases, the pain resolves spontaneously, but some patients may have lasting severe pain. The potential mechanism can be compression or stretching of the nerve or pain induced by the luxation of the cervix. Women with pudendal neuropathy usually improve during pregnancy due to the laxity of the ligaments under the specific hormonal environment. However, delivery is a critical event for the pudendal structures. It is not rare to have a patient with a characteristic perineal pain after the delivery. Fortunately, most of them will have a spontaneous recovery after few months. In our series we have had two women with prolonged pain. This situation is more complex because it is usually not only a pudendal nerve problem but also a coccygodynia. One of these two women is still in the early recovery phase but feels already a significant improvement. In the second case, the pudendal pain has resolved but the sacrococcygeal pain is still present.

Clinical Aspects

To understand the variety of the symptoms, it is important to remember that the artery, the vein, and the nerve can be compressed and create specific symptoms. It is well-known that pain is related to pudendal nerve compression. However, the feedback of the operated patients has revealed a wider range of potentially related symptoms. To understand this pathology, it is very important to operate on the patients with an efficient technique and to hear the clinical observations reported by them during the months of follow-up. Many unexplained syndromes may be associated with pudendal pathology, like sterile cystitis, chronic prostatitis, premature ejaculation, vesico-perineal dyssynergia, erectile dysfunction, and even bacterial urinary infection and many others [21]. Initially, the patients reported an unexpected improvement of specific symptoms after surgery. Later, we proposed the surgery for these new potential indications with good results.

The symptoms have a classical rhythm. Many patients have no or only mild symptoms at night. This peculiarity may explain why some patients search for psychiatric help. As an example, one of our patients urinated every 20 min during the day without nocturia. She was cured with simple postural correction. This diurnal variation is explained by the dynamic compression of the pudendal element by the pyriformis muscle. During night time the muscle is relaxed, and the pressure dissipates. Some patients place a cushion between the knees to sleep in a lateral flank position. The cushion increases the external rotation of the hips and allows a better relaxation of the pyriformis muscle, which runs posteriorly from the hip. Other patients prefer to sleep on the back in frog position, i.e., flexion of both hips and both knees, feet side by side, and hips completely in an external rotation.

Nocturnal symptoms may be present in case of severe compression, but in this situation, it is important to exclude a compression in the medulla. This compression can affect only the cauda equina, but it can be related to stenosis of the spinal canal or a herniated disc all along the vertebral column. If the patient presents with symptoms in the upper limb, an MRI scan of the cervical area is mandatory, and in case of symptoms of the lower limb, the lumbosacral part must be investigated.

The patients describe some worsening of the symptoms along the day with a recurrent rhythm. They know the moment when the symptoms will appear and the moment when they will be intolerable. At the beginning of the event, the symptoms occur from time to time to become more and more frequent (up and down symptomatology with unpredictable good and bad days) and finally to never relieve. The symptoms are dependent on the patient's position. They are worse in a seated position, better when standing up, and disappear when the patient is lying down. Some patients are completely unable to stay in a seated position and live only in a prone position. This simple issue creates many social life problems. They cannot go to a restaurant or stay seated to watch a movie, to travel, or simply to work. When a patient has a worsening in the seated position, she will prefer to be seated usually on a hard chair in case of pudendal neuralgia and a smooth cushion in case of clunealgia. The symptoms may be relieved after a few minutes seated on the toilet. In this situation, the perineum is pending in the toilet and the pressure on the nerve can disappear. Some patients need to stay longer on the toilet to wait for the effect of the decompression to help the relaxation of the sphincter.

Sexual activities will worsen the symptoms the day after. The most common are women who present with a cystitis (sterile or bacterial) 24 h after sexual intercourse. Many of them remark an association between sex and bladder pain, with worse symptoms when the sex is associated with an orgasm.

The symptoms are typically worse during a sport activity using a saddle. Some patients report an intolerance to bicycling. Joggers can feel improvement during the sport activity due to a stretching of the muscles during the exercise, but at each step, the unbalanced bone pelvis creates excessive tension on the muscle. They notice worsening of the symptoms 24 h later. Many patients report worsening of the symptoms when they are tired or stressed. This observation is classic in all neurologic diseases. They also remark an improvement of the symptoms when the temperature is higher. The best moment for them is when they are on holidays in a warmer climate country. Classically, patients observe an immediate relief of symptoms when they apply something warm on the perineum (e.g., a cushion heated in a microwave oven). The mechanism is to superpose the thermic stimulation over the painful sensation to reduce it. It is probably a similar effect to the electric stimulation of the posterior tibial nerve (sacral roots) to control urinary urgency and perineal pain.

Neurological Aspects

The pudendal nerve contains three different types of fibers: the sensory fibers, the motor fibers, and the sympathetic fibers. Each type can produce specific symptoms. The motor fibers are bigger than the sympathetic and the sensory fibers. The small fibers are more sensitive to compression. This explains why an electromyogram can be normal in a painful patient (like in sciatic pain). The intensity of compression can also modify the symptoms. A light compression will produce allodynia from the sensory fibers and a sphincteric spasm from the motor fibers. In the opposite case, a strong compression of the sensory fibers will create a numbness, and compression of the motor fibers will cause a palsy of the sphincter. The effect of compression can be completely opposite in function of the intensity. This difference will also potentially change the prognosis of the surgery. Allodynia and a hypertonic sphincter have a better chance of recovery after surgical decompression.

Sympathetic Fibers

These fibers are responsible for some odd symptoms: redness of the skin or the mucosa, swelling of the perineum, and sexual disorders. Premature ejaculation is commonly associated with a psychological problem by most specialists. In our experience, the history of this group of patients has the profile of pudendal neuropathy, and after surgery, this problem is improved or completely resolved [22]. If the systematic patient history reveals many small associated symptoms compatible with a pudendal neuropathy, surgery may be recommended. Similarly, women can present with an arousal syndrome. This involves experiencing unwanted sensations of arousal in their genitals that do not resolve with an orgasm. This female problem can be resolved with surgery but can also be observed temporarily in the recovery phase after the surgery. More unfrequently, the patient reports difficulty in reaching orgasm (probably related to a stronger compression). Female sexuality is complex, and the sexual preference and psychological aspect influence the quality of orgasms, but a part of this group may have a pudendal nerve compression as an underlying cause. Male patients may also report poor sensation during orgasm [23]. They describe, at the moment of the orgasm, a limited number of perineal contractions, a low volume of sperm, and a low pressure during the ejaculation. Globally, the intensity of the orgasm is reduced. In our experience, sexual disturbances, particularly premature ejaculation, and the arousal syndrome are highly specific of a pudendal nerve problem.

Sensory Fibers

The sensation of the perineum is controlled by several nerves, but some parts are only under pudendal innervation. A sensory symptom in these specific areas is pathognomonic to a pudendal nerve problem. The clitoris (or the glans penis in males), the urethra, and the vestibulum of the vagina are typically concerned. The description of the sensory symptoms is not always easy to understand (like all neurologic pain). The patient may report a sensation of burning, electricity (continuous or intermittent), needles, pressure, etc. The pain is not always present, and it may be one of the endpoints of this pathology. Many patients bothered with pain also report some functional symptoms, often becoming apparent years before the pain. If these symptoms are not specific to the pudendal nerve, some areas are specific to the pudendal nerve such as the clitoris or the glans penis, the urethra, the vaginal vestibulum, and probably the anal canal. As urologists, we have all seen patients with an abnormal hypersensitivity during cystourethroscopy or a simple digital rectal examination. We may consider this a psychological issue, but it may be related to a pudendal nerve problem. In this group of patients, a transurethral bladder catheter is impossible to tolerate (except sometime just after general anesthesia). In our experience, urethralgia and pain in the glans or the clitoris are highly specific to a pudendal nerve problem.

Urinary urgency is a common female complaint. Hypoestrogenic states may explain the symptom in a subgroup of these patients. Another subgroup has hypermobility of the urethra and commonly associated stress urinary incontinence. This group of patients describe better control when they are seated and urgency when they stand up. The pressure of the seat on the perineum compensates the mobility of the urethra. In this case, a sub-urethral sling may solve the problem. In the last subgroup of patients with urgency, it is common to prescribe an anticholinergic drug. During urodynamic exams, bladder instability may not always be present. In this case, urgency is a sensory problem. The patient has an urge to urinate. In our institution, we treat this symptom as a pudendal nerve problem with good results (except if it is associated with interstitial cystitis). This symptom can also appear after surgery in the lithotomy position. For example, de novo urgency incontinence after a sub-urethral sling is mainly related to pudendal nerve decompensation.

Dyspareunia is a common complaint [24]. The problem can be superficial at the intromission with a characteristic component of allodynia. For other patients the dyspareunia is deeper and may be related with direct pressure on some contracted sensitive muscle. In this case, the position adopted can influence the discomfort. Endometriosis must

be ruled out in all cases. The impression of a foreign body in the rectum or the vagina is a frequent symptom. Rectosigmoidoscopy must be done to exclude a true organic lesion in the rectum. An important question in the patient history is how often daily that she goes to the toilet to try to defecate [25]. If it is three times or more often, an unconscious impression of a foreign body in the rectum can be considered. This situation also explains the reported pseudo-diarrhea. The frequency of voiding of the rectum does not allow the formation of a normal stool. In the vagina, it is easy to confound a problem related with a vaginal prolapse and pudendal nerve symptoms. The authors have seen a few cases of patients who had undergone multiple surgeries for vaginal prolapse being ultimately cured by the release of the pudendal nerve.

Motor Fibers

In some cases, compression of the motor fibers causes a contraction of the perineum and the anal and urinary sphincters. These fibers are thicker and have a better resistance against compression. For this reason, a palsy of the sphincter is a rare condition but must be considered a more serious situation for which emergency surgery may be indicated. Dyschezia is caused by hypertonicity of the anal sphincter. This problem can be improved when the patient stays on the toilet for a longer time. When the perineum is pending in the toilet, the pressure on the nerve is reduced and the nerve less irritated. This allows a better sphincteric relaxation. A chronic hypertonic anal sphincter induces a reflex relaxation of the rectum. For this reason, patients with pudendal neuropathy can present with two opposite clinical situations: obstipation due to the relaxation of the rectum or pseudo-diarrhea when the rectal foreign body sensation is dominant.

Hypertonicity is also responsible for vaginismus and vesico-sphincteric dyssynergia. When patients are in a critical situation, they frequently complain of dysuria. Complete urinary retention can happen in extreme situations, sometimes in an acute manner. Vesico-sphincteric dyssynergia with high postvoid residual is improved with decompression (surgical or not) of the nerve. In our series, a woman was in complete urinary retention with a long history of dyspareunia. Six months after pudendal nerve release, the dyspareunia was resolved, and the patient returned to a normal life. She resumed urination without postvoid residual and recovered normal sexual function. Anecdotally, a patient presented in our clinic with obsessive-compulsive behavior related to a specific symptom such as hand washing. The most interesting was the potential relation between this symptom and the risk of bacterial cystitis [27].

Anal fissure is associated with a spasm of the anal sphincter. The fissure, the pain, and the spasm enter a vicious circle. The lesion of the anus is often suspected to be the first event; however, for some patients, a pudendal neuropathy is the origin of the problem. Indeed, both anal fissure and pudendal neuropathy can be treated using the nitric oxide effect (local cream with nitric oxide for the anal problem and inhibitor of degradation of nitric oxide for the nerve problem).

Arterial Aspects

The arterial issue was discovered with growing feedback from our patients. Some have spontaneously reported improvement of their erection or a longer penis in the flaccid position. These symptoms, associated with the impression of a cold glans, are the major complaints in some patients in our daily outpatient visits. These symptoms are not related to a neurological problem because the delay in recovery is much shorter than for other symptoms. The diagnosis is evident in case of a young patient. Erectile dysfunction is commonly assumed to be due to a neurologic sexual problem. However, erectile dysfunction can frequently be associated with a bilateral arterial compression [28]. Unilateral surgical release of the artery may cause some improvement, but to obtain full recovery, a bilateral decompression is mandatory. One of our patients has done a Doppler ultrasonography of the pudendal arteries. Before surgery one of the two arteries was completely occluded, and after the decompression, the flow was better on the operated side compared to the other. Finally, the patient was operated on the contralateral side and experienced complete recovery.

Patients older than 50 years with contraindication or side effects of phosphodiesterase-5 inhibitors (IPDE5i) may also obtain good results after surgical decompression. Certainly, most patients of this age group have other expectations than the patients in their 20 s or 30 s. For the oldest ones, it is more acceptable to take a pill once a week to improve the quality of the erection. Nevertheless, we believe that many of them probably have a pudendal artery compression related to a postural problem acquired with age more often than arteriosclerosis, a psychological, or an endocrinological problem. Erectile dysfunction can be dependent on body position and time of day. Patients can experience better function in the morning and in supine position compared with the evening and the standing position. The explanation is probably the relaxation of the pyriformis muscle and the reduction of the pressure on the artery after a night sleeping or lying down.

Venous Aspects

The pudendal venous pathology is not so evident, but many aspects are very interesting to understand some complaints of our patients [29, 30]. The venous system presents a high potential for anatomical variation with many connections between different venous systems. The occlusion of part of the venous drainage can create an upstream congestion. There is a high incidence of hemorrhoids reported by our patients. The interesting element is the drainage of the hemorrhoidal plexus, which is partly by the pudendal vein. Maybe the compression of the pudendal vein increases the pressure upstream and increases the risk of hemorrhoids.

A particular syndrome reported is the hard flaccid syndrome [31]. The patient observes a continuous tumescence of the penis, but when he wishes to have sexual intercourse, the erection is not sufficient. Upon reading the literature on that syndrome, we realize that the patients also present all the symptoms reported in pudendal neuropathy. Our theory is that this syndrome is a combination of two problems: the pudendal venous compression causing the tumescence and the arterial compression responsible for the erectile dysfunction. The prognosis concerning the erection is better and more predictable because we always increase the flow in the corpus cavernosum after surgery. However, we cannot be sure that the release of the pudendal vein will be adequate or enough to efficiently drain this increasing inflow.

Associated Pathology

A significant number of patients present with a problem of fibromyalgia [32]. If no clear explanation is found, a relationship involving a general myofascial syndrome in this group of patients, or a hypersensitivity of the nerves, should be suspected.

Another associated pathology observed or diagnosed in our clinic is the Ehlers-Danlos syndrome. The patient can present with different forms of the disease. The vascular, with the risk of aneurysm, and the articular forms, with the hyperlaxity, are well-known. The third one, the visceral form, is more often ignored by physicians. The collagen fiber abnormality damages the nerve receptors. The patient has difficulties walking straight in the darkness due to injury of the proprioceptors. They also have cold feet and sleep with warm socks on due to lack of vasomotor control. The last classical symptom is having the impression of electric shocks in the finger when they touch objects, which is due to hypersensitivity of the tactile receptors in the fingers.

Diagnosis

Patient History

The diagnosis is mainly based on the symptoms reported by the patients. A good history is usually enough to make the diagnosis. A complete analysis of the patient profile is fundamental. The environment is of potential clinical interest. Does the patient have a seated profession? Which sport activities is the patient engaged with? The research of a trigger event can be of significance: trauma, surgery, infection, childbirth, or an unusual sport activity. Potential postural problem(s) must be evaluated, such as a shorter leg and an unbalanced bone pelvis, or other may require treatment regularly by a physiotherapist or a chiropractor. Chronic knee or back pain, headache, or trochanteritis may be additional troubles. The rhythmic nature of the symptoms is also significant. There may be no or less symptoms at night; worsening along the day; better standing up, lying down, or seated on the toilet; worse sitting on a hard chair (compared with a smooth cushion); and worsening after sexual activity or defecation, in case of stress, fatigue, or cold weather. Some symptoms are very specific of pudendal compression: pain in the clitoris (or the glans), in the urethra, premature ejaculation (or an arousal syndrome), erectile dysfunction, or pseudo-sciatalgia [33]. Other functional problems that are significantly associated include recurrent urinary tract infections, obstipation, frequent need to defecate, urgency to urinate, and fluctuant dysuria.

The affected side can be spontaneously reported by the patient, but it is not always clear. Sciatic pain in a prolonged seated position is highly associated with the side of pudendal nerve compression. This symptom also localizes the point of compression, proximal to Alcock's canal, because it is the only location where both the root of the sciatic nerve and the pudendal nerve can be found. Nevertheless, a double compression scenario, that is, proximal to and inside Alcock's canal, cannot be excluded.

Clinical Exam of a Pudendal Pathology

The clinical exam begins already when the patient enters the clinical office, by observing the patient's gait. Many patients have an asymmetric step sometimes with a lateralized movement when they walk. This observation is highly correlated with a postural problem (Fig. 9). The aspect of the face is also suggestive of a higher risk of a postural problem [34]. Retrognathism and descending shoulders are signs of lower obstructive airways. This problem places the head more anteriorly and increases all the curvatures of the vertebral column. The increasing curvature of the lumbar spine rotates the bone pelvis anteriorly, and thus the pressure on the pudendal element caused by the pyriformis muscle increases. A visual impairment can lead to chronic rotation of the head. If the patient has a blind eye, he will turn his head to improve the angle of vision on the blind side, creating a rotation of the column, influencing the position of the bony pelvis. Some patients have an asymmetric growth of the face with one half bigger than the other. In this situation the eyes are not exactly horizontally placed in the skull. The patient usually tilts the head lightly to place both eyes on a good horizontal line and increases the risk of scoliosis. Finally, a disorder of the temporomandibular joint can also influence the skull position and be a risk factor for a postural problem.

Naturally, the patient adopts a comfortable position. Occasionally, the patient prefers to stand up during the consultation instead of taking a seat. This element is not specific of the pudendal neuralgia because it is also observed in case of clunealgia or other perinealgia. The lack of functional symptoms during the patient history taking and clinical exam can confirm this diagnosis. The position adopted when the patient is seated can give additional information. If she is seated on one side of the buttock, a contralateral perinealgia can be suspected. If the patient places her buttock on the edge of the seat, she may have a bilateral perinealgia but certainly not a coccygodynia. A quick postural evaluation can be done, like the position of both iliac crest and shoulder, the line of the vertebral column, and the examination of any sign of trauma or surgery on the inferior extremities. The evaluation should be done by a chiropodist specialized in postural disorders. The examination includes a static postural evaluation. An anatomical evaluation as well as a measurement of the pressure under the feet and the position of the center of gravity is important. The analysis is completed by a dynamic evaluation of the patient walking on a conveyer belt.

Our clinical exam is centered on around the perineum. The patient points to the locations of the symptoms. This part of the exam is certainly not the easiest because it can be confusing. The areas reported by the patients are usually not precise, and it is common to have more than one nerve involved in the problem. A patient with pudendal neuralgia can also have a pseudo-sciatic pain (not always representing the whole territory of the nerve and can be difficult to recognize) [35]. And, additionally, he can also have Maigne's syndrome related with a postural problem with irradiation to the iliac crest, the sacroiliac joint, and the inguinal area [19]. The palpation of the perineum must compare both sides as the normal feeling of the pelvic muscles is individual from patient to patient. In a standing position, we can search for a sign of contraction of the pyriformis muscle, by deeply palpating both sides of the buttock with the thumbs, starting up and going down. On a horizontal line, just above the anus, the patient can feel a sensitive deep point corresponding to the pyriformis muscle.

The patient is installed in lithotomy position. We evaluated the symmetry of the sensation of the simple touch of the finger on the skin and under a palpating rolling test. The test is done systematically to explore the perineum from the perianal to the suprapubic area. Some perineal deep points of pressure must be evaluated. The perianal points, localized just above the anus and under the ischiopubic branches, are pressed to evaluate the symmetry of the sensation. The ischiatic tuberosity is also explored. A sensitivity medial to the tuberosity is in favor of a pudendal nerve problem and a sensitivity lateral to the tuberosity is more in favor of a cluneal nerve problem.

Finally, a digital rectal and/or vaginal exam is performed. Most of the patients present with a hypertonic anal sphincter or contracted transverse perineal muscle. The sensitivity during the introduction of the finger can elicit an acute burning sensation. Digital examination must be performed very gently to avoid exacerbating the pain as well as attempting to find the most painful side of the anal area. Then the finger is introduced as deep as possible to feel the muscles of the perineum at

3 o'clock and 9 o'clock (Fig. 7). At that level, we can feel the arcus tendineus of the levator ani muscle covering the internal obturator muscle and check for any asymmetry of the muscle tonus. The second point to palpate is located posterolateral from the rectum, in the direction of the sciatic spine (Fig. 8). We evaluate for a possible asymmetry of sensation between the left and the right side. In some cases, the patients describe authentic pain that can be associated with a trigger effect, but in many cases, one side is just less comfortable. For women, the exam is completed by a vaginal prolapse evaluation, particularly to search for a potential descending perineum syndrome [36]. This pathology is a defect of the tonus of the muscle wall itself. The clinical exam can reveal a more superficially located anus between the buttocks, spontaneously or during Valsalva's maneuver. This sign is associated with a higher risk of traction on the pudendal nerve, particularly of the rectal branch. During the clinical exam, we can also search for signs of problems of other nerves, especially the sensitivity on the anterior iliac crest under the palpation for an iliohypogastric or ilioinguinal nerve entrapment, the sensitivity of the curvature of the sacrum during the digital rectal examination to search for pain from the impar ganglia, the sensation when the coccyx is mobilized, and the palpation of the lateral side of the ischiatic tuberosity for the cluneal nerve.

Complementary Exams

Many patients arrive to the clinic after a full diagnostic investigation done elsewhere, eventually with a wrong diagnosis such as vesico-perineal dyssynergia. Pelvic MRI is a classical exam that allows the exclusion of a compressive tumor in the pelvis or lesions of endometriosis. Sometimes, the radiologist reports inflammatory tissue around the pudendal nerve, but usually at that level, the exam is normal. The 3 Tesla MRI scan is able to detect lesions of the pudendal nerve entrapment when performed by highly experienced radiologists [37]. However, there is no consensus on these radiological findings, and many radiologists are still skeptical about the capacity of the imaging study to localize a point of compression of such a small nerve.

A dynamic pelvic MRI can exclude a descending perineum syndrome. It can be suspected when the anus descends more than 5 cm under the pubococcygeal line during straining (Fig. 8) [38]. In case of nocturnal symptoms, an MRI of the vertebral column is mandatory to exclude a compression in the vertebral column. Depending on some associated symptoms, a specific region of the vertebral column will be targeted (the lumbosacral in case of symptoms in the perineum with or without symptoms in the lower limbs) and the cervical and dorsal column (in case of symptoms in the upper limbs). If

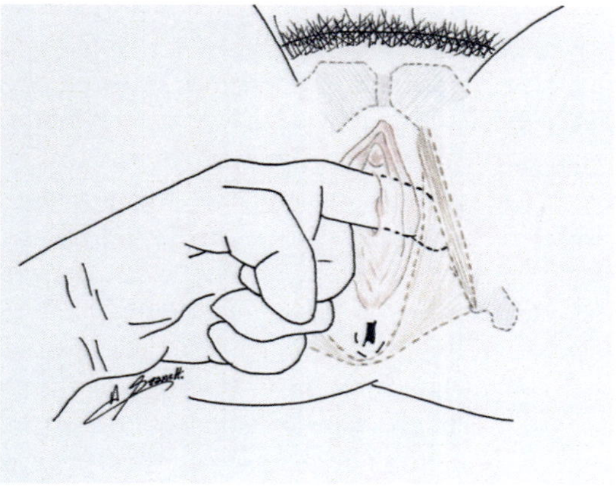

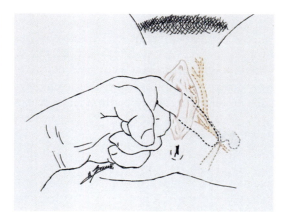

Fig. 7 Clinical exam: palpation of the arcus tendinues of the levatori muscle

Fig. 8 Clinical exam: palpation of the sciatic spine

the patient history is unclear, a complete evaluation of the vertebral column is recommended. If the neurologic history seems unusually complex, the patient should always be referred to a neurologist for a complete evaluation.

An electromyography (EMG) is the most common exam performed, but it is also the most confusing. The EMG tests only the motor fibers of the nerve. It is important to remember that these fibers are big compared to the sympathetic fibers and the sensory fibers. The big motor fibers are more resistant against compression. This explains why some patients may have a normal EMG and a lot of pain. When the EMG is abnormal, the compression is stronger, and the sensory and sympathetic fibers are also involved. However, some patients can have an abnormal EMG without complaints. The EMG is just indicative but can never exclude the diagnosis [39]. The speed conduction of the pudendal nerve is probably more specific, but it needs a specific research and is not, as the EMG, 100% specific or sensitive.

The Doppler ultrasonography of the pudendal artery is probably the most interesting exam [40]. The knowledge of the profile of a normal pudendal artery is fundamental to evaluate a potential compression. This exam provides a direct evaluation in case of erectile dysfunction but also an indirect sign of compression in case of pudendal neuropathy. One of our patients had a severe erectile dysfunction with a complete lack of flow on the Doppler ultrasound scan in one pudendal artery. He underwent surgery on that side and recovered partially in terms of erection. The control ultrasonography done postoperatively showed increased flow on the operated side. After surgery on the contralateral side, he recovered a normal erection.

The infiltration test can be valuable for an accurate diagnosis. It is important to understand the principles in defining a good strategy [41]. The infiltration can be done for different goals. If we want to prove the pudendal origin, we need to be most accurate to target only the pudendal nerve. In this case a CT scan is the most accurate (80% positive response). A mixture of contrast to localize the injection near the pudendal nerve, a local anesthetic (sufficient for few hours, maximum 1 day), and a corticosteroid is injected. After the infiltration the patient can experience a relapse of symptoms for up to 1 day. Also, during the first hours, a palsy of the sciatic nerve can occur, due to the proximity of the sciatic roots. During the following week, the symptoms can become worse than before the infiltration, as the effect of the local anesthesia wanes. After 1 week the liquid is resorbed and the patient returns to her baseline condition. One week later she can feel a progressive improvement for a few weeks or months due to the effect of the corticosteroid. Unfortunately, the corticosteroid effect produces a positive effect in only 15% of the cases. It is important to inform the patient about this evolution as many patients remember only the worsening of the symptoms and will assume a negative test. The infiltration test performed under ultrasonography is not so accurate (30% positive response) and even lower under finger guidance. The point of infiltration under ultrasonography or digital guidance is just to define the side of the compression. Indeed, an

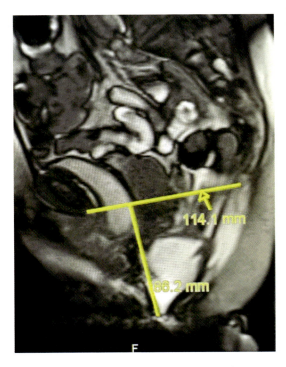

Fig. 9 Descending perineum syndrome: dynamic MRI

inaccurate injection can paralyze many nerves localized in the same area, like the cluneal nerve, and is not specific to the pudendal nerve.

Nantes Criteria

The Nantes criteria were published in 2008 to help diagnose pudendal neuralgia and include (1) pain in the territory of the pudendal nerve, (2) worsened by sitting, (3) not nocturnal, (4) without sensory loss, and (5) a positive pudendal nerve block. Hence, these criteria are based on pain only and do not include functional problems [42]. A clinical problem can be that neurologists see more patients with pain as their main complaint and urologists, gynecologists, and proctologists see more patients with functional problems. Unfortunately, many specialists never relate the functional symptoms to a potential pudendal origin, and the patients are usually stuck with an idiopathic diagnosis.

The pain is often the most difficult symptom to correctly diagnose the etiology, due to the unclear limits of the pudendal territory (first Nantes criterium). The patients can also present with many other sensory nerve problems associated with a postural problem. The myofascial syndrome related with a postural problem can cause compression of multiple nerves rendering it difficult to understand the etiology (pseudo-sciatic, ilioinguinal nerve, ilio-obturator nerve, and Maigne's syndrome). We have operated on a significant number of patients, previously rejected based on the Nantes criteria, with excellent results. When we discuss with our patients with pain, many of them describe a functional disorder years before the pain occurred. We see the pain as an endpoint of this pathology. The functional disorder reported by the patients is much more specific to a pudendal problem because all the other adjacent nerves are sensory. The presence of functional symptoms is always a sign of a pudendal component. For all the abovementioned reasons, we do not use the criteria of Nantes.

Treatment

Conservative Treatment

Our approach is opposite to the classical treatment proposed by many other authors. If drugs deliver comfort, the first line of treatment should target pudendal decompression. For other compressed nerves in the body, like in the carpal tunnel syndrome, the treatment is decompression. The pudendal nerve should not be an exception; otherwise the patient may in time develop an irreversible damage of the nerve.

An important point is to remove as many risk factors from the environment as possible. The patient must stop all sports at risk, particularly activities using a saddle, like bicycling [43]. If the patient refuses to cease the activity, he should choose a large saddle with a point of pressure localized on the sciatic tuberosity instead of a thin one pushing up into the smooth perineum. The patient must also avoid a seated position for a long time. We propose to use an alarm clock each hour to remember to stand up for 10 min. The office can be adapted with a specific desk that is movable up and down. The use of an ergonomic chair is also important, and a specific cushion can help. Some authors recommend cushions of donut or horseshoe shape (Fig. 10), but we prefer a neutral cushion to avoid increasing the pressure on other points of the perineum with a risk of causing other painful problems like clunealgia or a coccygodynia. This cushion must be thin and maintain a homogenous pressure (e.g., R/balanced seat, honeycomb technology). The patient also has to avoid all sport activities with reinforcement of the buttock like bodybuilding or specific exercises of CrossFit (steps, squats). Sports with a quick left-right movements (like squash, badminton, table tennis) should be avoided. All patients practicing a sport associated with running or walking long distances must have a postural evaluation done. If high-heeled shoes are not already prohibited, we advise to avoid wearing them all day long.

Postural Control and Postural Physiotherapy

A postural problem can be adapted with an orthopedic insole (Fig. 11) [44]. An unbalanced bone pelvis is the origin of a global myofascial syndrome associated with many muscle contractures [45]. One of these muscles is the pyriformis muscle responsible for the pressure on the pudendal elements. When we walk or run, at each step, the muscle is stimulated, particularly in case of an unbalanced bone pelvis. The patient can describe worsening of the symptoms during the exertion or the day after. The insoles cannot correct the postural problem in one step since a sudden modification will elicit potentially new pains in the joints or the back. The correction must be progressive and need multiple reassessments and adjustments. The patient has to wear the insole for 6–8 weeks to feel improvement. Sometimes the problem is not possible to solve when the disorder is too severe or when the patient cannot tolerate the insole.

Physiotherapy targets muscle relaxation of the perineum and the pelvis [46, 47]. The first option is the internal massage through the anus or the vagina. This approach can be efficient but difficult in many cases due to the hypersensitivity of the digital rectal or vaginal introduction. Elderly women also have some mucosal atrophy or vaginal adhesion. A major problem is the risk of worsening symptoms after the physiotherapy session because the pressure applied is not fully controlled. The second option is the external deep massage, particularly of the buttock to target the pyriformis muscle. The patient can reproduce this effect at home using a tennis ball placed on the floor. The patient sits on the ball and rolls it under the buttock. The third possibility is the external stretching exercise, particularly centered on the muscle of the buttocks attached on the trochanter. The physiotherapist must teach self-exercises, and the patient has to continue with a session of stretching every day. In every case we do not recommend electrostimulation on the perineum (either intrarectal or vaginal) because the electric current may stimulate the muscle and the nerves and significantly worsen the symptoms.

Fifteen percent of patients will be completely cured with the combination of postural physiotherapy and insoles to correct a postural problem. For instance, we have seen some patients who had urinary urgency and the need to urinate every 20 min. This problem can be completely solved

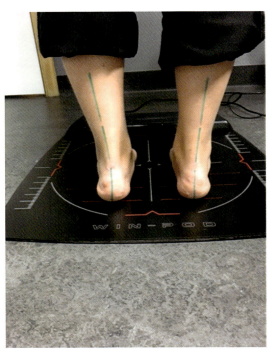

Fig. 11 Postural evaluation: measure of angle and position of the centre of gravity

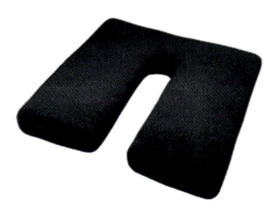

Fig. 10 Specific cushion

with this conservative treatment. Two thirds of patients will notice at least partial improvement (around 65% of symptoms, by their own evaluation). In case of an insufficient result, the next proposed treatment is surgical decompression.

Drugs

Drugs are just a type of palliative treatment. Drugs never change the pressure on the nerve; they only mask the pain problem. It is dangerous to let a patient with compression of the nerve mask the pain with drugs, as they run the risk of irreversible nerve damage. The majority of the patients arriving in our clinic is already under the classical treatment proposed for neuralgia like gabapentin, pregabalin, amitriptyline, and/or carbamazepine. Most of these treatments have a low efficiency rate or significant side effects judged incompatible with a normal social life by the patient. Paracetamol and the nonsteroidal anti-inflammatory drugs are usually insufficient. Tramadol can be used, but the associated obstipation can be counterproductive because straining usually increases the symptoms. More powerful opiates like oxycodone, fentanyl, or morphine are efficient but increase the sensitivity of the pain receptor. The patient has a risk of needing higher and higher doses to control the pain and end up in a dependency state. Patients on grade 3 opiates also have a worse prospect for recovery after surgery, probably because they have a more severe compression.

Many men with pudendal neuralgia also present with erectile dysfunction due to the compression of the arteries. For these patients we propose tadalafil 5 mg per day at the first consultation. The feedback from this group of patients has been impressive as they frequently report an improvement of other symptoms like the pain as well. This feedback was so common that we proposed tadalafil to women with a positive response in 50% of the cases. However, the mechanism remains unclear. We can suspect a myorelaxation effect related with the nitric oxide transmitter or an improvement of the oxygenation of the pudendal nerve and sciatic roots due to the increasing flow in the pudendal arteries [48]. This effect can also explain the efficiency of tadalafil for male patients with a small prostate presenting with

urinary symptoms. This group of men have poor outcomes and satisfaction rates after transurethral prostatic resection. In fact, these patients probably have a pudendal neuropathy with predominant urinary symptoms rather than a benign prostatic obstruction as etiology of their symptoms. The systematic patient history can usually uncover some symptoms suggestive of a pudendal problem like erectile dysfunction or premature ejaculation. The tolerance of tadalafil is much better than the classical drugs mentioned above. The main complaints are heartburn and headache at the beginning of the treatment. Tinnitus is a reason to stop the treatment because it can be an irreversible side effect. Hypersensitivity of the nervous fibers against pressure is a rarer condition. It is related to an abnormality of the sodium channel on the membrane of the nerve cells [1]. In this case, Lamotrigine® can be tried in progressively increasing doses.

Pudendal Nerve Infiltration

Pudendal nerve infiltration is not a treatment of pudendal compression but a diagnostic test. The effect is transitory. The exception is only when the patient arrives with an acute event directly in our clinic. If the infiltration is executed quickly after this trigger event, hopefully the condition will not progress to a chronic state. The infiltration in this case must contain a steroid to have a strong anti-inflammatory effect. Additionally, one patient had been placed on oral corticosteroids by his family doctor while waiting for a medical appointment. The characteristic symptoms of pudendal pathology had disappeared in the waiting period for an appointment at our clinic.

Psychiatric Support

Many physicians associate pelviperineal pain to a psychological or a sexual trauma in the past. Sexual abuse can be the origin of a lack of perineal muscle relaxation and a local myofascial disorder, but in our experience, this situation is uncommon compared with the number of patients presenting with this problem. We have seen only a few cases with clear sexual trauma in the past (sexual abuse, incest, prostitution). The majority of our patients refuse to see a psychiatrist because they feel a negation of the reality of their problem (they say "It's not in my head"). The dramatic situation and the psychological impact on their life may need psychological support, but first of all, they need recognition from the physicians of the reality of the problem. Hypnosis and sophrology can help in the control and perception of the pain. Some patients report self-capacity to introvert and do relaxation when they feel the crisis.

Laparoscopic Pudendal Decompression

We discovered this technique performed by Dr. Tibet Erdogu from Istanbul in 2014 during a live surgery event. We have developed a systematic approach to define a reproducible technique. At the beginning of our experience, Alcock's canal was not well accessible. However, with time, we have modified our technique to enable a complete dissection from the beginning of the sacrosciatic ligament, just behind the origin of the obturator vein, to the fat of the perineum. This access allows control of the passage of the rectal branch through the tuberous ligament. The distal branches of the pudendal nerve escape this access. This technique is minimally invasive, and the patients stay hospitalized for one night after surgery [1]. Some of them, if operated early in the morning, are discharged the same day.

Technique (Movies Available on YouTube; Renaud Bollens or Fabienne Absil Channels)

We place a bladder catheter and a nasogastric tube for the time of the surgery. The patient is placed in the classical supine position for pelvic surgery. An optical trocar of 11 mm is introduced just under the umbilicus. If you work with a 30° lens, it can be placed above the umbilicus. If you use a 0° lens, the optic placed too high will give you a tangential view on the sacrosciatic ligament which renders the dissection of the initial segment of the ligament very difficult. Two ports of 5 mm are placed on a line from the anterior iliac crest and the optical port. They are placed more medially (four fingers wide from the anterior iliac crest) on the side being operated. If the port is placed too laterally, the instrument will not reach the distal

part of the nerve dissection. A fourth trocar is placed in the right flank. To find the best position, we look in the direction of the site being operated (medial from the direction of the iliac vessels), and we try to have a triangulation between all the instruments. One difficulty with this surgery is the clashing between the instruments inside or outside the patient. Hence, we have to find a compromise in their positioning.

The patient is placed in Trendelenburg, and the intestinal loops are moved up, over the promontory. Sometimes the sigmoid colon can be fixed with a suture to the abdominal wall. In women, the presence of endometriotic lesions should always be searched for. If necessary, the lesions, particularly when they are located on the uterosacral ligament, should be excised. The first landmark is the umbilical artery. We incise lateral from the artery at the edge of the fat surrounding the vessels. The incision is extended from the anterior wall to the round ligament in women and the ureter in men. The vas deferens is freed from the peritoneum to allow a good aperture of the plane. In women, the incision is prolonged medially, parallel to the round ligament in the anterior layer of the broad ligament. Gentle traction helps when using monopolar coagulation to open the plane between the vessels and the lymphatic tissue laterally and the bladder medially. The dissection must be bloodless to avoid losing the landmarks. When approaching the obturator fossa, a fatty hernia can be observed in the foramen of the obturator elements. This hernia must be reduced to allow access to the distal part of the pudendal elements. At that level, the obturator vein can be found, which is the next important landmark. At the level of the vein, we change our anatomical plan. We stay close to the vein to go between the lymphatic tissue and the endopelvic fascia. This maneuver allows the possibility of removing this lymphatic tissue to find the edge of the sacrosciatic ligament behind the vein. Sometimes the origin of the vein is too far medially, and we have to proceed between the vein (with or without the artery) and the obturator nerves to see the beginning of the ligament. We may need to sacrifice the vein between clips (particularly if your optical material is sensitive to the overbrightness) to improve the view more than the access. The endopelvic fascia is freed from all the fat. At this level we can frequently see the arcus tendineus of the levator ani muscle. A small trick to localize it is the presence of a small fatty hernia between the arcus and the internal obturator muscle. The arcus is located medially from this hernia. When the arcus tendinous is followed on its lowest part, the sciatic spine can be palpated on a horizontal line, just behind the end of the arcus. The coccygeus muscle is the lowest part of the levator ani muscle and covers the distal part of the sacrosciatic ligament. This muscle is thick on the sciatic spine level and becomes thinner in the direction of the obturator vein. The muscle is coagulated using the bipolar grasp and cut with cold scissors. This maneuver frees the surface of the ligament itself. The ligament is coagulated and cut from the proximal edge to the sciatic spine. The first part must be done carefully because veins for the sciatic roots run just under the ligament. When the ligament is coagulated, the pudendal elements should be pushed down to reduce the exposure to the extreme heat induced by the bipolar grasp. The dissection is carried out close to the obturator muscle, particularly when we arrive at the level of the sciatic spine. If a small piece of muscle is left attached on the spine, it will be more difficult to turn around the spine. When this access becomes difficult, a hole is made just above the spine using monopolar coagulation. This hole must be created as lateral over the spine as possible to be sure to arrive laterally to the pudendal elements. It allows the surgeon double access and to completely open Alcock's canal. Distally, a small vein can usually be found crossing the pudendal elements transversally. This vein must be coagulated carefully because in case of accidental incision the stump of the vein disappears in the muscle. The surgeon should stop the dissection when he reaches the fat of the perineum with a sensation of complete freedom. In some patients the pudendal elements should also be mobilized from behind the spine if a potential point of pressure due to the spine is suspected. This maneuver can delay the recovery of the patient. If the patient presents with anorectal symptoms, the surgeon should also explore the rectal branch of the pudendal nerve. He should gently release the cut

ligament from the medial part of the pudendal elements and find the origin of these branches on the anterior aspect of the spine. The passage of the rectal nerve through the tuberous ligament can be stenotic. The passage along this small nerve should be enlarged. The dissection of this nerve is not easy because it is a small nerve, and the exact anatomical position can vary from patient to patient. At the end of the procedure, the surgeon should expect to see good pulsation in the pudendal artery as a sign of a good decompression. If you leave a drain, you can expect 200 cc of lymphorrhea due to the mobilization of the lymphatic tissue under the obturator vein. Before awakening the patient, the bladder catheter is removed. The pudendal neuropathy produces urethral pain, and the patients feel extreme discomfort if the catheter is left in place.

After surgery we prescribe tadalafil 5 mg daily for the first 3 postoperative months. The rationale is to increase the size of the pudendal artery to give more room around the pudendal elements when the fibrotic healing is forming over the released pudendal elements. Male patients are usually more difficult to operate than female patients, as the prostate can reduce the access aggravated by excess intra-abdominal fat, which is more common in obese men. The only significant perioperative complication we have experienced was injury of the pudendal artery in a young man. Ligation of the artery will cause irreversible erectile dysfunction. After trying hemostasis with pressure with a swab, we clamped the artery using small bulldog clamps. The suture was performed with a 5/0 Prolene®, and the patient did develop a sequela after this accident. For this reason, we recommend selecting female cases to start this technique.

Postoperative Recovery

Although the surgery is not very difficult, the knowledge of the postoperative recovery is fundamental to inform the patient about before surgery. Our patients have a follow-up visit at the first month postoperatively and every 3 months during the first year. In case of delayed recovery, the patient is seen every fourth to sixth month after the first year. The first week is marked by lack of symptoms. Some patients unable to be seated before surgery are able to stay seated the day after surgery. This impressive effect is not related to the surgery but is due to the general anesthesia. This phenomenon is well-known in facial neuralgia. When the patient is close to committing suicide, general anesthesia can suppress the pain for 7–10 days to give some time to reevaluate the treatment. After this first "honeymoon week," in 50% of the patients, the symptoms get back worse than before the surgery. The decompression of a nerve elicits an abnormal hypersignal in the nerve. The pain can be worse due to hypersignal of sensory fibers (allodynia), and urinary retention can occur due to stimulation of motor fibers. In our experience, a young patient was in urinary retention with a suprapubic catheter for 3 months. After 1 month the patient started to feel some improvement. Usually, it is an up and down evolution: the patient can wake up one day very well and to have the symptoms back the day after. For them, this evolution is socially difficult because they never know what they will be able to do the day after. The recovery is slow at the beginning to accelerate from the third until the sixth months. After 6 months the patient can expect 80% recovery. After 6 months the recovery is slower, and full recovery can take 18 months or more. The final result is expected between 6 months and 12 years after the surgery (Fig. 12). This is the most common evolution, but in the extreme, we have had some patients with 90% recovery after 1 month. Alternatively, other patients may need up to 2 years of delay before beginning to feel the recovery. During the recovery time, it is fundamental to support the patient and to search for signs of improvement. The frequency and the severity of the crisis improve further and further after the first month. Usually, we observe three phases: at the beginning the patient describes perineal numbness, followed by the allodynia, and finally normal sensation returns. The recovery usually starts at the anorectal level to extend in the direction of the anterior perineum to finish with the glans/clitoris and the pubic area. The rhythm along the day can also show a sign of recovery. Classically, the patient's symptoms appear at the same hours of the day. As they recover, they observe a progressive delay with the symptoms appearing later and later. These aspects of recovery must be stressed when informing patients before and after the surgery. When we operate on both pudendal nerves at the same time or the second side too early after the first one, we can have a transitory anesthesia of the anal canal. In our cohort, three patients presented with 3 months of fecal incontinence for this reason. Finally, one patient has reported a definitive lesion of the obturator nerve. We suppose that it was related to mechanical compression from the ipsilateral instrument when the trocar was placed

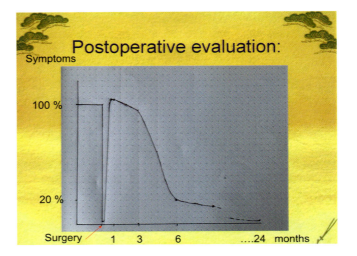

Fig. 12 Postoperative clinical evolution

too laterally or eventually an electric leak into the nerve.

Outcomes and Explanation of Failure

Our global success rate is around 80% of the patients who underwent surgery. This level is higher than in other centers, probably somewhat related to a selection bias. We advocate surgery as second-line treatment after failure of conservative decompression approaches. We also operate on many patients with functional problems only. These two elements lead to surgery earlier in the therapeutic algorithm and in a younger patient group presenting a better prognosis. The variety of symptoms in our group explains the difficulty in their evaluation. Some of the patients have pain predominantly; others present with sexual, urinary, or fecal disturbances. Finally, patients are asked to evaluate their satisfaction rate. The quality of the preoperative information also increases the global satisfaction rate because the patient knows what will happen after surgery. This parameter can also increase the global satisfaction rate. It is impossible to cure all patients with surgery. Certain case reports in our data help us to understand this pathology and so does the group in which surgery fails. We always try to understand the origin of the failure to propose a potential improvement to our patients.

Myofascial Pain

Some patients have an evolution of the symptoms. The symptoms related to the nerve, like allodynia and hypertonic sphincter, disappear, but the myofascial syndrome remains present. The muscle contracture of the perineum can be a reason for the persistence of some pain after surgery. Most of the cases are due to the patient not correcting their postural problem with insoles and physiotherapy. Some of them have an untreatable postural problem and will need lifelong physiotherapy or recurrent botulinum toxin injections for symptomatic improvement. A financial issue can be a drawback for some patients. Insoles in Belgium cost 200 euros and must be readapted every 2 years. The insoles are reimbursed only when they are prescribed by an orthopedic surgeon. Unfortunately, they only take care of the impact on the bone and joint, and they consider less than 8 mm of difference nonsignificant.

Contralateral Decompensation

Fifteen percent of our patients will be operated on both sides. We no longer operate prophylactically on the asymptomatic side. In case of failure on the pathological side and accident on the healthy side, the situation can be dramatic and the risk of prosecution very high. After unilateral surgery, some patients notice with time improved comfort on the operated side compared to the contralateral side. We assume that they initially had a bilateral problem with a dominant side. Another potential explanation is the increasing tension on the contralateral sacrosciatic ligament. In case of recurrence of symptoms, particularly when the patient cannot lateralize the problem, we must exclude this possibility.

Descending Perineum Syndrome

Although compression of the pudendal nerve is the most common situation, a stretching problem can also be the underlying cause in some specific situations. Women can present with a descending perineum syndrome. They describe mainly anorectal dyschezia and pain. They usually need to support the anus with the finger to stabilize the anus when trying to defecate. The stretching of the muscle of the perineum is a direct origin of the pain but can be also associated with pudendal symptoms due to constant traction. These patients describe that pain in the standing position improves when they support the perineum with the hand. Radiologically, the anus descends more than 5 cm under the pubococcygeal line. We recommend in these patients laparoscopic reconstruction of the perineum using mesh to reinforce the wall (video available on YouTube: Renaud Bollens Channel).

Hypersensitivity of Neurons

Two patients have reported a very strange syndrome in our clinic, associating perineal pain, facial symptoms with headache, and a sensation of dying. The symptoms were mainly nocturnal. They seem to be related with a hypersensitivity of neurons when they are compressed. The origin is an abnormality of the sodium channels of the membrane of the nerve [15]. In these patients we can try an antiepileptic drug specifically targeting the sodium channel (e.g., Lamictal).

Conclusion

After 8 years of intensive clinical and surgical work in our center, the pudendal nerve entrapment syndrome as well as other related perineal problems still remain unclear and poorly understood. The complexity of the symptoms and the lack of global approach and global view have hindered an easier and better clarification of this condition. The patient history and the feedback of our patients have been fundamental for the understanding of the mechanism of this pathologic entity. Once the etiology of this disease is understood, a more logical therapeutic approach can be suggested. The first line of treatment must be decompression of the nerve. It may be achieved by controlling the environment of the patient and the correction of a postural problem at the origin of the global myofascial syndrome. In this regard, physiotherapy helps and can break the vicious circle of muscle contracture, compression of the nerve, and pain. If this first line of treatment is inefficient, a surgical decompression should be proposed. All other treatments will just camouflage the symptoms, and the nerve will continue to be injured with a risk of irreversible lesion.

We have focused on the pudendal pain for several years. However, numerous functional symptoms are known to be associated with pudendal pathology [21–28]. A variety of symptoms result from the number of structures potentially interested in its pathophysiology: the pudendal nerve (sensory fibers, motor fibers, sympathetic fibers), the pudendal artery, and the pudendal vein. The association with functional problems is highly suggestive of pudendal pathology, much more than the pain. Treating these functional problems as a potential expression of pudendal pathology will completely change the approach to this syndrome. An etiological approach to these functional problems will avert their progression into a painful syndrome.

Lastly, we must continue to search for and understand the reasons of the nonresponding group of patients. New discoveries will probably emerge in the future if we keep searching for the origin of syndromes and failures that cannot yet be explained today.

Cross-References

▸ Bladder Dysfunction and Pelvic Pain: The Role of Sacral, Tibial, and Pudendal Neuromodulation
▸ Clinical Evaluation of the Female Lower Urinary Tract and Pelvic Floor
▸ Pathophysiology of Female Micturition Disorders
▸ Urodynamic Evaluation: Traditional, Video, and Ambulatory Approaches
▸ Voiding Dysfunction After Female Pelvic Surgery

References

1. Bollens R, Mjaess G, Sarkis J, et al. Laparoscopic transperitoneal pudendal nerve and artery release for pudendal entrapment syndrome. Surg Endosc. 2021;35 (11):6031–8. https://doi.org/10.1007/s00464-020-08092-4. Epub 2020 Oct 13
2. Erdogru T, Avci E, Akand M, et al. Laparoscopic pudendal nerve decompression and transposition combined with omental flap protection of the nerve (Istanbul technique): technical description and feasibility analysis. Surg Endosc. 2014;28(3):925–32. https://doi.org/10.1007/s00464-013-3248-1. Epub 2013 Oct 23
3. Bensignor-Le Henaff M, Labat JJ, Robert T, et al. Perineal pain and lesions of the internal pudendal nerves. Cah Anesthesiol. 1993;41(2):111–4.
4. Khoder W, Hale D. Pudendal neuralgia. Obstet Gynecol Clin N Am. 2014;41(3):443–52. https://doi.org/10.1016/j.ogc.2014.04.002. Epub 2014 Jul 9
5. Amarenco G, Savatovsky I, Budet C, et al. Perineal neuralgia and Alcock's canal syndrome. Ann Urol (Paris). 1989;23(6):488–92.
6. Robert R, Labat JJ, Riant T, et al. Neurosurgical treatment of perineal neuralgias. Adv Tech Stand Neurosurg. 2007;32:41–59. https://doi.org/10.1007/978-3-211-47423-5_3.
7. Cour F, Droupy S, Faix A, et al. Anatomy and physiology of sexuality. Prog Urol. 2013;23(9):547–61. https://doi.org/10.1016/j.purol.2012.11.007. Epub 2012 Dec 31
8. Kinter KJ, Newton BW. Anatomy, abdomen and pelvis, pudendal nerve. In: StatPearls [Internet]. Treasure Island: StatPearls Publishing; 2022.

9. Henry BM, Pękala PA, Vikse J, et al. Variations in the arterial blood supply to the penis and the accessory pudendal artery: a meta-analysis and review of implications in radical prostatectomy. J Urol. 2017;198(2):345–53. https://doi.org/10.1016/j.juro.2017.01.080. Epub 2017 Feb 12

10. Bookstein JJ, Lurie AL. Selective penile venography: anatomical and hemodynamic observations. J Urol. 1988;140(1):55–60. https://doi.org/10.1016/s0022-5347(17)41485-6.

11. Reese GE, von Roon AC, Tekkis PP. Haemorrhoids. BMJ Clin Evid. 2009;2009:0415.

12. Robert R, Labat JJ, Riant T, et al. Somatic perineal pain other than pudendal neuralgia. Neurochirurgie. 2009;55(4-5):470–4. https://doi.org/10.1016/j.neuchi.2009.07.002. Epub 2009 Sep 9

13. Sibert L, Rigaud J, Delavierre D, et al. Chronic pelvic pain: epidemiology and economic impact. Prog Urol. 2010;20(12):872–85. https://doi.org/10.1016/j.purol.2010.08.004. Epub 2010 Sep 29

14. Lacazio S, Foisy A, Tessier A, et al. Incidence of postural disorders in patients with chronic pelvic-perineal pain. Prog Urol. 2018;28(11):548–56. https://doi.org/10.1016/j.purol.2018.05.002. Epub 2018 Jun 6

15. Dib-Hajj SD, Geha P, Waxman SG. Sodium channels in pain disorders: pathophysiology and prospects for treatment. Pain. 2017;158(Suppl 1):S97–S107. https://doi.org/10.1097/j.pain.0000000000000854.

16. Bauer P. Chronic anoperineal pain: diagnosis and strategy for evaluation. J Chir (Paris). 2004 Jul;141(4):225–31. https://doi.org/10.1016/s0021-7697(04)95598-6.

17. Meister MR, Sutcliffe S, Badu A, et al. Pelvic floor myofascial pain severity and pelvic floor disorder symptom bother: is there a correlation? Am J Obstet Gynecol. 2019;221(3):235.e1–235.e15. https://doi.org/10.1016/j.ajog.2019.07.020. Epub 2019 Jul 15

18. Iacazio S, Foisy A, Tessier A, et al. Incidence of postural disorders in patients with chronic pelvic-perineal pain. Prog Urol. 2018;28(11):548–56. https://doi.org/10.1016/j.purol.2018.05.002. Epub 2018 Jun 6

19. Randhawa S, Garvin G, Roth M, et al. Maigne syndrome – a potentially treatable yet underdiagnosed cause of low back pain: a review. J Back Musculoskelet Rehabil. 2022;35(1):153–9. https://doi.org/10.3233/BMR-200297.

20. Fritel X. Pelvic floor and pregnancy. Gynecol Obstet Fertil. 2010;38(5):332–46. https://doi.org/10.1016/j.gyobfe.2010.03.008. Epub 2010 Apr 24

21. Vírseda Chamorro M, Salinas-Casado J, Zarza-Luciañez D, et al. Participation of the pudendal innervation in the detrusor overactivity of the detrusor and in the overactive bladder syndrome. Actas Urol Esp. 2012;36(1):37–41. https://doi.org/10.1016/j.acuro.2011.07.011. Epub 2011 Oct 15

22. Aoun F, Mjaess G, Assaf J, et al. Clinical effect of computed guided pudendal nerve block for patients with premature ejaculation: a pilot study. Scand J Urol. 2020;54(3):258–62. https://doi.org/10.1080/21681805.2020.1770855. Epub 2020 Jun 1

23. Aoun F, Mjaess G, Lilly E, et al. Is pudendal nerve entrapment a potential cause for weak ejaculation? Int J Impot Res. 2022;34(6):520–3. https://doi.org/10.1038/s41443-021-00443-6. Epub 2021 May 10

24. Aoun F, Alkassis M, Tayeh GA, et al. Sexual dysfunction due to pudendal neuralgia: a systematic review. Transl Androl Urol. 2021;10(6):2500–11. https://doi.org/10.21037/tau-21-13.

25. van Meegdenburg MM, Heineman E, Broens PM. Pudendal neuropathy alone results in urge incontinence rather than in complete Fecal incontinence. Dis Colon Rectum. 2015;58(12):1186–93. https://doi.org/10.1097/DCR.0000000000000497.

26. Afonso Ramos S, Guimarães T, Bollens R. Urethral leak: an unusual symptom of pudendal nerve entrapment. Cent European J Urol. 2020;73(1):46–8. https://doi.org/10.5173/ceju.2020.0024. Epub 2020 Mar 23

27. Aoun F, Semaan A, Mjaess G, et al. Pudendal nerve entrapment and recurrent urinary tract infection: is there a link? Turk J Urol. 2020;46(5):410–1. https://doi.org/10.5152/tud.2020.20148. Epub 2020 Jul 2

28. Aoun F, Mjaess G, Daher K, et al. Laparoscopic treatment of pudendal nerve and artery entrapment improves erectile dysfunction in healthy young males. Int J Impot Res. 2021;33(1):1–5. https://doi.org/10.1038/s41443-020-0287-8. Epub 2020 May 4

29. Nihon KK, Zasshi HG. Pathologic significance of the internal pudendal vein in the development of intrapelvic venous congestion syndrome. Jpn J Urol. 1996;87(11):1214–20. https://doi.org/10.5980/jpnjurol1989.87.1214.

30. Vin F. Vulvar varices. J Mal Vasc. 1990;15(4):406–9.

31. Abdessater M, Kanbar A, Akakpo W, et al. Hard flaccid syndrome: state of current knowledge. Basic Clin Androl. 2020;30:7. https://doi.org/10.1186/s12610-020-00105-5. eCollection 2020

32. Jones KD, King LA, Mist SD, et al. Postural control deficits in people with fibromyalgia: a pilot study. Arthritis Res Ther. 2011;13(4):R127. https://doi.org/10.1186/ar3432.

33. Park JW, Lee YK, Lee YJ, et al. Deep gluteal syndrome as a cause of posterior hip pain and sciatica-like pain. Bone Joint J. 2020;102-B(5):556–67. https://doi.org/10.1302/0301-620X.102B5.BJJ-2019-1212.R1.

34. Cuccia A, Caradonna C. The relationship between the stomatognathic system and body posture. Clinics (Sao Paulo). 2009;64(1):61–6. https://doi.org/10.1590/s1807-59322009000100011.

35. Delavierre D, Rigaud J, Sibert L, et al. Symptomatic approach to referred chronic pelvic and perineal pain and posterior ramus syndrome. Prog Urol. 2010;20(12):990–4. https://doi.org/10.1016/j.purol.2010.08.071. Epub 2010 Oct 13

36. Chaudhry Z, Tarnay C. Descending perineum syndrome: a review of the presentation, diagnosis, and management. Int Urogynecol J. 2016;27(8):1149–56. https://doi.org/10.1007/s00192-015-2889-0. Epub 2016 Jan 11

37. Wadhwa V, Hamid AS, Kumar Y, et al. Pudendal nerve and branch neuropathy: magnetic resonance neurography evaluation. Acta Radiol. 2017;58(6):726–33. https://doi.org/10.1177/0284185116668213. Epub 2016 Sep 23

38. Hilfiker PR, Debatin JF, Schwizer W, et al. MR defecography: depiction of anorectal anatomy and pathology. J Comput Assist Tomogr. 1998;22(5):749–55.

39. Lefaucheur JP, Labat JJ, Amarenco G, et al. What is the place of electroneuromyographic studies in the diagnosis and management of pudendal neuralgia related to entrapment syndrome? Neurophysiol Clin. 2007;37(4):223–8. https://doi.org/10.1016/j.neucli.2007.07.004. Epub 2007 Aug 2

40. Mollo M, Bautrant E, Rossi-Seignert AK, et al. Evaluation of diagnostic accuracy of colour duplex scanning, compared to electroneuromyography, diagnostic score and surgical outcomes, in pudendal neuralgia by entrapment: a prospective study on 96 patients. Pain. 2009;142(1-2):159–63. https://doi.org/10.1016/j.pain.2009.01.019. Epub 2009 Feb 4

41. Labat JJ, Riant T, Lassaux A, et al. Adding corticosteroids to the pudendal nerve block for pudendal neuralgia: a randomised, double-blind, controlled trial. BJOG. 2017;124(2):251–60. https://doi.org/10.1111/1471-0528.14222. Epub 2016 Jul 27

42. Labat JJ, Riant T, Robert R, et al. Diagnostic criteria for pudendal neuralgia by pudendal nerve entrapment (Nantes criteria). Neurourol Urodyn. 2008;27(4):306–10. https://doi.org/10.1002/nau.20505.

43. Silbert PL, Dunne JW, Edis RH, et al. Bicycling induced pudendal nerve pressure neuropathy. Clin Exp Neurol. 1991;28:191–6.

44. Christovão TC, Neto HP, Grecco LA, et al. Effect of different insoles on postural balance: a systematic review. J Phys Ther Sci. 2013;25(10):1353–6. https://doi.org/10.1589/jpts.25.1353. Epub 2013 Nov 20

45. Edwards J. The importance of postural habits in perpetuating myofascial trigger point pain. Acupunct Med. 2005;23(2):77–82. https://doi.org/10.1136/aim.23.2.77.

46. Berghmans B. Physiotherapy for pelvic pain and female sexual dysfunction: an untapped resource. Int Urogynecol J. 2018;29(5):631–8. https://doi.org/10.1007/s00192-017-3536-8. Epub 2018 Jan 9

47. Levesque A, Bautrant E, Quistrebert V, et al. Recommendations on the management of pudendal nerve entrapment syndrome: a formalised expert consensus. Eur J Pain. 2022;26(1):7–17. https://doi.org/10.1002/ejp.1861. Epub 2021 Oct 13

48. Tzadik A, Babin RW, Ryu JH. Hypotension-induced neuropraxia in the cat facial nerve. Otolaryngol Head Neck Surg. 1982;90(2):163–7. https://doi.org/10.1177/019459988209000203.

Retropubic Suspension Operations for Stress Urinary Incontinence

20

Jennifer A. Locke, Sarah Neu, and Sender Herschorn

Contents

Introduction 362
Pathophysiology and Anatomy as it Relates to Female Incontinence and Retropubic
Suspensions 362

Patient Selection for Retropubic Suspension Operations 363
Indications for Retropubic Suspension 363
Contraindications to Retropubic Suspension 363
Patient Factors 363

Retropubic Suspension Operation Types 364
Operative Types (Fig. 2) 364
Outcomes and Complications of the MMK Repair and
Burch Colposuspensions 364

Current Role of the Open Burch Colposuspension 365
Burch Colposuspension Compared to Mid-Urethral Sling 365
Burch Colposuspension Compared to Pubovaginal Sling 366
Burch Colposuspension: Open Compared to Laparoscopic 367

Steps of the Open Burch Colposuspension Operation (Fig. 3) 367

Cross-References 368

References 368

Abstract

Key Points:

1. The retropubic suspension acts to stabilize the bladder neck and proximal urethra to a fixed retropubic position during times of increased intra-abdominal pressure [3].

2. The Burch colposuspension has a durable effect with 5-year dry rates of 70% [21].
3. The Burch colposuspension remains a viable option for women with SUI, especially if vaginal access is limited, mesh is contraindicated, or when concurrent intra-abdominal surgery is planned [7].
4. The Burch colposuspension is contraindicated in women with inadequate vaginal length or mobility of vaginal tissues (i.e., due to prior vaginal surgery, radiotherapy, or prior vaginal incontinence procedure) and

J. A. Locke · S. Neu · S. Herschorn (✉)
Sunnybrook Health Sciences Centre, Toronto, ON, Canada
e-mail: s.herschorn@utoronto.ca

© Springer Nature Switzerland AG 2023
F. E. Martins et al. (eds.), *Female Genitourinary and Pelvic Floor Reconstruction*,
https://doi.org/10.1007/978-3-031-19598-3_21

where retropubic adhesions cannot be safely removed. It is not recommended in women with prior failed incontinence procedures and when the SUI is predominantly due to sphincteric deficiency.

5. The mid-urethral sling has modestly improved continence outcomes over the Burch colposuspension. However, the mid-urethral sling has higher rates of erosion and bladder perforation. The Burch colposuspension has higher rates of surgical wound infections, urinary tract infections, and de novo posterior prolapse.
6. The pubovaginal sling has improved continence outcomes over the Burch colposuspension but has higher rates of voiding dysfunction, such as urinary retention.
7. Laparoscopic Burch colposuspension takes longer but is associated with less blood loss, less pain, and quicker return to normal activities than the open approach.

Keywords

Retropubic suspension · Stress urinary incontinence · Burch colposuspension

Introduction

Pathophysiology and Anatomy as it Relates to Female Incontinence and Retropubic Suspensions

Stress urinary incontinence (SUI), defined as the complaint of any involuntary loss of urine on effort or physical exertion or on sneezing or coughing [1], accounts for the majority of women with urinary incontinence (29–75% of patients experiencing urinary incontinence have SUI) [2]. SUI is thought to occur secondary to the intra-abdominal pressure overcoming the urethral closure pressure [3]. The urethral closure pressure is dependent on the interaction of the striated and smooth muscle of the urethral sphincter, the urethral mucosa, and the periurethral blood vessels. These can be damaged during childbirth and aging leading to leakage with an increase in intra-abdominal pressures [4]. Furthermore, childbirth and aging can injure the pubourethral ligaments and muscles of the pelvic floor which normally help maintain continence (Fig. 1) [5].

The retropubic suspension acts to stabilize the bladder neck and proximal urethra to a fixed

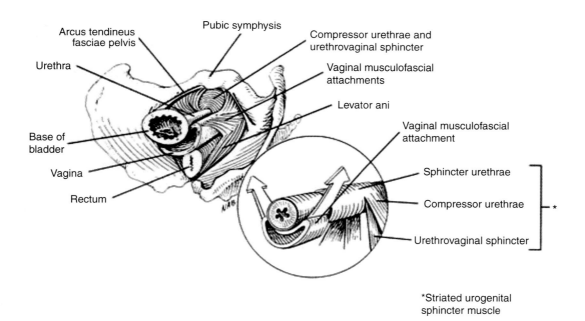

Fig. 1 Pelvic floor anatomy with muscular and fascial supports of the urethra

retropubic position during times of increased intra-abdominal pressure [3].

Patient Selection for Retropubic Suspension Operations

In a Cochrane review of 4738 women who underwent open retropubic suspension operations, the cure rate ranged from 68.9% to 88.0% [6]. To determine if the retropubic suspension operation is a reasonable option for your patient, it is essential to understand the procedure indications and contraindications as well as the influence of patient factors on outcomes.

Indications for Retropubic Suspension

Absolute

1. Laparotomy for concomitant abdominal surgery that cannot be performed vaginally
2. Limited vaginal access [7]

   Relative

1. Contraindication or adversity to mesh [7]

Contraindications to Retropubic Suspension

Absolute

1. Inadequate vaginal length or mobility of vaginal tissues (i.e., due to prior vaginal surgery, radiotherapy, or prior vaginal incontinence procedure)
2. Existence of retropubic adhesions that cannot be safely dissected

   Relative

1. Prior failed incontinence procedures
2. Existence of prominent sphincteric deficiency

Patient Factors

Age
Follow-up to 9 years has shown no difference in the success of retropubic suspensions regarding age [8] despite older women having a higher chance of sphincteric deficiency as an etiology for SUI and higher likelihood of previous incontinence procedures.

Comorbidities
The presence of multiple comorbidities may alter the long-term outcomes of retropubic suspensions; however, to date, the data are insufficient to draw conclusions.

Obesity
There is a correlation between obesity and SUI [9]. Obesity is linked to adverse outcomes during the retropubic suspension operation. In a series of 250 women undergoing retropubic suspension operations, 79 (32%) had a BMI of 30 or higher. Higher BMI was associated with higher estimated blood loss (344 mL vs. 284 mL p = 0.03) and longer mean length of surgery (15 min, p = 0.02) but no difference in length of hospital stay or postoperative complications when compared to patients with a BMI < 30 [10].

Previous SUI Surgeries
Women who have had previous surgeries for SUI have reduced efficacy rates from retropubic suspensions. Specifically, after one previous repair, the success rate of the Burch colposuspension is 81%, and this drops to 25% after two previous repairs and 0% after three previous repairs [11].

Concomitant Detrusor Overactivity
Women who have preoperative evidence of detrusor overactivity experience lower cure rates of SUI after Burch colposuspension than those women without detrusor overactivity (75% vs. 95% OR 0.1, 95% CI 0.01–0.9, p = 0.02) [12]. Furthermore, in those women who have pure SUI, there is a greater risk of developing detrusor overactivity after the Burch colposuspension than with other SUI procedures (~17.5% incidence at 6 months) [13].

Concomitant Prolapse

Retropubic suspension alone can treat mild anterior wall prolapse but does not treat moderate to severe anterior wall prolapse. SUI with moderate anterior wall prolapse is more amenable to treatment via a vaginal approach such as the pubovaginal sling or mid-urethral sling as it is possible to repair the concomitant anterior prolapse vaginally.

Additionally, if hysterectomy is indicated for prolapse or for another reason, there is no difference in efficacy between the Burch colposuspension and trans-obturator tape for SUI outcome; however, the Burch colposuspension has less blood loss and shorter operative time [14].

Lastly, during the retropubic suspension, the lateral vagina is elevated; this may aggravate posterior vaginal wall weakness predisposing to enterocele.

These are factors to consider when counseling the patient on the efficacy of the retropubic suspension in patients with concomitant prolapse.

Retropubic Suspension Operation Types

Operative Types (Fig. 2)

Paravaginal Repair and Vagino-obturator Shelf Repair

The paravaginal repair described in 1912 aimed to close the presumed fascial weakness laterally at the site of attachment of the pelvic fascia to the interior obturator fascia, essentially attaching the lateral vaginal sulcus to the arcus tendinous from the back of the lower edge of the symphysis pubis to the ischial spine [15]. The vagino-obturator shelf repair is a variant of the paravaginal repair in which the vagina is sutured to the internal obturator muscle with placement of the sutures laterally, anchored to the internal obturator fascia rather than hitching the vagina up to the iliopectoneal line [16].

Marshall-Marchetti-Krantz Repair

The Marshall-Marchetti-Krantz (MMK) procedure was described in 1949 [17]. In this approach, the anterolateral aspect of the urethra is elevated and fixed to the posterior aspect of the pubic symphysis and adjacent periosteum. This was initially done with a double-bite suture of the paraurethral tissue and vaginal wall but has been adapted to now exclude the tissue bite through the urethral wall because of concern with urethral injury. The aim was to provide retropubic elevation of the bladder neck through fixation of the endopelvic fascia at the pubic periosteum.

Burch Colposuspension

The first description of the Burch colposuspension was in 1961 [18]. In the initial descriptions, the paravaginal fascia was attached to the tendinous arch of the fascia pelvis or Cooper ligament with the use of two to four sutures on either side. Tanagho et al. modified the technique in 1978 to its current state where the paravaginal fascial sutures are placed further lateral from the urethra with a looser approximation of tissues [19].

Outcomes and Complications of the MMK Repair and Burch Colposuspensions

Although the MMK procedure had an 88.2% subjective cure rate in 2460 patients with 1–72 months follow-up, 21% of the cases had complications [20]. Placement of sutures through the pubic symphysis is associated with a 0.9–3.2% risk of osteitis pubis. Stone formation and erosion of the nonabsorbable cystourethropexy sutures into the bladder lumen can also occur.

In 5244 patients, the overall cure rate was 68.9–88.0% with the open Burch colposuspension; it has now become the best retropubic suspension available [21]. Complications include postoperative voiding difficulty, detrusor overactivity, and vaginal prolapse. Other less common complications include direct surgical injury to the urinary tract (0.3%), ureteral obstruction, and post-colposuspension syndrome, defined as pain in one or both groins at the site of suspension (occurs in up to 12% of patients).

The ICI committee concluded that the short-term results of MMK are comparable in cure to the

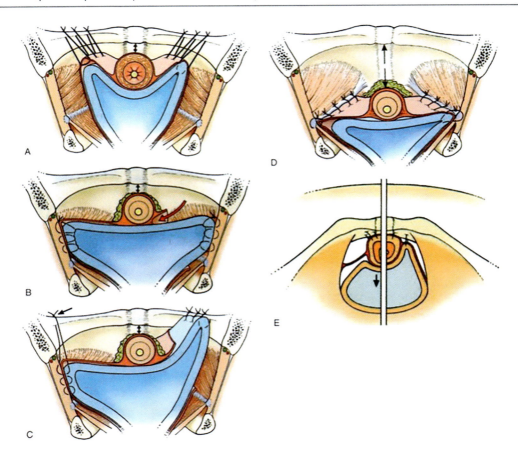

Fig. 2 Types of retropubic suspension operations. (**a**) Coronal view, diagram of a Burch colposuspension. (**b**) Coronal view, diagram of a vagino-obturator shelf procedure. (**c**) Coronal view, diagram of a vagino-obturator shelf procedure on the left, augmented by suturing to the iliopectineal line, and a Burch colposuspension on the right. (**d**) Coronal view, diagram of a paravaginal repair. (**e**) Diagram showing the sutures in a Marshall-Marchetti-Krantz procedure and their proximity to the urethra. (https://abdominalkey.com/retropubic-suspension-surgery-for-incontinence-in-women/)

Burch colposuspension, but the long-term outcomes are poorer after MMK and decline over time [22]. Thus, the MMK is no longer recommended.

Current Role of the Open Burch Colposuspension

The open Burch colposuspension has a durable effect with 5-year dry rates of 70% [21]. Several studies have compared outcomes of the Burch colposuspension to other surgical modalities for SUI.

Burch Colposuspension Compared to Mid-Urethral Sling

The mid-urethral sling was introduced in 1996 by Ulmsten and has gained widespread acceptance for the treatment of SUI given its low morbidity, short-term success rates, and the possibility for it to be done as an outpatient procedure under local anesthetic [23].

Efficacy

In a multicenter randomized controlled trial of 344 women with SUI, 81% of women in the mid-urethral sling group and 90% in the Burch colposuspension group reported negative 1-hour pad tests after 5 years (p = 0.21) [24]. In a retrospective matched cohort study of 1344 women with SUI, there was no significant difference in continence outcomes (83% Burch colposuspension vs. 85.1% mid-urethral sling, p = 0.38) with a mean follow-up of 13.1 years for the Burch colposuspension and 10.1 years for the mid-urethral sling [25].

In a meta-analysis of seven studies, including 531 patients, there was no significant difference between the Burch colposuspension and the mid-urethral sling regarding objective and subjective cure rates [26]. In another meta-analysis of 8 studies, including 246 patients, the cure rate with the mid-urethral sling was found to be significantly higher than the open Burch colposuspension (subjective OR, 0.59; 95% CI, 0.45–0.79; p = 0.0003; objective OR, 0.51; 95% CI: 0.34–0.76; p = 0.001) [27]. In another meta-analysis of 11 studies, including 1195 patients, the mid-urethral sling was associated with higher continence compared to the Burch colposuspension (OR, 0.61; 95% CI, 0.46–0.82; p = 0.00009) [28]. More recently a Cochrane review of 22 trials demonstrated better effectiveness with traditional slings (both mid-urethral and pubovaginal slings) in the medium and long term (RR, 1.35; 95% CI, 1.11–1.64 from 1 to 5 years follow-up; RR, 1.19; 95% CI, 1.03–1.37) [21].

In summary, the mid-urethral sling has better long-term efficacy than the open Burch colposuspension.

Complications

In the previously mentioned multicenter randomized controlled trial of 344 women, there were higher rates of subsequent enterocele and rectoceles with the Burch colposuspension group (49% vs. 32% mid-urethral sling, p = 0.023) [24]; indeed, 7.5% of the Burch colposuspension group underwent surgery for prolapse versus 1.8% in the mid-urethral group. Mesh-related erosions were seen in six women in the mid-urethral group. In the retrospective matched cohort study of 1344 women, there was also a higher need for future

prolapse surgery after Burch colposuspension compared to the mid-urethral sling (3.3% vs. 1.1%, p = 0.01) [25], particularly for the posterior compartment. No other differences in complications were noted in this study.

In the meta-analysis of seven studies, including 531 patients, the mid-urethral sling had higher rates of erosion (OR, 5.98; 95% CI, 1.16–30.67) and bladder perforation (OR, 2.74; 95% CI, 1.24–6.03), while the Burch colposuspension had higher rates of surgical wound complications (OR, 0.30; 95% CI, 0.10–0.90) and urinary tract infection (OR, 0.30; 95% CI, 0.14–0.63) [26]. In the meta-analysis of 11 studies, including 1195 patients, bladder perforation was significantly higher with the mid-urethral sling (OR, 4.94; 95% CI, 2.09–11.68; p = 0.00003) [28].

In a trial of 81 patients, there was no significant difference in overall sexual satisfaction between the mid-urethral sling and Burch colposuspension groups [29].

Burch Colposuspension Compared to Pubovaginal Sling

The pubovaginal sling has been an option for women with SUI since it was introduced in 1907 [30]. In the past, it was reserved for patients who had failed multiple incontinence procedures, had less prolapse, and had presumed sphincteric deficiency. It is now an option for all types of patients with SUI [31].

Efficacy

In a multicenter randomized clinical trial of 655 women with SUI, success rates were higher for women who underwent pubovaginal sling than for those who underwent Burch colposuspension, for both overall success (47% vs. 38%, P = 0.01) and rate of stress incontinence (66% vs. 49%, P < 0.001) at 2 years [32]. This conclusion held true at 5-year follow-up (24.1% continence rate for the Burch colposuspension (95% CI, 18.5–29.7) vs. 30.8% continence rate for the pubovaginal sling (95% CI, 24.7–36.9;

p = 0.002)). The 5-year reported continence rates were lower than the actual as more incontinent patients were enrolled than those continent patients in the follow-up study [33].

In a meta-analysis of three studies, including 744 patients, there was no significant difference in objective cure rates, but there was a significant difference favoring the pubovaginal sling in subjective cure rate (OR, 1.64; 95% CI, 1.10–2.44) [26].

In a recent Cochrane review, eight trials compared traditional suburethral (autologous and synthetic but not mid-urethral tapes) with open abdominal retropubic colposuspension [34]. Moderate-quality evidence shows that the traditional sub-urethral sling may lead to more continent women in the medium term (1–5 years) (69% vs. 59% after colposuspension: OR, 1.70; 95% CI, 1.22–2.37). Furthermore, the review included high-quality evidence supporting that women were less likely to need repeat continence surgery after a traditional sling operation than after Burch colposuspension (RR, 0.15; 95% CI, 0.05–0.42).

In summary, it appears that pubovaginal sling has better long-term efficacy than the open Burch colposuspension.

Complications

In the multicenter randomized clinical trial of 655 women, there were higher rates of voiding dysfunction in the pubovaginal sling group (14% vs. 2%, p < 0.001), and more patients in the pubovaginal group received treatment for postoperative urgency incontinence (27% vs. 20%, p = 0.04) [32] than those in the Burch colposuspension group. Furthermore, in the pubovaginal sling group, there were higher rates of urinary tract infections (48% vs. 32%).

The pubovaginal sling was associated with a higher rate of operations for retention (OR, 7.95; 95% CI, 3.34–18.94) in the meta-analysis of three studies (744 patients) [26].

In terms of sexual impact, in a prospective study of 94 women with SUI, the Burch colposuspension was associated with higher decrease in total sexual function score (23.6 ±

6.2 to 17.6 ± 7.7) compared to the pubovaginal sling (19.2 ± 10 to 17.2 ± 9.9) [35].

Burch Colposuspension: Open Compared to Laparoscopic

In a randomized surgical trial where 200 women underwent open or laparoscopic Burch colposuspension, there were no differences in continence outcomes [36]. Laparoscopic surgery took a longer time to perform (87 vs. 42 minutes, $P < 0.0001$) but was associated with less blood loss ($P = 0.03$), less pain ($P = 0.02$), and a quicker return to normal activities ($P = 0.01$).

Steps of the Open Burch Colposuspension Operation (Fig. 3)

The patient is placed in either a low or a modified dorsal lithotomy position using stirrups allowing access to the vagina during the procedure. A urethral catheter is placed. A Pfannenstiel or lower midline abdominal incision is made, and the retropubic space is developed to identify the bladder neck, anterior vaginal wall, and urethra. It is important to identify the lateral limits of the bladder as it reflects off the vaginal wall to avoid inadvertent suturing of the bladder itself.

The area for suture placement is identified by elevating the dissected anterolateral vaginal wall into the field using the surgeon's left vaginal examining fingers. The bladder is retracted to the opposite side, and two to four sutures are placed on each site, each suture taking a good bite of fascia and vaginal wall and avoiding perforation through the vaginal mucosa. The most distal suture is at the level of the bladder neck and no closer than 2 cm lateral to it. The sutures are then placed in the corresponding sites in the Cooper ligament, with the emphasis being on a mediolateral direction for the sutures. The assistant then elevates the appropriate portion of the vaginal wall when each suture is tied, and no attempt is made to tie the suture tightly. The

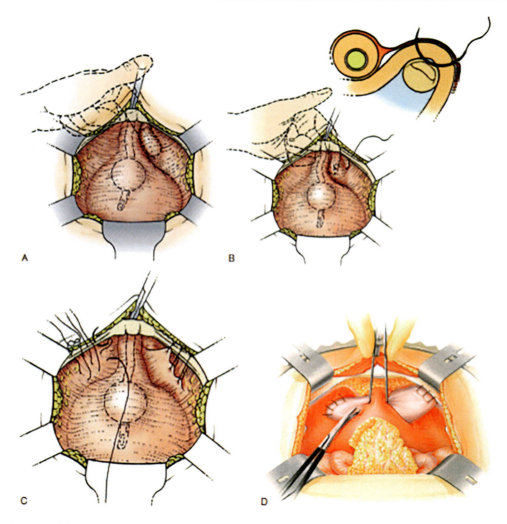

Fig. 3 Steps of the open Burch colposuspension operation

principle is to approximate the vaginal wall to the lateral pelvic wall, where it will heal and promote adhesion formation, thereby creating a broad support for the urethra and bladder neck.

Cross-References

▶ Sling Operations for Stress Urinary Incontinence and Their Historical Evolution: Autologous, Cadaveric, and Synthetic Slings

References

1. Abrams P, Cardozo L, Fall M, et al. The standardisation of terminology in lower urinary tract function: report from the standardisation sub-committee of the International Continence Society. Urology. 2003;61(1): 37–49. https://doi.org/10.1016/s0090-4295(02) 02243-4.
2. Hunskaar S, Burgio K, Diokno A, Herzog AR, Hjälmås K, Lapitan MC. Epidemiology and natural history of urinary incontinence in women. Urology. 2003;62(4 Suppl 1):16–23. https://doi.org/10.1016/ s0090-4295(03)00755-6.

3. Nikolaus Veit-Rubin JD, Ford A, Dubuisson J-B, Mourad S, Digesu A. Burch colposuspension. Neurourol Urodyn. 2019:553–62.
4. Cundiff GW. The pathophysiology of stress urinary incontinence: a historical perspective. Rev Urol. 2004;6(Suppl 3):S10–8.
5. Mostwin JL, Genadry R, Sanders R, Yang A. Anatomic goals in the correction of female stress urinary incontinence. J Endourol. 1996;10(3):207–12. https://doi.org/10.1089/end.1996.10.207.
6. Lapitan MC, Cody JD, Grant A. Open retropubic colposuspension for urinary incontinence in women: a short version Cochrane review. Neurourol Urodyn. 2009;28(6):472–80. https://doi.org/10.1002/nau.20780.
7. Sohlberg EM, Elliott CS. Burch Colposuspension. Urol Clin North Am. 2019;46(1):53–9. https://doi.org/10.1016/j.ucl.2018.08.002.
8. Sun MJ, Ng SC, Tsui KP, Chang NE, Lin KC, Chen GD. Are there any predictors for failed Burch colposuspension? Taiwan J Obstet Gynecol. 2006;45(1):33–8. https://doi.org/10.1016/S1028-4559(09)60187-X.
9. Lamerton TJ, Torquati L, Brown WJ. Overweight and obesity as major, modifiable risk factors for urinary incontinence in young to mid-aged women: a systematic review and meta-analysis. Obes Rev. 2018;19(12):1735–45. https://doi.org/10.1111/obr.12756.
10. Rogers RG, Lebküchner U, Kammerer-Doak DN, Thompson PK, Walters MD, Nygaard IE. Obesity and retropubic surgery for stress incontinence: is there really an increased risk of intraoperative complications? Am J Obstet Gynecol. 2006;195(6):1794–8. https://doi.org/10.1016/j.ajog.2006.07.012.
11. Petrou SP, Frank I. Complications and initial continence rates after a repeat pubovaginal sling procedure for recurrent stress urinary incontinence. J Urol. 2001;165(6 Pt 1):1979–81. https://doi.org/10.1097/00005392-200106000-00033.
12. Colombo M, Zanetta G, Vitobello D, Milani R. The Burch colposuspension for women with and without detrusor overactivity. Br J Obstet Gynaecol. 1996;103(3):255–60. https://doi.org/10.1111/j.1471-0528.1996.tb09715.x.
13. Ciećwież S, Chełstowski K, Brodowska A, Ptak M, Kotlęga D, Starczewski A. Association between the urinary bladder volume and the incidence of "de novo" overactive bladder in patients with stress urinary incontinence subjected to sling surgeries or Burch procedure. Biomed Res Int. 2019;2019:9515242. https://doi.org/10.1155/2019/9515242.
14. Seckin KD, Kadirogullari P, Kiyak H. Which anti-incontinence surgery option is better in patients undergoing total laparoscopic hysterectomy? Burch colposuspension or transobturator tape procedure. Eur J Obstet Gynecol Reprod Biol. 2020;249:59–63. https://doi.org/10.1016/j.ejogrb.2020.04.039.
15. McDermott CD, Hale DS. Abdominal, laparoscopic, and robotic surgery for pelvic organ prolapse. Obstet Gynecol Clin N Am. 2009;36(3):585–614. https://doi.org/10.1016/j.ogc.2009.09.004.
16. Turner-Warwick R. Turner-Warwick vagino-obturator shelf urethral repositioning procedure. In: Controversies and innovations in urological surgery. London: Springer; 1988. p. 195–200.
17. Marshall VF, Marchetti AA, Krantz KE. The correction of stress incontinence by simple vesicourethral suspension. Surg Gynecol Obstet. 1949;88(4):509–18.
18. Burch JC. Urethrovaginal fixation to Cooper's ligament for correction of stress incontinence, cystocele, and prolapse. Am J Obstet Gynecol. 1961;81:281–90. https://doi.org/10.1016/s0002-9378(16)36367-0.
19. Tanagho EA. Colpocystourethropexy: the way we do it. J Urol. 1976;116(6):751–3. https://doi.org/10.1016/s0022-5347(17)58997-1.
20. Mainprize TC, Drutz HP. The Marshall-Marchetti-Krantz procedure: a critical review. Obstet Gynecol Surv. 1988;43(12):724–9. https://doi.org/10.1097/00006254-198812000-00003.
21. Lapitan MCM, Cody JD, Mashayekhi A. Open retropubic colposuspension for urinary incontinence in women. Cochrane Database Syst Rev. 2017;7:CD002912. https://doi.org/10.1002/14651858.CD002912.pub7.
22. Smith AR, Chand D, Dmochowski R, et al. Committee 14: surgery for urinary incontinence in women. Health Publication; 2009.
23. Ulmsten U, Henriksson L, Johnson P, Varhos G. An ambulatory surgical procedure under local anesthesia for treatment of female urinary incontinence. Int Urogynecol J Pelvic Floor Dysfunct. 1996;7(2):81–5; discussion 85–6. https://doi.org/10.1007/BF01902378.
24. Ward KL, Hilton P. Group UaITT. Tension-free vaginal tape versus colposuspension for primary urodynamic stress incontinence: 5-year follow up. BJOG. 2008;115(2):226–33. https://doi.org/10.1111/j.1471-0528.2007.01548.x.
25. Karmakar D, Dwyer PL, Murray C, Schierlitz L, Dykes N, Zilberlicht A. Long-term effectiveness and safety of open Burch colposuspension vs retropubic midurethral sling for stress urinary incontinence-results from a large comparative study. Am J Obstet Gynecol. 2020. https://doi.org/10.1016/j.ajog.2020.11.043.
26. Oliveira LM, Dias MM, Martins SB, Haddad JM, Girão MJBC, Castro RA. Surgical treatment for stress urinary incontinence in women: a systematic review and meta-analysis. Rev Bras Ginecol Obstet. 2018;40(8):477–90. https://doi.org/10.1055/s-0038-1667184.
27. Fusco F, Abdel-Fattah M, Chapple CR, et al. Updated systematic review and meta-analysis of the comparative data on colposuspensions, pubovaginal slings, and midurethral tapes in the surgical treatment of female

stress urinary incontinence. Eur Urol. 2017;72(4):567–91. https://doi.org/10.1016/j.eururo.2017.04.026.

28. Novara G, Artibani W, Barber MD, et al. Updated systematic review and meta-analysis of the comparative data on colposuspensions, pubovaginal slings, and midurethral tapes in the surgical treatment of female stress urinary incontinence. Eur Urol. 2010;58(2):218–38. https://doi.org/10.1016/j.eururo.2010.04.022.

29. Demirkesen O, Onal B, Tunc B, Alici B, Cetinele B. Does vaginal anti-incontinence surgery affect sexual satisfaction? A comparison of TVT and Burch-colposuspension. Int Braz J Urol. 2008;34(2):214–9. https://doi.org/10.1590/s1677-55382008000200012.

30. Cespedes RD, Cross CA, McGuire EJ. Pubovaginal fascial slings. Tech Urol. 1997;3(4):195–201.

31. Bailly GG, Carlson KV. The pubovaginal sling: reintroducing an old friend. Can Urol Assoc J. 2017;11(6 Suppl 2):S147–51. https://doi.org/10.5489/cuaj.4611.

32. Albo ME, Richter HE, Brubaker L, et al. Burch colposuspension versus fascial sling to reduce urinary stress incontinence. N Engl J Med. 2007;356(21):2143–55. https://doi.org/10.1056/NEJMoa070416.

33. Brubaker L, Richter HE, Norton PA, et al. 5-year continence rates, satisfaction and adverse events of burch urethropexy and fascial sling surgery for urinary incontinence. J Urol. 2012;187(4):1324–30. https://doi.org/10.1016/j.juro.2011.11.087.

34. Saraswat L, Rehman H, Omar MI, Cody JD, Aluko P, Glazener CM. Traditional suburethral sling operations for urinary incontinence in women. Cochrane Database Syst Rev. 2020;1:CD001754. https://doi.org/10.1002/14651858.CD001754.pub5.

35. Cayan F, Dilek S, Akbay E, Cayan S. Sexual function after surgery for stress urinary incontinence: vaginal sling versus Burch colposuspension. Arch Gynecol Obstet. 2008;277(1):31–6. https://doi.org/10.1007/s00404-007-0418-1.

36. Carey MP, Goh JT, Rosamilia A, et al. Laparoscopic versus open Burch colposuspension: a randomised controlled trial. BJOG. 2006;113(9):999–1006. https://doi.org/10.1111/j.1471-0528.2006.01037.x.

Sling Operations for Stress Urinary Incontinence and Their Historical Evolution: Autologous, Cadaveric, and Synthetic Slings

21

Felicity Reeves and Tamsin Greenwell

Contents

Introduction 372

The History of Stress Incontinence Management 372

The History of Slings in Stress Urinary Incontinence 374

Autologous Slings 374

Cadaveric Slings 380

Xenografts 381

Synthetic Slings 382

Conclusions 388

Take-Home Message 388

Cross-References 389

References 389

Abstract

Stress urinary incontinence is common in women affecting up to 50% worldwide. The development of surgical techniques and materials has been informed and refined by improved understanding of physiology and anatomy (the hammock hypothesis and integral theory) as well as learning from failures in the past. Pubovaginal slings for stress urinary incontinence were first described in the 1900s with various materials and tissues including autograft, allograft, xenograft, and synthetic with varying results.

The mid-urethral synthetic sling became popular in the 1990s owing to properties of resistance to degradation, persistent tensile strength, resistance to transmissible diseases, and reduction in intraoperative and postoperative recovery time. Continence rates ranged from 70 to 80%. Concerns over vaginal and urinary tract exposure and extrusion related to mesh implants have led to caution and reviews over the use of mesh implants. This has driven

F. Reeves
Addenbrookes Hospital, Cambridge, UK
e-mail: felicity.reeves@nhs.net

T. Greenwell (✉)
University College London Hospitals, London, UK
e-mail: tamsin.greenwell2@nhs.net

© Springer Nature Switzerland AG 2023
F. E. Martins et al. (eds.), *Female Genitourinary and Pelvic Floor Reconstruction*,
https://doi.org/10.1007/978-3-031-19598-3_22

an increase in the use of the autologous pubovaginal sling and stimulated the potential need for further developments toward the ideal anti-stress urinary incontinence procedure.

In this chapter we explore the historical developments related to surgery for stress urinary incontinence in women, their risks, benefits, and published outcomes. The challenge exists to find the ideal method to treat stress urinary incontinence with optimum tensioning and anchoring technique.

Keywords

Stress urinary incontinence · Urodynamics · Pubovaginal sling · Rectus fascial sling · Mid-urethral sling · TVT · TVTO · Mini-sling · Complications · Outcomes

Introduction

Stress urinary incontinence (SUI) has been defined by the International Continence Society (ICS) as the involuntary loss of urine with impact on social factors and hygiene. Urodynamic stress incontinence refers to leakage of urine through an incompetent urethra in the absence of a detrusor contraction during urodynamic evaluation [1]. SUI is common and has been reported to affect between 4.5% and 53% of women worldwide [2, 3]. SUI affects quality of life due to psychological distress and can cause financial burden to both individual and the wider health service.

SUI can be further complicated by voiding dysfunction, pelvic organ prolapse, and/or detrusor overactivity. Conservative measures to improve leakage from stress urinary incontinence include pelvic floor physiotherapy, weight loss, and topical vaginal estrogen use. Drug therapy has not proved efficacious in stress urinary incontinence, so the mainstay of intervention is surgery to support the urethra at times of increased abdominal pressure. Pubovaginal slings can be placed vaginally or abdominally, open or via minimally invasive routes (laparoscopic or robotic).

Improved understanding of the anatomy and physiology related to stress urinary incontinence has informed and refined surgical developments over time. Approximately 200 different surgical techniques have been described for the management of SUI [4]. This chapter describes the history of the development of anti-stress incontinence surgery with the associated advances in understanding of physiology and anatomy. This is followed by the different tissues and materials utilized for slings in SUI treatment, their risks, benefits, and outcomes.

The History of Stress Incontinence Management

SUI was first classified by Green in 1961 based on radiological appearance of the bladder neck and urethra with loss of posterior urethrovesical angle (Type 1) and additional rotational urethral descent (Type 2) during raised abdominal pressure [5]. In 1980, McGuire included Type 3 SUI or intrinsic sphincter deficiency where the bladder neck was noted to be open at rest [6]. He found that these patients had high failure rates from urethropexy and better outcomes with autologous fascial sling surgery. In 1988, Blaivas and Olsen added Type 0 to the classification of SUI to represent those with a complaint of SUI, but no demonstrable SUI during urodynamic evaluation. They described Type 2B as those with apparent hypermobility, found to have a low-lying fixed scarred proximal urethra following previous surgery [7]. In the 1990s, through application of the leak point pressure, urethral sphincteric incontinence was grouped further into urethral hypermobility and intrinsic sphincter deficiency [8, 9]. Further research demonstrated that often these two conditions coexist without the inverse relationship between leak point pressure and urethral hypermobility [10, 11].

In the twentieth century, the bladder neck was felt to be the primary mechanism of continence, but this was challenged by the work of Petros and Ulmsten [12, 13]. They proposed that the mid-urethra, supported by the pubourethral ligaments anteriorly, was the primary mechanism of urinary continence. Through this "integral theory," they proposed that stress and urge incontinence had common causes [12–14]. Three synergistic mechanisms of support to the anterior vaginal wall were described involving anterior support by pubococcygeus, downward traction on the bladder neck, and voluntary lifting of the pelvic floor as a hammock of supportive tissue. Laxity of the anterior vaginal wall was thought to stimulate bladder neck and proximal urethral stretch receptions to simulate an overactive detrusor contraction [12]. From this understanding the tension-free vaginal tape was developed and was placed at the mid-urethra, with data showing short-term successful management of SUI [15–19]. The "integral theory" complemented the 1995 "hammock theory," proposed by John DeLancey, which described the maintenance of continence by urethral compression onto the musculofascial hammock of the pelvic floor and anterior vaginal wall [20]. Any weakness of the supportive layers contributing to the hammock was postulated to lead to incontinence as opposed to hypermobility or sphincteric deficiency.

Surgical treatments have evolved from aiming to achieve urethral compression, to restoring the bladder neck to a normal position, to preventing bladder neck descent, to reinforcing the back plate of the urethra to allow compression at times of raised abdominal pressure to prevent leakage. During this development, attention moved from placement of additional support from the bladder neck to the mid-urethral area.

Surgical procedures for SUI have developed initially from retropubic suspensions or urethropexy in 1909 by George White with an aim to enhance the support of the urethra surgically. This was part of a cystocele repair performed as a retropubic paravaginal repair aiming to reinforce and reposition the bladder neck [21]. In 1980, Richardson continued this technique to reattach the endopelvic fascia to the arcus tendinous fascia pelvis, and this was

reported to cure SUI; however, data concerning efficacy was lacking [22].

Vaginal plication was first described by Kelly in 1914 and later modified by Kennedy to include dissection of the urethra from the vaginal wall and plication of the sphincter at the urethrovesical junction [23, 24]. Despite poor long-term success (60%), these were widely utilized due to the simple approach, ability to perform concomitant prolapse repair, and minimal reported complications [25]. The Ball-Burch procedure combined a transvaginal imbrication of the urethra with a transabdominal Burch procedure; however, despite better continence rates, results were still not as good as for slings and retropubic techniques [25, 26].

The Marshall-Marchetti-Krantz (MMK) procedure reported in 1949 was based on observation in men with urinary retention following abdominoperineal resections. The first operation was performed on a man having noted that upward perineal elevation would relieve the retention. The suprapubic suspension of the vesical outlet with two sutures from the periurethral tissues to the periosteum of the pubic symphysis relieved the inability to void [27, 28]. In 1944, this operation was performed on a woman with SUI, and results demonstrated 21.1% overall complications with 2.5% suffering osteitis pubis [29]. In 1958, Burch described a bilateral three-suture attachment of the periurethral tissue to the iliopectineal ligament of Cooper, with Tanagho later stressing the importance of avoiding vaginal wall overelevation and excess tension to reduce the risk of voiding dysfunction [30, 31]. SUI cure rate from Burch colposuspension has been reported to be 69–93.7% over 10–15 years [32–34]. Laparoscopic Burch and MMK procedures have lower reported cure rates than the open method at 12-month follow-up (80% vs. 96%) [35].

Transvaginal needle suspension procedures introduced by Pereyra in 1959 aimed to elevate the proximal urethra and bladder neck. A ligature carrier suspended peri-cervical fascia from the rectus fascia with stainless steel sutures [35]. To prevent suture pull through, Thomas Stamey in 1973 passed the suture through Dacron pledgets and performed cystoscopy to minimize injury and identify the bladder neck and designed the Stamey needle [36]. In 1981, Raz made a modification to this technique by including the vaginal wall and pubocervical fascia reporting a 90% success rate, not reproduced by others [37]. An "incisionless suspension" by Gittes and Loughlin followed, with suprapubic puncture and blind needle passage from the vagina [38]. Complications were not reported, and there were no validated outcome measures other than a high rate of recurrent incontinence, and so these procedures were not recommended [25]. Raz developed a "four-corner suspension" in 1989 for the treatment of SUI and cystocele repair, with two additional sutures at the cystocele base. Initial subjective cure rates were reported as 94% for incontinence and 98% for cystocele; however, in the longer term there were high rates of cystocele recurrence [39].

Fixation techniques have modified over time, initially with pubic bone fixation in 1949, followed by Cooper's ligament for the Burch colposuspension, whilst for the needle suspension fixation was initially to the rectus fascia and then bony anchor fixation (of Leach) in 1998 [119].

The History of Slings in Stress Urinary Incontinence

Pubovaginal slings were first described nearly a century ago. Initially pubovaginal slings (PVS) were recommended for type 3 SUI or intrinsic sphincter deficiency. However, now there is supporting evidence that PVS can be utilized as a primary management of SUI in all cases [40–42]. One of the biggest challenges is that there is still a lack of evidence to guide women in making an informed choice about which anti-stress incontinence procedure is the best for them, to give the best outcome for them.

This chapter will move to explore in detail the history of slings to include autologous, synthetic, and cadaveric slings. It is important to be aware of the above historical developments that have led to a better understanding of urinary incontinence and

how the outcomes of the above procedures have led to the design of slings as a treatment for SUI.

Autologous Slings

The first autologous sling was described over a century ago, with a gracilis muscle graft described for use as a pubovaginal sling (1907). This was followed by use of pyramidalis tunnelled through the retropubic space, with fixation via sutures at the bladder neck [43]. The rectus fascia was then utilized to lengthen the sling in 1914, with a combined vaginal and abdominal approach described in 1917, followed by suturing of the rectus fascia and muscle around the urethra in 1923 [44]. The pubovaginal sling is said to restore the urethral resistance during times of increased abdominal pressure (stress maneuvers such as coughing and exercise) and to restore continence and coaptation at rest while allowing a physiological uninhibited void [59, 60].

The bulbocavernosus muscle and labial fat pad were discovered and used as a graft to interpose between the urethra and anterior vaginal wall through disconnection and tunnelling in 1929 (Martius) [45]. Though revolutionary, these techniques caused obstruction, voiding dysfunction, and fistulae. Use of the fascia lata for pubovaginal slings was first described in 1933 (Price), which was harvested, then passed antegrade around the urethra, and then fixed by suture to the rectus muscle [46]. Use of the fascia lata from the iliotibial tract was said to be beneficial in avoiding the morbidity associated with the abdominal incision, required to harvest the rectus fascia. Other benefits include the ability to gain more length compared to the rectus fascia and increased strength in virgin tissue. Complications include altered cosmesis, with scarring between the femoral greater trochanter and lateral epicondyle, pain, and additional time required for repositioning the patient. Urologists and gynecologists have limited experience with limb surgery, so despite the similar biocompatibility with rectus fascia as a sling choice, fascia lata is less often used. There are reports that after harvesting a fascia lata graft, two thirds of patients suffer from pain on walking for a week postoperatively [47]. This will impact recovery, mobility, quality of life, return to work, and increased venothromboembolic risks. The use of autologous fascial slings has been criticized for increased morbidity, due to extended operative time, complexity of harvesting the graft, and associated increased hospital stay.

Aldridge (1942) utilized rectus fascia and aponeurosis from external oblique, which remained attached medially, to pass as a sling tunnelled under the urethra via the retropubic space (Retzius) [48] (Fig. 1). However, the medial attachment meant the sling did not have the length required to pass around the urethra without tension. This led to bladder outlet obstruction, resultant voiding dysfunction, and ongoing complication despite modifications.

It was in 1978 that McGuire and Lytton modified the technique utilizing autologous rectus fascia for those patients with type 3 SUI. They dissected a 12×1 cm strip with one side left attached and then passed under the urethra and reattached on the other side of the rectus fascia [49]. Blaivas modified this to a free graft to allow the need for adjusting of tension and also published on use of the autologous fascial sling for all types of SUI with cure rates of 73–93%. This was at a time where they were seen to be primarily indicated for complex and recurrent SUI [50–54]. McGuire and Lytton reported 80% cure rates for use of autologous fascial pubovaginal sling in patients with intrinsic sphincter deficiency (type 3) [49].

Autologous PVS have also been noted to be successful in patients with neuropathic bladders and those with structural abnormalities (requiring repair such as urethral diverticulum), urethral loss in trauma, or complications of urogynecological surgery (urethral erosions from synthetic material such as mid-urethral slings as well as bladder neck artificial urinary sphincters that have eroded) [40–42, 55, 56]. Rectus fascia is the most commonly used autologous sling material. It has excellent biocompatibility with histological proof that the fascia embeds into host tissue, with microscopic connective tissue encroachment, ample fibroblast

numbers, and neovascularization, with minimal inflammatory reaction [57, 58].

Preoperatively patients should have had a detailed focused urogynecological history and examination including urodynamic assessment to confirm baseline bladder function and assess and quantify subjectively and objectively their stress urinary incontinence. Previous pelvic radiation and urethral or prolapse surgery will affect outcomes, through compromise of rectus fascia and vaginal dissection [2].

The technique for autologous rectus fascial pubovaginal sling includes lithotomy position in an appropriately anesthetized, counselled, and consented patient following a validated safety checklist. A vaginal incision is made in the midline of the anterior vaginal wall 2 cm below the urethral meatus toward the bladder neck, facilitated by a self-retaining vaginal retractor with tensioning hooks and a weighted vaginal speculum, after local anesthetic with adrenaline infiltration (hydro-dissection) (Fig. 2a). A Pfannenstiel incision is made 2 cm above the pubic symphysis, with attention given to previous scars and optimized access to a healthy piece of rectus fascia and for postoperative wound healing (Fig. 2b). Dissection proceeds to expose the rectus fascial sheath, and an 8×2 cm section is marked out (Fig. 2b) and dissected (Fig. 2c), and an absorbable (or nonabsorbable as per surgeon and/or patient preference) suture is placed at either end of the graft (Fig. 2d and e). Some recommend mobilization of the anterior bladder wall to reduce the risk of bladder perforation, whereas others will close the rectus sheath at this stage with no dissection. Urethral catheterization allows palpation of the bladder neck at the position of balloon. Dissection continues above the periurethral fascia to raise the lateral vaginal flaps, until the ischiopubic ramus is palpable, and the endopelvic fascia is perforated with scissors and gently opened at either side of the bladder neck immediately below and behind the pubic bones. The sutures are then attached to a needle guide or trocar and passed from the vagina to abdominal incision (Fig. 2f and g) with cystoscopic confirmation that there has been no bladder injury (Fig. 2h and i). The two sutures are pulled up

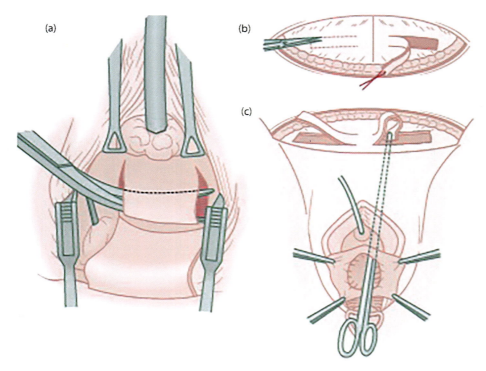

Fig. 1 Aldridge sling. (Republished with permission from: Lobel B, Manunta A and Rodriguez A. The management of female stress urinary incontinence using the sling procedure. BJUInt 2001; 88: 832–839 Fig. 3a–c), (**a**) Harvest of rectus fascia strip bilaterally keeping medial attachment. (**b**) Passage of lateral edge of rectus fascia strip retropubically to vaginal incision. (**c**) Dissection of subvaginal tunnel at the level of the bladder neck to allow passage of rectus fascia strips and attachment to each other

and sling placed at the mid-urethra tension-free (tied over a 16 Ch urethral catheter, a McIndoe scissor, and 2 assistant fingers) (Fig. 2j), the rectus sheath is closed (Fig. 2k), and the sling sutures are tied above the rectus fascia (Fig. 2l) followed by vaginal and abdominal closure (Fig. 2m and n).

Both the rectus fascia and fascia lata have been shown to be equally effective with minimal foreign body reaction and are viable up to 4 years at least from insertion [2]. The longest follow-up for outcomes following pubovaginal sling surgery is 10 years, with reported success rates of 46.9%–90% [61, 62]. A 10-year multicenter randomized controlled trial reported success (dry) rates that favored autologous pubovaginal sling over TVT and xenograft. None of the patients that had an autologous PVS suffered recurrent SUI and did not need further surgical intervention, so this was felt to be more durable than the TVT in the long term [61]. Morgan concurred that PVS was durable and effective in 247 patients (88% dry at 4 years) and demonstrated health-related quality-of-life improvement in type 2 and 3 SUI. 5.7% of patients required a further secondary surgical procedure for SUI in this study (bulking/PVS) [51]. Albo et al. through the SISTEr trial (n = 520 women) demonstrated higher success rates for autologous PVS compared to Burch colposuspension at 24 months [63]. Success was based on a negative pad test, no leakage reported on a 3-day bladder diary, no documented incontinence symptoms, and a negative cough test on examination [63]. Despite the higher success, there was a reported increase in voiding dysfunction, urge incontinence, and urinary tract infection in the autologous PVS group [63]. Voiding dysfunction after autologous PVS rates ranges from 2% to 20.8% [53, 64]. Risk factors for prolonged

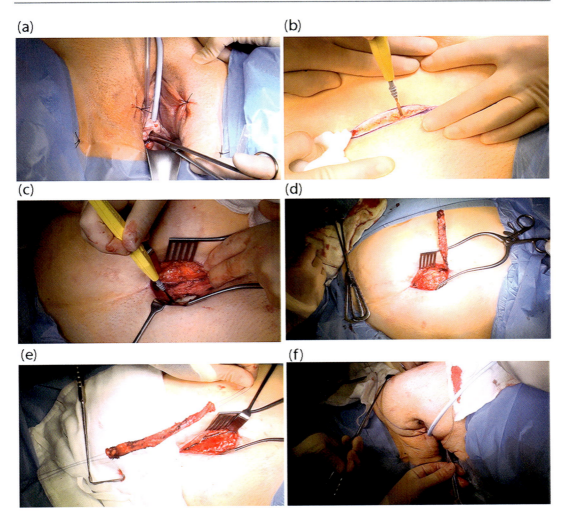

Fig. 2 Rectus fascial sling. (Original Photographs from Ms. Tamsin J Greenwell with patient permission). (**a**) Midline anterior vaginal wall incision over mid-urethra. (**b**) Small suprapubic Pfannenstiel skin incision. (**c**) Mobilization of 2 x 8 cm rectus fascia strip. (**d**) Rectus fascia strip remains attached at the left border and has had a 1 PDS whip stitch inserted on right edge. (**e**) Rectus fascia strip harvest complete with 1 PDS whip stitch inserted on the left edge. (**f**) Passage of needle containing both ends of the PDS suture attached to the right side of the rectus fascia, in retropubic space lateral to the bladder neck from the mid-urethra exit 2 cm lateral to the midline 1 cm above the upper border of the pubic ramus on the patient's right side. (**g**) Needle passage on the left side as per 2 f. (**h**) Loop pf rectus fascia sling seen below the urethra after passage of PDS sutures bilaterally to exit the rectus sheath 1 cm above the pubic rami and 2 cm lateral to the midline either side. (**i**) Post-insertion cystoscopy to ensure no egress into the bladder. (**j**) Site of suture exit from the rectus sheath after passage through retropubic space. (**k**) Closure of the rectus sheath with 1 PDS. (**l**) Sling sutures tied over the closed rectus sheath over two of the assistant's fingers (with a 16Ch urethral catheter in situ and McIndoe scissors between the sling and the urethra in the vagina). (**m**) Final appearance of the tension-free rectus sling in the vagina prior to vaginal closure. (**n**) Final appearance of suprapubic incision

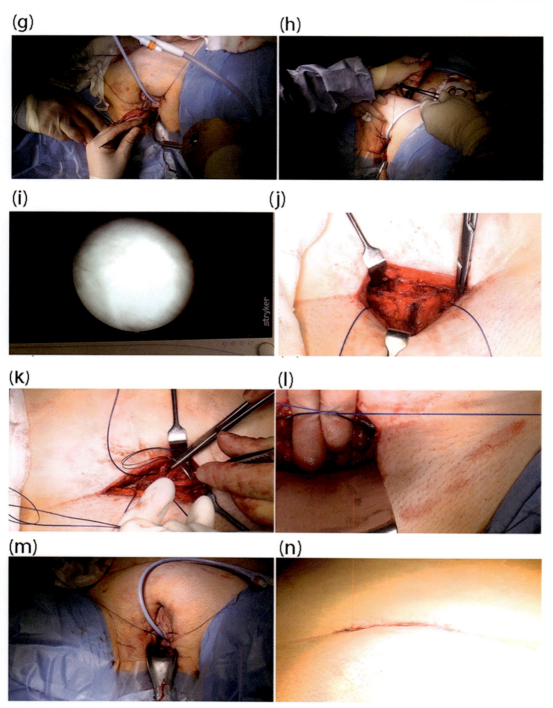

Fig. 2 (continued)

Fig. 3 Vaginal wall sling. (Republished with permission from: Lobel B, Manunta A and Rodriguez A. The management of female stress urinary incontinence using the sling procedure. BJUInt 2001; 88: 832–839 Fig. 7)

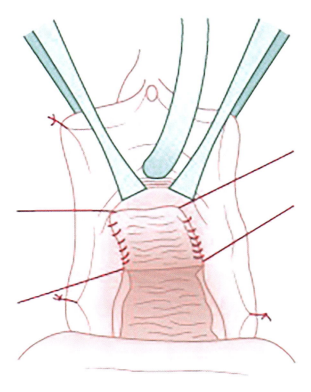

postoperative intermittent self-catheterization included a post-void residual urine measurement more than 100 mls and/or Qmax of less than or equal to 20 mls/sec in preoperative urodynamics [65]. The SISTEr trial secondary analysis demonstrated that 6% of those having a primary autologous PVS were retreated within 5 years for recurrent SUI [66].

Attempts have been made to pass an autologous fascial sling via the transobturator route with 80% success over 4 months in 10 patients, with the need for a larger longer-term study to determine further outcomes and its place in the urological armamentarium for SUI [67].

Autologous PVS has been utilized for secondary or recurrent SUI procedures particularly in post-mesh mid-urethral sling (MUS) excision for extrusion. There is debate whether PVS should be performed concomitantly with the MUS excision or delayed, as a secondary procedure. Most would advocate removal of MUS and repair of the urethra, allowing a period of time for full recovery and reassessment, prior to placing autologous PVS if required following further counselling. As a salvage procedure post-MUS removal, autologous PVS was reported to have cure rates for SUI in up to 69% of women [68]. Lee et al. demonstrated that over 7 years, functional outcomes for primary and secondary PVS were comparable with low morbidity [69].

Raz et al. developed an autologous sling utilizing the vaginal wall in 1989, where vaginal mucosa from a midline incision was harvested, and utilizing periurethral support, a sling was created. Long-term durability was dependent on the quality of supporting fascia and tissues. There was however a risk of shortening of the vagina with potential impact on sexual function [70–72] (Fig. 3).

Athanasopoulos et al. published on 3-year outcome results from 264 patients, treated with autologous rectus fascia PVS. 75.8% remained dry, and 9.1% reported improvement with a complication rate of 29.2% [73]. De novo urgency was the commonest complication; however, it is important to note that within this group, almost one third of patients (29.9%) had had previous mid-urethral sling surgery, with partial mesh removal during the sling procedure. These are a different group of patients, so perhaps should be compared with those undergoing secondary sling procedures within the subset group of those who had mesh removal surgery. This group is at risk of urethral loss and needs more extensive repair and potential Martius graft from the labia.

Lee et al. compared outcomes over 89 months of secondary (previous major continence surgery) versus primary PVS procedure demonstrating 69% versus 76% success, respectively [69]. Cure rates between the groups were deemed to be not significantly different. Three patients in the primary group and nine in the secondary group needed a further SUI procedure [69].

In a single surgeon study over 16 years ($n = 22$ women), results for autologous fascia lata sling for SUI due to intrinsic sphincter deficiency reported successful treatment in 63% of women at an average of 96 months. Four (18%) women required further surgery [74]. The women in this group were offered fascia lata as a PVS owing to patient-specific challenges with rectus fascia harvest, including obesity and previous complex abdominal surgery including abdominoplasty.

Operative technique includes placing a suitably counselled, consented, and anesthetized patient (following safety checklist) in a high lithotomy position (Fig. 4). The fascia lata is harvested with the leg straightened, via transverse incision two inches above the knee joint, along the line of fascia lata to harvest a 6×2 cm strip. The edges once the graft is removed are not closed, and skin closure is performed over a Penrose drain followed by compression bandage [74]. Vaginal incision is made on the anterior wall and endopelvic fascia perforated and procedure completed as for the rectus fascial sling with vaginal pack and urethral catheter placed for 24 h post procedure. Those having a primary PVS have been found to have better outcomes with 75% cure rate versus 69% in those having a secondary PVS, with no reported complications from the harvest site at the knee [74].

Other studies have reported improved success rates of 85% with the use of autologous fascia lata at a mean follow-up of 4 years ($n = 100$ patients)

and 92% in another study ($n = 251$ patients) [52, 75]. The reasons for the lower success rates described above at 63% were postulated to be due to many patients having secondary or salvage procedures and having a high body mass index, with the hypothesis that those having redo or salvage surgery have less optimal urethral function [74].

Cadaveric Slings

Allograft tissues from human donors are mostly cadaveric and hold the benefit to the patient of no requirement for graft harvest, in terms of operative time and absence of additional incisions with quicker potential recovery. With both autograft and allograft PVS, the sling sutures are directed and tied above the rectus fascia; however, despite the saving in time and recovery through use of allograft, there is increased cost in terms of purchasing the sling material and risk of increased infections [70].

Allograft tissue includes lyophilized dura mater, acellular dermis, and fascia lata. Lyophilized dura mater has been utilized in grafts in the bladder and urethra for augmentation repairs, with reported success in sling surgery of 89–92% cure rates [76, 77].

Cadaveric fascia lata was popularized in orthopedic and ophthalmic surgery initially and was first utilized in anti-stress incontinence sub-urethral sling surgery by Handa et al. in 1993 [78]. Allografts are held by a human tissue bank and undergo sterilization and serological screening. Despite these processes, allograft tissues still hold the possible risk of transfer of bacteria (DNA and protein), blood-borne viruses, and prion diseases including human immunodeficiency virus (HIV) (risk of one in eight million cases [79, 80]) and Creutzfeldt-Jakob disease (CJD) due to false-negative results [79,81–83]. Fatal CJD has been reported with use of dura graft, so it is not recommended for use; however, there have been no reports of CJD with use of cadaveric fascia lata [84].

Techniques for cadaveric fascia lata (CFL) preparation include use of gamma irradiation, freeze-drying, fresh frozen, and solvent dehydration followed by rehydration prior to use. Some

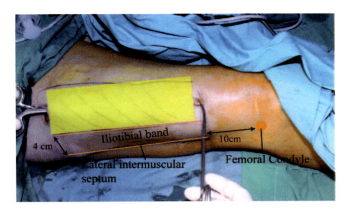

Fig. 4 Fascia lata harvest. (Republished with permission from: Tay VSL, Tan KS, Loh ICY. Minimally invasive fascia lata harvest: a new technique. PRS GO 2013;1: e74. Landmarks and boundaries for fascia lata harvest)

processes are felt to impair the tensile strength of the graft and lead to early failures. CFL from acellular cadaveric dermis is lyophilized (primary method of sterilization) and then treated with gamma irradiation as a method of secondary sterilization to reduce transmission of infectious disease [79]. Cure rates for SUI sling surgery utilizing CFL are reported to be between 62% and 98%, compared to autologous fascia; however, cure rate was shown to be short term with CFL and reduced at 6 months postoperatively in small studies [71, 85].

Acellular dermal allografts are said to maintain good tensile strength and integrate well into human tissue. They also rehydrate in half the time of CFL. In the reconstruction of the urinary tract, dermal allografts have been utilized in bladder augmentation, repair of cystocele, correction of Peyronie's disease, and congenital chordee, as well as hypospadias surgery for augmentation purposes [86].

Allogenic grafts were used for stress incontinence surgery with initial cure rates of 76%–98% starting in 1996 [87, 88]. In a small study of 21 patients utilizing solvent-dehydrated cadaveric dermis for sling surgery, despite cure rates of 86% over 9 months, there were around 50% that suffered with voiding dysfunction either with high post-void residuals needing self-catheterization ($n = 9$) or with de novo urge urinary incontinence ($n = 2$) [89]. Reasons for high failure rates in those requiring revision were postulated to be due to graft degradation, as seen in those removed with poor tissue remodelling. This was felt to be likely due to the freeze-drying technique, with concern that the proximal urethra was an unfavorable site to support graft remodelling [85]. Studies comparing cadaveric fascia lata to autologous fascia lata for pubovaginal sling surgery ($n = 121$ patients) demonstrated CFL to offer an acceptable alternative (cure 90% CFL vs. 83% AFL) with no significant difference in patient recorded outcome measures ($n = 49$ patients) using the incontinence impact questionnaire (IIQ-7) and the urogenital distress inventory (UDI-6) (79% success vs. 84% success $p > 0.05$) with patient satisfaction of 76% with their outcomes [87, 90].

Xenografts

Xenografts are tissues transferred to another species such as animals to humans. As with allografts, they require treatment to reduce risk of bacterial, protein, and DNA transfer by removing genetic material through the diisocyanate processing method [59]. Porcine corium treated with proteolytic enzymes was the first xenograft (from nonhuman animal tissue) utilized in sling surgery with reported cure rates of 78–90%, though wound infections were common [91–93]. Glutaraldehyde was utilized to reduce antigenicity; however, this was said to lead to graft mineralization. Other xenografts used for pubovaginal sling surgery include porcine bowel, porcine dermis, and bovine pericardium [59].

Donor-recipient immunogenic reaction and rejection and scarring were seen less with small intestine xenografts. This was felt to be due to the presence of rich growth factors in the intestinal submucosa; however, histologic results showed higher rates of inflammation with small intestinal submucosal grafts compared with copolymers and polypropylene mesh, with further mixed results related to inflammation [94, 95]. Porcine small intestine submucosa (SIS) was first described for use in pubovaginal sling surgery in 2003 ($n = 152$ patients), summarized to be durable and biocompatible with high tensile strength, with a success rate of 93% (improvement or resolution) over a 4-year follow-up period [96]. In comparison with synthetic slings (TVT), outcomes at 12 months were equivalent (89% PVS porcine dermis vs. 85% TVT) to comparable rates of de novo urge urinary incontinence postoperatively (6% PVS porcine dermis vs. 9% TVT) concluding that they were safe, effective, and non-inferior when compared with TVT [97, 98]. In contrast a comparison of the use of autologous rectus fascia for PVS ($n = 101$ patients) versus porcine dermis reported success rates of 80% versus 54%, respectively, from telephone questionnaires. In those deemed unsuccessful in each group, SUI was confirmed on urodynamic studies in just 6.5% of the rectus fascial sling group and in 90% of the porcine dermis group [99].

Stratasys® has also been utilized in sling surgery with cure rates of 94% at 36 months [96]. It is derived from porcine small intestinal submucosa with the sling attached to the pubic bone with infrapubic bone screws [96].

Synthetic Slings

Synthetic slings were first utilized in 1950, with nylon used in 1951 and then Perlon and Dacron [100–102]. Synthetic slings, though biocompatible, sterile, stronger, with no risk of transmissible disease, and noncarcinogenic, have an increased chance of infection and exposure or extrusion over allograft and autologous grafts [103]. Synthetic slings can be absorbable and non-absorbable. Initial use caused obstruction at the bladder neck resulting in urinary retention, fistulae, and suprapubic abscesses. Longer slings were

then developed (30 cm) with a diameter of 2.5 cm and again placed at the bladder neck with their ends secured to the rectus fascia, with a reported 81% cure rate [104, 105]. Polypropylene was utilized in 1970. It was monofilament with large pores. It was fixed to Coopers' ligament, requiring a vaginal and abdominal approach. Cure rate was reduced from 100% to 80% at 15 years, with 6% urethral extrusion, 5% overactivity, and 6% chronic retention reported [106, 107].

Silicone and Dacron were combined as a multifilament mesh to try and aid sling excision in cases of complications from extrusion, with 71% reported cured, but high complication rates which ultimately led to termination of its use [108]. Gore-Tex was first used in 1988; the polytetrafluoroethylene was thought to lead to less tissue reaction. However, the cure rate was only 61% with one third of patients suffering exposure, extrusion, and infection [109]. Despite modifications to the proportion of Gore-Tex and improved cure rates of 88–90%, 4% continued to suffer from exposure or extrusion, and up to 7% had urinary retention, so Gore-Tex usage was also discontinued [110–112]. Bovine collagen matrix was utilized by impregnation into nonabsorbable polyester in 1999; however, this was also discontinued following exposure and/or extrusion occurring in half of patients and reports of chronic pain [113].

The development of mid-urethral slings utilizing polypropylene monofilament, nonabsorbable mesh sited at the mid-urethra, as opposed to the bladder neck, occurred in 1994 [114, 115]. Other synthetic materials that have been utilized include multifilament polyester, polytetrafluoroethylene, silicone elastomer, and collagen-injected polyester. The concept was underpinned by the work of Petros and Ulmsten's "integral theory" of stress incontinence, with improved understanding of physiology, leading to the objective of creating a tension-free vaginal tape (TVT) to support the back plate posterior to the urethra [12, 13].

Polypropylene is a type 1 mesh and remains the most commonly used synthetic material for the surgical treatment of SUI. It has pore sizes which allow macrophages to pass through to encourage ingrowth of host tissues [2]. Increased fibroblasts

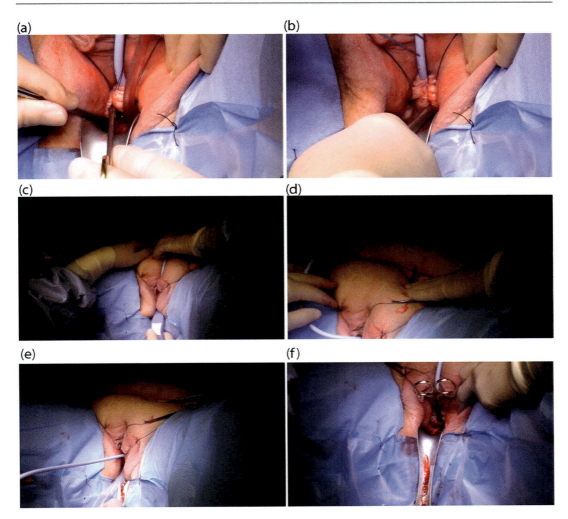

Fig. 5 Retropubic mid-urethral tape insertion. (Original photographs from Ms. Tamsin J Greenwell with patient permission). (**a**) Right paraurethral dissection under the vagina to the level of the undersurface of the endopelvic fascia immediately posterior to the pubic ramus lateral to the bladder neck. (**b**) Left paraurethral dissection as per 5a. (**c**) Passage of right-side trocar in retropubic space hugging the posterior aspect of the pubic bone to exit 1 cm above the superior margin of the pubic bone and 2 cm lateral to the midline on the right. (**d**) Same procedure on the left side. (**e**) Both trocars have been pulled through and lie on the abdominal wall with the loop of the TVT visible in the vagina. The urethral catheter is being removed to allow post-trocar insertion cystoscopy to ensure no egress into the bladder. (**f**) The trocars have been pulled through along with the distal ends of the retropubic tape within its plastic cover and the tape over the urethra tensioned loosely to allow a pair of McIndoe scissors to remain in place between the urethra and the tape, while the urethra has a 16Ch catheter in situ. (**g**) The trocars have been cut off, and two artery clamps are attached to the plastic covering of the tape to allow simultaneous removal. (**h**) The vaginal incision is closed with an absorbable suture. (**i**) The abdominal exit sites are closed with an absorbable suture and tissue glue

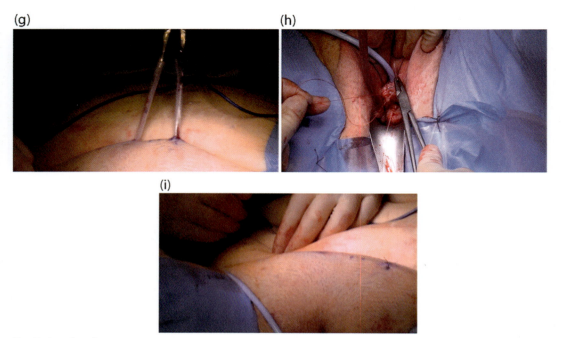

Fig. 5 (continued)

have been demonstrated in both the sling and neighboring normal tissues in comparison with the pubovaginal sling [2]. The technique described for the insertion of a tension-free vaginal tape (TVT) involves blind trocar placement through the retropubic space from the vagina to the abdomen, with the polypropylene sling attached passing either side of the urethra [116] (Fig. 5a–i). Over 10 years, up to 20 deaths occurred as a consequence of vascular or bowel injury, with reports of fistula formation and other visceral injuries including ureteric injury and extrusions (MAUDE database).

The aim of modifications was to allow slings to be placed in outpatient settings under local anesthetic via small anterior vaginal wall incision with trocars passed blind either top down (abdomen to vagina) or bottom up (vagina to abdomen). Raz revised the sling placement by perforation of the endopelvic fascia under direct vision to reduce the chance of visceral injury (bladder, neurovascular, bowel) [117]. Focus was also diverted to bringing the trocar to exit via the obturator foramen to avoid blind passage through the retropubic space, in an attempt to reduce complications from visceral injury and allow a more orthotopic support to the urethra, initially with trocar passing outside to inside (thigh to vagina) [118]. De Leval modified the direction of needle passage from outside (obturator) to inside (vagina) (Fig. 6a–d).

Ulmsten popularized the use of the synthetic mid-urethral sling which then replaced the autologous pubovaginal sling due to ease, local anesthesia, and shorter procedure with a more rapid recovery. The tension-free vaginal tape became the most common stress incontinence surgical procedure in Europe. TVT demonstrated equivalent efficacy over 4 years to an autologous fascial sling without the need to harvest a graft [16, 19].

Doo et al. report an overall success rate of 94.9% for TVT over 5 years, with patient satisfaction recorded at 86.6% [120]. Wadie et al. compared TVT ($n = 28$) to PVS procedures ($n = 25$) for SUI, with success rates of 92% in both groups. At 6 months postoperatively, one patient in each group had de novo urge urinary incontinence. Twice as many patients ($n = 7$) needed to catheterize for a week postoperatively in the PVS group, compared to the TVT group ($n = 3$) [121]. The team noted the economic impact,

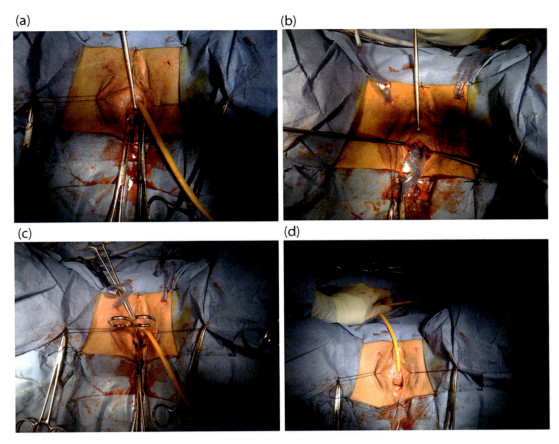

Fig. 6 Transobturator mid-urethral tape insertion. (Original photographs from Ms. Tamsin J Greenwell with patient permission). (**a**) Midline vaginal incision and dissection paraurethrally under the vagina to the inferior pubic ramus bilaterally. Two stab incisions as an exit guide have been made over the upper medial corner of the obturator foramen. (**b**) Both trocars have been passed under the inferior pubic ramus to exit via the stab incisions and pulled through. The tape can be seen in the vaginal wound and exiting the obturator region bilaterally. The urethral catheter has been removed to allow cystoscopy to exclude egress into the bladder. (**c**) The trocars have been pulled through along with the distal ends of the obturator tape within its plastic cover and the tape over the urethra tensioned loosely to allow a pair of McIndoe scissors to remain in place between the urethra and the tape, while the urethra has a 16Ch catheter in situ. The trocars have then been cut off and two artery clamps attached to the plastic covering in preparation for its removal. (**d**) The vaginal incision and stab exit site incisions have been closed with absorbable suture

which was that the PVS procedure was a lot less expensive than the TVT procedure [121].

When considering durability and degradation, samples of PVS material extracted (autologous, allograft, xenograft, and synthetic) were compared histologically. Histological structure revealed that the synthetic material had not degraded at all, with the highest concentration of fibroblast and infiltration of host tissue [58].

In a small randomized trial comparing Burch colposuspension to polytetrafluoroethylene (PTFE) mesh ($n = 36$) at 3 months, there was no difference in outcome; however, this is a very short follow-up period [122]. At one year follow-up, in a different study, the success of PTFE was found to be 61%; however, over one third of patients (40%) suffered a wound infection, and one fifth of patients required sling removal due to exposure/extrusion or infection

[109]. In a study of 176 patients utilizing Mersilene as the PVS material at 30 months, subjective and objective (stress test) cure rates were noted to be 90% and 93%, respectively. Complications were lower with 4% mesh erosion, 8.8% de novo urgency, and 3.5% suffering voiding dysfunction in the form of urinary retention [123]. A further study using Mersilene reported an exposure/extrusion rate of 8% ($n = 772$ patients) [124].

Bai et al. demonstrated that rectus fascial PVS outperformed both Burch colposuspension and TVT with 92.8% cure rate at 12 months postoperatively versus 87.8% for Burch colposuspension and 87% for TVT [125]. Meta-analysis has demonstrated equivalent continence rates for TVT and autologous pubovaginal slings.

Gynecare TVT® is described as the first dedicated mesh sling device for female stress urinary incontinence made of polypropylene mesh. Polythene sleeves cover the mesh with a perforation in the midline to allow smooth placement; the sleeves are then removed, allowing the tape to be placed tension-free at the mid-urethra [126]. The tape was placed vaginally upwards through the retropubic space. The SPARC™ sling system was designed to pass the mesh from a suprapubic incision downwards to the vagina; however, despite cure rates of 84%, there was a reported 7% risk of urinary tract perforation requiring cystoscopy and an 8% risk of voiding dysfunction (and overactive bladder), and it required a general anesthetic [16, 118].

The Monarc™ subfascial hammock mesh (transobturator) sling was brought out via the medial aspect of the obturator foramen, at the proximal inner thigh at the level of the clitoris. The benefits of this lateral route away from the bladder led to the reported outcomes of almost no bladder perforations and reduced rate of voiding dysfunction and de novo detrusor overactivity. This was believed to be due to a more anatomic, less obstructive support for the sub-urethral fascia [126]. A randomized controlled trial ($n = 170$ women with urodynamically proven SUI) over 18 months revealed the transobturator tape to be non-inferior to the retropubic tension-free vaginal tape [127].

Challenges with tape passage include the blind passage of the needle retropubically or transobturator, with risk of vascular and visceral injury, the requirement of a general anesthetic, inpatient stay, and vaginal and abdominal incision [128]. Complication rate overall is quoted at 8.2% with a full-length sling, whether via the retropubic or transobturator route [129]. In addition to the above risks, the transobturator approach has led to groin and lower limb neuropathy in up to 24% of patients in the short term and 4.75% in the long term. The risks were felt to be the highest with the in-out approach, owing to the less precise placement of the trocar when perforating the obturator membrane [130–134]. Cure rates of the transobturator procedure range from 51% to 95% [130, 135].

The above challenges led to the development of the mini-sling. The mini-sling (MiniArc™, Gynecare TVT Secur®) is a mesh sling designed to be placed via a single vaginal incision, under local anesthetic in the outpatient setting, avoiding the risks associated with blind needle passage. Instead of a long sling relying on fibrotic reaction to hold in place, there are paired anchors at each end of the tape which measures 8–14 cm and is inserted with a short needle introducer [126]. A push-fit technique is described, and the ends of the tape are designed to allow fixation and sit in indeterminate pelvic soft tissue. Initial results demonstrated a low morbidity and excellent tolerability under local anesthetic in the outpatient setting. However, efficacy was reported at 60%, well below a full-length sling [126]. As a result of this and due to a lack of long-term efficacy data, they have not been widely adopted. It is hypothesized that early failure is due to a lack of guaranteed reliable anchoring to strong tissues. Without this, they are not likely to allow good enough outcomes to succeed the full-length slings, despite their ease of placement and low morbidity [126].

In an attempt to offer improved anchoring to overcome the early failure of the mini-sling, the Minitape® was designed. It is made from the lightest weight polypropylene and is inserted via a single vaginal incision, with absorbable stay sutures attached, which remain for 3–10 days postoperatively. These stay sutures facilitate adjustment or release at this point of review. The retropubic version measures 12 cm, and the subfascial measures 8 cm in length. The stay sutures are passed with a carrying needle, finer than the previous trocar used, either retropubically to the suprapubic space or via the transobturator approach via the medial obturator foramen. The fine needle does not require a skin incision, and the smaller sutures are less traumatic if urinary tract perforation occurs. It is postulated that early mesh fixation occurs within 72 h, thus allowing the sutures to support the sling while the inflammation and fibroblast reaction occur to embed the sling. This aims to maintain the support required to offer acceptable cure rates for SUI comparable to full-length mesh slings or autologous PVS. The risk of groin symptoms with obturator membrane puncture is also felt to be reduced due to the fine needle puncture and absorbable 2/0 suture, as opposed to a piece of persisting mesh tape [126]. The effect of the ability to adjust the sling postoperatively is unstudied at present. At 21 weeks postoperatively, 1 study has reported a cure rate of 97% in 76 women with SUI utilizing the Minitape® [126]. These are short-term early results, and long-term outcomes are awaited.

There have been concerns about complications and governance of mesh surgery for pelvic organ prolapse and incontinence procedures in the United States, England, and Scotland. This led to a pause of mesh use in the United Kingdom pending completion of the required outcomes of the Cumberlege review [136] (establishment of national mesh centers for insertion and removal, a national implant registry and SUI surgery registry, and enhanced training and appraisal). The US Food and Drug Administration (FDA) issued a statement about long-term complications related to mid-urethral sling surgery in 2008 with recommendations on how to mitigate mesh-related risks and how to counsel patients with an ongoing review [137, 138]. This has led to a decline in use of the mid-urethral synthetic sling despite a joint statement from the American Urological Society and the American Urogynecological Society supporting its efficacy and safety.

The tissue reaction seen around a mesh involving increased fibroblasts does make removal more difficult with higher associated complication rates and a higher incidence of sling extrusion into the urinary tract and exposure into the vagina. The majority of exposures/extrusions are diagnosed around 18 months after surgery; however, some can present 10–20 years later [2]. Exposure/extrusion is more likely with a history of urethral or vaginal atrophy or radiation therapy as well as a consequence of technical factors such as over tensioning of the sling, skimming too close to the urethra during dissection, and urinary tract perforation at the time of insertion [139]. Compared with autologous, allograft, and xenograft slings, synthetic MUS are 14–15 times more likely to extrude into the urethra or become exposed into the vagina [139]. Extrusion often leads to urethral loss and exposure to vaginal length loss following complete excision of mesh and requires complex repair and reconstruction usually with a Martius labial fat pad flap, along with the requirement for secondary stress incontinence procedures, which had a reported success rate of only 56% in one study [139]. Longer-term complications include recurrent exposure/extrusion, chronic pain, and recurrent infection. One of the recommendations from the Cumberlege review involved the setting up of dedicated MESH removal centers in the United Kingdom due to the complexity and need for specialist skills in reconstruction [136]. Estimated complications from mesh surgery for pelvic organ prolapse and stress urinary incontinence range from 0 to 33% [140]. UK data from the NHS reported a 10% complication rate following mid-urethral sling surgery with mesh over a 5-year period with 3.3% requiring mesh removal over 9 years [141].

Alternatives to sling procedures for stress incontinence include the aforementioned colposuspension procedures, urethral bulking, the artificial urinary sphincter, or urinary diversion techniques including bladder neck closure with continent catheterizable channel (Mitrofanoff) or ileal conduit (incontinent diversion) with their own complications and risks.

Conclusions

Stress urinary incontinence is common, affecting up to half of women worldwide. There are economic as well as quality-of-life impacts on the individual. The pubovaginal sling was introduced in the early 1900s for stress urinary incontinence and has progressed through many developments and modifications, informed by better understanding of physiology and anatomy but also by learning from the mistakes and errors from the past. The hammock theory and in particular the integral theory have refined the modern approach to SUI surgery by proposing that a physiological backboard should be created through fixation of the mid-urethra via the pubourethral ligaments to the pubic bone [142]. Loss of the backboard is felt to inhibit normal urethral coaptation at times of raised intraabdominal pressure, causing urinary incontinence. Sling surgery has been modified by using different materials and techniques, and the move from placing interventions and slings at the bladder neck to the mid-urethra, to allow for more anatomic support.

Pubovaginal slings that are made out of autologous tissue, allograft tissue, xenograft tissue, and synthetic materials have been used with varying results, complications, and challenges related to their relative properties and tensile strength. The ideal sling should be chemically inert, biocompatible, and not carcinogenic, should not allow transmissible disease, and should resist degradation while maintaining tensile strength with minimal host reaction through inflammation.

There is a huge cost variation in the development of these different tissues from the additional cost of harvesting them versus the processes of sterilization and reconstitution to the development of synthetic materials and modifications to these.

The autologous PVS does offer the highest success rate and does not cause a tissue reaction with the benefit of lower complications than when using synthetic material. Allografts do risk transmissible disease, and though the risk is low, it is an unacceptable risk.

The tension-free vaginal tape was proven effective in randomized controlled trials and overtook the autologous pubovaginal sling in terms of popularity, but it still had problems with vascular and visceral injury plus voiding dysfunction. Transobturator tapes offered less risk of bladder perforation but had complications related to groin pain and lower limb neuropathy. Mini-slings are easy to place with a low morbidity but have poor efficacy with high early failure rates. The stabilized adjustable mini-sling in early short-term results has been shown to be effective, but long-terms results are awaited as well as governance plans around how to optimize the safe insertion of mesh.

The risk of exposure/extrusion and visceral injury has meant there are ongoing concerns with widespread use of mesh and the need for mesh excision and urethral repair and reconstruction to be managed in specialist centers to prevent further harm.

Challenges going forwards are to develop a sling or support for the treatment of SUI that does not have the risk of exposure, extrusion or other mesh-related complications, is simple, and has the potential to be placed under local anesthetic in the outpatient setting. Some of these challenges with regard to tensioning of slings and fixation to the bone or other fascial tissues continue, along with the uncertainty about the use of synthetic implants and materials. Counselling of patients to give options and choices is essential and should be tailored to individuals.

Take-Home Message

- Autologous rectus fascial slings are durable and readily available, with no tissue reaction and lower chance of exposure/extrusion and complications than synthetic mid-urethral slings.
- Autologous PVS do have a higher risk of voiding dysfunction and urinary tract infection than Burch colposuspension.
- Autologous PVS have similar efficacy and durability if used as primary or secondary SUI procedures.
- Synthetic pubovaginal slings show good efficacy and durability with a reported 8.4% risk of complications overall. Retropubic placement

holds the risks of visceral and vascular injury and voiding dysfunction. The transobturator route reduces the risk of voiding dysfunction and visceral injury and has specific risks of groin and lower limb neuropathy. Mini-slings have had high early failure rates owing to the challenges of reliable anchoring and are not currently recommended.

- Adjustable mini-slings have been developed with promising early outcomes; however, long-term results are awaited.

Cross-References

▶ Artificial Urinary Sphincter for Female Stress Urinary Incontinence
▶ Complications of Stress-Urinary Incontinence Surgery
▶ Historical Milestones in Female Genitourinary and Pelvic Floor Reconstruction
▶ Pathophysiology and Diagnostic Evaluation of Stress Urinary Incontinence: Overview
▶ Retropubic Suspension Operations for Stress Urinary Incontinence

References

1. Abrams P, Cardozo L, Fall M, Griffiths D, Rosier P, Ulmsten U, et al. The standardisation of terminology of lower urinary tract function: report from the standardisation sub-committee of the international continence society. Neurourol Urodyn. 2002;21(2): 167–78.
2. Wein A, Kavoussi L, Novick A, Partin A, Peters C. Campbell-Walsh urology. 10th ed. Saunders Elsevier; 2012.
3. Blaivas J, Groutz A. Urinary incontinence: pathophysiology, evaluation and management overview. Philadelphia: W.B. Saunders; 2002. p. 1027–52.
4. Demirci F, Yucel O. Comparison of pubovaginal sling and burch colposuspension procedures in type I/II genuine stress incontinence. Arch Gynecol Obstet. 2001;265(4):190–4.
5. Green TH. Development of a plan for the diagnosis and treatment of urinary stress incontinence. Am J Obstet Gynecol. 1962;83:632–48.
6. McGuire EJ, Lytton B, Kohorn EI, Pepe V. The value of urodynamic testing in stress urinary incontinence. J Urol. 1980;124(2):256–8.

7. Blaivas JG, Olsson CA. Stress incontinence: classification and surgical approach. J Urol. 1988;139(4): 727–31.
8. McGuire EJ, Fitzpatrick CC, Wan J, Bloom D, Sanvordenker J, Ritchey M, et al. Clinical assessment of urethral sphincter function. J Urol. 1993;150(5 Pt 1):1452–4.
9. Horbach NS, Ostergard DR. Predicting intrinsic urethral sphincter dysfunction in women with stress urinary incontinence. Obstet Gynecol. 1994;84(2):188–92.
10. Nitti VW, Combs AJ. Correlation of Valsalva leak point pressure with subjective degree of stress urinary incontinence in women. J Urol. 1996;155(1):281–5.
11. Fleischmann N, Flisser AJ, Blaivas JG, Panagopoulos G. Sphincteric urinary incontinence: relationship of vesical leak point pressure, urethral mobility and severity of incontinence. J Urol. 2003;169(3):999–1002.
12. Petros PE, Ulmsten UI. An integral theory of female urinary incontinence. Experimental and clinical considerations. Acta Obstet Gynecol Scand Suppl. 1990;153:7–31.
13. Petros PP, Ulmsten U. An anatomical classification--a new paradigm for management of female lower urinary tract dysfunction. Eur J Obstet Gynecol Reprod Biol 1998;80(1):87–94.
14. Constantinou CE, Govan DE. Contribution and timing of transmitted and generated pressure components in the female urethra. Prog Clin Biol Res. 1981;78:113–20.
15. Ulmsten U, Falconer C, Johnson P, Jomaa M, Lannér L, Nilsson CG, et al. A multicenter study of tension-free vaginal tape (TVT) for surgical treatment of stress urinary incontinence. Int Urogynecol J Pelvic Floor Dysfunct. 1998;9(4):210–3.
16. Nilsson CG, Kuuva N, Falconer C, Rezapour M, Ulmsten U. Long-term results of the tension-free vaginal tape (TVT) procedure for surgical treatment of female stress urinary incontinence. Int Urogynecol J Pelvic Floor Dysfunct. 2001;12(Suppl 2):S5–8.
17. Olsson I, Kroon U. A three-year postoperative evaluation of tension-free vaginal tape. Gynecol Obstet Investig. 1999;48(4):267–9.
18. Rezapour M, Ulmsten U. Tension-Free vaginal tape (TVT) in women with recurrent stress urinary incontinence – a long-term follow up. Int Urogynecol J Pelvic Floor Dysfunct. 2001;12(Suppl 2):S9–11.
19. Nilsson CG, Falconer C, Rezapour M. Seven-year follow-up of the tension-free vaginal tape procedure for treatment of urinary incontinence. Obstet Gynecol. 2004;104(6):1259–62.
20. DeLancey JO. Structural support of the urethra as it relates to stress urinary incontinence: the hammock hypothesis. Am J Obstet Gynecol. 1994;170(6): 1713–20. discussion 20-3
21. White G. A radical cure by suturing lateral sulci of vagina to white line of pelvic fascia. JAMA. 1909;21: 1707–8.

22. Richardson AC, Edmonds PB, Williams NL. Treatment of stress urinary incontinence due to paravaginal fascial defect. Obstet Gynecol. 1981;57 (3):357–62.

23. Kelly H, Dunn W. Urinary incontinence in women without manifest injury to the bladder. Sure Gynecol Obstet. 1914;18:444–50.

24. Kennedy W. Incontinence of urine in the female: the urethral sphincter mechanism, damage of function, and restoration of control. Am J Obstet Gynecol. 1937;34:576.

25. Leach GE, Dmochowski RR, Appell RA, Blaivas JG, Hadley HR, Luber KM, et al. Female stress urinary incontinence clinical guidelines panel summary report on surgical management of female stress urinary incontinence. The American Urological Association. J Urol. 1997;158(3 Pt 1):875–80.

26. Bergman A, Koonings PP, Ballard CA. The Ball-Burch procedure for stress incontinence with low urethral pressure. J Reprod Med. 1991;36(2):137–40.

27. Marshall VF, Marchetti AA, Krantz KE. The correction of stress incontinence by simple vesicourethral suspension. Surg Gynecol Obstet. 1949;88(4):509–18.

28. Marshall VF, Marchetti AA, Krantz KE. The correction of stress incontinence by simple vesicourethral suspension. 1949. J Urol. 2002;167(2 Pt 2):1109–14. discussion 15

29. Mainprize TC, Drutz HP. The Marshall-Marchetti-Krantz procedure: a critical review. Obstet Gynecol Surv. 1988;43(12):724–9.

30. Burch J. Urethrovesical fixation to Cooper's ligament for correction of stress incontinence, cystocele and prolapse. Am J Obstet Gynecol. 1961;81:281.

31. Tanagho EA. Colpocystourethropexy: the way we do it. J Urol. 1976;116(6):751–3.

32. Herbertsson G, Iosif CS. Surgical results and urodynamic studies 10 years after retropubic colpourethrocystopexy. Acta Obstet Gynecol Scand. 1993;72(4):298–301.

33. Alcalay M, Monga A, Stanton SL. Burch colposuspension: a 10-20 year follow up. Br J Obstet Gynaecol. 1995;102(9):740–5.

34. Langer R, Lipshitz Y, Halperin R, Pansky M, Bukovsky I, Sherman D. Long-term (10-15 years) follow-up after Burch colposuspension for urinary stress incontinence. Int Urogynecol J Pelvic Floor Dysfunct. 2001;12(5):323–6. discussion 6–7

35. Pereyra AJ. A simplified surgical procedure for the correction of stress incontinence in women. West J Surg Obstet Gynecol. 1959;67(4):223–6.

36. Stamey T. Cystoscopic suspension of the vesical neck for urinary incontinence. Surg Gynecol Obstet. 1973;136:547–54.

37. Raz S. Modified bladder neck suspension for female stress incontinence. Urology. 1981;17(1):82–5.

38. Gittes RF, Loughlin KR. No-incision pubovaginal suspension for stress incontinence. J Urol. 1987;138 (3):568–70.

39. Raz S, Klutke CG, Golomb J. Four-corner bladder and urethral suspension for moderate cystocele. J Urol. 1989;142(3):712–5.

40. Cross CA, Cespedes RD, McGuire EJ. Treatment results using pubovaginal slings in patients with large cystoceles and stress incontinence. J Urol. 1997;158(2):431–4.

41. Serels SR, Rackley RR, Appell RA. In situ slings with concurrent cystocele repair. Tech Urol. 1999;5(3):129–32.

42. Austin PF, Westney OL, Leng WW, McGuire EJ, Ritchey ML. Advantages of rectus fascial slings for urinary incontinence in children with neuropathic bladders. J Urol. 2001;165(6 Pt 2):2369–71. discussion 71–2

43. Ridley J. The Goebel-Stockel sling operation. In: Thompson J, Mattingly R, editors. TeLinde's operative gynaecology. Philadelphia: Lippincott; 1985.

44. Thompson R. A case of epispadias associated with complete incontinence treated by rectus transplantation. Br J Dis Child. 1923;20:146–51.

45. Martius H. Sphincter-und Harnrohrnplastik aus dem Musculus Bulbocavernosus. Chirurg. 1929;1:769.

46. Price P. Plastic operations for incontinence of urine and feces. Arch Surg. 1933;26:1043–8.

47. Wheatcroft SM, Vardy SJ, Tyers AG. Complications of fascia lata harvesting for ptosis surgery. Br J Ophthalmol. 1997;81(7):581–3.

48. Aldridge A. Transplantation of fascia for relief of urinary stress incontinence. Am J Obstet Gynaecol. 1942;44:398–411.

49. Mcguire EJ, Lytton B. Pubovaginal sling procedure for stress incontinence. J Urol. 1978;119(1):82–4.

50. Blaivas JG, Jacobs BZ. Pubovaginal fascial sling for the treatment of complicated stress urinary incontinence. J Urol. 1991;145(6):1214–8.

51. Morgan TO, Westney OL, McGuire EJ. Pubovaginal sling: 4-YEAR outcome analysis and quality of life assessment. J Urol. 2000;163(6):1845–8.

52. Chaikin DC, Rosenthal J, Blaivas JG. Pubovaginal fascial sling for all types of stress urinary incontinence: long-term analysis. J Urol. 1998;160(4):1312–6.

53. Mason RC, Roach M. Modified pubovaginal sling for treatment of intrinsic sphincteric deficiency. J Urol. 1996;156(6):1991–4.

54. McGuire EJ, Bennett CJ, Konnak JA, Sonda LP, Savastano JA. Experience with pubovaginal slings for urinary incontinence at the University of Michigan. J Urol. 1987;138(3):525–6.

55. Chancellor MB, Erhard MJ, Kiilholma PJ, Karasick S, Rivas DA. Functional urethral closure with pubovaginal sling for destroyed female urethra after long-term urethral catheterization. Urology. 1994;43(4):499–505.

56. Swierzewski SJ, McGuire EJ. Pubovaginal sling for treatment of female stress urinary incontinence complicated by urethral diverticulum. J Urol. 1993;149 (5):1012–4.

57. FitzGerald MP, Mollenhauer J, Brubaker L. The fate of rectus fascia suburethral slings. Am J Obstet Gynecol. 2000;183(4):964–6.
58. Woodruff AJ, Cole EE, Dmochowski RR, Scarpero HM, Beckman EN, Winters JC. Histologic comparison of pubovaginal sling graft materials: a comparative study. Urology. 2008;72(1):85–9.
59. Bayrak Ö, Osborn D, Reynolds WS, Dmochowski RR. Pubovaginal sling materials and their outcomes. Turk J Urol. 2014;40(4):233–9.
60. Govier FE, Kobashi K. Pubovaginal slings: a review of the technical variables. Curr Opin Urol. 2001;11 (4):405–10.
61. Khan ZA, Nambiar A, Morley R, Chapple CR, Emery SJ, Lucas MG. Long-term follow-up of a multicentre randomised controlled trial comparing tension-free vaginal tape, xenograft and autologous fascial slings for the treatment of stress urinary incontinence in women. BJU Int. 2015;115(6):968–77.
62. Bang SL, Belal M. Autologous pubovaginal slings: back to the future or a lost art? Res Rep Urol. 2016;8: 11–20.
63. Albo ME, Richter HE, Brubaker L, Norton P, Kraus SR, Zimmern PE, et al. Burch colposuspension versus fascial sling to reduce urinary stress incontinence. N Engl J Med. 2007;356(21):2143–55.
64. Zaragoza MR. Expanded indications for the pubovaginal sling: treatment of type 2 or 3 stress incontinence. J Urol. 1996;156(5):1620–2.
65. Mitsui T, Tanaka H, Moriya K, Kakizaki H, Nonomura K. Clinical and urodynamic outcomes of pubovaginal sling procedure with autologous rectus fascia for stress urinary incontinence. Int J Urol. 2007;14(12):1076–9.
66. Zimmern PE, Gormley EA, Stoddard AM, Lukacz ES, Sirls L, Brubaker L, et al. Management of recurrent stress urinary incontinence after Burch and sling procedures. Neurourol Urodyn. 2016;35(3):344–8.
67. Linder BJ, Elliott DS. Autologous transobturator urethral sling placement for female stress urinary incontinence. J Urol. 2015;193(3):991–6.
68. Milose JC, Sharp KM, He C, Stoffel J, Clemens JQ, Cameron AP. Success of autologous pubovaginal sling after failed synthetic mid urethral sling. J Urol. 2015;193(3):916–20.
69. Lee D, Murray S, Bacsu CD, Zimmern PE. Long-term outcomes of autologous pubovaginal fascia slings: is there a difference between primary and secondary slings? Neurourol Urodyn. 2015;34(1):18–23.
70. Roth CC, Holley TD, Winters JC. Synthetic slings: which material, which approach. Curr Opin Urol. 2006;16(4):234–9.
71. FitzGerald MP, Mollenhauer J, Bitterman P, Brubaker L. Functional failure of fascia lata allografts. Am J Obstet Gynecol. 1999;181(6):1339–44. discussion 44–6
72. Raz S, Siegel AL, Short JL, Snyder JA, Synder JA. Vaginal wall sling. J Urol. 1989;141(1):43–6.

73. Athanasopoulos A, Gyftopoulos K, McGuire EJ. Efficacy and preoperative prognostic factors of autologous fascia rectus sling for treatment of female stress urinary incontinence. Urology. 2011;78(5): 1034–8.
74. Lee D, Alhalabi F, Zimmern P. Long-term outcomes of autologous fascia lata sling for stress incontinence secondary to intrinsic sphincter deficiency in women. Urol Sci. 2017;28:135–8.
75. Latini JM, Lux MM, Kreder KJ. Efficacy and morbidity of autologous fascia lata sling cystourethropexy. J Urol. 2004;171(3):1180–4.
76. Enzelsberger H, Helmer H, Schatten C. Comparison of Burch and lyodura sling procedures for repair of unsuccessful incontinence surgery. Obstet Gynecol. 1996;88(2):251–6.
77. Rottenberg RD, Weil A, Brioschi PA, Bischof P, Krauer F. Urodynamic and clinical assessment of the Lyodura sling operation for urinary stress incontinence. Br J Obstet Gynaecol. 1985;92(8):829–34.
78. Handa VL, Jensen JK, Germain MM, Ostergard DR. Banked human fascia lata for the suburethral sling procedure: a preliminary report. Obstet Gynecol. 1996;88(6):1045–9.
79. Buck BE, Malinin TI. Human bone and tissue allografts. Preparation and safety. Clin Orthop Relat Res. 1994;303:8–17.
80. Wilson TS, Lemack GE, Zimmern PE. Management of intrinsic sphincteric deficiency in women. J Urol. 2003;169(5):1662–9.
81. Buck BE, Malinin TI, Brown MD. Bone transplantation and human immunodeficiency virus. An estimate of risk of acquired immunodeficiency syndrome (AIDS). Clin Orthop Relat Res. 1989;240:129–36.
82. Amundsen CL, Visco AG, Ruiz H, Webster GD. Outcome in 104 pubovaginal slings using freeze-dried allograft fascia lata from a single tissue bank. Urology. 2000;56(6 Suppl 1):2–8.
83. Malinin TI, Buck BE, Temple HT, Martinez OV, Fox WP. Incidence of clostridial contamination in donors' musculoskeletal tissue. J Bone Joint Surg (Br). 2003;85(7):1051–4.
84. Liščić RM, Brinar V, Miklić P, Barsić B, Himbele J. Creutzfeldt-Jakob disease in a patient with a lyophilized dura mater graft. Acta Med Croatica. 1999;53 (2):93–6.
85. Fitzgerald MP, Mollenhauer J, Brubaker L. Failure of allograft suburethral slings. BJU Int. 1999;84(7): 785–8.
86. Gallentine ML, Cespedes RD. Review of cadaveric allografts in urology. Urology. 2002;59(3):318–24.
87. Brown SL, Govier FE. Cadaveric versus autologous fascia lata for the pubovaginal sling: surgical outcome and patient satisfaction. J Urol. 2000;164(5): 1633–7.
88. Elliott DS, Boone TB. Is fascia lata allograft material trustworthy for pubovaginal sling repair? Urology. 2000;56(5):772–6.

89. Onur R, Singla A. Solvent-dehydrated cadaveric dermis: a new allograft for pubovaginal sling surgery. Int J Urol. 2005;12(9):801–5.

90. Onur R, Singla A, Kobashi KC. Comparison of solvent-dehydrated allograft dermis and autograft rectus fascia for pubovaginal sling: questionnaire-based analysis. Int Urol Nephrol. 2008;40(1):45–9.

91. Jarvis GJ, Fowlie A. Clinical and urodynamic assessment of the porcine dermis bladder sling in the treatment of genuine stress incontinence. Br J Obstet Gynaecol. 1985;92(11):1189–91.

92. Hilton P. A clinical and urodynamic study comparing the Stamey bladder neck suspension and suburethral sling procedures in the treatment of genuine stress incontinence. Br J Obstet Gynaecol. 1989;96(2):213–20.

93. Iosif CS. Porcine corium sling in the treatment of urinary stress incontinence. Arch Gynecol. 1987;240(3):131–6.

94. Wiedemann A, Otto M. Small intestinal submucosa for pubourethral sling suspension for the treatment of stress incontinence: first histopathological results in humans. J Urol. 2004;172(1):215–8.

95. John TT, Aggarwal N, Singla AK, Santucci RA. Intense inflammatory reaction with porcine small intestine submucosa pubovaginal sling or tape for stress urinary incontinence. Urology. 2008;72(5):1036–9.

96. Rutner AB, Levine SR, Schmaelzle JF. Processed porcine small intestine submucosa as a graft material for pubovaginal slings: durability and results. Urology. 2003;62(5):805–9.

97. Arunkalaivanan AS, Barrington JW. Randomized trial of porcine dermal sling (Pelvicol implant) vs. tension-free vaginal tape (TVT) in the surgical treatment of stress incontinence: a questionnaire-based study. Int Urogynecol J Pelvic Floor Dysfunct. 2003;14(1):17–23. discussion 1–2

98. Barrington JW, Edwards G, Arunkalaivanan AS, Swart M. The use of porcine dermal implant in a minimally invasive pubovaginal sling procedure for genuine stress incontinence. BJU Int. 2002;90(3):224–7.

99. Giri SK, Hickey JP, Sil D, Mabadeje O, Shaikh FM, Narasimhulu G, et al. The long-term results of pubovaginal sling surgery using acellular cross-linked porcine dermis in the treatment of urodynamic stress incontinence. J Urol. 2006;175(5):1788–92. discussion 93

100. BRACHT. Simplified operation for incontinence. Arch Gynakol. 1951;180:163–4.

101. Hohenfellner R, Petrie E. Sling procedure in surgery. In: Stanton S, editor. Surgery of female incontinence. Berlin: Springer; 1986. p. 105–13.

102. Williams TJ, Telinde RW. The sling operation for urinary incontinence using mersilene ribbon. Obstet Gynecol. 1962;19:241–5.

103. Niknejad K, Plzak LS, Staskin DR, Loughlin KR. Autologous and synthetic urethral slings for female incontinence. Urol Clin North Am. 2002;29(3):597–611.

104. Moir JC. The gauze-hammock operation. (a modified Aldridge sling procedure). J Obstet Gynaecol Br Commonw. 1968;75(1):1–9.

105. Nichols DH. The Mersilene mesh gauze-hammock for severe urinary stress incontinence. Obstet Gynecol. 1973;41(1):88–93.

106. Morgan JE, Farrow GA, Stewart FE. The Marlex sling operation for the treatment of recurrent stress urinary incontinence: a 16-year review. Am J Obstet Gynecol. 1985;151(2):224–6.

107. Morgan JE. A sling operation, using Marlex polypropylene mesh, for treatment of recurrent stress incontinence. Am J Obstet Gynecol. 1970;106(3):369–77.

108. Stanton SL, Brindley GS, Holmes DM. Silastic sling for urethral sphincter incompetence in women. Br J Obstet Gynaecol. 1985;92(7):747–50.

109. Weinberger MW, Ostergard DR. Long-term clinical and urodynamic evaluation of the polytetrafluoroethylene suburethral sling for treatment of genuine stress incontinence. Obstet Gynecol. 1995;86(1):92–6.

110. Choe JM, Staskin DR. Gore-Tex patch sling: 7 years later. Urology. 1999;54(4):641–6.

111. Norris JP, Breslin DS, Staskin DR. Use of synthetic material in sling surgery: a minimally invasive approach. J Endourol. 1996;10(3):227–30.

112. Staskin DR, Choe JM, Breslin DS. The Gore-tex sling procedure for female sphincteric incontinence: indications, technique, and results. World J Urol. 1997;15(5):295–9.

113. Kobashi KC, Dmochowski R, Mee SL, Mostwin J, Nitti VW, Zimmern PE, et al. Erosion of woven polyester pubovaginal sling. J Urol. 1999;162(6):2070–2.

114. Ulmsten U, Petros P. Intravaginal slingplasty (IVS): an ambulatory surgical procedure for treatment of female urinary incontinence. Scand J Urol Nephrol. 1995;29(1):75–82.

115. Petros PE. New ambulatory surgical methods using an anatomical classification of urinary dysfunction improve stress, urge and abnormal emptying. Int Urogynecol J Pelvic Floor Dysfunct. 1997;8(5):270–7.

116. Ulmsten U, Henriksson L, Johnson P, Varhos G. An ambulatory surgical procedure under local anesthesia for treatment of female urinary incontinence. Int Urogynecol J Pelvic Floor Dysfunct. 1996;7(2):81–5. discussion 5–6

117. Rodríguez LV, Raz S. Polypropylene sling for the treatment of stress urinary incontinence. Urology. 2001;58(5):783–5.

118. Delorme E, Droupy S, de Tayrac R, Delmas V. Transobturator tape (Uratape): a new minimally-invasive procedure to treat female urinary incontinence. Eur Urol. 2004;45(2):203–7.

119. Leach GE. Bone fixation technique for transvaginal needle suspension. Urology. 1988;31(5):388–90.

120. Lee KS, Han DH, Choi YS, Yum SH, Song SH, Doo CK, et al. A prospective trial comparing tension-free vaginal tape and transobturator vaginal tape inside-out for the surgical treatment of female stress urinary incontinence: 1-year followup. J Urol. 2007;177(1):214–8.

121. Wadie BS, Edwan A, Nabeeh AM. Autologous fascial sling vs polypropylene tape at short-term followup: a prospective randomized study. J Urol. 2005;174(3):990–3.

122. Sand PK, Winkler H, Blackhurst DW, Culligan PJ. A prospective randomized study comparing modified Burch retropubic urethropexy and suburethral sling for treatment of genuine stress incontinence with low-pressure urethra. Am J Obstet Gynecol. 2000;182(1 Pt 1):30–4.

123. Young SB, Howard AE, Baker SP. Mersilene mesh sling: short- and long-term clinical and urodynamic outcomes. Am J Obstet Gynecol. 2001;185(1):32–40.

124. Wohlrab KJ, Erekson EA, Myers DL. Postoperative erosions of the Mersilene suburethral sling mesh for antiincontinence surgery. Int Urogynecol J Pelvic Floor Dysfunct. 2009;20(4):417–20.

125. Bai SW, Sohn WH, Chung DJ, Park JH, Kim SK. Comparison of the efficacy of Burch colposuspension, pubovaginal sling, and tension-free vaginal tape for stress urinary incontinence. Int J Gynaecol Obstet. 2005;91(3):246–51.

126. Alinsod R. Recent advances in tape slings for female urinary stress incontinence. Rev Obstet Gynecol. 2009;2(1):46–50.

127. Barber MD, Kleeman S, Karram MM, Paraiso MF, Walters MD, Vasavada S, et al. Transobturator tape compared with tension-free vaginal tape for the treatment of stress urinary incontinence: a randomized controlled trial. Obstet Gynecol. 2008;111(3):611–21.

128. Ward K, Hilton P. Minimally invasive synthetic suburethral slings: emerging complications. Obstet Gynecol. 2005;7:223–32.

129. Stanford EJ, Paraiso MF. A comprehensive review of suburethral sling procedure complications. J Minim Invasive Gynecol. 2008;15(2):132–45.

130. Davila GW, Johnson JD, Serels S. Multicenter experience with the Monarc transobturator sling system to treat stress urinary incontinence. Int Urogynecol J Pelvic Floor Dysfunct. 2006;17(5):460–5.

131. Moore RD, Gamble K, Miklos JR. Tension-free vaginal tape sling for recurrent stress incontinence after transobturator tape sling failure. Int Urogynecol J Pelvic Floor Dysfunct. 2007;18(3):309–13.

132. Collinet P, Ciofu C, Cosson M, Jacquetin B. Safety of in-out transobturator approach for SUI: multi centre prospective study of 944 patients, French TVT-O registry. Int Pelvic Floor Dysfunction. 2006;17:103.

133. Lim J, Cornish A, Carey MP. Clinical and quality-of-life outcomes in women treated by the TVT-O procedure. BJOG. 2006;113(11):1315–20.

134. Roth TM. Management of persistent groin pain after transobturator slings. Int Urogynecol J Pelvic Floor Dysfunct. 2007;18(11):1371–3.

135. Juang CM, Yu KJ, Chou P, Yen MS, Twu NF, Horng HC, et al. Efficacy analysis of trans-obturator tension-free vaginal tape (TVT-O) plus modified Ingelman-Sundberg procedure versus TVT-O alone in the treatment of mixed urinary incontinence: a randomized study. Eur Urol. 2007;51(6):1671–8. discussion 9

136. Cumberlege J. First do no harm: the report of the Independent Medicines and Medical Devices Safety Review. 2020. Available from: www.immdsre-view.org.uk/Report.html.

137. Administration USFaD. FDA strengthens requirements for surgical mesh for the transvaginal repair of pelvic organ prolapse to address safety risks. 2016 [cited 2021 20th December]. Available from: https://www.fda.gov/newsevents/newsroom/pressannouncements/ucm479732.htm.

138. Lee D, Dillon B, Lemack G, Gomelsky A, Zimmern P. Transvaginal mesh kits – how "serious"' are the complications and are they reversible? Urology. 2013;81(1):43–8.

139. Blaivas JG, Sandhu J. Urethral reconstruction after erosion of slings in women. Curr Opin Urol. 2004;14(6):335–8.

140. Shah HN, Badlani GH. Mesh complications in female pelvic floor reconstructive surgery and their management: a systematic review. Indian J Urol. 2012;28(2):129–53.

141. Gurol-Urganci I, Geary RS, Mamza JB, Duckett J, El-Hamamsy D, Dolan L, et al. Long-term rate of mesh sling removal following midurethral mesh sling insertion among women with stress urinary incontinence. JAMA. 2018;320(16):1659–69.

142. Petros PE, Woodman PJ. The integral theory of continence. Int Urogynecol J Pelvic Floor Dysfunct. 2008;19(1):35–40.

Complications of Stress-Urinary Incontinence Surgery

22

Bilal Chughtai, Christina Sze, and Stephanie Sansone

Contents

Introduction	396
Urethral Bulking Agents	396
Individual Analyses of UBAs	396
Midurethral Sling	398
Intraoperative Complications	398
Postoperative Complications	399
Retreatment Rates	399
Autologous Fascia Pubovaginal Sling	399
Burch Colposuspension	400
Anti-incontinence Procedure at the Time of Prolapse Repair	401
Artificial Urinary Sphincter	401
Early Postoperative Complications	401
Late Postoperative Complications	401
Urethrolysis	402
Mesh Removal	402
Conclusion	403
Cross-References	403
References	403

B. Chughtai (✉) · S. Sansone
Department of Urology, Weill Cornell Medicine/New York
Presbyterian, New York, NY, USA

Department of Obstetrics and Gynecology, Weill Cornell
Medicine/New York Presbyterian, New York, NY, USA
e-mail: bic9008@med.cornell.edu

C. Sze
Department of Urology, Weill Cornell Medicine/New York
Presbyterian, New York, NY, USA

Abstract

Stress urinary incontinence (SUI) is a common and distressing symptom that affects up to 45% of women. There are several surgical treatment options for the management of women with SUI. As newer materials and less invasive techniques emerge, the prevalence of surgical treatment has increased (Jonsson Funk et al.,

© Springer Nature Switzerland AG 2023
F. E. Martins et al. (eds.), *Female Genitourinary and Pelvic Floor Reconstruction*,
https://doi.org/10.1007/978-3-031-19598-3_23

Obstet Gynecol 119:845, 2012). Although several Cochrane reviews and randomized controlled trials have attempted to compare the clinical effectiveness of each surgical approach, few have focused on adverse events and complications rates as an end point. This chapter details complications of surgery for SUI.

Keywords

Stress-urinary incontinence · Surgery · Complications · Sling · Artificial urinary sphincter · Suspension

Introduction

Stress-urinary incontinence (SUI) is the involuntary leakage of urine caused by increasing intra-abdominal pressure during exertion or on physical effort that affects 30–45% of women in their lifetime [1, 2]. Although SUI is non-life-threatening, it can cause significant health care burden in the aging population and lead to negative impacts on women's quality of life and mental well-being [3]. Since 2000, there has been 27% increase in the rate of surgical management of SUI with reoperation ranging from 5.3% to 11.2% by 8 years of follow-up [4, 5]. Thus, it is important to be well informed about the most common complications that are associated with SUI surgery, so they can be addressed and treated properly.

Urethral Bulking Agents

Urethral bulking agents (UBAs) are synthetic or natural substances that are injected into the urethral submucosa in order to improve coaptation of the urethra [6]. UBAs are primarily used in patients with SUI caused by intrinsic sphincter deficiency or in patients who are unfit for general anesthesia. UBAs are injected either transurethrally or periurethrally. In the transurethral technique, the bulking agent is injected submucosally via a needle inserted through a cystoscope under direct visual guidance. In the periurethral technique, the material is injected with a needle percutaneously from a perimeatal injection site. The goal is to inject the bulking agent into the urethral submucosal wall at the level of bladder neck or proximal urethra. Periurethral and transurethral methods of UBAs have demonstrated similar success rates, but there was a higher (but statistically insignificant) likelihood of early postoperative complications especially transient urinary retention in the periurethral group [7].

UBAs have an overall complication rate of 32% with onset that varies from several weeks to even several years postoperatively [7]. The onset of complications varies from 5 to 120 weeks, and most of them are mild, transient, and do not require surgical management. In a multicenter randomized clinical trial, UBAs compared to conventional sling surgery are associated with a lower rate of complications (63% vs 36%, respectively) [8]. Complications include urinary retention (8.4%), pain (dysuria, injection site pain, and pelvic pain) (6.4%), hematuria (3.7%), urinary tract or vaginal infection (5.5%), lower urinary tract symptoms (incontinence, frequency, and urgency) (7%), periurethral abscess (0.6%), mass formation (pseudocyst, pseudoabscess, and granuloma) (0.4%), migration of the injected material (0.03%), prolapse of the injected material (0.03%), and erosion of the urethral or vaginal wall (0.3%) [7].

A review consisting of 2095 complications in 79 studies demonstrated that most complications from injections were treated with noninvasive management such as oral antibiotics, anticholinergics, or urethral catheterization [7]. Retention was treated with an indwelling catheter in 9 cases and intermittent catheterization in 12 cases. Of the reported complications, 67 (3%) were considered major (Clavien grade III – requiring an additional procedure). Of the 67 complications that required an additional procedure, 46 (69%) required incision and drainage, and 21 (31%) required a more invasive procedure.

Individual Analyses of UBAs

There are several types of FDA-approved bulking agents currently on the market. Prior to these, a bovine collagen-based bulking agent was also available (Contigen®). This was the only non-permanent biodegradable option but was noted to have rates of allergic reactions as high as 2–5% [9]. In fact, it required skin testing prior to use. Ultimately, given it was absorbed, patients' symptoms would recur and they would need additional injections, which led to it being discontinued in 2011.

The most common UBAs used in children is dextranomer/hyaluronic acid (Zuidex™, Deflux™) which is used to correct vesicoureteral reflux. However, its application in female SUI has demonstrated significantly lower success rates in terms of the reduction of incontinence episodes when compared to collagen (53% vs 66.5%, respectively) [10]. Additionally due to high rates of abscess at the injection site, injection of dextranomer/hyaluronic acid was discontinued as a treatment option for SUI.

Currently, there are four bulking agents being offered for SUI. Three of them are particle based: carbon-coated beads (Durasphere®), spherical particles of calcium hydroxylapatite in a gel carrier (Coaptite®), and polydimethylsiloxane, or solid silicone, that is suspended in a carrier gel (Macroplastique®). The fourth bulking agent is a nonparticulate, nonresorbable cross-linked poly-acrylamide hydrogel called Bulkamid®. Unfortunately, few research articles have compared them. In fact, the most recent Cochrane review concluded that because of the small size and moderate quality of articles, a meta-analysis was not possible [11].

Carbon-coated zirconium (Durasphere™) was constructed with larger particles (251–300 μm) to provide more durable results and prevent migration. However, this relatively large size of Durasphere™ required greater pressures to inject the material which can lead to higher rates of postoperative de novo urgency and transient urinary retention when compared with collagen (25% vs 12% and 17% vs 3%, respectively). Overall treatment rates for Durasphere™ are comparable to collagen at 12 months (80% for Durasphere™ vs 69% for collagen) [12].

Coaptite™ consists of smooth calcium hydroxylapatite bioceramic which is similar to composition of bone and teeth. Coaptite™ particles are radiopaque; therefore, injection accuracy can be verified radiographically. Coaptite™ provides greater symptomatic improvement (statistically nonsignificant) in females with SUI, when compared with collagen. However transient urinary retention was insignificantly higher in the Coaptite™ group (41% vs 33%, P > 0.05) [13]. However, notable complications were encountered in two Coaptite™ patients from improper placement of the biomaterial-leading erosion. Additionally, urethral prolapse causing voiding difficulty was also reported in two patients requiring surgical treatment [14].

Macroplastique™ is the most studied of the synthetic injectable agents. Macroplastique™ consists of silicone polymers which is a larger particle diameter (>100 μm). Macroplastique™ has demonstrated significantly superior clinical improvement and dry/cure rates at 12 months follow-up when compared with collagen (61.5% and 36.9% for Macroplastique vs 48% and 24.8% for collagen, respectively) [15]. The same study concluded that the safety profiles and adverse events were similar between the two groups. Generally, the complications having been associated with Macroplastique™ usage were short-lived, mild, and easily managed without long-term sequelae: urinary tract infection (24%), dysuria and urgency (9%), frequency (8%), and transient urinary retention (7%).

Bulkamid® is the newest urethral bulking agent in the USA, approved by the FDA in 2020. In a multicenter noninferiority RCT, Bulkamid® was demonstrated to be noninferior to collagen in treating urinary incontinence. At 12 months, 77% of patients treated with Bulkamid® considered themselves cured or improved compared to 70% of patients treated with collagen.

Overall, UBAs have patient-reported improvement rates of 50–70%, however, and lack long-term durability. UBAs have traditionally been reserved for those patients with ISD without urethral hypermobility, but this landscape is changing given a relatively low complication rate, particularly for patients who may want to avoid mesh and mesh-related complications. Patients with recurrent SUI after a surgical intervention or those with rare, yet bothersome, symptoms may be ideal candidates. Given this procedure can be performed in the clinic setting and/or without anesthesia, this is also ideal for poor surgical candidates. Despite its minimally invasive and "low-risk" nature, UBAs are not without complications; however, these complications are less severe and do not warrant additional invasive treatment like other surgical alternatives of female SUI.

Midurethral Sling

With the evolution of surgical methods, midurethral sling (MUS) is the current gold standard surgical treatment of SUI [4]. There are three different types of MUSs: retropubic tension-free vaginal tape (TVT), transobturator (TOT), and single incision sling (SIS).

The TVT and TOT are full-length slings (~40 cm), whereas the SIS slings are much shorter (~8 cm). TVTs pass through the vagina, through the retropubic space and abdominal wall, and then exit the skin in the suprapubic area. The TOT, in contrast, passes through the vagina and bilateral obturator foramen prior to exiting the skin at the groin. Given these differing trajectories of the TVT and TOT slings, both methods have distinct complication profiles as described below. As an overview, the TVT is traditionally known to have bladder perforation, bowel injury, suprapubic pain, and voiding dysfunction, such as overactive bladder symptoms, as a complication given the trocar trajectory behind the pubic bone by the detrusor muscle and innervation. The TOT is traditionally known to have groin pain as a complication given its trajectory and less voiding dysfunction symptoms.

In terms of the shorter length SIS, these can be placed in a retropubic (attached to perineal membrane) or transobturator (attached to obturator internus muscle) fashion. It is believed that these pathways may lead to less dissection and lower risk of visceral injury. Yet, given their use is relatively new, there is a paucity of long-term data, and women undergoing primary midurethral

sling surgery should be recommended a full-length sling based on our available published studies. SISs may, however, be reserved for patients who opt for a shorter recovery and duration of postoperative pain. Surgeons are even able to perform SIS placement in the office under local anesthesia for the appropriate candidate.

Intraoperative Complications

Intraoperative complications include significant bleeding, and bladder and urethral injury.

Significant intraoperative bleeding requiring reintervention from MUS insertion is poorly reported, but it is estimated to occur in <1% of procedures [16]. A multicenter, randomized equivalence trial comparing outcomes with TVT and TOT demonstrated that vascular events are significantly more common in the TVT (p = 0.03); however, these did not require reintervention [17]. Because intraoperative bleeding is typically effectively managed by vaginal packing, it is advised to hold pressure and complete the procedure as quickly as possible [18].

The incidence of bladder perforation ranges from 2 to 10% [17]. Bladder perforation occurs more likely with TVT because of retropubic passage of trocars between the vagina and the abdomen [17]. In contrast, the TOT and SIS avoid the retropubic passage, thereby reducing the risk of bladder and bowel injury. In a review of sling complications consisting of 55 studies with 4188 participants, the authors noted that SIS had the lowest incidence of bladder perforation compared to TVT and TOT (0.7–2.9% vs 0.8–11.4% vs 0.8–10%, respectively) [19]. Most bladder perforations, if recognized intraoperatively, are treated by repositioning the needle and maintaining bladder drainage with a Foley catheter for 24–48 h [18]. Nevertheless, despite circumscribing the space of Retzius and thus reducing the risk of bladder injury, the TOT and SIS might potentially cause obturator neurovascular bundle injury. These injuries are typically managed conservatively in most cases [19].

Urethral injury rates range from 0.1% to 5.5% for TVT and 0–2.5% for TOT [20]. Urethral injury usually results from vaginal dissection too proximal to the urethra, and repair should be performed with periurethral fascia closure [18]. Additionally, placement of a synthetic sling following a urethral injury at the time of surgery is contraindicated and prolonged bladder drainage is recommended.

Bowel injury is rarely reported (0.03–0.7%) and has only been described with the retropubic technique. Treatment consists of exploratory laparotomy for bowel repair and sling removal [21].

Postoperative Complications

Early postoperative complications include voiding dysfunction, pain, and infection.

Bladder dysfunction (de novo overactive bladder and de novo urgency with/without incontinence) ranged from 5.9% to 25% for the TVT technique and from 0% to 15.6% for the TOT slings [19]. In a meta-analysis of randomized trials, TOT was associated with lower risks of long-term bladder dysfunction (OR 0.32, 95% CI 0.17–0.61) compared to TVT [22]. Postoperative lower urinary tract symptoms are common and typically resolve with conservative management. Persistent symptoms warrant further workup by excluding the possibility of sling erosion, local hematoma, or bladder outlet obstruction.

Postoperative pain in the groin and thighs may be noted 1–2 weeks after surgery. Most cases of groin pain resolved within the first 6 months following surgery. The TOMUS trial, a 12-month prospective series of 597 patients comparing the TOT and retropubic TVT techniques, showed a lower incidence of neurological symptoms (pain) for the TVTs (4.0%) compared to the TOTs (9.4%) [23]. In most cases, pain disappears within the first few weeks after surgery, but it may persist for more than 4 weeks in 1–2.7% of the patients [23]. If conservative treatments fail, ureterolysis or sling excision may be performed.

Complications such as mesh extrusion or erosion are more difficult to treat and are more common with TOT compared to TVT and SIS (1.9–10%, 0–5.7%, and 1.4–4.5%, respectively) [21]. Vaginal mesh erosion rates vary from 0% to 1.5% for TVT and from 0% to 10.9% for the TOT

[21]. Mesh erosions may be associated with symptoms affecting daily life: bleeding, discharge, discomfort, pain, or dyspareunia. Management of erosion can range from conservative (i.e., observation, vaginal estrogen therapy) to a more aggressive approach such as excision of the extruded segment (which is the preferred method), burying of the extruded segment, or removal of all graft materials (e.g., if infected or recurrent).

Erosion of slings into the urethra is uncommon (TVT 0.03–0.8% and TOT 0%) [24]. Late urethral erosion is caused by excessive tension of the sling under the urethra, leading to progressive atrophy and subsequent erosion. Missed urethral or bladder injury may be misclassified as bladder or urethral erosion. Treatment of urethral mesh erosion requires mesh removal and urethral repair.

Lastly, recurrent urinary traction infection may represent a complication secondary to the presence of a urethral/bladder erosion or bladder outlet obstruction. Therefore, full workup is needed to rule these causes out.

Retreatment Rates

A meta-analysis of 175 randomized controlled trials assessing a total of 21,598 women who underwent MUS demonstrated that retreatment rates of repeat surgeries were higher after TOT than after TVT at 12 months and more than 60 months.

Autologous Fascia Pubovaginal Sling

Autologous fascia slings, or pubovaginal slings (PVS), are used to support the proximal urethra and bladder neck using an autologous graft material. PVS have gained recent popularity given they are an option for primary treatment of intrinsic sphincter deficiency and/or SUI and does not involve synthetic mesh material. The procedure may also be used for recurrent SUI, urethral reconstruction (i.e., anomalies, repair of an injury, repair of a simultaneous diverticulum or fistula, etc.), or urethral obliteration. Those with a history of pelvic radiation or who have encountered complications (i.e., mesh erosion) from prior SUI surgeries are good candidates as well. The PVS procedure has a reported success rate of about 90% after 3–15 years of follow-up and has similar short-term outcomes as the MUS [25].

The reported overall complication rate for the PVS ranges from 14% to 45%. Acute intraoperative and postoperative complications from pubovaginal sling include bladder or urethral injury. These injuries typically occur during lateral dissection of the periurethral pockets and/or passage of the sling with Stamey needles or similar devices. These injuries should be repaired in several layers once the injury is noted, and patients should wear a catheter for 7–10 days. Ureteral injury and pelvic visceral injuries are rare. Of note, in contrast to synthetic sling placement, fascial slings can still be placed at time of injury following simultaneous repair. Wound infections, erosions, and hernias from the abdominal portion of the procedure are also rare.

The most common chronic complications following pubovaginal slings are related to voiding dysfunction. Urgency incontinence, de novo urgency, and obstructive symptoms are present in up to 25% of patients after 6 weeks, whereas urinary retention, which may occur in up to 20% of patients, tends to resolve after 2–4 weeks. Yet, very few patients require reoperation or urethrolysis (<3%) (see section on urethrolysis). To prepare for this possible complication, surgeons may choose to teach their patients how to perform intermittent self-catheterization preoperatively.

Burch Colposuspension

While there are have been several retropubic urethrovesical suspension procedures described, the Burch colposuspension procedure may be preferred. The procedure is not recommended for patients with intrinsic sphincter deficiency given higher failure rates.

Besides the minor complications typically associated with any surgery by the urinary tract, such as urinary tract or wound infections, it is very rare to have direct surgical injury to the urinary tract with a Burch colposuspension. While ureteral obstruction has been reported, given the potential for ureteral stretching or kinking with suspension, these are treated with suture removal and stenting. There have been no cases of ureteral transection, and fistulas are equally uncommon. Osteitis pubis, or inflammation of the bony and cartilaginous structures of the anterior pelvic girdle, is also rare following Burch colposuspension – it is more commonly seen following the Marshall-Marchetti-Krantz retropubic urethrovesical suspension procedure. This is typically diagnosed 2–12 weeks postoperatively by X-ray (evidence of bone destruction, symphysis pubis separation) and is characterized by suprapubic pain radiating to the thighs. Conservative therapy is recommended with resolution in weeks to months. With failure of conservative therapy, biopsy may be indicated with additional therapy, such as antibiotics, incision and drainage of a potential abscess, and debridement.

Other complications related to Burch colposuspension are the development of overactive bladder symptoms (de novo urgency) and voiding difficulties. Micturition patterns can change, introducing an element of obstruction with decreased flow rates, increased detrusor pressure at maximum flow rate, and increased urethral resistance. The mean number of days to complete voiding after an open Burch procedure is 7 days, which is longer than MUS. Risk factors for prolonged voiding include advanced age, prior incontinence surgery, increased first sensation to void, high postvoid residual volume, and postoperative cystitis [26, 27].

Finally, one other specific postoperative complication associated with a Burch procedure is the occurrence of posterior vaginal wall prolapse (rectocele, enterocele) [28]. While there is no true consensus among surgeons, there is general agreement that a Burch colposuspension may increase the risk of developing apical or posterior vaginal prolapse. Therefore, a procedure to obliterate the cul-de-sac is recommended at the time of Burch procedure to potentially prevent enterocele formation.

Anti-incontinence Procedure at the Time of Prolapse Repair

There is some controversy about the role of anti-incontinence procedures, namely, retropubic mid-urethral slings, at the time of prolapse repair. One review has suggested that combination surgery reduces de novo subjective SUI but is associated with short-term voiding difficulties, overactive bladder symptoms, and need for catheterization [29]. In contrast, another review suggested that a concomitant anti-incontinence procedure is not associated with an increased risk of complications and that medical comorbidity is strongly associated with complications after prolapse surgery [30]. Furthermore, a more recent database study assessed the impact of concurrent anti-incontinence procedures specifically at the time of abdominal sacrocolpopexy and only found higher rates of urinary tract infections in the 30-day postoperative period with no impact on readmission or reoperation [31].

Given these findings, it is prudent to perform comprehensive counseling about risks and benefits of anti-incontinence surgery at time of prolapse surgery, particularly knowing that up to half of women with prolapse also experience SUI and de novo SUI may occur in nearly a third of these patients as well.

Artificial Urinary Sphincter

Since the 1970s, the artificial urinary sphincter (AUS) has remained the gold standard treatment for moderate-to-severe male SUI. To date, the role for the artificial urinary sphincter (AUS) in adult female urinary incontinence has not been defined. However, AUS are usually performed as a last resort after other forms of treatment have failed or in certain patient groups, i.e., neurogenic. It is important to treat preexisting overactive bladder (OAB) in patients with mixed urinary incontinence before proceeding with AUS placement. In the largest cohort of 207 women with SUI who underwent AUS, 88.7% and 81.8% continence rates were reported in non-neurogenic and neurogenic causes of urinary incontinence,

respectively [32]. The 3-, 5-, and 10-year device survival rates were 92.0, 88.6, and 69.2%, respectively. One of the most concerning problems of AUS is the high rate of revision surgery (0–80%) [33]. Major risk factors for explantation are pelvic irradiation, age > 70 years, neurological pathology, and a history of pelvic surgery, including the Burch procedure and sacral colpopexy [34].

Early Postoperative Complications

Acute urinary retention (AUR) is the most common complication in the first 1–2 months following AUS implantation. AUR can usually be managed safely with confirmation of cuff deactivation followed by short-term catheterization with a low-diameter catheter. If AUR persists, an undersized cuff causing urethral coaptation may be the cause. Another early postoperative complication is unrecognized urethral injuries which can present with hematuria, dysuria, or AUR. Treatment usually includes device removal.

Late Postoperative Complications

Most cases of AUS failure occur late, after several years of SUI improvement. Therefore, lack of improvement in SUI after device activation requires immediate evaluation. One must rule out fluid loss first. Fluid loss presents with recurrent SUI and can occur at any point postoperatively. It should be suspected if the device does not cycle or there is a palpable abnormality when cycling the control pump.

Major AUS complications noted during long-term follow-up were prosthetic infections, urethral erosion, and urethral atrophy. Costa et al. reported a 4.8% risk of device infection in a series of female patients [32]. AUS infection can occur anytime in the postoperative period and is often associated with urethral cuff erosion. Superficial wound infections present with evidence of mild inflammation without purulent drainage and can usually be managed with antibiotics. Infections involving the deeper tissues around the device have a range of presentations from mild pain with pump fixation to severe deep tissue infection with a systemic inflammatory response. These infections of the deep tissue require complete device removal and antibiotic washout.

Urethral atrophy was previously thought to be a common cause of delayed nonmechanical failure. However, recent evidence has suggested that urethral atrophy may be due to urethral constriction due encapsulation at the cuff. The role of urethral atrophy in delayed AUS failure remains controversial. Urethral atrophy is a diagnosis of exclusion, and investigation of the device further is necessary to rule out other sources of AUS failure.

Urethrolysis

Iatrogenic bladder outlet obstruction is a potential complication of all stress incontinence procedures, leading to bothersome postoperative voiding dysfunction. The incidence of postoperative urethral obstruction varies widely in the literature, ranging from 2.5% to 24%, with the true incidence likely unknown. Urethrolysis is a procedure that has traditionally been the standard for management of complications after anti-incontinence surgery with success rate ranging from 65% to 80% [35, 36]. However, sling incision, with or without partial excision, is now preferred by many as a less aggressive option for managing obstruction from synthetic midurethral slings. Urethrolysis is usually performed after a failed partial excision of a synthetic sling, or for readjusting PVS. There are no guidelines regarding when to perform urethrolysis; however, expert opinion and most urethrolysis series recommend waiting a minimum of 3 months prior to intervention to allow for adequate retropubic scarification and fibrosis.

Complications for urethrolysis are poorly documented and reported. Heavy bleeding or entry into the bladder neck or urethra may occur during urethrolysis. Closure of any easily accessible lacerations and 2–3 weeks of catheter drainage for those that are not accessible usually enable complete healing. In the case of bleeding, rapidly finishing the procedure and packing the vagina

should allow the bleeding to tamponade and stop. Recurrent SUI occurs in up to 20% of patients. When it does occur, injection of a bulking agent may prove to be successful in treating the incontinence. If that approach fails, a resuspension or sling can be performed after the patient is reevaluated fully.

Mesh Removal

Mesh exposure rates range from 2% to 30% [37] following placement for repair of pelvic organ prolapse (POP) or for surgical correction of SUI [37]. If conservative or endoscopic treatment fails, partial or complete mesh removal can be used. In a large cohort of 112,152 women who underwent MUS for SUI, Mesh sling was removed in 1.4% of the women at 1 year, in 2.7% at 5 years, and in 3.3% at 9 years after the initial insertion. In the cohort, the risk of removal was higher (at all time points) in women who had a retropubic insertion than in those who had a transobturator insertion [37]. Reported intraoperative complications during complete mesh removal procedures include bowel injury, ureteric injury, bladder injury, and hemorrhage.

Postoperative complications from mesh removal include recurrent POP or SUI, wound infection, persistent vaginal or pelvic pain, and fistula formation. In a series of 277 patients, Rac et al. reported a 9% perioperatively mesh removal complication rate [38]. The most frequent complications were urinary tract infections and vaginal yeast infections in 37 patients (23.9%), followed by de novo SUI in 31 patients (20.0%), de novo urgency UI in 11 patients (7.1%), and de novo POP in 7 patients (4.5%). Overall, most complications tend to be minor and can typically be managed conservatively.

Most cases requiring mesh removal can be completed vaginally, particularly if a patient's complaints involve a vaginal mesh exposure. Providers may choose to expectantly manage small mesh exposures of macroporous monofilament material if the patient is not experiencing bothersome symptoms. The macroporous material may allow for tissue ingrowth, so smaller exposures

Conclusion

(0.5 cm or less) can have a trial of vaginal estrogen therapy for several months before pursuing more aggressive measures. Erosion into the bladder or urethra may be more challenging. If inside the bladder, adherent calculi may form over the mesh and require more extensive surgery for removal. For example, beyond vaginal or cystoscopic removal, open abdominal or laparoscopic removal may be necessary.

For laparoscopic removal, the retropubic space is entered above the bladder and dissected to open the space of Retzius. The bladder is reflected inferiorly to exposure of the urethra, bladder neck, and obturator neurovascular bundle. Once these important structures are identified, the arms of the mesh are isolated and the most proximal portion visible dissected off from the abdominal wall. A free edge is typically isolated and grasped while the surgeon dissects tissue off the mesh moving distally toward the vagina. The surgeon holds traction on the end of the sling arm as they move toward the vagina during this dissection. Once both arms are removed and hemostasis assured, the peritoneum is closed. There is very little data on laparoscopic removal of retropubic mesh slings, though it is feasible. Complications from laparoscopic removal of retropubic slings vary – from urinary tract infections to retropubic hematomas. In one series, development of a large retropubic hematoma required evacuation for two patients [29]. Other complications include surgical site infections and incisions hernias from the laparoscopic port sites. Given there are only small case series reporting on these complications, it is difficult to draw a larger conclusion on rates and severity of these setbacks. Although, with any sling removal procedure, it is imperative to counsel about the risk of recurrence of SUI. In the aforementioned case series of laparoscopic removal of retropubic midurethral slings, 71% of patients experienced recurrence of symptoms [29]. Yet, the majority of patients stated that they experienced improvement in pain, citing a 78% rate of cure or improvement in pain. Thus, a laparoscopic minimally invasive approach to sling removal could be offered after thorough counseling of risks and benefits of this procedure.

Conclusion

There is an increasing body of evidence to suggest that the number and severity of complications associated with SUI surgery are underestimated, by both surgeons and patients, because these complications are typically minor and managed conservatively. Nevertheless, proper diagnosis, evaluation, and realistic discussion of urinary symptom goals are paramount in selecting the appropriate surgical approaches to minimize surgical complications. Treatment of these complications start with physician awareness. Additionally, it is important to acknowledge that women aged 65 years and older have many unique age-related concerns that are critical to optimizing patient care and surgical outcomes.

Cross-References

▶ Artificial Urinary Sphincter for Female Stress Urinary Incontinence
▶ Retropubic Suspension Operations for Stress Urinary Incontinence

References

1. Abrams P, Cardozo L, Fall M, et al. The standardisation of terminology in lower urinary tract function: report from the standardisation sub-committee of the international continence society. Urology. 2003;61:37.
2. Komesu YM, Schrader RM, Ketai LH, et al. Epidemiology of mixed, stress, and urgency urinary incontinence in middle-aged/older women: the importance of incontinence history. Int Urogynecol J. 2016;27:763.
3. Coyne KS, Kvasz M, Ireland AM, et al. Urinary incontinence and its relationship to mental health and health-related quality of life in men and women in Sweden, the United Kingdom, and the United States. Eur Urol. 2012;61:88.
4. Jonsson Funk M, Levin PJ, Wu JM. Trends in the surgical management of stress urinary incontinence. Obstet Gynecol. 2012;119:845.
5. Trabuco EC, Carranza D, El Nashar SA, et al. Reoperation for urinary incontinence after retropubic and transobturator sling procedures. Obstet Gynecol. 2019;134:333.
6. Zoorob D, Karram M. Bulking agents: a urogynecology perspective. Urol Clin North Am. 2012;39:273.

7. de Vries AM, Wadhwa H, Huang J, et al. Complications of urethral bulking agents for stress urinary incontinence: an extensive review including case reports. Female Pelvic Med Reconstr Surg. 2018;24:392.

8. Corcos J, Collet JP, Shapiro S, et al. Multicenter randomized clinical trial comparing surgery and collagen injections for treatment of female stress urinary incontinence. Urology. 2005;65:898.

9. Lightner D, Rovner E, Corcos J, et al. Randomized controlled multisite trial of injected bulking agents for women with intrinsic sphincter deficiency: mid-urethral injection of Zuidex via the Implacer versus proximal urethral injection of Contigen cystoscopically. Urology. 2009;74:771.

10. Sokol ER, Karram MM, Dmochowski R. Efficacy and safety of polyacrylamide hydrogel for the treatment of female stress incontinence: a randomized, prospective, multicenter north American study. J Urol. 2014;192:843.

11. Casteleijn FM, Zwolsman S, Roovers JP, et al. Urethral bulking therapy for treating stress urinary incontinence in women. Cochrane Database Syst Rev. 2021

12. Hoe V, Haller B, Yao HH, et al. Urethral bulking agents for the treatment of stress urinary incontinence in women: a systematic review. Neurourol Urodyn. 2021;40:1349.

13. Lai HH, Hurtado EA, Appell RA. Large urethral prolapse formation after calcium hydroxylapatite (Coaptite) injection. Int Urogynecol J Pelvic Floor Dysfunct. 2008;19:1315.

14. Palma PC, Riccetto CL, Martins MH, et al. Massive prolapse of the urethral mucosa following periurethral injection of calcium hydroxylapatite for stress urinary incontinence. Int Urogynecol J Pelvic Floor Dysfunct. 2006;17:670.

15. Keegan PE, Atiemo K, Cody J, et al. Periurethral injection therapy for urinary incontinence in women. Cochrane Database Syst Rev. 2007;3:CD003881.

16. Kolle D, Tamussino K, Hanzal E, et al. Bleeding complications with the tension-free vaginal tape operation. Am J Obstet Gynecol. 2005;193:2045.

17. Richter HE, Albo ME, Zyczynski HM, et al. Retropubic versus transobturator midurethral slings for stress incontinence. N Engl J Med. 2010;362:2066.

18. Nitti VW. Complications of midurethral slings and their management. Can Urol Assoc J. 2012;6:S120.

19. Lin YH, Lee CK, Chang SD, et al. Focusing on long-term complications of mid-urethral slings among women with stress urinary incontinence as a patient safety improvement measure: a protocol for systematic review and meta-analysis. Medicine (Baltimore). 2021;100:e26257.

20. Morton HC, Hilton P. Urethral injury associated with minimally invasive mid-urethral sling procedures for the treatment of stress urinary incontinence: a case series and systematic literature search. BJOG. 2009;116:1120.

21. Gomes CM, Carvalho FL, Bellucci CHS, et al. Update on complications of synthetic suburethral slings. Int Braz J Urol. 2017;43:822.

22. Sun X, Yang Q, Sun F, et al. Comparison between the retropubic and transobturator approaches in the treatment of female stress urinary incontinence: a systematic review and meta-analysis of effectiveness and complications. Int Braz J Urol. 2015;41:220.

23. Latthe PM, Foon R, Toozs-Hobson P. Transobturator and retropubic tape procedures in stress urinary incontinence: a systematic review and meta-analysis of effectiveness and complications. BJOG. 2007;114:522.

24. Brubaker L, Norton PA, Albo ME, et al. Adverse events over two years after retropubic or transobturator midurethral sling surgery: findings from the trial of midurethral slings (TOMUS) study. Am J Obstet Gynecol. 2011;205:498e1.

25. Fusco F, Abdel-Fattah M, Chapple CR, et al. Updated systematic review and meta-analysis of the comparative data on colposuspensions, pubovaginal slings, and midurethral tapes in the surgical treatment of female stress urinary incontinence. Eur Urol. 2017;72:567.

26. Chai TC, Albo ME, Richter HE, et al. Complications in women undergoing Burch colposuspension versus autologous rectus fascial sling for stress urinary incontinence. J Urol. 2009;181:2192.

27. Kobak WH, Walters MD, Piedmonte MR. Determinants of voiding after three types of incontinence surgery: a multivariable analysis. Obstet Gynecol. 2001;97:86.

28. Wiskind AK, Creighton SM, Stanton SL. The incidence of genital prolapse after the Burch colposuspension. Am J Obstet Gynecol. 1992;167:399.

29. van der Ploeg JM, van der Steen A, Oude Rengerink K, et al. Prolapse surgery with or without stress incontinence surgery for pelvic organ prolapse: a systematic review and meta-analysis of randomised trials. BJOG. 2014;121:537.

30. Handa VL, Harvey L, Cundiff GW, et al. Perioperative complications of surgery for genital prolapse: does concomitant anti-incontinence surgery increase complications? Urology. 2005;65:483.

31. Boysen WR, Adamsky MA, Cohen AJ, et al. Thirty-day morbidity of abdominal sacrocolpopexy is influenced by additional surgical treatment for stress urinary incontinence. Urology. 2017;109:82.

32. Costa P, Poinas G, Ben Naoum K, et al. Long-term results of artificial urinary sphincter for women with type III stress urinary incontinence. Eur Urol. 2013;63:753.

33. Islah M, Cho SY, Son H. The current role of the artificial urinary sphincter in male and female urinary incontinence. World J Mens Health. 2013;31:21.

34. Tricard T, Jochum F, Bergerat S, et al. Outcomes of open artificial urinary sphincter in women with stress

urinary incontinence: long-term follow up. Ther Adv Urol. 2019;11:1756287219874676.

35. Drain A, Enemchukwu E, Shah N, et al. Current role of urethrolysis and partial excision in patients seeking revision of anti-incontinence sling. Female Pelvic Med Reconstr Surg. 2019;25:409.

36. Starkman JS, Scarpero H, Dmochowski RR. Methods and results of urethrolysis. Curr Urol Rep. 2006;7:384.

37. Gurol-Urganci I, Geary RS, Mamza JB, et al. Long-term rate of mesh sling removal following midurethral mesh sling insertion among women with stress urinary incontinence. JAMA. 2018;320:1659.

38. Rac G, Greiman A, Rabley A, et al. Analysis of complications of pelvic mesh excision surgery using the Clavien-Dindo classification system. J Urol. 2017;198:638.

Artificial Urinary Sphincter for Female Stress Urinary Incontinence

23

Amélie Bazinet, Emmanuel Chartier-Kastler, and Stéphanie Gazdovich

Contents

Introduction	408
History and Development of Devices	409
Mechanism of Device Action	410
Evaluation and Diagnosis	411
History	411
Patient-Reported Measures	412
Physical Examination	412
Paraclinical Testing	413
Cystoscopy	413
Urodynamic Studies	413
Imaging	414
Indications for Surgery	415
Indications	415
Contraindications	415
The Place of AUS for Female Non-neurologic Stress Incontinence in the Guidelines	415
Technique of Device Implantation	416
Patient Preparation	416
Material	416

A. Bazinet · S. Gazdovich
Department of Urology, Maisonneuve-Rosemont Hospital,
University of Montreal, QC, Canada
e-mail: amelie.bazinet@umontreal.ca;
stephanie.gazdovich@umontreal.ca

E. Chartier-Kastler (✉)
Department of Urology, Sorbonne Université, Academic
Hospital Pitié-Salpêtrière, Paris, France
e-mail: emmanuel.chartier-kastler@aphp.fr

© Springer Nature Switzerland AG 2023
F. E. Martins et al. (eds.), *Female Genitourinary and Pelvic Floor Reconstruction*,
https://doi.org/10.1007/978-3-031-19598-3_24

Open Transabdominal Implantation	418
Open Transvaginal Implantation	420
Laparoscopic Implantation	421
Robotic-Assisted Implantation	421
Postoperative Care	425
Complications	425
Perioperative Complications	425
Early Postoperative Complications	429
Long-Term Complications	429
Results	430
Evaluation of Persistent or Recurrent Urinary Incontinence After AUS Implantation	432
Future Perspectives	433
Summary	433
Cross-References	434
References	434

Abstract

Stress urinary incontinence (SUI) is a very common condition in women. Indeed, SUI affects nearly 25% of women during their lifetime and has a major impact on the patient's health status, quality of life, and expenses. Treatment options are varied and range from behavioral therapy to surgery. However, when SUI is due to intrinsic sphincter deficiency, several therapeutic options, including surgery, tend to fail, making this affliction difficult to treat. An efficient solution for these women is the implantation of an artificial urinary sphincter (AUS). The high success rate of this procedure outweighs the potential drawbacks. Indeed, the principal complication of AUS is mechanical failure, which occurs on average 10 years after implantation in female patients. The first successful AUS surgery in women dates to 1972, and, since then, the technique and device have greatly improved. Multiple surgical approaches are possible for AUS implantation, the newest being the robotic-assisted laparoscopic implantation. In this chapter, we will review the indications, the preoperative evaluation, the surgical technique, as well as the complications and results of AUS implantation in women with non-neurological SUI.

Keywords

Artificial urinary sphincter · Urinary stress incontinence · Intrinsic urethral deficiency · Female urology

Introduction

Urinary incontinence (UI) is defined as any involuntary leakage of urine [1]. It is a common symptom affecting one in two [2] women over the course of a lifetime. Of these women, it is estimated that nearly half of them will have stress urinary incontinence (SUI) [3]. Results from an American population survey showed that 49.8% of women complained of pure SUI versus 34.4% for mixed UI (MUI) and 15.9% for pure urge UI (UUI) [4]. SUI is defined by the loss of urine during effort, exertion, sneezing, or coughing due to insufficient bladder neck support (increased urethral mobility) and/or because of poor sphincter function: intrinsic sphincter deficiency (ISD) [1].

In younger women, SUI is generally associated with pregnancy and postpartum. Between the ages of 40 and 50, there is a second peak in SUI prevalence. Following menopause, the SUI prevalence decreases, while the prevalence of UUI and MUI increases [4]. In addition to pregnancy, obesity, oral hormonal therapy, pelvic floor dysfunction, family history, smoking, and diabetes are considered risk factors for the development of SUI [2].

Although SUI is not a life-threatening disease, it may genuinely compromise the patient's quality of life (QoL). Nearly 50% of women with SUI suffer from distress resulting in social isolation, loss of self-esteem, sexual dysfunction, anxiety, and depression [5]. Moreover, negative impact on QoL is one of the main reasons why women seek surgical intervention as this treatment may significantly improve their QoL [6].

Beyond the impact of QoL, SUI has a significant cost burden on patients and society. Indeed, Subak et al. reported that severely incontinent women spend, on average, 900 US dollars annually on incontinence supplies and routine care [7]. It was further demonstrated that surgical treatment can lower the societal and individual expense by 72% [7].

Many treatments are available for women with SUI. Initial treatment of female SUI consists of appropriate lifestyle interventions, pelvic floor muscle or bladder training, a scheduled voiding regimen, behavioral therapy, and/or medication [8]. When these first-line measures fail, surgical interventions can be considered, with nearly 20% of women requiring an incontinence correction surgery by the age of 80 [12]. These included urethral bulking agents, synthetic mid-urethral slings such as tension-free vaginal tapes (TVT) and trans-obturator tapes (TOT, TVT-O), non-synthetic bladder neck slings, open or laparoscopic colposuspension, as well as the implantation of an artificial urinary sphincter (AUS) [8].

Since the beginning of the twenty-first century, the use of AUS for SUI in women has escalated in Europe [9], and studies so far show promising outcomes [10, 11]. The AUS is an implantable, fluid-filled, solid silicone elastomer device. In women, it is placed circumferentially around the bladder neck to reproduce normal sphincteric function. To urinate, the patient controls the opening and closure of the artificial sphincter with a manual pump placed in the labium major. The AUS is indicated in severe and refractory SUI when an intrinsic sphincter deficiency is present or following failed anti-incontinence surgeries [12]. In such cases, restoring urethral support alone may be insufficient to ensure optimal continence.

In this chapter, we will thus review the indications, the preoperative evaluation, the surgical technique, as well as the complications and results of AUS implantation for women with non-neurologic SUI.

History and Development of Devices

Since 1880, men have attempted to develop a surgical device to address UI [13]. Wanting to create new strategies for treating urinary incontinence, Brantley Scott started working with the American Medical System (AMS) company. Together, they designed the first modern AUS model and implemented it for the first time in 1972 in a female patient. The first version of AUS, the AMS-721 model (American Medical Systems, Minnetonka, MN), consisted of four elements: a reservoir, an inflatable cuff, an inflatable bulb, and a deflate bulb [13]. Rapidly, the device was abandoned due to high mechanical failure and erosion rates approaching 100% [14].

Over the next decade, many design modifications and adjustments were brought to the AUS model. In 1974, the second generation (AMS-742) was simplified to include a single pump, a pressure balloon, and a compressive cuff. Thus, this was the first AUS model to provide an automatic cuff closure after cuff decompression [14].

In 1979, the connection mechanism was modified, and the original Dacron-reinforced cuff was replaced by a dip-coated silicone rubber cuff, the AMS-791 (bulbar urethra insertion) and the AMS-792 (bladder neck insertion). Though easier to place surgically, the erosion rate was still high. In 1983, a significant development in design led to the introduction of a deactivation button within the control pump (AMS-800). The erosion rate decreased significantly by delaying sphincter activation, thus allowing the urethra to heal without compressive pressure during the first weeks after implantation. In 1987, the cuff was narrowed from 2 to 1.5 cm, which further decreased the rate of atrophy and erosion by improving the pressure transmission from the cuff to the urethral tissue [14].

The AMS-800™ is still the current model used today. It consists of three components: the control pump, the pressure-regulating balloon (PRB), and the cuff (Fig. 1). The control pump consists of two valves, a resistor, and a deactivation button. In women, this pump is commonly placed in the subcutaneous tissue of the major labium on the patient's hand-dominant side. The balloon reservoir comes in multiple sizes that accommodate various degrees of pressure range: 41–50, 51–60, 61–70, 71–80, 81–90, and 91–100 cmH$_2$O. For bladder neck AUS implantation, the most widely used PBR is 61–70 cmH$_2$O. The silicone cuff is available in 12 different sizes ranging from 3.5 to 11-cm-long and is 1.8 cm in width. Those three components are connected with coiled kink-resistant tubing [15].

In 2008, AMS introduced the InhibiZone™ coating, which consists of an antibiotic surface treatment process of the AMS-800™ components. However, this latest modification failed to demonstrate lower infection rates compared to the non-coated version [16].

Mechanism of Device Action

In women, AUS operates by creating a circumferential zone of compression around the bladder neck within a low physiologic pressure range, usually around 60 cm H$_2$O. The degree of mechanical compression can be modulated by the emptying and filling the cuff. When the cuff is filled, generated compression pressure is predetermined by the balloon reservoir compliance. To avoid urethral atrophy secondary to chronic compression and subsequent urethral tissue hypoxia, the surgeon must choose the smallest PRB range that grants effective urethral closure. The 61–70 cm H$_2$O pressure balloon is most widely used in female patients. When the cuff is open, the compressive pressure around the urethra is negligible, allowing the patient to void normally without excessive straining.

The AUS thus reproduces the normal sphincteric function by means of manual activation. When the cuff is in its resting position, the circumferential compression around the bladder neck provides continence. When the patient needs to urinate, she must deflate the urethral cuff manually by squeezing and releasing the bottom half of the control pump several times. Through pumping, the valves in the pump transfer the fluid from the cuff to the balloon reservoir, thus depressurizing the cuff and allowing urine to pass easily through the urethra. The cuff is open for a period of 1–11 min (depending on the cuff and balloon size), after which the fluid returns passively into the cuff until the pressure between the different components is stable, closing the urethra and restoring continence. The resistor in the upper part of the pump slows down the refilling process. The deactivation button is also

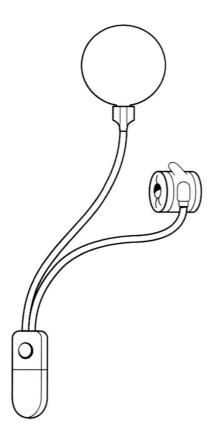

Fig. 1 AMS-800™ model

located in the superior part of the control pump. When activated, this button stops the fluid from being transferred from one component to another. This feature allows the cuff to be set in an open/empty position which is especially useful during the postoperative healing period or when performing intraurethral procedures to decrease complications [15, 17].

Evaluation and Diagnosis

Before considering surgical management, each female patient presenting with SUI requires an initial evaluation. This evaluation mandatorily includes a detailed history, physical examination to confirm SUI, post-void residual (PVR) urine measurement, and urinalysis [18]. Cystoscopy and pressure-flow urodynamic studies are not done routinely in the initial SUI workup. However, these exams are helpful to evaluate complex clinical situations, and since AUS is often indicated for refractory SUI, these tests are usually performed preoperatively.

AUS is primarily indicated in women with intrinsic sphincter deficiency (ISD). These women present with SUI because they cannot seal the urethral lumen entirely due to weak outlet resistance. On the other hand, SUI with urethral hypermobility is due to an underlying lack of urethral support by the surrounding pelvic floor muscles, which can be treated surgically with AUS or slings. Therefore, to adequately diagnose ISD and establish the indication of surgery, one must rely on distinct clinical features and urodynamic criteria [19].

History

A focused medical history should be the first step of every UI evaluation [18]. It provides valuable information helping the clinician confirm and characterize the type and severity of UI, identify potential underlying comorbidities, and measure the impact of UI on QoL to guide appropriate treatment selection. Patients should also provide a detailed medical and surgical history, with an in-depth inquiry into previous UI treatments (Kegel exercise, pelvic floor muscle training) and past history of pelvic surgery, especially prior incontinence or organ prolapse surgery. Furthermore, it is important to assess the patient's obstetric history and menopausal status. Finally, special considerations should be taken to exclude any underlying neurological disease and evaluate if any accompanying symptoms such as pelvic pain, sexual dysfunction, or constipation are present.

Symptom history helps to elucidate the type of UI present. Women reporting a positive clinical history of urine leakage during physical effort (coughing, sneezing, lifting, walking, or running) have roughly 75% chance of suffering from SUI, compared to 15% if the clinical history is negative [20]. It is important to distinguish UUI from SUI, knowing both forms can also coexist. When both UI subtypes are present, it is crucial to evaluate which one is predominant or has the highest impact on QoL as it may guide the treatment offered. Patients with MUI and overactive bladder can undergo AUS implantation after thorough preoperative counselling and only if their overactive bladder symptoms are well managed preoperatively, knowing that these symptoms can persist or even worsen postoperatively [21].

The severity of UI and its impact on the patient's daily activity and QoL must be assessed during a patient interview. Voiding diaries and pad-weighing tests are valuable tools to quantify urine leakage during the day. The degree by which UI alters QoL will weigh in the therapeutic decision-making process, with nonsurgical therapy being strongly considered when there is low QoL bother [18].

Before any AUS implantation surgery, clinicians must evaluate specific requirements, including surrounding tissue quality, patient's cognitive status, and manual dexterity. Patient tissue characteristics can be affected by lack of estrogen associated with menopause, external radiation therapy, local surgery, or previous local infection. Though poor tissue integrity does not constitute an absolute contraindication for AUS placement, the clinician must choose the cuff size accordingly and, if needed, modify postoperative care such as delaying sphincter activation.

The patient must possess the physical and cognitive capacities to use the AUS device correctly to avoid potential complications such as urinary retention, infection, erosion, or failure. Advanced age is not a contraindication to surgery; the AUS can theoretically be implanted at any age. However, a large retrospective cohort showed that men over the age of 80 had a higher risk of AUS erosion and infection [22]. Even if AUS female patients tend to be younger than their male counterparts, mean age of 55 compared to 72, special care must still be taken to evaluate their physical and cognitive function [12, 55].

A wide variety of comorbidities, such as arthritis, diabetes, and neurological disorders, can lead to joint problems or loss of peripheral sensation or motor function and influence the patient's manual dexterity. More so, the patient's inability to physically reach the pump can represent a significant obstacle to AUS placement. In the clinical setting, the handgrip test, consisting of the patient firmly shaking the examiner's hand, can be used as a short and practical screening tool to assess a patient's manual dexterity and coordination [23]. However, this test is purely qualitative, and if the physician suspects a reduced handgrip, a further assessment by a physical or functional therapist may be required [23].

History of dementia, mood disorder, autonomy, and frailty levels are essential to assess [24]. For example, gait speed measurements may predict the risk of future cognitive impairments and can quickly be done in the outpatient clinic setting by observing patients as they enter the examination room [24]. When indicated, the physician may rely on more objective evaluations such as the mini-mental state exam (MMSE), the Montreal Cognitive Assessment test (MoCA) or the clock-drawing test [23].

There is no specific guideline requirement regarding the minimum manual dexterity level and cognitive function needed to support an AUS implantation. Thus, clinicians must rely on their judgment and experiences. However, when dealing with a complex patient, a multidisciplinary team including surgeons, geriatricians, nurses, and therapists may be involved [24].

Patient-Reported Measures

Patient-reported measures can be useful supplements to clarify the presence and severity of UI symptoms. The International Continence Society (ICS) standardized pad weight test offers a means to qualify and quantify UI [39]. For the 1 h pad test, a urine leak of 1–10 g represents mild incontinence, 11–50 g represents moderate incontinence, and >50 g represents severe incontinence [71]. According to the Society of Urodynamics, Female Pelvic Medicine and Urogenital Reconstruction (SUFU) guideline, the 1-or the 48-h pad test can confirm the presence and severity of UI but does not help to distinguish the type of incontinence; thus, it does not alleviate the importance of history and physical examination [18].

Physical Examination

Physical examination should include a focused abdominal assessment, a pelvic exam to evaluate the presence of organ prolapse or vaginal atrophy, as well as a focused neurological exam including anal and pelvic floor muscle tone. Evaluation of urethral mobility and performing a stress test with a comfortably full bladder are also part of the initial evaluation [18].

To evaluate urethral mobility, the patient needs to cough or perform a Valsalva maneuver while in supine or lithotomy position. Traditionally to detect urethral hypermobility, a rigid Q-tips was inserted into the urinary meatus, after which the patient was asked to cough. At the same time, the physician inspected the motion and angle range of the Q-tips. The test was considered positive if the Q-tips moved by more than 30°. Nowadays, simple visual examination is preferred. When performed by experienced clinicians, this noninvasive method strongly correlates with the Q-tip test findings [19]. Nevertheless, clinicians must remember that on its own, such clinical results do not confirm with certainty the diagnosis of

SUI since SUI may exist without hypermobility and hypermobility may be present without SUI [25].

The cough stress test (CST) referred by the ICS involves observing urine loss during coughing or Valsalva maneuver. Though no standardization of the performance of CST exists, the ICS recommends the patient be in a supine or lithotomy position with 200–400 ml of fluid in the bladder filled either naturally or retrogradely [27]. The patient should cough forcefully up to four times. The examiner spreads the labia and directly inspects urine leakage from the meatus. Witnessing involuntary urine loss concurring with increased abdominal pressure is sine qua non to diagnose SUI. If leakage does not occur in the supine position, the test can be repeated while standing, thus increasing the test's sensitivity [28]. Therefore, a positive CST, especially when performed in the supine and standing position, has high sensitivity and specificity for detecting SUI on urodynamics [28].

The Marshall/Bonney test consists of applying fingers on either side of the proximal urethra and elevating it to artificially restore the anterior vaginal wall hammock effect providing support to the urethra and bladder neck. If the patient still leaks during the CST despite urethral support, the test is negative, which might suggest an underlying ISD. The clinical application of such a test is controverted, but some studies support nonetheless its use in predicting surgical outcomes [26].

As such, physical examination aids the clinician in identifying potential individuals that could benefit from AUS implantation, knowing that a positive CST without urethral hypermobility and a negative Marshall/Bonney maneuver is strongly suggestive for ISD [29].

Paraclinical Testing

PVR and urinalysis are included in the diagnostic evaluation of SUI and should be done prior to any surgical correction [8, 18]. Assessment of PVR serves many purposes. First, it can unveil an underlying voiding dysfunction that would cause overflow incontinence. More so, an elevated PVR can indicate bladder hypocontractility, which may influence the postoperative risk of retention after SUI treatment.

The urinalysis is useful to assess the differential diagnosis of UI. If microhematuria is detected, a full workup including cystoscopy and upper tract imaging may be warranted. In the presence of bacteriuria with urinary tract infection (UTI) symptoms, UI should be reevaluated after appropriate treatment [18].

Furthermore, a sterile urinary analysis is desirable before AUS placement.

Cystoscopy

Routine cystoscopy is not recommended for index patients, which, according to SUFU, represents any healthy women, including women with low-grade pelvic organ prolapse, who wish to undertake a surgical treatment for the first time to correct their pure SUI or stress-predominant MUI [18].

However, cystoscopy should be done in whom a bladder pathology is suspected based on clinical history or paraclinical findings such as hematuria. It is also recommended if the patient has a history of prior anti-incontinence or pelvic prolapse surgery. An endoscopic exam allows the clinician to assess the quality of the urethra and rule out mesh erosion or suture perforation and provide a visual evaluation of the degree of residual external sphincter function and closure [18].

Urodynamic Studies

Urodynamic studies (UDS) are often used to determine if SUI is caused by a pathological condition, such as ISD, by measuring maximal urethral closure pressure (MUCP) and Valsalva leak point pressure (VLPP). The urodynamic definition of ISD varies in the literature, but a MUCP of less than 20–35 cm H_2O and a VLPP of less than 60 cm H_2O should raise suspicion for this pathology [1].

In return, ISD diagnosis cannot be made solely with urodynamic testing. Indeed, the ICS subcommittee believes urethral pressure measurement has an unclear clinical utility since it does not discriminate urethral incompetence from other disorders or measure its severity and cannot offer a reliable indicator of surgical success [30]. For instance, decreased urethral pressure is more likely to be caused by urethral hypermobility in younger women compared to tissue fibrosis in older women. Furthermore, the outcome of urodynamic testing can vary between and within tests. Moreover, it is difficult to establish the exact normal limits for VLPP and MUCP since these measures depend on other variables such as a woman's age, physical condition, etc. Indeed, a MUCP less than 30 cm H_2O strongly suggests ISD in a younger woman while it can be physiological in an 80-year-old woman. Most importantly, not every woman with IDS urodynamic suggesting findings is incontinent [31]. Therefore, the evaluation and diagnostic of the ISD must be based on the combination of history, physical exam, cystoscopy, and UDS.

Video urodynamics might add value over standard urodynamic to assess the bladder neck and urethra mobility using fluoroscopic images [19]. The ISD is hence suggested by the presence of severe SUI, a fixed "lead-pipe" urethra on physical examination or less than 20 degree urethra hypermobility, a negative Marshall/Bonney test, or an open bladder neck at cystoscopy or voiding cystourethrogram (VCUG) [32].

UDS also evaluates bladder capacity, contractility, and detrusor overactivity. In cases of SUI associated with decreased bladder contractility, AUS may be a better option since it will not significantly increase the urethral resistance during voiding, contrary to other methods [33]. Detrusor overactivity (DO) is not a contra-indication to AUS, but patients must receive realistic counselling regarding surgical success and the potential need for adjuvant treatments addressing this issue.

Overall, there is no formal recommendation to support mandatory UDS before AUS implantation in the current guidelines. However, urodynamic evaluation is recommended in the non-index SUI patients, including those with previous anti-incontinence or pelvic prolapse surgery [18]. Therefore, most patients undergoing an AUS placement will have completed a UDS beforehand.

Imaging

Different imaging modalities can help identify ISD. However, morphological imaging does not always correlate with the clinical sphincteric function, making it an adjunction test rather than a diagnostic one. The imaging options described in the literature are the retrograde voiding cystourethrography (VCUG), the dynamic and static magnetic resonance (MRI), and the perineal ultrasound.

ISD definition on VCUG is opening of the bladder neck during Valsalva without any urethral mobility on the lateral view, giving the appearance of a funnel or a beak. However, the bladder neck may open secondary to bladder contractions, or it may remain closed even in the presence of ISD, making it neither a sensitive nor a specific study for its diagnosis [34].

MRI can identify sphincter thinning, small urethral length, and urethral support abnormalities. Yet, no urodynamic correlation has been described with these findings. That said, static MRI studies in SUI women detected more puborectalis muscle asymmetry and periurethral ligament distortion than in incontinent women [34].

Trans-perineal sphincter ultrasound has been evaluated in many studies. A loss in sphincter volume, sphincter thickness, and suboptimal vascularity of the urethra on Doppler is suggestive of ISD. Still, no consensus exists regarding normal ultrasound urethral values. Moreover, ultrasound examination offers no prognostic value in terms of surgical success [34].

Therefore, the correlation between imaging and clinical SUI with ISD is modest. Thus, imaging modalities are considered non-discriminant when diagnosing ISD, but they may help comfort history, physical exam, and urodynamic studies.

Indications for Surgery

Indications

The main female candidate for AUS implantation is the patient with bothersome SUI due to ISD. Be that as it may, there are currently no universally accepted characteristics to define this clinical entity. The ISD definition is therefore a combination of clinical and urodynamic criteria: demonstrable SUI on cough or Valsalva stress tests without urethral mobility, negative Marshall/Bonney test, fixed urethra, and low MUCP and VLPP. Thus, the indication for an AUS in females highly depends on the physician's clinical judgment and expertise. Other clinical criteria such as failed previous anti-incontinence procedure, high SUI scores, constant urinary leakage during any daily activity, or urinary leakage with abdominal straining can reinforce the clinical suspicion of ISD [19]. AUS is generally recommended a second-line or last-resort treatment of SUI. Indeed, a recent series demonstrated that up to 87% of women had a prior history of pelvic surgery and 84% had undergone at least one anti-incontinence surgery before being treated with an AUS [35].

Few studies evaluated the role of AUS as a first-line surgical treatment for SUI. However, Costa et al. presented the widest series of first intention AUS implantation for female patients with ISD. There data showed encouraging short- and long-term results with 86% of patients remaining dry and satisfied at 10 years [12]. The fact that other surgical approaches have lower success rates than AUS and that AUS implantation following multiple prior surgery is associated with higher complications rates, such as erosion and infection due to the tissue quality impairment, supports the indication of first intention AUS in severe and isolated ISD [34]. However, we must keep in mind that the mean AUS survival in women is approximately 10 years [29], so when used as a first intention procedure, younger patients must be informed of the non-negligible risk of AUS revision.

Contraindications

AUS implantation is contraindicated in women with urogynecological malformation and mono-symptomatic UUI. Traditionally, a history of pelvic radiotherapy was considered a contraindication to surgical correction of SUI since it the increased the risk of erosion and infection [19]. Relative contraindications are uncontrolled detrusor overactivity or poor bladder compliance, skin infection, and urethral and vaginal pathology [31]. More so, the risk of AUS failure increases with the number of previous pelvic surgery, prior pelvic radiation, and advancing age [36].

Prior to surgery, clinicians should identify patients with poor cognition and manual dexterity since it will compromise AUS safety and consequently its survival.

The InhibiZone™ AUS is also contraindicated in patient reporting allergies to the tetracycline family of antibiotics [15].

The Place of AUS for Female Non-neurologic Stress Incontinence in the Guidelines

Contrary to the male incontinence treatment algorithm, given the lack of evidence-based data, AUS is not yet recognized as a gold-standard surgical treatment of female SUI but is rather considered an optional or a second-line treatment. National records showed that nearly 900 AUS cases were performed in France in 2011, and of those, only 9% were implanted in women [37]. In the United States, a survey reported that only 1% of women with incontinence were treated with an AUS in 2005. Since the AUS in female patients is currently not approved by the US Food and Drug Administration (FDA), the American Urology Association (AUA) guidelines make no mention of it [18].

According to the European Association of Urology guidelines (EAU), AUS should be implanted only as a last-resort procedure and only in expert centers [8]. The National Institute for Health and Care Excellence (NICE) guidelines recommend against AUS as an option to manage female SUI unless another previous surgery has failed [38]. The International Consultation on Incontinence (ICI) of the International Continence Society (ICS) guidelines recommends use of AUS only in highly selected individuals, usually those with recurrent SUI [39]. The Canadian Urology Association (CUA) guideline states that AUS is an option for ISD particularly when previous surgery has failed [40]. All guidelines advocate in favor of an appropriate counselling regarding the high likelihood of surgical revision over time and lack of long-term randomized control trial (RCT) data.

Therefore, most international scientific societies recommend the AUS as an optional or second-line treatment for female SUI (Table 1). However, first intention AUS implantation in carefully selected women had demonstrated favorable long-term outcomes [12].

Technique of Device Implantation

The AUS implantation in female patients is different from implantation in male patients. It is considered a more complex surgical technique, since it requires the AUS cuff to be inserted around the bladder neck, compared to placement around the bulbous urethra. Multiple approaches to AUS implantation are used worldwide, and the method has evolved over time, the newest one being the transabdominal robotic-assisted approach.

Dissecting the bladder neck represents a true surgical challenge. The lack of a natural plane between the anterior vaginal wall and the bladder and its deep pelvic localization make the bladder neck challenging to dissect. The open method was the predominant approach for decades but yielded higher complication outcomes with nearly 45% bladder neck injury, 25% vaginal injury, and high explantation rates of 45% [41]. The first laparoscopic AUS implantation in women was performed in 2005 by Ngninkeu's team, hoping that a minimally invasive approach would be associated with lower complication rates [42]. Laparoscopic implantation showed encouraging outcomes, primarily when an experienced surgeon performs the surgery [41]. More recently, multiple series reported that robotic-assisted AUS implantation in women was safe and feasible and showed reproducible and favorable outcomes [43].

Patient Preparation

Surgery is conducted under general anesthesia with the patient in the lithotomy position. Prophylactic intravenous antibiotics with activity against Gram-negative rods and *Staphylococcus aureus* must be administered within 60 min before skin incision. Best practice recommends an aminoglycoside with a second- or third-generation cephalosporin or vancomycin [44]. First-generation cephalosporin does not offer adequate anaerobic vaginal germ coverage if need be [44].

The operative site is completely shaved in the operating room. The device manufacturer recommends scrubbing the surgical area for 10 min using povidone-iodine soap or the approved hospital preoperative scrub preparation [15]. A single-center randomized controlled trial evaluating the preoperative skin preparation protocols before genitourinary prosthesis implantation showed that chlorhexidine-alcohol scrub, even though superior in terms of skin germs eradication, had similar postoperative prosthesis infection rates compared with povidone-iodine [45]. For bladder neck cuff placement, the patient must be draped for an abdominal incision while maintaining access to the perineum. A Foley catheter is then placed to help identify the urethra and empty the bladder during the procedure.

Overall, strict adherence to sterile techniques is essential to minimize potential infections.

Material

The AMS-800™ AUS model is the gold standard used in men as well as in women. The main three components of the AMS-800™ device are the occlusive cuff, the pressure-regulating balloon and the control pump (Fig. 2). The cuff size will be determined intraoperatively by measuring the circumference of the tissue around the bladder neck.

Table 1 Indication of female AUS in the current international guidelines

Guidelines	Recommendations	Grade of recommendation
American Urology Association (AUA)/ Society of Urodynamic and Female Pelvic Medicine and Urogenital Reconstruction (SUFU)	Not mentioned for women	–
Canadian Urology Association (CUA)	Consider for nonfunctioning urethras secondary to trauma to the pelvic nerves, severe intrinsic sphincter deficiency with multiple prior failed surgical procedures and significant SUI with poor bladder contractility	Level of evidence 3, Grade B
European Association of Urology (EAU)	Complicated SUI as a last option treatment in high-volume centers	Grade 3: weak
French Association of Urology (AFU)	Gold-standard treatment for SUI due to ISD especially with the lack of urethral hypermobility	NR
International Continence Society (ICS)	In highly selected individual, especially those with recurrent SUI	Grade C
National Institute for Health and Care Excellence (NICE)	Only in case of previous failed surgery	NR

SUI stress urinary incontinence, *ISD* intrinsic sphincter deficiency, *NR* not reported

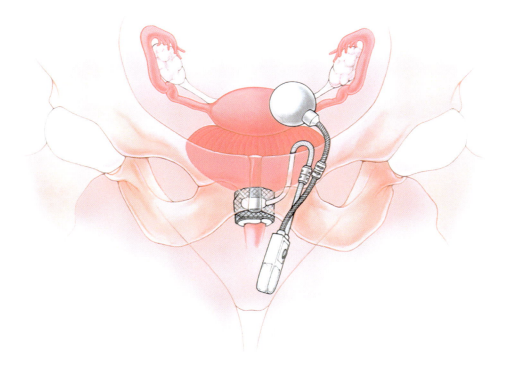

Fig. 2 AUS placement in women

The balloon size partly depends on the size of the cuff chosen, but usually, the surgeon will select the lowest pressure range required to keep the bladder neck closed. The 60–71 cm H_2O balloon is routinely chosen for bladder neck implantation in female patients. The connecting tubes are color-coded to help make the appropriate connections between the control pump and the other components: clear tubing to connect the cuff and black tubing to connect the balloon. The manufacture packaging includes a quick connect assembly kit with either quick or suture-tie connectors.

Every surgeon must be familiar with each component and its preparation. To this effect, the manufacturer provides a detailed, informative manual. The AMS-800™ must be correctly prepared to ensure that any excess of air is drained out of the components and replaced with an isotonic solution. Normal saline is usually recommended to fill the prosthesis. If desired, an isotonic contrast solution can be used instead to facilitate follow-up radiologically. Contrast solutions are contraindicated if the patient reports a history of adverse reactions to iodine or contrast products.

Once correctly filled, the components are submerged in a storage basin filled with the filling solution until implantation. Nevertheless, caution should be taken not to submerge in saline InhibiZone-treated component to prevent the antibiotic coating from diffusing into the solution, turning it orange, and, thus, diluting the antibiotic concentration on the device.

For the complete AMS-800™ preparation, please refer to the device manual instruction [15].

Open Transabdominal Implantation

The open abdominal technique was the traditional approach used in female patients when the intended site for AUS implantation was at the bladder neck [46]. However, it has since given way to minimally invasive techniques.

By using a suprapubic approach, either through a low transverse abdominal midline incision or a Pfannenstiel incision, the surgeon can access the pelvis without breaching the peritoneum. The bladder is swiped from the abdominal wall medially to allow the bladder to drop down inferiorly and expose the space of Reitzius, which is dissected until the endopelvic fascia is visualized on both sides of the bladder neck.

A finger or povidone-iodine-soaked spongestick is placed in the vaginal cul-de-sac pushing upward and laterally to put tension on the vaginal wall and facilitate identification of the vesicovaginal plane. Once the vesicovaginal plane has been found, the surgeon dissects the posterior aspect of the bladder neck with scissors using his finger as a guide. This dissection is completed precociously to avoid inadvertently entering the bladder or vagina. The same maneuver is done on the contralateral side, and the two dissected planes are joined together. Such a dissection can be complicated in patients who had previous pelvic surgery (Figs. 3 and 4), in which case, it might be necessary to perform an anterior cystostomy away from the bladder neck to facilitate the dissection [46]. If a tear is detected in the bladder or vaginal wall, it must be closed in two layers, using absorbable sutures. The circumferential dissection around the bladder neck should be at least 2 cm in width to ensure the cuff placement is not restricted.

The Foley catheter should be removed before measuring the circumference of the bladder neck using the provided calibrated measuring tape to determine the cuff size (Fig. 5). This step is crucial as an oversized cuff might not compress the bladder neck enough during the filing phase leading to urine leakage, and an undersized cuff might be associated with an increased risk of retention and erosion. Usually, the bladder neck in women measures 6–8 cm. The cuff is passed and secured around the bladder neck, with the tubing exiting laterally on the side of the future pump (Fig. 6). The tubing is passed through the rectus muscle and anterior fascia via an inguinal incision performed near the internal inguinal ring.

A pressure-regulating balloon of 61–70 cmH_2O is routinely placed in the prevesical space ipsilateral to the location of the pump. The tubing is exteriorized in the same manner next to the cuff tubing. The balloon is filled with 22 ml of

Fig. 3 The dissection plan between the bladder neck and the vagina

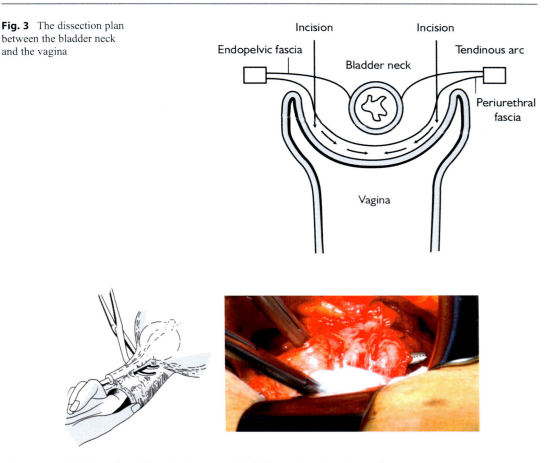

Fig. 4 (**a** and **b**) Dissection of the plane between the bladder neck and anterior vagina

filling solution, and to avoid fluid loss, the balloon tubing is clamped with a single click using silicone-shod Hemostat clamps [15].

The pump is placed in a subcutaneous pouch created with a Hegar dilator in the labium majus on the patient's dominant side. The pump is installed in the dependent portion of the pocket, with the deactivation button facing outward to be easily accessed.

The surgeon connects the black tubing (balloon to pump) and the clear tubing (cuff to pump) using the different connectors. Afterward, the tubing can be fixed to the external oblique aponeuroses to lower the risk of skin erosion. The skin incision is closed. A 14 Fr Foley catheter is inserted in the urethra and left in place for 3–5 days. At the end of the procedure, the device is cycled and inactivated. The cuff is set in the open/empty position for the remaining postoperative period.

Pressurization of the cuff may be necessary for wider cuffs since they may require more fluid to be fully occlusive or functional. To do so, the surgeon makes a temporary connection between the balloon and cuff after having filled the balloon with 22 ml of filling solution. A 1 min waiting time allows the fluid pressure to equilibrate. The balloon is then disconnected from the cuff, and the remaining solution is emptied. The surgeon refills the balloon with 20–21 ml and makes the final connections [15].

The retropubic approach is technically more challenging in obese patients due to difficult deep pelvis access rendering poor visibility and making it difficult to dissect the bladder neck and position the cuff, increasing the possibility of

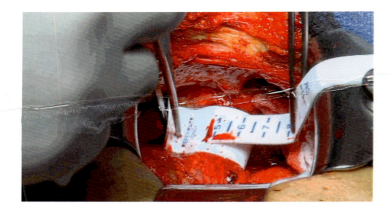

Fig. 5 Measurer tape around the bladder neck. The cuff must be tight enough to compress the urethra during filling, but not too much to avoid the risk of retention and erosion

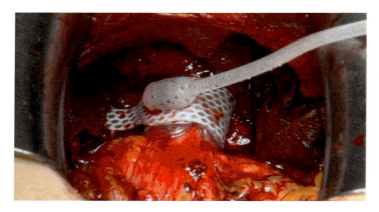

Fig. 6 Cuff position around the bladder neck

vaginal or urinary tract trauma. The open approach is associated with elevated rates of vaginal (25%) and bladder neck injury (46%) and device explantation (45%) [41].

Open Transvaginal Implantation

Appell described in 1998 a technique in which the bladder neck is accessed through a vaginal incision [72]. This technique mimics the combined perineal and abdominal approach done in male patients whereby the vaginal incision allows the surgeon to insert the cuff around the bladder neck and the abdominal incision permits placement of the balloon reservoir.

The patient is placed in a dorsal lithotomy position. The skin preparation includes the lower third of the abdomen and the perineum with a specific iodophor preparation for the vagina. Draping is done to expose the abdomen and vagina. To maximize visualization of the anterior vaginal wall, the labia minora should be retracted laterally with temporary sutures, and a weighted vaginal speculum should be used. To help identify an important anatomical landmark, the surgeon can gently pull on the Foley catheter and palpate the balloon to determine the bladder neck [46]. Using a semicircular incision, a flap of vaginal mucosa is created. The apex of the incision is midway between the urethra meatus and the bladder neck. The anterior vaginal wall is dissected free from the urethra toward the bladder neck. Keeping a good flap thickness will prevent future material erosion. If desired, the dissection can be facilitated by injecting normal saline solution for hydrodissection.

The retropubic space is entered on each side of the bladder neck by perforating the endopelvic fascia using scissors while pointing them toward the ipsilateral shoulder. The surgeon bluntly dissects the bladder neck off the pubic bone with a fingertip. Once the Foley catheter is removed, the calibrated measuring tape is applied around the bladder neck to determine the cuff size. The cuff is inserted and snapped into place with the tubing exiting laterally on the side of the future pump and reservoir placement. A cystoscopy can be done to confirm the sphincter's good position and verify that the ureteral orifices are not compromised by the cuff [46].

Once the cuff is in place, an abdominal incision is made laterally in the lower quadrant to allow the balloon and pump insertion. The external and transverse fasciae are open near the external inguinal ring to allow the insertion of the balloon in the prevesical space. The balloon is filled with 22 ml of filling solution, and the extremities of the tubing are clamped. The cuff tubing is transferred from the vaginal incision into the abdominal incision by passing along the posterior aspect of the pubic bone up until reaching the rectus muscle.

After which, the remaining procedure is done in the same fashion. The pump is placed in a subcutaneous pocket in the labia majora, and the connections are made. Pressurization of the cuff can be done at this moment if wanted (see abdominal approach for more details). The abdominal and vaginal incisions are closed, and the vagina is packed for a couple of hours. The system is cycled and then deactivated as per usual. The Foley catheter is removed after 3–5 days [46].

This technique requires a longer surgical time and is more prone to complications than the abdominal approach. Due to the increased risk of infection and erosion, the vaginal route is no longer recommended and has largely been abandoned [47].

Laparoscopic Implantation

The patient is positioned in dorsal lithotomy with 30 degrees of Trendelenburg. Arms are placed along the body, and a catheter is inserted into the bladder. A $0°$ laparoscopic camera is inserted through a 10 mm trocar at the level of the umbilicus. A second 10 mm trocar is positioned midway between the umbilicus and the pubic symphysis, and two 5 mm trocars are placed

medial and cranial to the anterior superior iliac spines (Fig. 7).

The parietal peritoneum of the abdominal cavity is incised to access the retropubic space leading to the bladder neck. The urethral catheter balloon can aid the surgeon in identifying the bladder neck during this step. The pelvic fascia is incised bilaterally, and the urethra is dissected from the vaginal wall. The assistant can move the index finger inserted in the vagina to facilitate the dissection. The lack of blood in the vaginal cavity confirms the absence of vaginal injury. More so, urethral integrity is confirmed if no leakage occurs during bladder filling [35].

A lateral low abdominal wall incision is made through the external oblique fascia. This incision will be used to assemble the AUS connections. The cuff is positioned circumferentially around the urethra while the balloon reservoir is inserted in the Retzius space. Both connecting tubes are exteriorized through the lateral incision. The trocars are removed once the abdomen has been deflated. A pocket in the labium majus is created to allocate the AUS control pump. If needed, the cuff pressurization can be done. The AUS components are connected, and the tubing is fixed to the aponeurosis. The AUS is cycled and deactivated. The abdominal incisions are closed, and a 14 Fr catheter is left in place [35].

The first laparoscopic AUS implantation in women was reported in the late 2000s [42]. This approach improved visualization and dissection of pelvic structures compared to the open retropubic approach. The magnified vision and high definition of laparoscopy allow for an accurate urethrovaginal dissection minimizing urinary tract or genital injury. Long-term results are satisfactory with low postoperative complication rates, mostly Clavien-Dindo grade I complications [35].

Robotic-Assisted Implantation

The patient is placed in a dorsal lithotomy position with exaggerated Trendelenburg. The patient's abdomen, perineum, and vagina are adequately scrubbed and draped. A sterile catheter is inserted into the bladder.

Fig. 7 Laparoscopic trocar insertion

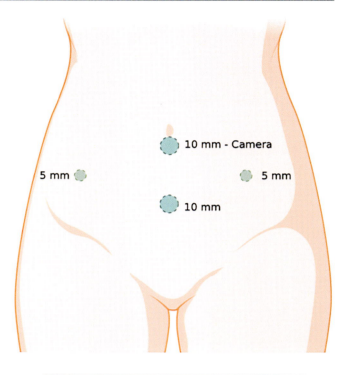

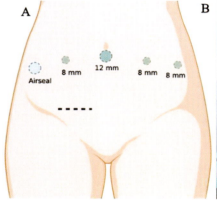
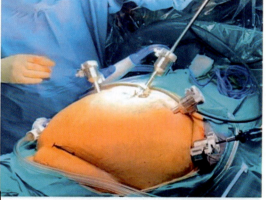

Fig. 8 (**a** and **b**) Robotic-assisted trocar position

Five ports are positioned: a 12 mm camera port at the umbilicus, three 8 mm robotic ports, and an AirSeal® 12 mm assistant port on the left side. Ideally, a minimum of 7 cm between each port is respected (Fig. 8).

The vesicovaginal plane is dissected with the bladder still fully attached to the abdominal wall. Inserting a malleable retractor anteriorly into the vagina helps identify the plane between the bladder and the anterior vaginal wall. The retractor is pushed down and toward the head of the patient. Dissection is initiated with cold scissors and pursued bluntly until the bladder neck is reached to minimize the risk of adjacent organ injury. Once the plane has sufficiently been developed, dissection is pursued on each side of the bladder neck using the Prograsp forceps. The blades are opened tangential to the plane while

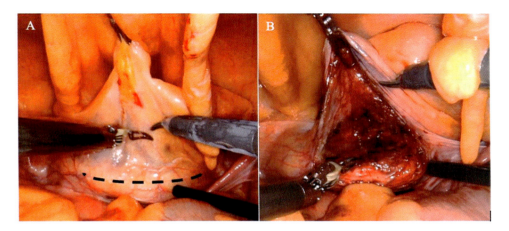

Fig. 9 Dissection of the vesicovaginal plane. (**a**) Malleable retractor reflection, (**b**) the dissected plane between the bladder and the anterior vagina

"sliding" on the vaginal wall to separate the bladder neck from the vaginal wall. The assistant must ensure with his finger that the vaginal wall is intact and fill the bladder with normal saline or methylene blue to verify the integrity of the bladder neck (Fig. 9).

The anterior bladder wall is dissected from the abdominal wall, but the bladder remains partially suspended by leaving the urachus attachment intact. The Retzius space is dissected until the bladder neck and endopelvic fascia are reached. When dissecting laterally, the surgeon must be particularly cautious not to penetrate the anterior vaginal wall or the lateral bladder wall.

Once the bladder neck is thoroughly dissected, the measuring tape is inserted in the abdomen via the AirSeal® trocar. A suture can be placed beforehand on one of its extremities to facilitate tape handling intra-abdominally. The Prograsp forceps is passed behind the bladder neck, and the tape is grabbed on the right-side lateral. The forceps are retracted to drag the tape posteriorly. The tape is then brought anteriorly to encircle the bladder neck and measure its circumference to determine the size of the AUS cuff (Fig. 10). Once the cuff is prepared with an occlusive cork placed on the tubing extremity, it is inserted via the AirSeal® access port. The free extremity of the cuff is sutured to the posterior end of the measuring tape. This will serve as a traction mechanism to facilitate the passage of the cuff around the bladder neck. The cuff is then snapped in place, and the measurer is removed from the abdomen. The device must be manipulated cautiously to avoid any damage (Fig. 11).

A separate inguinal incision is done on the lateral side where the future pump will be placed. The incision is carried to the external oblique fascia. A Zenker clamp is used to perforate the aponeurosis near the pubic bone next to the paravesical space. The cuff's tubing is grabbed with the Zenker and exteriorized from the pelvis. Two rubber clamps are placed on the extremity of the tubing to discard the occlusive cork.

After placing an occlusion cork on the tubing extremity, the 60–71 cmH$_2$O pressure balloon is inserted by the AirSeal® port and positioned in the paravesical space. In the same manner, the balloon tubing is exteriorized through the inguinal incision. The balloon can then be filled with 22 ml of isotonic filling solution. If cuff pressurization is required, it must be done ideally after deflating the pneumoperitoneum.

Once proper hemostasis is confirmed, barbed sutures are used to close the peritoneum on either side of the bladder. Special care must be taken during this step to avoid perforating the balloon or tubing with the needle. The pneumoperitoneum is evacuated before removing trocars. Via the inguinal incision, the subcutaneous pocket in the

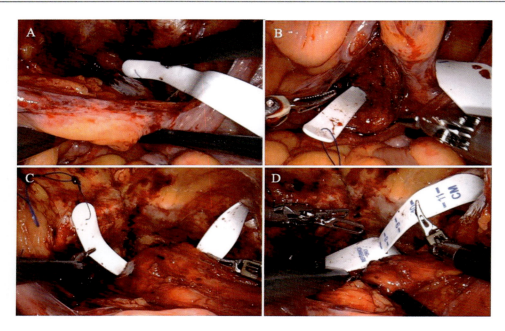

Fig. 10 Measuring tape placement. (**a**) The Prograsp forceps is passed behind the bladder neck, and the tape is grabbed on the right-side lateral (**b**). The forceps are retracted to drag the tape posteriorly (**c**). The tape is then brought anteriorly to encircle the bladder neck and measure its circumference to determine the size of the AUS cuff (**d**)

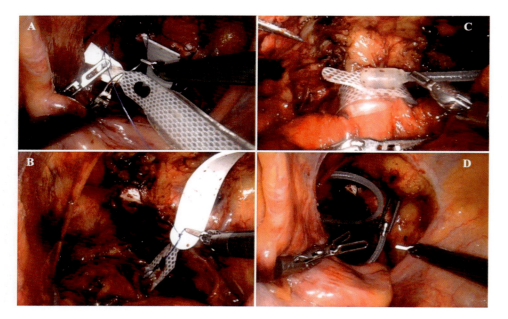

Fig. 11 Placement of the bladder cuff. The free extremity of the cuff is sutured to the posterior end of the measuring tape (**a**). This will serve as a traction mechanism to facilitate the passage of the cuff around the bladder neck (**b**). The cuff is then snapped in place (**c**). The cuff's tubing is grabbed with the Zenker and exteriorized from the pelvis (**d**)

labium majus is created and the pump placed. After the connections are made, the tubing is fixed to the external oblique fascia, and skin incisions are closed. The AUS is cycled and locked in the open/empty cuff position. A 14 Fr catheter is left in place [43].

The main advantages of robotic-assisted surgery include greater movement precision with robotic arms, high-definition 3D visualization, and the endowrist instrumentation technology facilitating suturing, particularly in the narrow pelvis space [43]. Compared to open AUS implantation, the robotic-assisted approach has lower perioperative morbidity, including decreased blood loss and length of stay, and similar functional outcomes [48].

Postoperative Care

The catheter is left in place for a short period since patients have an increased risk of postoperative urinary retention. Indeed, postoperative tissue edema resulting from the dissection can lead to temporary acute urinary retention in the days following surgery. In our center, the catheter is usually removed on postoperative day 5 with a bladder ultrasound confirming adequate voiding. However, if the patient was already on intermittent self-catheterization (ISC) prior to the surgery, the catheter can be removed sooner, and the patient can resume her ISC.

Postoperative prophylactic antibiotics are not generally recommended since they fail to prevent postoperative material infection [43].

Patients should be advised to limit physical activity until 6 weeks postoperative.

To limit erosion risk, activation of the AUS is performed four to 6 weeks after implantation in an outpatient setting. After an AUS replacement or revision, the timing of activation may be adjusted based on the clinical situation and patient comfort. After catheter removal, the patient must void to ensure adequate bladder emptying. It is also advisable to review the AUS functioning with the patients and observe how they manipulate the pump the first time around. A patient's

information booklet from the manufacturing company should also be given to the patient.

Patients must be informed to forewarn healthcare professionals in the event of catheterization. In addition, they should avoid perineal pressure and be instructed to wear a *MedicAlert or similar type* bracelet [47].

The patient is usually followed at 3 and 6 months and then once a year. The follow-up visits include a clinical interview, physical examination, uroflowmetry, and PVR. Proper use of the device is also verified at each visit. Radiography of the artificial sphincter in the open and closed position can be prescribed if AUS malfunction is suspected [43].

Complications

Perioperative Complications

The two most severe complications relating to the AUS surgery in women are bladder neck and vaginal wall injuries. In the literature, the mean range of bladder or vaginal injury is 11% (0–46) [11]. However, several series demonstrated that the perioperative outcomes differ depending on which surgical technique is used for implanting an AUS. The rate of intraoperative bladder neck injury ranges from 5.8% to 43.8% in the open group, vs. 0% to 40% in the laparoscopic group, vs. 0% to 22.2% in robotic group (Tables 2, 3, and 4). The rate of intraoperative vaginal injury ranges from 0% to 25%, 0% to 20%, and 0% to 25% in the open, laparoscopic, and robotic-assisted group, respectively (Tables 2, 3, and 4). More so, retrospective analysis showed a trend toward lower intraoperative complication rates (37.5 vs. 62.5%; $p = 0.25$) and decreased blood loss (17 vs. 275 ml; $p = 0.22$) in the robotic-assisted group compared with the open group [48].

Early recognition of vaginal or bladder injury is important to prevent early AUS infection and erosion and therefore AUS explantation. In one of the widest AUS cohort series, intraoperative injuries were not strongly associated with lower device survival, probably because of their

Table 2 Open AUS implantation outcomes studies

Study	Study type	Number of patients (n)	Mean age	Previous incontinence surgery (%)	Mean cuff size (cm)	Preoperative bladder neck injury (%)	Pre-operative vaginal injury (%)	Mean operative time (min)	Mean bladder cathe-terization duration (days)	Length of stay (days)	Postoperative complication (%)/C-D ≥3 (%)	Mean follow-up (months)	Explantation rate (%)	Revision rate (%)	Continence rate = 0 pad (%)
Thomas et al. (2002) [57]	Retrospective, single center	68	51	81	NR	46		NR	NR	NR	NR	144	45.6	17.6	81
Chung et al. (2010) [53]	Retrospective, single center	47	51	74.4	NR	NR	NR	141	NR	NR	4.2/0	162	17	42.6	59
Vayleux et al. (2011) [36]	Retrospective, single center	240	62.8	88.8	7	10.7		NR	NR	NR	24.7/–	72	7	15.3	65
Costa et al. (2013) [12]	Retrospective, single center	344	57.2	69.1	NR	5.8	4.7	NR	NR	NR	NR/4.9	115	NR	14	94
Peyronnet et al. (2016) [48]	Retrospective single center (comparison robot vs. open, open arm)	16	69.1	93.8	7.3	43.8	25	214	NR	9.3	75/25	28.1	18.8	12.5	68.8
Tricard et al. (2019) [54]	Retrospective, single center	63	58	17.5	NR	6.3	4.8	NR	NR	9	31.7/3.2	168	31.7	46	74.5

C-D Clavien-Dindo, UTI urinary tract infection, NR not reported

Table 3 Laparoscopic AUS implantation outcomes studies

Study	Study type	Number of patients (n)	Mean age	Previous incontinence surgery (%)	Mean cuff size (cm)	Preoperative bladder neck injury (%)	Preoperative vaginal injury (%)	Mean operative time (min)	Mean bladder catheterization duration (days)	Length of stay (days)	Postoperative complication (%)/C-D ≥3 (%)	Mean follow-up (months)	Explantation rate (%)	Revision rate (%)	Continence rate = 0 pad (%)
Ngninkeu et al. (2005) [42]	Retrospective, single center	4	68.5	75	NR	0	0	NR	7	8	0/0	6	0	25	75
Rouprêt et al. (2009) [58]	Retrospective, single center	12	56.7	83.3	6.5	16.7 (all converted to open procedure)	16.7 (all converted to open procedure)	181	10	7	45/0	12.1	0	0	83.3
Mandron et al. (2010) [59]	Retrospective, single center	25	66.8	100	6.5	0	4	92	NR	4	44/8	26.1	8	0	76
Trolliet et al. (2013) [60]	Retrospective, single center	25 18 initial placements 8 revisions	64	88	6	20 (3 converted to open procedure)	0	149 160 120	3	5	44/12	20	4	20	64
Peyronnet et al. (2016) [48]	Retrospective single center (comparison robot vs. open, laparoscopic arm)	5	NR	NR	NR	40	20	242	NR	6.8	60/40	NR	40	NR	60
Ferreira et al. (2017) [61]	Retrospective, single center	49	69.1	79.6	6.5	0	12	128	NR	2	18.4/4.1	37.5	22.4	14.3	77.6
Bracchitta et al. (2019) [35]	Retrospective, single center	74	66.9	83.8	6.5	1.4	1.4	120	NR	2.7	20.3/8.1	44.5	21.6	13.5	78.3

AUS artificial + urinary sphincter, *C-D* Clavien-Dindo, *UTI* urinary tract infection, *NR* not reported

Table 4 Robotic-assisted AUS implantation outcomes studies

Study	Study type	Number of patients (n)	Mean age	Previous incontinence surgery (%)	Cuff size (cm)	Preoperative bladder neck injury (%)	Preoperative vaginal injury (%)	Mean operative time (min)	Mean bladder catheterization duration (days)	Length of stay (days)	Postoperative complication (%)/C-D ≥3 (%)	Mean follow-up (months)	Explantation rate (%)	Revision rate (%)	Continence rate = 0 pad (%)
Fournier G et al. (2014) [52]	Retrospective, single center	6	65	83	8	0	0	210	7	6	16.7/0	14.3	0	0	83.3
Biardeau et al. (2015) [47]	Retrospective, single center	11	66	100	6.5	18.2	18.2	142	3	4	45/9	17.6	27.3	0	87.5
		9 initial placements			6.5	22.2	22.2		4	5			22		
		2 revisions			6	0	0		2	3.5			50		
Peyronnet et al. (2016) [48]	Retrospective single center (comparison robot vs. open, robotic arm)	8	64	88	7	12.5	25	211	–	3.5	25/12.5	5	12.5	0	75
Peyronnet et al. (2019) [43]	Retrospective, five institutions	49	70.5	85.7	7	10.2	6.1	180	7–10	4	18.3/4.1	18.5	2	6.1	81.6
Kourban-houssen et al. (2019) [62]	Retrospective, single center	19	67.9	NR	6	20	0	NR	3	4.1	21.1/15.6	22	0	16	85
		10 initial placements	66.4		6.5	40 (2 had laparotomy conversion)								10	70
		9 revisions	68.5		5.5	0								22	100
Gondran-Tellier et al. (2019) [63]	Retrospective, single center	8	64	62.5	8	0	0	244	NR	NR	37.5/0	12	0	0	67.5
Peyronnet et a. (2020) [64]	Retrospective, 14 centers	123	68	87	7.5	9.8	6.5	170	NR	3.5	18/3.3	13	4.1	5.5	80.5
Chartier-Kastler et al. (2020) [65]	Prospective, single center	27 initial placements	68	73	7.5	11	18.5	130	NR	7	44/0	19	0	11	84

C-D Clavien-Dindo, *UTI* urinary tract infection, *NR* not reported

perioperative recognition and repair [12]. The best way to detect vaginal defects is for the surgeon or the assistant to insert a finger into the patient's vagina once the bladder neck dissection is completed. If blood is detected on the glove after this maneuver or if the surgical glove is visible on the video screen, the surgeon must suspect an underlying vaginal injury. Once located, the injury is closed in two layers, using absorbable sutures. To rule out a bladder neck injury, the bladder is filled with normal saline or methylene blue. If a leak is detected, the defect is closed in two layers, using absorbable sutures.

Bladder neck and vaginal injuries are relative contraindications to AUS implantation unless the surgical team can address them properly intraoperatively.

Early Postoperative Complications

Early postoperative complications include acute urinary retention, labial hematoma, hematuria, urinary tract infection, wound infection or dehiscence, early device infection and herniation, and deep venous thrombosis. The rates of postoperative complications vary widely, ranging from 16.7% to 45% in robotic series, 0% to 60% in laparoscopic series, and 4.1% to 75% in open series (Tables 2, 3, and 4). Most of them are Clavien-Dindo complications grade <3. Clavien-Dindo complications grade ≥ 3 occur in 0–25% of open procedures, 0–40% of laparoscopic procedures, and 0–15.6% of robotic procedures (Tables 2, 3, and 4). Once more, a trend in fewer postoperative complications is seen in the robotic-assisted group compared to the open one (75% vs. 25%, $p = 0.02$) [48].

Urinary retention in the postoperative period should be managed by inserting a small transurethral catheter (10-Fr or 12-Fr). The surgeon should confirm the cuff is deactivated before catheterization. If the patient fails to void after 1 week, ISC should be initiated. When patients are unable to self-catheterize, a suprapubic cystostomy drainage is preferable to indwelling urethral catheter to reduce the risk of erosion. To avoid puncturing the device, such a procedure is best done under ultrasound or fluoroscopic guidance. Prolonged retention beyond several weeks may require a reoperation to undersize the cuff. Choosing the best course of action in such instances depends largely on preoperative urodynamic findings.

Long-Term Complications

Long-term complications include prosthetic infection, mechanical failure, urethral or vaginal erosion, and development of DO. Recurring UI, hematuria, de novo dysuria, retention, or recurrent UTI warrants subsequent investigation to rule out any of these complications. In a meta-analysis, the mean time before device implantation and first complication was 42.1 months [11].

Late onset of urinary retention may result from urethral stenosis, erosion, or detrusor hypocontractility; thus an endoscopic evaluation and UDS are necessary.

Infection is a serious complication of AUS implantation surgery. Infection should be suspected in the occurrence of perineal pain, erythema, or edema of the labium majus, with or without the presence of fever or purulent discharge. Moreover, in case of urethral, vaginal, or cutaneous erosion, the surgeon should presume the underlying device is infected. The infection with initial AUS surgery varies between 2% and 26% in women [10]. Many postulated the introduction of the InhibiZone surface treatment combining rifampin and minocycline to the AUS cuff and pump would lead to a reduction in postoperative infection rates. Unfortunately, the InhibiZone failed to demonstrate a superiority in this matter over the non-coated version [16, 47]. Infected or eroded AUS cannot be treated solely with antibiotic therapy and require total device explantation [50]. In men, studies of immediate salvage of the infected non-eroded AUS had demonstrated feasibility. This procedure consists of completely removing the infected device, performing extensive antiseptic irrigation, and immediately reimplanting a new prosthetic [50]. In a retrospective study, Bryan et al. salvaged seven of eight infected non-eroded AUS with an overall success rate of 87%. Contraindications to prosthesis salvage include sepsis, ketoacidosis, necrotizing infection, device erosion, immunosuppression, and the finding of gross purulent material at the time of explantation [50].

Delayed activation of the sphincter has greatly decreased the rate of urethral erosion [17]. Previous radiotherapy is now the principal risk factor for AUS erosion in the female population [36]. Overall, AUS erosion in females ranges between 0.5% and 27% [10]. In case of erosion, the entirety of the AUS is considered infected, and complete device removal is recommended [49].

After AUS removal, reimplantation should be delayed 3–6 months to allow sufficient time for the urethral tissue to heal properly. Before reimplantation, a cystoscopy must be done to assess the patency and quality of the urethra and bladder neck [49]. To decrease the risk of secondary erosion after reimplantation, certain authors recommend nightly deactivation of the AUS [51].

Results

Open AUS implantation for SUI was first reported by Scott et al. in 1973. Subsequently, Ngninkeu et al. introduced the laparoscopic AUS implantation in 2005 with a satisfactory continence rate (75%) and a very low-operative complications rate [42]. In 2014, Fournier et al. presented promising result with robotic-assisted AUS implantation in SUI women. Indeed, they yield a complete continence of 83.3% and had a Clavien-Dindo ≥ 3 complication rate of 0% [52].

AUS implantation in SUI women has since been reported in many retrospective cohort studies. However, no RCT compares AUS efficiency and safety to other SUI surgical treatments (Burch, aponeurosis sling, etc.). This total absence of comparative data in the literature makes it impossible to draw robust conclusions as to where AUS might be placed in the surgical armamentarium for recurrent or persistent SUI in female patients and to build an evidenced-based therapeutic algorithm in this specific population [10].

Moreover, no RCT compares the open vs. the laparoscopic vs. the robotic AUS implantation.

One retrospective study did; however, compare the open vs. robotic approach. Mean operative time was similar in both groups (214 vs. 211 min; $p = 0.90$). Postoperative complication rate was significantly lower in the robotic-assisted group (25% vs. 75%; $p = 0.02$). There was a trend toward a lower intraoperative complication rate (37.5% vs. 62.5%; $p = 0.25$), decreased blood loss (17 vs. 275 ml; $p = 0.22$), and shorter length of stay (3.5 vs. 9.3 days; $p = 0.09$) in the robotic-assisted group. Continence rates were comparable in both groups (75% vs. 68.8%; $p = 0.75$). Three AUS explantations were required in the open approach group (18.8%) and one in the robotic-assisted group (12.5%; $p = 0.70$) [48].

Tables 2, 3, and 4 presented studies on AUS implantation in women suffering from SUI. None of those studies is RCT nor prospective. Only two studies were multicenter [43, 64] and assessed the robotic-assisted approach. Only one study retrospectively compared the open vs. robotic approach [48]. The mean age varied between 49 and 71 years. Most of the women (63–100%) had at least one previous SUI surgery. The mean bladder cuff size varied between 6 and 8 cm.

The trial with the larger cohort as well as the longer follow-up is the one evaluating the open approach, probably because it was the standard of care for many years. The mean follow-up time varied between 28 and 168 months (14 years). The continence rate defined as use of 0 pads varied between 59% and 94%. The revision and explantation rate varied across the studies with the highest rate reported with longer follow-up. The studies on laparoscopic implantation reported a 0-pad rate ranging between 64% and 83%. The mean follow-up varied between 6 and 45 months. The revision and explantation rate seem lower than in the open approach, but it is probably accountable to the shorter follow-up. The robotic-assisted approach was evaluated in seven retrospective studies. The continence rate varies between 68% and 88%, and the mean follow-up time varies between 5 and 22 months. Once more, shorter follow-up may be responsible for the low rate of explantation and revision (0–27%). Comparing performance and safety outcomes between the different approaches at this point would thus be premature. Indeed, the total number of patients operated varies between the surgical approach, the mean follow-up is significantly lower in the laparoscopic and robotic approach, the surgical techniques were not standardized, and the surgeon learning curve evolved since the earliest cohorts. All those variables may have caused results heterogeneity in the same AUS implantation approach and thus make it impossible to adequately compare the three different implantation approaches.

According to a meta-analysis, the complete continence rate after AUS implantation, defined as 0-pad use, varied between 80% [11] and 83% [10], all approaches included. The one-pad rate outcome was not reported in all studies but ranged between 7% and 17%. The outcome of 0–1-pad rate ranged between 58% and 100% [10]. As stated earlier, the revision rate varies across study, with higher revision rates with longer follow-up. The mean time before the first revision secondary to device failure varies between studies; it was 88 months for Chung et al. [53], 105.2 months for Vayleux et al., 176 months for Costa et al., and 108 months for Tricard et al. [54]. According to a meta-analysis, the mean time before revision was 11.2 years, and at 3, 5, and 10 years, 92.0%, 88.6%, and 69.2% of devices, respectively, were still in place [10]. Two risk factors that affected device survival after multivariate analyses were identified: the number of previous surgeries for UI and the cause of UI. The number of incontinence surgeries before the implantation reduced the longevity of the device; a statistically significant difference was found comparing the population with one or no previous surgery for UI against the population with two or more procedures ($p = 0.04$). Survival of the device in patients with a non-neurogenic bladder was significantly longer than in patients with neurogenic bladder ($p < 0.001$) [12].

Explantation rates varied between 2% and 31% across studies. The reasons were mostly infection (2–26%) and erosion (1–27%) [10]. On multivariate analysis, predisposing factors for AUS explantation were a history of pelvic radiotherapy (OR: 6; 95% CI, 1.13–31.9)

and a concomitant surgical procedure during AUS implantation ($p < 0.055$; OR: 4.59; 95% CI, 0.96–21.9), including sacral colpopexy or bladder augmentation surgery. Likewise, radiotherapy (OR: 26; 95% CI, 4.45–161) was associated with an increased risk of erosion [36].

The main causes of continence failure after AUS implantation are poor dexterity of the sphincter pump (27.5%), permanent explantation (23.5%), and de novo detrusor overactivity (21.6%). Lack of dexterity may result in poor bladder emptying with high PVR, frequent urinary tract infections, UI, and obstruction leading to detrusor overactivity. Patients older than 70 years and those with poor dexterity with the AUS were significantly associated with device failure ($p < 0.004$). De novo detrusor overactivity was observed in 22% of the patient following AUS implantation. Up to 15% of the failures were related to persistent UUI in patients with MUI before AUS [36].

The AUS survival in women is longer than the device longevity observed in men. Petero et al. did a comparison of the long-term outcomes between incontinent men and women treated with AUS [55]. The proportion of device failures across time using Kaplan-Meier analysis showed that men have a significantly shorter AUS device duration before failure than women in terms of nonmechanical ($p < 0.021$) and iatrogenic causes ($p < 0.003$). The proportion of mechanical failures across time was comparable ($p < 0.218$). Median duration of the original implanted device in men is 5.0 years and in women is 11.2 years ($p < 0.001$) [55].

The difference in AUS survival between men and women is explained by many factors. First, the anatomic bladder neck location of the cuff in women is more secure compared to the peribulbar placement of the cuff in men which is a more superficial structure and consequently more prone to injuries. As a matter of fact, a higher postoperative surgical complication rate in males (20%) compared to female patients (10%) was reported in the latest systematic review. Secondly, the cuff size inserted in women is larger (6 cm on average) than the 4–4.5 cm cuff routinely used in men. Finally, the control pump is more mobile and prone to skin erosion or kinks in the scrotum than in the labium majus [56].

Evaluation of Persistent or Recurrent Urinary Incontinence After AUS Implantation

UI may recur after AUS implantation. In a retrospective study of 240 open AUS implantations, the three main causes of UI recurrence were poor dexterity that leads to poor bladder emptying, permanent explantation, and de novo DO [36]. Other causes of recurrent UI included inadvertent deactivation of the pump, cuff oversizing with insufficient bladder neck compression, mechanical failure secondary to fluid loss, kinked or obstructed tubing, cuff erosion, bladder storage failure, and bladder neck atrophy [66].

The evaluation of patients with recurrent or persistent UI after AUS implantation must include clinical history and physical examination. Other investigations such as cystoscopy, UDS, or radiographic may be necessary depending on the context [49].

Mechanical failure or inadvertent deactivation is suggested by the sudden loss of continence. During physical exam, actively cycling and pumping the device may exclude deactivation. Pelvic X-ray of the contrasted fluid balloon or balloon ultrasound can suggest a mechanical failure due to fluid lost (Fig. 12).

Atrophy is suggested by the recurrence of UI with a normally filled balloon on radiographic exams. A cystoscopy is then useful to evaluate the urethral aspect and its compression during the cycling of the AUS. In addition, cystoscopy can exclude AUS erosion and urethral strictures [49].

When a bladder storage failure is suspected to be the cause of UI, a UDS should be performed. It has been reported that 22% of female patients develop de novo DO after AUS implantation [36].

Median duration of the originally implanted device in women varies between 7 and 15 years across long-term follow-up studies [10]. Mechanical failure accounts for 2–41% of AUS revisions [10]. Mechanical failure can be addressed by the replacement of an isolated malfunctioning component or by all the AUS components. A partial revision may be feasible if it occurs within 3 years of implantation and when there is no erosion or infection [67]. If there is any doubt on which component is defecting during the revision, all components must be changed. After 3 years, it is recommended to replace all the device

Fig. 12 Pelvic X-ray of a closed/filled cuff AUS

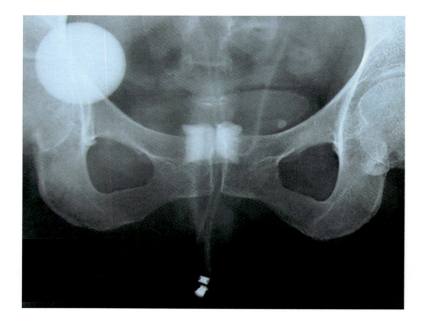

components because of the increased risk of remaining component failure [67].

Future Perspectives

The AMS-800™ version of the AUS was launched on the market in 1983, and no revolutionizing improvements have been made since. According to the Report of the 2015 ICS Consensus Conference on AUS, the ideal device must be simple, affordable, and easily manipulated and inactivated [68]. Manual dexterity is one of the main limitations of device implantation and one of the main causes of device failure. Thus, remotely controlled devices may eventually bypass this problem. A remotely controlled AUS could indeed help skill deprived patients and their caregivers. Furthermore, it may also allow easier AUS deactivation for patients before transurethral manipulation and during nighttime, to decrease the risk of atrophy by limiting the continuous urethral pressure.

The ideal AUS should also be able to adjust in real time the pressure of the cuff after the implantation. This may archive several goals. First, it should be interesting to adjust the cuff pressure in real time according to the abdominal pressure to effectively control SUI with high abdominal pressure but also improve safety by decreasing the cuff pressure when abdominal pressure is lower, like at rest or when the patient is lying down. In addition, persistent SUI may be caused by an insufficient cuff compression after the implantation. To be able to upgrade the compression without the need for a cuff revision may be helpful.

The ideal AUS should finally be robust. Indeed, mechanical failure is the leading cause of AUS revision rate in the long term. The multiple components of the device and the hydraulic mechanism are often implicated in the device failure. Multiple components multiply the risk of device failure because of the numbers of connections needed and by augmenting the number of components that may fail. The present hydraulic mechanism is also prompt to failure, by loss of fluid or by PRB expansion and gain of compliance. Having a more simple, robust, and non-hydraulic device may thus improve AUS longevity.

According to the AUS consensus statement of 2015, a total of nine AUS models have been reported in development. Among the latest developments, AUS using electromagnetically or Bluetooth-controlled devices are currently in development. For example, a collective work between McGill University and École Polytechnique de Montreal experimented with an ex vivo remotely activated AUS on pigs with promising success. Their device uses the same tubing, connector, PRB, and cuff, but the pump is changed for a small electronic pump implanted besides the PRB. The device integrity can also be checked remotely [69].

Another innovation in the field of AUS is the arrival of the VICTO® and VICTO PLUS® (Promedon, Austria) on the European market. This device includes a self-sealing port that allows for in-office pressure adjustment. The device is also able to increase the cuff pressure, while abdominal pressure increases and decrease it when the pressure is lower, decreasing the risk of urethral atrophy and perforation. Preliminary results in human implantation are available and promising [70].

Summary

AUS implantation in female patients suffering from SUI must be considered as a treatment option, particularly when the principal cause is ISD. Evaluation of the patient and of the continence mechanism is mandatory before implantation. Cognitive status and dexterity of the patient are also corner stones of the preimplantation evaluation. Multiple surgical approaches for AUS implantation have been described; the newest and probably the more promising one is the robotic-assisted implantation. Robotic implantation allows for more range of instrument mobility, a better visualization of the dissection plan, and a trend in fewer perioperative complications. Overall, AUS implantation has a low postoperative complication rate, and, thus, it is a safe treatment option. The more frequent complication is mechanical failure, which occurred approximately 10 years after implantation in the female patient. Thus, the device longevity is longer than what is seen in men. Other rare, but serious complications are AUS infection and erosion which are normally addressed by device explantation. The efficacy of the AUS is high, and nearly 80% of the female patients do not wear pads after the implantation. New developments in the AUS device are currently ongoing. Real-life cuff pressure adjustment and remote-controlled devices seem to be the future of the AUS and are now being evaluated in clinical trials.

Cross-References

▶ Clinical Evaluation of the Female Lower Urinary Tract and Pelvic Floor
▶ Sling Operations for Stress Urinary Incontinence and their Historical Evolution: Autologous, Cadaveric, and Synthetic Slings

References

1. Abrams P, Cardozo L, Fall M. The standardization of terminology of the lower urinary tract function: report for the standardization Sub-committee of the International Continence Society. Neurourol Urodyn. 2002;21:167–78.
2. Minassian VA, Stewart WF, Wood GC. Urinary incontinence in women: variation in prevalence estimates and risk factors. Obstet Gynecol. 2008;111:324–31.
3. Reynolds WS, Dmochowski RR, Penson DF. Epidemiology of stress urinary incontinence in women. Curr Urol Rep. 2011;12:370.
4. Dooley Y, Kenton K, Cao G, et al. Urinary incontinence prevalence: results from the National Health and Nutrition Examination Survey. J Urol. 2007;179(2): 656–61.
5. Karin L, Coyne S, Kvasz M, et al. Urinary incontinence and its relationship to mental health and health-related quality of life in men and women in Sweden, the United Kingdom, and the United States. J Eur Urol. 2011;61(1):88–95.
6. Gil KM, Somerville AM, Cichowski S, et al. Distress and quality of life characteristics associated with seeking surgical treatment for stress urinary incontinence. Health Qual Life Outcomes. 2009;7:8.
7. Subak LL, Goode PS, Brubaker L, et al. Urinary incontinence management costs are reduced following Burch or sling surgery for stress incontinence. Am J Obstet Gynecol. 2014;211(2):171.e1–7.
8. Harding CK, Lapitan MC, Arlandis S et al. EAU guideline: non-neurogenic Female LUTS. 2021. https://uroweb.org/guideline/non-neurogenic-female-luts/#4. Accessed 21 Dec 2021.
9. Richard F, Lefort J, Bitker M, et al. Female incontinence with primary sphincter deficiency: results of artificial urinary sphincter (AMS 800) with long-term follow-up. J Urol. 1996;20(Suppl 2):155–60.
10. Reus CR, Phe V, Dechartres A, et al. Performance and safety of the artificial urinary sphincter (AMS 800) for non-neurogenic women with urinary incontinence secondary to intrinsic sphincter deficiency: a systematic review. Eur Urol Focus. 2020;6(2):327–38.
11. Barakat B, Franke K, Hijazi S, et al. A systematic review and meta-analysis of clinical and functional outcomes of artificial urinary sphincter implantation in women with stress urinary incontinence. Arab J Urol. 2020;18(2):78–87.
12. Costa P, Mottet N, Rabut B, et al. The use of an artificial urinary sphincter in women with type III incontinence and a negative Marshall test. J Urol. 2001;165(4): 1172–6.
13. Schultheiss D, Hofner K, Oelke M, et al. Historical aspects of the treatment of urinary incontinence. Eur Urol. 2000;38:352–62.
14. Siegel SW. History of the prosthetic treatment of urinary incontinence. Urol Clin North Am. 1989;16:99–104.
15. Boston Scientific Corporation. AMS 800™, Système de contrôle urinaire pour les hommes, les femmes et les enfants. Manuel opératoire. 2016. https://www.bostonscientific.com/content/dam/elabeling/uro-ph/pr/1002534_AMS_800_ORM_fr_w_s.pdf. Assessed 21 Dec 2021.
16. De Cogan M, Elliott D. The impact of InhibiZone® on artificial urinary sphincter infection rate. J Urol. 2013;190(1):113–7.
17. Petrou SO, Elliott DS, Barrett DM. Artificial urethral sphincter for incontinence. Urology. 2000;56(3):353–9.
18. Kobashi KC, Albo ME, Dmochowski RR, et al. Surgical treatment of female stress urinary incontinence: AUA/SUFU guideline. J Urol. 2017;198(4):875–83.
19. Peyronnet B, Greenwell T, Gary G, et al. Current use of the artificial urinary sphincter in adult females. Curr Urol Rep. 2020;21(12):53.
20. Martin JL, Williams KS, Sutton AJ, et al. Systematic review and meta-analysis of methods of diagnostic assessment for urinary incontinence. Neurourol Urodyn. 2006;25:674.
21. Roupret M, Chartier-Kastler E, Almeras C, et al. Sacral neuromodulation for refractory detrusor overactivity in women with an artificial urinary sphincter. J Urol. 2004;172(1):236–9.
22. Ziegelmann MJ, Linder BJ, Rivera ME, et al. Outcomes of artificial urinary sphincter placement in octogenarians. Int J Urol. 2016;23(5):419–23.

23. Lavi A, Boone TB, Cohen M, et al. The patient beyond the sphincter – cognitive and functional considerations affecting the natural history of artificial urinary sphincters. Urology. 2020;137:14–8.
24. Chan SP, Ip KY, Irwin MG. Peri-operative optimisation of elderly and frail patients: a narrative review. Anaesthesia. 2019;74(Suppl 1):80–9.
25. Bergman A, McCarthy TA, Ballard CA, et al. Role of the Q-tip test in evaluating stress urinary incontinence. J Reprod Med. 1987;32(4):273–5.
26. Quiboeuf E, Fritel X. Bonney maneuver and its derivatives: history, technique, significance, and prognostic value. Prog Urol. 2020;30(16):1014–21.
27. Guralnick ML, Fritel X, Tarcan T, et al. ICS Educational Module: Cough stress test in the evaluation of female urinary incontinence: introducing the ICS-Uniform Cough Stress Test. Neurourol Urodyn. 2018;37(5):1849–55.
28. Patnam R, Edenfield AL, Swift SE. Standing vs supine; does it matter in cough stress testing? Female Pelvic Med Reconstr Surg. 2017;23(5):315–7.
29. Roupret M, Chartier-Kastler E, Richard F. Sphincters urinaires artificiels chez la femme: indications, techniques, résultats. Prog Urol. 2005;15(3):489–93.
30. Lose G, Griffiths D, Hosker G, et al. Standardisation of urethral pressure measurement: report from the Standardisation Sub-Committee of the International Continence Society. Neurourol Urodyn. 2002;21(3):258–60.
31. Chartier-Kastler E, Van Kerrebroeck P, Olianas R, et al. Artificial urinary sphincter (AMS 800) implantation for women with intrinsic sphincter deficiency: a technique for insiders? BJU Int. 2011;107(10):1618–26.
32. Woodman PJ. Pathophysiology of intrinsic sphincteric deficiency. 2015. https://www.ics.org/Workshops/HandoutFiles/000523.pdf. Accessed 21 Dec 2021.
33. Comiter CV. Surgery insight: surgical management of postprostatectomy incontinence: the artificial urinary sphincter and male sling. Nat Clin Pract Urol. 2007;4(11):615–24.
34. Cour F, Le Normand L, Lapray JF, et al. Insuffisance sphinctérienne et incontinence urinaire de la femme. Prog Urol. 2015;25:437–54.
35. Bracchitta D, Costa P, Borojeni S, et al. Laparoscopic artificial urinary sphincter implantation in women with stress urinary incontinence: update on 13 years' experience in a single centre. BJU Int. 2019;123:14–9.
36. Vayleux B, Rigaud J, Luyckx F, et al. Female urinary incontinence and artificial urinary sphincter: study of efficacy and risk factors for failure and complications. Eur Urol. 2011;59:1048–53.
37. Phé V, Rouprêt M, Mozer P, et al. Trends in the landscape of artificial urinary sphincter implantation in men and women in France over the past decade. Eur Urol. 2013;63(2):407–8.
38. National Guideline Alliance (UK). Urinary incontinence and pelvic organ prolapse in women: management. London: National Institute for Health and Care Excellence (NICE); 2019.
39. Burkhard C, Bosch JL, Cruz F, et al. EAU guidelines on urinary incontinence in adults. 2020. Available online at: https://uroweb.org/guideline/urinary-incontinence/. Accessed 15 Dec 2021.
40. Bettez M, Tu le M, Carlson K, et al. Guidelines for adult urinary incontinence collaborative consensus document for the Canadian Urological Association. Can Urol Assoc J. 2012;6(5):354–63.
41. Peyronnet B, O'Connor E, Khavari R, et al. AMS-800 artificial urinary sphincter in female patients with stress urinary incontinence: a systematic review. Neurourol Urodyn. 2019;38:S28–41.
42. Ngninkeu BN, Van Heugen G, Di Gregorio M, et al. Laparoscopic artificial urinary sphincter in women for type III incontinence: preliminary results. Eur Urol. 2005;47:793–7.
43. Peyronnet B, Capon G, Belas O, et al. Robot-assisted AMS-800 artificial urinary sphincter bladder neck implantation in female patients with stress urinary incontinence. Eur Urol. 2019;75:169–75.
44. Lightner DJ, Wymer K, Sanchez J, et al. Best practice statement on urologic procedures and antimicrobial prophylaxis. J Urol. 2020;203:351–6.
45. Yeung LL, Grewal S, Bullock A, et al. A comparison of chlorhexidine-alcohol versus povidone-iodine for eliminating skin flora before genitourinary prosthetic surgery: a randomized controlled trial. J Urol. 2013;189:136–40.
46. Elliot DS, Barret M. The artificial urinary sphincter in the female: indications for use, surgical approach, and results. Int Urogynecol J Pelvic Floor Dysfunct. 1998;9(6):409–15.
47. Biardeau X, Aharony S, AUS Consensus Group. Artificial urinary sphincter: report of the 2015 consensus conference. Neurourol Urodyn. 2015;35(Suppl 2):S8–S24.
48. Peyronnet B, Vincendeau S, Tondut L, et al. Artificial urinary sphincter implantation in women with stress urinary incontinence: preliminary comparison of robot-assisted and open approaches. Int Urogynecol J. 2016;27(3):475–81.
49. Sandhu JS, Breyer B, Comiter C, et al. Incontinence after prostate treatment: AUA/SUFU guideline. J Urol. 2019;202(2):369–78.
50. Bryan DE, Mulcahy JJ, Simmons GR. Salvage procedure for infected noneroded artificial urinary sphincters. J Urol. 2002;168(6):2464–6.
51. Frank I, Elliott DS, Barrett DM. Success of de novo reimplantation of the artificial genitourinary sphincter. J Urol. 2000;163:1702–3.
52. Fournier G, Callerot P, Thoulouzan M, et al. Robotic-assisted laparoscopic implantation of artificial urinary sphincter in women with intrinsic sphincter deficiency incontinence: initial results. Urology. 2014;84:1094–8.
53. Chung E, Cartmill RA. 25-Year experience in the outcome of artificial urinary sphincter in the treatment of female urinary incontinence. BJU Int. 2010;106(11):1664–7.
54. Tricard T, Jochum F, Bergerat S, et al. Outcomes of open artificial urinary sphincter in women with stress

urinary incontinence: long-term follow up. Ther Adv Urol. 2019;11:1756287219874676.

55. Petero VG, Diokno AC. Comparison of the long-term outcomes between incontinent men and women treated with artificial urinary sphincter. J Urol. 2006;175(2):605–9.

56. McGuire EJ, Fitzpatrick CC, Wan J, et al. Clinical assessment of urethral sphincter function. J Urol. 1993;150:1452–4.

57. Thomas K, Venn SN, Mundy AR. Outcome of the artificial urinary sphincter in female patients. J Urol. 2002;167:1720–2.

58. Rouprêt M, Misraï V, Vaessen C, et al. Laparoscopic approach for artificial urinary sphincter implantation in women with intrinsic sphincter deficiency incontinence: a single-centre preliminary experience. Eur Urol. 2010;57(3):499–504.

59. Mandron E, Bryckaert PE, Papatsoris AG, et al. Laparoscopic artificial urinary sphincter implantation for female genuine stress urinary incontinence: technique and 4-year experience in 25 patients. BJU Int. 2010;106(8):1194–8.

60. Trolliet S, Mandron E, Lang H, et al. Laparoscopic approach for artificial urinary sphincter implantation for women with severe stress urinary incontinence. Prog Urol. 2013;23:877–83.

61. Ferreira C, Brychaert PE, Menard J, et al. Laparoscopic implantation of artificial urinary sphincter in women with intrinsic sphincter deficiency: mid-term outcomes. Int J Urol. 2017;24(4):308–13.

62. Kourbanhoussen K, Cecchi M, Chevrot A, et al. Laparoscopic robot-assisted artificial urinary sphincter in women: first approach. Prog Urol. 2019;29(7):371–7.

63. Gondran-Tellier B, Boissier R, Baboudjian M, et al. Robot-assisted implantation of an artificial urinary sphincter, the AMS-800, via a posterior approach to the bladder neck in women with intrinsic sphincter deficiency. BJU Int. 2019;124(6):1077–80.

64. Peyronnet B, Capon G, Belas O, et al. Robot-assisted artificial urinary sphincter implantation in female patients: an international multicenter study. Eur Urol. 2020;19:604–5.

65. Chartier-Kastler E, Vaessen C, Rouprêt M, et al. Robot-assisted laparoscopic artificial urinary sphincter insertion in women with stress urinary incontinence: a pilot single-centre study. BJU Int. 2020;126:722–30.

66. Montague DK, Angermeier KW. Artificial urinary sphincter troubleshooting. Urology. 2001;58(5):779–82.

67. Srivastava A, Joice GA, Patel HD, et al. Causes of artificial urinary sphincter failure and strategies for surgical revision: implications of device component survival. Eur Urol Focus. 2019;5(5):887–93.

68. Biardeau X, Aharony S, AUS Consensus Group, et al. Artificial urinary sphincter: report of the 2015 consensus conference. Neurourol Urodyn. 2015;35:S3–S22.

69. Biardeau X, Hached S, Loutochin O, et al. Montreal electronic artificial urinary sphincters: our futuristic alternatives to the AMS800™. Can Urol Assoc J. 2017;11(10):E396–404.

70. Giammò A, Falcone M, Blecher G, et al. A novel artificial urinary sphincter (VICTO®) for the management of postprostatectomy urinary incontinence: description of the surgical technique and preliminary results from a multicenter series. Urol Int. 2021;105(5–6):414–20.

71. O'Sullivan R, Karantanis E, Stevermuer TL, et al. Definition of mild, moderate, and severe incontinence on the 24-hour pad test. BJOG. 2004;111(8):859–62.

72. Appel RA. Techniques and results in the implantation of the artificial urinary sphincter in women with type III stress urinary incontinence by a vaginal approach. Neurourol Urodyn. 1988;7:613–9.

Urethral Bulking Agents

24

Quentin Alimi, Béatrice Bouchard, and Jacques Corcos

Contents

Introduction	438
History of Urethral Bulking Agents	438
Mechanism of Action	439
Injection Techniques	440
Bulkamid	441
Results	441
Adverse Events	442
Durasphere	442
Results	442
Adverse Events	442
Coaptite	442
Results	443
Adverse Events	443
Urolastic	443
Results	443
Adverse Events	443
Macroplastique	443
Results	444
Adverse Events	444
Conclusion	444
Cross-References	445
References	445

Q. Alimi (✉) · B. Bouchard · J. Corcos
Department of Urology, McGill University, Jewish
General Hospital, Montreal, QC, Canada
e-mail: quentin.alimi@gmail.com;
beatrice.bouchard@umontreal.ca; jcorcosmd@gmail.com

© Springer Nature Switzerland AG 2023
F. E. Martins et al. (eds.), *Female Genitourinary and Pelvic Floor Reconstruction*,
https://doi.org/10.1007/978-3-031-19598-3_25

Abstract

Urethral bulking agents (UBA) has been used for decades to treat stress urinary incontinence (SUI). After being first described in the 1930s, several agents have been introduced to the market with varying profiles of safety, durability, and efficacy. Currently available agents include polyacrylamide hydrogel (Bulkamid®), calcium hydroxyl apatite (Coaptite®), carbon-coated zirconium (Durasphere®), polydimethylsiloxane elastomer (Macroplastique®), and PDMS-U (Urolastic®). Considered safe and minimally invasive procedures, UBA benefit from a renewed interest from patients and practitioners, regarding the growing controversies surrounding the use of mid-urethral synthetic slings. After describing the mechanisms of action and injection techniques, this chapter looks at currently available UAB and their own safety and efficacy profile based on the most relevant data found in the literature.

Keywords

Urethral bulking agents · Stress urinary incontinence · Urinary incontinence

Introduction

Stress urinary incontinence (SUI) is a common and potentially debilitating condition that predominantly affects women [1]. The current gold standard treatment for SUI is the insertion of a mid-urethral sling (MUS), via the retropubic or the transobturator route [2]. With the sling acting as a hammock, MUS provides support at the level of the mid-urethra and prevents the urethra from dropping.

However, concerns regarding the safety of SUI surgical procedures have been raised. Indeed, mesh has been associated with complications such as chronic pain, infection, and erosion. This has led to court action in the USA, Canada, the UK, as well as some other European countries. For this reason, vaginal slings and tapes have now become under great scrutiny, and some countries have even banned their use.

Patients are becoming more informed of the potential side effects of MUS, and this has led to a greater demand of less invasive treatments with fewer side effects, even if this may be associated with a lower cure rate [3]. Therefore, there has

been an increase in the use of conservative and alternative approaches to avoid the complications and side effects of surgery.

An alternative technique that avoids surgical treatment is, for instance, the injection of urethral bulking agents (UBA). In this chapter, we will describe the available UBAs, their mechanism of action, the injection technique, as well as their efficacy and side effects, based on a review of the literature.

History of Urethral Bulking Agents

UBAs have been part of the therapeutic arsenal for female SUI for many decades. Murless first reported sodium morrhuate injections around the urethra in 1938 [4]. The following attempts, realized with paraffin wax by Quackels [5] and sclerosing agents by Sachse [6], led to poor results and significant complications, such as urethral sloughing and pulmonary emboli. Since then, several agents were introduced to the market but subsequently withdrawn secondary to clinical safety or economic concerns [7].

Autologous fat was initially thought to be attractive because of its hypothesized reduced immunogenicity. However, it was abandoned due to rapid digestion and potential migration [8]. Polytetrafluoroethylene, a derivative of Teflon™, has also been used as a UBA. First introduced in the 1970s, it was not FDA approved due to particle migration to lymph nodes and distant organs, granuloma formation, and its carcinogenic potential [9].

On the other hand, glutaraldehyde cross-linked bovine collagen (GAXcollagen or Contigen®) was the first UBA to be approved by the FDA in 1993. It was the most widely used injectable in clinical practice and has been used as the control arm in many trials. It consists of 95% type-1 collagen and 1–5% of type-3 collagen. Initial results were promising, with cure rates as high as 85–94%, but long-term success rates declined to approximatively 25–65%. Complications included urinary tract infections, hematuria, and de novo urgency. Immunogenic complications, such as delayed skin reactions and arthralgia, led to discontinuation of its production worldwide in 2011 [11, 12].

Ethylene vinyl alcohol copolymer (Uryx™) was withdrawn from the market 2 years after its introduction, possibly as a result of high rates of urethral erosion [13]. Due to concerns about high levels of pseudo-abscess formation, hyaluronic acid with dextranomer (Zuidex™) was also withdrawn from the market [14, 15].

Mechanism of Action

SUI results from failure of the urethra to remain closed during urine storage. It can be divided into two categories. Types 1 and 2 are extrinsic and related to poor anatomic support of the urethra and bladder neck, leading to incontinence with urethral hypermobility. This, therefore, responds well to pelvic floor resuspension. Alternatively, type 3 urethral failure may be intrinsic. Also called intrinsic sphincter deficiency, this type of urethral failure may respond to sphincter augmentation procedures. However, these processes may often coexist to a variable degree, and urethral hypermobility alone does not necessarily lead to SUI. The difference between women with urethral hypermobility who leak and those who do not is probably more related to urethral resistance to intra-abdominal stressors.

Urethral injections, by adding bulk to the proximal urethra, improve coaptation of the urethral wall and ultimately result in increasing resistance to the passive outflow of urine in patients with SUI [16, 17]. Initially, it was believed that the mechanism of action of UBAs was through obstruction, thus preventing the opening of the bladder neck under stress. However, other investigations have also reported an increased area of pressure transmission ratio in the proximal urethra after bulking agent injections [18]. Proper placement of the bulking agent, below the bladder neck or at the mid-urethra, improves intrinsic sphincter deficiency (Figs. 1 and 2).

The AUA guidelines recommend that bulking agents should be reserved for patients with SUI and a fixed, immobile urethra [19]. However, because ISD can coexist with hypermobility, injectables have been administered to patients with hypermobility to improve the ISD component of their incontinence. Some bulking agent trials have grouped all types of SUI together, regardless of measured sphincteric function. These studies did not demonstrate a significant difference between

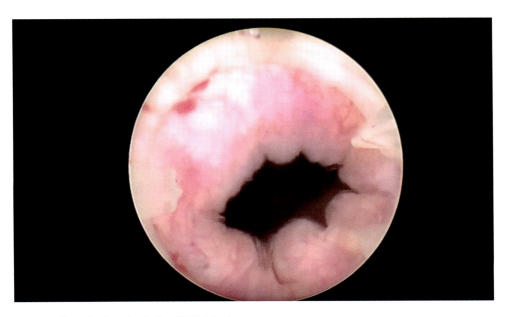

Fig. 1 Aspect of proximal urethra before UAB injection

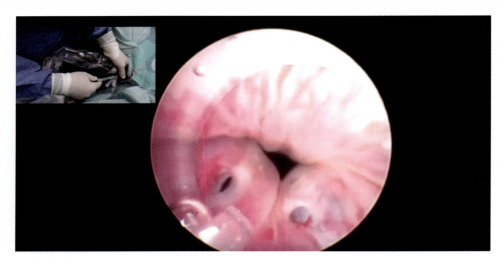

Fig. 2 Aspect of proximal urethra coaptation after UAB injection (Bulkamid®)

successful injections according to the degree of urethral hypermobility [20].

Injection Techniques

The ideal agent should be easily injectable and should maintain its volume with time. It should also be biocompatible, nonimmunogenic, noncarcinogenic, hypoallergenic, and nonmigratory (particle size greater than 80 μm), with minimal scarring and good wound healing properties [21].

UBAs can be administered under local anesthesia as an outpatient procedure. Usually, a urinary tract infection (UTI) is ruled out by carrying out a urinalysis, and the procedure should be canceled in case of suspected or demonstrated UTI.

Both periurethral and transurethral methods can be used to inject UBAs. It can be realized using ultrasound or under direct vision with cystoscopy or an Implacer™-guided device implantation. Local anesthesia is realized with 1% or 2% lidocaine, injected 3–4 mm lateral to the urethral meatus, often at the 3 and 9 o'clock or 4 and 8 o'clock positions.

Periurethral injection requires a 30° cystoscope to allow injection lateral to the urethral meatus in the area of the proximal urethra and bladder neck, which may lead to reduced local urethral trauma [22].

Care must be taken to prevent the needle from entering or getting too close to the urethral lumen, as rupture of the mucosa and extravasation will occur. The quantity injected is usually decided by the operator to obtain an adequate bulking effect. The substance is usually injected bilaterally, at the 3 and 9 o'clock positions, but might as well be injected in three or four points to obtain a satisfying coaptation.

The transurethral route allows direct visualization with a cystoscope and injection of the bulking agent 2 cm distal to the bladder neck into the urethral wall. This technique requires less volume of the material for the injection [22]. The urethral bulking agent can also be administered with the Implacer™-guided implantation device. This technique does not require a cystoscope, but instead uses a three-angled channel inserted into the urethra with the bladder neck identified when fluid drains out [22] (Fig. 3).

Periurethral and transurethral routes seem comparable in terms of subjective and objective outcomes, but periurethral injections might lead to a higher rate of acute postoperative retention compared to the transurethral route [23].

The site of the injection (i.e., bladder neck or mid-urethra) has also been a matter of debate. Traditional (proximal) bladder neck injection was compared to mid-urethral injection using collagen in 30 women. At 10 months, the reported

Fig. 3 Periurethral route for UBA injection using the Implacer™ device

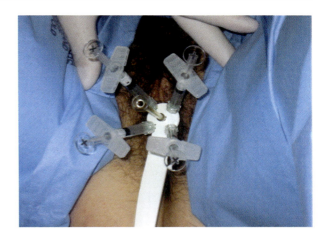

cure rates were similar in both groups, but there was a higher rate of postoperative urinary retention in the mid-urethral route [24].

Currently marketed UBAs include polyacrylamide hydrogel (Bulkamid®), polydimethylsiloxane (Macroplastique®), carbon-coated zirconium oxide (Durasphere®), and calcium hydroxylapatite (Coaptite®) with the latest product being a polydimethylsiloxane silicone gel that polymerizes when injected (Urolastic®).

Bulkamid

Bulkamid® is a polyacrylamide hydrogel, made up of 2.5% cross-linked polyacrylamide and 97.5% water which Has Been Available since 2006 in the United Kingdom, Europe, North America, and Australia. It Received FDA Approval in 2020

Results

Definition of treatment success differs considerably between studies, resulting in great variability in the reported success rates. In addition, only a few studies have reported long-term outcomes (>36 months).

Lose et al. followed 135 women with either SUI or mixed urinary incontinence (MUI) and reported a subjective response rate of 66% after 12 months (patients considering themselves "cured" or "improved"), with reduction of median International Consultation on Incontinence Questionnaire (ICIQ) score of approximately 50%. Similar efficacy was found between patients with MUI and SUI. About 35% of the patients had a reinjection [25].

On the other hand, Toozs-Hobson et al. reported an overall 64% response rate (improved or cured patients) after 24 months in 135 women. Repeat injections were realized in 35% of the patients [26].

In a group of 25 patients suffering from SUI followed retrospectively, Mouritsen et al. reported a cure or improvement rate of 44% after 96 months. Seven (28%) patients underwent a mid-urethral sling placement, and two (8%) had a reinjection [27].

A randomized controlled trial comparing Bulkamid® to Contigen® injections in 345 women with untreated SUI or MUI demonstrated that Bulkamid® was non-inferior to Contigen®. In both groups, the success rate (cured or improved urinary incontinence) approached approximatively 70% after 12 months [28].

Zivanovic et al. reported results of Bulkamid® injections for recurrent SUI or MUI after previous MUS surgery. Sixty patients were prospectively included with a cure/improvement rate of 83.6% at 12 months [29].

Bulkamid® injections were found to be inferior to tension-free vaginal tape (TVT) in a randomized control trial involving 224 women with primary SUI. At 1 year, primary outcome (satisfaction score of 80 or greater on visual analogue scale) was reached in 95% for TVT patients, as compared to 59.8% for Bulkamid® injections [30].

Adverse Events

The most common side effects with Bulkamid® injections are acute urinary retention (AUR), urinary tract infections (UTI), and de novo urgency. AUR usually ranges between 0% and 20%, while rates of UTIs range between 1.6% and 40%, and de novo urgency between 0% and 10% [25–30]. Across studies, injection site rupture was noticed in three patients, without evidence of erosion [25, 29, 31]. A higher rate of complications (44.6%) was reported in TVT patients when compared to Bulkamid® (19.6%). Indeed, 6.0% of TVT patients required a reoperation due to complications such as hematoma, acute urinary retention (AUR), and erosion, as compared to 0% in Bulkamid® patients [30].

Durasphere

Durasphere (Carbon Medical Technologies) is a synthetic nonabsorbable urethral bulking (UBA) agent that was designed to be nonreactive, permanent, and nonmigratory [32]. It is made of carbon-coated zirconium oxide beads suspended in a polysaccharide gel made of 2.8% glucan. The particles are smaller (95–200 um), which allows for a lower pressure injection while maintaining the target size threshold of 80 um [33]. It has been FDA approved since 1999 and is available in the United States and Europe [33].

Results

The duration of follow-up greatly varies among studies, ranging from 9.4 to 37 months [34]. The short-term efficacy rate varies between 33.3% and 65.5% [34]. On the other hand, two studies evaluated the long-term success rate, and this has been reported to be 21% at 36 months in the first study

compared to 80% at 31.6 months in the second one [35, 36]. In a randomized controlled, multicenter trial, Lightner et al. compared Durasphere to Contigen in 355 women. After Durasphere injections in 176 women, 80.3% reported improvement of one or more Stamey incontinence grades 12 months after the last injection compared to 69.1% of the 188 women who were injected with Contigen ($P = 0.162$) [32]. Pannek et al. had a 15.4% reinjection rate reported in one study [37].

Adverse Events

Lightner et al. also demonstrated a higher rate of AUR and de novo urinary urgency in the Durasphere group in comparison to Contigen [32]. These events all resolved spontaneously and were attributed to the larger needle size that was required for Durasphere injections [2]. A downside that has been noted is that the carbon beads can become clogged in the syringe with loss of the carrier gel, resulting in higher injection pressure, making the injection process more difficult as well as creating a greater risk of extrusion [38]. A more serious complication was reported by Pannek et al. where the Durasphere beads migrated to regional or distant lymph nodes in one woman [37]. This was detected on routine X-ray 3 months postoperatively and was associated with declining success rates from 6 to 12 months [37].

Coaptite

Coaptite (Boston Scientific), another synthetic nonabsorbable UBA, consists of spherical calcium hydroxylapatite that is suspended in a carboxymethyl cellulose gel carrier [39]. The particles are uniform in shape and size (between 75 and 125 um) [3]. Calcium hydroxylapatite is the main constituent of bones and teeth and remains pliable after injection into soft tissues. It is neither immunogenic nor inflammatory, is easily injected, and is radiopaque, which allows for radiographic follow-up of injection [32]. It has gained FDA approval in 2005 and is available in the United States and Turkey [33].

Results

In a randomized controlled trial (RCT) comparing Coaptite to Contigen in 296 women with ISD, Mayer et al. did not show a significant difference in improvement in both materials [40]. Indeed, at 12 months, 63% of the Coaptite patients had an improvement of at least one Stamey grade or more of their stress incontinence compared to 57% in the Contigen group. However, women in the Coaptite group were less likely to need repeat injections, and a lower volume of material was injected compared to the Contigen group [40]. A total of four studies have evaluated the reinjection rate, and this varies between 15.6% and 70% [39]. Long-term success rates have also been evaluated in other studies, and these vary between 60% and 74.7% [39].

Adverse Events

AUR (11.7% to 50%), UTI (0% to 30%), and de novo urgency (0% to 5.7%) have all been reported as adverse events [39]. More severe complications include vaginal wall erosion with apparent dissection of the material into the distal urethra, large urethral mucosa prolapses, as well as dissection of the bulking material beneath the bladder mucosa resulting in difficult visualization of one ureteric orifice, without any evidence of clinically significant ureteric obstruction (1 event each) [39].

Urolastic

Urolastic (Urogyn BV) is one of the more recent UBAs in the market. It is a biomaterial made of vinyl dimethyl terminated dimethylsiloxane (PDMS) polymer [1]. It differs from the other UBAs in that it polymerizes in situ into a uniform elastomer, therefore retaining its flexibility and

adapting to its environment [38]. This is thought to reduce the risk of migration. It has been available in Europe since 2012.

Results

Due to its relatively recent introduction, no long-term data exists for Urolastic. Follow-up duration in studies is between 6 and 25 months with reported success rates of 32.7% to 85.3% [39]. Hoe et al. reported a mean improvement of number of incontinence episodes of −4.5 to −16.6, a mean improvement in pad weight test of −10 to −16.8 g, and reinjection rates of 16.9% to 35% [39].

Adverse Events

Complications include AUR (from 15% to 40%), UTI (2.9% to 5%), de novo urgency (20%), and dyspareunia (3.8% to 10%) [5]. Five patients had migration of the material into the bladder, and this was removed cystoscopically. Exposure or erosion of the implant through the tissue was observed in one study (26.2% of patients) and required removal of the implant in 21.5% of patients [39].

Macroplastique

Macroplastique (Uroplasty Ltd.) is made of polydimethylsiloxane particles (silicone) suspended in a water-soluble carrier gel (polyvinylpyrrolidone) [38]. It is a flexible, highly texturized irregularly shaped implant. It is a large particle (usually greater than 100 um) and therefore has a lower likelihood of migration, and manufacturers claim that this leads to longer results for patients [33]. However, particle size is variable from less than 50 um to greater than 400 um [33]. It acts by getting surrounded by fibroblasts and forming collagen nodules [33]. It was FDA approved in 2006 and is commonly used in the United Kingdom, Europe, and the United States [39].

Results

In a meta-analysis, Ghoniem and Miller demonstrated improvement in 75% of patients at short-term follow-up (<6 months), 73% at midterm follow-up (6–18 months), and 64% at long-term follow-up (>18 months) [41]. The authors also found that Macroplastique reduced urine loss by >50% in 79% of patients according to the 1-hour pad test [41]. In another study, Maher et al. compared Macroplastique injections to pubovaginal sling in a prospective RCT of 45 women with SUI and ISD [34]. After 62 months, patient satisfaction rates were comparable, but objective success rates were significantly greater following sling treatment (81% vs. 9%) [34]. The authors also demonstrated that Macroplastique also had significantly lower morbidity compared to sling with reduced operating time (median 22 vs. 60 min), blood loss (0 vs. 200 mL), inpatient stay (1 vs. 4 days), duration of catheterization (1 vs. 5 days) and time to resume normal activities (2.8 vs. 4 days) [34].

In a systematic review of UBAs for SUI in women, Hoe et al. reported a reinjection rate between 7.4% and 52.2% [5].

Adverse Events

In another meta-analysis of UBAs for female SUI, Siddiqui et al. reported the most common adverse effects of 651 women treated with Macroplastique [34]. These included AUR (9%), UTI (9%), de novo urgency (11%), dysuria (7%), hematuria (3%), implantation site pain (2%), and persistent urge urinary incontinence (2%). Even though the material is thought to be inert, there have been two reported cases of rapid failure after initial success that was attributed to an immune rejection [34]. Two cases of urethral erosion have also been reported, as well as a suburethral mass formation requiring excision [34].

Conclusion

UBAs were initially designed as an alternative, second-line treatment to slings or colposuspension for SUI in women. However, growing concerns about the use of mesh, in addition to the ageing population, have led to an increased interest for minimally invasive procedures. Although less efficacious than open surgery, UBAs remain an attractive alternative because of their improved tolerability, low morbidity, and favorable adverse event profile.

Obviously, patient involvement in the decision-making process, as well as choice of treatment that respects their personal goals and expectations, remains of utmost importance.

In a study based on a questionnaire completed by women attending a tertiary referral urodynamic clinic, Robinson et al. showed that while 43% of patients expected a good improvement in symptoms where the latter would no longer interfere with life, only 17% of them expected a complete cure of all bladder symptoms [3]. When considering the acceptability of treatments for SUI, a clinical procedure with a 60% improvement rate and no long-term risks would be acceptable in 57% of patients compared with only 23% for a major operation with a cure rate of 85% [3].

When given the option, patients have a general preference for less invasive treatments for SUI. Indeed, many are willing to trade a lower success rate for a less invasive procedure and lower risks of complications [42, 43]. About 64% and 75% of patients would prefer to have a UBA as a second-line therapy between conservative treatment and more invasive surgery [44].

The few trials that have compared UBAs to surgical procedures have shown better overall objective cure rates in the surgical groups [34]. Corcos et al., in a randomized study, compared the efficacy, quality of life, and complication rates between collagen injections and open surgery. In the surgical group, 29 slings, 19 Burch colposuspensions, and 6 bladder neck suspensions were reviewed [45]. After a follow-up period of 12 months, the success rate was 53.1% in the collagen group compared to 72.2% in the surgical group. Women were more satisfied after open surgery group (79.6%) than those in the collagen group (67.2%), but the difference was not statistically significant. Complications occurred more frequently in the open surgery group (84 events in 34 women in the open surgery group compared to 36 events in 23 women in the collagen group). There were a high number of women who refused their allocated treatment of open surgery post-randomization, and this might have led to potential bias. Nonetheless, this study highlighted the importance of involving patients in the decision-making process.

Dray et al. performed a retrospective review of 75 patients treated with UBAs for a primary complaint of SUI following a failed prior sling procedure (mid-urethral or fascial pubovaginal sling). They found that after UBA treatment, 67.1% of patients reported at least a moderate improvement in incontinence (24.7% reported total resolution) and 32.9% reported only minimal or no improvement. The type of previous sling and the UAB used did not impact the results [46].

Numerous agents have been tried in the context of urethral bulking therapies, but available evidence hinders an objective choice between them in terms of efficacy or safety [10]. UBAs, although minimally invasive and with a low morbidity profile, are not exempt of complications. Approximatively one third of the patients experience some degree of complications after UBA injection. That being said, a majority of UBA-associated complications are mild and transient and do not need additional invasive treatment [47].

The search for the ideal agent remains ongoing, with a growing interest on regenerative injection therapies. With the use of stem cells, these treatments aim at restoring sphincteric function. Despite over a decade of investigations and promising results in preclinical animal studies, these studies remain small and show only mild to modest efficacy in human trials, without adequate long-term data [48, 49].

The lack of standardized outcome measures, the multitude of agents available, as well as the risk of bias in some studies have made it difficult to draw firm conclusions from the available data. What these studies have shown, however, is that patient goals and expectations should be at the center of the decision-making process.

In conclusion, although less effective and definitive, UBAs remain a safe and convenient alternative to open surgery and should be included in the treatment options for women with SUI, when appropriate. Larger-scale studies are needed to determine their exact role in the treatment algorithm for SUI.

Cross-References

▶ Sling Operations for Stress Urinary Incontinence and Their Historical Evolution: Autologous, Cadaveric, and Synthetic Slings
▶ Stem Cell and Tissue Engineering in Female Urinary Incontinence

References

1. Minassian VA, Drutz HP, Al-Badr A. Urinary incontinence as a worldwide problem. Int J Gynaecol Obstet. 2003;82(3):327–38.
2. Brazzelli M, Javanbakht M, Imamura M, Hudson J, Moloney E, Becker F, Wallace S, Omar MI, Shimonovich M, MacLennan G, Ternent L, Vale L, Montgomery I, Mackie P, Saraswat L, Monga A, Craig D. Surgical treatments for women with stress urinary incontinence: the ESTER systematic review and economic evaluation. Health Technol Assess. 2019;23(14):1–306.
3. Robinson D, Anders K, Cardozo L, et al. What women want – their interpretation of the concept of cure. Neurourol Urodyn. 2002;21:429–30.
4. Murless BC. The injection treatment of stress incontinence. J Obstet Gynaecol Br Emp. 1938;45:67–73.
5. Quackles R. Deux incontinences après adénomectomie guéries par injection de paraffine dans le périnée. Acta Urol Belkg. 1955;23:259–62.
6. Sachse H. Treatment of urinary incontinence with sclerosing solutions. Indications, results, complications. Urol Int. 1963;15:225–44.
7. Mamut A, Carlson KV. Periurethral bulking agents for female stress urinary incontinence in Canada. Can Urol Assoc J. 2017;11:S152–4.
8. Lee PE, Kung RC, Drutz HP. Periurethral autologous fat injection as treatment for female stress urinary incontinence: a randomized double-blind controlled trial. J Urol. 2001;165(1):153–8.
9. Kiilholma PJ, Chancellor MB, Makinen J, Hirsch IH, Klemi PJ. Complications of Teflon injection for stress urinary incontinence. Neurourol Urodyn. 1993;12: 131–7.
10. Kirchin V, Page T, Keegan PE, Atiemo K, Cody JD, McClinton S. Urethral injection therapy for urinary incontinence in women. Cochrane Database Syst Rev. 2017;37:2286–7.
11. Appell RA. Collagen injection therapy for urinary incontinence. Urol Clin North Am. 1994;21:177–82.

12. Cross CA, English SF, Cespedes RD, et al. A follow-up on transurethral collagen injection therapy for urinary incontinence. J Urol. 1998;159:106–8.
13. Hurtado EA, Appell RA. Complications of Tegress injections. Int Urogynecol J Pelvic Floor Dysfunct. 2009;20(1):127; author reply 129. https://doi.org/10.1007/s00192-008-0674-z. Epub 2008 Jul 5.
14. Hilton P. Urethrovaginal fistula associated with 'sterile abscess' formation following periurethral injection of dextranomer/hyaluronic acid co-polymer (Zuidex) for the treatment of stress urinary incontinence: a case report. BJOG. 2009;116(11):1527–30.
15. Loisel C, Secco M, Rocher-Barrat A, Caremel R, Grise P. Periurethral pseudocysts following urethral injections of Zuidex: review of the literature. Prog Urol. 2008;18(13):1038–43. French
16. Herschorn S, Randomski SB, Steele DJ. Early experience with intraurethral collagen injections for urinary incontinence. J Urol. 1992;148:1797–800.
17. Richardson TD, Kennelly MJ, Faerber GJ. Endoscopic injections of glutaraldehyde cross-linked collagene for the treatment of intrinsic deficiency in women. Urology. 1995;46:378–81.
18. Monga AK, Robinson D, Stanton SL. Periurethral collagens injections for genuine stress incontinence. Br J Urol. 1995;76:156–60.
19. Kobashi KC, Albo ME, Dmochowski RR, et al. Surgical treatment of female stress urinary incontinence: AUA/SUFU guideline. J Urol. 2017;198:875.
20. Bent AE, Foote J, Siegel S, et al. Collagen implant for treating stress urinary incontinence in women with urethral hypermobility. J Urol. 2001;166:1354–7.
21. Kotb AF, Campeau L, Corcos J. Urethral bulking agents: techniques and outcomes. Curr Urol Rep. 2009;10:396–400.
22. Ghoniem G, Boctor N. Update on urethral bulking agents for female stress urinary incontinence due to intrinsic sphincter deficiency. J Urol Res. 2014;1:1009.
23. Schulz JA, Nager CW, Stanton SL, Baessler K. Bulking agents for stress urinary incontinence: short-term results and complications in a randomized comparison of periurethral and transurethral injections. Int Urogynecol J. 2004;15(4):261–5.
24. Kuhn A, Stadlmayr W, Lengsfeld D, Mueller MD. Where should bulking agents for female urodynamic stress incontinence be injected? Int Urogynecol J Pelvic Floor Dysfunct. 2008;19:817–21.
25. Lose G, Sørensen HC, Axelsen SM, Falconer C, Lobodasch K, Safwat T. An open multicenter study of polyacrylamide hydrogel (Bulkamid®) for female stress and mixed urinary incontinence. Int Urogynecol J. 2010;21(12):1471–7.
26. Toozs-Hobson P, Al-Singary W, Fynes M, Tegerstedt G, Lose G. Two-year follow-up of an open-label multicenter study of polyacrylamide hydrogel (Bulkamid®) for female stress and stress-predominant mixed incontinence. Int Urogynecol J. 2012;23(10):1373–8.
27. Mouritsen L, Lose G, Møller-Bek K. Long-term follow-up after urethral injection with polyacrylamide hydrogel for female stress incontinence. Acta Obstet Gynecol Scand. 2014;93(2):209–12.
28. Sokol ER, Karram MM, Dmochowski R. Efficacy and safety of polyacrylamide hydrogel for the treatment of female stress incontinence: a randomized, prospective, multicenter North American study. J Urol. 2014;192 (3):843–9.
29. Zivanovic I, Rautenberg O, Lobodasch K, von Bünau G, Walser C, Viereck V. Urethral bulking for recurrent stress urinary incontinence after midurethral sling failure. Neurourol Urodyn. 2017;36(3):722–6.
30. Itkonen Freitas AM, Mentula M, Rahkola-Soisalo P, Tulokas S, Mikkola TS. Tension-free vaginal tape surgery versus polyacrylamide hydrogel injection for primary stress urinary incontinence: a randomized clinical trial. J Urol. 2020;203(2):372–8.
31. Martan A, Masata J, Svabik K, Krhut J. Transurethral injection of polyacrylamide hydrogel (Bulkamid®) for the treatment of female stress or mixed urinary incontinence. Eur J Obstet Gynecol Reprod Biol. 2014;178: 199–202.
32. Lightner DJ. Review of the available urethral bulking agents. Curr Opin Urol. 2002;12:333–8.
33. Li H, Westney OL. Injection of urethral bulking agents. Urol Clin N Am. 2019;46:1–15. https://doi.org/10.1007/s00192-021-04937-1.
34. Maher CF, O'Reilly BA, Dwyer PL, Carey MP, Cornish A, Schluter P. Pubovaginal sling versus transurethral Macroplastique for stress urinary incontinence and intrinsic sphincter deficiency: a prospective randomized controlled trial. BJOG. 2005;112(6):797–801.
35. Andersen RC. Long-term follow-up comparison of Durasphere and Contigen in the treatment of stress urinary incontinence. J Low Genit Tract Dis. 2002;6 (4):239–43.
36. Chrouser KL, Fick F, Goel A, Itano NB, Sweat SD, Lightner DJ. Carbon coated zirconium beads in beta-glucan gel and bovine glutaraldehyde cross-linked collagen injections for intrinsic sphincter deficiency: continence and satisfaction after extended followup. J Urol. 2004;171(3):1152–5.
37. Pannek J, Brands FH, Senge T. Particle migration after transurethral injection of carbon coated beads for stress urinary incontinence. J Urol. 2001;166(4):1350–3.
38. Hussain SM, Bray R. Urethral bulking agents for female stress urinary incontinence. Neurourol Urodyn. 2019:1–6.
39. Hoe V, Haller B, Yao HH, O'Connel HE. Urethral bulking agents for the treatment of stress urinary incontinence in women: a systematic review. Neurourol Urodyn. 2021:1–40.
40. Mayer RD, Dmochowski RR, Appell RA. Multicenter prospective randomized 52-week trial of calcium hydroxylapatite versus bovine dermal collagen for treatment of stress urinary incontinence. Urology. 2007;69:976–880.

41. Ghoniem G, Corcos J, Comiter C, Westney OL, Hershorn S. Durability of urethral bulking agent injection in for female stress urinary incontinence: 2-year multicenter study results. J Urol. 2010;183(4):1444–9.
42. Chapple CR, Brubaker L, Haab F, van Kerrebroeck P, Robinson D. Patient-perceived outcomes in the treatment of stress urinary incontinence: focus on urethral injection therapy. Int Urogynecol J. 2006;18:199–205.
43. Casteleijn FM, Zwolsman SE, Kowalik CR, Roovers J-PPWR. Patients' perspectives on urethral bulk injection therapy and mid-urethral sling surgery for stress urinary incontinence. Int Urogynecol J. 2018;29(9): 1249–57.
44. Cox SJ. A study of factors that influence the choice of primary surgical procedure for stress urinary incontinence from the perspective of patients and clinicians. Master's thesis. 2019; University of Manchester, England.
45. Corcos J, Collet JP, Shapiro S, Herschorn S, Radomski SB, Schick E, Gajewski JB, Benedetti A, MacRamallah E, Hyams B. Multicenter randomized clinical trial comparing surgery and collagen injections for treatment of female stress urinary incontinence. Urology. 2005;65(5):898–904.
46. Dray E, Cameron A, Hall M, Clemens JQ, Stoffel J. Can urethral bulking agents salvage failed slings? Neurourol Urodyn. 2017;36
47. Kocjancic E, Mourad S, Acar Ö. Complications of urethral bulking therapy for female stress urinary incontinence. Neurourol Urodyn. 2018:1–9.
48. Sèbe P, Doucet C, Cornu JN, Ciofu C, Costa P, de Medina SG, Pinset C, Haab F. Intrasphincteric injections of autologous muscular cells in women with refractory stress urinary incontinence: a prospective study. Int Urogynecol J. 2011;22(2):183–9.
49. Hillary CJ, Roman S, MacNeil S, Aicher WK, Stenzl A, Chapple CR. Regenerative medicine and injection therapies in stress urinary incontinence. Nat Rev Urol. 2020;17(3):151–61. https://doi.org/10.1038/s41585-019-0273-4.

Laparoscopic Burch

25

Tamara Grisales and Kathryn Goldrath

Contents

Introduction 450

Stress Urinary Incontinence 450

History of Burch Colposuspension 450

Surgical Technique 451

Outcomes of Burch Colposuspension 452

Complications 454

Conclusion 454

References 454

Abstract

Burch colposuspension is a widely accepted surgical technique for management of stress urinary incontinence. It is a transabdominal retropubic approach aimed at treating stress incontinence by restoring support to the urethra. Traditionally, Burch procedures were performed via laparotomy. However, due to invasive nature of the open approach, they have been largely replaced by retropubic slings over the last several decades. However, laparoscopic and robotic approaches to the retropubic space can offer a minimally invasive surgical technique for management of stress urinary incontinence. This chapter will review the history of Burch colposuspension, describe minimally invasive surgical techniques, and discuss clinical outcomes of laparoscopic approaches.

Keywords

Stress incontinence · Burch colposuspension · Retropubic · Cooer's ligament

T. Grisales (✉) · K. Goldrath
University of California Los Angeles, Los Angeles, CA, USA
e-mail: tgrisales@mednet.ucla.edu;
Kgoldrath@mednet.ucla.edu

© Springer Nature Switzerland AG 2023
F. E. Martins et al. (eds.), *Female Genitourinary and Pelvic Floor Reconstruction*,
https://doi.org/10.1007/978-3-031-19598-3_26

Introduction

Stress urinary incontinence is a common condition estimated to affect 17–45% of adult women worldwide and can significantly affect quality of life. Burch colposuspension is a widely accepted technique for surgical management of SUI and was previously considered the gold standard treatment. It was originally described as an open technique and, due to its invasive nature, was largely replaced by midurethral sling (MUS) in the late 1990s and the early 2000s. However, as mesh slings have come under scrutiny and even been withdrawn from the market in certain countries, Burch colposuspension has re-emerged as an alternative surgical option for management of SUI. The continued refinement of laparoscopic- and robotic-assisted approaches to the Burch procedure allows it to remain minimally invasive in nature.

Stress Urinary Incontinence

Stress urinary incontinence is defined as the involuntary loss of urine associated with increased intraabdominal pressure such as cough, sneeze, or physical exertion [1]. Surgical correction of SUI is aimed at stabilizing the bladder neck and urethra and increasing the outlet resistance of the urethra. Burch colposuspension is retropubic urethral suspension that stabilizes the urethra and bladder neck by fixing them between the anterior abdominal wall and the posterior aspect of the pubic bone. This has been shown to improve the urethral pressure during elevations in intraabdominal pressure [2]. Urethral length and resting urethral pressure by urodynamic assessment remain unchanged, suggesting that the intrinsic function of the urethral is not changed by retropubic colposuspension [2].

History of Burch Colposuspension

Burch colposuspension was first described in 1961 by Dr. John Burch who was a revered professor at Vanderbilt Medical School, a former dean of the medical school and chairman of Vanderbilt Obstetrics and Gynecology Department,

and a prolific gynecologic surgeon and researcher [3] (photo of Burch?). Burch originally developed this suspension procedure as a modification to the first retropubic suspension, the Marshall-Marchetti-Krantz (MMK) operation, to provide improved treatment for surgical management of stress urinary incontinence and correction of cystocele [4]. The MMK procedure, first developed in 1949 by Marshall et al., sought to address stress urinary incontinence by fixing the periurethral tissue to the periosteum of the pubis symphysis with sutures [5]. Burch found while performing the MMK procedure that the periosteum was not a stable structure to hold sutures. Initially he promoted attaching endopelvic fascia to the tendinous arch of the pelvis; however, he found similar issues with maintaining suture durability. In later iterations, he discovered the utilization of Cooper's (iliopectineal) ligament as the point of fixation for the endopelvic fascia and retropubic elevation of the bladder neck [4]. Burch's procedure historically had similar cure rates for SUI as the MMK procedure, ranging from 65% to 91%, at 2–7 years follow-up [6], but without running the risk of osteitis pubis (0.7%) seen in MMK complications [7, 8]. Eventually, the International Consultation on Incontinence Committee determined in 2009 that there was no evidence to continue MMK procedure because of potentially harmful infection risk [9]. In 1978, the Burch procedure was further modified by Dr. Emil A. Tanagho to its current technique [10]. Adjustments included placing paravaginal sutures further lateral to the bladder neck (2 cm) in the endopelvic fascia to minimize injury to neurovascular tissue adjacent to the urethra and looser approximation of sutures from vaginal tissue to Cooper's ligament by leaving a 2–4 cm bridge to avoid overlifting the bladder neck which ultimately could cause bladder neck obstruction and urinary retention [3, 8].

In 1991, the first laparoscopic Burch procedures were performed by Vancaillie and Schuessler in response to trends toward minimally invasive surgery to achieve shorter hospital stays, less pain and morbidity, and faster overall recovery [8, 11]. Although initial studies in the early 2000s proved difficult for laparoscopic approach due to high learning curve and trends toward higher complication rates and longer operative times [9, 12], outcomes have improved for laparoscopy with similar objective cure rates to open approach up to 5 years follow-up with the additional benefits of reduced blood loss, improvement in postoperative pain, faster discharge from hospital, and overall association with minimally invasive surgery [13, 14]. Not long after the first laparoscopic Burch procedure, the earliest mention of robotic-assisted Burch colposuspension was cited in a 1995 paper as a part of a feasibility study of 17 urologic laparoscopic procedures that were performed with the use of one or two robotic arms as a substitute for surgical assistants [15]. A complete robotic-assisted Burch procedure was first reported in 2007 by Khan et al. [16] in a paper of two case reports. Another minimally invasive variant of the Burch procedure proposed by Lind et al. in 2004 advocated the use of 1.5–2.5 cm Pfannenstiel mini-incision technique under spinal anesthesia and a suturing device to allow suture passage and retrieval in one motion [17].

Burch colposuspension was considered the gold standard surgical treatment of stress urinary incontinence until the urethral sling gained widespread acceptance. Transvaginal tape was first described in 1995 by Ulmsten and Petros [18], and the first midurethral sling was approved by the FDA in 1998 [19]. Since then, midurethral slings have become the dominant form of surgical treatment for SUI over the last 20 years, accounting for 80% of surgical corrections in 2009 [19]. However, negative publicity toward synthetic mesh for any procedure after the 2011 FDA warning of complications from transvaginal mesh for surgical treatment of pelvic organ prolapse [20] has kept Burch procedure as a relevant alternative option for treatment of SUI for patients who have failed a prior incontinence procedure and decline mesh implantation or where suburethral mesh slings are not available.

Surgical Technique

The iliopectineal line is contained within the retropubic space. Therefore, understanding the anatomy of the retropubic space is critical to performing a Burch procedure safely. The retropubic space, also known as the space of Retzius, is bordered by the pubic bone anteriorly and the bladder posteriorly. It is laterally bounded by the obturator internus muscle, levator muscles, and the arcus tendineus fascia pelvis. The space contains several nerves and vascular structures. The iliopectineal ligament runs along the superior aspect of the ischiopubic rami bilaterally. The obturator canal, containing the obturator neurovascular bundle, is located 5–6 cm from the pubic symphysis and 1–2 cm inferior to the iliopectineal line. Lateral to the proximal bladder neck lies a plexus of veins called the veins of Santorini as well as nerves that innervate the urethra and bladder. Familiarity with these structures is paramount to the placement of Burch sutures through the periurethral fascia and the iliopectineal line accurately and safely.

Laparoscopic and robotic Burch procedure is initiated with identification of the bladder. This is typically performed by backfilling the bladder with at least 200 mL of fluid in order to identify the site of entry into the retropubic space. Once this is performed, the medial umbilical ligaments are identified, and a transverse incision is created in the anterior abdominal wall peritoneum about 2–3 cm above the edge of the bladder to enter the retropubic space. Staying medial to the medial umbilical ligaments avoids injury to the inferior epigastric vessels, which course laterally. Pneumodissection from the insufflated abdomen facilitates the opening of the retropubic space. The bladder is reflected inferiorly by dissecting through the adventitial tissue of this area with careful attention to hemostasis. Dissection should be carried out in the midline toward the pubic symphysis. Once the pubic bone is identified, dissection is continued laterally toward the obturator internus muscles. Cooper's ligament is cleared off with mostly blunt dissection. Dissection in the retropubic space is continued caudally through the adventitial tissue to expose the periurethral tissue. Overlying adipose tissue is then cleared off bluntly, ideally while an assistant elevates the periurethral tissue on either side of the Foley catheter balloon to expose the glistening white periurethral fascia. Upward periurethral pressure with a vaginal hand or instrument is used to identify the location of Burch sutures at the proximal urethral and bladder neck. A suture is placed through the ligament, then through the periurethral tissue 1–2 cm lateral to the proximal urethral, and then back through the ligament. The suture is then cut and held. A second suture is placed in a similar fashion through the ligament, then just lateral to the bladder neck, and back through the ligament. This is repeated on the contralateral side. Placement of the periurethral sutures is performed with an assistant hand in the vagina with the index and middle fingers straddling the urethra. In some cases a sterile thimble or other instrument has been described to protect the surgeons finger. The Foley balloon is palpated in order to identify the bladder neck. Once all four sutures are placed, the sutures are tied down such to stabilize the urethra. Typically permanent suture is used. Both monofilament and polyfilament sutures have been described. The authors utilize No. 0 permanent Prolene or Gore-Tex suture on an SH needle. The sutures are tied leaving a suture bridge such that the urethral is elevated toward but not all the way to Cooper's ligament. Postoperatively, cystourethroscopy is performed to assess integrity of the bladder and urethra. A voiding trial is recommended postoperatively to evaluate for postoperative urinary retention.

Outcomes of Burch Colposuspension

From the time when Burch colposuspension was first described in 1961, there have been a plethora of observational and comparative studies published in the literature regarding outcomes for the procedure. The most current Cochrane review from 2017 of 55 trials involving a total of 5417 women reported overall continence rate of 85–90% 1 year after open retropubic colposuspension with a decline to about 70% continence rate 5 years postoperatively [21] and similar success rates of about 65–70% continence after 20 years follow-up [22]. This stability in success makes Burch colposuspension one of the most effective long-term surgical options for stress urinary incontinence.

Since the surgical paradigm shifted toward minimally invasive techniques, many trials have been conducted comparing laparoscopic to open approach for Burch procedure. The initial Cochrane review in 2002 demonstrated similar subjective but poorer objective outcomes of laparoscopic compared to open Burch procedure likely secondary to surgical inexperience and longer operative times associated with laparoscopy [12]. Some early studies described several modifications that affected postoperative continence outcomes in laparoscopic cases; laparoscopic clips and mesh and staples for fixation of periurethral tissue were trialed to offer easier, more accessible laparoscopic option to surgeons, yes both were found to be inferior to suture-based repairs [14, 23, 24]. One study also showed that two laparoscopic sutures on each paravaginal side were more effective than placement of only one suture per side from a curative standpoint and risk of voiding dysfunction [8, 25]. Limited studies have also been performed comparing extraperitoneal laparoscopy to transperitoneal approach with overall nonsignificant differences in short-term cure rates [26, 27].

The most recent 2019 Cochrane review of 13 trials concluded, with high-quality evidence, similar subjective and objective cure rates between laparoscopic colposuspension with sutures and open colposuspension within short-term follow-up of 18 months (RR 1.04, 95% CI 0.99–1.08, 755 women; 6 trials). Two long-term trials that followed patients for 3–5 years and 2 years respectively reported no difference in subjective or objective cure rates between laparoscopic and open colposuspension [13, 28]. Although laparoscopic colposuspension took significantly longer to perform compared to open surgery, women reported significantly less pain with fewer postoperative analgesia needs, lower estimated blood loss, shorter duration of catheterization, and shorter hospital stays with faster return to normal activity level [29]. (Dumville et al.'s LSC approach is not cost-effective compared to open approach during the first 6 months, but it may be at 24 months.) Given the overall similar subjective and objective cure rates between open and minimally invasive approach to Burch colposuspension, it is recommended that surgeons should perform the procedure with which they feel most comfortable.

There are limited studies assessing the effectiveness of robotic-assisted Burch colposuspension. Although the cost to perform a Burch procedure robotically is significant, this approach may be worthwhile in the setting of performing concomitant robotic surgery [8]. A small case study of 20 individuals compared robotic-assisted Burch procedure during robotic hysterectomy to open colposuspension with abdominal hysterectomy and noted similar incontinence subjective cure rates at 6 months postoperatively, though data may be confounding by concurrent hysterectomy [30]. While robotic-assisted approach for Burch colposuspension has observed similar treatment success rates (85%) with a short mean follow-up (134 days) in a case series [31], no comparative studies between robotic and laparoscopic approach exist.

Numerous studies have compared laparoscopic Burch colposuspension with tension-free vaginal tape (TVT), though comparisons can be challenging due to variation of outcome measures and nonstandard definition of continence. In Ward and Hilton's 2008 seminal randomized controlled trial comparing TVT to open colposuspension, the study did not detect a significant difference between TVT and colposuspension for cure of stress incontinence at 5 years follow-up, and both groups maintained subjective cure rates as well and sustained improvement in quality of life. The study did demonstrate an increase in enterocele and rectocele in the colposuspension group and several cases of tape erosion in the TVT group [32]. A systematic review and meta-analysis of multiple randomized controlled trials compared urethral slings to various operative techniques of laparoscopic Burch colposuspension (i.e., suture, mesh) and found general favorability toward midurethral slings for "any definition of continence" but did not meet statistical significance [33]. However, the improved subjective and objective cure rates in urethral slings may be offset by increased risk of urinary tract infections, postoperative de novo urge incontinence, voiding dysfunction, and reoperation as noted in the SISTEr trial [34]. At 5-year follow-up for the SISTEr trial, more women who had a Burch retropubic colposuspension underwent retreatment for stress urinary incontinence compared to fascial sling patients, 12% versus 2%, $P < 0.0001$ [35].

Paraiso et al. performed a randomized controlled trial comparing laparoscopic Burch with sutures to TVT and noted objective and subjective higher incontinence rates at 1 year and longer operative times for Burch compared to TVT; however, the 4–8 year follow-up of this study demonstrated similar long-term efficacies between the two procedures (58% vs. 48% respectively reported any incontinence symptoms) [36, 37]. In the 2019 Cochrane review of 4 trials (256 women), a little difference was noted between laparoscopic colposuspension using sutures and TVT for subjective cure within 18 months, though evidence was low-quality data. Summary from the Cochrane review also deduced a similar risk of perioperative complications between the two procedures and a little difference in terms of developing de novo detrusor overactivity or voiding dysfunction; however, conclusions are uncertain due to a wide confidence intervals among studies [29]. TVT is associated with shorter operating times, hospital stays, and time to returning to normal activities [38].

Laparoscopic Burch colposuspension has demonstrated to be an effective and safe secondary treatment for stress urinary incontinence or intrinsic sphincter deficiency after failed incontinence surgery with objective cure rates ranging from 54.5% to 90% (24 and 18 months) and subjective cure rates up to 92.9% [39, 40]. Though TVT procedures are more commonly performed in the context of failed anti-incontinence procedures, when a revision or reoperation is required due to prior mesh-related complications, Burch colposuspension or fascial sling would be favorable options [41]. One randomized controlled trial demonstrated similar effectiveness at 6 months between laparoscopic Burch colposuspension and TVT for secondary surgical management [42]. Amaye-Obu and Drutz did note however that the cure rate of open colposuspension declines to 81%, 25%, and 0% as the numbers of previous anti-incontinence operations increased to 1, 2, and 3, respectively. According to this study, one should probably avoid colposuspension if the patient has received two or more anti-incontinence surgeries [43]. No studies have yet compared Burch colposuspension with other incontinence surgery as salvage procedures [41].

Complications

As with any type of surgery, the Burch procedure can be associated with risks and complications. The main intraoperative complications seen include bleeding or urinary tract injuries. It is important for surgeons to be comfortable with the retropubic space and knowledgeable about the vascular anatomy. Bleeding is typically caused from injury to paravaginal veins (plexus of Santorini) within the adipose tissue overlying the endopelvic fascia or injury to the obturator or anomalous obturator vessels that can lead to hemorrhage or hematoma [8]. Blood transfusion rates have been quoted in small studies to be about 0.7–3% for open colposuspension, and general consensus is an overall lower risk of bleeding with laparoscopic Burch colposuspension [8, 13]. Bladder injuries can range from 0.4% to 9.6% (depending on prior surgical history and are usually incurred from a suture placement in the bladder which can simply be removed and replaced). Ureteral injury is rarer given the location of surgery. It is recommended to perform universal cystoscopy after Burch colposuspension to best identify bladder or ureteral kinking injury. Both bleeding and bladder injury can be reduced with careful and diligent dissection of the bladder edge and endopelvic fascia.

With regard to postoperative complications, rates of urinary tract infection range from 4 to 40%, and wound infections range from 4% to 10.8%. It is not uncommon to have temporary urinary retention with about 22% of patients that experience dysfunction postoperatively, though retention typically resolves spontaneously with risk of long-term catheterization (>1 month) usually <3% in most studies [8, 22]. De novo detrusor overactivity can occur (5–27%), but the overall incidence of voiding dysfunction is less

compared to TVT, for which retention can be very common and should be factored into preoperative counseling [38]. Reports of dyspareunia or pelvic pain have also been reported. Longer-term complications of Burch colposuspension include its association with pelvic organ prolapse formation with rectocele formation documented in about 11–25% and enterocele in 4–10% of patients at 10–20 years follow-up [22, 38].

Conclusion

Burch colposuspension is a widely accepted surgical technique for management of stress incontinence. While the Burch procedure has been largely replaced by midurethral sling as the gold standard surgery, it has re-emerged as an alternative option for women who are not candidates for MUS or prefer to avoid mesh or for surgeons in countries in which mesh products have been completely removed from the market.

References

1. Haylen BT, de Ridder D, Freeman RM, Swift SE, Berghmans B, Lee J, et al. An International Urogynecological Association (IUGA)/International Continence Society (ICS) joint report on the terminology for female pelvic floor dysfunction. Int Urogynecol J. 2010;21(1):5–26.
2. Penttinen J, Lindholm EL, Käär K, Kauppila A. Successful colposuspension in stress urinary incontinence reduces bladder neck mobility and increases pressure transmission to the urethra. Arch Gynecol Obstet. 1989;244(4):233–8.
3. Marquini GV, Bella Z, Sartori MGF. Burch procedure: a historical perspective. Rev Bras Ginecol Obstet. 2022;44(5):511–518. https://doi.org/10.1055/s-0042-1744312
4. Burch JC. Urethrovaginal fixation to Cooper's ligament for correction of stress incontinence, cystocele, and prolapse. Am J Obstet Gynecol. 1961;81:281–90.
5. Marshall VF, Marchetti AA, Krantz KE. The correction of stress incontinence by simple vesicourethral suspension. Surg Gynecol Obstet. 1949;88(4):509–18.
6. Colombo M, Scalambrino S, Maggioni A, Milani R. Burch colposuspension versus modified Marshall-Marchetti-Krantz urethropexy for primary genuine

stress urinary incontinence: a prospective, randomized clinical trial. Am J Obstet Gynecol. 1994;171(6):1573–9.

7. Kammerer-Doak DN, Cornella JL, Magrina JF, Stanhope CR, Smilack J. Osteitis pubis after Marshall-Marchetti-Krantz urethropexy: a pubic osteomyelitis. Am J Obstet Gynecol. 1998;179(3 Pt 1):586–90.

8. Sohlberg EM, Elliott CS. Burch colposuspension. Urol Clin North Am. 2019;46(1):53–9.

9. Green J, Herschorn S. The contemporary role of Burch colposuspension. Curr Opin Urol. 2005;15(4):250–5.

10. Tanagho EA. Colpocystourethropexy: the way we do it. J Urol. 1976;116(6):751–3.

11. Vancaillie TG, Schuessler W. Laparoscopic bladderneck suspension. J Laparoendosc Surg. 1991;1(3):169–73.

12. Moehrer B, Ellis G, Carey M, Wilson PD. Laparoscopic colposuspension for urinary incontinence in women. Cochrane Database Syst Rev. 2002;1:Cd002239.

13. Carey MP, Goh JT, Rosamilia A, Cornish A, Gordon I, Hawthorne G, et al. Laparoscopic versus open Burch colposuspension: a randomised controlled trial. BJOG. 2006;113(9):999–1006.

14. Dean NM, Ellis G, Wilson PD, Herbison GP. Laparoscopic colposuspension for urinary incontinence in women. Cochrane Database Syst Rev. 2006;3:Cd002239.

15. Partin AW, Adams JB, Moore RG, Kavoussi LR. Complete robot-assisted laparoscopic urologic surgery: a preliminary report. J Am Coll Surg. 1995;181(6):552–7.

16. Khan MS, Challacombe B, Rose K, Dasgupta P. Robotic colposuspension: two case reports. J Endourol. 2007;21(9):1077–9.

17. Lind LR, Gunn GC, Mattox TF, Stanford EJ. Miniincisional Burch urethropexy: a less invasive method to accomplish a time-tested procedure for treatment of genuine stress incontinence. Int Urogynecol J Pelvic Floor Dysfunct. 2004;15(1):20–4. discussion 4

18. Ulmsten U, Petros P. Intravaginal slingplasty (IVS): an ambulatory surgical procedure for treatment of female urinary incontinence. Scand J Urol Nephrol. 1995;29(1):75–82.

19. Jonsson Funk M, Levin PJ, Wu JM. Trends in the surgical management of stress urinary incontinence. Obstet Gynecol. 2012;119(4):845–51.

20. Drain A, Khan A, Ohmann EL, Brucker BM, Smilen S, Rosenblum N, et al. Use of concomitant stress incontinence surgery at time of pelvic organ prolapse surgery since release of the 2011 notification on serious complications associated with transvaginal mesh. J Urol. 2017;197(4):1092–8.

21. Lapitan MCM, Cody JD, Mashayekhi A. Open retropubic colposuspension for urinary incontinence in women. Cochrane Database Syst Rev. 2017;7(7):Cd002912.

22. Alcalay M, Monga A, Stanton SL. Burch colposuspension: a 10-20 year follow up. Br J Obstet Gynaecol. 1995;102(9):740–5.

23. Zullo F, Morelli M, Russo T, Iuzzolino D, Palomba S. Two techniques of laparoscopic retropubic urethropexy. J Am Assoc Gynecol Laparosc. 2002;9(2):178–81.

24. Ankardal M, Milsom I, Stjerndahl JH, Engh ME. A three-armed randomized trial comparing open Burch colposuspension using sutures with laparoscopic colposuspension using sutures and laparoscopic colposuspension using mesh and staples in women with stress urinary incontinence. Acta Obstet Gynecol Scand. 2005;84(8):773–9.

25. Persson J, Wølner-Hanssen P. Laparoscopic Burch colposuspension for stress urinary incontinence: a randomized comparison of one or two sutures on each side of the urethra. Obstet Gynecol. 2000;95(1):151–5.

26. Wallwiener D, Grischke EM, Rimbach S, Maleika A, Bastert G. Endoscopic retropubic colposuspension: "Retziusscopy" versus laparoscopy – a reasonable enlargement of the operative spectrum in the management of recurrent stress incontinence? Endosc Surg Allied Technol. 1995;3(2–3):115–8.

27. Bulent Tiras M, Sendag F, Dilek U, Guner H. Laparoscopic burch colposuspension: comparison of effectiveness of extraperitoneal and transperitoneal techniques. Eur J Obstet Gynecol Reprod Biol. 2004;116(1):79–84.

28. Kitchener HC, Dunn G, Lawton V, Reid F, Nelson L, Smith AR. Laparoscopic versus open colposuspension – results of a prospective randomised controlled trial. BJOG. 2006;113(9):1007–13.

29. Freites J, Stewart F, Omar MI, Mashayekhi A, Agur WI. Laparoscopic colposuspension for urinary incontinence in women. Cochrane Database Syst Rev. 2019;12(12):Cd002239.

30. Ulubay M, Dede M, Öztürk M, Keskin U, Fidan U, Alanbay I, et al. Comparison of robotic-assisted and abdominal hysterectomy with Concomitant Burch Colposuspension: preliminary study. J Minim Invasive Gynecol. 2015;22(6s):S242–s3.

31. Lee TG, Unlu BS, Petruzzi VA, Borahay MA, Dursun F, Saad AF, et al. Safety and efficacy of robotic-assisted Burch for pure stress urinary incontinence: a large case series. J Obstet Gynaecol. 2021;41(5):803–6.

32. Ward KL, Hilton P. Tension-free vaginal tape versus colposuspension for primary urodynamic stress incontinence: 5-year follow up. BJOG. 2008;115(2):226–33.

33. Fusco F, Abdel-Fattah M, Chapple CR, Creta M, La Falce S, Waltregny D, et al. Updated systematic review and meta-analysis of the comparative data on colposuspensions, pubovaginal slings, and midurethral tapes in the surgical treatment of female stress urinary incontinence. Eur Urol. 2017;72(4):567–91.

34. Albo ME, Richter HE, Brubaker L, Norton P, Kraus SR, Zimmern PE, et al. Burch colposuspension versus fascial sling to reduce urinary stress incontinence. N Engl J Med. 2007;356(21):2143–55.

35. Brubaker L, Richter HE, Norton PA, Albo M, Zyczynski HM, Chai TC, et al. 5-year continence

rates, satisfaction and adverse events of burch urethropexy and fascial sling surgery for urinary incontinence. J Urol. 2012;187(4):1324–30.

36. Paraiso MF, Walters MD, Karram MM, Barber MD. Laparoscopic Burch colposuspension versus tension-free vaginal tape: a randomized trial. Obstet Gynecol. 2004;104(6):1249–58.

37. Jelovsek JE, Barber MD, Karram MM, Walters MD, Paraiso MF. Randomised trial of laparoscopic Burch colposuspension versus tension-free vaginal tape: long-term follow up. BJOG. 2008;115(2):219–25. discussion 25

38. Veit-Rubin N, Dubuisson J, Ford A, Dubuisson JB, Mourad S, Digesu A. Burch colposuspension. Neurourol Urodyn. 2019;38(2):553–62.

39. Moore RD, Speights SE, Miklos JR. Laparoscopic Burch colposuspension for recurrent stress urinary incontinence. J Am Assoc Gynecol Laparosc. 2001;8(3):389–92.

40. De Cuyper EM, Ismail R, Maher CF. Laparoscopic Burch colposuspension after failed sub-urethral tape procedures: a retrospective audit. Int Urogynecol J Pelvic Floor Dysfunct. 2008;19(5):681–5.

41. Kwon J, Kim Y, Kim DY. Second-line surgical management after midurethral sling failure. Int Neurourol J. 2021;25(2):111–8.

42. Laparoscopic colposuspension or tension-free vaginal tape for recurrent stress urinary incontinence and/or intrinsic sphincter deficiency-a randomised controlled trial. Neurourol Urodyn 2004;23(5–6):433.

43. Amaye-Obu FA, Drutz HP. Surgical management of recurrent stress urinary incontinence: a 12-year experience. Am J Obstet Gynecol. 1999;181(6):1296–307. discussion 307–9

Management of Urinary Incontinence in the Female Neurologic Patient

26

Oluwarotimi S. Nettey, Katherine E. Fero, and Ja-Hong Kim

Contents

Introduction	458
Neurologic Control of Micturition	459
Lower Urinary Tract Dysfunction After Nervous System Damage	459
Suprapontine Lesions	459
Suprasacral Cord Lesions	459
Sacral Lesions	461
Epidemiology	461
Suprapontine Lesions	461
Suprasacral Lesions	463
Sacral and Peripheral Nervous System Lesions	464
Disseminated Central Disease: Multiple Sclerosis	465
Evaluation of the Female Neurologic Patient	465
History	465
Questionnaires	465
Physical Examination	466
Diagnostic Workup	466
Surveillance	468
Management	468
Reversible Causes of Incontinence	469

O. S. Nettey
Scott Department of Urology, Baylor College of Medicine,
Houston, Texas, USA

K. E. Fero
Department of Urology, David Geffen School of Medicine
at UCLA, Los Angeles, CA, USA

J.-H. Kim (✉)
Division of Pelvic Medicine and Reconstructive Surgery,
David Geffen School of Medicine at UCLA, Los Angeles,
CA, USA

Department of Urology, David Geffen School of Medicine
at UCLA, Los Angeles, CA, USA
e-mail: jhkim@mednet.ucla.edu

© Springer Nature Switzerland AG 2023
F. E. Martins et al. (eds.), *Female Genitourinary and Pelvic Floor Reconstruction*,
https://doi.org/10.1007/978-3-031-19598-3_27

Management of Storage Dysfunction 469
The Bladder Outlet 474
Combined Storage and Emptying Disorders 479
Other Considerations 479

Conclusions 481

Cross-References 482

References 482

Abstract

The dual functions of the bladder are low-pressure storage of urine and volitional emptying. This is accomplished in a neurologically intact individual via a complex interplay of somatic, sympathetic, and parasympathetic pathways. There are a number of neurologic conditions – congenital and acquired – that have the potential to disrupt this coordinated control of micturition. Of particular interest here is a discussion of urinary continence. Unintended, non-volitional leakage of urine has significant quality-of-life implications and can also put individuals at risk of complications related to the threat to the skin and soft tissue due to moisture. As is the case in the general population, patients with neurologic etiologies of their voiding dysfunction can present with either stress incontinence, or symptoms related to overactive bladder (detrusor instability), or both. Symptomatology and presentation are characteristically predicted by the level of the neurologic lesion and its extent; however, every patient requires an individualized approach to management given each person's unique non-urologic clinical, functional, and social context. A comprehensive management approach, which may change over time as a patient's disease state changes, will allow for patient-centered care in the management of urinary incontinence in the female neurologic patient.

Keywords

Neurogenic bladder · Neurogenic lower urinary tract dysfunction · Female · Urinary incontinence

Introduction

Micturition is dependent on the coordinated interplay of neuromuscular events resulting in voiding in a manner that is volitional and socially appropriate and upholds desired quality of life. Neurogenic lower urinary tract dysfunction (NLUTD) and neurogenic bladder (NGB) encompass a spectrum of disorders and/or injuries resulting in end organ bladder and lower urinary tract dysfunction as a sequela of neurologic disease and is commonly encountered by urologists [1]. Acquired conditions including multiple sclerosis (MS), spinal cord injury (SCI), transverse myelitis, and Parkinson's disease (PD), as well as congenital malformations of the vertebrae and spinal cord such as spina bifida/myelomeningocele (SB/MM), fall under this umbrella [2]. The site of the neurologic injury or insult generally determines the pattern of lower urinary tract dysfunction and patient symptoms.

Complications arising from neurogenic bladder and associated lower urinary tract dysfunction (LUTD) include urinary incontinence; recurrent urinary tract infections (UTI), which can lead to renal scarring and loss of function; urinary retention; and elevated bladder pressures which similarly result in renal failure [3–5]. Furthermore, women with NLUTD remain vulnerable to the same risk factors for urinary incontinence as neurologically intact women such as birth trauma, parity, and estrogen loss with advancing age. These patients pose unique management considerations which the modern-day urologist should be prepared to address with a combination of behavioral, pharmacologic, and surgical interventions.

Neurologic Control of Micturition

Control of voiding and storage is complex and modulated by parasympathetic, sympathetic, and somatic pathways working in concert to effect the storage function of the bladder (detrusor smooth muscle), internal sphincter (bladder neck), and external striated sphincter function of the urethra. During the storage or continence phase, the low pressure inside the bladder allows the ureters to fill the bladder continuously with urine produced by the kidneys, and the urethra remains closed even during stressful events. Sympathetic-mediated inhibition of the detrusor promotes low-pressure bladder storage [6]. The urinary sphincter is composed of both autonomic and somatic elements which help to mediate its tonicity. The internal urinary sphincter is composed of smooth muscle fibers controlled by hypogastric sympathetic postganglionic nerve fibers which innervate the bladder neck and a portion of the urethra proximal to the mid-urethra. The external urinary sphincter is located at the level of the mid-urethra and under the influence of somatic control through pudendal nerve fibers. Activation of sympathetic and pudendal nerve fibers during bladder filling and storage results in the contraction of the internal and external sphincter to maintain continence, commonly known as the guarding reflex. Female continence is further influenced by a complex network of subepithelial tissue within the pelvic floor ligaments and striated muscle structures innervated by somatic pudendal nerve fibers. The pelvic floor musculature contributes to continence via direct compression of the urethra against the anterior vaginal wall.

Voiding is initiated by conscious decision, requiring higher cortical elements, and is determined by the perceived state of bladder fullness and an assessment of the social appropriateness of doing so. The detrusor contracts in response to parasympathetic stimulation, and the sphincters (external and internal), along with the pelvic floor, relax resulting in bladder emptying [7]. Coordination of each of these individual neuromuscular components is essential for successful and synergistic voiding. Neurologic injury consequently results in impairment of bladder storage mechanisms and voiding or loss of coordination in one or more of these elements.

Lower Urinary Tract Dysfunction After Nervous System Damage

Lesions of the nervous system, both central and peripheral, result in lower urinary tract dysfunction that is influenced by the location and extent of the lesion (Fig. 1) [7].

The sixth International Consultation on Incontinence (ICI) proposed a classification system for patients with neurogenic urinary incontinence using four groups [8]. Group 1 includes patients with peripheral lesions, for example, following a major pelvic surgery such as abdominal hysterectomy, and lesions of the cauda equina (not shown in Fig. 1). Group 2 includes patients with spinal cord lesions involving the sacral micturition center. Group 3 includes patients with spinal cord lesions situated above the sacrum (infrapontine-suprasacral). Group 4 includes patients with central brain and brain stem lesions [8].

Suprapontine Lesions

Suprapontine and higher cortical lesions affect the storage phase of micturition resulting in reduced bladder capacity, detrusor overactivity, and hyperreflexia. Clinically, the patient may have varying degrees of urgency, frequency, nocturia, and urgency urinary incontinence. On urodynamic studies these patients may have detrusor overactivity and detrusor overactivity incontinence.

Suprasacral Cord Lesions

Acute spinal cord injury is characterized by an initial phase of spinal shock during which the detrusor is hypocontractile or acontractile resulting in poor bladder emptying. Duration of this phase varies but thought to last about 6 weeks; however, reports up to 2 years exist, and it precedes the onset of detrusor overactivity. Recovery

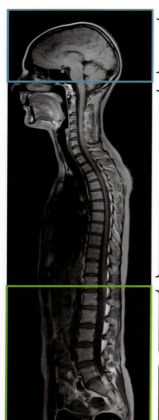
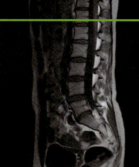

Suprapontine lesion
- **History:** predominantly storage symptoms
- **Ultrasound:** insignificant PVR urine volume
- **Urodynamics:** detrusor overactivity

Normo-active

Spinal (infrapontine–suprasacral) lesion
- **History:** both storage and voiding symptoms
- **Ultrasound:** PVR urine volume usually raised
- **Urodynamics:** detrusor overactivity, detrusor–sphincter dyssynergia

Overactive

Sacral/infrasacral lesion
- **History:** predominantly voiding symptoms
- **Ultrasound:** PVR urine volume raised
- **Urodynamics:** hypocontractile or acontractile detrusor

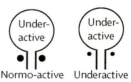
Normo-active   Underactive

Fig. 1 The pattern of lower urinary tract dysfunction is determined by the site of neurologic insult. PVR, post-void residual. (Obtained with permission from Elsevier)

from spinal shock is manifested by the return of reflex bladder activity and deep tendon reflexes in the lower extremities. Detrusor overactivity from spinal cord injury results from increased sensitization of afferent C-fibers which drive involuntary detrusor contractions emerging from the sacral reflex arc.

Injury to the suprasacral spinal cord also results in loss of coordinated activation of the detrusor and inhibition of the urethral sphincter during voiding. Instead, there is a simultaneous contraction of the detrusor and urethral sphincter, a condition known as detrusor-sphincter dyssynergia (DSD). DSD is a form of voiding phase dysfunction that results in incomplete bladder emptying and high pressures in the bladder. High intravesical pressures can lead to end-stage morphological changes in the bladder such as trabeculations, sacculations, diverticula, and fibrosis and can ultimately be transmitted to the upper urinary tract resulting in renal failure.

A study by McGuire et al. [9] suggested that bladder leakage at detrusor pressures greater than 40 cmH$_2$0 is indicative of increased risk of upper tract deterioration; however, various studies have challenged the generalizability of these findings to other neurologic conditions. Patients with spinal cord injury or neural tube defects including spina bifida have a substantially increased risk of renal failure compared with the general population [4]. In contrast, the prevalence of upper urinary tract damage and renal failure is low in patients with slowly progressive nontraumatic neurologic disorders, such as multiple sclerosis and Parkinson's disease, for unclear reasons [4].

Sacral Lesions

Damage to the sacral cord results in voiding phase dysfunction associated with acontractile detrusor activity and a fixed, open, non-relaxing urethral sphincter.

Epidemiology

Prevalence estimates of various neurourological disorders vary globally and in the general population. Table 1 describes typical lower urinary tract symptoms and urodynamic findings associated with specific neurologic disorders, some of which are detailed below [10].

Suprapontine Lesions

Cerebrovascular Accidents (CVA)

In the United States, approximately 795,000 people experience a CVA every year with 28–79% having symptoms of urinary incontinence post-CVA. Up to 15% of patients remain incontinent one-year post-stroke; hence, urinary incontinence remains the greatest prognostic marker of stroke severity and functional outcome [11]. The most frequent urinary symptom is nocturia (76%) followed by urgency (70%) and daytime frequency (59%) [11].

Dementia

Globally, dementias affect over 6% of adults over 65 [10]. Incontinence is often a prominent symptom in the late stages of dementia, but the timing varies based on underlying disease etiology. Incontinence tends to occur early in normal-pressure hydrocephalus, dementia with Lewy bodies, vascular dementia, and frontotemporal dementia, whereas generally it occurs late in the course of Alzheimer's disease or Parkinson's disease with dementia. Furthermore, there is a threefold increased frequency of incontinence in geriatric patients with dementia compared to those without.

Parkinson's Disease (PD)

The most common neurodegenerative motor disorder, PD, presents with tremor, rigidity, bradykinesia/akinesia, and postural instability. Nonmotor symptoms include cognitive impairment as well as lower urinary tract symptoms. It is associated with neurogenic detrusor overactivity (70%) and underactive bladder (50%). Bladder symptoms are typically not responsive to levodopa, a dopaminergic agent and primary mainstay of PD treatment. Novel interventions, such as deep brain stimulation, are expected to improve bladder dysfunction in patients with PD however remain investigational.

PD differs from multiple system atrophy (MSA), another progressive neurodegenerative condition characterized by progressive autonomic dysfunction, Parkinsonian features, and cerebellar and pyramidal symptoms. Patients have urinary urge incontinence or retention, orthostatic hypotension, inspiratory stridor, motor rigidity, and gait instability. No specific treatment for MSA exists; however, patients are managed based on their symptoms. Patients with MSA suffer from incontinence resulting from detrusor overactivity and external sphincter weakness and have an open bladder neck on videourodynamics.

Cerebral Palsy

Cerebral palsy is an umbrella designation referring to conditions affecting the cerebral motor cortex resulting in problems with movement, balance, and posture. Patients with cerebral palsy have abnormal development of the cerebral motor cortex in utero and may have sustained an anoxic insult in the peripartum period. Over 55% of these patients have lower urinary tract symptoms. Storage symptoms tend to be more prevalent; however, patients with voiding phase dysfunction and pelvic floor overactivity are more prone to progress to upper urinary tract deterioration as adults. Spastic subtypes of cerebral palsy are associated with more severe

Table 1 Neurologic conditions grouped by location. Disease prevalence, symptoms, and urodynamic findings are described

Suprapontine lesions		
Neurologic disease	Lower urinary tract symptoms	Urodynamics study (UDS) findings
Cerebrovascular accident (stroke) [11, 18]	Nocturia, overactive bladder, urge urinary incontinence 57–83% of symptoms occur within 1 month post-stroke 71–80% achieve spontaneous recovery at 6 months Persistent urinary symptoms correlate to poor prognosis	Detrusor overactivity
Dementias: Alzheimer's disease (80%) Vascular dementia (10%) Others (10%)	Overactive bladder, urge urinary incontinence	Detrusor overactivity
Parkinsonian syndrome [19, 20] Idiopathic Parkinson's disease (IPD 75–80%) Non-IPD (18%): multiple system atrophy (MSA), Lewy body dementia, secondary Parkinson's (2%), corticobasal degeneration, progressive supranuclear palsy	Urgency, nocturia Urinary symptoms affect 50% at disease onset; early presentation associated with worse disease progression	Impaired detrusor contractility + PVR >150 ml distinguishes MSA from IPD MSA patients exhibit inhibited external sphincter relaxation and bladder neck dysfunction during filling and DSD during voiding
Brain tumors	Urge urinary incontinence associated with frontal lobe tumors	Lacking data
Cerebral palsy [12]	Urge urinary incontinence 46% of patients with cerebral palsy suffer from urgency urinary incontinence	Neurogenic detrusor overactivity (59%), DSD (11%) 85% of patients have abnormal urodynamic studies 2.5% progress to upper tract deterioration
Traumatic brain injury [21]	44% storage dysfunction, 38% voiding dysfunction Storage dysfunction associated with poor functional outcome	60% urodynamic abnormalities, typically associated with motor deficits
Normal-pressure hydrocephalus [22]	Triad of gait and cognitive disturbance and urinary incontinence Urgency urinary incontinence affects >98% of patients Storage dysfunction improved after cerebrospinal fluid shunt surgery	Detrusor overactivity (77%), detrusor underactivity (75%) Elevated post-void residual or reduced peak flow rate (60%)
Suprasacral spinal cord lesions		
Spinal cord injury (SCI) [23]	Urinary retention, overflow incontinence during spinal shock Overactive bladder	Neurogenic detrusor overactivity Detrusor sphincter dyssynergia (95%), detrusor underactivity (83%) depending on level of lesion
Spina bifida/myelomeningocele [24]	Bladder function is impaired in as many as 96% of SB patients Over 50% of patients are incontinent	Detrusor overactivity, detrusor underactivity or impaired bladder compliance Fixed external urethral sphincter depending on level or cord involvement or detrusor sphincter dyssynergia

(continued)

26 Management of Urinary Incontinence in the Female Neurologic Patient

Table 1 (continued)

Suprapontine lesions		
Neurologic disease	Lower urinary tract symptoms	Urodynamics study (UDS) findings
Peripheral nervous system lesions		
Lumbar spine degenerative disease Disc prolapse [25] Lumbar stenosis	Overactive bladder	Acontractile detrusor in 26%, 83% with detrusor underactivity Elevated post-void residual Patients with Tarlov cysts experience early filling sensation (70%), neurogenic detrusor overactivity (33/%), stress urinary incontinence (33%)
Iatrogenic pelvic nerve lesions (or injury) Rectal cancer Cervical cancer Endometriosis, radical hysterectomy surgeries	50% rate of urinary retention after abdominoperineal resection 10–30% voiding dysfunction after total mesorectal excision	Elevated post-void residual Detrusor underactivity or atony
Peripheral neuropathy Diabetes [14] Others: alcohol abuse, lumbosacral zona and genital herpes, Guillain-Barre syndrome	Urgency, frequency, urgency urinary incontinence Reduced bladder sensation Incomplete bladder emptying Overflow incontinence	Hyposensitive during filling and detrusor underactivity Elevated post-void residual
Disseminated central disease		
Multiple sclerosis (MS) [26]	Urgency, frequency, urgency incontinence, urinary retention, stranguria 10% of MS patients present with voiding dysfunction at disease onset; 75% of patients will develop it after 10 years of MS	Detrusor overactivity (86%), DSD (35–43%) Detrusor underactivity (25%) No UDS findings (10%) Elevated post-void residual

functional and cognitive impairment and tend to have the worst urinary outcomes [12].

Suprasacral Lesions

Spinal Cord Injury (SCI)

According to the National Spinal Cord Injury Statistical Center [13], there are approximately 54 cases per one million people in the United States, which equals about 17,900 new SCI cases each year. SCI patients are predominantly male, and age of peak incidence occurs in patients younger than 30 years old. Traffic accidents are typically the most common cause of SCI, followed by falls in the elderly. Traumatic SCI results in loss of sensation, motor ability, and autonomic function. The majority of patients with a SCI have some degree of NLUTD with greater than 80% requiring use of a catheter

(e.g., condom, intermittent, indwelling) post-injury. The epidemiology of nontraumatic spinal cord diseases is less known; however, it includes etiologies such as spinal stenosis, tumor compression, vascular ischemia, and infections. There is emerging data that the incidence of nontraumatic manifestations may in fact be higher than traumatic insults, a number that is sure to rise with an increasingly aging population.

In the initial post-injury phase, spinal shock occurs resulting in an atonic, areflexic detrusor with preserved urethral sphincter tone. Patients present with urinary retention and overflow incontinence typically managed with catheter decompression. The initial phase is of variable duration with reports indicating that it can last up to 2 years post-injury. Following recovery from spinal shock, as spinal reflexes return, patients experience detrusor overactivity and dyssynergistic voiding due to a lack of coordination between the urethral sphincter and detrusor. Sustained high intravesical pressures can result; hence, these patients are at the greatest risk for upper tract damage.

SCI at or above the sixth thoracic (T6) spinal cord segment often results in autonomic dysreflexia (AD). AD is precipitated by noxious visceral or somatic stimulation below the level of injury. Common triggers include overdistension of the bowel or bladder, urinary tract infections, sexual activity, and lower urinary tract procedures. This potentially life-threatening disorder is characterized by >20 mm Hg increase in blood pressure above baseline, headache, flushing, piloerection, stuffy nose, sweating above the level of the lesion, vasoconstriction below the level of the lesion, and dysrhythmias. AD is treated with vasoactive drugs intended to stymie the acute hypertensive crises rather than preventing them from occurring.

Spina Bifida/Myelomeningocele (SB/MM)

Over 90% of children with spina bifida have lower urinary tract symptoms; however, the level of the lesion does not always correlate well with urodynamic findings. Symptoms usually start in infancy or childhood, although occasionally they are delayed until adulthood and present as occult tethered cord. Videourodynamic studies (VUDS) can identify a variety of features, such as detrusor overactivity, detrusor underactivity, or low compliance with poor contractility. Findings at the bladder outlet include DSD or a static or fixed external urethral sphincter. Young patients with sudden-onset severe urinary incontinence should be worked up for spinal cord tethering with a lumbosacral MRI and monitored regularly by urologists, given the increased risk of developing upper urinary tract complications [7].

Sacral and Peripheral Nervous System Lesions

Lower motor neuron injury in patients with sacral lesions or peripheral neuropathy results in reduced or absent detrusor contractions. Patients report reduced sensation of bladder fullness, inability to initiate micturition voluntarily, and bladder distension, to the point of overflow incontinence. However, in a subset of patients, there might be detrusor overactivity.

Diabetes

34.2 million Americans, or 10.5% of the total population, had diabetes in 2018. Globally, the prevalence of pharmacologically managed diabetes is 8.3%. Up to 80% of diabetics experience some type of lower urinary tract complication during their lifetime. Diabetic cystopathy is described as a triad of decreased bladder sensation, increased bladder capacity, and poor bladder emptying; however, emerging data points to prevalence of overactive bladder symptoms in these patients (22.5%) and urinary incontinence (48.0%) [14, 15]. Diabetic cystopathy is a two-stage process: In the early compensated stage, storage problems with a urodynamic finding of overactive bladder dominate. In the later decompensated stage, voiding dysfunction with urinary retention and urodynamic finding of atonic bladder are characteristic.

Lumbar Disc Herniation

Up to 40% of patients with lumbar disc disease have abnormal urodynamic testing. The most common finding is detrusor areflexia; however, detrusor overactivity related to early nerve root stretch injury has been reported.

Cauda Equina Syndrome (CES)

CES is most commonly caused by lumbar disc herniation but can also be related to malignancy. CES manifests as bilateral sacral, buttock, perineal, and posterior leg pain, tingling, and numbness as well as urinary retention and overflow urinary incontinence, with variable motor and sensory involvement of the lower extremities. Progressive neurologic symptoms may necessitate acute surgical intervention. Surgical treatment within 48 hours of onset has a 70% probability that lost bladder function may be recovered at 2 years compared to 40% seen with delayed care [16].

Disseminated Central Disease: Multiple Sclerosis

Multiple sclerosis (MS) is an autoimmune disease which affects myelinated neurons throughout the central nervous system resulting in muscle weakness, visual disturbance, sensory aberration, cognitive decline, and lower urinary tract symptoms. Traditionally, it is viewed as a two-stage disease, with early inflammation responsible for relapsing-remitting disease and delayed neurodegeneration causing non-relapsing progression. Globally, MS affects 2.5 million individuals and has an estimated prevalence ranging from 288 to 309 per 100,000 in the United States. It is a disease of the middle-aged adult with onset between 20 and 40 years and a 2:1 predilection for females [17]. Although genitourinary manifestations of MS are rarely life-threatening, they significantly impact quality of life. The location of MS plaques determines unique features of patient symptoms – spinal or suprapontine nervous system involvement results in storage phase dysfunction and loss of coordination between the detrusor and urethral sphincter during voiding. Lesions of the sacral cord result in detrusor areflexia and a non-relaxing sphincter. Nearly 90% of patients with MS experience some degree of voiding dysfunction and/or incontinence with initial presentation of urinary symptoms occurring roughly 6–8 years after MS diagnosis.

Evaluation of the Female Neurologic Patient

History

When approaching the female neurologic patient, a thorough history assessing urinary symptoms, neurologic abnormalities, prior urogenital complications, treatment, and reconstructive surgery as well as urinary tract, sexual, bowel (fecal incontinence, mode of bowel emptying, and rectal sensation), gynecologic, and neurologic function is important. Urinary symptoms should be classified by type (storage vs emptying), frequency, and severity. If incontinent, assess not only for urgency and stress urinary incontinence but also for functional incontinence (i.e., limited mobility or neurologic deficits preventing timely toileting). Urinary symptoms should be interpreted in the context of concomitant bowel function and neurologic status. A medication history should be performed. Drugs with anticholinergic properties (antipsychotic drugs, antidepressants, and anticholinergic respiratory agents) and alpha-adrenergic agonists can cause voiding dysfunction. Lifestyle factors such as smoking, alcohol, or addictive drugs, as well as a patient's physical and mental abilities, may affect quality of life and impact treatment outcomes.

It is important to understand the impact of bladder symptoms on patient quality of life. In spinal cord patients, evidence of autonomic dysreflexia, including triggers and typical symptoms, should be considered. A bladder diary (catheterization log for patients who cannot void) quantifying frequency of micturition, voided volumes, and incontinence episodes can provide objective data regarding patient-reported lower urinary tract (LUT) symptoms and functional bladder capacity and can serve as a useful adjunct to history taking or questionnaire use.

Questionnaires

Questionnaires may aid clinical assessment by providing additional insight into severity and impact of symptoms or be used to evaluate the effectiveness of treatments over time. The Neurogenic Bladder Symptom Score has been validated for use in the MS, spinal cord injury, and congenital neurogenic bladder populations. This 22-item questionnaire is used by patients to report severity of urinary incontinence, storage and emptying symptoms, urinary complications, and urinary-specific quality of life [27, 28]. Condition-specific questionnaires such as Qualiveen (MS, SCI populations), Quality Life Index/Spinal Cord Injury (SCI population), and Incontinence-Quality of Life (I-QoL) have also been validated for neurourological patients. Evidence remains lacking as to which questionnaire is most appropriate to use in assessment of patients with neurologic urinary tract dysfunction.

Physical Examination

Physical examination consists of examining the abdomen, flanks, and pelvic and genital organs and, when appropriate, assessing urogenital sensation, sacral spinal cord reflexes (bulbocavernosus and anal reflex), pelvic floor contraction, and anal sphincter tone. Reduced mobility can cause pressure ulcers that should be identified and documented. All patients with an indwelling catheter should routinely have a genital or pelvic exam to identify and manage impending urethral erosion or in the suprapubic region evaluate for pressure necrosis. Urinary incontinence can cause dermatitis and yeast infections, and as such, dependent regions such as the perineum and inguinal skin folds should be directly examined.

Cognitive function can be assessed through brief mental status exams. A focused neurologic exam directed at gait, extremity strength, sensation, and spasticity is paramount especially as it may affect management decisions and treatment options which require manual dexterity.

According to the American Urological Association (AUA) guidelines (Table 2 and Fig. 2) [29], risk stratification should occur after the initial evaluation of the female neurourological patient to determine further need for diagnostic testing and develop a plan for appropriate surveillance over time. Stratification can be done based on the location of the neurologic disease or insult. Typically, patients with suprapontine lesions or lesions

below the spinal cord, or who spontaneously void, are considered low risk, while patients with supra-sacral cord lesions would be placed in the unknown-risk category until further diagnostic evaluation.

Diagnostic Workup

Urinalysis is performed for all patients in the initial evaluation to assess for hematuria, pyuria, glucosuria, and proteinuria which may prompt further evaluation. Abnormalities should be interpreted in the context of the patient's underlying comorbidities and presence or absence of a urinary catheter.

Low-Risk Patients

Post-void residual (PVR) should be performed in all patients that spontaneously void. Defined as the volume of urine left in the bladder after micturition, an elevated PVR value may suggest abnormalities in bladder emptying due to detrusor underactivity, bladder outlet obstruction, or both. A normal value does not preclude lower urinary tract dysfunction or risk to the upper tracts. While no universally agreed-upon definition of an elevated PVR either as an absolute value or percentage of bladder emptying exists, volumes upwards of 300 cc have been put forth as indicative of non-neurogenic chronic urinary retention [30, 31]. NLUTD patients with urinary symptoms in the setting of a symptomatic elevated PVR, recurrent UTIs, hematuria, or progressive refractory incontinence should be further evaluated with upper tract imaging and multichannel

Table 2 Adapted from AUA/SUFU Guideline on Adult Neurogenic Lower Urinary Tract Dysfunction [29]

Diagnostic evaluation	Low-risk	Moderate-risk	High-risk
Renal function	Normal/ stable	Normal/stable	Abnormal/unstable
Urinary tract imaging	Normal/ stable	Normal findings	Hydronephrosis, new renal scarring, loss of renal parenchyma, staghorn, or large renal stone burden
Urodynamics	Synergistic voiding	Neurogenic retention Detrusor overactivity with incomplete emptying	Poor compliance Vesicoureteral reflux (if UDS performed with fluoroscopy) High storage pressures with detrusor overactivity and detrusor sphincter dyssynergia

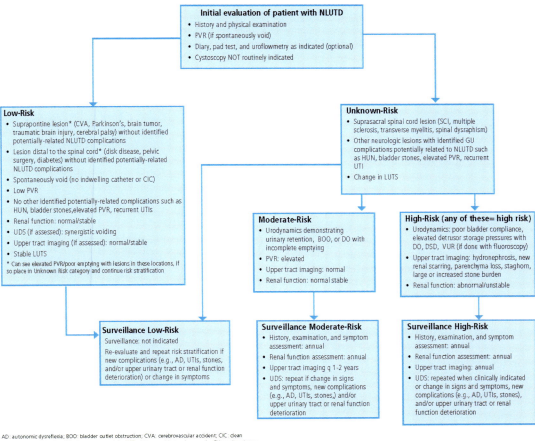

Fig. 2 Obtained with permission from AUA Office of Education

urodynamics. PVRs can be measured using a transabdominal bladder scanner or ultrasound or urethral catheterization. A single elevated PVR may not be diagnostic. Values should be checked periodically to monitor for changes in bladder emptying instead.

Uroflowmetry may be combined with measurement of PVR to detect voiding dysfunction. It is limited in utility for discriminating between underlying mechanisms for voiding dysfunction which would require urodynamic testing.

At initial evaluation, clinicians should not routinely obtain upper tract imaging, renal function assessment, or urodynamic studies as they are unlikely to add significant value given low intravesical storage pressures and subsequent favorable urologic prognosis in these patients.

Unknown-Risk Patients

Unknown-risk patients are at risk of developing high detrusor storage pressures and should undergo upper tract assessment with a combination of serum chemistry, imaging, and multichannel urodynamics studies. Renal function can be estimated with serum creatinine or in patients with poor muscle mass and cystatin C-based glomerular filtration rate [32]. These patients may present with widely variable symptoms and UDS findings (detailed in Table 1 by neurologic condition). Initial evaluation should not occur in the acute phase following a neurologic insult as the short-term changes in lower urinary tract function are not prognostically valuable or predictive of future function. Risk stratification should be postponed until the neurologic condition of these patients has stabilized [33].

Multichannel UDS assess bladder storage pressures as well as detrusor leak point pressures to determine if the upper urinary tracts are safe from deterioration. Sustained bladder pressures in excess of 40 cmH20 are associated with increased risk of renal failure [9]. When combined with fluoroscopy, structural information such as vesicoureteral reflux (VUR), morphological changes to the bladder, and outlet abnormalities help to assess prognosis and direct treatment. Urodynamics should not be performed in the acute phase following a neurologic insult as initial changes in lower urinary tract function do not always predict future function. For patients with spinal shock particularly following spinal cord injury, tumor, vascular infarct, or transverse myelitis, urodynamic evaluation should be deferred after evidence of recovery and stabilization, typically in the realm of 6–12 months after the inciting event.

Renal and bladder ultrasound can evaluate the upper urinary tract for dilation, stones, and other pathology. If technical or anatomical factors preclude reliable ultrasonography, cross-sectional imaging with computed tomography or magnetic resonance imaging is warranted.

Cystoscopy should not be routinely performed and instead be reserved for evaluation of anatomic abnormalities [29, 34]. Routine cystoscopy is invasive, costly, and not without morbidity. In the neurourological patient who utilizes indwelling catheters, it may lead to overdetection of benign lesions and furthermore has not been shown to increase detection of bladder cancer when performed routinely [34, 35]. Endoscopic evaluation is indicated in cases of hematuria, pyuria, suspected urethral pathology, recurrent urinary tract infections, stones, or known or suspected bladder cancer [34].

Patients are reclassified as moderate-risk if after initial evaluation they have normal renal function and intact upper tracts with urodynamic evidence of detrusor overactivity with incomplete emptying or neurogenic retention. Urodynamic findings in high-risk patients include poor bladder compliance, high intravesical storage with DO and DSD, and evidence of reflux to the upper tracts. Any evidence of hydronephrosis, new renal scarring or parenchymal loss, and significant nephrolithiasis also confers a high-risk status.

Surveillance

Following initial evaluation, low-risk patients with stable urinary symptoms can be managed expectantly with education on signs and symptoms that would prompt re-evaluation and subsequent risk re-stratification [29]. Clinical signs which warrant repeat evaluation include new incontinence or difficulty emptying, recurrent UTIs, stones, or evidence of upper tract deterioration.

Patients who are deemed to be of moderate risk and with stable urinary symptoms should undergo annual focused history, exam, symptom assessment, renal function assessment, and annual or biennial upper tract imaging. High-risk patients with stable urinary symptoms similarly follow the same care pathway except for the addition of multichannel urodynamic studies which can be repeated when clinically indicated and annual upper tract imaging [29]. Moderate- or high-risk patients who experience a change in urinary symptoms or complications, such as worsening incontinence, autonomic dysreflexia, recurrent UTIs, stones, or evidence of upper tract deterioration, should have multichannel urodynamics performed [36].

Management

The goals of management are to maximize social continence, facilitate bladder emptying, and avoid urinary tract infections in addition to preserving upper tract function. Further considerations include the patient's disability, medical comorbidities, and goals for maximizing quality of life. Management strategies should address reversible causes of incontinence, as well as storage or bladder level dysfunction, and voiding or outlet level abnormalities.

Reversible Causes of Incontinence

Worsening urinary incontinence in the neurourological patient may be driven by recurrent urinary tract infection. The diagnosis of a UTI in the neurourological patient is especially challenging, as patients may have altered sensation and manage their bladders with catheters which inevitably introduce bacteriuria. The classic symptoms of UTI such as dysuria, urgency, and frequency may not apply to these patients, especially if they have suprasacral lesions that may alter sensation. Potential signs and symptoms of UTI, as defined by the International SCI UTI Basic Dataset, include fever, urinary incontinence, leaking around an indwelling catheter, increased spasticity, malaise, lethargy, cloudy and/or malodorous urine, back and/or bladder pain, dysuria, and autonomic dysreflexia [37]. In patients with MS, a relapse or progression of disease may be the only sign of a UTI.

Regular bladder emptying is protective against UTIs as it reduces accumulation of bacteria from urinary stasis. In patients who do not void, frequent catheterization is beneficial. The use of hydrophilic catheters has been shown to reduce UTI risk. There is insufficient evidence to recommend single-use catheters over multiuse devices. In SB patients with prior bladder augmentation, use of high-volume (>240 ml) intravesical instillation has been shown to decrease stone formation and symptomatic UTIs. Unfortunately these results have not been confirmed in other neurourological populations. Aggressive bowel management with fiber products, suppositories, and bowel stimulants, as well as perineal care, in patients who also have fecal incontinence are important interventions for decreasing UTI risk.

Recurrent UTIs in the female neurourological patient may be indicative of changes in bladder dynamics or the presence of foreign bodies such as stones. Appropriate management includes treatment of the urinary tract infection followed by multichannel urodynamics, cystoscopic evaluation, and cross-sectional imaging of the urinary tract.

The initiation of vaginal estrogen therapy for postmenopausal women may decrease UTI risk, although its benefit has not been explicitly demonstrated in women with neurogenic lower urinary tract dysfunction [37, 38]. Overall, cranberry supplementation, use of bacteriostatic agents such as methenamine hippurate, and bladder irrigation have not been shown to have long-term efficacy among neurourological patients [39–41]. Long-term use of prophylactic oral antibiotics is discouraged in nonpregnant neurologic patients due to increased risk of antibiotic resistance.

Management of Storage Dysfunction

Overactive Bladder
Goals of treatment are to convert a high-pressure, overactive bladder to a low-pressure reservoir. Reduction of detrusor storage pressures contributes to urinary continence however, depending on the neurologic insult, may result in residual urine. Patients who are incontinent may have involuntary loss of urine due to urgency urinary incontinence (inability to postpone void) or, in patients who do not void, neurogenic detrusor overactivity incontinence. Patients can also experience overflow urinary incontinence if storage dysfunction coexists with bladder outlet abnormalities.

Conservative Measures
Noninvasive assisted bladder emptying measures, including Crede or Valsalva maneuvers to cause a reflex sphincteric contraction, have long since fallen out of favor as they may increase bladder outlet resistance and diminish efficient emptying resulting in high intravesical pressures [42].

For patients who void, timed and complete bladder emptying remains paramount for management of urinary symptoms. Pelvic floor physiotherapy may be offered as an adjunctive intervention. Several studies obtained from patients with MS and CVA have established the utility of pelvic floor muscle strengthening in urinary symptom reduction and improvement on various quality-of-life questionnaires. Pelvic floor exercises work by enhancing the inhibitory effect of pelvic floor contraction on detrusor overactivity. A randomized controlled trial of 74 MS patients assigned to pelvic floor training, pelvic floor training and electromyography (EMG) biofeedback, or pelvic floor training, EMG biofeedback, and neuromuscular electrical stimulation showed improvement in mean episodes of incontinence and 24-hour pad test after 9 weeks, with the greatest benefit seen when pelvic floor training was combined with neuromuscular electrical stimulation and EMG biofeedback [43]. A study of 26 female CVA patients randomized to standard rehabilitation vs standard rehabilitation plus pelvic floor muscle training and bladder education saw improvement after 12 weeks in daytime frequency, 24-hour pad test, and pelvic floor strength compared to controls, with a follow-up study 6 months later demonstrating continued effect [44, 45]. Among patients with spinal cord injury or congenital spinal dysraphisms, the data is even more sparse, and while pelvic floor exercises may improve quality-of-life measures [46, 47], these are best included as part of a multimodal approach. Overall, due to minimal associated risks, pelvic floor physiotherapy may provide some benefit in treating lower urinary tract symptoms in selected patients, particularly those with suprapontine lesions.

Pharmacology

Antimuscarinic Agents
Antimuscarinic medications competitively bind to M3 receptors widely distributed in the detrusor and urothelium to effect detrusor relaxation, lower intravesical pressures, and reduce storage symptoms. They are a first-line option for increasing bladder capacity and reducing episodes of urinary incontinence among patients with neurogenic detrusor overactivity (NDO) [48]. Since the introduction of oxybutynin, several newer anticholinergic agents have appeared on the market; however, there is no consensus regarding the

superiority of one agent over others [49, 50]. The only difference between drugs is their individual side effect profiles [50], which may include adverse effects such as dry mouth, blurred vision, constipation, and occasional tachycardia. Side effects may be mitigated by use of controlled-release formulations or other routes of administration, such as intravesical use.

Oxybutynin, trospium, tolterodine, propiverine, solifenacin, and darifenacin are well established and tolerated treatments for neurourological patients [49, 51–53]. No published clinical evidence for use of fesoterodine exists in management of neurourological disorders. Higher doses of a single antimuscarinic, or combination therapy with two antimuscarinics or a beta3-adrenergic agonist, have been shown to improve outcomes [54, 55]. The use of antimuscarinics however remains fraught with high rates of discontinuation [56], not to mention emerging data that cognitive effects from anticholinergics may be deleterious and likely irreversible [57]. Agents that do not readily cross the blood-brain barrier or have increased affinity for bladder level muscarinic receptors may have less effect on cognition; however, caution should be used when using these agents in neurologic patients. Serial measurement of PVRs before and during treatment with antimuscarinic should be performed among patients who void. In patients with impaired bladder emptying, antimuscarinic therapy combined with intermittent catheterization facilitates appropriate bladder management.

Beta-3-Adrenergic Receptor Agonists
The role of mirabegron, a beta-3 selective receptor agonist which acts by relaxing the detrusor muscle, in neurourological patients is still not well established. A multicenter RCT of 78 patients with SCI or MS showed improvement in bladder compliance and bladder volume at first detrusor contraction but no significant effect on detrusor pressure or cystometric capacity [58], while a smaller study reported no significant improvement in aforementioned parameters [59]. A systematic review of 302 patients with neurourological conditions found that mirabegron may have a role as a second-line option for

patients with storage symptoms unresponsive to antimuscarinic therapy [60].

Because of its high selectivity, mirabegron remains better tolerated due to a favorable side effects profile. There remains no high-level data for its use in the neurourological patient.

Other Drugs

Cannabinoids and desmopressin have been reported to be effective and safe in treating frequency and nocturia in MS patients [61, 62]. Desmopressin reduces urine production by promoting water reabsorption at the distal and collecting renal tubules and is particularly indicated for managing nocturnal polyuria. There is evidence to suggest that it can be safely used in combination with mirabegron in MS patients [62]. It should be prescribed with caution in geriatric patients or patients with pedal edema because of the risk of hyponatremia or congestive heart failure.

Catheterization

Incomplete bladder emptying can worsen detrusor overactivity and render pharmacotherapeutic interventions less effective. Intermittent catheterization remains the preferred mode of bladder management for patients who are unable to empty their bladders effectively or safely. Neurologic lesions resulting in poor manual dexterity, weakness, spasticity, rigidity, and impaired visual acuity or cognition may hamper the patient's ability to perform self-catheterization. Frequency of bladder catheterizations varies (typically every 4–6 hours); however, bladder volumes should not exceed 400–500 ml, and a regimen can be constructed by reviewing urodynamics results or catheter logs. Regularly performed catheterizations have been shown to reduce UTI risk [63]. Intermittent catheterization is not without the risk of complications, however, including UTI and sequelae of chronic urethral trauma such as stricture and hematuria. Hydrophilic catheters are associated with lower rates of UTI and urethral trauma [64, 65].

Indwelling catheters are associated with several complications as well as increased risk of UTI, encrustation, and stone formation [66]. Silicone catheters are less susceptible to encrustation and may be preferred in this population given the high incidence of latex allergies [66]. Suprapubic tubes are a good option for those not amenable to urethral catheterization. They carry similar UTI risk to indwelling catheterization with the additional technical risk associated with placement and revision but may help to reduce the burden of patient dependence on caregivers and avoid the sequelae of urethral loss and erosion.

Prolonged use of indwelling urethral and suprapubic catheters may increase a patient's risk of bladder stone formation and bladder malignancy. Moreover, SCI patients and patients with neuropathic bladders and prior history of enterocystoplasty reconstruction have been shown to have increased risk of aggressive bladder cancer [67, 68].

Chemodenervation

In 2000, Schurch et al. [69] reported on the successful use of intradetrusor onabotulinumtoxinA in 21 spinal cord injury patients. These patients had decreased intravesical pressure, improved continence, and decreased use of anticholinergic medication [69]. OnabotulinumtoxinA has since revolutionized the management of neurogenic detrusor overactivity. In 2011, onabotulinumtoxinA was approved for patients with neurogenic detrusor overactivity after spinal cord injury by the US Food and Drug Administration (FDA). OnabotulinumtoxinA causes a long-lasting, reversible chemical denervation which may arrest the hyperexcitability of sensory afferents in the urothelium and detrusor overactivity; however, its exact mechanism of action remains unknown [70]. Toxin injections are mapped out over the detrusor and can be repeated without loss of efficacy [71].

The strongest evidence for clinical use in NDO comes from the DIGNITY (Double-Blind Investigation of Purified Neurotoxin Complex in Neurogenic Detrusor Overactivity) trials which compared response to onabotulinumtoxinA to placebo in patients with NDO due to SCI or MS with intolerance or failure of anticholinergics, at doses of 200 U or 300 U or placebo. While these studies showed no differences in efficacy between the 200 U and 300 U doses, administration of onabotulinumtoxinA significantly improved the number of urinary urge incontinence episodes, involuntary detrusor contractions, maximum cystometric capacity, and the maximum detrusor pressure during involuntary contractions [72–74]. There is an increasing dose-dependent relationship regarding risk of retention and need for CIC. A de novo self-catheterization rate of up to 42% has been reported, which is particularly important to note when counseling patients who void. In non-catheterized MS patients randomized to 100 U of onabotulinumtoxinA, CIC rates due to urinary retention were 15.2% compared to 31.4% and 47.1% in MS patients who received 200 U and 300 U, respectively [72–75]. In clinical practice, neurourological patients who void and do not require catheterization to facilitate bladder emptying may be initiated at a dose of 100 units. All patients should be counseled thoroughly about the risk of urinary retention which is still relatively modest at low doses.

No standardized injection template exists; however, the DIGNITY trials utilized a trigone-sparing template. Studies examining submucosal vs intradetrusor injection templates have shown no differences in urodynamic parameters [76], and trials with trigone-including templates have shown improvements in efficacy based on detrusor pressure and episodes of incontinence without an appreciable increase in complications [72]. UDS studies should be performed within a few weeks (6 weeks) of onabotulinumtoxinA administration, especially in patients with unsafe intravesical filling pressures, to evaluate for efficacy of response to onabotulinumtoxinA.

Botulism syndrome, or neuromuscular weakness of the upper trunk, face, mouth, and throat, is listed as a black box warning and must be discussed in preoperative counseling with neurologic patients, particularly those with MS. Other side effects include hematuria, urinary tract infection (51.8–56%), and increased risk of retention. These effects can be pronounced among MS patients who void. While onabotulinumtoxin A may leave up to 42.9% dry [77], as many as 88% of patients with MS may need to initiate

CIC [78]. Furthermore there is a considerable risk of post-procedural UTI which is significant in this particularly vulnerable group of patients. UTIs worsen urinary symptoms and may promote disease progression among MS patients in addition to negatively impacting quality of life [79, 80].

For spinal cord injury patients with NDO, the DIGNITY trials showed improved clinical outcomes and UDS parameters after onabotulinumtoxinA injection. Another important consideration for SCI patients is its favorable effect on the frequency and severity of autonomic dysreflexia and possible benefits in UTI risk reduction [80].

No high-level evidence currently exists for onabotulinumtoxinA efficacy or dosage among patients with Parkinson's disease or cerebrovascular accident (CVA) although it has been used in small case series. The International Continence Society guidelines have indicated that it may be used for intractable urinary incontinence among PD patients [81]. Caution must be used with CVA patients, who tend to be older with underlying medical comorbidities which may make them more frail, due to increased risk of urinary retention.

Among patients with spina bifida, studies have indicated the use of onabotulinumtoxinA therapy to delay or prevent progression to augmentation cystoplasty particularly after failure of anticholinergic therapy at doses of 10–12 U/kg in the pediatric setting and a maximum 300 U for adults with good results [82, 83]. Studies suggest that onabotulinumtoxinA may have a lower efficacy in patients with poor bladder compliance; however, high-level evidence is lacking [84].

While onabotulinumtoxinA is widely regarded as a successful measure for treating neurogenic detrusor overactivity and associated incontinence, in the longest follow-up study of the use of onabotulinumtoxinA (15 years), the overall discontinuation rate among all neurogenic patients (SCI, MS, spina bifida) was 40%, and only 14% of MS patients continued with the treatment [85]. The reasons for patient dissatisfaction over time are many and may relate to the high incidence of post-procedural UTI, finite duration of efficacy, and need for catheterization. It may best serve those MS patients who already perform CIC as the adverse effects (UTI, retention, need for CIC) may stymie adherence to therapy among MS patients who are able to empty their bladders.

Neuromodulation

Electrical stimulation of peripheral nerves such as the sacral nerve roots, tibial nerve, pudendal nerve, and dorsal genital nerves has an established role in managing idiopathic overactive bladder; however, its application to patients with underlying neurourological conditions is less established.

Transcutaneous/Percutaneous Options

Tibial nerve stimulation and transcutaneous electrical nerve stimulation (TENS) might be effective and safe for treating neurogenic LUT dysfunction; however, more reliable higher-level evidence is lacking [86]. Percutaneous tibial nerve stimulation (PTNS) has been shown to improve storage symptoms and urodynamic parameters in patients with multiple sclerosis, Parkinson's disease, and CVA who void volitionally [87]. A typical treatment course includes stimulation of the tibial nerve using a fixed-frequency electrical signal, once weekly for 30 minutes, over an 8–12-week period. PTNS is a minimally invasive option for managing patients with mild or moderate overactive bladder symptoms, and while it is associated with few adverse effects, its effects are short lived. Transcutaneous tibial nerve stimulation (TTNS) is an alternative that can be done at home and has proved to be safe and effective in treating urgency incontinence in patients with multiple sclerosis or who are post-stroke [88, 89].

Sacral Neuromodulation

Sacral neuromodulation (SNM) has well-established efficacy in the management of idiopathic overactive bladder, urge urinary incontinence, nonobstructive urinary retention, and fecal incontinence. Its role in the management of patients with neurogenic lower urinary tract dysfunction is less clear although various emerging studies point to its applicability to select groups of neurourological patients. Several observational studies show that SNM can improve urinary frequency, incontinence episodes, and voiding (for patients with retention) with minimal adverse events in MS patients [90, 91]. SNM is an attractive option for patients with MS given the high prevalence of lower urinary tract symptoms and fecal incontinence (75% and 29%, respectively). While MS patients may appear to benefit most from this modality, there are legitimate concerns for using SNM in patients with a progressive neurologic condition. Chaabane et al. reported that three out of seven patients with MS (43%) failed SNM after an MS prolapse [75]. While follow-up studies have demonstrated that SNM is safe in patients with progressive MS, in practice, this technology should be used in patients with disease stability over the preceding 6–12 months [92].

SNM has been utilized successfully in other neurourological conditions. A pooled study of 107 patients with neurogenic bladder including those with SCI, spinal dysraphism, and neurologic injury resulting from pelvic surgery, diabetes, and PD showed a 58.5% rate of progression to full device implantation after successful lead testing. Significant improvements in urinary frequency, urgency, nocturia, daily urine volume, daily urinary leakage, and residual urine persisted at a mean follow-up of 20.1 months [93]. Kessler et al. similarly reported a test success rate of 68% (256 patients) and a permanent success rate of 92% (206 patients) [94], with a follow-up meta-analysis evaluating 887 patients across 21 studies demonstrating a pooled success rate of 84.2% with mean follow-up of 61 months [95]. The highest test success rates were achieved in patients with back surgery, MS, and pelvic surgery (84.1%, 76.6%, and 77.8%, respectively), suggesting a higher likelihood for preservation of nerve plasticity or reversibility [95].

Although complete SCI is considered a general contraindication for SNM, Sievert et al. showed that early bilateral SNM, during the phase of spinal shock, seems to prevent the subsequent development of neurogenic detrusor overactivity and urinary incontinence in patients with complete SCI [96]. Use however remains investigational. For patients with incomplete SCI, several studies have demonstrated improvement in detrusor sphincter dyssynergia and maximum detrusor pressures during storage [97].

Prior limitation of SNM included the device's MRI incompatibility and fixed battery life which necessitated device revision. However, newer devices are MRI compatible and have a longer battery life with rechargeable battery options, thereby improving opportunities for utilization.

Underactive Bladder

Underactive bladder is a symptom complex characterized by detrusor underactivity; prolonged urination time; reduced sensation on filling; a sensation of incomplete bladder emptying, usually with hesitancy; and slow stream. The International Continence Society (ICS) defines detrusor underactivity (DU) as a bladder contraction of reduced strength and/or duration, resulting in prolonged bladder emptying and/or failure to achieve complete bladder emptying within a normal time span [98]. Pressure-flow urodynamic testing is necessary to help differentiate DU from other conditions such as OAB; however, no universally accepted criteria exist. In the neurourological patient, patients with underactive bladder will present with incomplete bladder emptying, urinary retention, or overflow incontinence. Well-recognized mechanisms include myogenic dysfunction from fibrosis and the disruption of efferent neural pathways from traumatic neurologic injury or disease.

Treatment options are limited and include behavioral modifications (timed voiding, double voiding), continuous bladder drainage via indwelling or suprapubic catheter, and clean intermittent catheterization (CIC) to facilitate complete bladder emptying and mitigate the likelihood of overflow incontinence. Cholinergic drugs such as bethanechol or distigmine were considered in the past to enhance detrusor contractility and promote bladder emptying but are not recommended in practice today. Intravesical prostaglandin E2 instillations to increase detrusor tonicity as well as the use of alpha blocker agents to decrease tonicity of the internal urinary sphincter have also been described.

Sacral neuromodulation has been shown in small prospective studies to reduce the need for catheterization among patients with refractory nonobstructive urinary retention; however, applicability to patients with underlying neurologic conditions remains investigational [99].

Other surgical options include intrasphincteric onabotulinumtoxinA injection and transurethral incision of the bladder neck, both of which are targeted at decreasing urethral sphincter resistance. These options are described in more detail in the overactive outlet section.

End-Stage Bladder Dysfunction

In patients with severe incontinence, poor bladder compliance, fibrosis, or evidence of upper tract deterioration, augmentation cystoplasty with de-tubularized portions of the ileum may be offered as an ameliorative solution to improve bladder capacity and maintain a low-pressure reservoir for urine storage. A catheterizable channel may need to be performed simultaneously for patients who are unable to catheterize via the native urethra or with poor manual dexterity. If bladder capacity is adequate, autoaugmentation (detrusor myomectomy) can also be performed to reduce detrusor overactivity and improve bladder compliance with minimal morbidity to the patient.

High-quality long-term studies evaluating efficacy of augmentation cystoplasty are lacking. A meta-analysis by Hoen et al. [100] evaluating 511 patients found an 87% rate of continence. Long-term complications measured up to 10 years postoperatively included bowel dysfunction (15%), bladder stone formation (10%), bladder perforation (1.9%), mucus production (12.5%), metabolic abnormalities (3.35%), and one bladder cancer.

The Bladder Outlet

The bladder outlet in the female patient consists of the smooth muscle of the bladder neck under sympathetic control and the striated muscle of the urinary sphincter at the level of the mid-urethra modulated by somatic elements. When approaching the management of a female patient with neurologic disease, it is important to reflect on the level of the underlying lesion and the predictable implications based on this location. Suprapontine insults (those of the brain and brainstem, including tumors, Parkinson's disease, normal-pressure hydrocephalus, cerebrovascular accidents, and traumatic brain injury) tend to allow for synergistic voiding, and as such patients have low PVRs. Patients with Parkinson's disease and Parkinsonism may be at risk of sphincter bradykinesia. Lesions of the suprasacral spinal cord, including multiple sclerosis and spinal cord injuries, can lead to detrusor external-sphincter dyssynergia (DESD). DESD can present as a concomitant involuntary contraction of the detrusor and the striated sphincter with uncontrolled subsequent relaxation of the sphincter at peak detrusor contraction leading to incontinence or ongoing (or intermittent) sphincter contraction despite volitional detrusor contraction leading to urinary retention. For patients with more distal neurologic insults, at the sacral level, which can be the result of neurovascular damage due to uncontrolled diabetes mellitus, or iatrogenic injury to the pudendal nerve as a sequela of pelvic surgery, underactivity of the sphincter is the result of interrupting the baseline tonicity of the bladder outlet. Women with neurologic disorders may also become pregnant and undergo traumatic vaginal deliveries which disrupt the pelvic floor supportive structures, thereby affecting sphincteric competence. Direct injury of the urethral sphincter is also a common problem among patients with neurogenic lower urinary tract dysfunction and typically occurs in patients with chronic indwelling urethral catheters placed for bladder management. Due to altered sensation and chronicity, the catheter erodes through and damages the continence mechanism.

Pragmatically, management of the bladder outlet can be efficiently summarized by dichotomizing patients by their phenotypic presentation: is the bladder outlet underactive or overactive? Additional patient characteristics must be considered when managing the bladder outlet, in particular manual dexterity and implications for intermittent catheterization.

Underactive Outlet

Patients with underactive outlets clinically present with an open bladder neck due to a flaccid denervated external sphincter and dysfunctional reflexes to increases in intra-abdominal pressure resulting in stress urinary incontinence. Patients may also have stress urinary incontinence due to direct urethral injury, loss, or destruction. In patients managed with a chronic indwelling catheter, repetitive pressure from the Foley balloon on the bladder neck may result in pressure necrosis. Similarly, repetitive dislodgment of the Foley catheter from the urethra can devastate the outlet. The sequelae of chronic incontinence include maceration of the perineal skin which may promote the development of decubitus ulcers and osteomyelitis. Externalized female catheters such as the PureWick™ female external catheter which, when connected to suction, can keep a patient dry. While attractive because it can be applied noninvasively, as it requires suction, use of externalized female catheters is not a feasible option for many active patients or an affordable option for home use.

Pharmacologic Therapies

Pharmacologic therapies that act to increase urethral sphincter contractions include duloxetine, imipramine, and midodrine. Duloxetine is a serotonin-norepinephrine reuptake inhibitor, and its implication for the lower urinary tract is due to its central action at the level of the sacral spinal cord [101–103]. Duloxetine, at a dose of 40 mg BID, has been demonstrated among non-neurogenic patients with SUI to decrease incontinence episodes and improve patient-reported outcomes [104]. Imipramine, a tricyclic antidepressant, has been used for decades in the management of nocturnal enuresis and has some evidence in animal models that it increases urethral sphincter tone. However, both pharmacologic options are generally not accepted to be an appropriate management strategy for women with stress urinary incontinence [105].

Surgical Management

Depending on the severity of the neurologic insult, many patients will require more invasive procedures or surgical intervention to increase outlet resistance and improve continence. Urodynamic assessment should be performed prior to surgical treatment of stress incontinence as coexisting detrusor overactivity or poor bladder compliance may compromise the efficacy of surgical outcomes. In patients with storage dysfunction and concomitant sphincteric incompetence, a bladder outlet procedure to increase resistance may lead to overflow incontinence or upper tract deterioration due to the loss of the safety valve or pop off mechanism provided by an underactive urethral sphincter. Furthermore surgical intervention on the outlet may result in difficulty with intermittent catheterization in patients who catheterize per urethra due to changes in urethral anatomy.

Urethral Bulking

Urethral bulking agents can be injected either in a procedure room in-office or in a surgery center setting with sedation depending on local capabilities and patient preference. Urethral bulking, while associated with a lower risk of complications, has a higher failure rate than surgical procedures. A variety of bulking agents exist, including glutaraldehyde cross-linked bovine collagen (GAX), dextranomer/hyaluronic acid (Deflux), and polydimethylsiloxane (Macroplastique) which have been evaluated with suboptimal outcomes among neurologic patients. Results, the bulk of which comes from studies of pediatric subjects, are mixed with short-term improvement and long-term SUI recurrence; however, data is lacking for newer agents such as polyacrylamide gel (Bulkamid). One study of 12 adult subjects with SUI caused by spinal injury or myelomeningocele showed a failure rate of 36.3% after GAX treatment with no observable increase in abdominal leak pressure in those who failed bulking therapy [106]. Other studies have evaluated the utility of bulking agents as a second-line agent to augment continence after prior sling with equally dismal results. A study of 27 patients treated with endoscopic periurethral bulking after a prior fascial sling procedure resulted in a continence rate of 7% after a sling bulking treatment at

a median follow-up of 8 years. Approximately, 59% of the patients managed with bulking agent eventually required further surgical intervention to treat their incontinence [107]. Data remains lacking as to whether the type of bulking agent used has an impact on outcome among neurourological patients with SUI. Furthermore, it is unclear if the need for intermittent catheterization compromises the efficacy of bulking agents in patients with incomplete bladder emptying.

Urethral Slings

Urethral slings increase bladder outlet resistance by urethral compression and offer the possibility of long-term durability compared to periurethral bulking. When compared to urethral bulking, slings have a higher success rate, measured both by decreased incontinence and quality-of-life outcomes [108, 109]. Autologous fascial slings, in particular, remain a commonly utilized management approach to the underactive outlet in NLUTD. Notably, often the postoperative goal after sling placement is to increase outlet resistance sufficiently to result in intentional urinary retention, necessitating intermittent catheterization. Consideration must be given to the feasibility of CIC in each individual patient. In neurologically intact women, cure rates of 67–93% [30] have been reported after placement, and women with neurogenic stress incontinence have generally been found to have comparable outcomes. De novo OAB symptoms however have been found to be higher in women with neurologic disease (21.05%) compared to neurologically intact women (5.26%). A study by Athanasopoulos et al. [110] of 33 female patients with myelomeningocele and SCI who underwent autologous rectal fascia sling placement had a dry rate of 75.8% and a complication rate of 15.2% over a mean follow-up period of 52 months. Furthermore, over 90% of the patients deemed the intervention to be satisfactory.

Synthetic mid-urethral slings have been shown to significantly ameliorate neurogenic stress incontinence with a pooled success rate of 87% reported by a recent meta-analysis of 852 neurourological patients undergoing surgical management of neurogenic SUI [111]. Of these women, 42% underwent transobturator tape, 53% retropubic, and 5% single-incision sling approaches, with a dry rate approaching 79% over a mean duration ranging from 3.5 to 10 years. The need to commence intermittent catheterization was reported to occur at a frequency of 7–35% depending on the study, and very few mesh complications were observed [111].

In a prospective nonrandomized pilot study comparing outcomes between patients with sacral lesions undergoing retropubic synthetic sling vs pubovaginal sling placement, cure rates were 80 and 85%, respectively. Failure was defined as leakage on cough stress test at a 250 ml intravesical volume. Patients reported similar a reduction in urinary symptoms on validated symptom questionnaires with failure rates of 41.8% in the retropubic sling group vs 25.4% in the pubovaginal sling group at 4 years. The prevalence of de novo urge incontinence was higher in the retropubic sling group (30%) compared to PVS (10%). Authors noted that whereas all patients undergoing pubovaginal sling required clean intermittent catheterization postoperatively, only 47% of patients undergoing retropubic sling placement required CIC, thereby suggesting that retropubic slings may be a viable option for mitigating the risk of postoperative CIC in patients who void [112].

Adjustable Continence Devices

Adjustable continence devices (ProACT™ and ACT™), which consist of a minimally invasively implanted peri-urethral balloon system placed to exert pressure on the bladder neck with adjustable volume metrics, have also been utilized to manage neurogenic stress urinary incontinence; however, long-term data is lacking. Study results (which also evaluated men with neurogenic stress urinary incontinence) showed a complete cure rate of 12% (mean follow-up 1.4–3.16 years) with improvements >50% reported in 17% of patients. The studies did not stratify outcomes by patient gender or report urodynamic results after device

implantation. Reimplantation occurred in 27% of patients due to infection (19%), migration (30%), perforation (15%), and urethral (18%) or cutaneous exposure (18%) [111].

Artificial Urinary Sphincters (AUS)

Artificial urinary sphincters (AUS) are less commonly used in female patients compared to males with neurogenic SUI. Similar to adjustable continence devices, they have the advantage of dynamic influence on the outlet (as opposed to the fixed resistance generated by a sling or bulking agent), which can allow patients with preserved manual dexterity to spontaneously void without need for intermittent catheterization. Several studies demonstrate satisfactory continence rates among patients with neurogenic SUI (71.4–90.7%) which is comparable to patients who are neurologically intact [112, 113]. However, revision rates of AUS among patients with NULTD are as high as 85%, twice as high as neurologically intact women and notably higher than when used in the post-prostatectomy setting (50%) [109].

Bladder Neck Closure

The most invasive, and arguably the most definitive, management of refractory stress urinary incontinence secondary to an underactive outlet is bladder neck closure and urinary diversion. Bladder neck closure can be performed abdominally or vaginally when AUS is not feasible or prior outlet procedures have failed. It remains the single most definitive option for patients with significant urethral erosion, loss, or severe damage. A transvaginal approach is associated with a lower perioperative morbidity and a shorter operative time and hospital stay and may be considered in patients for whom supravesical urinary diversion is not being contemplated. To minimize the risk of failure and/or fistula formation, patients should be counseled about maintaining proper bladder drainage either with suprapubic tube, catheterization via channel, or other urinary diversion so that low bladder pressures are maintained. Surgical principles of a multilayer, tension-free, water-tight closure remain key to successful outcomes. The most effective way to minimize fistulization or recanalization of the bladder to the urethra is tissue interposition with flaps to help with neovascularization and wound healing. The choice of flap depends on surgical approach. Omental flaps or pedicled rectus abdominis muscle flaps can be utilized during transabdominal approaches. Fibrofatty labial flaps, also known as Martius flaps, can be employed transvaginally.

Data is sparse regarding surgical outcomes after bladder neck closure; however, Shpall et al. report vesicourethral fistula rate of 31% in patients with bladder neck closure and concomitant augmentation and catheterizable channel, suprapubic tube, or ileovesicostomy resulting in persistent incontinence [114]. Bladder neck closure results in loss of urethral access which makes options for future endoscopic evaluation of the bladder more limited. Bladder neck closures should be performed in carefully selected patients with continent native bladder reconstruction (i.e., augmentation cystoplasty with catheterizable channel) who will be compliant due to the potentially life-threatening complications associated with a closed outlet, risk of bladder perforation, and inability to catheterize per native urethra. Patients with good social support, reliable clinic follow-up, and reasonable access to tertiary care are most ideal.

Overactive Outlet

Patients with an overactive bladder outlet present with elevated post-void residual volumes. They may be continent albeit in urinary retention, or they may suffer from overflow urinary incontinence. Patients unable to empty their bladders can be managed with catheter drainage: intermittent catheterization is preferred over chronically indwelling urethral catheters or suprapubic tubes. Many patients are unable to completely empty their bladders, and as such pharmacologic or procedural approaches may be employed.

Pharmacologic Therapies

Alpha-blockers (prazosin, doxazosin, alfuzosin, terazosin, tamsulosin, and silodosin) have been reported to be useful for treating voiding dysfunction by decreasing urethral resistance, but their value with NLUTD is still controversial. In particular, long-term tamsulosin treatment (0.4–0.8 mg once daily) seems to be effective and well tolerated in patients with NLUTD, suggesting that it improves bladder storage and emptying, and decreases symptoms of autonomic dysreflexia. Alpha-blockers have been demonstrated to decrease post-void residual volumes, decrease maximal urethral pressure, and increase voided urinary volume. In an open-label phase of an RCT in the population of interest, alpha-blocker use also improved patient-reported QOL. Overall adverse effects of alpha-blockers were transient with <5% discontinuation rate overall [115].

Baclofen, an antispasmodic and GABA-B receptor agonist commonly used to decrease muscle spasticity in neurologic patients, has also been shown to decrease external urethral sphincter resistance by depressing pudendal nerve reflexes. It may be helpful in the treatment of dyssynergistic voiding typical of patients with DSD; however, no randomized trial data exists.

Intrasphincteric Botox

Intrasphincteric onabotulinumtoxinA injection therapy is a procedural intervention used to decrease outlet resistance. For patients who void, it may increase feasibility of emptying with aid of abdominal straining or reduce the need for catheterization. OnabotulinumtoxinA is a paralytic that acts by blocking presynaptic release of the acetylcholine at the neuromuscular junction. Commonly used in the treatment of detrusor overactivity, investigations into its use for sphincter hypertonicity have demonstrated that injections into the external urethral sphincter might improve bladder emptying in patients with spinal cord injury. However, its use in patients with MS did not result in decreased post-void residual volumes [116]. In a study of female SCI patients with urinary retention who struggled with CIC, those who underwent urethral injection of 100 U of onabotulinumtoxinA were found to have self-reported increased satisfaction, decreased PVR (70%), fewer episodes of autonomic dysreflexia (50%), and fewer urinary tract infections (67%).

Not surprisingly, incontinence episodes increased in 45% of patients [117]. Repeat injections of onabotulinumtoxinA are required to maintain its beneficial effects on the striated muscle fibers of the external sphincter, which typically last in the 3–4 month range but may wane sooner.

Transurethral Incision of the Bladder Neck (TUIBN)

For patients with dyssynergic voiding who are motivated to reduce catheter dependence or usage, more aggressive management options include transurethral incision of the bladder neck (TUIBN). TUIBN is a bladder outlet procedure which may improve voiding efficiency and decrease post-void residuals or the need for catheterization in patients with an overactive outlet or impaired coordination between the detrusor and external sphincter. It can also be utilized in patients with detrusor underactivity. While the mechanisms have yet to be clearly defined, ablation of the bladder neck may decrease sympathetic outflow, which inhibits detrusor contractility in patients with underactive bladder, in addition to decreasing bladder outlet resistance for patients with an overactive outlet. Bladder neck incision may be performed using a holmium laser or a urethrotome. While there is no standard recommended approach to bladder neck incision, some utilize an interior incision at 12 o'clock, others have incised the bladder neck at 5 and 7 o'clock, and yet still other studies have reported incisions at 3, 6, 9, and 12 o'clock. Overall despite the technique used, outcomes have remained favorable [117]. Care must be taken to avoid a significant disruption to the sympathetic nerve fibers innervating the internal sphincter which are concentrated at the 4 and 8 o'clock positions.

Patients should be counseled about the risk of de novo SUI resulting from incompetency of the bladder neck and overflow urinary incontinence during sleep due to disruption of sensory afferents. TUIBN may damage neural fibers important for maintaining the guarding reflex during micturition by inhibiting neural control of bladder contraction. Unilateral incision can mitigate these sequelae but at the risk of less satisfactory results in terms of improved bladder emptying and/or catheter dependence. TUIBN remains limited in use with pilot studies performed primarily in neurologically intact women and men with bladder outlet obstruction.

Combined Storage and Emptying Disorders

Neurologic conditions can be responsible for many different phenotypes of bladder storage and emptying dysfunction. Patients may have detrusor overactivity, detrusor underactivity, detrusor-external sphincter dyssynergia, or combinations of the above disorders. Elucidating the type of storage and outlet dysfunction, typically with urodynamics and the combination of fluoroscopy, is essential to treating the patient as well as understanding the patient's goals for improved quality of life. Shared decision-making between patient and doctor may help to prioritize whether the patient ultimately desires to be continent at the expense of urinary retention and need for catheterization or have improved bladder emptying with some degree of incontinence.

Other Considerations

Caring for female neurourological patients can be challenging; however, these patients most benefit from ongoing urologic care that is complemented by coordination across multiple disciplines. Numerous barriers to care exist for these patients particularly due to the complexity of their underlying neurologic injury and associated medical comorbidities. As such patients tend to seek care at tertiary or safety net institutions or get lost entirely to follow-up. Many institutions and physician offices also lag in their ability to accommodate these patients; they lack appropriate equipment such as lifts, ramps, and exam tables optimized for patients with neurourological injury and physical disability. A study of 49 neurourological patients undergoing complex urologic reconstruction found nonclinical factors such as unmarried status, poor health literacy, and marked distance from quaternary care to be especially prevalent in this population than reported in other urologic literature for patients undergoing major reconstructive operations [118].

A patient-centered approach that harnesses iterative discourse between medicine, nephrology, gynecology, neurology, neurosurgery, gastroenterology, physiatry, physical therapy, orthopedics, social work, and psychiatry, among other specialties, most optimizes health for these patients throughout their lifetime. The process of transitioning care from office to inpatient setting to home is critical to minimizing preventable hospital admissions as well as equipping both patients and community-based providers with resources and knowledge to best serve the patient in her home environment. For patients with congenital neurologic disorders, they often require major genitourinary reconstructive surgery in childhood, which has important sequelae and necessitates longitudinal care. As these patients age out of pediatric care, it is important that they are cared for by multidisciplinary teams that can coordinate this especially vulnerable transition and, at the same time, serve as a preemptive rather than reactionary health safety net.

Cognition

Intact cognition is important to optimize patient independence and enlist patient engagement in treatment decisions. The neurourological patient is particularly vulnerable, and cognitive function may be further hampered by pharmacotherapeutic interventions. Cognitive function also declines over time as patients age or underlying neurologic disease progresses. Patients may struggle with executive function and complex tasks such as self-catheterization and decision-making, and many depend on the input and supervision of caregivers.

Social Support and Caregivers

An assessment of a patient's social support structure may be insightful in understanding patient behavior and attitudes towards taking an active role in medical decision-making.

Several studies have shown that higher levels of social support positively affect cognitive function. Conversely caregivers of patients with neurologic condition disorders report a significant

burden including decline in overall satisfaction with life, exhaustion, reduced cognitive function, and increased levels of psychological disorders, such as depression, anxiety, and distress, and social isolation. These burdens may be compounded by the additional burden and stigma attached to caring for incontinent dependents. The cost of informal care and associated continence products for patients with urinary incontinence in the United States exceeds $286.2 billion annually in 2021 [119]. The confluence of increased care tasks and financial burden further compounds the risk of neglect, abuse, and potential placement in nursing care facilities.

Clinicians should support both patients and caregivers by providing education about incontinence care and help to align patient and caregiver expectations in a way that reinforces dignity for both parties and promotes independence for the patient, as well as coping strategies and respite care for caregivers. Enlisting social workers may help with finding financial resources to offset lost income and high costs associated with incontinence products in addition to bolstering social support networks.

Manual Dexterity

While various tests to assess manual dexterity exist, the ultimate goal is to evaluate fine motor skills by requiring extensive use of the finger tips. Decline of this skill is associated with progression of neurodegenerative disease states. In clinical practice, assessing if patients can simply hold a pen or grasp a pencil as though poised to write is a rapid and facile proxy for determining manual dexterity, which may limit the applicability of certain urologic interventions.

Obesity

Patients with neurologic injury may also be physically less active due to their disability and face unique challenges in food and economic security which may predispose them to weight gain. This is particularly notable in the SCI and SB population. Undernutrition is a risk factor for poor clinical outcomes and, along with obesity, may increase complications in the perioperative period.

Perioperative Considerations

Patients with neurologic conditions may have other associated comorbidities that may increase their risk of perioperative complications. Patients with suprasacral cord lesions in particular are most vulnerable to postoperative ileus which may ensue after major reconstructive surgery involving intestinal harvest or a general anesthetic. While no high level evidence exists to support the use of mechanical bowel preparation prior to reconstructive procedures, a retrospective study of 80 pediatric SB patients found no significant difference in postoperative complications for patients who did not undergo a preoperative bowel preparation [120]. Alvimopan, a mu-opioid receptor antagonist that promotes early gut motility after enteric motility following bowel resection, may have a limited role in patients with neurologic conditions. A study of patients undergoing urologic reconstruction for benign indications found that patients with neurogenic bowel who used alvimopan ($n = 4$) had shorter time to bowel movement (4.0 vs 5.5 days, $p < 0.001$) and shorter length of hospitalization (6.0 vs 9.0 days, $p < 0.001$) than those who did not ($n = 8$) [121]. Although higher-level data regarding applicability of alvimopan to this population is lacking, enhanced recovery protocols and use of non-narcotic analgesics and regional anesthetics are other strategies which may help to reduce narcotic use and subsequent rates of postoperative ileus.

The optimal approach to caring for spina bifida or hydrocephalus patients with ventriculoperitoneal shunts preoperatively remains controversial. Some authors have reported conversion to ventriculoatrial shunt or shunt ligation, if nonfunctional. Pinto et al. reported that the incidence of postoperative ventriculoperitoneal shunt infections after augmentation cystoplasty could be kept low when prophylactic antibiotics and short-term drains are used [122]. Other authors advocate for preoperative sterilization of urinary tract with antibiotics prior to intra-abdominal and bowel surgery.

No consensus exists regarding antibiotic prophylaxis for intravesical onabotulinumtoxinA injection in patients with neurogenic bladder, and it is conventionally accepted that bacteriuria may hamper the efficacy of the toxin and cause UTI. Paradella et al. [123] found that patients who were treated with antibiotics for more than 3 days prior to their procedure trended towards a higher rate of identified cases of UTI. Leitner et al. [124] examined 154 patients undergoing 273 consecutive treatment cycles and found no association between treatment-related adverse events and presence of bacteriuria.

Conclusions

Micturition depends on the tightly orchestrated coordination of neuromuscular events in cortical centers, parasympathetic, sympathetic, and somatic elements resulting in volitional voiding that is socially appropriate. Involuntary loss of urine can be a devastating sequela of neurologic injury. The level of the lesion determines the extent of injury and typically results in dysfunction of bladder storage, emptying, or both. Assessment strategies center on localizing the neurologic injury and performing risk stratification based on the level of injury and the patient's voiding status. Patients who spontaneously void or have suprapontine lesions or lesions below the spinal cord are considered low-risk, while patients with suprasacral cord lesions are considered unknown-risk until further diagnostic evaluation. Low-risk patients can be managed expectantly unless progressive urinary symptoms including worsening incontinence, evidence of upper tract pathology or deterioration, or difficulty emptying prompt re-stratification. Moderate- and high-risk patients should be evaluated with adjunctive assessments of renal function and urodynamics at regular intervals. Worsening urinary symptoms in moderate- and high-risk patients should be evaluated with multichannel urodynamics.

The goals of management are to maximize social continence, facilitate bladder emptying, and avoid urinary tract infections in addition to preserving upper tract function and maximizing the patient's quality of life goals. Treatment should be individualized to the patient and offered based on the understanding of whether the patient suffers from storage disorders, outlet dysfunction, or both. Careful attention should be paid to the patient's support system, cognitive function, overall health status, and dexterity to determine her ability to fully engage with and self-direct care.

Cross-References

▶ Neuroanatomy and Neurophysiology
▶ Pathophysiology of Female Micturition Disorders

References

1. Jamison J, Maguire S, McCann J. Catheter policies for management of long term voiding problems in adults with neurogenic bladder disorders. Cochrane Database Syst Rev. 2013:CD004375.
2. Ruffion A, Castro-Diaz D, Patel H, Khalaf K, Onyenwenyi A, Globe D, Lereun C, Teneishvili M, Edwards M. Systematic review of the epidemiology of urinary incontinence and detrusor overactivity among patients with neurogenic overactive bladder. Neuroepidemiology. 2013;41:146–55.
3. Basiri A, Shakhssalim N, Hosseini-Moghddam SM, Parvaneh MJ, Azadvari M. Renal transplant in patients with spinal cord injuries. Exp Clin Transplant. 2009;7:28–32.
4. Lawrenson R, Wyndaele J-J, Vlachonikolis I, Farmer C, Glickman S. Renal failure in patients with neurogenic lower urinary tract dysfunction. Neuroepidemiology. 2001;20:138–43.
5. de Viv MJ, Stuart Krause J, Lammertse DP. Recent trends in mortality and causes of death among persons with spinal cord injury. Arch Phys Med Rehabil. 1999;80:1411–9.
6. Fowler CJ, Griffiths D, de Groat WC. The neural control of micturition. Nat Rev Neurosci. 2008;9: 453–66.
7. Panicker JN, Fowler CJ, Kessler TM. Lower urinary tract dysfunction in the neurological patient: clinical assessment and management. Lancet Neurol. 2015;14:720–32.
8. Gajewski JB, Schurch B, Hamid R, Averbeck M, Sakakibara R, Agrò EF, Dickinson T, Payne CK, Drake MJ, Haylen BT. An International Continence Society (ICS) report on the terminology for adult neurogenic lower urinary tract dysfunction (ANLUTD). Neurourol Urodyn. 2018;37:1152–61.
9. McGuire EJ, Woodside JR, Borden TA, Weiss RM. Prognostic value of urodynamic testing in myelodysplastic patients. J Urol. 1981;126:205–9.
10. European Association of Urology (EAU) Guidelines on Neuro-Urology; 2019.
11. Mehdi Z, Birns J, Bhalla A. Post-stroke urinary incontinence. Int J Clin Pract. 2013;67:1128–37.
12. Samijn B, van Laecke E, Renson C, Hoebeke P, Plasschaert F, vande Walle J, van den Broeck C. Lower urinary tract symptoms and urodynamic findings in children and adults with cerebral palsy: a systematic review. Neurourol Urodyn. 2017;36:541–9.
13. National Spinal Cord Injury Statistical Center. Spinal cord injury: facts and figures at a glance. 2021. https://www.nscisc.uab.edu/Public/Facts%20and%20Figures%20-%202021.pdf.
14. Yuan Z, Tang Z, He C, Tang W. Diabetic cystopathy: a review 综述:糖尿病性膀胱病. J Diabetes. 2015;7: 442–7.
15. Liu R-T, Chung M-S, Lee W-C, Chang S-W, Huang S-T, Yang KD, Chancellor MB, Chuang Y-C. Prevalence of overactive bladder and associated risk factors in 1359 patients with type 2 diabetes. Urology. 2011;78:1040–5.
16. Bednar DA. Cauda equina syndrome from lumbar disc herniation. Can Med Assoc J. 2016;188:284.
17. Klocke S, Hahn N. Multiple sclerosis. Mental Health Clin. 2019;9:349–58.
18. Rotar M, Blagus R, Jeromel M, Škrbec M, Tršinar B, Vodušek DB. Stroke patients who regain urinary continence in the first week after acute first-ever stroke have better prognosis than patients with persistent lower urinary tract dysfunction. Neurourol Urodyn. 2011;30:1315.
19. Kim M, Jung JH, Park J, Son H, Jeong SJ, Oh S-J, Cho SY. Impaired detrusor contractility is the pathognomonic urodynamic finding of multiple system atrophy compared to idiopathic Parkinson's disease. Parkinsonism Relat Disord. 2015;21:205–10.
20. Yamamoto T, Asahina M, Yamanaka Y, Uchiyama T, Hirano S, Fuse M, Koga Y, Sakakibara R, Kuwabara S. Postvoid residual predicts the diagnosis of multiple system atrophy in Parkinsonian syndrome. J Neurol Sci. 2017;381:230–4.
21. Kulaklı F, Koklu K, Ersoz M, Ozel S. Relationship between urinary dysfunction and clinical factors in patients with traumatic brain injury. Brain Inj. 2014;28:323–7.
22. Aruga S, Kuwana N, Shiroki Y, Takahashi S, Samejima N, Watanabe A, Seki Y, Igawa Y, Homma Y. Effect of cerebrospinal fluid shunt surgery on lower urinary tract dysfunction in idiopathic normal pressure hydrocephalus. Neurourol Urodyn. 2018;37: 1053–9.
23. Weld KJ, Dmochowski RR. Association of level of injury and bladder behavior in patients with post-traumatic spinal cord injury. Urology. 2000;55:490–4.
24. Wiener JS, Suson KD, Castillo J, Routh JC, Tanaka ST, Liu T, Ward EA, Thibadeau JK, Joseph DB. Bladder management and continence outcomes in adults with spina bifida: results from the National

Spina Bifida Patient Registry, 2009 to 2015. J Urol. 2018;200:187–94.

25. Bartolin Z, Savic I, Persec Z. Relationship between clinical data and urodynamic findings in patients with lumbar intervertebral disk protrusion. Urol Res. 2002;30:219–22.

26. de Sèze M, Ruffion A, Denys P, Joseph P-A, Perrouin-Verbe B. The neurogenic bladder in multiple sclerosis: review of the literature and proposal of management guidelines. Mult Scler J. 2007;13:915–28.

27. Welk B, Morrow S, Madarasz W, Potter P, Sequeira K. The conceptualization and development of a patient-reported neurogenic bladder symptom score. Res Rep Urol. 2013;5:129.

28. Welk B, Lenherr S, Elliott S, Stoffel J, Presson AP, Zhang C, Myers JB. The Neurogenic Bladder Symptom Score (NBSS): a secondary assessment of its validity, reliability among people with a spinal cord injury. Spinal Cord. 2018;56:259–64.

29. Ginsberg DA, Boone TB, Cameron AP, et al. The AUA/SUFU guideline on adult neurogenic lower urinary tract dysfunction: diagnosis and evaluation. J Urol. 2021;206:1097–105.

30. Kobashi KC, Albo ME, Dmochowski RR, et al. Surgical treatment of female stress urinary incontinence: AUA/SUFU guideline. J Urol. 2017;198:875–83.

31. Stoffel JT, Peterson AC, Sandhu JS, Suskind AM, Wei JT, Lightner DJ. AUA white paper on non-neurogenic chronic urinary retention: consensus definition, treatment algorithm, and outcome end points. J Urol. 2017;198:153–60.

32. Dangle PP, Ayyash O, Kang A, Bates C, Fox J, Stephany H, Cannon G. Cystatin C-calculated glomerular filtration rate—a marker of early renal dysfunction in patients with neuropathic bladder. Urology. 2017;100:213–7.

33. Khanna R, Sandhu A, Doddamani D. Urodynamic management of neurogenic bladder in spinal cord injury. Med J Armed Forces India. 2009;65:300–4.

34. Welk B, McIntyre A, Teasell R, Potter P, Loh E. Bladder cancer in individuals with spinal cord injuries. Spinal Cord. 2013;51:516–21.

35. Cameron AP, Rodriguez GM, Schomer KG. Systematic review of urological followup after spinal cord injury. J Urol. 2012;187:391–7.

36. Kavanagh A, Akhavizadegan H, Walter M, Stothers L, Welk B, Boone TB. Surveillance urodynamics for neurogenic lower urinary tract dysfunction: a systematic review. Can Urol Assoc J. 2018;13:133. https://doi.org/10.5489/cuaj.5563.

37. Goetz LL, Cardenas DD, Kennelly M, Bonne Lee BS, Linsenmeyer T, Moser C, Pannek J, Wyndaele J-J, Biering-Sorensen F. International spinal cord injury urinary tract infection basic data set. Spinal Cord. 2013;51:700–4.

38. Chen Y-Y, Su T-H, Lau H-H. Estrogen for the prevention of recurrent urinary tract infections in postmenopausal women: a meta-analysis of randomized controlled trials. Int Urogynecol J. 2021;32:17–25.

39. Gallien P, Amarenco G, Benoit N, et al. Cranberry versus placebo in the prevention of urinary infections in multiple sclerosis: a multicenter, randomized, placebo-controlled, double-blind trial. Mult Scler J. 2014;20:1252–9.

40. Lee BSB, Bhuta T, Simpson JM, Craig JC. Methenamine hippurate for preventing urinary tract infections. Cochrane Database Syst Rev. 2012;10:CD003265. https://doi.org/10.1002/14651858.CD003265.pub3.

41. Waites KB, Canupp KC, Roper JF, Camp SM, Chen Y. Evaluation of 3 methods of bladder irrigation to treat bacteriuria in persons with neurogenic bladder. J Spinal Cord Med. 2006;29:217–26.

42. Wyndaele JJ, Kovindha A, Madersbacher H, Radziszewski P, Ruffion A, Schurch B, Castro D, Igawa Y, Sakakibara R, Wein A. Neurologic urinary incontinence. Neurourol Urodyn. 2010;29:159–64.

43. McClurg D, Ashe RG, Lowe-Strong AS. Neuromuscular electrical stimulation and the treatment of lower urinary tract dysfunction in multiple sclerosis— a double blind, placebo controlled, randomised clinical trial. Neurourol Urodyn. 2008;27:231–7.

44. Tibaek S, Gard G, Jensen R. Is there a long-lasting effect of pelvic floor muscle training in women with urinary incontinence after ischemic stroke? Int Urogynecol J. 2007;18:281–7.

45. Tibaek S, Gard G, Jensen R. Pelvic floor muscle training is effective in women with urinary incontinence after stroke: a randomised, controlled and blinded study. Neurourol Urodyn. 2005;24:348–57.

46. Khan F, Amatya B, Ng L, Galea M. Rehabilitation outcomes in persons with spina bifida: a randomised controlled trial. J Rehabil Med. 2015;47:734–40.

47. Elmelund M, Biering-Sørensen F, Due U, Klarskov N. The effect of pelvic floor muscle training and intravaginal electrical stimulation on urinary incontinence in women with incomplete spinal cord injury: an investigator-blinded parallel randomized clinical trial. Int Urogynecol J. 2018;29:1597–606.

48. Madersbacher H, Mürtz G, Stöhrer M. Neurogenic detrusor overactivity in adults: a review on efficacy, tolerability and safety of oral antimuscarinics. Spinal Cord. 2013;51:432–41.

49. Madhuvrata P, Singh M, Hasafa Z, Abdel-Fattah M. Anticholinergic drugs for adult neurogenic detrusor overactivity: a systematic review and meta-analysis. Eur Urol. 2012;62:816–30.

50. Buser N, Ivic S, Kessler TM, Kessels AGH, Bachmann LM. Efficacy and adverse events of antimuscarinics for treating overactive bladder: network meta-analyses. Eur Urol. 2012;62:1040–60.

51. Ethans KD, Nance PW, Bard RJ, Casey AR, Schryvers Ol. Efficacy and safety of Tol Terodine in

51. people with neurogenic detrusor overactivity. J Spinal Cord Med. 2004;27:214–8.

52. Bycroft J, Leaker B, Wood S, Knight S, Shah G, Craggs M. The effect of darifenacin on neurogenic detrusor overactivity in patients with spinal cord injury; 2003.

53. Amarenco G, Sutory M, Zachoval R, Agarwal M, del Popolo G, Tretter R, Compion G, de Ridder D. Solifenacin is effective and well tolerated in patients with neurogenic detrusor overactivity: results from the double-blind, randomized, active- and placebo-controlled SONIC urodynamic study. Neurourol Urodyn. 2017;36:414–21.

54. Horstmann M, Schaefer T, Aguilar Y, Stenzl A, Sievert KD. Neurogenic bladder treatment by doubling the recommended antimuscarinic dosage. Neurourol Urodyn. 2006;25:441–5.

55. Nardulli R, Losavio E, Ranieri M, Fiore P, Megna G, Bellomo RG, Cristella G, Megna M. Combined antimuscarinics for treatment of neurogenic overactive bladder. Int J Immunopathol Pharmacol. 2012;25:35–41.

56. Tijnagel MJ, Scheepe JR, Blok BFM. Real life persistence rate with antimuscarinic treatment in patients with idiopathic or neurogenic overactive bladder: a prospective cohort study with solifenacin. BMC Urol. 2017;17:30.

57. Coupland CAC, Hill T, Dening T, Morriss R, Moore M, Hippisley-Cox J. Anticholinergic drug exposure and the risk of dementia. JAMA Intern Med. 2019;179:1084.

58. Krhut J, Borovička V, Bílková K, Sýkora R, Míka D, Mokriš J, Zachoval R. Efficacy and safety of mirabegron for the treatment of neurogenic detrusor overactivity-prospective, randomized, double-blind, placebo-controlled study. Neurourol Urodyn. 2018;37:2226–33.

59. Welk B, Hickling D, McKibbon M, Radomski S, Ethans K. A pilot randomized-controlled trial of the urodynamic efficacy of mirabegron for patients with neurogenic lower urinary tract dysfunction. Neurourol Urodyn. 2018;37:2810–7.

60. el Helou E, Labaki C, Chebel R, el Helou J, Abi Tayeh G, Jalkh G, Nemr E. The use of mirabegron in neurogenic bladder: a systematic review. World J Urol. 2020;38:2435–42.

61. Abo Youssef N, Schneider MP, Mordasini L, Ineichen BV, Bachmann LM, Chartier-Kastler E, Panicker JN, Kessler TM. Cannabinoids for treating neurogenic lower urinary tract dysfunction in patients with multiple sclerosis: a systematic review and meta-analysis. BJU Int. 2017;119:515–21.

62. Zachariou A, Filiponi M, Baltogiannis D, Giannakis J, Dimitriadis F, Tsounapi P, Takenaka A, Sofikitis N. Effective treatment of neurogenic detrusor overactivity in multiple sclerosis patients using desmopressin and mirabegron. Can J Urol. 2017;24:9107–13.

63. Woodbury MG, Hayes KC, Askes HK. Intermittent catheterization practices following spinal cord injury: a national survey. Can J Urol. 2008;15:4065–71.

64. Rognoni C, Tarricone R. Intermittent catheterisation with hydrophilic and non-hydrophilic urinary catheters: systematic literature review and meta-analyses. BMC Urol. 2017;17:4.

65. Cardenas DD, Moore KN, Dannels-McClure A, Scelza WM, Graves DE, Brooks M, Busch AK. Intermittent catheterization with a hydrophilic-coated catheter delays urinary tract infections in acute spinal cord injury: a prospective, randomized, multicenter trial. PM&R. 2011;3:408–17.

66. Hollingsworth JM, Rogers MAM, Krein SL, Hickner A, Kuhn L, Cheng A, Chang R, Saint S. Determining the noninfectious complications of indwelling urethral catheters. Ann Intern Med. 2013;159:401.

67. Rove KO, Husmann DA, Wilcox DT, Vricella GJ, Higuchi TT. Systematic review of bladder cancer outcomes in patients with spina bifida. J Pediatr Urol. 2017;13:456.e1–9.

68. Ismail S, Karsenty G, Chartier-Kastler E, Cussenot O, Compérat E, Rouprêt M, Phé V. Prevalence, management, and prognosis of bladder cancer in patients with neurogenic bladder: a systematic review. Neurourol Urodyn. 2018;37:1386–95.

69. Schurch B, Stöhrer M, Kramer G, Schmid DM, Gaul G, Hauri D. Botulinum-A toxin for treating detrusor hyperreflexia in spinal cord injured patients: a new alternative to anticholinergic drugs? Preliminary results. J Urol. 2000;164:692–7.

70. Weckx F, Tutolo M, de Ridder D, van der Aa F. The role of botulinum toxin A in treating neurogenic bladder. Transl Androl Urol. 2016;5:63–71.

71. Ni J, Wang X, Cao N, Si J, Gu B. Is repeat Botulinum Toxin A injection valuable for neurogenic detrusor overactivity-A systematic review and meta-analysis. Neurourol Urodyn. 2018;37:542–53.

72. Cruz F, Herschorn S, Aliotta P, Brin M, Thompson C, Lam W, Daniell G, Heesakkers J, Haag-Molkenteller C. Efficacy and safety of onabotulinumtoxinA in patients with urinary incontinence due to neurogenic detrusor overactivity: a randomised, double-blind, placebo-controlled trial. Eur Urol. 2011;60:742–50.

73. Ginsberg D, Cruz F, Herschorn S, et al. OnabotulinumtoxinA is effective in patients with urinary incontinence due to neurogenic detrusor activity regardless of concomitant anticholinergic use or neurologic etiology. Adv Ther. 2013;30:819–33.

74. Ginsberg D, Gousse A, Keppenne V, Sievert K-D, Thompson C, Lam W, Brin MF, Jenkins B, Haag-Molkenteller C. Phase 3 efficacy and tolerability study of onabotulinumtoxinA for urinary incontinence from neurogenic detrusor overactivity. J Urol. 2012;187:2131–9.

75. Hui C, Keji X, Chonghe J, et al. Combined detrusor-trigone BTX-A injections for urinary incontinence

secondary to neurogenic detrusor overactivity. Spinal Cord. 2016;54:46–50.

76. Chartier-Kastler E, Rovner E, Hepp Z, Khalaf K, Ni Q, Chancellor M. Patient-reported goal achievement following onabotulinumtoxinA treatment in patients with neurogenic detrusor overactivity. Neurourol Urodyn. 2016;35:595–600.

77. Kalsi V, Gonzales G, Popat R, Apostolidis A, Elneil S, Dasgupta P, Fowler CJ. Botulinum injections for the treatment of bladder symptoms of multiple sclerosis. Ann Neurol. 2007;62:452–7.

78. Metz LM, McGuinness SD, Harris C. Urinary tract infections may trigger relapse in multiple sclerosis. Axone (Dartmouth, NS). 1998;19:67–70.

79. Phé V, Pakzad M, Curtis C, Porter B, Haslam C, Chataway J, Panicker JN. Urinary tract infections in multiple sclerosis. Mult Scler J. 2016;22:855–61.

80. Fougere RJ, Currie KD, Nigro MK, Stothers L, Rapoport D, Krassioukov A, v. Reduction in bladder-related autonomic dysreflexia after onabotulinumtoxinA treatment in spinal cord injury. J Neurotrauma. 2016;33:1651–7.

81. Sakakibara R, Panicker J, Finazzi-Agro E, Iacovelli V, Bruschini H. A guideline for the management of bladder dysfunction in Parkinson's disease and other gait disorders. Neurourol Urodyn. 2016;35: 551–63.

82. Hassouna T, Gleason JM, Lorenzo AJ. Botulinum toxin A's expanding role in the management of pediatric lower urinary tract dysfunction. Curr Urol Rep. 2014;15:426.

83. Gamé X, Mouracade P, Chartier-Kastler E, et al. Botulinum toxin-A (Botox®) intradetrusor injections in children with neurogenic detrusor overactivity/neurogenic overactive bladder: a systematic literature review. J Pediatr Urol. 2009;5:156–64.

84. Peyronnet B, Even A, Capon G, et al. Intradetrusor injections of botulinum toxin a in adults with spinal dysraphism. J Urol. 2018;200:875–80.

85. Leitner L, Guggenbühl-Roy S, Knüpfer SC, Walter M, Schneider MP, Tornic J, Sammer U, Mehnert U, Kessler TM. More than 15 years of experience with intradetrusor onabotulinumtoxinA injections for treating refractory neurogenic detrusor overactivity: lessons to be learned. Eur Urol. 2016;70:522–8.

86. Schneider MP, Gross T, Bachmann LM, et al. Tibial nerve stimulation for treating neurogenic lower urinary tract dysfunction: a systematic review. Eur Urol. 2015;68:859–67.

87. de Sèze M, Raibaut P, Gallien P, Even-Schneider A, Denys P, Bonniaud V, Gamé X, Amarenco G. Transcutaneous posterior tibial nerve stimulation for treatment of the overactive bladder syndrome in multiple sclerosis: results of a multicenter prospective study. Neurourol Urodyn. 2011;30:306–11.

88. Monteiro ÉS, de Carvalho LBC, Fukujima MM, Lora MI, do Prado GF. Electrical stimulation of the posterior tibialis nerve improves symptoms of post-stroke neurogenic overactive bladder in men: a randomized controlled trial. Urology. 2014;84:509–14.

89. Andretta E, Simeone C, Ostardo E, Pastorello M, Zuliani C. Usefulness of sacral nerve modulation in a series of multiple sclerosis patients with bladder dysfunction. J Neurol Sci. 2014;347:257–61.

90. Chaabane W, Guillotreau J, Castel-lacanal E, Abu-Anz S, de Boissezon X, Malavaud B, Marque P, Sarramon J-P, Rischmann P, Game X. Sacral neuromodulation for treating neurogenic bladder dysfunction: clinical and urodynamic study. Neurourol Urodyn. 2011;30:547–50.

91. Engeler DS, Meyer D, Abt D, Müller S, Schmid H-P. Sacral neuromodulation for the treatment of neurogenic lower urinary tract dysfunction caused by multiple sclerosis: a single-centre prospective series. BMC Urol. 2015;15:105.

92. Zhang P, Wang J, Zhang Y, et al. Results of sacral neuromodulation therapy for urinary voiding dysfunction: five-year experience of a retrospective, multicenter study in China. Neuromodulation. 2019;22: 730–7.

93. Kessler TM, la Framboise D, Trelle S, Fowler CJ, Kiss G, Pannek J, Schurch B, Sievert K-D, Engeler DS. Sacral neuromodulation for neurogenic lower urinary tract dysfunction: systematic review and meta-analysis. Eur Urol. 2010;58:865–74.

94. van Ophoven A, Engelberg S, Lilley H, Sievert K-D. Systematic literature review and meta-analysis of Sacral Neuromodulation (SNM) in patients with Neurogenic Lower Urinary Tract Dysfunction (nLUTD): over 20 years' experience and future directions. Adv Ther. 2021;38:1987–2006.

95. Sievert K-D, Amend B, Gakis G, Toomey P, Badke A, Kaps HP, Stenzl A. Early sacral neuromodulation prevents urinary incontinence after complete spinal cord injury. Ann Neurol. 2010;67:74–84.

96. Lombardi G, Musco S, Celso M, del Corso F, del Popolo G. Sacral neuromodulation for neurogenic non-obstructive urinary retention in incomplete spinal cord patients: a ten-year follow-up single-centre experience. Spinal Cord. 2014;52:241–5.

97. Abrams P, Cardozo L, Fall M, Griffiths D, Rosier P, Ulmsten U, van Kerrebroeck P, Victor A, Wein A. The standardisation of terminology of lower urinary tract function: report from the standardisation sub-committee of the International Continence Society. Neurourol Urodyn. 2002;21:167–78.

98. U.S. Food and Drug Administration. Premarket approval supplement number P970004/S4. Implantable Electrical Stimulator for Incontinence. 2019. https://www.accessdata.fda.gov/scripts/cdrh/cfdocs/cfpma/pma.cfm?ID=P970004.

99. Hoen L'T, Ecclestone H, BFM B, et al. Long-term effectiveness and complication rates of bladder augmentation in patients with neurogenic bladder dysfunction: a systematic review. Neurourol Urodyn. 2017;36:1685–702.

100. Fraser MO, Chancellor MB. Neural control of the urethra and development of pharmacotherapy for stress urinary incontinence. BJU Int. 2003;91:743–8.

101. Bymaster F. Comparative affinity of duloxetine and venlafaxine for serotonin and norepinephrine transporters in vitro and in vivo, human serotonin receptor subtypes, and other neuronal receptors. Neuropsychopharmacology. 2001;25:871–80.

102. Thor KB, Katofiasc MA. Effects of duloxetine, a combined serotonin and norepinephrine reuptake inhibitor, on central neural control of lower urinary tract function in the chloralose-anesthetized female cat. J Pharmacol Exp Ther. 1995;274:1014–24.

103. Millard RJ, Moore K, Rencken R, Yalcin I, Bump RC, Group DUIS. Duloxetine vs placebo in the treatment of stress urinary incontinence: a four-continent randomized clinical trial. BJU Int. 2004;93:311–8.

104. National Institute for Health and Care Excellence Do Not Do Recommendation. In: https://www.nice.org.uk/donotdo/do-not-use-duloxetine-as-a-firstline-treatment-for-women-with-predominant-stress-urinary-incontinence.

105. Bennett JK, Green BG, Foote JE, Gray M. Collagen injections for intrinsic sphincter deficiency in the neuropathic urethra. Paraplegia. 1995;33:697–700.

106. de Vocht TF, Chrzan R, Dik P, Klijn AJ, de Jong TPVM. Long-term results of bulking agent injection for persistent incontinence in cases of neurogenic bladder dysfunction. J Urol. 2010;183:719–23.

107. Farag F, Koens M, Sievert K-D, de Ridder D, Feitz W, Heesakkers J. Surgical treatment of neurogenic stress urinary incontinence: a systematic review of quality assessment and surgical outcomes. Neurourol Urodyn. 2016;35:21–5.

108. Myers JB, Mayer EN, Lenherr S, (NBRG.org) NBRG. Management options for sphincteric deficiency in adults with neurogenic bladder. Transl Androl Urol. 2016;5:145–57.

109. Athanasopoulos A, Gyftopoulos K, McGuire EJ. Treating stress urinary incontinence in female patients with neuropathic bladder: the value of the autologous fascia rectus sling. Int Urol Nephrol. 2012;44:1363–7.

110. Musco S, Ecclestone H, Hoen L't, et al. Efficacy and safety of surgical treatments for neurogenic stress urinary incontinence in adults: a systematic review. Eur Urol Focus. 2021; https://doi.org/10.1016/j.euf.2021.08.007.

111. El-Azab AS, El-Nashar SA. Midurethral slings versus the standard pubovaginal slings for women with neurogenic stress urinary incontinence. Int Urogynecol J. 2015;26:427–32.

112. Costa P, Poinas G, ben Naoum K, Bouzoubaa K, Wagner L, Soustelle L, Boukaram M, Droupy S. Long-term results of artificial urinary sphincter for women with type III stress urinary incontinence. Eur Urol. 2013;63:753–8.

113. Shpall AI, Ginsberg DA. Bladder neck closure with lower urinary tract reconstruction: technique and long-term followup. J Urol. 2004;172:2296–9.

114. Abrams P, Amarenco G, Bakke A, et al. Tamsulosin: efficacy and safety in patients with neurogenic lower urinary tract dysfunction due to suprasacral spinal cord injury. J Urol. 2003;170:1242–51.

115. Naumann M, So Y, Argoff CE, et al. Assessment: botulinum neurotoxin in the treatment of autonomic disorders and pain (an evidence-based review) [RETIRED]. Neurology. 2008;70:1707–14.

116. Kuo H-C. Satisfaction with urethral injection of Botulinum Toxin A for detrusor sphincter dyssynergia in patients with spinal cord lesion. Neurourol Urodyn. 2008;27:793–6.

117. King AB, Goldman HB. Bladder outlet obstruction in women: functional causes. Curr Urol Rep. 2014;15:436.

118. Sosland R, Kowalik CA, Cohn JA, Milam DF, Kaufman MR, Dmochowski RR, Reynolds WS. Nonclinical barriers to care for neurogenic patients undergoing complex urologic reconstruction. Urology. 2019;124:271–5. https://doi.org/10.1016/j.urology.

119. Langa KM, Fultz NH, Saint S, Kabeto MU, Herzog AR. Informal caregiving time and costs for urinary incontinence in older individuals in the United States. J Am Geriatr Soc. 2002;50:733–7.

120. Farber NJ, Davis RB, Grimsby GM, et al. Bowel preparation prior to reconstructive urologic surgery in pediatric myelomeningocele patients. Can J Urol. 2017;24:9038–42.

121. Hensley P, Higgins M, Rasper A, Ziada A, Strup S, Coleman C, Ruf K, Gupta S. Efficacy and safety of alvimopan use in benign urinary tract reconstruction. Int Urol Nephrol. 2021;53:77–82.

122. Pinto K, Jerkins GR, Noe HN. Ventriculoperitoneal shunt infection after bladder augmentation. Urology. 1999;54:356–8.

123. Paradella AC, de A Musegante AF, Brites C. Comparison of different antibiotic protocols for asymptomatic bacteriuria in patients with neurogenic bladder treated with botulinum toxin A. Braz J Infect Dis. 2016;20:623–6.

124. Leitner L, Sammer U, Walter M, Knüpfer SC, Schneider MP, Seifert B, Tornic J, Mehnert U, Kessler TM. Antibiotic prophylaxis may not be necessary in patients with asymptomatic bacteriuria undergoing intradetrusor onabotulinumtoxinA injections for neurogenic detrusor overactivity. Sci Rep. 2016;6:33197.

Stem Cell and Tissue Engineering in Female Urinary Incontinence

27

Elisabeth M. Sebesta and Melissa R. Kaufman

Contents

Introduction	488
Current Management of Stress Urinary Incontinence	488
Cell-Based Therapy for Stress Urinary Incontinence in Women	488
Types of Stem Cells	489
Animal Models for the Study of Stress Urinary Incontinence	489
Cell-Based Therapies for Female Stress Urinary Incontinence	490
Conclusions	501
References	501

Abstract

Stress urinary incontinence (SUI) is a common condition, which affects the quality of life of female patients. There is a need for effective and durable treatment options that confer minimal morbidity to the patients. The newest frontier of treatment for SUI includes regenerative medicine with the use of cell-based therapies to restore the native continence mechanism via regeneration of the urethral sphincter complex. Cell-based therapies have thus far proven to be a promising option with increasing experimental, both in animal and human studies, and clinical investigations. The most extensively studied cell type being autologous muscle-derived cells (AMDCs). The literature to date has revealed this to be safe for the treatment of SUI in women, with larger clinical trials currently underway. Continued investigation regarding the mechanisms, effectiveness, and durability of injected cells will be necessary in order to make this innovative therapy option commercially available for use in patients.

Keywords

Stress urinary incontinence · Stem cells · Regenerative medicine · Cell-based therapy

E. M. Sebesta · M. R. Kaufman (✉)
Department of Urology, Vanderbilt University Medical Center, Nashville, TN, USA
e-mail: elisabeth.sebesta@vumc.org;
melissa.kaufman@vumc.org

© Springer Nature Switzerland AG 2023
F. E. Martins et al. (eds.), *Female Genitourinary and Pelvic Floor Reconstruction*,
https://doi.org/10.1007/978-3-031-19598-3_28

Introduction

Stress urinary incontinence (SUI) is defined as the involuntary loss of urine on effort or physical exertion [1]. Urinary incontinence is an extremely common condition, with SUI affecting up to one in four women and accounting for an estimated $12 billion annually in healthcare costs [2]. Additionally, SUI has substantial effect on women's quality of life (QOL) with significant psychosocial overlap. In a case-control study demonstrated in women with incontinence, the odds ratios for depression and anxiety were 1.64 and 1.59, respectively [3]. Therefore, considering the substantial healthcare resources and dollars spent on managing patients with SUI, in addition to the profound effect on patients' QOL, there is a need to develop durable treatments for these patients. Using tissue engineering and novel cell-based therapies for treatment of SUI is a compelling option and an exciting new frontier of SUI management with the possibility to offer a minimally invasive treatment option with minimal morbidity. Such cell-based therapies use autologous patient tissues to regenerate the native continence mechanism. In this chapter we will review the different types of stem cells and their properties, the available animal models used for study of SUI, and a discussion of the currently available preclinical and human trials on the use of cell-based regenerative therapies for the management of SUI in women.

Current Management of Stress Urinary Incontinence

The classic pathophysiology of SUI is postulated to involve the loss of anatomic hammock-like support of the urethra and/or a loss of urethral mucosal coaptation [4]. The current management options for women with SUI range widely, from conservative therapy to invasive surgical procedures [5]. Conservative measures are recommended prior to offering invasive surgery and encompass such measures include weight loss, behavioral management, fluid management, pelvic floor physical therapy, pelvic floor electrical stimulation, biofeedback, and incontinence pessaries or vaginal inserts [5, 6]. Although recommended prior to undergoing invasive surgical procedures, the outcomes of conservative therapies are understandably limited [6, 7].

More invasive treatments for women with SUI include injection of urethral bulking agents and surgical procedures including retropubic suspensions and both synthetic mid-urethral and autologous fascial pubovaginal slings [5]. Overall, slings have acceptable long-term improvement rates, which is why they are considered the gold standard for surgical treatment of SUI in women; however, there are numerous short- and long-term complications which may confer great morbidity to patients affected.

The use of synthetic mid-urethral slings (MUS) is the most common procedure currently performed for female SUI in the United States [8, 9]. While there are favorable long-term outcomes for managing SUI, there are also many risks of the procedure which should not be discounted, including voiding dysfunction, obstruction, mesh erosions or extrusions, urinary tract infections, bladder perforations, chronic pain, and vascular and nerve injuries [8, 9]. The injection of urethral bulking agents appears to be an attractive alternative option for management of women with SUI, due to its less invasive nature and fewer complications. However, injectable urethral bulking agents lack the durability of slings, and women can expect to require repeat injections in order to achieve the desired result; thus bulking agents may be difficult to sustain as a long-term management strategy for patients [10]. Therefore, with the large number of patients suffering from SUI and its effect on overall QOL, there is a clear clinical need for less invasive yet highly effective and durable management strategies for women with SUI.

Cell-Based Therapy for Stress Urinary Incontinence in Women

The newest frontier with regard to treatment of SUI in women includes regenerative medicine with the use of cell-based therapies. The goal of regenerative medicine technologies includes replacing, engineering, or regenerating human cells or tissues in order to restore normal function [11]. Regenerative technologies harness the body's native repair mechanisms to functionally restore tissues. Such therapies rely on the use of stem cells, which are unique in their ability to self-renew and thereby produce a population of differentiated progeny [12]. Stem cells have been used for the purpose of regenerating injured tissues in a variety of pathologic conditions. For over 40 years, stem cells have been used in the treatment of hematologic conditions; however, the real spotlight on their multi-therapeutic potential started in the late 1990s [3]. With regard to incontinence in women, stem cell therapies have been investigated with the goal of restoring the external sphincter (striated muscle), internal sphincter (smooth muscle), the neuromuscular synapse, and blood supply [13]. Most clinical trials for urinary incontinence involve the injection of stem cells into the striated urethral sphincter with the goals of regenerating the native continence mechanism and thereby truly reversing the primary pathophysiology of intrinsic sphincter deficiency (ISD). This is distinct as compared to most current treatments for female SUI which only temporize symptoms [14, 15].

According to the American Urologic Association (AUA) Guidelines on the management of SUI in women, cell-based therapy is an exciting option on the leading edge of SUI management; however, at the time of guideline publication, it recommends these therapies only be offered to patients as part of a clinical trial [5]. With continued research in this area, we hope in the near future this can be recommended as a part of the treatment algorithm for female patients with SUI.

Types of Stem Cells

Stem cells are classified into one of four main categories: embryonic stem cells, amniotic fluid stem cells, induced pluripotent stem cells, and adult somatic stem cells [16–18]. Embryonic stem cells have the ability to differentiate into any human cell form and are derived from a human blastocyst [16, 18]. They have expansive therapeutic potential as they are the least differentiated. There remains a continued ethical concern regarding the use of embryonic stem cells, in addition to questions regarding potential allogenicity and oncogenesis. Therefore, the use of embryonic stem cells in regenerative medicine for urologic applications is limited.

Induced pluripotent stem cells are pluripotent cells that can be reprogrammed to differentiate into various cell lines with different transcription factors [18]. Similar to embryonic stem cells, they have a wide differentiation potential; however, they preclude the necessity of an embryo [12]. Their use is again limited by concerns with oncogenesis and the required time to induce them.

Amniotic fluid stem cells are isolated from the amniotic fluid or placental membrane of a developing fetus [16]. Their potential for differentiation is intermediate, but they are hypothesized to have lower tumorigenicity [19]. The available data on their use in SUI will be discussed below.

The majority of current cell-based therapies utilize somatic multipotent adult stem cells derived from various tissue types. Such cells are terminally differentiated and serve as progenitor cells for the regeneration and renewal of local tissues. We will discuss all the different types of adult somatic stem cells below, along with the currently available literature regarding their use in SUI.

Animal Models for the Study of Stress Urinary Incontinence

Over the last 50 years, many animal models for SUI have emerged. The majority of the research regarding cell-based therapy for SUI has been carried out in small animals including rabbits and rodents; however, larger animals such as pigs and dogs have also been used. There are numerous animal models in the literature for inducing urethral dysfunction. These include vaginal distension, pudendal nerve injury or transection, urethrolysis, periurethral cauterization, and urethral sphincterotomy [20].

Many of the first animal models aimed to replicate the mechanisms of SUI associated with childbirth. This was first done by Lin et al. in rats using a intravaginal balloon to induce vaginal distension [21]. They found a significant decrease in periurethral striated and smooth muscle in this model, in addition to various markers indicating nerve injury. Although a widely employed model, the results are temporary, with most animals displaying a recovery of urethral function between 10 days and 6 weeks [22, 23]. This is a simple model in which one can effectively study the pathophysiology of childbirth-induced SUI and the recovery; however, it is challenging to use for testing the efficacy of SUI treatments beyond 6 weeks. In humans, however, nearly half of women who have a full remission of SUI after childbirth redevelop SUI in 5 years [24]. The long-term and age-induced effects of simulated childbirth injury have not yet been studied in animals. Similar to vaginal distension models, pudendal nerve crush injury animal models have been used to simulate childbirth-induced SUI. Again, although useful in the investigation of neuromuscular recovery after childbirth, as the effects are generally temporary, it is not an ideal model for investigating the longer-term effects of cell-based therapies [20].

More durable animal models for studying cell-based therapies for SUI consist of simulating periurethral sphincter damage with the goal of producing a longer-lasting SUI either directly or indirectly. Transabdominal urethrolysis first performed in rats was found to induce neuromuscular and functional dysfunction that simulated SUI, as measured by a decrease in leak point pressure (LPP). This was shown to be more durable and persistent than previously mentioned models, with the persistence of low LPP to around 24 weeks [25]. Periurethral electrocauterization achieves a similar outcome for simulating SUI via heat destruction, as opposed to physical destruction, of tissues. In this model, the periurethral tissues are cauterized from the bladder neck to the upper face of the pubic symphysis at elevated temperatures [26]. The differences observed in LPP in rats that underwent this periurethral cauterization were maintained for up to

16 weeks. Finally, direct sphincter damage via sphincterotomy has been used to simulate SUI and seems to be quite durable lasting up to 7 months after surgery in a canine model [27]. It is believed that these models are representative of surgically induced incontinence. However, these animal models are still not necessarily indicative of the complex etiology associated with the SUI seen with aging in women [20].

Finally, researchers have utilized indirect injury including pudendal nerve transection with or without pubourethral ligament transection to simulate SUI. Pudendal nerve transections have been performed either uni- or bilaterally, with bilateral transection resulting in a more significant decrease in LPP and striated muscle atrophy in rats [28]. This model has also been used in other non-rodent and larger animal models including cats, dogs, and nonhuman primates. The applicability of this method of inducing SUI to a human-like animal model makes it seem to be highly promising in the study of SUI to most accurately replicate the pathophysiology observed in humans.

To date, the majority of preclinical animal studies for cell-based regenerative therapy for SUI have been performed in murine models, which do not necessarily recapitulate the characteristics of SUI seen in humans. However, using larger animals to study SUI, while perhaps more accurately replicating the loss of sphincter function seen in humans, is also limited by their rate of growth and the special facilities often required to perform such research [14]. Currently available animal studies have implemented all of the above models for inducing SUI in animals; therefore it is important to be familiar with the different strengths and weaknesses of each animal model in order when reviewing this literature.

Cell-Based Therapies for Female Stress Urinary Incontinence

Autologous Muscle-Derived Cells for Urethral Sphincter Regeneration

The vast majority of research both preclinical animal and human clinical trials regarding cell-based therapies for SUI has involved autologous muscle-derived cells for urethral sphincter regeneration (AMDC-USR). Autologous cells are harvested from skeletal muscle, expanded ex vivo, and reinjected into the external urethral sphincter with the goal of regenerating the sphincteric muscle to restore continence.

Background

Skeletal muscle, unlike smooth muscle, has the ability to undergo constant repair due to the presence of satellite cells, and muscle-derived cells used in sphincter regeneration are considered the precursors to satellite cells [29]. Satellite cells are mononucleated myogenic cells located between the basement membrane and the sarcolemma of terminally differentiated muscle fibers [30]. In adult skeletal muscle, these cells are a quiescent reserve, which can become activated for tissue regeneration in response to injury. Once activated, satellite cells have the ability to regenerate into more satellite cells or into a variety of cell types, including myogenic, endothelial, adipogenic, or osteogenic [31–33]. In muscle regeneration, the satellite cells will fuse and form myotubes. The myotubes subsequently develop into myofibers which are capable of muscle contraction or fuse with damaged segments of muscle fibers.

In the development of AMDC-USR for treatment of SUI, the first feasibility studies aimed at demonstrating the ability to reliably harvest AMDCs containing satellite cells and myoblasts from a skeletal muscle biopsy [34]. Additionally, using AMDCs in muscular regeneration relies on demonstrating the fusion of implanted cells with host myofibers, which also had not been previously been accomplished. Prior to the efforts in developing AMDC-USR, only the use of myogenic cell lines and primary muscle cultures had been previously attempted, each of which had significant problems. Myogenic cell lines have significant tumorigenic potential, and muscle cultures contain a substantial proportion of non-myogenic cells which demonstrated difficulty fusing with host fibers; therefore neither is really ideal for muscular regeneration in this manner.

A new modified pre-plate technique was developed for the purpose of expanding myogenic cells based on their adherence characteristics in order to overcome these previous difficulties. After mechanical and enzymatic digestion, the cells were subjected into a series of platings on collagen-coated flasks of non-adherent cells until the cultures were contained the desired cells with the myogenic marker, desmin. There were two distinct cell populations found in the platings, which were subsequently termed "early" and "late" plates. The early plates contained the cells that adhered early, in the first 4 days after plating, and were found to be primarily fibroblasts and conventional myoblasts. In contrary, late plates were morphologically and functionally distinct, with stem cell-like properties.

The first studies on these late-plate cells were performed in the treatment of muscular dystrophies (MD). In MD models, late-plate cell populations were able to improve the efficiency of myoblast transplantation in dystrophin-deficient mice. This was further investigated by evaluating their capacity for self-renewal, proliferation over time, multipotent differentiation potential, and immune-privileged behaviors [35]. Ninety days after injection of the cells, a significantly high number of dystrophin-positive myofibers were observed in late-plate muscles as compared to the very few observed in early-plate muscles. These investigations helped to strengthen the hypothesis that early- and late-plate cells are truly two distinct cell populations of satellite cells and that the late-plate cells have the ability to persist and integrate in the long term for successful transplantation.

These preliminary studies established that AMDCs could easily be harvested and reliably expanded in vitro and laid the groundwork for the animal and human studies on AMDC-USR. The next steps in the development of this technology included verifying the feasibility and effect of transplanting AMDCs in various animal models for the treatment of SUI.

Animal Studies

As previously discussed, there is no animal model that perfectly replicates the complex pathology that results in SUI in adult women; however, there are several useful models each with distinct strengths and weaknesses, which have been used in the development of AMDC-USR technology. Furthermore, the data obtained from animal studies demonstrated tissue integration with neuroregeneration, neovascularization, and ultimately improvement in sphincteric function when injected in these animal models [29]. These studies also allowed for further investigation into the mechanism of action, including direct incorporation into the muscular sphincter complex, secretion of chemokines and growth factors, and paracrine effects from adjacent tissues [14].

The initial studies using muscle cell injection for SUI used myoblasts tagged with a fluorescent marker transduced with an adenovirus vector carrying the *lacZ* reporter gene [36]. These cells were then injected into the urethra of adult rats. Two to 4 days after injection, tissue was harvested and histologically examined. A large population contained the *lacZ* marker as evidenced by the expression of beta-galactosidase. This indicated the survival of the myoblasts injected into the urethral tissue. Subsequently, in order to examine long-term survival, again myoblasts transduced with *lacZ* gene were injected into the bladder and proximal urethra of mice with severe combined immunodeficiency [37]. The tissues were then examined for beta-galactosidase activity at multiple time points after injection up to 6 months. At all time points, many myofibers with beta-galactosidase were observed, which demonstrated the long-term survival of myoblasts being injected into urothelial tissue.

Next, the durability of injected AMDCs was compared to that of bovine collagen using a rat model [38]. Muscle-derived cells were obtained via gastrocnemius biopsy in six rats and then injected into the urethra at a concentrations of 1 to 1.5×10^6 cells per 20 µL. Commercially available bovine collagen was injected into the urethras of three rats to serve as controls. At 3 and 30 days after injection, tissue was harvested for histological examination. At 3 days, the presence of the muscle-derived cells in the urothelial tissue was similar to that of collagen. At 30 days, however, the concentration of muscle-derived

cells was much higher than that of the collagen, with the concentration of muscle-derived cells at 88% of what it was at day 3 as compared to almost no collagen persistent in the tissues. With this study, the authors demonstrated the feasibility of injecting AMDCs into the urethra in a rat model, in addition to displaying the superior durability of these cells as compared to collagen.

Subsequent studies utilizing various animal models focused on examining the functional restoration of the urinary sphincter following AMDC injection. Using a rat model of SUI simulating postsurgical incontinence with urethral electrocauterization performed via laparotomy, authors examined the effect of AMDC injection [39]. After urethral cauterization, AMDCs were obtained via foot muscle biopsy and subsequently injected into the injured urethra at a concentration 5×10^6 cells per 10 µL. Outcomes included sphincter contractility and LPP with a vertical tilt table system to simulate the erect posture of humans more accurately. The LPP was determined on cystometrogram when combined with a sneeze test in which the rat was stimulated by tickling a whisker. Histological evaluation was also performed. The rats injected with AMDCs were compared to rats that received sphincteric injury but no injections and to controls that received no sphincteric injury at all. After sphincter injury, the measured LPP was low, indicating urethral sphincter damage as desired. One month after AMDC injection, the LPP recovered to 41% of the control value with no injury. On histological examination, the authors observed after sphincteric injury, there was atrophy and fibrosis of urethral cells. In rats treated with AMDCs, the cells had fused and formed multinucleated myotubes. Additionally, at the junction between injured and normal cells, the regenerated myotubes were intermingled with the normal non-injured myofibers. The results obtained from this trial demonstrated that AMDCs from adult rats when injected into injured urethral sphincters had the capability to induce the formation of contracting muscle fibers and restore at least partial sphincter function after 1 month.

Several other groups conducted subsequent studies in animal models of adult female rats that underwent denervation of the sciatic or pudendal nerves to induce sphincteric injury [40, 41]. With the objective of examining whether periurethral injection of AMDCs could increase the LPP, denervated rats injected with either AMDCs or a saline vector alone were compared to controls without urethral injury [33]. After denervation, the LPP was appropriately decreased to indicate sphincteric injury. After 1 and 4 weeks, the injection of AMDCs increased the LPP as compared to the injection of saline alone. This study demonstrated a true regeneration effect with the urethral injection of AMDCs that was distinct from a possible bulking effect from injecting saline alone. A similar study examined the contractility of urethral sphincter muscle in denervated rats after periurethral injection of AMDCs as compared to controls [41]. Again, urethral denervation decreased the sphincteric contractility appropriately, measured to be 8% of the controls, indicating urethral injury. After urethral injection of AMDCs, contractility was restored to 87% of normal. Histological examination revealed the formation of new skeletal muscles in the urethral tissue of the rats injected with AMDCs.

In another study examining the effects of urethral injection of AMDCs as compared to other cells, authors evaluated effects of injecting AMDCs that were isolated and expanded ex vivo specifically to retain the capacity to fuse and form postmitotic multinucleated myotubes as compared to fibroblasts [42]. Denervated rats were injected with these AMDCs or fibroblasts. The outcome measures included LPP and urethral muscle contractility, with the additional objectives of differentiating from possible bulking effect of fibroblast injection. As expected, LPP increased after AMDC and fibroblast injection in denervated rats as compared to controls which were injected with only saline. The increase in LPP occurred in a dose-response manner, and was similar between the two cell populations. However, only rats injected with the highest density of fibroblasts experienced urinary retention, whereas rats injected with high-dose AMDCs did not display any adverse events. Electrical stimulation in vitro of urethral muscles demonstrated that after AMDC injection, muscle contraction was 73% of controls, whereas after fibroblast injection, muscle contraction was only 46% of controls. This study strengthened the observations of previously discussed studies that the benefit of AMDC injection is not simply a bulking effect but a function of true muscle regeneration.

Finally, an animal model utilizing cauterization of the mid-urethra of rats to induce rhabdosphincter damage was used to investigate AMDC injection [43]. On histological examination, 4 weeks after intraurethral injection of AMDCs, the cells had integrated into the striated muscle of the damaged urethra. Additionally, neuroregeneration was enhanced as compared to controls injected with only saline. The LPP was measured at 4 and 6 weeks after injection, and in rats injected with AMDCs, the LPP was increased significantly as compared to rats injected with only saline and not significantly different from non-cauterized controls. Authors concluded this muscular regeneration, and neuroregeneration suggests that AMDCs have the capability for multipotent differentiation and/or to elicit a paracrine effect such that the muscle-nerve complex is able to successfully regenerate.

After numerous studies on animal models demonstrating not only the feasibility of urethral injection of AMDCs but also the effectiveness of improving urethral contractility and muscle cell regeneration, clinical trials were developed to examine the use of AMDCs in humans with SUI.

Human Trials on Autologous Muscle-Derived Cells for Urethral Sphincter Regeneration

Human clinical trials on AMDC injections first began reporting results in the late 2000s. In 2007, an Austrian group published the first clinical trial on autologous myoblast and fibroblast injection for use in patients with SUI [44]. In 2008, however, the publication of this trial was officially retracted by the journal due to numerous ethical concerns regarding the trial design and data interpretation [45]. This was a setback in the overall development of AMDCs and undoubtedly resulted in a delay in further advancement of this promising technology.

Subsequently in 2008, the first North American pilot study on the use of AMDCs to treat SUI was published [46]. In this trial, eight women with urodynamic-documented SUI who had failed conservative therapies underwent quadriceps biopsy to isolate 18 to 22 $\times$ 10^6 AMDCs. These cells were then injected using local anesthesia in a clinic-based setting via both a transurethral and periurethral approach into the external urethral sphincter. Three of the eight patients received repeat injection using a periurethral approach after 3 months of follow-up. The patients were followed for a mean of 16.5 months (range 3–24 months), with three women withdrawing after only 1 month. In the remaining five women who were followed longer than 1 month, all women observed clinical improvement in SUI between 3 and 8 months, which was sustained to a median follow-up of 10 months. One of the five women achieved complete continence and was subjectively dry through trial completion at 12 months. Importantly, there were no adverse side effects observed, as this phase I trial was primarily designed to demonstrate safety. Additionally, two patients who later went on to undergo suburethral sling surgery for persistent incontinence had no evidence of changes to their tissues that negatively impacted their surgical treatment. The results of this pilot study were extremely encouraging and paved the way for further advances by demonstrating clear safety and possible clinical efficacy of AMDC-USR in the management of female SUI.

Following this successful pilot study, the next undertaking was a multiphase, prospective, randomized, blinded feasibility study to explore different doses of AMDC injections [47]. Thirty-eight women with SUI were randomized to undergo a low-dose (1, 2, 3, 8, or 16 $\times$ 10^6) AMDC periurethral injection in phase I, followed by nine sequentially enrolled patients undergoing a high-dose (32, 64, or 128 $\times$ 10^6) AMDC injection in phase II. Finally in phase III, nine women were treated with 16, 32, or 64 $\times$ 10^6 AMDC injection under transvaginal ultrasound (TVUS) guidance. Ultimately, the use of TVUS guidance did not appear to effect outcomes at all, and therefore the data was analyzed from this study independent of the method of injection. All women enrolled in the study were given the option to undergo repeat injections, with a second dose 3 months after their first. Thirty-two patients elected to receive a second treatment. Outcome measures included pad tests, incontinence diaries, and patient-reported symptom questionnaires. Thirty-three of the 38 women completed the study with 18-month follow-up, 4 of whom underwent 1 treatment and 29 who underwent 2 treatments. In the 29 women who completed 2 treatment injections, high-dose injections were associated with 50% or greater improvement in pad weight in 89% and 50% or greater reduction in subjective diary-reported leakage in 78%. The authors concluded a dose-dependent response, as significantly more women receiving high-dose injections reported experiencing 0–1 leaks in a 3-day period at the trial end of 18 months as compared to women receiving a low-dose injection. Greater improvements in QOL were also observed on standardized questionnaires. There were no serious treatment-related adverse events observed. Mild bruising or pain at the muscle biopsy site and/or urethral injection site or mild increase in lower urinary tract symptoms after injection was observed but resolved without other interventions within 30 days.

Due to the increased efficacy of the high-dose injections in this trial, subsequent trials focused on the higher dose range. By including additional patients, an expanded analysis was completed by pooling data from two phase I/II trials with identical inclusion criteria with the goal of assessing safety and efficacy of AMDC-USR at 12 months of follow-up [48]. A total of 80 women with SUI were included in this analysis and received peri- or transurethral injections of 10 ($n = 16$), 50 ($n = 16$), 100 ($n = 24$), or 200 $\times$ 10^6 ($n = 24$) AMDCs obtained via quadriceps femoris biopsy. Outcome measures included adverse events, 3-day voiding diary, 24-hour pad tests, and the validated patient questionnaires including Urogenital Distress Inventory (UDI-6) and Incontinence Impact Questionnaire (IIQ-7). Seventy-four of the 80 women completed 12 months of follow-up. All dose groups in this study reported fewer stress leak events on voiding diary at 1–3 months from injection. Only patients receiving the higher doses of 100 or 200 × 10⁶ AMDCs demonstrated significant reduction in 24-hour pad weight, with 60% and 64% of patients achieving a 50% or greater reduction in the 100 and 200 × 10⁶ dose groups, respectively. All patients regardless of dose had improvements in UDI-6 and IIQ-7 scores at 12 months. Adverse events were mild and transient. Four of 74 women had mild biopsy site events. Additionally, 18% of women experienced injection-related events, all after transurethral injections, which included dysuria (7/14), pelvic/abdominal pain (4/14), pruritus (3/14) urinary urgency (2/14), and self-limited hematuria (2/14). Across all treatment doses, there was no urinary retention observed – a risk observed in all other procedural treatment options for female SUI. From this study, the authors concluded that injections in the examined dose range were safe, and again they confirmed the dose-response relationship, with great efficacy seen at the highest doses of 100 and 200 × 10⁶ AMDC injections.

With the promising results and clear safety demonstrated in the aforementioned trials, a multicenter double-blind, randomized, placebo-controlled clinical trial was designed to determine the efficacy of ADMC-USR [49]. The target enrollment for this trial was 246 women with primary SUI, who would be randomized 2:1 to undergo transurethral injection of either 150 × 10⁶ AMDCs or placebo. Within the treatment group, the patients were randomized 1:1 to undergo either one or two injections. In this trial, participants underwent an office-based biopsy (Fig. 1a) of the vastus lateralis muscle under local anesthesia. The tissue obtained from the biopsy was placed in a hypothermic solution and shipped to a central laboratory where the AMDCs were expanded in culture and cryopreserved in 2% human serum albumin (Fig. 1b). At a mean time of 13 weeks from muscle biopsy (range 8–21 weeks), the patient returned for an in-office transurethral sphincteric injections of AMDCs or placebo, which consisted of the cryopreservation medium alone. The injection was performed using a multi-injection needle (Cook Medical), which deploys three 25 gauge needles simultaneously into the urethra. This specialized injection needle

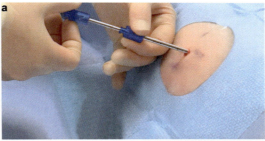
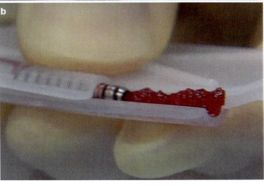

Fig. 1 (**a**) In-office biopsy procedure under local anesthesia of the vastus lateralis (**b**) from which the autologous muscle-derived cells for later intraurethral injection are obtained after culture expansion

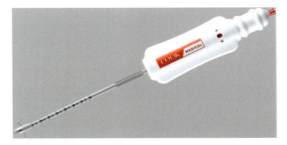

Fig. 2 The multi-injection needle used for intraurethral injection of autologous muscle-derived cells deploys three 25 gauge needles simultaneously which allows for standardized circumferential injection of the cells

allowed for standardized circumferential injection (Fig. 2). At 12 months, all patients were unblinded, and those in the placebo group had the option to electively undergo AMDC injection. Outcome measures for the trial included 3-day voiding diaries, 24-hour pad tests, in-office pad tests, and various validated patient questionnaires (UDI-6, IIQ-7, Incontinence Quality of Life Scale

[IQOL], Global Quality of Life Assessment [GQOL], and Severity Index for Urinary Incontinence in Women [ISI]). Safety via adverse events was also assessed. With regard to adverse events, AMDC-USR was once again demonstrated to be safe, without any significant adverse events reported. However, due to an unexpectedly high response rate observed in the placebo group, enrollment for this trial was unfortunately halted at 150 women.

A post hoc analysis of the data from this trial was performed, and the authors concluded that making the endpoint for efficacy more stringent (>75% reduction in incontinence episodes as opposed to >50% reduction) more effectively differentiated the treatment group from the placebo group at all time points, showing a trend toward an increased benefit in the treatment group. Additionally, an analysis was performed on the subpopulation of patients with recurrent or persistent SUI with a history of prior anti-incontinence procedure, and using the more stringent endpoints, the authors found a significantly increased effect in the treatment group over the placebo group. This study did exclude patients with primary urethral hypermobility as measured by the clinician to be greater than 30 degrees on a Q-tip test; however, these subgroup findings suggest AMDC-USR may particularly benefit in patients with sphincteric deficiency after prior pelvic floor surgery. Because of the exclusion criteria, it is unknown how these therapies may benefit patients with primarily or isolated urethral hypermobility. While having to halt the trial prematurely was an unfortunate setback in the development of this exciting technology, there were still several valuable lessons learned from these efforts. The experience with this trial informed subsequent study designs, and the next iteration focused on more strict inclusion criteria and more rigorous efficacy endpoints.

Therefore, using these lessons, a second double-blind, randomized, placebo-controlled, phase III clinical trial completed enrollment of 311 patients in November 2020 (NCT01893138). Data from this trial is currently undergoing statistical analysis. Additionally, using a combined analysis from trials focusing on patients who have had prior pelvic surgery, AMDC-USR was granted the Regenerative Medicine Advanced Therapy (RMAT) designation by the Food and Drug Administration (FDA) in January 2021. This designation acknowledges the seriousness of refractory SUI on patients and is a step toward FDA approval of this technology. Additionally, a confirmatory adaptive, two-stage, double-blind, stratified, randomized, placebo-controlled trial began enrollment in 2019 with a target of 320 participants with the ultimate goal of obtaining regulatory approval and commercial use of AMDC-USR for women with SUI (NCT03104517).

Other Case Series in Humans on Autologous Muscle-Derived Cells

Aside from these large trials on AMDC-USR, there have been several other small investigational case series regarding the use of AMDC in women with SUI. These studies are quite heterogeneous, and due to variability in techniques, dosing, and outcome measures, it is difficult to compare these efforts to each other and to the ADMC-USR trials [50–56].

One study examined transurethral ultrasound (TUUS)-guided injection of autologous fibroblasts into the urethral submucosa and myoblasts into the external sphincter in 123 women with SUI [57]. Cells were obtained from biceps biopsy. After 12 months, 79% of women were subjectively cured, 13% were substantially improved, and 7% slightly improved. On TUUS, there was an increase in thickness of the rhabdosphincter after injection, in addition to increased contractility as measured by EMG. Another study examined a much lower dose of AMDCs [47]. Sixteen women with SUI underwent transurethral sphincter injection of 0.6 to 25×10^6 cells obtained from deltoid biopsy. After 2 years, 50% of women were dry and 25% were improved. They observed a mean time from injection to improvement of 4.7 months, suggesting the benefit is due to regenerative effect over time as opposed to an immediate bulking effect.

In a prospective study with longer follow-up, 12 women with SUI underwent injection of autologous muscle progenitor cells obtained from deltoid biopsy into the external urethral sphincter [52, 58]. Eleven of the 12 women in this series had recurrent SUI after anti-incontinence surgery. Two patients were fully continent at 1 and 6 years, which suggests the potential durability of this therapy. Five women were improved at 1 year, but their response worsened over time. However, at 6 years, three of these five women remained at least satisfied with their response. The authors did not determine what conferred a better and more durable response in some women over others.

In an attempt to avoid the expensive cell preparation techniques required for the AMDC-USR trials and other cell-based therapies, one study tested a urethral injection of minced autologous skeletal muscle tissue in 35 women with complicated and uncomplicated SUI [55]. Previous investigations by this group suggested that when the tissue is minced, while the muscle cells themselves die, some satellite cells survive, and the authors hypothesized these surviving satellite cells would then be able to divide into proliferating myoblasts. Twelve months after injection, cure was observed in 25% of the women with uncomplicated SUI and improvement in 63%. The improvement was less profound in women with complicated SUI. While this approach is different, the benefits seen by patients appear to be somewhat comparable to other, more expensive cell preparation techniques and therefore possibly warrant further investigation.

Finally, in a phase I/II open, single-center clinical trial, 38 women with moderate urodynamic-confirmed SUI without hypermobility had injection into the external sphincter of very low-dose 0.2×10^6 AMDCs per 2 mL obtained via biceps or pectoralis muscle biopsy injected under TUUS guidance [56]. With the hypothesis that pelvic floor muscle exercise in the immediate postinjection period would enhance cell integration, as an adjuvant, 25 patients underwent electrical stimulation of the pelvic floor with an intravaginal device for the 4 weeks immediately after injection. At 1 year, there was improvement in questionnaire scores and pad usage in the patients who underwent electrical stimulation as compared to those who did not. Additionally, 79% of the patients who underwent electrical stimulation were very much or much improved as compared to 38% of those who did not. The authors concluded that overall AMDC injection was safe and that pelvic floor muscle therapy immediately postinjection could have a dramatic effect on improving results via enhanced cell integration into host tissues.

Although the efficacy of the injection of AMDCs for the treatment of female SUI will continue to undergo investigation and rigorous clinical testing, the safety and feasibility have been clearly and repeatedly demonstrated in these numerous trials. Comparing these smaller clinical trials and case series to the AMDC-USR clinical trials is difficult, as there is a lack of standardized techniques, dosing, or outcomes; however, the science behind the use of muscle progenitor cell for regeneration of urethral continence is sound. The trials necessary for FDA approval and more widespread use of AMDC-USR are currently underway and showing promising results.

Autologous Adipose-Derived Stem Cells

Adipose tissue as a source of multipotent cells has been extensively evaluated over the years. Cells derived from adipose tissue possess the ability to differentiate into multiple different cells lines including adipocytes, osteoblasts, chondrocytes, myocytes, and neuronal cells [59]. Additionally, adipose-derived stem cells (ADSCs) have also been shown to promote angiogenesis via secretion of different growth factors, including hepatocyte growth factor and vascular endothelial growth factor (VEGF). Adipose-derived stem cells can be harvested in a simple, noninvasive manner in humans via subcutaneous adipose tissue sites such as the anterior abdominal wall, making them potentially an ideal candidate for regenerative medicine technologies [60].

There have been numerous preclinical trials in animal models investigating the use of ADSCs for the treatment of SUI. In 2010, the first animal trial used rats that underwent vaginal balloon dilation to induce SUI [61]. The rats also underwent bilateral oophorectomy, and ADSCs were harvested from the periovarian fat. Twelve rats underwent urethral injection of ADSCs, and their response was compared to 10 rats that had urethral injection of saline and six rats that received intravenous injection of ADSCs via the tail vein. After 4 weeks the authors observed a significant increase in LPP in rats injected both transurethral and intravenously with ADSCs as compared to controls. The differentiation of ADSCs into myoblasts has also been performed in vitro and then subsequently injected into the urethra of 20 SUI model rats [53]. At 1 and 3 months after injection, the LPP in rats that received ADSC injection increased significantly as compared to controls. Histologically, the authors observed an increased numbers of myoblasts in the urethras of rats that were treated with ADSCs.

A few studies have examined the effect of growth factors along with ADSCs to enhance their regenerative effects. One group designed a stem cell transplantation system containing controlled release nerve growth factor (NGF) using polylactic-co-glycolic acid (PLGA) microspheres [62]. Adipose-derived stem cells were injected along with NGF periurethrally in rats after pudendal nerve transection. Forty rats total were included in the study and allocated to one of five groups receiving urethral injections of saline, ADSCs, ADSCs with PLGA, ADSC with NGF, or ADSC with NGF in PLGA. The authors reported that the addition of NGF to ADSCs increased cell proliferation and survival. Additionally, after 8 weeks, the most significant improvement in LPP was seen in the rats that received the controlled release system of ADSCs with NGF in PLGA microspheres. Increased muscle and neuron density was observed on histologic examination. The authors concluded from these results that NGF has the capability to enhance the survival of ADSCs in vivo, in addition to inducing neuronal regeneration of the ADSC-based muscle fibers which may further enhance restoration of the urethral continence mechanism. Similarly, a more recent study examined the paracrine effects of ADSC injection via the ability of ADSC-based microtissues to secrete VEGF and NGF [63]. Forty SUI model rats received periurethral injection of saline, ADSCs, or ADSC-based microtissues. Both injection of ADSC and the microtissues increased LPP as compared to controls. However, the microtissue injection increased LPP significantly as compared ADSC injection. On histologic examination, both ADSC and microtissue injection increased the smooth muscle of the rat urethra. However, in the rats injected with microtissues, there was significantly increased expression of VEGF and NGF, which suggests increased angiogenesis and neurogenesis as hypothesized.

Another study compared bulking agent injection and ADSC injection in rats that underwent pudendal denervation [64]. After 4 weeks, both injection of bulking agent (silk fibroin microspheres) and ADSCs resulted in improvements in LPP. By 8 weeks, however, rats injected with a combination of bulking agent and ADSCs had significantly increased LPP as compared to those injected with bulking agent alone. This suggests the perhaps a regenerative effect of the ADSC outlived the bulking effects alone.

There have been several small human clinical trials using ADSCs for SUI; however, the majority of these have been conducted in men with post-prostatectomy incontinence [65–67]. In women with SUI, there have been two human trials in the literature. The first was a small pilot study in five women with either SUI or stress-predominant mixed urinary incontinence (MUI) who were treated with transurethral injection a mixture of 2.5 to 8.5 $\times$ 10^6 ADSCs mixed with 2.1 mL of collagen [68]. After 6 months, only one patient was continent on cough stress test; however, after 12 months, additional two patients were continent. All patients experienced subjective improvement as assessed via questionnaires, and two of the three patients who achieved objective continence reported that they were so satisfied with their treatment that they did not desire further treatment of incontinence. No serious adverse events occurred in this series. As the ADSCs were mixed with collagen in this trial, it is difficult to differentiate the potential regenerative effect of the ADSCs as compared to a bulking effect with the collagen alone. The fact that a few women had an increase in continence over time may suggest at actual tissue regeneration. However, the authors did demonstrate the safety of injecting ADSCs for SUI in humans.

A more recent phase I clinical trial included ten women with SUI who underwent periurethral injection of ADSCs [69]. Patients included in the trial had primarily urethral hypermobility as assessed by a positive Q-tip test. Women underwent transurethral and transvaginal periurethral injection of 1.2×10^6 ADSCs. After 24 weeks, all ten women were significantly improved as assessed on 24-hour pad tests. Interestingly, at the 2-week mark, pad tests were improved; however, at 6 weeks, the effect was no longer seen. The authors hypothesize that this suggests a bulking effect immediately after the injection, with a subsequent regenerative effect observed by 24 weeks. Self-reported leakage followed a similar pattern. One patient in this trial required catheterization immediately after the procedure, which has not been observed in other cell-based therapy trials. There were no other adverse outcomes observed. There are a few issues with the methodology of this trial, including that all pad tests were performed at home and not under supervision, there was no urodynamic testing, and 60% of the women in this study also had pelvic organ prolapse which could have affected outcomes [11].

The few human clinical trials of ADSC injection have demonstrated their safety, and their use in SUI is attractive as the stem cells are quite easy to harvest from patients with minimal morbidity. However, it is difficult to draw any meaningful conclusions from the limited and heterogeneous clinical data. There are currently ongoing phase I and II trials to further evaluate the use of ADSCs in SUI treatment.

Bone Marrow-Derived Stem Cells

Bone marrow contains both hematopoietic and non-hematopoietic stem cells. The non-hematopoietic stem cells contained in bone marrow are multipotent mesenchymal cells [11]. Such mesenchymal cells have the ability to differentiate into the muscle, bone, cartilage, adipose tissue, hepatocytes, and neural cells both in vitro and in vivo.

Bone marrow-derived stem cells (BMSCs) were first investigated over a decade ago for their use in SUI [70]. The initial studies were performed in female rats that underwent urethrolysis. When BMSCs were injected in the rats with SUI and compared to rats injected with placebo, there was no change in urethral closing pressure or LPP observed. However, on histological examination, the BMSCs were noted to have differentiated into skeletal muscle cells and peripheral nerves. While the desired outcome was not reached, this study did provide some evidence for the potential use for BMSCs. Subsequently, 12 rats that underwent pudendal nerve transection were periurethrally injected with BMSCs and their responses compared to six SUI controls and six rats that received placebo injections [71]. In vivo, the BMSCs expressed both smooth and striated muscle cell markers. In the rats injected with BMSCs, LPP was significantly increased as compared to the two other groups. Finally, to investigate the ability of BMSCs to work synergistically with a bulking agent, rats with SUI were injected with BMSCs along with calcium alginate as a composite gel [72]. No significant difference was observed in LPP after 4 and 8 weeks between groups that received the cells and those that received bulking agent injection alone.

The results observed in rat studies with BMSCs have been quite variable. Because of this, one group hypothesized that the true regenerative mechanism of action of mesenchymal cells is via their paracrine capabilities to stimulate progenitor cells and angiogenesis [73]. To examine this, the authors co-cultured mouse BMSCs with muscle cells in vitro and found that the BMSCs promoted the regeneration of muscle cells while remaining undifferentiated themselves.

Finally, a recent study hypothesized that birth-related trauma resulting in decreased collagen in the anterior vaginal wall, pelvic fascia, and ligaments contributes to SUI and that the secretory effects of BMSCs could induce collagen regeneration in the vaginal wall and surrounding tissues and therefore improve continence [74]. They employed rats that underwent vaginal distension to simulate birth trauma-related SUI followed by urethral injection with BMSCs. The authors found that after BMSC injection, the LPP increased to the levels controls. Additionally, histological examination revealed increased fibroblasts and collagen fibers in the anterior vaginal wall, which the authors believe confirms the paracrine effects of BMSC injection on fibroblasts in the vaginal wall and surrounding tissues which may aid in improving continence.

While some animal model studies on BMSCs have been promising, there are no human clinical studies as of yet examining BMSCs for SUI. Additionally, harvesting bone marrow cells which must be obtained via bone marrow biopsy is much more morbid than undergoing a percutaneous muscle biopsy, and therefore their use in treating SUI in humans has not gained traction.

Amniotic Fluid Stem Cells

Amniotic fluid stem cells (AFSCs) have been viewed as a potential source of mesenchymal stem cells. They are multipotent cells and have demonstrated the ability to differentiate into adipogenic, osteogenic, myogenic, endothelial, neuronal, and hepatic cell lineages [75].

There are a few animal studies available on the use of human AFSCs for SUI. The majority of the literature comes from the same group, who used early differentiation of human AFSCs into different cell lineages to then inject the progenitor cells [76]. Human AFSCs are obtained via amniocentesis. In the studies, AFSCs underwent early differentiation into muscle, neuron, and endothelial progenitor cells. Periurethral injections in 30 female mice with pudendal nerve transection was performed and compared to five control mice. The injections consisted of saline, undifferentiated human AFSCs, muscle progenitor cells, muscle and endothelial progenitor cells, muscle and neuron progenitor cells, or all three cell types. After 4 weeks, the mice injected with all three cell lineages had significantly higher LPP as compared to all other groups and improved sphincter regeneration observed histologically.

While this data seems encouraging, there is really minimal literature examining the use of human AFSCs for SUI. Additionally, their use remains an ethical controversy due to the need to obtain cells from human amniocentesis. Finally, there are continued concerns regarding their clinical use, as the cells are, by definition, allogenic. There are, therefore, no human studies using this cell type in SUI.

Umbilical Cord Blood Stem Cells

Umbilical cord blood stem cells are the most primitive type of mesenchymal stem cell. These cells have a very high proliferative capacity which makes them a desirable cell type in regenerative medicine.

There has been some limited literature on their use in SUI. In 28 rats that underwent urethral cauterization, after periurethral injection with human umbilical cord blood cells, their response was compared to 22 controls injected with saline [77]. After 4 weeks, LPP was significantly improved in the rats that received cell injection as compared to controls, in addition to improved urethral sphincter muscle on histological examination.

There has been one human trial examining the use of umbilical cord blood stem cells for use in women with SUI [78]. In the trial, 39 women with SUI (including women with urethral hypermobility, ISD, or MUI) underwent a transurethral injection of a 2 mL suspension including human umbilical cord blood stem cells in saline. After 12 months, 26 (72.2%) were subjectively cured or improved, and 10 (27.8%) were unchanged. Five patients with ISD and five patients with MUI underwent urodynamics after 3 months. The mean maximum urethral closing pressure (MUCP) in this group was 45 cmH$_2$O as compared to 20 cmH$_2$O prior to the procedure.

Again, while these results are promising, the use of umbilical cord blood as a source of stem cells has significant ethical controversies, and therefore implementation or further investigation on their use in human trials has been limited.

Autologous Ear Chondrocytes

Autologous ear chondrocytes were one of the first cell types investigated in regenerative medicine for their use in SUI. Chondrocytes are harvested from the ear and suspended in calcium alginate gel for urethral injection. After the gel dissolves, it is hypothesized that the chondrocytes are able to promote new collage formation.

There have been a few studies examining autologous chondrocyte injection in animal models for the treatment of vesicourethral reflux [79–81]. With regard to the use of chondrocytes in SUI, there is limited data. A clinical trial was designed to investigate the safety and feasibility of urethral injection of autologous ear chondrocytes for the treatment of SUI [82]. Chondrocytes were harvested from the auricular cartilage in 32 women with ISD. These cells were then expanded in culture and mixed with calcium alginate to form an injectable gel. This was then transurethrally injected into the bladder neck. After 12 months, 16 women were subjectively cured and 10 were improved, as assessed via questionnaires. Additionally, there were fewer incontinence episodes after chondrocyte injection. Importantly there were no adverse side effects observed in this trial. The authors concluded the injection of autologous chondrocytes is feasible and safe, in addition to possibly demonstrating benefit for the treatment of SUI in women.

After this trial, however, there were no further investigations regarding the use of autologous ear chondrocytes in female SUI. Chondrocytes are different from other cell-based therapies discussed in this chapter, as the goal of injecting chondrocytes is really to provide a stable and durable bulking effect with the generation of collagen. This is opposed to the other regenerative medicine therapies which have the goal of muscle regeneration of the urethral sphincter to re-establish the native continence mechanism.

Conclusions

Stress urinary incontinence is a common condition that greatly affects the QOL of patients, and there is a need for effective, durable treatments which confer minimal morbidity on patients. Clinical trials have been ongoing since for the last 15 years on the use of cell-based therapies for SUI and have shown substantial promise. With the ultimate goal of these therapies being

restoration of the native continence mechanism, the treatment has the potential to be highly durable and could theoretically outlive any currently available surgical correction of female SUI in patients. The feasibility and safety for cell-based therapies have been repeated demonstrated in these clinical trials. However, the trials have significant variability in the cells used, dosages injected, routes of injections, patient populations, and outcomes measures. The reported efficacies also vary significantly across the trials, which is likely a function of all these heterogenous variables. Besides the ongoing further clinical trials on the efficacy of these treatments, there is also a need to streamline the investigation of these technologies, including animal models for SUI; consistent harvesting, processing, and dosing of cells; and consistent inclusion criteria to determine the patients for which these therapies will show the greatest benefit.

Of all the different cell types, AMDCs are the most extensively studied to date and have been deemed safe. The pending results of large randomized clinical trials will be critical in determining the true efficacy of the treatment and to gain the necessary approvals to integrate this technology into our clinical practices. Additionally, it will be key to continue to further understand the mechanism of action of injected cells, in addition to their survival, proliferation, differentiation, paracrine effects, and roles of growth factors and chemokines.

References

1. Haylen BT, De Ridder D, Freeman RM, Swift SE, Berghmans B, Lee J, et al. An International Urogynecological Association (IUGA)/International Continence Society (ICS) joint report on the terminology for female pelvic floor dysfunction. Neurourol Urodyn. 2010;29(1):4–20.
2. Chong EC, Khan AA, Anger JT. The financial burden of stress urinary incontinence among women in the United States. Curr Urol Rep. 2011;12(5):358.
3. Felde G, Bjelland I, Hunskaar S. Anxiety and depression associated with incontinence in middle-aged women: a large Norwegian cross-sectional study. Int Urogynecol J. 2012;23(3):299–306.
4. Petros PE, Ulmsten UI. An integral theory of female urinary incontinence. Experimental and clinical

considerations. Acta Obstet Gynecol Scand Suppl. 1990;153:7–31.

5. Kobashi KC, Albo ME, Dmochowski RR, Ginsberg DA, Goldman HB, Gomelsky A, et al. Surgical treatment of female stress urinary incontinence: AUA/SUFU guideline. J Urol. 2017;198(4):875–83.

6. Dumoulin C, Cacciari LP, Hay-Smith EJC. Pelvic floor muscle training versus no treatment, or inactive control treatments, for urinary incontinence in women. Cochrane Database Syst Rev. 2018;10:CD005654.

7. Ford AA, Rogerson L, Cody JD, Aluko P, Ogah JA. Mid-urethral sling operations for stress urinary incontinence in women. Cochrane Database Syst Rev. 2017;7:CD006375.

8. Anger JT, Weinberg AE, Albo ME, Smith AL, Kim JH, Rodriguez LV, et al. Trends in surgical management of stress urinary incontinence among female Medicare beneficiaries. Urology. 2009;74(2):283–7.

9. Richter HE, Albo ME, Zyczynski HM, Kenton K, Norton PA, Sirls LT, et al. Retropubic versus transobturator midurethral slings for stress incontinence. N Engl J Med. 2010;362(22):2066–76.

10. Kirchin V, Page T, Keegan PE, Atiemo KO, Cody JD, McClinton S, et al. Urethral injection therapy for urinary incontinence in women. Cochrane Database Syst Rev. 2017;(7).

11. Zambon JP, Williams KJ, Bennington J, Badlani GH. Applicability of regenerative medicine and tissue engineering for the treatment of stress urinary incontinence in female patients. Neurourol Urodyn. 2019;38:S76–83.

12. Gill BC, Sun DZ, Damaser MS. Stem cells for urinary incontinence: functional differentiation or cytokine effects? Urology. 2018;117:9–17.

13. Hart ML, Izeta A, Herrera-Imbroda B, Amend B, Brinchmann JE. Cell therapy for stress urinary incontinence. Tissue Eng Part B Rev. 2015;21(4):365–76.

14. Williams JK, Dean A, Badlani G, Andersson K-E. Regenerative medicine therapies for stress urinary incontinence. J Urol. 2016;196(6):1619–26.

15. Gill BC, Damaser MS, Vasavada SP, Goldman HB. Stress incontinence in the era of regenerative medicine: reviewing the importance of the pudendal nerve. J Urol. 2013;190(1):22–8.

16. Thomson JA, Itskovitz-Eldor J, Shapiro SS, Waknitz MA, Swiergiel JJ, Marshall VS, et al. Embryonic stem cell lines derived from human blastocysts. Science. 1998;282(5391):1145–7.

17. Wagers AJ, Weissman IL. Plasticity of adult stem cells. Cell. 2004;116(5):639–48.

18. Klapper-Goldstein H, Tamam S, Sade S, Weintraub AY. A systematic review of stem cell therapy treatment for women suffering from stress urinary incontinence. Int J Gynaecol Obstet. 2022;157(1):19–30.

19. Hipp J, Atala A. Sources of stem cells for regenerative medicine. Stem Cell Rev. 2008;4(1):3–11.

20. Herrera-Imbroda B, Lara MF, Izeta A, Sievert K-D, Hart ML. Stress urinary incontinence animal models as a tool to study cell-based regenerative therapies targeting the urethral sphincter. Adv Drug Deliv Rev. 2015;82:106–16.

21. Lin AS, Carrier S, Morgan DM, Lue TF. Effect of simulated birth trauma on the urinary continence mechanism in the rat. Urology. 1998;52(1):143–51.

22. Pan HQ, Kerns J, Lin DL, Liu S, Esparza N, Damaser MS. Increased duration of simulated childbirth injuries results in increased time to recovery. Am J Physiol Regul Integr Comp Physiol. 2007;292(4):R1738–R44.

23. Woo LL, Hijaz A, Pan HQ, Kuang M, Rackley RR, Damaser MS. Simulated childbirth injuries in an inbred rat strain. Neurourol Urodyn. 2009;28(4):356–61.

24. Viktrup L. The risk of lower urinary tract symptoms five years after the first delivery. Neurourol Urodyn. 2002;21(1):2–29.

25. Rodríguez LV, Chen S, Jack GS, de Almeida F, Lee KW, Zhang R. New objective measures to quantify stress urinary incontinence in a novel durable animal model of intrinsic sphincter deficiency. Am J Physiol Regul Integr Comp Physiol. 2005;288(5):R1332–R8.

26. Chermansky CJ, Cannon TW, Torimoto K, Fraser MO, Yoshimura N, de Groat WC, et al. A model of intrinsic sphincteric deficiency in the rat: electrocauterization. Neurourol Urodyn. 2004;23(2):166–71.

27. Eberli D, Andersson K-E, Yoo JJ, Atala A. A canine model of irreversible urethral sphincter insufficiency. BJU Int. 2009;103(2):248–53.

28. Peng CW, Chen JJJ, Chang HY, De Groat WC, Cheng CL. External urethral sphincter activity in a rat model of pudendal nerve injury. Neurourol Urodyn. 2006;25(4):388–96.

29. Yokoyama T, Pruchnic R, Lee JY, Chuang Y-C, Jumon H, Yoshimura N, et al. Autologous primary muscle-derived cells transfer into the lower urinary tract. Tissue Eng. 2001;7(4):395–404.

30. Morgan JE, Partridge TA. Muscle satellite cells. Int J Biochem Cell Biol. 2003;35(8):1151–6.

31. Cao Y, Zhao Z, Gruszczynska-Biegala J, Zolkiewska A. Role of metalloprotease disintegrin ADAM12 in determination of quiescent reserve cells during myogenic differentiation in vitro. Mol Cell Biol. 2003;23(19):6725–38.

32. Lee JY, Qu-Petersen Z, Cao B, Kimura S, Jankowski R, Cummins J, et al. Clonal isolation of muscle-derived cells capable of enhancing muscle regeneration and bone healing. J Cell Biol. 2000;150(5):1085–100.

33. Peng H, Huard J. Muscle-derived stem cells for musculoskeletal tissue regeneration and repair. Transpl Immunol. 2004;12(3–4):311–9.

34. Rando TA, Blau HM. Primary mouse myoblast purification, characterization, and transplantation for cell-mediated gene therapy. J Cell Biol. 1994;125(6):1275–87.

35. Qu-Petersen Z, Deasy B, Jankowski R, Ikezawa M, Cummins J, Pruchnic R, et al. Identification of a novel population of muscle stem cells in mice potential for muscle regeneration. J Cell Biol. 2002;157(5):851–64.

36. Chancellor MB, Yokoyama T, Tirney S, Mattes CE, Ozawa H, Yoshimura N, et al. Preliminary results of myoblast injection into the urethra and bladder wall: a possible method for the treatment of stress urinary incontinence and impaired detrusor contractility. Neurourol Urodyn. 2000;19(3):279–87.
37. Yokoyama T, Chancellor MB, Watanabe T, Ozawa H, Yoshimura N, de Groat WC, et al. Primary myoblasts injection into the urethra and bladder as a potential treatment of stress urinary incontinence and impaired detrusor contractility; long-term survival without significant cytotoxicity. J Urol. 1999;161(4S):307
38. Yokoyama T, Yoshimura N, Dhir R, Qu Z, Fraser MO, Kumon H, et al. Persistence and survival of autologous muscle derived cells versus bovine collagen as potential treatment of stress urinary incontinence. J Urol. 2001;165(1):271–6.
39. Yiou R, Yoo JJ, Atala A. Restoration of functional motor units in a rat model of sphincter injury by muscle precursor cell autografts. Transplantation. 2003;76(7):1053–60.
40. Lee J, Cannon T, Pruchnic R, Fraser M, Huard J, Chancellor M. The effects of periurethral muscle-derived stem cell injection on leak point pressure in a rat model of stress urinary incontinence. Int Urogynecol J. 2003;14(1):31–7.
41. Cannon TW, Lee JY, Somogyi G, Pruchnic R, Smith CP, Huard J, et al. Improved sphincter contractility after allogenic muscle-derived progenitor cell injection into the denervated rat urethra. Urology. 2003;62(5):958–63.
42. Kwon D, Kim Y, Pruchnic R, Jankowski R, Usiene I, De Miguel F, et al. Periurethral cellular injection: comparison of muscle-derived progenitor cells and fibroblasts with regard to efficacy and tissue contractility in an animal model of stress urinary incontinence. Urology. 2006;68(2):449–54.
43. Chermansky CJ, Tarin T, Kwon D-D, Jankowski RJ, Cannon TW, de Groat WC, et al. Intraurethral muscle-derived cell injections increase leak point pressure in a rat model of intrinsic sphincter deficiency. Urology. 2004;63(4):780–5.
44. Strasser H, Marksteiner R, Margreiter E, Pinggera GM, Mitterberger M, Frauscher F, et al. RETRACTED: autologous myoblasts and fibroblasts versus collagen for treatment of stress urinary incontinence in women: a randomised controlled trial. Elsevier; 2007;369 (9580):2179–2186
45. Kleinert S, Horton R. Retraction–autologous myoblasts and fibroblasts versus collagen [corrected] for treatment of stress urinary incontinence in women: a [corrected] randomised controlled trial. Lancet (London, England). 2008;372(9641):789–90.
46. Carr L, Steele D, Steele S, Wagner D, Pruchnic R, Jankowski R, et al. 1-year follow-up of autologous muscle-derived stem cell injection pilot study to treat stress urinary incontinence. Int Urogynecol J. 2008;19(6):881–3.

47. Carr LK, Robert M, Kultgen PL, Herschorn S, Birch C, Murphy M, et al. Autologous muscle derived cell therapy for stress urinary incontinence: a prospective, dose ranging study. J Urol. 2013;189(2):595–601.
48. Peters KM, Dmochowski RR, Carr LK, Robert M, Kaufman MR, Sirls LT, et al. Autologous muscle derived cells for treatment of stress urinary incontinence in women. J Urol. 2014;192(2):469–76.
49. Jankowski RJ, Tu LM, Carlson C, Robert M, Carlson K, Quinlan D, et al. A double-blind, randomized, placebo-controlled clinical trial evaluating the safety and efficacy of autologous muscle derived cells in female subjects with stress urinary incontinence. Int Urol Nephrol. 2018;50(12):2153–65.
50. Blaganje M, Lukanović A. Intrasphincteric autologous myoblast injections with electrical stimulation for stress urinary incontinence. Int J Gynaecol Obstet. 2012;117(2):164–7.
51. Blaganje M, Lukanović A. Ultrasound-guided autologous myoblast injections into the extrinsic urethral sphincter: tissue engineering for the treatment of stress urinary incontinence. Int Urogynecol J. 2013;24(4):533–5.
52. Sèbe P, Doucet C, Cornu J-N, Ciofu C, Costa P, de Medina SGD, et al. Intrasphincteric injections of autologous muscular cells in women with refractory stress urinary incontinence: a prospective study. Int Urogynecol J. 2011;22(2):183–9.
53. Elmi A, Kajbafzadeh A-M, Tourchi A, Talab SS, Esfahani SA. Safety, efficacy and health related quality of life of autologous myoblast transplantation for treatment of urinary incontinence in children with bladder exstrophy-epispadias complex. J Urol. 2011;186(5):2021–6.
54. Stangel-Wojcikiewicz K, Jarocha D, Piwowar M, Jach R, Uhl T, Basta A, et al. Autologous muscle-derived cells for the treatment of female stress urinary incontinence: a 2-year follow-up of a polish investigation. Neurourol Urodyn. 2014;33(3):324–30.
55. Gräs S, Klarskov N, Lose G. Intraurethral injection of autologous minced skeletal muscle: a simple surgical treatment for stress urinary incontinence. J Urol. 2014;192(3):850–5.
56. Blaganje M, Lukanović A. The effect of skeletal muscle-derived cells implantation on stress urinary incontinence and functional urethral properties in female patients. Int J Gynaecol Obstet. 2022;157(2):444–51.
57. Mitterberger M, Marksteiner R, Margreiter E, Pinggera GM, Colleselli D, Frauscher F, et al. Autologous myoblasts and fibroblasts for female stress incontinence: a 1-year follow-up in 123 patients. BJU Int. 2007;100(5):1081–5.
58. Cornu J-N, Lizée D, Pinset C, Haab F. Long-term follow-up after regenerative therapy of the urethral sphincter for female stress urinary incontinence. Eur Urol. 2013;65(1):256–8.

59. Forcales S-V. Potential of adipose-derived stem cells in muscular regenerative therapies. Front Aging Neurosci. 2015;7:123.
60. Vinarov A, Atala A, Yoo J, Slusarenco R, Zhumataev M, Zhito A, et al. Cell therapy for stress urinary incontinence: present-day frontiers. J Tissue Eng Regen Med. 2018;12(2):e1108–e21.
61. Lin G, Wang G, Banie L, Ning H, Shindel AW, Fandel TM, et al. Treatment of stress urinary incontinence with adipose tissue-derived stem cells. Cytotherapy. 2010;12(1):88–95.
62. Zhao W, Zhang C, Jin C, Zhang Z, Kong D, Xu W, et al. Periurethral injection of autologous adipose-derived stem cells with controlled-release nerve growth factor for the treatment of stress urinary incontinence in a rat model. Eur Urol. 2011;59(1):155–63.
63. Li M, Li G, Lei H, Guan R, Yang B, Gao Z, et al. Therapeutic potential of adipose-derived stem cell-based microtissues in a rat model of stress urinary incontinence. Urology. 2016;97:277.e1–7.
64. Shi LB, Cai HX, Chen LK, Wu Y, Zhu SA, Gong XN, et al. Tissue engineered bulking agent with adipose-derived stem cells and silk fibroin microspheres for the treatment of intrinsic urethral sphincter deficiency. Biomaterials. 2014;35(5):1519–30.
65. Choi JY, Kim T-H, Yang JD, Suh JS, Kwon TG. Adipose-derived regenerative cell injection therapy for postprostatectomy incontinence: a phase I clinical study. Yonsei Med J. 2016;57(5):1152.
66. Gotoh M, Shimizu S, Yamamoto T, Ishizuka O, Yamanishi T, Mizokami A, et al. Regenerative treatment for male stress urinary incontinence by periurethral injection of adipose-derived regenerative cells: outcome of the ADRESU study. Int J Urol. 2020;27(10):859–65.
67. Yamamoto T, Gotoh M, Kato M, Majima T, Toriyama K, Kamei Y, et al. Periurethral injection of autologous adipose-derived regenerative cells for the treatment of male stress urinary incontinence: report of three initial cases. Int J Urol. 2012;19(7):652–9.
68. Kuismanen K, Sartoneva R, Haimi S, Mannerström B, Tomás E, Miettinen S, et al. Autologous adipose stem cells in treatment of female stress urinary incontinence: results of a pilot study. Stem Cells Transl Med. 2014;3(8):936–41.
69. Arjmand B, Safavi M, Heidari R, Aghayan H, Bazargani ST, Dehghani S, et al. Concomitant transurethral and transvaginal-periurethral injection of autologous adipose derived stem cells for treatment of female stress urinary incontinence: a phase one clinical trial. Acta Med Iran. 2017;55:368–74.
70. Kinebuchi Y, Aizawa N, Imamura T, Ishizuka O, Igawa Y, Nishizawa O. Autologous bone-marrow-derived mesenchymal stem cell transplantation into injured rat urethral sphincter. Int J Urol. 2010;17(4):359–68.
71. Yu A, Campeau L. Bone marrow mesenchymal stem cell therapy for voiding dysfunction. Curr Urol Rep. 2015;16(7):49.
72. Du XW, Wu HL, Zhu YF, Hu JB, Jin F, Lv RP, et al. Experimental study of therapy of bone marrow mesenchymal stem cells or muscle-like cells/calcium alginate composite gel for the treatment of stress urinary incontinence. Neurourol Urodyn. 2013;32(3):281–6.
73. Gunetti M, Tomasi S, Giammò A, Boido M, Rustichelli D, Mareschi K, et al. Myogenic potential of whole bone marrow mesenchymal stem cells in vitro and in vivo for usage in urinary incontinence. PLoS One. 2012;7(9):e45538.
74. Jiang M, Liu J, Liu W, Zhu X, Bano Y, Liao H, et al. Bone marrow stem cells secretome accelerates simulated birth trauma-induced stress urinary incontinence recovery in rats. Aging (Albany NY). 2021;13(7):10517.
75. De Coppi P, Bartsch G, Siddiqui MM, Xu T, Santos CC, Perin L, et al. Isolation of amniotic stem cell lines with potential for therapy. Nat Biotechnol. 2007;25(1):100–6.
76. Chun SY, Kwon JB, Chae SY, Lee JK, Bae JS, Kim BS, et al. Combined injection of three different lineages of early-differentiating human amniotic fluid-derived cells restores urethral sphincter function in urinary incontinence. BJU Int. 2014;114(5):770–83.
77. Lim J-J, Jang J-B, Kim J-Y, Moon S-H, Lee C-N, Lee K-J. Human umbilical cord blood mononuclear cell transplantation in rats with intrinsic sphincter deficiency. J Korean Med Sci. 2010;25(5):663.
78. Lee CN, Jang JB, Kim JY, Koh C, Baek JY, Lee KJ. Human cord blood stem cell therapy for treatment of stress urinary incontinence. J Korean Med Sci. 2010;25(6):813.
79. Atala A, Cima LG, Kim W, Paige KT, Vacanti JP, Retik AB, et al. Injectable alginate seeded with chondrocytes as a potential treatment for vesicoureteral reflux. J Urol. 1993;150(2 Part 2):745–7.
80. Atala A, Kim W, Paige KT, Vacanti CA, Retik AB. Endoscopic treatment of vesicoureteral reflux with a chondrocyte-alginate suspension. J Urol. 1994;152(2):641–3.
81. Cozzolino DJ, Cendron M, DeVore DP, Hoopes PJ. The biological behavior of autologous collagen–based extracellular matrix injected into the rabbit bladder wall. Neurourol Urodyn. 1999;18(5):487–95.
82. Bent AE, Tutrone RT, McLennan MT, Lloyd K, Kennelly MJ, Badlani G. Treatment of intrinsic sphincter deficiency using autologous ear chondrocytes as a bulking agent. Neurourol Urodyn. 2001;20(2):157–65.

Part IV

Pelvic Organ Prolapse

Etiology, Diagnosis, and Management of Pelvic Organ Prolapse: Overview

28

Connie N. Wang and Doreen E. Chung

Contents

Introduction	508
Definition	508
Classification	508
Staging	508
Etiology	510
Incidence and Prevalence	510
Risk Factors	510
Diagnosis	510
Symptoms/Presentation	510
Workup	511
Management	512
Observation	512
Pelvic Floor Muscle Exercises	512
Pessaries	512
Surgery	512
Conclusion	516
Cross-References	516
References	516

Abstract

Pelvic organ prolapse (POP) is a common condition that adversely impacts quality of life for women. The etiology of POP is multifactorial but risk factors for development include higher parity, history of vaginal delivery, older age, and higher body mass index. POP can occur in younger women, but peak incidence of symptoms is in women aged 70–79. Symptoms include vaginal bulge and pressure, voiding dysfunction, defecatory dysfunction, and/or sexual dysfunction. POP is measured with the Pelvic Organ Prolapse Quantification (POP-Q) system and can be assigned an ordinal stage to guide evaluation and management. Management of POP is varied. Asymptomatic POP

C. N. Wang (✉) · D. E. Chung
Department of Urology, Columbia University Irving Medical Center, New York, NY, USA
e-mail: cnw2123@cumc.columbia.edu; dec2154@cumc.columbia.edu

© Springer Nature Switzerland AG 2023
F. E. Martins et al. (eds.), *Female Genitourinary and Pelvic Floor Reconstruction*,
https://doi.org/10.1007/978-3-031-19598-3_29

does not require treatment and mild POP can be managed with conservative treatment including pessaries and pelvic floor exercises. Symptomatic or advanced POP can be treated with surgical intervention, which can be transvaginal or transabdominal, obliterative, open, laparoscopic, or robotic and may involve use of biologic or synthetic grafts.

Keywords

Pelvic organ prolapse · Cystocele · Rectocele · Enterocele · Pelvic floor dysfunction

Introduction

Understanding the risk factors for proper diagnosis, staging, workup, and initial management of pelvic organ prolapse is vitally important for providers who care for aging female patients, especially as the population of the United States continues to age.

Definition

Pelvic organ prolapse (POP) encompasses a heterogeneous group of conditions in which pelvic floor musculature and connective tissue weakness result in the descent of one or more pelvic organs, such as bladder, bowel, or uterus, into the vaginal canal that can be associated with the feeling or visualization of a bulge from the vagina during daily activities [29].

Classification

POP can be classified by vaginal compartment. In anterior vaginal wall prolapse, the bladder and/or urethra bulges into the vaginal canal. This is clinically termed *as cystocele or urethrocele.* Urethroceles represent distal anterior compartment defects and usually result in urethral hypermobility. In apical vaginal prolapse, disruption in the uterosacral/cardinal ligament complex results in protrusion of the uterus or vaginal cuff (after hysterectomy) into the vaginal canal. This type of pelvic organ prolapse is known as uterine prolapse or vaginal vault prolapse. Apical compartment defects can also result in prolapse of the peritoneum cul-de-sac with or without bowel contents into the vaginal canal, which is clinically termed an *enterocele.* In posterior vaginal wall prolapse, the rectum, small bowel, and/or sigmoid colon bulges into the vaginal canal. This is clinically termed as *rectocele.* While prolapse of the anterior vaginal wall is the most common form of prolapse, many women present with POP in multiple compartments [30].

POP can also be classified as symptomatic or asymptomatic. Not all POP is clinically significant, and asymptomatic patients do not require intervention. Treatment is only indicated if POP is causing bothersome bulge and/or pressure symptoms, sexual dysfunction, lower urinary tract dysfunction, or defecatory dysfunction.

Staging

Several grading/staging systems have been developed to measure POP, but the most widely used system in clinical settings to date is the International Continence Society's Pelvic Organ Prolapse Quantification (POP-Q) system [27]. The POP-Q system is a reproducible, standardized method of quantifying and describing extent of prolapse for clinicians and researchers and has been shown to have good interobserver and intraobserver reliabilities [17].

The POP-Q system is applied during physical examination of the external genitalia and vaginal canal and describes the locations of six vaginal sites (representing the anterior, apical, and posterior vaginal compartments) relative to the hymen [8]. The POP-Q system does not use terms such as "cystocele" and "rectocele," as the organ that lies behind prolapsed vaginal epithelium is difficult to ascertain based on physical exam alone. Instead, the POP-Q system describes prolapse in terms of "prolapsed segment" – i.e., anterior wall, posterior wall, and apical wall. It is recommended to perform and document a POP-Q exam before treatment of POP to establish an objective record of the extent of POP at initial presentation to facilitate comparison of physical exam between different providers and to compare physical exam before and after intervention.

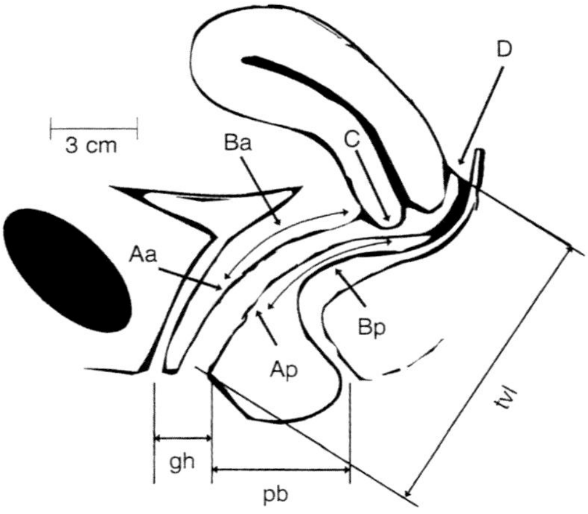

Anterior wall **Aa**	Anterior wall **Ba**	Cervix or cuff **C**
Genital hiatus **gh**	Perineal body **pb**	Total vaginal length **tvl**
Posterior wall **Ap**	Posterior wall **Bp**	Posterior fornix **D**

Fig. 1 Pelvic Organ Prolapse Quantification (POP-Q) System. Nine defined points measured in the midline and relative to the hymen assessed during maximal Valsalva except for TVL: Aa, 3 cm proximal to the external urethral meatus; Ba, most prolapsed portion of the anterior vaginal wall; C, leading edge of the cervix or vaginal cuff; gh, middle of the urethral meatus to the midline of the posterior hymen; pb, middle of the posterior hymen to the middle of the anal opening; tvl, maximum depth of the vagina with prolapse reduced; Ap, 3 cm proximal to the posterior hymen; Bp, most prolapsed portion of the posterior vaginal wall; D, posterior fornix in a woman who has a cervix. (Reprinted with permission from Elsevier from Bump RC, Mattiasson A, Bo K, Brubaker L, DeLancey J, Klarskov P, et al. The standardization of terminology of female pelvic organ prolapse and pelvic floor dysfunction. Am J Obstet Gynecol. 1996;175:10–17)

The six points that are measured in the POP-Q system are (see Fig. 1):

- *Point Aa*: a point in the midline of the anterior vaginal wall, 3 cm proximal to external urethral meatus.
- *Point Ba*: a point on the anterior vaginal wall that represents the most distal/dependent position of the upper anterior vaginal wall from vaginal cuff or anterior vaginal fornix to point Aa. In the absence of prolapse, point Ba would be at the level of Aa and measured at −3 cm.
- *Point C*: a point on the superior vagina that represents the most distal/dependent edge of cervix or the leading edge of the vaginal cuff after hysterectomy.
- *Point D*: a point on the superior vagina that represents the location of the posterior fornix in a woman who still has a cervix. This point is omitted in the absence of the cervix.
- *Point Ap*: a point in the midline of the posterior vaginal wall, 3 cm proximal to the hymen.
- *Point Bp*: a point on the posterior vaginal wall that represents the most distal/dependent position of the upper posterior vaginal wall from vaginal cuff or posterior vaginal fornix to point Ap. In the absence of prolapse, point Bp would be measured at −3 cm.

The six points are described in centimeters above/proximal to hymen (negative number) or in centimeters below/distal to hymen (positive number), with the hymen defined as zero. For example, a cervix that protrudes 2 cm distal to the hymen would be described as +2 cm while a cervix that protrudes to 1 cm proximal to the hymen would be described as −1 cm.

Other measurements included in the POP-Q system are the total vaginal length (tvl) measured as the greatest depth of the vagina when point C or D is reduced to its full normal position, the genital hiatus (gh) measured from the middle of the external urethral meatus to the posterior midline hymen, and the perineal body (pb) measured from the posterior margin of the genital hiatus to the mid-anal opening.

All measurements should be taken at the point of maximal degree of prolapse, which can be confirmed by patient report based on maximal protrusion noted during her daily activities. Other important factors to include in the quantitative description and staging of pelvic organ prolapse include the position of the patient at time of measurements/examination, the type of examination table or chair used, the type of vaginal speculum or retractor used, the type of straining (e.g., Valsalva maneuver, cough) used to maximally develop prolapse, fullness of bladder, content of rectum, and method by which any quantitative measurements were taken [8].

POP-Q measurements can be converted to ordinal stages of POP, based on the most severely prolapsed vaginal segment when full extent of protrusion has been demonstrated. Staging is based on relationship of vaginal compartments to the hymen. POP is typically symptomatic once the most distal extent of POP reaches the hymenal ring, or Stage II or higher.

The stages of POP are:

- Stage 0: No prolapse demonstrated (anterior and posterior points are all at -3 cm and C or D is --between -TVL and – (TVL-2) cm)
- Stage I: Most distal portion of prolapse is >1 cm above the level of the hymen (less than −1 cm)
- Stage II: Most distal portion of prolapse is ≤1 cm proximal to or distal to the plane of the hymen (at least one point is −1, 0, or +1)
- Stage III: Most distal portion of prolapse is >1 cm below plane of hymen but protrudes no further than 2 cm less than the total vaginal length in centimeters
- Stage IV: Complete eversion of the total length of the lower genital tract. Distal portion of prolapse protrudes to at least 2 cm less than total vaginal length

Etiology

Incidence and Prevalence

Peak incidence of POP symptoms in women is between 70 and 79 years, although POP can occur in younger women [18]. As the population of the United States ages, it is anticipated that by 2050 the number of women experiencing POP will increase by approximately 50% [36].

The true incidence and prevalence of POP is difficult to know, as many women with anatomical POP on physical exam are asymptomatic and may go undiagnosed. One systematic review found that the prevalence of POP when defined by symptoms alone is 3–6%, while the prevalence of POP based on physical examination was 41–50% [3]. Overall, women in the United States have a 13% lifetime risk of undergoing surgery for POP [37].

Risk Factors

The etiology of POP is likely multifactorial. The interplay of genetics and anatomy, lifestyle, and reproductive history likely all contribute in part to the pelvic floor dysfunction that results in POP. One systemic review identified higher parity, history of vaginal delivery, older age, and higher body mass index (BMI) as significantly associated with primary POP and pre-operative stage as significantly associated with POP recurrence [33]. Other risk factors that have been associated with POP include connective tissue disorders, menopausal status, and chronic constipation. There is conflicting data on whether hysterectomy status is a risk factor for POP [26].

Diagnosis

Symptoms/Presentation

Symptoms of POP can include sensation of pressure with or without a vaginal bulge, sexual dysfunction, lower urinary tract symptoms, needing to splint (reduce the bulge) to urinate or have a bowel movement, or bowel dysfunction. The most specific symptoms of POP are sensation of vaginal bulging or protrusion, seeing or feeling a vaginal bulge, and vaginal heaviness or pressure, but women usually present with a combination of symptoms. In addition, women with severe prolapse may present with vaginal bleeding or spotting secondary to erosions of the vaginal and/or cervical epithelium [2]. It is important to note that POP often exists in conjunction with other pelvic floor disorders, and there may be overlap of symptoms from multiple etiologies. A cross-sectional study of 237 women evaluated for POP found 73% with concurrent urinary incontinence, 86% with urinary urgency/frequency, 34–62% with other voiding dysfunction, and 31% with fecal incontinence [13]. Other than vaginal bulging, these associated symptoms are not specific to POP and can be attributable to other pelvic floor disorders and/or primary bladder or bowel dysfunction. It is important to assess for and document the nature of and degree of bother of patient's pelvic symptoms.

Workup

The recommended initial evaluation for a woman with suspected POP includes a thorough medical, surgical, obstetric, gynecologic, urologic, and defecatory history and physical examination. The clinician should perform an assessment of the nature of, severity of, and degree of bother of symptoms. It is also important to discuss the patient's goals of treatment, to appropriately guide management and/or intervention.

In assessing patient symptoms, clinicians should specifically ask if POP-related symptoms are limiting physical activity and/or sexual function and whether symptoms are becoming progressively worse or bothersome. Not all anatomical POP is bothersome to patients and asymptomatic POP does not require treatment. Lower urinary tract function should be assessed by evaluating for presence and type (urge, stress, mixed) of urinary incontinence, urinary urgency/frequency, weak urinary stream, use of positional changes to start/complete voiding, adequacy of bladder emptying, use of splinting to void, and any relationship between urinary symptoms and severity of prolapse (based on patient position throughout the day). All women with significant apical or anterior wall prolapse should undergo preoperative evaluation for occult stress urinary incontinence, with cough stress testing or

urodynamic testing with the prolapse reduced. Bowel function should be assessed to determine any history of straining to defecate, use of splinting to defecate, incontinence of flatus or stool, urgency to defecate, and/or incomplete rectal emptying. Sexual dysfunction should be assessed by identifying sexual activity status of the patient, symptoms of dyspareunia, decreased sensation, decreased arousal or orgasm, or incontinence of urine or stool during coitus. Pain in the vagina, bladder, rectum, pelvis, or lower back should be identified and quantified [2, 19].

Physical examination should include an abdominal and pelvic examination to rule out pelvic masses. The external genitalia and vagina should be evaluated for vaginal atrophy, skin irritation, or ulceration. Exam for prolapse should be done by spreading the patient's labia and using a split speculum while the patient is in a supine position, to allow for evaluation of maximum descent of prolapse. A split speculum, created by separating a bivalve speculum and using only the posterior blade, should be used to examine the apex and anterior vaginal wall while the patient is asked to strain. Turning the blade to hold up the anterior vaginal wall allows for examination of the posterior vaginal wall and perineal body while the patient performs Valsalva maneuvers and/or coughing to evaluate for posterior wall prolapse. If prolapse is not confirmed in the supine position, repeating a physical exam in the standing position is recommended. POP-Q measurements should be documented at initial evaluation, prior to any treatment of POP. Pelvic floor muscle tone should also be assessed by asking the patient to contract and relax pelvic floor muscles volitionally, and strength of contractions can be described as "absent," "weak," "normal," or "strong" [2, 26].

Additional assessments beyond a thorough history and physical may be needed if patients report voiding symptoms. If a patient reports urinary urgency, hematuria, or other lower urinary tract symptoms, a urinalysis with culture and microscopy should be obtained. A post void residual should be measured either with straight catheterization or ultrasound measurement in any patient who has prolapse beyond the hymen and/or reports difficulty urinating. Urodynamic testing may guide further patient management for patients with POP and urinary incontinence, storage symptoms, or other voiding dysfunction. In patients with high-grade POP but without symptoms of stress urinary incontinence (SUI), clinicians should perform stress testing with reduction of prolapse. In patients with high-grade POP and associated lower urinary tract symptoms, mutichannel urodynamics with prolapse reduction may be used to assess for occult SUI and detrusor dysfunction [34]. Defecography, anal manometry, and endoanal ultrasound can be considered for women with fecal incontinence or outlet constipation. Finally, if there is a mismatch between degree of prolapse on physical exam and patient's reported symptoms, further imaging (ultrasonography, magnetic resonance imaging) may be required [1].

Management

Observation

Women with clinically asymptomatic POP do not require intervention. Reassurance and education on the manifestation of POP symptoms (urinary and defecatory), risk factors for, and preventative measures to prevent progression of POP should be offered to patients. Lifestyle modifications can be offered to patients to alleviate and/or prevent symptoms of POP, including management of constipation, elevation of lower extremities to decrease bulge symptoms, weight loss to reduce abdominal pressure on pelvic organs, and pelvic muscle exercises to strengthen pelvic floor musculature [26].

Pelvic Floor Muscle Exercises

The performance of pelvic floor muscle exercises can improve symptoms of POP. It is important to provide thorough education to patients on the correct form of pelvic floor muscle exercises to achieve maximal benefit. Referrals can be made to physical therapists with specialty training in pelvic floor dysfunction and use of biofeedback may

be useful for patients to learn appropriate technique for independent exercise at home. Several randomized trials have demonstrated that patients with mild to moderate POP who received regular, supervised pelvic floor physiotherapy with a trained physiotherapist that included education, manual feedback to ensure correct pelvic floor muscle contraction, and individualized home exercise regimens, had improvement in POP symptoms through 12 months after start of treatment [5, 15, 16].

Pessaries

Pessaries are mechanical devices inserted into the vagina to reduce prolapsed tissue and reduce pressure on the bladder and bowel. They are available in different shapes and sizes (ring, ring with support, Gellhorn, doughnut, etc.), Vaginal pessaries represent an effective, conservative option for treatment of POP for patients who are not interested in or who are not candidates for surgical intervention. Pessaries should be offered to women with symptomatic POP who wish to become pregnant in the future. Pessaries can be fitted successfully for up to 92% of women [10]. Women who are able to learn how to independently change their pessaries should be followed annually to assess pessary fit, comfort, and effectiveness. For those that are unable to remove and replace their own pessary, regular follow-up is needed for pessary exchange every 3–4 months. Risks of pessary use include sustained pressure on the vaginal wall that may result in local devascularization of erosion (2–9% of cases) or in rare instances, fistula [28]. In cases of erosion or devascularization of vaginal wall tissue, treatment entails removal of the pessary for 2–4 weeks and local estrogen therapy. Recurrent tissue erosion may require more frequent pessary exchanges or fitting of a different pessary.

Surgery

Surgery is indicated for treatment of bothersome POP for women who have failed or declined conservative, nonsurgical treatments. About one in eight women in the United States with POP undergo surgery by age 80 [36]. Of those who undergo POP surgery, 13% require repeat surgery within 5 years and up to 29% of women will undergo another POP surgery at some point in their lifetime [9, 25].

The goal of POP surgery is to restore normal pelvic support and anatomy and to reduce or eliminate symptoms of POP. Many women with POP have prolapse of multiple compartments and surgery for these patients should correct all areas of prolapse. The type and route (transvaginal vs. transabdominal approach) of surgery offered to patients should consider location and severity of prolapse, the patient's most bothersome symptoms, the patient's general age and health, the patient's preference, and the surgeon's experience.

Different types of surgeries for treatment of POP are summarized in Table 1. Anterior compartment prolapse can be repaired via anterior colporrhaphy, native tissue repair, or graft-augmented repair. Apical compartment prolapse can be repaired with uterosacral ligament suspension, sacrospinous ligament fixation, iliococcygeus suspension, sacrocolpopexy, Manchester procedure, hysterectomy with vaginal apex suspension and/or McCall culdoplasty, supracervical hysterectomy and sacrocervicocolopopexy, hysteropexy for uterine preservation, or colpocleisis. Posterior compartment prolapse can be repaired transvaginally, transperineally, or transanally with posterior colporrhaphy with or without concurrent perineorrhaphy. Surgical technique, indications, success rates, and potential complications of different surgical approaches for POP repair will be further detailed in subsequent chapters of this textbook.

Abdominal Versus Vaginal Approach

Transvaginal approaches to POP surgery include vaginal hysterectomy, vaginal apex suspension for repair of apical compartment prolapse, anterior colporrhaphy for anterior vaginal wall prolapse, and posterior colporrhaphy for posterior vaginal wall prolapse.

Abdominal approaches to POP surgery include abdominal sacrocolpopexy and/or abdominal hysterectomy. Abdominal sacrocolpopexy involves suspension of the apex of the vagina to the anterior longitudinal ligament of the sacrum with placement of a synthetic mesh or biologic graft.

Transvaginal surgical repair of POP is an effective option for most women with POP, and based on ICD-9 data, nearly 80% of POP surgery in the United States is performed transvaginally [6]. However, there is growing evidence to suggest that in a subset of patients with POP, an abdominal approach to POP repair may be more efficacious and durable. A literature review of randomized or quasi-randomized controlled trials of surgical operations for POP found that for uterine or vault vaginal prolapse, compared to vaginal sacrospinous colpopexy, abdominal sacrocolpopexy was associated with lower rate of postoperative recurrent prolapse and painful intercourse. However, the abdominal approach is associated with longer operating time, longer time to return to daily activities, and increased cost [7]. The reduced short-term morbidity of transvaginal POP surgery must be balanced with the risk of increased prolapse recurrence [11].

Individual patient characteristics such as age, future desire for pregnancy, sexual activity level, vaginal size, general health, and life expectancy, patient preference, and the surgeon's training and experience should guide selection of surgical approach. Patient characteristics that would favor an abdominal approach to POP repair include patients with a shortened vaginal length, intra-abdominal pathology, or risk factors for recurrent POP. Risk factors for recurrent POP include young age (<60 years), advanced prolapse (stage 3 or 4), and obesity (BMI > 26 kg/m^2) [19, 26].

Grafts

Anterior compartment prolapse repairs can be performed with autologous or biologic grafts, such as porcine dermis. A recent Cochrane review of surgical management of POP concluded that for anterior compartment prolapse repairs, objective failure rates were higher with anterior colporrhaphy alone compared to use of

Table 1 Types of pelvic organ prolapse surgery

Surgery	Technique	Approach
Anterior compartment repairs		
Anterior colporrhaphy	Plication of pubocervical fascia in the midline anterior vaginal wall to repair central compartment defects (often combined with paravaginal repair)	Transvaginal
Paravaginal repair	Reattachment of pubocervical fascia to the arcus tendineus fasciae pelvis to repair lateral compartment defects (often combined with anterior colporrhaphy)	Transvaginal or abdominal
Anterior repair with cadaveric fascia lata	Cadaveric fascia lata anchored to the arcus tendineus fasciae pelvis bilaterally and the cardinal and ureterosacral ligament apically	Transvaginal
Anterior repair with porcine dermis	Porcine dermis anchored to the arcus tendineus fasciae pelvis	Transvaginal
Apical compartment repairs		
Uterosacral ligament suspension	Suture attachment of apex of vagina to uterosacral ligaments, preserving natural vaginal axis	Transvaginal or abdominal
Sacrospinous ligament fixation	Suture attachment of apex of vagina to sacrospinous ligament, altering vaginal axis; can be done unilaterally or bilaterally	Transvaginal
Iliococcygeus suspension	Suture attachment of vaginal vault to fascia of the iliococcygeus muscle	Transvaginal
Sacrocolpopexy	Use of synthetic mesh or autologous fascia to fixate apex of vagina to the anterior longitudinal ligament of the sacral promontory	Transvaginal or abdominal (open, laparoscopic, or robotic assisted)
Manchester procedure	Amputation of cervix, cardinal and uterosacral ligament plication, and anterior and posterior colporrhaphy	Transvaginal
McCall (posterior) culdoplasty or vaginal apex suspension after hysterectomy	Closing the peritoneal cul-de-sac of Douglas posteriorly to prevent enterocele formation (culdoplasty) and attachment of vaginal apex to the uterosacral ligaments in the midline	Transvaginal
Hysteropexy: (sacrospinous hysteropexy, uterosacral ligament hysteropexy, abdominal sacrohysteropexy)	Suture or graft attachment of uterus/cervix to the uterosacral ligaments, sacrospinous ligament, or sacral promontory	Transvaginal or abdominal (open, laparoscopic, or robotic assisted
Colpocleisis	Suturing of vaginal walls together to close the vagina	Transvaginal
Posterior compartment repairs		
Posterior colporrhaphy	Plication of rectovaginal fascia in the midline posterior vaginal wall, decreasing width of the posterior vaginal wall	Transvaginal
Perineorrhaphy	Often performed concurrently with posterior colporrhaphy to reconstitute muscles of the urogenital diaphragm and recreate approximation of rectovaginal connective tissues to the central tendon of the perineum	Transvaginal

polypropylene mesh or biologic graft. However, there was no difference in subjective cure rates between the two groups [20]. Mesh-related complications after use of synthetic mesh for anterior wall prolapse repair include mesh extrusion at a rate of 11.4%, with 6.8% requiring surgical intervention, dyspareunia, and increased prolapse recurrence and de novo stress urinary incontinence rates compared to repair with native tissue repair [19].

Apical compartment prolapse repairs, such as sacrocolpopexy, can be performed with synthetic mesh, native tissue, or biologic grafts. Randomized control trials have shown a significantly higher rate of anatomic success with mesh abdominal sacrocolpopexy compared to vaginal apex repair with native tissue, but use of synthetic mesh is associated with more postoperative complications including ileus or small bowel obstruction, thromboembolic events, mesh or suture complications, and a significantly higher reoperation rate due to mesh-related complications such as vaginal erosion, visceral erosions, mesh exposure, and sacral osteitis [24]. Unfortunately, there is limited literature to date on the efficacy of biologic grafts for apical compartment prolapse repair, but studies have not demonstrated superiority of biologic grafts over native tissue repairs for POP [22].

Posterior compartment prolapse repairs are not routinely performed with graft augments.

Mesh Complications

Patients with synthetic mesh complications may present with mesh extrusion, vaginal bleeding, pelvic pain, dyspareunia, or bladder or bowel dysfunction. The increased rate of mesh-related complications resulted in the US Food and Drug Administration issuing a public health notification in 2011 that identified serious safety concerns about the use of transvaginal mesh for POP treatment [32]. Subsequently, many transvaginal mesh products were removed from the market. The current FDA guideline is that no intervention is needed for asymptomatic patients who received transvaginal mesh for surgical repair of POP who are not experiencing any complications. These patients should continue routine

follow-up and should be encouraged to report any new gynecologic or urologic symptoms [31]. Of note, these FDA announcements and health warnings do not apply to use of transvaginal mesh for stress urinary incontinence or use of transabdominal mesh for POP repair due to lower risk of mesh complications when used intra-abdominally. Of the ongoing research on long-term efficacy and safety of transvaginal mesh procedures, the Study of Uterine Prolapse Procedures Randomized Trial (SUPeR trial) notably found no difference at 3 years in treatment failure (defined as need for retreatment, anatomically defined prolapse recurrence, or recurrence of bulge symptom) between patients who underwent vaginal hysterectomy and patients who underwent hysteropexy for uterovaginal prolapse. Additionally, there was no significant difference in overall rates of adverse effects, de novo dyspareunia, or pelvic pain between the two groups. Although the trial observed an 8% rate of mesh exposure, no patients required surgical intervention [23].

Women who are chronic steroid users, current smokers, or otherwise immunocompromised are at increased risk of synthetic mesh-related complications and should be offered biologic grafts, autologous grafts, or native tissue repair of POP [26].

Hysterectomy or Hysteropexy

For women with uterine prolapse, either hysterectomy or hysteropexy can be performed. For women who wish to preserve their uterus, a uterine suspension or hysteropexy should be performed. Options for hysteropexy include vaginal sacrospinous hysteropexy, transvaginal, laparoscopic, or robotic-assisted uterosacral ligament hysteropexy, and open, laparoscopic, or robotic-assisted abdominal sacrohysteropexy [4, 35]. Benefits of hysteropexy compared to hysterectomy include reduced operative time, blood loss, and risk of mesh exposure. In a systematic review and meta-analysis of the literature, there was no significant difference in short-term prolapse outcomes between uterine preserving POP surgeries and POP surgeries with concomitant hysterectomy [21].

Hysterectomy alone is not an adequate treatment of uterine prolapse, and vaginal apex suspension should be performed at time of hysterectomy to reduce the risk of recurrent POP [12].

Colpocleisis

Women with symptomatic POP who wish to avoid hysterectomy, who have significant comorbidities precluding more extensive surgeries, and who are no longer interested in vaginal intercourse or vaginal preservation can be offered a colpocleisis. Colpocleisis is an obliterative surgery in which the vaginal walls are sutured together to close the vagina and correct vaginal vault prolapse. It represents an effective treatment for POP with high patient satisfaction rate and success rate with low risk of POP recurrence, but patients should be counseled that this is an irreversible surgery. Colpocleisis can be performed under local or regional anesthesia and represent a good option for treatment of symptomatic POP in women with significant medical comorbidities that are not good candidates for general anesthesia or prolonged surgeries. Elective hysterectomy is not associated with improvement in outcomes. If the uterus is still present at time of colpocleisis, cervical cytology, human papillomavirus testing, and endometrial evaluation should be obtained and documented prior to surgery, as the uterus becomes difficult to access after colpocleisis. The surgeon should consider a sub-urethral plication or mid-urethral sling and perineorrhaphy at the time of colpocleisis to decrease risk of de novo postoperative stress urinary incontinence and recurrent posterior wall prolapse [14].

Conclusion

Pelvic organ prolapse (POP) represents a common group of conditions that urologists, gynecologists, and primary care providers will encounter in their clinical practice with increasing frequency as the population of the United States continues to age. Clinicians who regularly see the demographic of patients at risk for POP should be familiar with the modifiable risk factors, spectrum of presenting symptoms, accepted measurements, and staging, and both conservative and surgical treatment options for POP. Clinicians should become familiar with prescription of pessaries and/or pelvic floor muscle exercises for patients with asymptomatic POP or refer those patients to specialists as needed. Individual patient characteristics such as age, future desire for pregnancy, sexual activity level, vaginal size, general health and life expectancy, patient preference, and the surgeon's training and experience should guide selection of surgical approach.

Cross-References

- ▶ Clinical Evaluation of the Female Lower Urinary Tract and Pelvic Floor
- ▶ Complications of the Use of Synthetic Mesh Materials in Stress Urinary Incontinence and Pelvic Organ Prolapse
- ▶ Laparoscopic Paravaginal Repair
- ▶ Management of Vaginal Posterior Compartment Prolapse: Is There Ever a Case for Graft/Mesh?
- ▶ Measurement of Urinary Symptoms, Health-Related Quality of Life, and Outcomes of Treatment of Genitourinary and Pelvic Floor Disorders
- ▶ Minimally Invasive Approaches in the Treatment of Pelvic Organ Prolapse: Laparoscopic and Robotic
- ▶ Minimally Invasive Sacrocolpopexy
- ▶ Open Abdominal Sacrocolpopexy
- ▶ Role of Vaginal Hysterectomy in the Treatment of Vaginal Middle Compartment Prolapse
- ▶ Transvaginal Repair of Cystocele
- ▶ Vaginal Vault Prolapse: Options for Transvaginal Surgical Repair

References

1. Abrams P, Andersson KE, Birder L, et al. Fourth International Consultation on Incontinence recommendations of the International Scientific Committee: evaluation and treatment of urinary incontinence, pelvic organ prolapse, and fecal incontinence. Neurourol Urodyn. 2010;29:213–40.

2. Barber MD. Pelvic organ prolapse. BMJ. 2016;354: i3853. https://doi.org/10.1136/bmj.i3853.
3. Barber MD, Maher C. Epidemiology and outcome assessment of pelvic organ prolapse. Int Urogynecol J. 2013;24:1783–90.
4. Bradley S, Gutman RE, Richter LA. Hysteropexy: an option for the repair of pelvic organ prolapse. Curr Urol Rep. 2018;19:15. https://doi.org/10.1007/s11934-018-0765-4.
5. Braekken IH, Majida M, Engh ME, et al. Can pelvic floor muscle training reverse pelvic organ prolapse and reduce prolapse symptoms? An assessor-blinded, randomized, controlled trial. Am J Obstet Gynecol. 2010;203:170.e1–7.
6. Brown JS, Waetjen LE, Subak LL, Thom DH, Van den Eeden S, Vittinghoff E. Pelvic organ prolapse surgery in the United States, 1997. Am J Obstet Gynecol. 2002;186(4):712–6. https://doi.org/10.1067/mob.2002.121897.
7. Brubaker L. Controversies and uncertainties: abdominal versus vaginal surgery for pelvic organ prolapse. Am J Obstet Gynecol. 2005;192(3):690–3. https://doi.org/10.1016/j.ajog.2004.10.633.
8. Bump RC, Mattiasson A, Bo K, Brubaker L, DeLancey JOL, Klarscov P, et al. The standardization of terminology of female pelvic organ prolapse and pelvic floor dysfunction. Am J Obstet Gynecol. 1996;175:10–7.
9. Clark AL, Gregory T, Smith VJ, Edwards R. Epidemiologic evaluation of reoperation for surgically treated pelvic organ prolapse and urinary incontinence. Am J Obstet Gynecol. 2003;189:1261–7. https://doi.org/10.1067/S0002-9378(03)00829-9. pmid:14634551.
10. Cundiff GW, Amundsen CL, Bent AE, et al. The PESSRI study: symptom relief outcomes of a randomized crossover trial of the ring and Gellhorn pessaries. Am J Obstet Gynecol. 2007;196:405.e1–8.
11. Diez-Itza I, Aizpitarte I, Becerro A. Risk factors for the recurrence of pelvic organ prolapse after vaginal surgery: a review at 5 years after surgery. Int Urogynecol J Pelvic Floor Dysfunct. 2007;18:1317–24.
12. Eilber KS, Alperin M, Khan A, et al. Outcomes of vaginal prolapse surgery among female Medicare beneficiaries: the role of apical support. Obstet Gynecol. 2013;122:981–7.
13. Ellerkmann RM, Cundiff GW, Melick CF, Nihira MA, Leffler K, Bent AE. Correlation of symptoms with location and severity of pelvic organ prolapse. Am J Obstet Gynecol. 2001;185:1332–7; discussion 1337–8. https://doi.org/10.1067/mob.2001.119078. pmid:11744905.
14. FitzGerald MP, Richter HE, Siddique S, Pelvic Floor Disorders Network, et al. Colpocleisis: a review. Int Urogynecol J Pelvic Floor Dysfunct. 2006;17:261–71.
15. Hagen S, Stark D. Conservative prevention and management of pelvic organ prolapse in women [Systematic review]. Cochrane Database Syst Rev. 2011;12: CD003882.

16. Hagen S, Stark D, Glazener C, POPPY Trial Collaborators, et al. Individualised pelvic floor muscle training in women with pelvic organ prolapse (POPPY): a multicentre randomised controlled trial. Lancet. 2014;383:796–806.
17. Hall AF, Theofrastous JP, Cundiff GC, Harris RL, Hamilton LF, Swift SE, et al. Interobserver and intraobserver reliability of the proposed International Continence Society, Society of Gynecologic Surgeons, and the American Urogynecologic Society Pelvic organ prolapse classification system. Am J Obstet Gynecol. 1996;175:1467–71.
18. Luber KM, Boero S, Choe JY. The demographics of pelvic floor disorders: current observations and future projections. Am J Obstet Gynecol. 2001;184:1496–501; discussion 1501–1503.
19. Maher C, Feiner B, Baessler K, Schmid C. Surgical management of pelvic organ prolapse in women. Cochrane Database Syst Rev. 2013;4:CD004014. https://doi.org/10.1002/14651858.CD004014.pub5. Published 2013 Apr 30.
20. Maher C, Feiner B, Baessler K, Christmann-Schmid C, Haya N, Marjoribanks J. Transvaginal mesh or grafts compared with native tissue repair for vaginal prolapse. Cochrane Database Syst Rev. 2016;2(2):CD012079. https://doi.org/10.1002/14651858.CD012079. Published 2016 Feb 9.
21. Meriwether KV, Antosh DD, Olivera CK, et al. Uterine preservation vs hysterectomy in pelvic organ prolapse surgery: a systematic review with meta-analysis and clinical practice guidelines. Am J Obstet Gynecol. 2018;219(2):129–146.e2. https://doi.org/10.1016/j.ajog.2018.01.018.
22. Merriman AL, Kennelly MJ. Biologic grafts for use in pelvic organ prolapse surgery: a contemporary review. Curr Urol Rep. 2020;21(12):52. https://doi.org/10.1007/s11934-020-01013-x. Published 2020 Oct 24.
23. Nager CW, Visco AG, Richter HE, et al. Effect of vaginal mesh hysteropexy vs vaginal hysterectomy with uterosacral ligament suspension on treatment failure in women with uterovaginal prolapse: a randomized clinical trial. JAMA. 2019;322(11):1054–65. https://doi.org/10.1001/jama.2019.12812.
24. Nygaard I, Brubaker L, Zyczynski HM, et al. Long-term outcomes following abdominal sacrocolpopexy for pelvic organ prolapse. JAMA. 2013;309:2016–24.
25. Olsen AL, Smith VJ, Bergstrom JO, Colling JC, Clark AL. Epidemiology of surgically managed pelvic organ prolapse and urinary incontinence. Obstet Gynecol. 1997;89:501–6. https://doi.org/10.1016/S0029-7844(97)00058-6. pmid:9083302.
26. Pelvic Organ Prolapse. Obstet Gynecol. 2019;134 (5):e126–42. https://doi.org/10.1097/AOG.0000000000003519.
27. Pham T, Burgart A, Kenton K, et al. Current use of pelvic organ prolapse quantification by AUGS and ICS members. Female Pelvic Med Reconstr Surg. 2011;17: 67–9.

28. Robert M, Schulz JA, Harvey MA, et al. Urogynaecology committee. Technical update on pessary use. J Obstet Gynaecol Can. 2013;35:664–74.

29. Sung VW, Hampton BS. Chapter 7: Epidemiology and psychosocial impact of female pelvic floor disorders. In: Walters MD, Karram MM, editors. Urogynecology and reconstructive pelvic surgery. 4th ed. Saunders/Elsevier; 1999. p. 98–101.

30. Swift S, Woodman P, O'Boyle A, et al. Pelvic Organ Support Study (POSST): the distribution, clinical definition, and epidemiologic condition of pelvic organ support defects. Am J Obstet Gynecol. 2005;192:795–806.

31. U.S. Food and Drug Administration. FDA takes action to protect women's health, orders manufacturers of surgical mesh intended for transvaginal repair of pelvic organ prolapse to stop selling all devices. Silver Spring: FDA; 2019. Available at: https://www.fda.gov/NewsEvents/Newsroom/PressAnnouncements/ucm636114.htm

32. US Food and Drug Administration, authors. Urogynecologic surgical mesh: update on the safety and effectiveness of transvaginal placement for pelvic organ prolapse. 2011. www.fda.gov/downloads/MedicalDevices/Safety/AlertsandNotices/UCM262760.pdf

33. Vergeldt TF, Weemhoff M, IntHout J, Kluivers KB. Risk factors for pelvic organ prolapse and its recurrence: a systematic review. Int Urogynecol J. 2015;26(11):1559–73. https://doi.org/10.1007/s00192-015-2695-8.

34. Winters JC, Dmochowski RR, Goldman HB, et al. Urodynamic studies in adults: AUA/SUFU guideline. J Urol. 2012;188(6 Suppl):2464–72.

35. Winters JC, Krlin RM, Hallner B. Vaginal and abdominal reconstructive surgery for pelvic organ prolapse. In: Campbell MF, Kavoussi LR, Wein AJ, editors. Campbell-Walsh-Wein urology. 12th ed. Philadelphia: Elsevier Saunders; 2021. p. 2776–829.

36. Wu JM, Vaughan CP, Goode PS, et al. Prevalence and trends of symptomatic pelvic floor disorders in U.-S. women. Obstet Gynecol. 2014a;123:141–8.

37. Wu JM, Matthews CA, Conover MM, et al. Lifetime risk of stress urinary incontinence or pelvic organ prolapse surgery. Obstet Gynecol. 2014b;123:1201–6.

Transvaginal Repair of Cystocele

29

Rita Jen, Atieh Novin, and David Ginsberg

Contents

Introduction	520
Anatomy and Etiology	520
Presentation and Diagnosis	521
Additional Preoperative Evaluation	522
Dynamic Imaging	522
Urodynamics	522
Cystoscopy	523
Transvaginal Surgical Techniques	523
Anterior Colporrhaphy	523
Transverse Defect Repair	524
Paravaginal Repair	524
Outcomes of Repair	524
Complications	525
Conclusion	525
References	530

Abstract

Pelvic organ prolapse increases in risk with parity and as women age. The most commonly found defect is in the anterior compartment with the finding of a cystocele on exam. Patients may be asymptomatic or could describe vaginal pressure or bladder symptoms. Cystocele repair with native tissue usually involves repair of central and lateral defects, otherwise known as anterior colporrhaphy and paravaginal repair, respectively. The repair is more durable when apical suspension is performed at the same time. In patients with occult stress urinary incontinence, an anti-incontinence procedure can be performed concomitantly as well. Patient counseling on bladder and sexual functional outcomes prior to surgery is extremely

---

R. Jen · A. Novin · D. Ginsberg (✉)
USC Institute of Urology, Los Angeles, CA, USA
e-mail: ginsberg@med.usc.edu

© Springer Nature Switzerland AG 2023
F. E. Martins et al. (eds.), *Female Genitourinary and Pelvic Floor Reconstruction*,
https://doi.org/10.1007/978-3-031-19598-3_30

important for setting expectations of surgical repair. Overall, patient-reported outcomes and satisfaction are greater than anatomic success rates postoperatively.

Keywords

Bladder · Cystocele · Prolapse

Introduction

Pelvic organ prolapse (POP) is a common condition in women as they age. In the Women's Health Initiative studies [1], 41% of women aged 50–79 years showed some degree of POP, with cystoceles being the most common at 34% followed by rectoceles at 19%, and apical prolapse at 14%. However, the true prevalence of a cystocele or anterior vaginal wall prolapse among women is not clear. The anterior compartment is particularly significant because it is the most common site of prolapse and the most common site of operative failure with recurrences of up to 42% [2]. Anterior wall prolapse also has significant association with urinary symptoms given the defect can be at the location of the urethrovesical junction. For these reasons management of this compartment can be challenging. Several theories regarding the pathophysiology as well as surgical methods have been proposed which will be outlined in this chapter.

Anatomy and Etiology

POP refers to descent of one or more of the vaginal compartments or the apex. Systematic descriptions have been used for classification of POP for the purposes of documentation and research and establishing guidelines with standardized techniques. The classification was first established by Baden [3] in 1968 followed by the Pelvic Organ Prolapse Quantification (POP-Q) by Bump in 1996 [4]. Prolapse of any compartment is associated with risk factors such as obesity, age, and parity. Other risks factors include increased intraabdominal pressure, collagen abnormalities,

family history, or prior pelvic surgeries [5]. Compared to other compartments, the increased prevalence of anterior compartment prolapse has been noted in several studies, such as Handa's follow-up [6] of the Women's Health Initiative study. Some theories that make this compartment more challenging are the lack of direct support of this compartment by the levator plate as compared to the posterior compartment, possible increased injury of this compartment during childbirth, and possible higher elasticity of the anterior compartment.

DeLancey [7] described the connective tissue support of the pelvis in various levels, which are important in choosing the correct surgical method and will be described later. The connective tissues of the pelvis connect the vagina and uterus laterally to the pelvic walls, and these supportive structures can be divided into three levels. In Level I, the cervix and the upper third of the vagina are attached to the pelvic walls by the cardinal and uterosacral ligaments. In Level II, the middle third of the vagina is attached laterally to fascial structures, i.e., the arcus tendineus fascia pelvis (ATFP), also called the white line. Distally in Level III, the vagina is fused anteriorly to the urethra and posteriorly with the surrounding structures, the levator ani muscles and the perineal body [7]. The pelvis can also be divided into three compartments to describe prolapse – the anterior compartment containing the bladder and urethra, the middle compartment with the uterus and cervix (or vaginal cuff if there was a prior hysterectomy), and the posterior compartment with the rectum. It is important to consider all levels of support and the sites of defects when choosing a method not only for anterior compartment repair but also for POP repair in general.

A cystocele results from a defect in the anterior compartment, which can be midline, lateral, or both. Midline defects, also called central defects, arise from vertical defects in the endopelvic fascia extending anteriorly to posteriorly. The bladder, bladder neck, and urethra can expand through the defect resulting in the characteristic bulge of a cystocele with loss of rugae anteriorly. Not surprisingly, disruption of this region can result in stress urinary incontinence (SUI) as it is the main area of support of the urethrovesical junction [8]. As first described by White [9], lateral defects, also called paravaginal defects, are thought to be due to disruption of the ATFP; the lateral vaginal sulci descend, but the vaginal rugae is preserved on the anterior vagina in the midline [10].

Another potential anterior site-specific defect includes transverse defects, which occur when the pubocervical fascia separates from its insertion into the ring of connective tissue around the cervix and uterosacral ligaments, creating a transverse support defect and loss of the anterior support of the cervix. On examination, these defects often result in a large anterior vaginal wall defect, which appears to originate high on the anterior vaginal wall or near the cervix, although the urethra may remain well supported [8, 11]. Distal defects are the least common forms of anterior vaginal wall defects. They are due to a break in the fibromuscular support of the anterior vaginal wall, just before the insertion into the pubic symphysis. These defects are usually associated with urethral hypermobility and stress urinary incontinence [12].

Additionally, there is evidence that the apex provides some degree of anterior support. Lowder et al. [13] measured prolapse using the POP-Q in 197 women with at least stage 2 prolapse, both with simulated apical support and without. They simulated apical support by using the posterior blade of a speculum to suspend the vaginal apex. On remeasurement of prolapse, the authors found a statistically significant improvement in both anterior and posterior prolapse. Specifically, they found that 55% of women had point Ba improved to either stage 0 or stage 1 [13].

Presentation and Diagnosis

Symptoms of anterior wall prolapse can vary depending on severity and location of the defect. Women may present with vaginal pressure or urinary symptoms such as incontinence or urgency; they may also be completely asymptomatic [2]. The Pelvic Floor Impact Questionnaire (PFIQ) can be used to assess pelvic prolapse-related symptoms [14]. Women may complain of a feeling of pressure or sensation of a bulge or that something is coming out of the vagina. Often, symptoms develop when the prolapse is at the level of the hymen or beyond.

Urinary symptoms range from stress incontinence to frequency and urgency as well as trouble initiating urination and the feeling of incomplete evacuation. The prevalence of urinary incontinence with cystocele can be up to almost 50%, and urgency symptoms range from 14% to 68% [15]. With advanced stages of anterior wall prolapse, women may experience bladder outlet obstruction due to kinking at the level of the outlet or detrusor underactivity due to prolonged obstruction. Some women may report a need to press on the anterior vaginal wall to void [16]. Patients may also have discharge, bleeding, or vaginal pain. Sexual dysfunction can also be present and can be due to physical, psychological, or partner-related factors [17].

Pelvic examination is standard and includes inspection of the quality of the vaginal epithelium, presence of SUI and occult SUI (done by having the patient cough or strain with the bladder both prolapsed and reduced), quantification of cystocele severity, and presence of prolapse in other compartments. Should the patient have urinary complaints at presentation, a post-void residual should be obtained.

Characterizing a cystocele is completed with the hymen as the point of reference. The examination is done with the patient straining or by placing gentle traction on the most dependent portion of the prolapse. The patient may be in dorsal lithotomy or standing for the exam. The points of reference most associated with anterior wall prolapse are points Aa and Ba in the POP-Q classification system. Point Aa is the point located in the midline of the anterior vaginal wall 3 cm proximal to the external urethral meatus. Point Ba represents the most dependent portion of the anterior vaginal wall from the cuff to point Aa [4]. It is important to note that apical descent can sometimes give the impression of a cystocele, and thus quantifying the cervix or cuff position, Point C, and the posterior fornix, Point D, is essential.

Additional Preoperative Evaluation

While the pelvic examination is the foundation of diagnosis and treatment of cystoceles, additional studies may be used for diagnosis of concomitant pelvic floor disorders and operative preparation and may be helpful for predicting postoperative outcomes.

Dynamic Imaging

In the 1990s, surgeons, gastroenterologists, and radiologists began using dynamic magnetic resonance imaging (MRI) to understand and evaluate various pelvic floor disorders including defecatory dysfunction, POP, and incontinence [18–22]. Dynamic MRI of the pelvis, specifically, MR defecography, captures real-time images of the pelvic organs as the patient performs various maneuvers like relaxing the pelvic floor muscles or defecation after the distal rectum is filled with contrast gel [23]. The study not only provides anatomic detail of the soft tissues in all three compartments but also functional elements.

Attenberger et al. [24] compared their findings and diagnoses on conventional pelvic examination to the findings in MR defecography in 63 women with pelvic floor dysfunction. In the 50 women who underwent both MR defecography and pelvic examination successfully, the authors found MR defecography necessary for proper diagnosis in 22 patients, and management was altered in 19 patients [24]. All of the differences in MR and pelvic exam findings involved the posterior and/or the middle compartment, specifically, with diagnosis of enteroceles. They concluded that imaging was a less useful adjunct to the physical exam for diagnosis of anterior compartment disorders [24].

In another study by Al-Najar et al. [25], findings on MR defecography were correlated to patients' initial complaints and symptoms. Out of the 70 women in the study, 62% initially presented with constipation and 21.1% with obstructed defecation; other complaints included urinary incontinence, fecal incontinence, rectal prolapse, and blood per rectum [25]. On imaging, the majority of the women had posterior compartment disorders (85.7%); and of those with a posterior compartment abnormality, more than 50% had concomitant cystocele on imaging [25]. Nineteen percent of women had a middle compartment abnormality, and 72% of those patients also had a cystocele on imaging.

These studies suggest MR defecography is most useful in the patient with suspected prolapse that was not elicited on exam, in the patient with descent of multiple compartments, or in the patient with defecatory complaints. In a patient with an isolated cystocele on exam without any other complaints or pelvic surgical history, MR defecography would be an invasive, superfluous, and expensive test for the patient.

Urodynamics

There is no consensus recommendation for urodynamics (UDS) prior to cystocele repair, and there is limited evidence that UDS is helpful in preoperative planning in those with POP other than to assess for occult SUI [26]. However, it may be reasonable that UDS is employed in patients with multicompartment defects with complaints of difficulty emptying for counseling purposes if they have not committed to POP repair already [15, 27].

Wolter and colleagues [15] assessed the usefulness of preoperative UDS in predicting urinary outcomes in post-hysterectomy women with mixed urinary incontinence (MUI) and cystocele undergoing surgical repair. The authors retrospectively reviewed 111 women who had undergone both an anterior compartment repair and a concomitant sling. Depending on the presence of apical descent or posterior compartment complaints, the authors also performed simultaneous apical suspension or posterior repair. All of the subjects also had UDS testing with prolapse present and reduced before surgery. Sixty of the 111 patients presented with MUI, and 10 had urgency urinary incontinence (UUI) with occult stress incontinence on UDS. The investigators had at least an 88% cure rate in patients' preoperative urinary symptoms and 89% cure rate for prolapse [15]. Cure for incontinence was defined as a negative cough stress test or no incontinence recorded on the voiding diary; prolapse was cured if the patient had an asymptomatic grade II defect or better. They did not find that preoperative UDS findings, like detrusor overactivity, were associated with urinary outcomes like de novo UUI or sling failure. They concluded that UDS was not useful in surgical planning in patients with cystocele and presentation with MUI but was helpful in identifying occult SUI in patients with cystocele. However, only a fraction of their patients was in the latter category.

Glass et al. [27] made similar conclusions in their study evaluating the influence of preoperative UDS on patients undergoing POP repair. They retrospectively identified patients with POP who elected surgical repair and subsequently also had preoperative UDS to determine whether any concomitant procedures would be performed at the time of the prolapse repair [27]. Only 11 of 316 women identified had change in their treatment plan or preoperative counseling due to findings on UDS. Five women were counseled or started on medications for overactive bladder, and an additional five were diagnosed with incomplete emptying or findings of detrusor underactivity that changed the decision for sling placement [27]. Finally, another patient underwent lysis of prior urethral sling due to UDS findings [27]. The authors concluded UDS in patients already planning on undergoing POP surgery would only be beneficial in those with occult SUI that was not seen on exam or in patients with additional incomplete emptying or voiding symptoms [27].

It should be noted that none of these studies evaluated the utility of UDS in patients with isolated cystoceles.

Cystoscopy

Cystoscopy is not indicated in patients with cystoceles unless there are additional concerning signs or symptoms such as hematuria or refractory recurrent urinary tract infections. Cystoscopy may be helpful in distinguishing a cystocele from an enterocele, but this could also be done at the time of prolapse repair, should that be planned.

Transvaginal Surgical Techniques

Various transvaginal surgical techniques exist for cystocele repair and continue to evolve given the Food and Drug Administration's removal of polypropylene mesh kits for vaginal prolapse from the market. This chapter will focus on native tissue repair.

The transvaginal approaches for cystocele repair can be largely categorized by the sites of defects being addressed, in other words, midline or lateral defects. The choice of which repair to perform is dependent on both the location of the defect and surgeon preference and experience. Not all cystoceles have the same defects and often involve other compartments as described earlier. Thus, the varying techniques for cystocele repair often overlap in their application. All repairs begin with preoperative prophylactic antibiotics, patient positioning in dorsal lithotomy, and use of a weighted speculum and/or self-retaining vaginal retractor to expose the cystocele. A urethral catheter is placed, and the bladder is drained.

Anterior Colporrhaphy

Anterior colporrhaphy or plication of the fibromuscular tissues in the anterior vaginal wall has been a timeless approach to cystocele repair. A midline incision is made in the anterior vaginal wall, and the vaginal epithelium is carefully dissected from the pubocervical fascia proximally to the cuff, laterally to expose the pelvic side wall, and distally to the bladder neck. If planning a sling at the same time, the dissection for the sling is usually spared from this incision and dissection. Kelly plication of the bladder neck and proximal urethra can be performed through the same incision. After dissection, interrupted sutures, either absorbable or nonabsorbable, are placed bilaterally through the pubocervical fascia and re-approximated in the midline to reduce the cystocele. Cystoscopy is performed to ensure patent ureters and no injuries to the urinary tract. Excess vaginal epithelium can be excised and then re-approximated with absorbable suture. As such, this repair addresses a central or midline defect as the cause of the cystocele. Vaginal packing is left in place to prevent hematoma formation. Patients are usually able to be discharged the same day of surgery and are usually able to pass a voiding trial prior to leaving. The vaginal packing is removed before patient discharge.

Transverse Defect Repair

As in anterior colporrhaphy, repair of the transverse defect also starts with a midline incision and dissection of the anterior vaginal epithelium from the pubocervical fascia. The redundant, transverse points of the pubocervical fascia are then sutured superiorly to the cervical stroma as in a cervicopexy [11]. Thereafter, midline plication of the pubocervical fascia is performed as in anterior colporrhaphy.

Paravaginal Repair

Repair of lateral defects, often called paravaginal repair and first reported by White [9], involves restoring the ATFP or plication sutures placed through the obturator fascia [28]. Similar to anterior colporrhaphy, the anterior vaginal epithelium is dissected off the pubocervical fascia as described above. However, dissection is carried further laterally to reach the retropubic space, which is developed laterally enough to palpate bony structures of the ischial spine, the pubic symphysis, and the ischiopubic rami. The bladder is retracted medially to expose the ATFP, lateral pelvic sidewall, and the obturator fascia. After identifying the ATFP, a series of four to six interrupted sutures are placed around the ATFP from just the anterior to the ischial spine down to the level of the urethrovesical junction [10]. These sutures can be placed through the obturator fascia instead if the ATFP is thought to be insubstantial. The needles are left in place so that

each suture can then be passed through the pubocervical fascia and the undersurface of the dissected vaginal epithelium at the lateral sulcus, this time starting at the urethrovesical junction and proceeding proximally. After all sutures are placed bilaterally, they are tied sequentially from the urethrovesical junction to the last suture at the ischial spine. This repair not only restores the lateral support but also the vaginal sulci bilaterally. Once all sutures are tied, cystoscopy is performed to rule out urinary tract injury. Then the vaginal epithelium is trimmed and re-approximated. Postoperative care is the same as for anterior colporrhaphy.

As cystoceles can involve both midline and lateral defects, both techniques can be used at the same time. To reduce cystocele recurrence, modifications of these approaches have involved both synthetic and biologic grafts over the years.

Outcomes of Repair

For over a century, surgeons have struggled with recurrent cystocele [28]. Although there are numerous studies seeking a durable cure, most of them are smaller series, have a short follow-up of 1–2 years, and have variable definitions of success. For example, investigators may define success by anatomic standards, reoperation rates, by patients' sensation of a bulge, or patients' report of vaginal pressure. Patients seeking surgical repair often do not have isolated cystoceles and may also have urinary complaints. Additionally, randomized controlled trials of cystocele repair often compared native tissue repair with surgeries involving various types of grafts or mesh. As such, comparison of studies and outcomes is difficult.

In 1994, Shull et al. [29] described their paravaginal defect repairs via the vaginal route in 62 consecutive women; the reported success rate at 6 weeks was 94%, but 34% of women had some support defect observed on follow-up thereafter. Complications included a proctotomy repaired at the time of surgery and ureteral obstruction that required removal of a culdoplasty suture; other significant complications, like hematoma formation and need for blood transfusion, were observed in a similar study of 100 consecutive women by Young and colleagues [29, 30].

Although the true prevalence is unknown, women with apical prolapse often also have anterior vaginal wall prolapse. Furthermore, as mentioned previously, the apex does lend support to the anterior compartment [13]. Eilber et al. [31] reported higher reoperation rates in women undergoing anterior repair alone (20.2%) compared to those having concomitant apical repair (11.6%). Given this logic, treatment of only the apex in some patients may result in resolution of any anterior compartment prolapse as well. In one observational study seeking to compare rates of recurrent cystocele after abdominal sacrocolpopexy (SCP), Shippey et al. [32] reported that SCP alone was as effective as SCP combined with paravaginal repair. The comparison was between 28 patients who had SCP alone and 77 patients who underwent paravaginal repair at the time of SCP. Anterior vaginal wall failure, defined as stage 2 POP or worse after at least 6 months post-op, was 21% in the first group and 26% in the second group, which was not statistically significant.

Similarly, van Zanten et al. [33] found a 20% failure rate in the anterior compartment (grade II or worse) of patients undergoing robotic SCP or robotic supracervical hysterectomy with sacrocervicopexy at least 1 year postoperatively [33]. Ninety-six percent of patients had no apical recurrence at 50-month follow-up, and only one patient underwent anterior repair for recurrence.

Interestingly, Padoa et al. [34] reported that an anterior compartment defect of point Ba at +3 or worse preoperatively was independently related to POP recurrence after robotic SCP. Their anatomic failure rate in the anterior compartment was 34.4%.

Recently, more focus has been placed on outcomes of patient satisfaction, urinary function, and sexual function, instead of anatomical success. Several studies are summarized in Table 1. Overall, patient success rates for anterior repair appear satisfactory, and concomitant apical repair contributes to its durability.

Complications

Although not common, potential intraoperative complications during cystocele repair include blood loss and injury to the urinary tract or other surrounding structures. Hematoma formation is reported between 0% and 4% among various studies and was more likely in paravaginal repairs with aggressive lateral and retropubic dissection [36, 45, 47, 49]. The majority of studies had a very low incidence of blood transfusion after cystocele repair, less than 1% [51]. However, one study by Young et al. [30] reported a transfusion rate of 16%. Although the authors posited that their transfusion rate may have been higher than expected due to their low threshold for transfusion, they did describe a significant venous bleeding in three patients that occurred during retropubic dissection [30].

Any injuries to the urinary tract, like cystotomy, should be repaired in multiple layers and immediately at the time of injury. Bladder decompression with an indwelling catheter for 1–2 weeks is standard for the bladder to heal. If a urinary tract injury is missed, the patient could develop a urinary tract to vagina fistula, so cystoscopy is crucial during cystocele repair. Likewise, injury to the ureters must also be ruled out. One study [52] noted a 2% incidence of ureteral obstruction during 346 cystocele repairs, which was thought to be kinking of the ureters due to lateral plication sutures.

Other postoperative complications include urinary tract and surgical site infections.

Long-term functional complications involve sexual function (dyspareunia) and bladder function, namely, de novo stress incontinence, overactive bladder, and urinary retention. The table summarizing surgical outcomes includes these complications as well, if reported in the original study.

Conclusion

Often accompanied by apical prolapse, cystoceles are the most common site of defect in patients complaining of prolapse symptoms. Central and

Table 1 Studies evaluating outcomes of cystocele repair

Author, year	Type of study	Single or multiple	Type of repair	Additional procedure(s), if indicated	Number of patients	Mean follow-up (months)	Success definition	Success rate	Other reported outcomes
Shull, 1994 [29]	Prospective study	Single center	Paravaginal repair	Hysterectomy, culdoplasty, suspension, posterior colporrhaphy	62 consecutive	19.2	Baden-Walker halfway 1	93.5%	1 patient with cul-de-sac prolapse to hymen on follow-up
Kohli, 1996 [35]	Retrospective review	Single center	Anterior colporrhaphy with or without needle bladder neck suspension	Hysterectomy, posterior colporrhaphy, enterocele repair	67 (40 with, 27 without)	13.1	Baden-Walker halfway 0	67.5% (with) 92.6% (without)	4 patients underwent reoperation in the bladder neck suspension group
Mallipeddi, 2001 [36]	Retrospective review	Single center	Paravaginal repair	Anterior/posterior colporrhaphy, hysterectomy, enterocele repair, McCall's culdoplasty, sacrospinous suspension	45	20.18	Baden-Walker halfway 0	97.1% success with cystocele; 20% recurrent enterocele	57% persistent SUI
Sand, 2001 [37]	Randomized clinical trial	Single center	Compared anterior colporrhaphy with and without mesh	Hysterectomy, culdoplasty, enterocele repair, posterior colporrhaphy with or without mesh	160 (80 with mesh and 80 without mesh)	12	Modified Baden-Walker 0	57% in anterior colporrhaphy alone 75% in mesh group	
Weber, 2001 [38]	Randomized clinical trial	Single center	Compared standard anterior colporrhaphy, anterior colporrhaphy with mesh, and ultralateral anterior colporrhaphy	Hysterectomy, posterior colporrhaphy, enterocele repair, vault suspension	109	23.3 (median)	POP-Q Aa and Ba stage 1 or stage 0	30% in anterior colporrhaphy alone 42% in anterior colporrhaphy with mesh	Only 83 patients returned for follow-up No statistical difference in success rates

Young, 2001 [30]	Retrospective review	Single center	Paravaginal repair	Hysterectomy, enterocele repair, culdoplasty, Burch, anterior or posterior colporrhaphy, sling	100 consecutive	10.6	Baden-Walker halfway 0	46% in ultralateral anterior colporrhaphy; Paravaginal 98% Midline 78%	16% blood transfusion rate
Gandhi, 2005 [39]	Randomized clinical trial	Single center	Compared anterior colporrhaphy (ultralateral) with and without dehydrated fascia lata	Hysterectomy, culdoplasty, suspension, posterior colporrhaphy, Cooper's ligament sling	78 anterior colporrhaphy alone 76 anterior colporrhaphy with fascia lata	12	POP-Q < stage 2 No pelvic pressure No vaginal bulge	71% 69% 89% (Only reporting for anterior colporrhaphy alone)	Concomitant bladder neck slings associated with reduced risk of recurrence
Nieminen, 2010 [40]	Randomized clinical trial	Multicenter	Compared anterior colporrhaphy with and without mesh	Hysterectomy, enterocele repair, posterior colporrhaphy	97 no mesh 105 with mesh	36	POP-Q < stage 2 No pelvic pressure	59% anatomic 72% symptoms	Reoperation rate 18%
Valenčić, 2010 [41]	Retrospective review	Single center	Modified anterior colporrhaphy with incorporation of cardinal ligament and endopelvic fascia laterally		76	60.14	Anatomic cure	95%	Urinary urgency 4%, de novo SUI 5%
Altman, 2011 [42]	Randomized clinical trial	Multicenter	Compared anterior colporrhaphy with and without mesh		189 colporrhaphy alone 200 colporrhaphy with mesh	12	POP-Q stage 0 or 1 without symptoms	34.5%	47.5% anatomic success 62.1% no bulge symptoms 6.3% de novo SUI

(continued)

Table 1 (continued)

Author, year	Type of study	Single or multiple	Type of repair	Additional procedure(s), if indicated	Number of patients	Mean follow-up (months)	Success definition	Success rate	Other reported outcomes
Vollebregt, 2011 [43]	Randomized clinical trial	Multicenter	Compared anterior colporrhaphy with transobturator mesh	Sacrospinous suspension, posterior colporrhaphy	125 (64 anterior colporrhaphy and 61 mesh)	12	No reoperation for anatomic failure (POP-Q ≥ grade 2)	95% in anterior colporrhaphy alone 0% in mesh group	
Song, 2012 [44]	Retrospective review	Single center	Purse-string anterior colporrhaphy	Suspension, hysterectomy, sling	69	48	Baden-Walker halfway ≥ grade 2	98%	
Chen, 2013 [45]	Retrospective review	Single center	Ultralateral anterior repair	Sacrospinous suspension, mesh sling	135	111	Reported symptoms Anterior wall < stage 2 POP-Q No reoperation	74.1% 54.7% 92.6%	
Wong, 2014 [46]	Retrospective review	Multicenter	Compared anterior colporrhaphy alone with anterior colporrhaphy with mesh		183	48	POP-Q < stage 2 Bladder descent <1 cm below pubic symphysis on ultrasound No symptoms of bulge	45% in anterior colporrhaphy alone 67% in anterior colporrhaphy with mesh	

29 Transvaginal Repair of Cystocele

Study	Study type	Center	Intervention	Other procedures	N	Follow-up	Outcome measure	Success	Patient-reported
Balzarro, 2017 [47]	Retrospective review	Single center	Anterior colporrhaphy	Hysterectomy 14, sacrospinous suspension 6, posterior colporrhaphy 7, mesh sling 18, others 3	42	108.5	Anterior wall with < stage 2 POP-Q	81.0%	Patient-reported satisfaction 95.2%
Serati, 2017 [48]	Prospective study	Single center	Transverse cystocele repair, anterior colporrhaphy, uterine suspension		102	31	No prolapse symptoms PGI-I score $\leq$ 2 Prolapse stage <2 No further surgery	95.1%	
Arenholt, 2019 [49]	Prospective study	Single center	Paravaginal repair (unilateral if bilateral not indicated)	Sacrospinous suspension, posterior colporrhaphy	46	6	POP-Q $\leq$ 2 without symptoms	61%	
Rude, 2021 [50]	Prospective study	Single center	Paravaginal repair	Suspension 10, posterior colporrhaphy 9	109	12	POP-Q Ba <1 No bothersome vaginal bulge	89.0% 94.5%	Transient urinary retention 19% De novo SUI 5.5%

Source: Amin K and Lee U. Surgery for Anterior Compartment Vaginal Prolapse: Suture-Based Repair. Urol Clin North Am. 2019 Feb;46(1):61–70. https://doi.org/10.1016/j.ucl.2018.08.008

Maher C. Anterior vaginal compartment surgery. Int Urogynecol J (2013) 24:1791–1802. https://doi.org/10.1007/s00192-013-2170-3

lateral defects are often the cause of cystoceles, and native tissue repair of these areas includes anterior colporrhaphy and paravaginal defect repair. Concomitant apical suspension provides additional longevity to the repair. Patient satisfaction with surgical repair is higher than anatomic success rates. Patients with higher-grade cystoceles are more likely to have occult SUI, which can be evaluated with UDS although often not necessary. Patients must be counseled on postoperative bladder and sexual function outcomes.

References

1. Hendrix SL, Clark A, Nygaard I, Aragaki A, Barnabei V, McTtiernan A. Pelvic organ prolapse in the Women's Health Initiative: gravity and gravidity. In: American journal of obstetrics and gynecology. Mosby Inc; 2002. p. 1160–6.
2. Maher C, Feiner B, Baessler K, Christmann-Schmid C, Haya N, Brown J. Surgery for women with anterior compartment prolapse. Cochrane Database Syst Rev. 2016;2017:CD004014. https://doi.org/10.1002/14651858.CD004014.pub6.
3. Baden WF, Walker TA, Lindsey JH. The vaginal profile. Texas Med. 1968;64:56–8.
4. Bump RC, Mattiasson A, Bø K, Brubaker LP, DeLancey JOL, Klarskov P, Shull BL, Smith ARB. The standardization of terminology of female pelvic organ prolapse and pelvic floor dysfunction. Am J Obstet Gynecol. 1996;175:10–7.
5. MacLennan AH, Taylor AW, Wilson DH, Wilson D. The prevalence of pelvic floor disorders and their relationship to gender, age, parity and mode of delivery. BJOG Int J Obstet Gynaecol. 2000;107:1460–70.
6. Handa VL, Garrett E, Hendrix S, Gold E, Robbins J. Progression and remission of pelvic organ prolapse: a longitudinal study of menopausal women. Am J Obstet Gynecol. 2004;190:27–32.
7. DeLancey JOL. Anatomic aspects of vaginal eversion after hysterectomy. Am J Obstet Gynecol. 1992;166:1717–28.
8. Richardson AC, Lyon JB, Williams NL. A new look at pelvic relaxation. Am J Obstet Gynecol. 1976;126:568–71.
9. White GR. Cystocele. J Am Med Assoc. 1909;LIII:1707.
10. Walters MD, Paraiso MFR. Anterior vaginal wall prolapse: innovative surgical approaches. Cleve Clin J Med. 2005;72:S20.
11. Huffaker RK, Kuehl TJ, Muir TW, Yandell PM, Pierce LM, Shull BL. Transverse cystocele repair with uterine preservation using native tissue. Int Urogynecol J. 2008;19:1275–81.
12. Brincat CA, Larson KA, Fenner DE. Anterior vaginal wall prolapse. Clin Obstet Gynecol. 2010;53:51–8.

13. Lowder JL, Park AJ, Ellison R, Ghetti C, Moalli P, Zyczynski H, Weber AM. The role of apical vaginal support in the appearance of anterior and posterior vaginal prolapse. Obstet Gynecol. 2008;111:152–7.
14. Barber MD, Walters MD, Bump RC. Short forms of two condition-specific quality-of-life questionnaires for women with pelvic floor disorders (PFDI-20 and PFIQ-7). Am J Obstet Gynecol. 2005;193:103–13.
15. Wolter CE, Kaufman MR, Duffy JW, Scarpero HM, Dmochowski RR. Mixed incontinence and cystocele: postoperative urge symptoms are not predicted by preoperative urodynamics. Int Urogynecol J. 2011;22:321–5.
16. Tan JS, Lukacz ES, Menefee SA, Powell CR, Nager CW. Predictive value of prolapse symptoms: a large database study. Int Urogynecol J. 2005;16:203–9.
17. Handa VL, Cundiff G, Chang HH, Helzlsouer KJ. Female sexual function and pelvic floor disorders. Obstet Gynecol. 2008;111:1045–52.
18. Maubon A, Aubard Y, Berkane V, Camezind-Vidal M-A, Marès P, Rouanet JP. Magnetic resonance imaging of the pelvic floor. Abdom Imaging. 2003;28:217–25.
19. Kirschner-Hermanns R, Wein B, Niehaus S, Schaefer W, Jakse G. The contribution of magnetic resonance imaging of the pelvic floor to the understanding of urinary incontinence. Br J Urol. 1993;72:715–8.
20. Fletcher J, Busse R, Riederer S, Hough D, Gluecker T, Harper C, Bharucha A. Magnetic resonance imaging of anatomic and dynamic defects of the pelvic floor in defecatory disorders. Am J Gastroenterol. 2003;98:399–411.
21. Comiter CV, Vasavada SP, Barbaric ZL, Gousse AE, Raz S. Grading pelvic prolapse and pelvic floor relaxation using dynamic magnetic resonance imaging. Urology. 1999;54:454–7.
22. Yang A, Mostwin JL, Rosenshein NB, Zerhouni EA. Pelvic floor descent in women: dynamic evaluation with fast MR imaging and cinematic display. Radiology. 1991;179:25–33.
23. del Salto LG, de M Criado J, del Hoyo LFA, Velasco LG, Rivas PF, Paradela MM, de las Vacas MIDP, Sanz AGM, Moreno EF. MR imaging-based assessment of the female pelvic floor. Radiographics. 2014;34:1417–39.
24. Attenberger UI, Morelli JN, Budjan J, et al. The value of dynamic magnetic resonance imaging in interdisciplinary treatment of pelvic floor dysfunction. Abdom Imaging. 2015;40:2242–7.
25. Al-Najar MS, Ghanem AF, AlRyalat SAS, Al-Ryalat NT, Alhajahjeh SO. The usefulness of MR defecography in the evaluation of pelvic floor dysfunction: our experience using 3T MRI. Abdom Radiol. 2017;42:2219–24.
26. Winters JC, Dmochowski RR, Goldman HB, Herndon CDA, Kobashi KC, Kraus SR, Lemack GE, Nitti VW, Rovner ES, Wein AJ. Urodynamic studies in adults: AUA/SUFU guideline. J Urol. 2012;188:2464–72.
27. Glass D, Lin FC, Khan AA, van Kuiken M, Drain A, Siev M, Peyronett B, Rosenblum N, Brucker BM, Nitti

VW. Impact of preoperative urodynamics on women undergoing pelvic organ prolapse surgery. Int Urogynecol J. 2020;31:1663–8.

28. White GR. An anatomical operation for the cure of cystocele. In: Transaction of the American Association of Obstetricians and Gynecologists for the year 1911. New York: The Maple Press; 1912. p. 323–6.

29. Shull BL, Benn SJ, Kuehl TJ. Surgical management of prolapse of the anterior vaginal segment: an analysis of support defects, operative morbidity, and anatomic outcome. Am J Obstet Gynecol. 1994;171:1429–39.

30. Young SB, Daman JJ, Bony LG. Vaginal paravaginal repair: one-year outcomes. Am J Obstet Gynecol. 2001;185:1360–7.

31. Eilber KS, Alperin M, Khan A, Wu N, Pashos CL, Clemens JQ, Anger JT. Outcomes of vaginal prolapse surgery among female medicare beneficiaries. Obstet Gynecol. 2013;122:981–7.

32. Shippey SH, Quiroz LH, Sanses TVD, Knoepp LR, Cundiff GW, Handa VL. Anatomic outcomes of abdominal sacrocolpopexy with or without paravaginal repair. Int Urogynecol J. 2010;21:279–83.

33. van Zanten F, Lenters E, Broeders IAMJ, Schraffordt Koops SE. Robot-assisted sacrocolpopexy: not only for vaginal vault suspension? An observational cohort study. Int Urogynecol J. 2021;33:377. https://doi.org/10.1007/s00192-021-04740-y.

34. Padoa A, Shiber Y, Fligelman T, Tomashev R, Tsviban A, Smorgick N. Advanced cystocele is a risk factor for surgical failure following robotic-assisted laparoscopic sacrocolpopexy. J Minim Invasive Gynecol. 2021;29:409. https://doi.org/10.1016/j.jmig.2021.11.002.

35. Kohli N, Sze EHM, Roat TW, Karram MM. Incidence of recurrent cystocele after anterior colporrhaphy with and without concomitant transvaginal needle suspension. Am J Obstet Gynecol. 1996;175:1476–82.

36. Mallipeddi PK, Steele AC, Kohli N, Karram MM. Anatomic and functional outcome of vaginal paravaginal repair in the correction of anterior vaginal wall prolapse. Int Urogynecol J. 2001;12:83–8.

37. Sand PK, Koduri S, Lobel RW, Winkler HA, Tomezsko J, Culligan PJ, Goldberg R. Prospective randomized trial of polyglactin 910 mesh to prevent recurrence of cystoceles and rectoceles. Am J Obstet Gynecol. 2001;184:1357–64.

38. Weber AM, Walters MD, Piedmonte MR, Ballard LA. Anterior colporrhaphy: a randomized trial of three surgical techniques. In: American journal of obstetrics and gynecology. Mosby Inc; 2001. p. 1299–306.

39. Gandhi S, Goldberg RP, Kwon C, Koduri S, Beaumont JL, Abramov Y, Sand PK. A prospective randomized trial using solvent dehydrated fascia lata for the prevention of recurrent anterior vaginal wall prolapse. Am J Obstet Gynecol. 2005;192:1649–54.

40. Nieminen K, Hiltunen R, Takala T, Heiskanen E, Merikari M, Niemi K, Heinonen PK. Outcomes after anterior vaginal wall repair with mesh: a randomized,

controlled trial with a 3 year follow-up. Am J Obstet Gynecol. 2010;203:235.e1–8.

41. Valenčić M, Maričić A, Oguić R, Rahelić D, Sotošek S, Grškoviċ A. Modified extensive anterior vaginal wall repair for cystocoele. Coll Antropol. 2010;34:191–4.

42. Altman D, Väyrynen T, Engh ME, Axelsen S, Falconer C. Anterior colporrhaphy versus transvaginal mesh for pelvic-organ prolapse. N Engl J Med. 2011;364:1826–36.

43. Vollebregt A, Fischer K, Gietelink D, van der Vaart C. Primary surgical repair of anterior vaginal prolapse: a randomised trial comparing anatomical and functional outcome between anterior colporrhaphy and trocar-guided transobturator anterior mesh. BJOG Int J Obstet Gynaecol. 2011;118:1518–27.

44. Song H-S, Choo GY, Jin L-H, Yoon S-M, Lee T. Transvaginal cystocele repair by purse-string technique reinforced with three simple sutures: surgical technique and results. Int Neurourol J. 2012;16:144.

45. Chen Z, Wong V, Wang A, Moore KH. Nine-year objective and subjective follow-up of the ultra-lateral anterior repair for cystocele. Int Urogynecol J Pelvic Floor Dysfunct. 2014;25:387–92.

46. Wong V, Shek KL, Goh J, Krause H, Martin A, Dietz HP. Cystocele recurrence after anterior colporrhaphy with and without mesh use. Eur J Obstet Gynecol Reprod Biol. 2014;172:131–5.

47. Balzarro M, Rubilotta E, Porcaro AB, Trabacchin N, Sarti A, Cerruto MA, Siracusano S, Artibani W. Long-term follow-up of anterior vaginal repair: a comparison among colporrhaphy, colporrhaphy with reinforcement by xenograft, and mesh. Neurourol Urodyn. 2018;37:278–83.

48. Serati M, Braga A, Cantaluppi S, Caccia G, Ghezzi F, Sorice P. Vaginal cystocele repair and hysteropexy in women with anterior and central compartment prolapse: efficacy and safety after 30 months of follow-up. Int Urogynecol J. 2018;29:831–6.

49. Arenholt LTS, Pedersen BG, Glavind K, Greisen S, Bek KM, Glavind-Kristensen M. Prospective evaluation of paravaginal defect repair with and without apical suspension: a 6-month postoperative follow-up with MRI, clinical examination, and questionnaires. Int Urogynecol J. 2019;30:1725–33.

50. Rude T, Sanford M, Cai J, Sevilla C, Ginsberg D, Rodriguez L, v. Transvaginal paravaginal native tissue anterior repair technique: initial outcomes. Urology. 2021;150:125–9.

51. le Teuff I, Labaki M, Fabbro-Peray P, Debodinance P, Jacquetin B, Marty J, Letouzey V, Eglin G, de Tayrac R. Perioperative morbi-mortality after pelvic organ prolapse surgery in a large French national database from gynecologist surgeons. J Gynecol Obstet Human Reprod. 2019;48:479–87.

52. Kwon CH, Goldberg RP, Koduri S, Sand PK, Adam R. The use of intraoperative cystoscopy in major vaginal and urogynecologic surgeries. In: American journal of obstetrics and gynecology. Mosby Inc; 2002. p. 1466–72.

Laparoscopic Paravaginal Repair

30

Nikolaos Thanatsis, Matthew L. Izett-Kay, and Arvind Vashisht

Contents

Introduction 534

Anatomy of Pelvic Floor Support 535

Pathogenesis of Anterior Vaginal Wall Defects 536

Evolution of the Procedure 537

Preoperative Assessment and Considerations 538
History 538
Clinical Examination 538
Diagnostic Tests 539
Patient Counselling 540

Description of the Procedure 541
Preoperative Steps 541
Cystoscopic Insertion of Ureteric Catheters 541
Entry into the Peritoneal Cavity 542
Evaluation of the Abdominal Cavity and Concomitant Abdominal or
Apical Prolapse Surgery 542
The Technique of Paravaginal Repair 543
Repeat Cystoscopy and Abdominal Closure 544
Postoperative Care 544

Efficacy and Safety of Laparoscopic Paravaginal Repair 545

N. Thanatsis (✉) · A. Vashisht
Urogynaecology and Pelvic Floor Unit, University College
London Hospital, London, UK
e-mail: nikolaos.thanatsis@nhs.net;
arvind.vashisht@nhs.net

M. L. Izett-Kay
Department of Urogynaecology, The John Radcliffe
Hospital, Oxford University Hospitals, Oxford, UK

Nuffield Department of Women's and Reproductive
Health, Women's Centre, Oxford University, Oxford, UK
e-mail: m.izett@nhs.net; matthew.izett@doctors.net.uk

© Springer Nature Switzerland AG 2023
F. E. Martins et al. (eds.), *Female Genitourinary and Pelvic Floor Reconstruction*,
https://doi.org/10.1007/978-3-031-19598-3_31

Alternative Surgical Approaches to Anterior Compartment Prolapse	546
Apical Suspension Procedures	546
Anterior Colporrhaphy With or Without Graft Reinforcement	546
Conclusion	548
Cross-References	549
References	549

Abstract

The surgical management of anterior compartment prolapse remains a challenge, particularly in women with isolated anterior wall descent. In clinical practice, anterior compartment prolapse usually coexists with a concomitant Level I defect. Surgical correction of descent of the latter is often enough to treat the former as well, while at the same time reducing the risk of prolapse recurrence. The traditional approach of isolated anterior colporrhaphy for midline fascial defects carries a high risk of failure, reported to vary between 30% and 88%. Hence, its role in contemporary practice has been re-evaluated. Following the description of the four anatomic sites of anterior vaginal support defects by Richardson, the technique of paravaginal repair was introduced in an effort to address lateral defects. The procedure was initially performed through a vaginal route; its open abdominal counterpart was described only in 1976, and it has grossly been replaced by the laparoscopic approach in modern clinical practice due to the well-established advantages of laparoscopy with regard to improved visualization, precise dissection and suture placement, and reduced blood loss and postoperative pain. This chapter describes the surgical technique of laparoscopic paravaginal repair as employed in our unit. As with every surgical technique, several modifications have been proposed in an effort to improve outcomes, the main being the tissue used to anchor the pubocervical fascia. Key concepts such as patient selection, preoperative assessment and counselling, safety and efficacy data, as well as alternative surgical options are also presented and remain common irrespective of the surgical technique.

Keywords

Pelvic organ prolapse · Cystocele · Urogynecology · Laparoscopy · Paravaginal defect repair · Anterior colporrhaphy · Anterior vaginal support defects

Introduction

According to the International Continence Society, anterior compartment prolapse is defined as the descent of the anterior vaginal wall, so that a point 3 cm proximal to the external urethral meatus or any anterior point proximal to this is less than 3 cm above the level of the hymen [1]. Most commonly the descending structure is the urinary bladder (cystocele); however, the bulge may as well include a prolapsed urethra (urethrocele).

Similarly to apical and posterior compartment prolapse, it is difficult to estimate accurately the exact prevalence of anterior compartment prolapse due to the large number of asymptomatic women who do not seek any medical assistance. Regardless, it is a very common condition; 40–60% of parous women are diagnosed with some degree of pelvic organ prolapse (POP) during a routine gynecological examination, and the most frequent site is the anterior vaginal wall, followed by the posterior vaginal wall and the apex [2, 3]. The Women's Health Initiative (WHI) study, the largest study utilizing an objective diagnosis of POP to date, concluded that 34.3% out of the 16,616 participants with a uterus in situ and 32.9% out of the 10,727 hysterectomized participants, aged 50–79 years, had a cystocele. The incidence of anterior compartment prolapse was higher than the prevalence of rectocele (18.6% and 18.3% in non-hysterectomized and hysterectomized women, respectively) and uterine prolapse (14.2% in non-hysterectomized participants) [4]. A population-based study by Samuelsson et al. confirmed that the anterior vaginal wall is the most common single site for prolapse in a younger population of women 20–59 years old [5]. It should be highlighted, however, that in clinical practice, isolated anterior compartment prolapse is not common, and it usually coexists with some degree of apical descent.

In common with the management of posterior and apical prolapse, the management of anterior vaginal wall descent follows an escalating individualized approach from the least to the most invasive option. Asymptomatic women and especially those with a first- or second-degree prolapse should be encouraged to manage expectantly. Should women experience symptoms, then first line interventions would include pelvic floor muscle training and vaginal support pessaries [3]. Surgery is usually reserved for symptomatic patients who fail or decline conservative management. Approximately 11–19% of women will undergo primary prolapse surgery by the age of 80–85 years old, and almost one third of them will need a repeat operation [3, 6]. Surgical interventions for anterior compartment prolapse are therefore common and may become more frequent in the future given the rising obesity rates and the aging population.

Various surgical techniques to treat anterior compartment prolapse have been employed so far. In cases of concurrent apical descent, elevation of the vaginal apex is of paramount importance, as it may suffice to correct some degree of anterior compartment prolapse as well. The traditional surgical approach for isolated anterior compartment prolapse has been vaginal; anterior colporrhaphy is still the most popular procedure, especially in patients with central (midline) defects of the pubocervical fascia of the anterior vaginal wall. Nevertheless, success rate of isolated native tissue anterior colporrhaphy is poor and varies between 30% and 88%, which generates a need for innovation and alternative approaches [3, 7]. In an effort to improve clinical outcomes, a number of tissue-augmenting grafts have been used over the last few decades. Polypropylene mesh has been the most widely trialled, as either a custom inlay or branded device. Yet high-quality prospective randomized studies have shown minimal advantages with respect to efficacy, and mesh-augmented vaginal colporrhaphy is associated with a high risk of mesh-related adverse events, which has been estimated at 12% over 2 years [8]. At present a number of national and international guidelines advise against the use of transvaginal mesh in anterior vaginal compartment surgery [9, 10].

Moving beyond the conventional approach of anterior colporrhaphy and following the description of the four anatomic sites of anterior vaginal support defects in the pubocervical fascia by Richardson et al., the paravaginal repair gained popularity in an attempt to address lateral defects [11]. Although the vaginal route was first described more than 100 years ago, the abdominal paravaginal repair was introduced only in 1976, and, initially, it was performed through a laparotomy [11–13]. More recently the advent of minimal access surgery (MAS) in gynecology has inspired new approaches in pelvic floor disorders with many abdominal procedures being undertaken laparoscopically or even robotically. The ultimate aim of any prolapse surgery is to restore anatomy, reduce symptoms of prolapse, and potentially improve bladder, bowel, and sexual function, while minimizing morbidity and providing long-term efficacy. As technology has advanced, laparoscopic surgery has been established as the gold-standard route for abdominal prolapse procedures due to the improved visualization of pelvic organs, reduced blood loss and postoperative pain, shorter hospitalization, and faster return to daily activities.

This chapter serves to review the surgical technique of laparoscopic paravaginal repair. We will consider aspects of patient selection, preoperative assessment, and counselling, and we will present the latest safety and efficacy data.

Anatomy of Pelvic Floor Support

Knowledge of the structures that support the anterior vaginal wall is essential in order to understand the pathogenesis of anterior wall defects and, subsequently, appreciate which patients would benefit from a paravaginal repair. The well-illustrated reports by DeLancey based on cadaver dissections suggest three integrated levels of anatomical vaginal support. In particular:

- The upper portion of the vagina (cephalic 2–3 cm of the vagina) is supported by the uterosacral and cardinal ligaments through their attachments to the cervix and the upper vagina (Level I).
- The middle portion of the vagina is supported along its length laterally by the fascial attachment of the pubocervical fascia to the arcus tendineus fascia pelvis (ATFP) (Level II).
- The distal portion of the vagina (caudal 2–3 cm above the hymenal ring) is supported by the perineal body and the levator ani muscle complex (Level III) [14].

The following structures play a crucial role within the complex system that is responsible for the normal anatomical support of the anterior vaginal wall:

- Apical support: Apex (Level I) constitutes a key factor in orchestrating anterior vaginal wall support. Initially proposed by DeLancey, this has been since confirmed by numerous other studies, which established a significant association between apical and anterior compartment prolapse. It has been estimated that, in 53–77% of women, anterior compartment descent is attributable to loss of apical support [3, 15, 16].
- Fascial support: Stretched between the right and the left AFTP, the pubocervical fascia serves as a base upon which the bladder rests and, thus, prevents its descent.
- Muscular support: The levator ani muscle complex (pubococcygeus, puborectalis, and iliococcygeus) plays a crucial role in anterior vaginal compartment support. A magnetic resonance imaging (MRI) study by Berger et al. found that levator ani defects can be found in about 70% of patients with POP [17].

Failure of the support structures at each one of the three levels will cause descent of a different vaginal compartment. Isolated loss of Level I support will lead to apical prolapse and likely an enterocele formation, whereas isolated failure of the Level II suspensory structures will result in the development of an anterior compartment prolapse. With regard to Level III support, its failure may contribute to both an anterior and a posterior vaginal wall prolapse and an enlarged genital hiatus and/or a perineal descent [14]. A combined failure of the suspensory structures at Level I and II is common in clinical practice, and it will present with different degrees of apical, anterior, and posterior wall prolapse [14].

Pathogenesis of Anterior Vaginal Wall Defects

Contemporary theories suggest that the pathogenesis of anterior compartment prolapse is attributable to specific defects in the abovementioned suspensory structures rather than a gradual thinning/stretching process of the anterior vaginal wall and its supportive structures [11, 12, 18]. Richardson focused on Level II failure and described four different anatomic sites of anterior vaginal support defects [11, 13]:

- Midline (central) defects. These are vertical defects at the central portion of the triangular plate of the endopelvic fascia, which may extend from the base of the fascial triangle up to the apex. The former defects will present as a large anterior vaginal wall bulge with intact lateral vaginal fornices, whereas the latter defects may cause loss of urethral support and, possibly, urethral hypermobility and stress urinary incontinence.
- Paravaginal (lateral) defects, which are unilateral or bilateral detachments of the triangular plate of pubocervical fascia from the ATFP. Such defects may result in descent of the lateral vaginal sulcus and may present clinically as a mild to moderate anterior wall bulge

(cystourethrocele) along with loss of support of the urethrovesical junction and stress urinary incontinence. Paravaginal defects are common; they are noticed in 88.7% (on the right side) and 87.3% (on the left side) of women undergoing retropubic procedures for cystourethrocele and stress urinary incontinence [18]. A recent study of 3D analysis of anterior compartment prolapse using MRI confirmed the presence of significant paravaginal defects in women with anterior wall prolapse compared to control women without any prolapse, highlighting the importance of lateral vaginal attachment in pelvic support [19].

- Transverse defects, which are generated from the detachment of the base of the triangular plate of fascia from the cervix. Such defects will present as a large anterior wall bulge near the cervix (high cystocele); however, the support of the urethrovesical junction will not be influenced, and therefore there is theoretically a lower risk of stress urinary incontinence.
- Distal defects, which are detachments of the apex of the triangular plate of fascia from the pubic symphysis. Women with distal defects will usually present with a small anterior wall bulge near the introitus and possibly with urethral hypermobility and stress urinary incontinence.

Clinical assessment and detection of the structures that are implicated in anterior compartment descent are a key component for surgical planning; however, distinguishing between the abovementioned defects can be challenging, and there is little in the way of quality data to suggest it has a meaningful impact on symptomatic outcome after surgical repair. The clinical examination described by Richardson et al. and Shull for identification of paravaginal defects has not been validated, and studies have shown inconsistent findings [11, 20–22]. The former two defects have gained the most attention, as they are more common, and they account for the majority of cases of anterior wall prolapse. This chapter focuses on the lateral (paravaginal) defects,

which can be addressed by the technique of laparoscopic paravaginal repair.

Evolution of the Procedure

The technique of paravaginal repair was first introduced by White in 1909. Following his cadaver research on the structures that support the anterior vaginal wall, he described a vaginal procedure to treat anterior compartment prolapse. Instead of plicating the fibromuscular tissue of the anterior vaginal wall, as would happen during an anterior colporrhaphy, White proposed attaching the vaginal sulci to a fascia overlying the pelvic muscles, which he named as "white line of pelvic fascia" [12]. This approach, however, did not gain much attention until Richardson et al. and Shull and Baden published their work many decades later.

Based on the description of the four sites of anterior vaginal support defects, Richardson suggested an abdominal retropubic procedure to treat patients with lateral defects of the anterior vaginal wall and stress urinary incontinence in 1976. His approach included elevation of the superior lateral aspect of the vaginal sulci with a finger in the vagina and placement of four to six sutures between the ATFP and the pubocervical fascia on each side [11]. The outcomes of a cohort of 233 patients undergoing the procedure were published in 1981; it was found that more than 95% of them had functionally satisfactory results at 2- to 8-year follow-up [13]. Richardson's technique of abdominal paravaginal repair conceptually confirmed and set the foundation for what would ultimately become the approach used in contemporary practice.

There have been subsequent adaptations of White's vaginal and Richardson's abdominal paravaginal repair techniques [23, 24]. The weakness of ATFP and the associated risk of prolapse recurrence were recognized by Shull and Baden. Therefore, they advocated anchoring some of the middle pubocervical fascia-ATFP sutures through the Cooper's ligament as a safety mechanism but only after they had been tied and immobilized at the ATFP or the obturator fascia [23]. The use of Cooper's ligaments to anchor the pubocervical fascia instead of the potentially atrophic ATFP or the obturator internus muscle has been suggested by other authors as well [25]. Shull et al. also proposed utilizing the iliococcygeus fascia, the strong insertion point of the iliococcygeus muscle to the ATFP near the ischial spines, as a robust anchor point [26]. More recently, a modified technique of graft-augmented paravaginal repair with the use of a polypropylene mesh was described; however, it was not popularized, possibly due to the wider moves to avoid surgical applications of nonabsorbable materials [27]. Most of the variations of the procedure within the literature are related to the tissue used to suspend the pubocervical fascia; others include changes in the dissection technique, suture placement, the intra- and postoperative use of a Foley catheter, as well as differences in the number and material of sutures used.

Advances in MAS over the last decade of the twentieth century led to the introduction of laparoscopic surgery in modern urogynecological practice. Soon afterward, laparoscopy became the gold-standard route for almost every abdominal procedure. Vancaillie and Schuessler performed the first laparoscopic retropubic procedure in 1991. This was a modification of the Marshall-Marchetti-Kranz bladder neck suspension technique, during which the vagina was suspended on either side of the bladder neck to the pubic symphysis using two nonabsorbable sutures. In 1993, Liu and Paek described the first laparoscopic Burch colposuspension. Subsequently, the laparoscopic approach of paravaginal defect repair was also employed, grossly based on the concept of its open counterpart as outlined by Richardson et al. [28, 29]. The procedure gained popularity over the last 20 years. Although published prospective data are limited, the advantages of laparoscopy with respect to improved visualization within the restricted space of Retzius, sharper delineation of anatomy, more precise dissection, less blood loss, and less postoperative pain have resulted in laparoscopic approaches superseding the open alternatives, which are now less commonly performed in clinical practice.

Preoperative Assessment and Considerations

A thorough history, assessment of all pelvic floor symptoms and their impact on the quality of life, and a comprehensive clinical examination constitute crucial steps of the preoperative work-up.

History

The majority of POP coexists with some degree of urinary incontinence, voiding, defecatory, or sexual dysfunction. A study using the validated Pelvic Floor Distress Inventory (PFDI) questionnaire found that 96% of women with POP report some lower urinary tract symptoms (LUTS), with 72% of the study population complaining of mixed urinary incontinence (MUI) (57% among them had stress predominant MUI, and 43% had urge predominant MUI), 24% complaining of urinary urgency, and less than 1% reporting stress urinary incontinence (SUI) [30].

Such questionnaires are useful to identify the extent of patient reported symptoms and their adverse impact on quality of life. Prolapse itself, while not life threatening, may significantly impair a woman's day-to-day life. It is important that the nuances of this are appreciated by the surgeon; it is the extent of symptoms bother that should chiefly drive patient's management plan rather than the extent of the prolapse per se. In addition, it is important that the surgeon takes a holistic view of the patient, considering any medical or surgical comorbidities that may impact efficacy and morbidity of any proposed intervention.

Clinical Examination

Central to assessment is a comprehensive vaginal examination. Most women do not have isolated anterior wall prolapse but rather involving more than one vaginal compartment. It is imperative that a concurrent apical descent is identified preoperatively and addressed accordingly at the time of surgery with an apical suspension procedure. This may be often enough to correct anterior compartment prolapse without the need for a paravaginal repair; additionally, a concomitant apical and anterior prolapse surgery decreases the risk of anterior wall prolapse recurrence compared to anterior prolapse surgery alone [16].

Standardized methods of examination should be adopted such as the Baden-Walker or Pelvic Organ Prolapse Quantification (POP-Q) systems. Their utility is the obligation of the examiner to specifically document the extent of prolapse in all vaginal sites. They also serve as a useful numerical representation of the extent of prolapse that can be interpreted by fellow specialists as well as a defined objective measure useful in determining changes following surgery.

A modification of the standard vaginal examination for the diagnosis of paravaginal defects in women with anterior compartment prolapse has been described by Richardson et al. and modified by Shull [11, 20]. With the patient in supine position, a Sims speculum is used to retract the posterior vaginal wall. Subsequently, an open sponge forceps is applied to each vaginal corner, imitating the ATFP-pubocervical fascia attachment, followed by elevation of the vagina up to the level of the inferior margin of the symphysis pubis. Then, the patient performs a Valsalva maneuver:

- If no anterior wall prolapse is observed (i.e., the previously noticed anterior wall prolapse is eliminated by the paravaginal support provided by the open sponge forceps), then the defect is classified as paravaginal.
- If the anterior wall prolapse persists despite the paravaginal support and descends between the two open sponge forceps, then the defect is classified as midline.

Nevertheless, the prognostic value of the above-described technique has been questioned. It has a poor intra- and inter-examiner reliability, as shown by Whiteside et al. [31]. In addition, a comparison of the preoperative clinical examination results to the perioperative findings during vaginal surgery for anterior compartment prolapse has led to inconsistent findings; Barber et al. found a good sensitivity and negative predictive value of the clinical assessment (94% and 91%, respectively) with a poor specificity and positive predictive value (50% and 57%, respectively) [21]. On the other hand, a prospective study by Segal et al. demonstrated a very poor sensitivity (23.5%) with a specificity of 80% [22]. It could be argued that this form of assessment is a poor predictor for the actual presence of paravaginal defects and its findings should be interpreted with caution; in the authors' opinion, the real-world clinical utility of such an assessment is limited.

Diagnostic Tests

The next step of the preoperative work-up may include further diagnostic tests. The limited prognostic value of the above-described examination technique along with the recent advances in technology has led to the use of various imaging modalities such as pelvic floor ultrasound and MRI to assess the normal anatomical support structures and identify possible paravaginal defects. It has been proposed that such defects alter the axial image of vagina, so that the normal H-shape of the vagina (due to the pubocervical-ATFP attachment) will be "sagging" on the side of defect. Nevertheless, published data are not particularly encouraging; pelvic floor ultrasound does not seem to correlate well with clinical assessment for the detection of paravaginal defects [32]. In addition, the "missing H configuration" sign on ultrasound and MRI imaging can be observed in 37–84% of women with prolapse but also in 4–32% of women without any prolapse [32–34].

More recently, a stress 3D MRI technique was introduced. It allows direct visualization and measurement of the distance between the lateral margin of the vagina and the normal location of the ATFP at maximal Valsalva. Hence, anterior vaginal wall deformation can be objectively assessed, and defects can be classified as paravaginal, in case of separation of the vaginal wall from the ATFP, or midline, when the vaginal wall is wider [19]. Although such studies are promising, stress 3D MRI has mainly been used in a research context. The clinical utility of the abovementioned imaging modalities has to date been limited. It is likely, however, that with the technology advances and the need for objective preoperative assessment, they will become an integral part of daily practice in the future. At present their routine use is not supported by international guidance [3].

Other diagnostic tests that may be needed, especially in women with concurrent lower urinary tract or defecatory symptoms, include urodynamic studies (UDS) and dynamic MRI or MRI defecatory proctogram. The role of UDS and their prognostic value in predicting postoperative lower urinary tract symptoms (LUTS) such as "occult SUI" has been questioned [35]. Invasive UDS have not been shown to be clinically superior to an office evaluation prior to surgical management of stress urinary incontinence [36]. As a result, there is no consensus about the role of invasive bladder function testing prior to a paravaginal repair or any POP surgery, and clinical practice varies significantly [9]. Nevertheless, it is important that voiding parameters are adequately assessed prior to a laparoscopic paravaginal repair especially in patients who report voiding symptoms; if preoperative invasive UDS are not deemed necessary, then a noninvasive free uroflowmetry and assessment of postvoid residual of urine should be considered.

In conclusion, the aim of diagnostic tests is to objectively quantify anatomical and functional status that may correlate to symptom status; however, their routine use has been questioned, and there remain questions over their clinical utility in many cases. Therefore, such investigations should be performed on an individual basis depending on symptoms and findings from clinical assessment and according to local resource availability. Their role in decision-making should be approached with caution.

Patient Counselling

Women with prolapse may present with a wide range of symptoms, and this, combined with the complexities of decision-making due to the myriad of surgical options, makes a shared decision-making process imperative. Patient decision aids can be used to promote informed choices, although they lack any published evidence base with respect to utility and satisfaction. In addition, a multidisciplinary team-based approach should be encouraged; patients will benefit from the expertise of different specialties, such as urogynecologists, gastroenterologists, colorectal surgeons, urologists, nurse specialists, and pelvic floor physiotherapists, contributing to the ultimate objective management plan.

Preoperative counselling regarding surgical options therefore needs to happen within the context of the aforementioned factors. Women needing surgery for isolated anterior compartment prolapse in our unit are generally offered a laparoscopic paravaginal repair or a native tissue anterior colporrhaphy. If a concurrent apical descent is identified during the preoperative work-up, then patients are offered an apical suspension procedure with the provision of a laparoscopic paravaginal repair or a native tissue anterior colporrhaphy, if there is any residual prolapse once the apical descent has been corrected. All the available surgical techniques for apical suspension with or without uterine conservation through an abdominal laparoscopic approach are discussed with the patients (e.g., laparoscopic mesh or suture sacrohysteropexy, laparoscopic uterosacral hysteropexy, laparoscopic hysterectomy with uterosacral ligament plication and vaginal vault suspension, laparoscopic mesh sacrocolpopexy in cases of post-hysterectomy vault prolapse, suture vault suspension, and autologous fascial repair). Patients also have the options of a vaginal approach (e.g., vaginal hysterectomy and McCall culdoplasty, uterosacral ligament suspension or sacrospinous ligament fixation, vaginal sacrospinous hysteropexy, Manchester-Fothergill procedure). Women who no longer wish to be sexually active are also given the option of an obliterative procedure (partial or total colpocleisis), although this approach is mainly reserved for frail patients, who cannot undergo a lengthy operation. The risks and benefits of the surgical procedures are explained in detail.

A paravaginal repair should be considered when the preoperative assessment has raised the suspicion of lateral defects of the anterior vaginal wall. This would be the absolute indication for the procedure; if the anterior wall prolapse is thought to be due a midline defect, then another surgical technique may need to be followed. Other factors that may influence the decision- making are both patient-related and surgeon-related. Patients' symptoms, age, fertility wishes, surgical history, medical comorbidities, the need for a concomitant abdominal surgery, as well as women's own personal view on the kind of procedure should be taken into account. From a surgeon's perspective, appropriate training and surgical skills may influence their decision-making. A contemporary pelvic floor surgical team should endeavor to offer the full range of procedures and treatments to patients presenting with pelvic floor disorders.

A discussion about the expectations from surgery constitutes an important part of preoperative counselling. The surgical goals should be agreed in advance and they should be realistic. It is likely that physicians and patients have different perceptions of surgical success. Although the former may prioritize the anatomical success, i.e., the postoperative restoration of anatomy, the latter may consider symptomatic relief and improvement of quality of life as more important parameters. Due to the different definitions of success, success rates of POP surgery in general vary from 19.2% to 97.2% with the absence of vaginal bulge correlating the best with postoperative improvement from patient's perspective [37]. Hence, outcome measures should include both objective anatomic (POP-Q) and subjective criteria with the aid of quality of life questionnaires.

Having considered their surgical options and following a case review at the multidisciplinary meeting, patients return for a surgical consent as well as consenting to inclusion within a national database, which is an NHS England requirement.

Description of the Procedure

In the current section, we will describe the technique of laparoscopic paravaginal repair as employed in our unit. The procedure is grossly based on the steps of its open abdominal counterpart. Nevertheless, multiple modifications have been incorporated throughout the years as a result of a growing experience; some of them lack a solid evidence-based background and may as well alter in the future.

Preoperative Steps

The basic preoperative steps include:

- Antimicrobial prophylaxis with administration of a single dose of a broad-spectrum intravenous antibiotic immediately prior to operating. The most common regimes are gentamicin and co-amoxiclav. The choice of the appropriate antibiotic is based on the local hospital guidelines and, of course, should be in line with the patient's allergy history.
- Appropriate positioning of the patient on the operating table, once intubated, and general anesthesia has been administered. The patient should be placed supine without any table tilt, and legs should be placed in a dorsal lithotomy position at an angle of 30° at the hips.
- Insertion of anti-embolism stockings and use of intermittent pneumatic compression as a thromboprophylactic strategy in accordance with the local hospital guidelines.
- Skin preparation with application of a chlorhexidine or Betadine solution to the operative field for cutaneous disinfection followed by appropriate draping.
- Insertion of a size 14 Foley catheter into the bladder. The catheter is then left on free drainage. The choice of the catheter's size is a compromise to provide relative patient comfort postoperatively while allowing free drainage of urine following the manipulation of the bladder during the procedure.

Cystoscopic Insertion of Ureteric Catheters

Prior to laparoscopic entry into the peritoneal cavity, we routinely perform a cystoscopic insertion of ureteric Pollack catheters. This practice is not informed by any literature evidence; however, our experience suggests that it is a simple, safe, and quick intervention, which only adds minimally into the total operating time and enables easy visualization of the ureters throughout the procedure and prompt identification of any possible ureteric injury or kinking [38]. This step promotes not only surgical ease but also patient's safety, especially in complex cases where intraoperative difficulties are anticipated.

Entry into the Peritoneal Cavity

We usually utilize the classic closed technique with the use of a Veress needle to obtain a pneumoperitoneum. Once we confirm that the patient is placed supine with no tilt, a small umbilical wound incision is made. Then, the abdominal wall below the umbilicus is lifted for counter traction, and a Veress needle is inserted in the midline in sagittal plane at a 45° angle to the spine. In this position the tip of the needle is directed toward the sacral promontory, anterior to the sacrum but inferior to the bifurcation of the aorta and proximal aspects of the vena cava. Once the two characteristic clicks of passing through the layers are felt and heard, then we stop advancing the needle. The correct intraperitoneal positioning of the needle is confirmed by routine safety checks (aspiration test, saline drop test, and low initial insufflation pressure).

The abdomen is then insufflated with CO_2; the maximum insufflation pressure is set at 20 mmHg for insertion of the main trocar and then reduced to a maximum of 15 mmHg throughout the procedure. The main 11 mm trocar is placed through the subumbilical skin incision. Subsequently, the laparoscope is inserted, and the visceral organs are examined to exclude any injury. Once the patient has been placed in a Trendelenburg's position, the auxiliary ports are inserted under direct vision to avoid injury to viscera or vessels. Due attention should be given to the inferior epigastric vessels, which should be identified and avoided during the insertion of the lateral ports. We utilize two lateral 5 mm ports, which are inserted 8 cm lateral to the midline at the level of the umbilicus, and one 11 mm suprapubic port. The latter is inserted

after the space of Retzius has first been dissected and allows for passage of sutures into the abdominal cavity.

We employ a different entry technique in the following cases:

- If the patient is very thin, then we choose the open Hasson entry technique to reduce the risk of vascular injury. During the open Hasson entry, first a small umbilical incision is made, followed by dissection of the subcutaneous fat tissue and incision of the rectus sheath and the peritoneum under direct vision. The laparoscopic port without its trocar is inserted into the peritoneal cavity, which is then insufflated.
- If the patient has a history of previous abdominal surgeries and carries a high risk of bowel or omental adhesions around the umbilicus, then we employ a Palmer's point entry (3 cm below the costal margin in the left midclavicular line). Prior to inserting the Veress needle, a palpation should be performed to identify the spleen, and a nasogastric tube should be inserted to minimize the risk of perforating an inflated stomach. Following insufflation of the peritoneal cavity, a 5 mm port is inserted at the Palmer's point. Should the inspection of the peritoneal cavity with the use of a 5 mm laparoscope do not reveal any evidence of periumbilical adhesions, then the main subumbilical port can be inserted under direct vision. Sometimes, the port at the Palmer's point can be utilized further during the procedure without the need for inserting an extra left lateral port.

Evaluation of the Abdominal Cavity and Concomitant Abdominal or Apical Prolapse Surgery

The next step includes a thorough evaluation of the abdominal cavity and assessment of the abdominopelvic organs. This is performed in a systematic way, and any possible abnormality that may compromise the surgical field (e.g., adhesions) is dealt with simultaneously.

If any additional surgery is needed (such as hysterectomy or adnexal procedure), this is routinely performed prior to the paravaginal repair. This also applies to concomitant apical prolapse surgery. As discussed previously, isolated anterior compartment prolapse is not common. If the preoperative work-up has identified a concurrent apical descent, this should be addressed prior to the paravaginal repair. The most common apical suspension procedures in our unit are a laparoscopic mesh or suture sacrohysteropexy, a laparoscopic hysterectomy and vaginal vault suspension, and a laparoscopic mesh sacrocolpopexy in women with post-hysterectomy vault prolapse. In such cases, the initial steps of the abovementioned procedures (i.e., the hysterectomy, the preparation of the sacral promontory and uterosacral ligaments, or the dissection of uterovesical and rectovaginal spaces in case of a mesh sacrohysteropexy) are carried out before we proceed to the dissection of the space of Retzius. The final steps, such as sacral promontory fixation in vault elevation surgery, are performed after the paravaginal repair; otherwise, the latter becomes technically more challenging due to the ensuing reduced vaginal mobility on the (now well-supported) vaginal apex and proximal vaginal walls.

The Technique of Paravaginal Repair

In accordance with its open counterpart, the first step of a laparoscopic paravaginal repair is the installation of 200–300 mL of normal saline within the urinary bladder in order to delineate it and identify the superior border of the bladder dome.

We then proceed with entrance into the space of Retzius, which is achieved by a transperitoneal approach using an energy source. The markers for entry into the retropubic space are the obliterated median umbilical ligaments, which are incised 2–4 cm cephalad to the bladder dome. Identification of the loose areolar tissue at the point of incision confirms the appropriate plane of dissection. With regard to the energy source used, we routinely use an ultrasonic scalpel with bipolar; alternative options include a monopolar hook diathermy or monopolar scissors on 60 W coagulation. All the above options allow bloodless tissue

dissection. The space of Retzius is then dissected toward the Cooper's ligaments utilizing a combination of blunt dissection and the energy source. Once the retropubic space has been entered and the pubic rami visualized, the bladder is then drained to prevent any inadvertent damage. Due attention during the dissection is given to the urethra, the dorsal vein of the clitoris in the midline, and the obturator neurovascular bundle and external iliac vessels laterally. The dissection is continued until the retropubic anatomy is clearly visualized. At completion, the pubic symphysis should be exposed, and the bladder neck should be identified in the midline as well as the ATFP and the Cooper's ligaments laterally along the pelvic sidewall.

The paravaginal space is identified by medial dissection of the bladder with the use of a pledget on a grasper with a marker thread. The dissection can be aided further by inserting a finger within the vagina to elevate the anterior vaginal wall and the pubocervical fascia up to the ATFP. The finger should later be replaced by a rectal probe or large Hagar during suturing to prevent any sharp injury.

The attachment of the pubocervical fascia and anterior vaginal wall to the ATFP is assessed from the pubic symphysis to the ischial spine on both sides to identify any paravaginal defects. These can usually be recognized as detachments of the pubocervical fascia from the pelvic sidewall at the ATFP and may be unilateral or bilateral.

Following anatomical exposure and identification of the paravaginal defects, suture repair is undertaken. Several variations have been described regarding not only suture material and gauge but also the tissue used to anchor the pubocervical fascia. The traditional approach of paravaginal repair utilized the ATFP as an anchor point. However, previous publications as early as 1989 questioned this practice, as the ATFP is a weak and, hence, not an optimal support structure [23]. This has also been confirmed by our experience. We therefore advocate utilizing Cooper's ligaments to anchor the pubocervical fascia, as done in Burch colposuspension. As far as the choice of suture material is concerned, both delayed absorbable and permanent options have been used over the years. Currently, there is a growing trend toward the use of dissolvable surgical materials in an effort to avoid complications such as extrusion into other organs. This is grossly based on the theory that it is not the strength of the sutures per se but the development of fibrosis around the approximated tissues that provides long-term surgical efficacy. Significant differences also exist in the number of sutures placed, which can vary between two and six per side [25, 39, 40].

In our practice, we usually use a permanent suture No. 0 Ethibond®; the first suture is placed at the level of the urethrovesical junction and includes a double bite of the fibromuscular tissue of the pubocervical fascia, which is then anchored with one bite to the ipsilateral Cooper's ligament. Extra care should be taken to avoid the vaginal mucosa, while at the same time the suture should be placed deeply through the vaginal fascia so as to include a volume of pubocervical fascial tissue. The suture is then tied with limited only tension using an extracorporeal surgical knot. In our experience, a distance of about 2 cm between the fascia and the ligament is sufficient, and further tension should be avoided. The tighter the suture is, the more anterior anchoring will be achieved, but also the greater the risk of postoperative voiding difficulties will be. It is important that voiding parameters are assessed preoperatively and patients will be counselled appropriately regarding postoperative voiding problems, including preparing particularly high-risk patients for the possibility of requiring prolonged postoperative catheterization. The same process is repeated on the contralateral side, as the sutures should be alternated on the left and right to maintain vaginal symmetry. Following this pattern, two to four sutures are usually placed on each side sequentially along the paravaginal defects from the urethrovesical junction toward the ischial spine.

Repeat Cystoscopy and Abdominal Closure

Once the paravaginal defect has been repaired, we routinely perform a cystoscopy using a 120° cystoscope to exclude any unintentional suture penetration and confirm ureteric patency. Should any suture be seen within the bladder, this should be removed and, if needed, replaced. With regard to ureteric patency, this is usually assessed with the ease that the Pollack catheters are removed and, chiefly, with the subsequent visualization of a urine jet from ureteric orifices.

After the cystoscopy has been performed, the next step includes assessment of hemostasis in the space of Retzius. Again, the absolute direct vision afforded by the laparoscope, particularly with advances in technology and visual enhancement, allows precise dissection, identification of the vasculature and, hence, hemostasis. Unless blood loss during dissection has been above average, we do not routinely leave a surgical drain in the retropubic space. The anterior peritoneal defect over the space of Retzius is then closed using continuous or interrupted absorbable sutures to minimize the risk of bowel adhesions, which could make future surgery in this space more technically challenging.

The final step of the procedure is closure of any sheath defects of more than 10 mm to prevent postoperative hernia formation. We use an absorbable No. 1 Vicryl® suture utilizing an Endoclose® device for the rectus sheath at the suprapubic port, and, once the excess gas has been expelled, we close the sheath at the umbilical port with a No. 1 Vicryl® suture on a "J" needle under direct vision. Finally, the skin is closed using No. 2/0 Monocryl®, No. 2/0 Vicryl Rapide® or surgical glue.

Postoperative Care

Besides a single dose of a broad-spectrum intravenous antibiotic given prior to the start of the procedure, there is no routine need for further antimicrobial prophylaxis. Of course, this is variable, and it should be altered if there are the appropriate clinical indications. As per the local hospital guidelines, postoperative thromboprophylaxis with low-molecular-weight heparin is administered.

Usually, the indwelling urethral catheter inserted at the start of the procedure is removed on the second postoperative day, once the patient can mobilize comfortably. Nevertheless, this is individualized and varies from overnight to

7 days. Following removal of the Foley catheter, a trial of void protocol is performed as per the local hospital guidelines. The patient voids twice, the voided volume is measured, and the postvoid residual of urine is assessed with a bladder scan after the patient voids for the second time. Should the residual of urine be less than 150 ml, then the patient does not usually need re-catheterization. Otherwise, they are discharged home with an indwelling catheter and attend the outpatient clinic for a further trial of void in 1 week.

Efficacy and Safety of Laparoscopic Paravaginal Repair

Literature data on paravaginal repair are quite scarce, and most of the efficacy and safety outcomes come from the open abdominal or the vaginal procedure. In general, success rates of paravaginal repair for anterior compartment prolapse vary between 75% and 97% for the open abdominal approach and 67% and 100% for the vaginal approach [24, 41–43].

The lack of a standardized surgical technique of laparoscopic paravaginal repair (i.e., attachment of pubocervical fascia to the ATFP versus Cooper's ligaments, differences in the number of sutures, addition of a graft) as well as the heterogeneity between the reported subjective and objective definitions of surgical success makes it even harder to draw any robust conclusions. In addition, no randomized controlled trials have directly compared outcomes of isolated laparoscopic versus vaginal or open paravaginal repair.

Behnia-Willison et al. conducted one of the few studies to assess the efficacy and morbidity of laparoscopic bilateral paravaginal repair for anterior compartment prolapse [25]. A cohort of 212 women was followed up prospectively over an average period of 14.2 months. According to the author's description of their surgical technique, each suture was initially passed from the lateral pubocervical fascia and subepithelial vagina to the ATFP and obturator internus muscle and then to the Cooper's ligaments. Four to six permanent sutures No. 0 Ethibond® were usually placed on each side; a concurrent apical descent or

posterior fascia defect was treated with a simultaneous laparoscopic uterosacral hysteropexy or colpopexy and laparoscopic supralevator repair, respectively. The objective cure rate following laparoscopic paravaginal repair (defined as a POP-Q grade <2 during follow-up) was 76.4% (95% CI 70.7–82.1%). Nine patients (4.2%) sustained a major complication (bladder injury, blood loss greater than 1 l, bowel injury, and unintended laparotomy), whereas 61 patients had a minor complication, the most common being prolonged (more than 7 days) urinary retention requiring catheterization (10.4%).

Another prospective study of 223 patients undergoing a laparoscopic paravaginal repair along with a concurrent apical suspension procedure, if needed, found that 26% of women developed a recurrent anterior compartment prolapse beyond the hymen and 28.3% of women had a repeat procedure for anterior compartment prolapse at a median follow-up of 5.2 years (range: 1–12 years) [40]. The authors utilized a similar surgical technique to Behnia-Willison et al. The most common major complication was cystotomy (3.1%) followed by blood loss more than 500 ml (2.2%), while one patient had a bowel injury, ureteric ligation, and unintended laparotomy. Minor complications such as urinary tract infections and need for suprapubic catheter for more than 7 days were more frequent (6.7% and 5.3%, respectively).

A recent smaller prospective study by Duraisamy et al. assessed 44 women following a laparoscopic or robotic paravaginal repair during a period of 12 months [39]. The authors approximated the pubocervical fascia to the Cooper's ligaments without incorporating the ATFP in their sutures. Objective success rate (defined as prolapse stage 0 or 1 according to the Baden-Walker system) was 97.7%, and subjective symptomatic improvement rate was also high (93.2% at 12-month follow-up). No major intra- or postoperative complication was noted in this cohort. According to a publication by Banerjee and Noe, their modified technique of laparoscopic paravaginal repair utilizing a combination of sutures and mesh had an anatomical success rate of 96% at a mean 30 month follow-up; no cases of mesh extrusion were noted, and, again, the most common complications were urinary tract infection (10.5%), prolonged catheter use (5.8%), and bladder injury (1.1%) [27].

In summary, the major complications that have been reported following a laparoscopic paravaginal repair include damage to the bladder and other organs (e.g., bowel), intraoperative bleeding and retropubic hematoma, neuropathy, vaginal abscess, ureteric/urethral obstruction, fistula, and emergency laparotomy. Other possible complications are urinary tract infection, need for prolonged use of catheter, voiding difficulty, de novo detrusor overactivity, and chronic pain. Prompt identification of a urinary tract injury is essential in order to reduce long-term morbidity. Bladder injuries are usually repaired laparoscopically in one or two layers using a dissolvable suture, with a period of catheterization and a postoperative cystogram at the time of catheter removal subjectively determined dependent on the size of defect and repair.

Alternative Surgical Approaches to Anterior Compartment Prolapse

In addition to the paravaginal repair, an anterior compartment prolapse can be addressed by other surgical approaches, such as (i) apical suspension procedures, (ii) native tissue anterior colporrhaphy, and (iii) anterior colporrhaphy with graft reinforcement.

Apical Suspension Procedures

As previously outlined, the role of apex (Level I) in pelvic floor support is crucial and, in clinical practice, anterior wall prolapse coexists very often with apical descent. It has been estimated that around 60% of patients with stage 2 or greater cystocele have a clinically significant apical prolapse (defined as point C-3 or greater). Furthermore, the higher the grade of cystocele is, the more likely is that the patient will have a clinically significant concurrent apical prolapse [44]. Rooney et al. found that should the anterior vaginal wall be at least 2 cm below the hymen,

then 80% of women will have a vaginal apex to at least 2 cm above the hymen, and 55% of women will have a vaginal apex more than 2 cm below the hymen [16].

An apical suspension procedure may suffice to address anterior wall descent without the need for a concomitant anterior wall surgery. Even if an anterior compartment surgery is required, correction of apical descent is critical to reduce prolapse recurrence. In a national cohort study of more than 2700 women, Eilber et al. found that isolated anterior wall surgery carries a significantly higher 10-year reoperation rate compared to a combined anterior and apical procedure (20.2% vs. 11.6%; $P < 0.01$) [45]. Thus, it is essential for surgical planning that an apical descent is identified preoperatively and addressed accordingly at the time of anterior prolapse repair.

Anterior Colporrhaphy With or Without Graft Reinforcement

Since its first description in literature in 1886, native tissue anterior colporrhaphy popularized and has been established as the most common procedure for anterior compartment prolapse. It is defined as the repair of the fibromuscular tissue of the anterior vaginal wall; this may include the midline plication of the entire pubocervical fascia, or it may be limited to a specific site in case of a specific site defect.

In summary, the surgical steps of native tissue anterior colporrhaphy are as follows:

- A longitudinal midline incision is made at the anterior vaginal wall starting from the urethrovesical junction up to the most distal aspect of the prolapse.
- The vaginal epithelium is mobilized and separated from the pubocervical fascia.
- The pubocervical fascia is plicated.
- The excess vaginal skin is removed and the vaginal epithelium is sutured [3].

If a graft is used at the time of an anterior colporrhaphy, then a more extended dissection between the vaginal epithelium and the fibromuscular tissue is required; the graft is then placed within the vesicovaginal space and sutured in place or fixated to its attachment points (e.g., ATFP, obturator membrane/muscles, or sacrospinous ligament), occasionally with the aid of a mesh kit. Unfortunately, despite its popularity the published success rates for native tissue anterior colporrhaphy are varied; literature data report conflicting results with success rates fluctuating between 30% and 88% [3, 7, 8]. Although these inconsistent findings may be due the different criteria and definitions of success used in the studies, it is now well-established that isolated anterior colporrhaphy carries a high risk of recurrence. Undoubtedly, this is partially attributable to a missed concurrent apical descent, which has not been identified at preoperative assessment and, hence, not addressed at the time of surgery [45]. Again, this highlights the significance of attention to the apex in preventing prolapse recurrence. Additionally, it is likely that the paucity of residual robust fascial tissue also contributes to the high published failure rates.

The high failure rates of isolated native tissue anterior colporrhaphy generated the need for innovation and led to the use of grafts. These are either synthetic or biological in nature. The former can be made from materials such as polypropylene, polyglactin, prolene, and polyethylene, and they may be dissolvable or permanent, whereas the latter can be autografts (rectus fascia, tensor fascia lata), allografts (fascia lata and acellular dermal matrix from human cadavers), or xenografts (porcine or bovine acellular extracts from dermis, pericardium, and submucosa of intestines).

A 2015 Cochrane meta-analysis compared safety and efficacy of native tissue anterior colporrhaphy versus anterior colporrhaphy using biological grafts and dissolvable or non-dissolvable meshes [46]. The authors concluded that biological grafts and absorbable meshes offer only minimal benefits compared to isolated anterior colporrhaphy. Compared to biological grafts, native tissue repair has a slightly higher risk of prolapse recurrence (risk ratio [RR] 1.32, 95% CI 1.06–1.65), but no significant difference in repeat prolapse surgery (RR 1.02,

95% CI 0.53–1.97). Compared to absorbable meshes, native tissue repair has a slightly increased risk of prolapse recurrence (RR 1.50, 95% CI 1.09–2.06), but no difference in reoperation rates was found (RR 2.13, 95% CI 0.42–10.82). With regard to permanent polypropylene mesh, the meta-analysis demonstrated a lower risk of recurrence of anterior wall prolapse (RR 3.01, 95% CI 2.52–3.60), surgery for recurrent anterior wall prolapse (RR 2.03, 95% CI 1.15–3.58), and awareness of POP (RR 1.77, 95% CI 1.37–2.28) compared to native tissue repair; however, the nonabsorbable mesh carries higher risk of de novo SUI, bladder injury, repeat surgery for prolapse, stress urinary incontinence, and mesh exposure (composite outcome) as well as longer operating time and greater blood loss. The rates of mesh erosion and reoperation for mesh extrusion reach 11.5% and 7.0%, respectively [46]. Subsequent to this meta-analysis, the PROSPECT study showed that mesh- or graft-augmented vaginal repair does not lead to improved subjective outcomes with regard to effectiveness and quality of life. In addition, 12% of women (cumulative number) exposed to a synthetic mesh suffer a mesh complication over 2 years [8]. Due to the increased mesh-related morbidity and questionable advantages, most guidelines do not recommend mesh-augmented anterior colporrhaphy for the surgical treatment of anterior compartment prolapse [9, 10]. More recently, the abovementioned safety concerns resulted in governmental bodies prohibiting the sale of vaginal mesh kits for POP surgery (US Food and Drug Administration 2019) and effectively pausing any vaginal mesh surgery (United Kingdom 2018) [47, 48].

In some units, anterior colporrhaphy may be combined with a concomitant Kelly-Kennedy bladder neck plication in women with concurrent SUI. It should be noted, however, that anterior colporrhaphy is not a widely recognized effective treatment of SUI; 38% of patients undergoing anterior colporrhaphy for SUI experience persistent or recurrent incontinence symptoms at medium- and long-term follow-up, according to a Cochrane meta-analysis [49]. The authors therefore do not advocate anterior repair of cystocele with or without bladder neck support with the sole objective of improving SUI.

Conclusion

The surgical management of anterior compartment prolapse remains a clinical challenge, particularly in the less common scenario of isolated anterior wall descent. In clinical practice anterior compartment prolapse is usually accompanied by a simultaneous Level I defect. Irrespective of the approach, surgical correction of the latter can be enough to treat the former as well, but it is also important to balance the risk of repeat or further surgery.

For situations where apical correction is not needed or does not resolve the presence of a symptomatic cystocele, the examination of anatomical defects of the anterior wall may guide surgical decision-making and potentially lead to contemplation of laparoscopic paravaginal repair. Richardson's cadaver studies and description of the different anatomic sites of anterior vaginal support defects offered an insight into the pathogenesis of anterior compartment prolapse; we can now identify which support structures have failed for a patient and should, subsequently, be addressed. While the prognostic value of the examination technique described to distinguish between midline and lateral anterior wall defects has been questioned, a thorough clinical examination along with a detailed history remains the cornerstones of management.

It is now well-established that the conventional approach of isolated anterior colporrhaphy for midline fascial defects carries a high risk of failure, which varies between 30% and 88%. As such, its role in contemporary practice must be re-evaluated. Moving beyond the classic technique of anterior colporrhaphy, the paravaginal repair was described to focus on the lateral defects of the pubocervical fascia. Initially undertaken through a vaginal and then open abdominal route, the procedure gained popularity over the last 50 years. The advances in MAS led to the establishment of laparoscopy as the gold-standard route to perform a paravaginal repair, and it has now replaced the open abdominal approach in contemporary clinical practice.

Undoubtedly, the laparoscopic paravaginal repair requires a surgeon competent in minimally invasive surgery as well as urogynecology. However, in addition to the well-recognized advantages of laparoscopy with regard to improved visualization, precise dissection and suture placement, reduced blood loss, and postoperative pain, it offers other procedure-specific advantages, including the ability to undertake higher apical concurrent repair, and avoidance of vaginal scar tissue and allows for correction of site specific paravaginal defects.

As with every surgical technique, several modifications have been proposed in an effort to improve outcomes, the main being the tissue used to anchor the pubocervical fascia. Whereas the initial description of the technique utilized the ATFP, clinical experience has confirmed its weak nature. Many authors, including us, favor the use of Cooper's ligaments, as done in Burch colposuspension, as they provide a robust support structure.

Data on the efficacy of laparoscopic paravaginal repair are very sparse with no direct comparisons between the procedure and its open abdominal or vaginal counterparts. Anatomical success rates in literature vary between 74% and 98%; however, the heterogeneity between the surgical techniques used does not allow us to draw solid conclusions. Further large prospective studies are needed to provide clarification and guide clinical management; ideally, these would be prospective comparative studies against the routinely performed anterior colporrhaphy. This would however require clarity over the optimal approach with respect to different surgical routes (laparoscopic versus open abdominal versus vaginal) but also the specific surgical techniques of the laparoscopic paravaginal repair, so that a clear standardized approach can be utilized for high-quality prospective studies. This lack of uniformity of procedure continues to beset difficulties for absolute objective comparison for most pelvic floor repair procedures.

Cross-References

► Etiology, Diagnosis, and Management of Pelvic Organ Prolapse: Overview
► Laparoscopic Burch
► Minimally Invasive Approaches in the Treatment of Pelvic Organ Prolapse: Laparoscopic and Robotic
► Retropubic Suspension Operations for Stress Urinary Incontinence
► Transvaginal Repair of Cystocele

References

1. Abrams P, Cardozo L, Fall M, Griffiths D, Rosier P, Ulmsten U, et al. The standardisation of terminology of lower urinary tract function: report from the Standardisation Sub-committee of the International Continence Society. Neurourol Urodyn. 2002;21(2): 167–78.
2. Handa VL, Garrett E, Hendrix S, Gold E, Robbins J. Progression and remission of pelvic organ prolapse: a longitudinal study of menopausal women. Am J Obstet Gynecol. 2004;190(1):27–32.
3. Abrams P, Cardozo L, Wagg A, Wein A, editors. Incontinence. 6th ed. Bristol: ICI-ICS (International Continence Society); 2017.
4. Hendrix SL, Clark A, Nygaard I, Aragaki A, Barnabei V, McTiernan A. Pelvic organ prolapse in the Women's Health Initiative: gravity and gravidity. Am J Obstet Gynecol. 2002;186(6):1160–6.
5. Samuelsson EC, Victor FT, Tibblin G, Svärdsudd KF. Signs of genital prolapse in a Swedish population of women 20 to 59 years of age and possible related factors. Am J Obstet Gynecol. 1999;180(2 Pt 1): 299–305.
6. Wu JM, Matthews CA, Conover MM, Pate V, Jonsson FM. Lifetime risk of stress urinary incontinence or pelvic organ prolapse surgery. Obstet Gynecol. 2014;123(6):1201–6.
7. Weber AM, Walters MD, Piedmonte MR, Ballard LA. Anterior colporrhaphy: a randomized trial of three surgical techniques. Am J Obstet Gynecol. 2001;185(6):1299–304. Discussion 304–6
8. Glazener CMA, Breeman S, Elders A, Hemming C, Cooper KG, Freeman RM, et al. Mesh, graft, or standard repair for women having primary transvaginal anterior or posterior compartment prolapse surgery: two parallel-group, multicentre, randomised, controlled trials (PROSPECT). Lancet. 2017;389(10067): 381–92.
9. National Institute for Health and Care Excellence: Clinical Guidelines. Urinary incontinence and pelvic organ prolapse in women: management. London:

National Institute for Health and Care Excellence (UK); 2019. Copyright © NICE 2019
10. Chapple CR, Cruz F, Deffieux X, Milani AL, Arlandis S, Artibani W, et al. Consensus statement of the European Urology Association and the European Urogynaecological Association on the use of implanted materials for treating pelvic organ prolapse and stress urinary incontinence. Eur Urol. 2017;72(3): 424–31.
11. Richardson AC, Lyon JB, Williams NL. A new look at pelvic relaxation. Am J Obstet Gynecol. 1976;126(5): 568–73.
12. White GR. Cystocele – a radical cure by suturing lateral sulci of the vagina to the white line of pelvic fascia. 1909. Int Urogynecol J Pelvic Floor Dysfunct. 1997;8(5):288–92.
13. Richardson AC, Edmonds PB, Williams NL. Treatment of stress urinary incontinence due to paravaginal fascial defect. Obstet Gynecol. 1981;57 (3):357–62.
14. DeLancey JO. Anatomic aspects of vaginal eversion after hysterectomy. Am J Obstet Gynecol. 1992;166 (6 Pt 1):1717–24. Discussion 24–8
15. Lee MH, Kim BH, Na ED, Jang JH, Kim HC. Correlation between the posterior vaginal wall and apex in pelvic organ prolapse. Obstet Gynecol Sci. 2018;61(4):505–8.
16. Rooney K, Kenton K, Mueller ER, FitzGerald MP, Brubaker L. Advanced anterior vaginal wall prolapse is highly correlated with apical prolapse. Am J Obstet Gynecol. 2006;195(6):1837–40.
17. Berger MB, Morgan DM, DeLancey JO. Levator ani defect scores and pelvic organ prolapse: is there a threshold effect? Int Urogynecol J. 2014;25(10): 1375–9.
18. Delancey JO. Fascial and muscular abnormalities in women with urethral hypermobility and anterior vaginal wall prolapse. Am J Obstet Gynecol. 2002;187(1): 93–8.
19. Larson KA, Luo J, Guire KE, Chen L, Ashton-Miller JA, DeLancey JO. 3D analysis of cystoceles using magnetic resonance imaging assessing midline, paravaginal, and apical defects. Int Urogynecol J. 2012;23 (3):285–93.
20. Shull BL. Clinical evaluation of women with pelvic support defects. Clin Obstet Gynecol. 1993;36(4):939–51.
21. Barber MD, Cundiff GW, Weidner AC, Coates KW, Bump RC, Addison WA. Accuracy of clinical assessment of paravaginal defects in women with anterior vaginal wall prolapse. Am J Obstet Gynecol. 1999;181 (1):87–90.
22. Segal JL, Vassallo BJ, Kleeman SD, Silva WA, Karram MM. Paravaginal defects: prevalence and accuracy of preoperative detection. Int Urogynecol J Pelvic Floor Dysfunct. 2004;15(6):378–83. Discussion 83
23. Shull BL, Baden WF. A six-year experience with paravaginal defect repair for stress urinary incontinence.

Am J Obstet Gynecol. 1989;160(6):1432–9. Discussion 1439–40

24. Shull BL, Benn SJ, Kuehl TJ. Surgical management of prolapse of the anterior vaginal segment: an analysis of support defects, operative morbidity, and anatomic outcome. Am J Obstet Gynecol. 1994;171(6):1429–36. Discussion 1436–9

25. Behnia-Willison F, Seman EI, Cook JR, O'Shea RT, Keirse MJ. Laparoscopic paravaginal repair of anterior compartment prolapse. J Minim Invasive Gynecol. 2007;14(4):475–80.

26. Shull BL, Capen CV, Riggs MW, Kuehl TJ. Bilateral attachment of the vaginal cuff to iliococcygeus fascia: an effective method of cuff suspension. Am J Obstet Gynecol. 1993;168(6 Pt 1):1669–74. Discussion 1674–7

27. Banerjee C, Noé KG. Endoscopic cystocele surgery: lateral repair with combined suture/mesh technique. J Endourol. 2010;24(10):1565–9. Discussion 9

28. Ross JW. Techniques of laparoscopic repair of total vault eversion after hysterectomy. J Am Assoc Gynecol Laparosc. 1997;4(2):173–83.

29. Ostrzenski A. Genuine stress urinary incontinence in women. New laparoscopic paravaginal reconstruction. J Reprod Med. 1998;43(6):477–82.

30. Lowder JL, Frankman EA, Ghetti C, Burrows LJ, Krohn MA, Moalli P, et al. Lower urinary tract symptoms in women with pelvic organ prolapse. Int Urogynecol J. 2010;21(6):665–72.

31. Whiteside JL, Barber MD, Paraiso MF, Hugney CM, Walters MD. Clinical evaluation of anterior vaginal wall support defects: interexaminer and intraexaminer reliability. Am J Obstet Gynecol. 2004;191(1):100–4.

32. Dietz HP, Pang S, Korda A, Benness C. Paravaginal defects: a comparison of clinical examination and 2D/3D ultrasound imaging. Aust N Z J Obstet Gynaecol. 2005;45(3):187–90.

33. Athanasiou S, Chaliha C, Toozs-Hobson P, Salvatore S, Khullar V, Cardozo L. Direct imaging of the pelvic floor muscles using two-dimensional ultrasound: a comparison of women with urogenital prolapse versus controls. BJOG. 2007;114(7):882–8.

34. Tillack AA, Joe BN, Yeh BM, Jun SL, Kornak J, Zhao S, et al. Vaginal shape at resting pelvic MRI: predictor of pelvic floor weakness? Clin Imaging. 2015;39(2):285–8.

35. Visco AG, Brubaker L, Nygaard I, Richter HE, Cundiff G, Fine P, et al. The role of preoperative urodynamic testing in stress-continent women undergoing sacrocolpopexy: the Colpopexy and Urinary Reduction Efforts (CARE) randomized surgical trial. Int Urogynecol J Pelvic Floor Dysfunct. 2008;19(5):607–14.

36. Nager CW, Brubaker L, Litman HJ, Zyczynski HM, Varner RE, Amundsen C, et al. A randomized trial of

urodynamic testing before stress-incontinence surgery. N Engl J Med. 2012;366(21):1987–97.

37. Barber MD, Brubaker L, Nygaard I, Wheeler TL 2nd, Schaffer J, Chen Z, et al. Defining success after surgery for pelvic organ prolapse. Obstet Gynecol. 2009;114(3):600–9.

38. Merritt AJ, Crosbie EJ, Charova J, Achiampong J, Zommere I, Winter-Roach B, et al. Prophylactic pre-operative bilateral ureteric catheters for major gynaecological surgery. Arch Gynecol Obstet. 2013;288(5):1061–6.

39. Duraisamy KY, Balasubramaniam D, Kakollu A, Chinnusamy P, Periyasamy K. A prospective study of minimally invasive paravaginal repair of cystocele and associated pelvic floor defects: our experience. J Obstet Gynaecol India. 2019;69(1):82–8.

40. Bedford ND, Seman EI, O'Shea RT, Keirse MJ. Long-term outcomes of laparoscopic repair of cystocoele. Aust N Z J Obstet Gynaecol. 2015;55(6):588–92.

41. Bruce RG, El-Galley RE, Galloway NT. Paravaginal defect repair in the treatment of female stress urinary incontinence and cystocele. Urology. 1999;54(4):647–51.

42. Scotti RJ, Garely AD, Greston WM, Flora RF, Olson TR. Paravaginal repair of lateral vaginal wall defects by fixation to the ischial periosteum and obturator membrane. Am J Obstet Gynecol. 1998;179(6 Pt 1):1436–45.

43. Young SB, Daman JJ, Bony LG. Vaginal paravaginal repair: one-year outcomes. Am J Obstet Gynecol. 2001;185(6):1360–6. Discussion 1366–7

44. Elliott CS, Yeh J, Comiter CV, Chen B, Sokol ER. The predictive value of a cystocele for concomitant vaginal apical prolapse. J Urol. 2013;189(1):200–3.

45. Eilber KS, Alperin M, Khan A, Wu N, Pashos CL, Clemens JQ, et al. Outcomes of vaginal prolapse surgery among female Medicare beneficiaries: the role of apical support. Obstet Gynecol. 2013;122(5):981–7.

46. Maher C, Feiner B, Baessler K, Christmann-Schmid C, Haya N, Brown J. Surgery for women with anterior compartment prolapse. Cochrane Database Syst Rev. 2016;11(11):CD004014.

47. Urogynecologic Surgical Mesh Implants. U.S. Food and Drug Administration. 2019. www.fda.gov/MedicalDevices/ProductsandMedicalProcedures/ImplantsandProsthetics/UroGynSurgicalMesh/default.htm. Accessed 18 Apr 2019.

48. Mesh letter to acute trust CEOs and medical directors. July 2018. https://i.emlfiles4.com/cmpdoc/9/7/2/8/1/1/files/47633_mesh-letter-to-acute-ceos-and-mds.pdf. Accessed 12 August 2019

49. Glazener CM, Cooper K, Mashayekhi A. Anterior vaginal repair for urinary incontinence in women. Cochrane Database Syst Rev. 2017;7(7):CD001755.

Minimally Invasive Approaches in the Treatment of Pelvic Organ Prolapse: Laparoscopic and Robotic

31

Justina Tam, Dena E. Moskowitz, Katherine A. Amin, and Una J. Lee

Contents

Introduction/Background	553
Open Abdominal Prolapse Surgery Versus Minimally Invasive Prolapse Surgery	553
Laparoscopic Versus Robotic Surgery for Pelvic Organ Prolapse	553
Prevalence of Laparoscopic and Robotic Surgeries for Pelvic Organ Prolapse	554
Trends in the Usage of Minimally Invasive Surgery	554
Laparoscopic and Robotic Procedures for Pelvic Organ Prolapse	555
Patient Selection	555
Minimally Invasive Prolapse Surgery in Older Women	555
Cost-Effectiveness	556
Availability, Access, and Efficiency of Robotic Versus Laparoscopic Surgery	556

J. Tam
Section of Urology and Renal Transplantation, Virginia Mason Franciscan Health, Seattle, WA, USA

Urogynecology, Stony Brook Medicine, Stony Brook, NY, USA
e-mail: justina.tam@stonybrookmedicine.edu

D. E. Moskowitz
Department of Urology, University of California Irvine, Irvine, CA, USA

K. A. Amin
Department of Urology, University of Miami Miller School of Medicine, Miami, FL, USA
e-mail: katherine.amin@med.miami.edu

U. J. Lee (✉)
Section of Urology and Renal Transplantation, Virginia Mason Franciscan Health, Seattle, WA, USA
e-mail: Una.Lee@virginiamason.org

© Springer Nature Switzerland AG 2023
F. E. Martins et al. (eds.), *Female Genitourinary and Pelvic Floor Reconstruction*,
https://doi.org/10.1007/978-3-031-19598-3_32

Ergonomics for Surgeons	556
ERAS Protocols for Minimally Invasive Approaches for Pelvic Organ Prolapse Surgery	556
Laparoscopic and Robotic Paravaginal Repair for Anterior Vaginal Wall Prolapse	557
Laparoscopic and Robotic Uterosacral Ligament Suspension	559
Laparoscopic Pectopexy	561
Laparoscopic and Robotic Supracervical Hysterectomy and Total Hysterectomy	562
Trends and Future Directions in Utilization of Laparoscopy and Robotics in POP Surgery	564
Conclusions	565
References	566

Abstract

Pelvic organ prolapse is a common disease process in women as the descent of the pelvic organs is a multifactorial process. Approximately 40% of women have some degree of prolapse on exam. However, when examined by degree of bother, the prevalence of symptomatic prolapse is less – ranging from 3% to 6% of parous women. For women who are symptomatic and bothered by prolapse, the treatment options are conservative management, pelvic floor physical therapy, pessary use, and surgery. Surgery for prolapse has remained an important option for women to restore pelvic anatomy, improve prolapse symptoms, and maintain quality of life. With the advancement of minimally invasive surgical techniques, the morbidity of pelvic organ prolapse surgery has decreased. Minimally invasive surgery (MIS) approaches have revolutionized and advanced contemporary pelvic organ prolapse surgery. Minimally invasive prolapse surgeries, both laparoscopic and robotic-assisted laparoscopic, have benefited women by facilitating apical support through smaller incisions and with improved visualization. With the advancement of minimally invasive surgical techniques, the morbidity of pelvic organ prolapse surgery has decreased.

Surgery for prolapse has remained an important option for women to restore pelvic anatomy, improve prolapse symptoms, and maintain quality of life.

Keywords

Minimally invasive prolapse surgery · Paravaginal repair · Pectopexy · Hysterectomy · Uterosacral ligament suspension

Abbreviations

ASC	Open abdominal sacrocolpopexy
ATFP	Arcus tendineus fascia pelvis
ERAS	Enhanced recovery after surgery
FDA	Food and Drug Administration
LSC	Laparoscopic sacrocolpopexy
MIS	Minimally invasive surgery
POP	Pelvic organ prolapse
POP-Q	POP quantification
RSC	Robotic-assisted sacrocolpopexy
SDD	Same-day discharge
TLH-USLS	Total laparoscopic hysterectomy
TVH-USLS	USLS and total vaginal hysterectomy
US	United States
USLS	Uterosacral ligament suspension

Introduction/Background

Minimally invasive surgery (MIS) approaches have revolutionized and advanced contemporary pelvic organ prolapse surgery. Minimally invasive prolapse surgeries, both laparoscopic and robotic-assisted laparoscopic, have benefited women by facilitating apical support through smaller incisions and with improved visualization. Compared to open abdominal surgery, this approach and the associated technology are associated with less morbidity and shorter recovery times. The improved postoperative recovery and excellent anatomic outcomes associated with minimally invasive prolapse surgery makes it an attractive and feasible option for women with symptomatic prolapse. Additionally, MIS approaches are well suited to the pelvic anatomy and repair of prolapsed vaginal tissues, due to the ability to visualize and safely access these tissue planes using laparoscopy.

Pelvic organ prolapse (POP) is a common disease process in women as the descent of the pelvic organs is a multifactorial process. Approximately 40% of women have some degree of prolapse on exam. However, when examined by degree of bother, the prevalence of symptomatic prolapse is less – ranging from 3% to 6% of parous women. For women who are symptomatic and bothered by prolapse, the treatment options are conservative management, pelvic floor physical therapy, pessary use, and surgery. Surgery for prolapse has remained an important option for women to restore pelvic anatomy, improve prolapse symptoms, and maintain quality of life. The objective of this chapter is to discuss and review data on minimally invasive approaches to POP surgery.

Open Abdominal Prolapse Surgery Versus Minimally Invasive Prolapse Surgery

Open abdominal sacrocolpopexy (ASC) represents the "gold-standard" treatment for apical POP as it restores and supports the vaginal apex which is fundamental to a durable repair. While associated with excellent anatomic outcomes and performed since the 1950s, ASC is also associated with increased length of stay, need for more analgesia, and higher cost compared with transvaginal procedures. MIS is defined as surgery through incisions and approaches less morbid than an open abdominal incision. The two most common MIS approaches include laparoscopy and robotic-assisted laparoscopy. Laparoscopic sacrocolpopexy (LSC) was introduced in the 1990s, and robotic-assisted sacrocolpopexy (RSC) gained popularity in the mid-late 2000s as the da Vinci robotic surgical systems subsequently became more available and widespread.

Laparoscopic Versus Robotic Surgery for Pelvic Organ Prolapse

ASC has long been considered the gold standard for POP surgery. However, this operation can be associated with significant operative time, blood loss, and a difficult postoperative recovery. As such, minimally invasive strategies have become increasingly popular in order to provide surgical correction of POP. Indeed, the minimally invasive approach, whether robotic or laparoscopic, has been shown to be associated with decreased blood transfusion, shorter hospitalization, decreased 30-day complications, and decreased hospital readmission as compared to ASC [1].

Given the absence of an open abdominal incision, LSC and RSC are associated with shorter postoperative recovery while maintaining equivalent rates of cure. The laparoscopic approach and robotic-assisted laparoscopic approach for prolapse repair and reconstruction are appropriate and excellent applications of these technologies. LSC and RSC achieve and emulate the surgical principles of open ASC, with the advantages of laparoscopic tissue handling and hemostasis as well as the increased degrees of freedom of the robotic surgical instrumentation. The minimally invasive approach, whether robotic or laparoscopic, has been shown to be associated with decreased blood transfusion, shorter hospitalization, decreased 30-day complications, and decreased hospital readmission as compared to ASC [1]. The advantages of LSC and RSC compared to open ASC have made minimally invasive prolapse surgery the contemporary gold standard for over 20 years.

Prevalence of Laparoscopic and Robotic Surgeries for Pelvic Organ Prolapse

Based on the POP quantification (POP-Q) system, there are four stages of prolapse severity, with stages III–IV representing the most advanced/severe cases of POP [2]. Most data regarding the distribution of pelvic organ support in women are based on gynecologic clinic populations, and prevalence is often believed to be underestimated. The frequency of high-grade POP (stage $\geq$III) was estimated to be 0.6–2.6% based on three observational studies [3–5]. Advanced POP is often due to multi-compartment defects and is generally treated with surgery, especially if the patient has failed conservative treatment and has bothersome symptoms.

In one review of laparoscopic surgery for treatment of advanced uterine prolapse, vaginally assisted LSC was the most common procedure performed for the treatment of severe uterovaginal prolapse, followed by LSC combined with laparoscopic supracervical hysterectomy [6]. Uterine-preserving techniques include laparoscopic inguinal ligament suspension with mesh, combined trachelectomy with laparoscopic uterosacral ligament suspension (USLS), and vaginally assisted laparoscopic uterine sacropexy. All procedures resulted in an anatomical cure rate of >90%, within a range of 91.4–100% and no significant differences reported based on procedure type. Nezhat et al. described the first case series of 15 patients who underwent LSC which was published in 1994 [7] and demonstrated an objective cure rate of 100%.

The first use of the da Vinci Surgical System (Intuitive Surgical, Inc.) for RSC was described in 2004 by Di Marco et al. [8]. Robotic-assisted surgery received US Food and Drug Administration (FDA) approval in 2005 and since then has gained popularity and is used in US hospital systems and worldwide. Case series of LSC and RSC have been published to report learning curves, complications, and outcomes. A large compilation of data evaluated LSC, RSC, and ASC [9]. A total of 11 patient series utilizing LSC were reviewed demonstrating an objective cure of 91% and satisfaction rate of 92% with 26-month follow-up. Six patient series utilizing RSC were reviewed with a mean follow-up of 28 months, mean operative time of 202 min, objective cure rate of 94%, and subjective success rate 95%. Three studies were reviewed comparing LSC and ASC, but all were short-term, with follow-up either less than 12 months or unreported.

Trends in the Usage of Minimally Invasive Surgery

A nationwide analysis of minimally invasive hysterectomy procedures performed between 2007 and 2012 reported robotic utilization in 45% of all US cases [10]. This high utilization of robotic surgery is multifactorial including surgeon training and preference, patient choice, commercial marketing, and reimbursement for robotic procedures. In Europe and the United Kingdom, the implementation of robotic-assisted gynecologic surgery is steadily increasing in line with a global trend toward increased minimally invasive surgery [11]. Data from a population-based Swedish registry for benign hysterectomy between 2009 and 2015 reported 7.5% of hysterectomies were performed with robotic assistance [12]. In comparison, the majority of robotic-assisted procedures in 2016 in Australia represent 31% of gynecological procedures, with hysterectomy for endometrial cancer being the most common [13].

A study using the data from the American College of Surgeons National Surgical Quality Improvement Program database from 2010 to 2015 compared patients who underwent USLS and total vaginal hysterectomy (TVH-USLS) and USLS and total laparoscopic hysterectomy (TLH-USLS) [14]. TVH-USLS was performed in 87.4%, whereas TLH-USLS was performed in 12.6% of patients from this cohort. Patients who underwent TLH-USLS were younger, more likely to smoke, more likely to be African American, and had lower rates of hypertension compared to patients who underwent TVH-USLS. Both vaginal approaches and laparoscopic/robotic approaches remain excellent surgical options for women with prolapse. The optimal surgical approach is multifactorial. Having increased in the last two decades, MIS surgery for prolapse is certainly one of the gold standards for addressing apical support.

Laparoscopic and Robotic Procedures for Pelvic Organ Prolapse

The management of POP may be approached through either vaginal or abdominal approaches. However, apical and/or multi-compartment prolapse can be successfully treated through an abdominal approach [15] such as through a laparotomy or laparoscopic and robotic techniques. While laparoscopic techniques have been described as having less blood loss, less pain, and shorter hospital stays compared to laparotomy, this approach also has a steeper learning curve and longer operative times compared to a robotic approach possibly owing to the limited degrees of freedom of movement and two-dimensional vision during laparoscopic procedures [16]. Access to laparoscopic surgery is more favorable than robotic surgery, so in lower resource areas or smaller hospitals, this may be a significant factor. The advantages of the robotic approach, despite the higher costs for its use [16], have resulted in increased adoption of this technique compared to laparoscopic approaches. The ergonomics of robotic surgery for the surgeon are also more favorable. Surgeon access to robotic surgery could also be a contributing factor as not all hospitals are equipped with robotic surgical systems. However, published data suggest that robotic and laparoscopic sacrocolpopexy are equally effective in the management of POP [17]. Additionally, the introduction of robotic techniques has resulted in a shift away from vaginal approaches of apical prolapse repair such as uterosacral ligament suspension, toward abdominal approaches such as sacrocolpopexy [18].

Patient Selection

For any patient with POP desiring surgery, multiple factors should be considered in choosing the surgical approach. These include degree of prolapse, presence of the uterus, prior surgeries, and medical comorbidities. Although vaginal surgery is generally considered to be the least invasive, a recent case series demonstrated good outcomes for patients older than 75 who underwent LSC [19]. In general, the authors recommend laparoscopic (with or without robotic assistance) sacrocolpopexy over vaginal native tissue repair in patients with recurrent prolapse and those with high-grade ($\geq$ stage III) prolapse, in patients who are not candidates for colpocleisis.

Considering these basic principles, however, some patients are not good candidates for laparoscopic surgery regardless. These include patients with restrictive lung disease, who may not tolerate prolonged insufflation, particularly in a steep Trendelenburg position. In addition, patients who have had multiple prior abdominal surgeries may require an extensive lysis of adhesions, making a minimally invasive approach less desirable than a vaginal approach. Obesity should not be considered a contraindication; however, surgeons should be aware of the possibilities of higher rates of conversion to open surgery, infection, longer operative duration, and increased blood loss in obese women, even with open surgery [20].

Minimally Invasive Prolapse Surgery in Older Women

The feasibility of robotic technologies for older patients is being debated, with the long operating time and steep Trendelenburg positioning of highest concern. Sanci et al. looked at the safety and effectiveness of RSC in patients with symptomatic apical pelvic organ prolapse who were over 65 years old [21]. The open abdominal technique was used on 44 patients, whereas the robotic approach was used on 30 others, with mean ages of 68 and 69 years, respectively. The authors concluded that anatomical outcomes and adverse events in elderly patients receiving open vs RSC are similar.

Cost-Effectiveness

Several studies have compared outcomes of RSC to LSC, but only two of these review the costs of the procedure. In one randomized study, the robotic group had higher initial hospital costs that remained higher over 6 weeks. However, when the cost of purchasing the robot was taken out of the comparison, costs were similar [22]. In the other randomized trial, the robotic approach was more costly than the laparoscopic approach, and this extra expense was driven entirely by the difference in operating room costs [23]. In this trial, the operating time was longer for robotic as compared to laparoscopic, while the operating times were the same in study by Anger et al. Therefore, one could conclude that in a hospital where the robot is already present, and with a surgeon who is more adept at robotic surgery than laparoscopic surgery, costs are similar.

Availability, Access, and Efficiency of Robotic Versus Laparoscopic Surgery

Over time, the use of minimally invasive sacrocolpopexy has increased, while use of ASC has decreased [24]. As mentioned previously, the robotic and laparoscopic approaches have both been associated with excellent patient outcomes, though with possibly increased cost using the robotic approach. Because much of this cost is incurred in the purchase of the surgical robot, many surgeons may not have access to this technology.

Another significant consideration is the operative time for each of the approaches. The two randomized studies comparing laparoscopic versus robotic showed differing results. Paraiso et al. found that the total operating time for the sacrocolpopexy-only (subtracting out time to dock/undock the robot) was lower for laparoscopic than robotic [23]. Anger et al. demonstrated equivalence in the sacrocolpopexy-only time, with a longer total operating time for the robotic approach [22]. We suspect the differences in these findings are at least in part due to the learning curve associated with robotic surgery, as the first study was published in 2011 and the second in 2014.

Ergonomics for Surgeons

The surgical robot improves surgeon comfort as the console is highly customizable to accommodate surgeons of different sizes. One study examined the ergonomics of laparoscopic versus robotic sacrocolpopexy [25]. The authors used pre- and postoperative surveys to evaluate discomfort after each type of surgery. They found that surgeons performing RSC had less neck, shoulder, and back discomfort than those who did the surgery laparoscopically. The ergonomics of surgery is an important factor to take into account to promote workplace safety, prevention of surgeon injuries and strain, and the longevity of surgeons, who will perform many procedures over their careers.

ERAS Protocols for Minimally Invasive Approaches for Pelvic Organ Prolapse Surgery

Enhanced recovery after surgery (ERAS) protocols, first developed for colorectal surgery, utilize a multidisciplinary approach to enhance recovery and improve perioperative outcomes [26, 27]. The elements included in ERAS protocols include patient education, preoperative optimization, avoidance of preoperative fasting, carbohydrate loading, intraoperative euvolemia, opioid sparing anesthesia, prevention of postoperative pain and nausea, and early mobilization [26, 28]. While the benefits of implementing ERAS guidelines have been demonstrated in surgical procedures that generally have had longer inpatient hospitalizations, its benefits are less clear in pelvic organ prolapse procedures that may only require 24-h observation [29]. However, implementation of an ERAS protocol in a urogynecology population has been shown to result in an increase in same-day discharge from 25.9% to 91.7% in one study [29], suggesting that even in POP procedures with a short length of stay, ERAS protocols can further decrease length of stay. Another study from the same authors demonstrated that the decrease in length of stay and reduction in opioid usage do not appear to be impacted by age [30].

Furthermore, a systematic literature review evaluated ERAS components used in ASC, and, based on their findings, suggested a best practice guideline describing recommended ERAS elements for ASC, such as preoperative counseling and education, optimizing the use of non-opioid analgesics, early mobilization, and early oral diet (Table 1) [31]. ERAS protocols have demonstrated promising results in surgical outcomes, highlighting that even in POP surgeries which are increasingly performed as outpatient procedures [32], ERAS protocols may further improve postoperative recovery [31].

Laparoscopic and Robotic Paravaginal Repair for Anterior Vaginal Wall Prolapse

Anterior vaginal wall prolapse is difficult to treat as it may result from lateral defects with detachment of the fascia from the arcus tendineus fascia pelvis (ATFP), apical defects from fascial detachment from the apex of the anterior vaginal wall, and/or centrally which results from midline defects in the pubocervical fascia [33]. Central defects are often repaired with plication of the pubocervical fascia, often through a vaginal

approach. A "paravaginal defect" refers to a defect in the lateral support of the anterior vaginal tissue, caused by detachment of the pubocervical fascia from the ATFP [34, 35]. Repair of this defect has been described as suturing of the vagina to lateral surface of ATFP or tendinous arch of pelvis [34, 35]. It is believed that the majority of anterior vaginal wall prolapse is caused by paravaginal defects; however, identification of paravaginal defects is challenging. Site-specific repair of this defect has been described through a minimally invasive approach with 60–89% success rates [36–39] and has been reported to be more anatomic, to reduce the risk of vaginal shortening compared to conventional colporrhaphy, and can be performed at the same time as other laparoscopic abdominal procedures such as hysterectomy, vault suspension, or sacrocolpopexy [40]. One small study suggests that vaginal and abdominal approaches to paravaginal defect repair had better short-term outcomes than laparoscopic approaches [41]. Some authors have advocated for performing concurrent paravaginal repair at the time of sacrocolpopexy if anterior wall prolapse is present after appropriate mesh tensioning, as over-tensioning of mesh to treat concurrent apical and anterior wall prolapse may result in apical pain or dyspareunia [40].

The technique for a laparoscopic paravaginal repair involves placement of trocars at the midline for the camera and to the left and right lower quadrants of the abdomen. Additional trocars may be placed to aid in laparoscopic suturing. The space of Retzius is then accessed via a transperitoneal or preperitoneal approach. With a Foley catheter in place, the urethra and bladder neck are identified. The bladder and urethra are mobilized, and paravaginal tissues are identified and elevated. After bladder mobilization, the arcus tendineus fasciae pelvis is identified along the obturator internus muscle running from the pubic ramus to the ischial spine. The surgeon's hand may be placed into the vagina to elevate the anterior vaginal wall and pubocervical fascia to the normal attachment along the ATFP [40]. Permanent suture is then used to reattach the

Table 1 ASC best practices for ERAS

ERAS single item	Specifics for ASC/other surgery	Evidence level ASC/other surgeries	Grade of recommendation
Preoperative counseling and education	Patients should routinely receive dedicated preoperative counseling and education	Na/low	Strong
Preoperative medical optimization	Smoking and alcohol consumption should be stopped 4 weeks before surgery	Na/moderate–high	Strong
	Correction of anemia	Na/moderate	
	Nutritional support for malnourished patients	Moderate/high	
	Maximizing functional status of patient before surgery	Moderate	
	Need not exclude older or more obese individuals	Moderate	
Oral mechanical bowel preparation	Preoperative bowel preparation can be omitted	Moderate/high	Strong
Preoperative carbohydrate loading	Carbohydrate loading reduces insulin resistance and should be administered to all nondiabetic patients	Na/low–moderate	Strong
Preoperative fasting	Intake of clear fluids up until 2 h and solids up until 6 h before anesthesia induction	Na/moderate	Strong
Preanesthesia medication	Avoid long-acting sedatives	Na/low–moderate	Strong
	Preoperative IV acetaminophen might not be necessary	Moderate	
Thrombosis prophylaxis	Mechanical and pharmacological prophylaxis with LMWH and extended prophylaxis for patients at risk	Na/high	Strong
Epidural analgesia	Spinal analgesia with general anesthesia is superior to general anesthesia alone at reducing postoperative analgesics	Moderate/high	Strong
Minimally invasive approach	Laparoscopic and robotic surgeries are comparable to open approach and recommended for appropriate patients	High/moderate	Strong
Antimicrobial prophylaxis and skin preparation	Single-dose antimicrobial prophylaxis within 1 h of surgery is sufficient for preventing postoperative infection	Low/high	Strong
Standard anesthetic protocol	Maintain adequate hemodynamic control, central and peripheral oxygenation, muscle relaxation, depth of anesthesia	Na/moderate	Strong
	Injection of liposomal bupivacaine into laparoscopic and vaginal incisions can be omitted	Low	
Perioperative fluid management	Fluid balance must be optimized to the individual	Na/high	Strong
Preventing intraoperative hypothermia	Maintenance of normal body temperature throughout the perioperative period	Na/high	Strong
Urinary drainage	Same-day voiding trials might be done, but patients should be monitored for incomplete emptying and UTI	Low/low	Weak
Prevention of postoperative ileus	We recommend a multimodal approach to maximize gut function	Moderate/high	Strong
Prevention of PONV	Should use a multimodal approach with at least two antiemetic agents	Na/moderate	Strong
Postoperative analgesia	Recommend multimodal postoperative analgesia with NSAIDS/acetaminophen, gabapentin, and dexamethasone when appropriate	Na/low–high	Strong

(continued)

Table 1 (continued)

ERAS single item	Specifics for ASC/other surgery	Evidence level ASC/other surgeries	Grade of recommendation
Early mobilization	Encourage early mobilization with liberal postoperative activity	Low/low	Strong
Early oral diet	Encourage oral nutrition started 4 h postoperatively	Na/moderate	Strong
Audit	Patients to be audited for protocol compliance and outcomes	Na/low	Strong

ASC abdominal sacrocolpopexy, *ERAS* enhanced recovery after surgery, *Na*, no data found for ASC. (Reprinted with permission from John Wiley and Sons: Nemirovsky et al. [31])

previously identified lateral superior vaginal sulcus and overlying pubocervical fascia to the ATFP overlying the obturator internus and pelvic sidewall (Fig. 1). Full thickness bites of vaginal tissue, excluding epithelium, are taken. The first suture is placed 1 cm caudal to the ischial spine, with subsequent sutures placed 1–2 cm apart, and the final suture placed as close as possible to the pubic ramus [43]. These sutures are placed bilaterally if bilateral defects are identified, and cystoscopy is performed at the completion of the procedure. If a transperitoneal approach was performed, the anterior peritoneum is closed. Modifications to this technique have been described, including suture placement into Cooper's ligament rather than ATFP [33, 44], fixation to the ischial periosteum and obturator membrane [45], and use of mesh secured with surgical staples to the lateral vagina and Cooper's ligament [39]. Another technique utilizing a reversed T-shaped anterior mesh has been described during sacrocolpopexy, which allows repair of a paravaginal defect to be performed at the same time and with the same piece of mesh used during sacrocolpopexy [46]. Some studies suggest that vaginal surgery and dissection can worsen perineal neuropathy in those with pelvic relaxation and stress urinary incontinence [47], but pelvic floor prolapse itself has also been linked with pudendal neuropathy, and pelvic floor surgery involving vaginal dissection produces neuropathy of the pudendal nerve [48]. The neuropathy may have an effect on muscle strength and integrity of muscular tissue support and may also be related to lower urinary tract

dysfunction [49]. Neuropathy has been suggested to play a role in failed reconstructive surgery [50]. Reported complications of laparoscopic paravaginal repair include major complications in 4.2% such as laparotomy for bleeding or small bowel strangulation and bowel or bladder injury. Minor complications including urinary tract infection were reported in 8.5%, and prolonged urinary retention with post-void residuals greater than 100 ml by 7 days after surgery were reported in 10.4% [36].

Laparoscopic and Robotic Uterosacral Ligament Suspension

Descent of the apex of the vagina may be treated through vaginal or abdominal approaches by suspending the vaginal apex to the uterosacral ligament. Laparoscopic and robotic uterosacral ligament suspension may be performed in women without a uterus as well as in a uterine-preserving procedure. In this procedure, a uterine manipulator may be used to aid in the identification of the uterosacral ligaments, and sutures are passed on either side of the upper portion of the ligament, lateral to the rectosigmoid, where the ligaments are furthest away from the uterus [51]. The distal end of the sutures is passed through the pubocervical and rectovaginal fascia (Fig. 2). An incision in the peritoneum is made to avoid kinking of the ureter [53]. Permanent suture is commonly used to attach the uterus or vaginal cuff to more proximal portions of the uterosacral

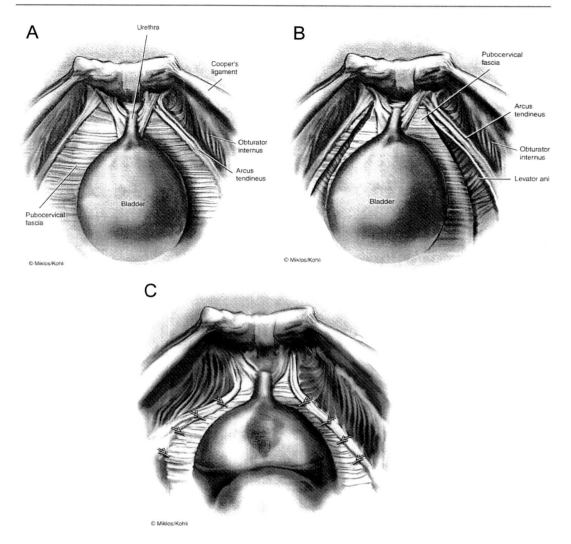

Fig. 1 (**a**) Normal anatomy of space of Retzius. (**b**) Separation of arcus tendineus fascia pelvis (ATFP) away from levator ani muscle resulting in loss of support to anterolateral vaginal wall and a paravaginal defect. (**c**) Sutures placed to reattach vaginal sulcus to ATFP and pelvic sidewall. (Reprinted from Miklos and Kohli [42], Copyright 2000 with permission from Elsevier)

ligaments [54] (Fig. 3), although some studies suggest that absorbable suture has similar surgical success rates with less suture exposure/erosion and suture removal compared to permanent suture [56]. A systematic review in 2019 found that that 95.5% of women reported their condition was "very much better" or "much better" after laparoscopic uterosacral ligament suspension [53]. Short-term retrospective data has shown no significant difference in 1 year postoperative results between robotic-assisted laparoscopic uterosacral ligament suspension (92% success) compared to vaginal uterosacral ligament suspension (85% success), defined as prolapse with leading edge of 0 or less, apex of ½ total vaginal length, no POP symptoms, and no prolapse reoperations or pessary use [51]. In this study, the rate of postoperative complications for patients who underwent robotic uterosacral ligament repair included persistent pelvic pain in

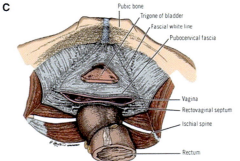
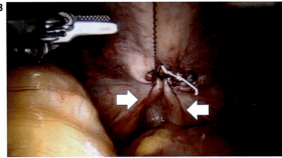
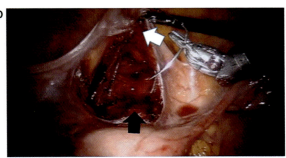

Fig. 2 Uterosacral ligament (USL) and pubocervical fascia (PCF) identification during robotic-assisted laparoscopic apical suspension. (**a**) Posterior view of the uterus and relation to right/left USL, (**b**) after completing right USL suspension, left USL is attached to the right. White arrows: left/right USL, (**c**) identification of the PCF and relation to the trigone of the bladder, and (**d**) holding the bladder up (white arrow), in preparation for the PCF plication (black arrow). (Reprinted by permission from Springer Nature: Davila et al. [52], Copyright 2019)

3.8%, and 92.3% of patients were able to pass a voiding trial on postoperative day 1. No ureteral, bowel, or bladder injuries occurred in either patient group.

When compared to LSC, the overall success rate of laparoscopic uterosacral ligament suspension has not been demonstrated to be significantly different (95.9% vs. 89.7% respectively); however, sacrocolpopexy resulted in better anterior compartment support [55]. Patients undergoing uterosacral ligament suspension developed significantly more abnormal granulation tissue at follow-up (6.9% vs. 0%) without risk of mesh erosion which was noted in 1.2% of patients undergoing sacrocolpopexy [55]. These results suggest that sacrocolpopexy may be better than laparoscopic uterosacral ligament suspension to correct anterior compartment prolapse with low rates of mesh erosion [55].

Laparoscopic Pectopexy

Laparoscopic pectopexy has been described as an alternative to sacrocolpopexy for repair of POP. In this repair, the lateral aspects of the iliopectineal ligament are used as the anchor point for mesh fixation of prolapsed structures, following the round and broad ligaments without crossing near bowel or ureter and avoiding the need for sacral dissection (Fig. 4) [57]. During this procedure, the peritoneal layer around the right-sided round ligament is opened toward the pelvic sidewall until the external iliac vein is visualized, and the soft tissue in this region is opened to allow visualization of the iliopectineal ligament [57]. This procedure is then repeated on the left side. The peritoneal layers are then opened bilaterally toward the vaginal apex. The peritoneum at the

Fig. 3 Placement of uterosacral ligament sutures after hysterectomy and closure of vaginal cuff. (Reprinted by permission from Springer Nature: Filmar et al. [55], Copyright 2014)

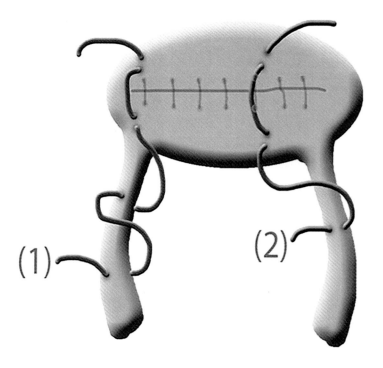

anterior and posterior vaginal apex is dissected free, and mesh is secured to bilateral iliopectineal ligaments and vaginal apex in a tension-free fashion. If the uterus is to be left in place, the anterior peritoneum of the uterus is dissected, and the mesh is secured to the lower anterior segment of the uterus. The peritoneum above the mesh is then closed. Short-term results have been reported and have been compared to sacrocolpopexy [58], with no intraoperative or postoperative complications and no recurrence of prolapse at 6-month follow-up reported in either group [57, 58]. When laparoscopic pectopexy is compared to vaginal sacrospinous fixation, de novo cystocele rates were higher in the sacrospinous fixation group. However, there were no significant differences in rates of de novo rectocele nor treatment satisfaction rates (93% in sacrospinous fixation vs. 91.7% in pectopexy) with a mean follow-up of 13 months [59].

Laparoscopic and Robotic Supracervical Hysterectomy and Total Hysterectomy

POP is the third most common reason for hysterectomy overall and is indicated for the treatment of uterine prolapse [60]. Hysterectomy may be performed through vaginal and abdominal approaches. The American College of Obstetrics and Gynecology recommends performing a vaginal apex suspension at the time of hysterectomy to prevent subsequent POP [61]. In addition, long-term follow-up data of up to 17 years suggest that the technique by which hysterectomy is performed has no impact on the risk of subsequent POP [61]. A systematic review and meta-analysis demonstrated no statistical differences in the rate of postoperative complications, length of hospital stay, total operative time, conversion to laparotomy, blood loss, or surgical outcomes between robotic and laparoscopic techniques in

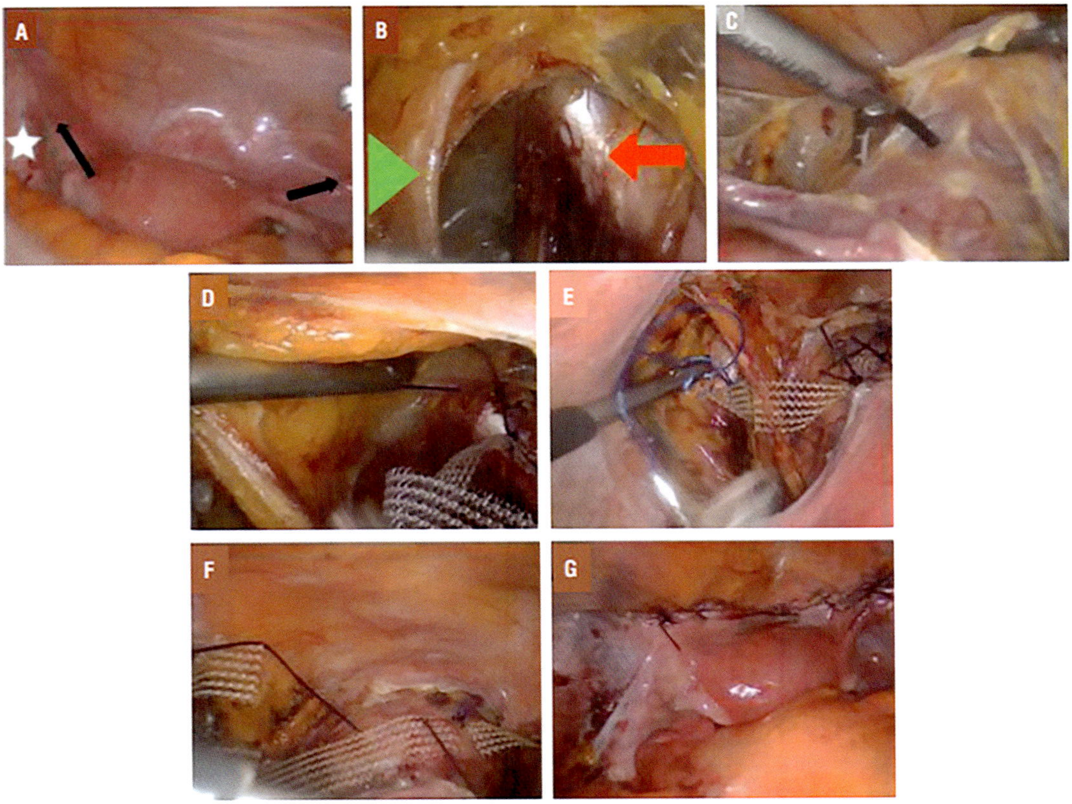

Fig. 4 (**a**) Determination of the round ligaments (arrows) and external iliac vessels (star). (**b**) The peritoneal layer is opened along the right round ligament toward the pelvic sidewall. The iliopectineal ligament (arrow) and the medial umbilical ligament (triangle) are demonstrated. The same procedure is then repeated on the left side of the patient. (**c**) The peritoneal layers on both sides are opened toward the cervix. (**d** and **e**) After completion of dissections, the ends of the mesh are sutured to both iliopectineal ligaments via the intracorporeal suture technique, using nonabsorbable sutures. (**f**) The middle of the mesh is fixed at the lower anterior segment of the uterus with three stitches. (**g**) The peritoneum above the mesh is sutured with an absorbable suture material. (Reprinted from Kale et al. [57]. This is an Open Access article distributed under the terms of the Creative Commons Attribution License, which permits unrestricted use, distribution, and reproduction in any medium, provided the original work is properly cited)

hysterectomy for benign disease [62]. These data suggest no clear benefit of the robotic approach over the laparoscopic approach in hysterectomy for benign disease.

Preoperative counseling regarding concomitant salpingectomy has also been recommended by the American College of Obstetrics and Gynecology to reduce the risk of ovarian cancer, as the most common subtype of ovarian cancer is believed to originate in the distal fallopian tube [63]. Therefore, salpingectomy is commonly performed at the time of hysterectomy, and in 2016, 46.8% of women undergoing vaginal hysterectomy for POP also underwent salpingectomy [63].

The rate of postoperative complications associated with robotic or laparoscopic hysterectomy for benign disease has been reported to be 5.2%, including urinary tract infection (2.1%), superficial surgical site infection (1%), blood transfusion (1%), and vaginal dehiscence (0.64–1.35% in laparoscopic approaches and 1.64% in robotic approaches) [64].

Hysterectomy may be performed before a sacrocolpopexy, and if this is planned, a supra-cervical hysterectomy should be considered because preservation of the cervix and avoidance of amputation at the level of the vagina may decrease risk of future mesh erosion [65]. However, endometrial assessment preoperatively should be considered in all postmenopausal patients undergoing intra-abdominal uterine morcellation regardless of risk factors. If vaginal hysterectomy is indicated, a double-layered closure of the vaginal cuff should be performed before minimally invasive abdominal repair and care taken to avoid suturing mesh to the vaginal apex to minimize risk of mesh erosion into vagina. However, electrosurgical current spread to vaginal apex tissues may predispose patients to mesh erosion.

Women with in situ uterus should be evaluated for postmenopausal or abnormal uterine bleeding, should undergo transvaginal ultrasonography as indicated to rule out a suspicious mass, and should have clearly documented Pap smear history. Appropriate candidates may be considered for sacrohysteropexy or may elect to undergo concomitant supracervical hysterectomy at the time of sacrocolpopexy [66].

During laparoscopic or robotic hysterectomy, a uterine manipulator may be placed to allow mobilization of the uterus to aid in identification of the vagina, uterus, bladder, and ureters [67]. During initial anatomic evaluation, both ureters and uterine vessels should be identified. The adnexa are first separated from the uterus to allow ease of visualization of the broad ligament. The round ligaments are then identified, coagulated, and transected away from the body of the uterus to avoid bleeding from ascending uterine vessel branches. The anterior and posterior leaves of the broad ligament are then separated with blunt dissection. This dissection of the broad ligament is carried toward the cervix and then continued in the midline along the vesicouterine reflection to create a bladder flap and allow identification of the cervix. The dissection will allow bilateral skeletonization of the uterine vessels, which should then be coagulated and transected bilaterally, at a right angle to prevent vessel shearing. Care should be taken not to lateralize the uterine vessels excessively as the ureters often run within 1.5–2 cm of the internal cervical os. If a subtotal hysterectomy is to be performed, monopolar shears may be used to amputate the uterine corpus below the internal os. The cervical stump may be left open if hemostatic or closed with interrupted sutures. The endocervical canal should be fulgurated to reduce cervical stump bleeding risk.

If total hysterectomy is to be performed, the cardinal and uterosacral ligaments are divided bilaterally. Pneumoperitoneum is maintained during total hysterectomy with various techniques of vaginal occlusion such as a vaginal pneumo-occluder, or even a sterile glove filled with gauze. A colpotomy ring may be used to assist in completing the anterior or posterior colpotomy. Care should be taken to prevent devascularization of the cuff to prevent risk of vaginal cuff dehiscence. The edges of the vaginal cuff are reapproximated using either barbed sutures or figure-of-eight sutures.

If the fallopian tubes and ovaries are to be maintained, the utero-ovarian ligament and tube are sealed and transected proximally. If salpingectomy is to be performed, the mesosalpinx is transected at the distal end of the tube. If the fallopian tubes and ovaries are to be removed, the infundibulopelvic ligaments are skeletonized, and these vascular pedicles are sealed and transected.

Specimens may be removed through the vagina, or if too large to be removed vaginally, a cold knife may be used to debulk the specimen after placing it into a specimen bag. They may also be removed abdominally through an extended umbilical incision.

Trends and Future Directions in Utilization of Laparoscopy and Robotics in POP Surgery

Originally, the implementation of minimally invasive procedures for POP surgery was aimed to decrease morbidity and length of hospital stay. Historically, following robotic or laparoscopic procedures, patients are discharged home the next day. Current trends are aiming to achieve same-day discharge (SDD) for minimally invasive prolapse surgery. The literature supports the safety and feasibility of SDD following minimally invasive prolapse procedures as a way to improve patient satisfaction without increasing postoperative complications or healthcare utilization. A study of 272 patients undergoing RSC discharged 80 of 272 (29.4%) patients on the same day and demonstrated no differences in unplanned provider visits, emergency department visits, or readmission between SDD patients and those admitted overnight [68]. Another prospective study of 47 SDD patients following minimally invasive sacrocolpopexy showed a readmission rate of 4.3% [69]. Based on current literature, SDD appears to result in high patient satisfaction with no increased risk of complications or changes in the postoperative course.

Despite the popularity of robotic approaches for POP surgery, existing literature has not shown robotic approaches to be superior to laparoscopic, and long-term outcomes data for robotic approaches are lacking. Advances in techniques for minimally invasive approaches such as nerve sparing sacral promontory dissection [70], retroperitoneal sacrocolpopexy [71], single-site surgeries [72, 73], and natural orifice vaginal sacrocolpopexy have been described and may improve patient outcomes [74]. Alternative techniques for apical suspension which avoid sacral promontory dissection and thus avoid the complications of hemorrhage, discitis, and ureteral injury, such as laparoscopic pectopexy in which vaginal apex is suspended using two mesh arms to the lateral iliopectineal ligaments [57, 74, 75], and lateral suspension in which lateral mesh arms are passed through the lateral anterior abdominal wall where the round ligament exists the peritoneal cavity [72, 74, 76] have also been described. In addition, given the risks related to synthetic mesh use in the repair of POP, further study on the use of autologous fascia or development of resorbable grafts [77] should be encouraged [78]. As technological advances in robotics, innovative techniques, and bioengineering of graft materials will undoubtedly continue to progress and improve, so too will patient outcomes in POP surgery.

Single-port LSC has been described in case reports [79]; however, it is associated with substantially longer mean operation times and a higher level of difficulty compared to multi-port LSC. Single-port robotic surgery is the latest trend in the evolution of minimally invasive procedures and is still undergoing implementation. The appeal of single-port access lies within the potential reduced morbidity for patients and improved cosmetic results. However, the availability and learning curve for single-port surgical techniques limit its popularity. Lauterbach et al. demonstrated a significant decrease in operative time from the first 15 to the subsequent 15 single-port RSC and similar short-term outcomes between multi-port and single-port RSC [80]. A single-center randomized controlled trial of 70 women randomized to undergo single-port or multi-port RSC demonstrated longer operative time for single-port RSC, with a difference of 23.8 min, however demonstrated similar intraoperative complication rates, short-term outcomes, and quality-of-life parameters [81].

Lastly, manufacturers of robotic devices continue to improve visual and tactile technology. New innovations are underway to improve the haptic feedback loop for the surgeon by improving the perception of palpation and the ability to react to cues on the surgical field. The challenge is to integrate kinematic precision, minimize distortion perceived by the surgeon, and decrease temporal lags [82].

Conclusions

Minimally invasive prolapse surgery is here to stay and offers surgical and postoperative benefits for women. Over 20 years of data and outcomes have shown that LSC or RSC is safe, effective, and durable in treating symptomatic POP. Our field will continue to innovate to improve the care that we provide to our patients.

References

1. Linder BJ, Occhino JA, Habermann EB, Glasgow AE, Bews KA, Gershman B. A national contemporary analysis of perioperative outcomes of open versus minimally invasive sacrocolpopexy. J Urol. 2018;200:862–7.
2. Bump RC, Mattiasson A, Bo K, Brubaker LP, DeLancey JO, Klarskov P, Shull BL, Smith AR. The standardization of terminology of female pelvic organ prolapse and pelvic floor dysfunction. Am J Obstet Gynecol. 1996;175:10–7.
3. Seo JT, Kim JM. Pelvic organ support and prevalence by Pelvic Organ Prolapse-Quantification (POP-Q) in Korean women. J Urol. 2006;175:1769–72.
4. Swift S, Woodman P, O'Boyle A, Kahn M, Valley M, Bland D, Wang W, Schaffer J. Pelvic Organ Support Study (POSST): the distribution, clinical definition, and epidemiologic condition of pelvic organ support defects. Am J Obstet Gynecol. 2005;192:795–806.
5. Swift SE. The distribution of pelvic organ support in a population of female subjects seen for routine gynecologic health care. Am J Obstet Gynecol. 2000;183:277–85.
6. Rountis A, Zacharakis D, Athanasiou S, Kathopoulis N, Grigoriadis T. The role of laparoscopic surgery in the treatment of advanced uterine prolapse: a systematic review of the literature. Cureus. 2021;13:e18281.
7. Nezhat CH, Nezhat F, Nezhat C. Laparoscopic sacral colpopexy for vaginal vault prolapse. Obstet Gynecol. 1994;84:885–8.
8. Di Marco DS, Chow GK, Gettman MT, Elliott DS. Robotic-assisted laparoscopic sacrocolpopexy for treatment of vaginal vault prolapse. Urology. 2004;63:373–6.
9. Lee RK, Mottrie A, Payne CK, Waltregny D. A review of the current status of laparoscopic and robot-assisted sacrocolpopexy for pelvic organ prolapse. Eur Urol. 2014;65:1128–37.
10. Desai VB, Guo XM, Fan L, Wright JD, Xu X. Inpatient laparoscopic hysterectomy in the United States: trends and factors associated with approach selection. J Minim Invasive Gynecol. 2017;24:151–158.e1.
11. Cameron-Jeffs R, Yong C, Carey M. Robotic-assisted gynaecological surgery in Australia: current trends, challenges and future possibility. ANZ J Surg. 2021;91:2246–9.
12. Billfeldt NK, Borgfeldt C, Lindkvist H, Stjerndahl JH, Ankardal M. A Swedish population-based evaluation of benign hysterectomy, comparing minimally invasive and abdominal surgery. Eur J Obstet Gynecol Reprod Biol. 2018;222:113–8.
13. Nicklin J. The future of robotic-assisted laparoscopic gynaecologic surgery in Australia – a time and a place for everything. Aust N Z J Obstet Gynaecol. 2017;57:493–8.
14. Chapman GC, Slopnick EA, Roberts K, Sheyn D, Wherley S, Mahajan ST, Pollard RR. National analysis of perioperative morbidity of vaginal versus laparoscopic hysterectomy at the time of uterosacral ligament suspension. J Minim Invasive Gynecol. 2021;28:275–81.
15. Maher C, Feiner B, Baessler K, Schmid C. Surgical management of pelvic organ prolapse in women. Cochrane Database Syst Rev. 2013;2013:CD004014.
16. Callewaert G, Bosteels J, Housmans S, Verguts J, Van Cleynenbreugel B, Van der Aa F, De Ridder D, Vergote I, Deprest J. Laparoscopic versus robotic-assisted sacrocolpopexy for pelvic organ prolapse: a systematic review. Gynecol Surg. 2016;13:115–23.
17. Alas AN, Anger JT. Management of apical pelvic organ prolapse. Curr Urol Rep. 2015;16:33.
18. Carroll AW, Lamb E, Hill AJ, Gill EJ, Matthews CA. Surgical management of apical pelvic support defects: the impact of robotic technology. Int Urogynecol J. 2012;23:1183–6.
19. Sato H, Abe H, Ikeda A, Miyagawa T, Sato K, Tsukada S. Laparoscopic sacrocolpopexy for pelvic organ prolapse in the elderly: safety and outcomes. J Obstet Gynaecol. 2021;42:1–6.
20. Wen Q, Zhao Z, Wen J, Yang Y, Wang L, Wu J, Miao Y. Impact of obesity on operative complications and outcome after sacrocolpopexy: a systematic review and meta-analysis. Eur J Obstet Gynecol Reprod Biol. 2021;258:309–16.
21. Sanci A, Akpinar C, Gokce MI, Suer E, Gulpinar O. Is robotic-assisted sacrocolpo(hystero)pexy safe and effective in women over 65 years of age? Int Urogynecol J. 2021;32:2211–7.
22. Anger JT, Mueller ER, Tarnay C, Smith B, Stroupe K, Rosenman A, Brubaker L, Bresee C, Kenton K. Robotic compared with laparoscopic sacrocolpopexy: a randomized controlled trial. Obstet Gynecol. 2014;123:5–12.
23. Paraiso MFR, Jelovsek JE, Frick A, Chen CCG, Barber MD. Laparoscopic compared with robotic sacrocolpopexy for vaginal prolapse: a randomized controlled trial. Obstet Gynecol. 2011;118:1005–13.
24. Slopnick EA, Petrikovets A, Sheyn D, Kim SP, Nguyen CT, Hijaz AK. Surgical trends and patient factors associated with the treatment of apical pelvic organ prolapse from a national sample. Int Urogynecol J. 2019;30:603–9.
25. Tarr ME, Brancato SJ, Cunkelman JA, Polcari A, Nutter B, Kenton K. Comparison of postural ergonomics between laparoscopic and robotic sacrocolpopexy: a pilot study. J Minim Invasive Gynecol. 2015;22:234–8.
26. Kalogera E, Dowdy SC. Enhanced recovery pathway in gynecologic surgery: improving outcomes through evidence-based medicine. Obstet Gynecol Clin N Am. 2016;43:551–73.
27. Kehlet H. Fast-track colorectal surgery. Lancet. 2008;371:791–3.
28. Ljungqvist O. ERAS – enhanced recovery after surgery: moving evidence-based perioperative care to practice. JPEN J Parenter Enteral Nutr. 2014;38:559–66.
29. Carter-Brooks CM, Du AL, Ruppert KM, Romanova AL, Zyczynski HM. Implementation of a urogynecology-specific enhanced recovery after

surgery (ERAS) pathway. Am J Obstet Gynecol. 2018;219:495.e1–e10.

30. Carter-Brooks CM, Romanova AL, DeRenzo JS, Shepherd JP, Zyczynski HM. Age and perioperative outcomes after implementation of an enhanced recovery after surgery pathway in women undergoing major prolapse repair surgery. Female Pelvic Med Reconstr Surg. 2021;27:e392–8.

31. Nemirovsky A, Herbert AS, Gorman EF, Malik RD. A systematic review of best practices for the perioperative management of abdominal sacrocolpopexy. Neurourol Urodyn. 2020;39:1264–75. https://doi.org/10.1002/nau.24411.

32. Sammarco AG, Swenson CW, Kamdar NS, Kobernik EK, DeLancey JOL, Nallamothu B, Morgan DM. Rate of pelvic organ prolapse surgery among privately insured women in the United States, 2010–2013. Obstet Gynecol. 2018;131:484–92.

33. Duraisamy KY, Balasubramaniam D, Kakollu A, Chinnusamy P, Periyasamy K. A prospective study of minimally invasive paravaginal repair of cystocele and associated pelvic floor defects: our experience. J Obstet Gynaecol India. 2019;69:82–8.

34. Richardson AC, Lyon JB, Williams NL. A new look at pelvic relaxation. Am J Obstet Gynecol. 1976;126: 568–73.

35. White GR. Cystocele – a radical cure by suturing lateral sulci of the vagina to the white line of pelvic fascia. 1909. Int Urogynecol J Pelvic Floor Dysfunct. 1997;8:288–92.

36. Behnia-Willison F, Seman EI, Cook JR, O'Shea RT, Keirse MJ. Laparoscopic paravaginal repair of anterior compartment prolapse. J Minim Invasive Gynecol. 2007;14:475–80.

37. Rivoire C, Botchorishvili R, Canis M, Jardon K, Rabischong B, Wattiez A, Mage G. Complete laparoscopic treatment of genital prolapse with meshes including vaginal promontofixation and anterior repair: a series of 138 patients. J Minim Invasive Gynecol. 2007;14:712–8.

38. Seman EI, Cook JR, O'Shea RT. Two-year experience with laparoscopic pelvic floor repair. J Am Assoc Gynecol Laparosc. 2003;10:38–45.

39. Washington JL, Somers KO. Laparoscopic paravaginal repair: a new technique using mesh and staples. JSLS. 2003;7:301–3.

40. Chinthakanan O, Miklos JR, Moore RD. Laparoscopic paravaginal defect repair: surgical technique and a literature review. Surg Technol Int. 2015;27:173–83.

41. Hosni MM, El-Feky AE, Agur WI, Khater EM. Evaluation of three different surgical approaches in repairing paravaginal support defects: a comparative trial. Arch Gynecol Obstet. 2013;288:1341–8.

42. Miklos JR, Kohli N. Laparoscopic paravaginal repair plus burch colposuspension: review and descriptive technique. Urology. 2000;56(6 Suppl 1):64–9.

43. Nguyen JK. Current concepts in the diagnosis and surgical repair of anterior vaginal prolapse due to paravaginal defects. Obstet Gynecol Surv. 2001;56:239–46.

44. Bai SW, Jeon JD, Chung KA, Kim JY, Kim SK, Park KH. The effectiveness of modified six-corner suspension in patients with paravaginal defect and stress urinary incontinence. Int Urogynecol J Pelvic Floor Dysfunct. 2002;13:303–7.

45. Scotti RJ, Garely AD, Greston WM, Flora RF, Olson TR. Paravaginal repair of lateral vaginal wall defects by fixation to the ischial periosteum and obturator membrane. Am J Obstet Gynecol. 1998;179:1436–45.

46. Ichikawa M, Sekine M, Ono S, Mine K, Akira S, Takeshita T. Hybrid laparoscopic sacrocolpopexy for pelvic organ prolapse with severe cystocele. J Minim Invasive Gynecol. 2015;22:S117.

47. Zivkovic F, Tamussino K, Ralph G, Schied G, Auer-Grumbach M. Long-term effects of vaginal dissection on the innervation of the striated urethral sphincter. Obstet Gynecol. 1996;87:257–60.

48. Benson JT, McClellan E. The effect of vaginal dissection on the pudendal nerve. Obstet Gynecol. 1993;82: 387–9.

49. Benson JT, Lucente V, McClellan E. Vaginal versus abdominal reconstructive surgery for the treatment of pelvic support defects: a prospective randomized study with long-term outcome evaluation. Am J Obstet Gynecol. 1996;175:1418–21. Discussion 1421–2

50. Welgoss JA, Vogt VY, McClellan EJ, Benson JT. Relationship between surgically induced neuropathy and outcome of pelvic organ prolapse surgery. Int Urogynecol J Pelvic Floor Dysfunct. 1999;10:11–4.

51. Vallabh-Patel V, Saiz C, Salamon C. Subjective and objective outcomes of robotic and vaginal high uterosacral ligament suspension. Female Pelvic Med Reconstr Surg. 2016;22:420–4.

52. Davila HH, Brown K, Dara P, Bruce L, Goodman L, Gallo T. Robotic-assisted laparoscopic apical suspension: description of the spiral technique. J Robot Surg. 2019;13(3):519–23. https://doi.org/10.1007/s11701-018-0879-1.

53. Szymczak P, Grzybowska ME, Wydra DG. Comparison of laparoscopic techniques for apical organ prolapse repair – a systematic review of the literature. Neurourol Urodyn. 2019;38:2031–50.

54. Frick AC, Paraiso MF. Laparoscopic management of incontinence and pelvic organ prolapse. Clin Obstet Gynecol. 2009;52:390–400.

55. Filmar GA, Fisher HW, Aranda E, Lotze PM. Laparoscopic uterosacral ligament suspension and sacral colpopexy: results and complications. Int Urogynecol J. 2014;25:1645–53.

56. Peng L, Liu YH, He SX, Di XP, Shen H, Luo DY. Is absorbable suture superior to permanent suture for uterosacral ligament suspension? Neurourol Urodyn. 2020;39:1958–65.

57. Kale A, Biler A, Terzi H, Usta T, Kale E. Laparoscopic pectopexy: initial experience of single center with a new technique for apical prolapse surgery. Int Braz J Urol. 2017;43:903–9. https://doi.org/10.1590/S1677-5538.IBJU.2017.0070.

58. Chuang FC, Chou YM, Wu LY, Yang TH, Chen WH, Huang KH. Laparoscopic pectopexy: the learning curve and comparison with laparoscopic sacrocolpopexy. Int Urogynecol J. 2021;33(7): 1949–56.

59. Astepe BS, Karsli A, Koleli I, Aksakal OS, Terzi H, Kale A. Intermediate-term outcomes of laparoscopic pectopexy and vaginal sacrospinous fixation: a comparative study. Int Braz J Urol. 2019;45:999–1007.

60. Jeppson PC, Sung VW. Hysterectomy for pelvic organ prolapse: indications and techniques. Clin Obstet Gynecol. 2014;57:72–82.

61. Gabriel I, Kalousdian A, Brito LG, Abdalian T, Vitonis AF, Minassian VA. Pelvic organ prolapse after 3 modes of hysterectomy: long-term follow-up. Am J Obstet Gynecol. 2021;224:496.e1–e10.

62. Albright BB, Witte T, Tofte AN, Chou J, Black JD, Desai VB, Erekson EA. Robotic versus laparoscopic hysterectomy for benign disease: a systematic review and meta-analysis of randomized trials. J Minim Invasive Gynecol. 2016;23:18–27.

63. Slopnick EA, Sheyn DD, Chapman GC, Mahajan ST, El-Nashar S, Hijaz AK. Adnexectomy at the time of vaginal hysterectomy for pelvic organ prolapse. Int Urogynecol J. 2020;31:373–9.

64. Catanzarite T, Saha S, Pilecki MA, Kim JY, Milad MP. Longer operative time during benign laparoscopic and robotic hysterectomy is associated with increased 30-day perioperative complications. J Minim Invasive Gynecol. 2015;22:1049–58.

65. Paraiso MF. Robotic-assisted laparoscopic surgery for hysterectomy and pelvic organ prolapse repair. Fertil Steril. 2014;102:933–8.

66. White WM, Pickens RB, Elder RF, Firoozi F. Robotic-assisted sacrocolpopexy for pelvic organ prolapse. Urol Clin North Am. 2014;41:549–57.

67. Simpson KM, Advincula AP. The essential elements of a robotic-assisted laparoscopic hysterectomy. Obstet Gynecol Clin N Am. 2016;43:479–93.

68. Kisby CK, Polin MR, Visco AG, Siddiqui NY. Same-day discharge after robotic-assisted sacrocolpopexy. Female Pelvic Med Reconstr Surg. 2019;25:337–41.

69. Hickman LC, Paraiso MFR, Goldman HB, Propst K, Ferrando CA. Same-day discharge after minimally invasive sacrocolpopexy is feasible, safe, and associated with high patient satisfaction. Female Pelvic Med Reconstr Surg. 2021;27:e614–9.

70. Serbetcioglu GC, Simsek SY, Alemdaroglu S, Aytac PC, Kalayci H, Celik H. Outcomes of nerve-sparing laparoscopic sacropexy on one hundred fifteen cases. J Gynecol Obstet Hum Reprod. 2020;49:101795.

71. Onol FF, Kaya E, Kose O, Onol SY. A novel technique for the management of advanced uterine/vault prolapse: extraperitoneal sacrocolpopexy. Int Urogynecol J. 2011;22:855–61.

72. Giannini A, Russo E, Mannella P, Simoncini T. Single site robotic-assisted apical lateral suspension (SS R-ALS) for advanced pelvic organ prolapse: first case reported. J Robot Surg. 2017;11:259–62.

73. Iavazzo C, Minis EE, Gkegkes ID. Single-site port robotic-assisted hysterectomy: an update. J Robot Surg. 2018;12:201–13.

74. Schachar JS, Matthews CA. Robotic-assisted repair of pelvic organ prolapse: a scoping review of the literature. Transl Androl Urol. 2020;9:959–70.

75. Banerjee C, Noe KG. Laparoscopic pectopexy: a new technique of prolapse surgery for obese patients. Arch Gynecol Obstet. 2011;284:631–5.

76. Dubuisson JB, Yaron M, Wenger JM, Jacob S. Treatment of genital prolapse by laparoscopic lateral suspension using mesh: a series of 73 patients. J Minim Invasive Gynecol. 2008;15:49–55.

77. Aghaei-Ghareh-Bolagh B, Mukherjee S, Lockley KM, Mithieux SM, Wang Z, Emmerson S, Darzi S, Gargett CE, Weiss AS. A novel tropoelastin-based resorbable surgical mesh for pelvic organ prolapse repair. Mater Today Bio. 2020;8:100081.

78. Oliver JL, Kim JH. Robotic sacrocolpopexy – is it the treatment of choice for advanced apical pelvic organ prolapse? Curr Urol Rep. 2017;18:66.

79. Kaouk JH, Haber GP, Goel RK, Desai MM, Aron M, Rackley RR, Moore C, Gill IS. Single-port laparoscopic surgery in urology: initial experience. Urology. 2008;71:3–6.

80. Lauterbach R, Mustafa-Mikhail S, Matanes E, Amit A, Wiener Z, Lowenstein L. Single-port versus multi-port robotic sacrocervicopexy: establishment of a learning curve and short-term outcomes. Eur J Obstet Gynecol Reprod Biol. 2019;239:1–6.

81. Matanes E, Boulus S, Lauterbach R, Amit A, Weiner Z, Lowenstein L. Robotic laparoendoscopic single-site compared with robotic multi-port sacrocolpopexy for apical compartment prolapse. Am J Obstet Gynecol. 2020;222:358.e1–e11.

82. Alip SL, Kim J, Rha KH, Han WK. Future platforms of robotic surgery. Urol Clin North Am. 2022;49:23–38.

Complications of the Use of Synthetic Mesh Materials in Stress Urinary Incontinence and Pelvic Organ Prolapse

32

Michelle E. Van Kuiken and Anne M. Suskind

Contents

Introduction	570
A Note on Terminology	570
Overview of Synthetic Mesh Materials Used for SUI and POP	571
A Brief History of Synthetic Mesh Materials and Rationale for Use in Pelvic Organ Prolapse	571
Current State of Synthetic Mesh Materials for SUI and POP Internationally	571
Types of Synthetic Mesh and Mesh Characteristics Used in SUI and POP Surgery	572
Use and Trends of Synthetic Mesh Materials for POP	574
Vaginally Inserted Transvaginal Mesh for Repair of POP	574
Abdominally Inserted Synthetic Mesh for POP	574
Synthetic Mesh Materials for Stress Urinary Incontinence	575
Complications of Synthetic Midurethral Slings: Urinary Tract Infection and Voiding Dysfunction	577
Evaluation of Women Who Present with Mesh Complications	577
History	578
Physical Examination	578
Cystoscopy	578
Imaging Studies	578
Management of Mesh Complications	579
Dyspareunia and Pain	580
Vaginal Mesh Exposure	580
Infection	581
Visceral Injury	581
Ureter	584
Mesh Exposure into Rectum	585
Complications After Mesh Removal	586
Recurrent SUI After Synthetic Midurethral Sling Removal	586
Persistent or Worsening Pain	587

M. E. Van Kuiken (✉) · A. M. Suskind
Department of Urology, University of California, San
Francisco, CA, USA
e-mail: michelle.vankuiken@ucsf.edu;
anne.suskind@ucsf.edu

© Springer Nature Switzerland AG 2023
F. E. Martins et al. (eds.), *Female Genitourinary and Pelvic Floor Reconstruction*,
https://doi.org/10.1007/978-3-031-19598-3_33

Recurrent Prolapse 587
Recurrent Vaginal Mesh Exposure 588
Loss of Vaginal Length or Vaginal Canal Stenosis 588

Future Directions 589

Conclusions 589

Cross-References 589

References 590

Abstract

Synthetic mesh materials for the surgical management of stress urinary incontinence (SUI) and pelvic organ prolapse (POP) have been in use for decades. However, these materials have come under scrutiny due to high complication rates including vaginal and pelvic pain, vaginal mesh exposure, infection, and exposure into pelvic viscera, with many women suffering from both short- and long-term sequela of these complications. Due to these issues, the practice of mesh insertion for SUI and POP has changed over the years with evolution of mesh materials and advances in surgical technique. Additionally, the availability of mesh products remains variable around the world. Despite practice location, surgeons who specialize in treatment of women with pelvic floor disorders including SUI and POP should be well versed in the evaluation and management of women with a history of synthetic mesh placement who present with concerns for mesh complications.

Keywords

Mesh erosion · Mesh exposure · Mesh removal · Mesh excision · Pain due to mesh

Introduction

One of the main goals of pelvic reconstructive surgery is to provide durable relief of symptoms from pelvic floor disorders such as stress urinary incontinence (SUI) and pelvic organ prolapse (POP). Synthetic mesh materials were introduced

with the intention of increasing the efficacy and durability of surgical repair of POP, along with creating a simpler surgical approach to management of SUI with minimal incisions or postoperative convalescence. While synthetic mesh materials still have an important role in the surgical management of SUI and POP, they also carry a history of significant and occasionally serious health consequences for women who received these implants. All surgeons who specialize in the care of women with pelvic floor disorders should be familiar with mesh-related complications and management.

The purpose of this chapter is to describe both short- and- long-term complications that can result from the insertion of synthetic mesh materials for both SUI and POP along with operative and nonoperative management strategies.

A Note on Terminology

In 2010, the International Urogynecological Association (IUGA) and then International Continence Society (ICS) released the "Joint Terminology and Classification of the Complications Related Directly to the Insertion of Prostheses (Meshes, Implants, Tapes) & Grafts in Female Pelvic Floor Surgery" [24]. More recently, in 2020, the American Urogynecological Association (AUGS) and IUGA released the "Joint Position Statement on the Management of Mesh-Complications for the FPRMS Specialist," which re-emphasized the use of this standardized terminology surrounding mesh complications and mesh removal [29]. The terminology used in this chapter is consistent with the terminology introduced in the 2010 IUGA/ICS document and re-emphasized in the 2020 AUGS/IUGA position statement as follows:

Exposure: *A condition of displaying, revealing, exhibiting, or making accessible (e.g., mesh exposure).*

Extrusion: *Passage gradually out of a body structure or tissue.*

The term "erosion," while commonly used to describe mesh complications, is not supported by the ICS, IUGA, or AUGS and therefore is not used in this chapter.

Overview of Synthetic Mesh Materials Used for SUI and POP

A Brief History of Synthetic Mesh Materials and Rationale for Use in Pelvic Organ Prolapse

The use of mesh materials in surgical repair is not a new concept and dates back to the late nineteenth century when German surgeon Dr. Theodor Billroth envisioned the use of a prosthetic graft to aid in inguinal hernia repair. In 1900, a mesh made of silver filigrees was introduced by Oscar Witzel and R. Goepel for repair of inguinal hernia until the 1960s. This silver mesh had significant complications, such as chronic pain and drainage from the operative site, promoting the need for new and better graft materials. Synthetic mesh materials were subsequently developed and introduced for the repair of surgical hernias in the 1950s [48].

Synthetic mesh, in the form of polyethylene terephthalate (Mersilene®) and polypropylene, revolutionized the repair of both inguinal and abdominal hernias. Subsequently in the 1970s, surgeons began using surgical mesh for abdominal repair of POP with good success. As vaginal native tissue repairs for POP were known to be associated with high rates of recurrence, surgeons began using synthetic mesh materials via the transvaginal route to provide greater strength and durability. The initial practice of transvaginal

mesh placement involved surgeons cutting their own mesh from larger sheets and placing into the compartment with attachment sites of their choice.

Given initial favorable outcomes and good surgeon experience, the first transvaginal mesh for the repair of POP was cleared for use by the Food and Drug Administration (FDA) in the United States as a class II moderate-risk device in 2002. Following FDA approval, implantation of transvaginal mesh for POP increased significantly. From 2005 to 2010 in the United States, the number of vaginal mesh surgeries for POP increased from 36.7 per 100,000 person-years to 60.8 per 100,00 person-years, respectively ($p < 0.001$). By 2010, 74.9% of all mesh used for POP repair was implanted via vaginal route, as opposed to abdominally instated mesh for POP [31].

Initial outcomes of this practice were favorable with use of transvaginal mesh demonstrating decreased risk of anatomic failure compared to use of native tissue and/or xenografts, particularly in the anterior compartment [37, 49]. A 2016 Cochrane Review compared transvaginal native tissue repair to mesh-augmented repairs and found that there was a decreased risk of patient awareness of prolapse, objective prolapse on examination, and reoperation for prolapse at 1–3 years follow-up [35]. However, these higher rates of anatomic success came with more, and sometimes, devastating complications.

Current State of Synthetic Mesh Materials for SUI and POP Internationally

United States and Canada

Insertion of transvaginal mesh for prolapse became standard practice for many years until there were increasing reports of significant complications associated with mesh inserted via transvaginal approach. Less than 10 years after formal FDA approval, the FDA began issuing warnings about transvaginal mesh for POP with the first notice entitled "Serious Complications Associated with Transvaginal Placement of Surgical

Mesh for Pelvic Organ Prolapse" issued in October of 2008. This was followed by an updated warning issued in July 2011 after a systematic review found that serious complications were "not rare." In 2016, the FDA reclassified transvaginal mesh for POP into class III (high risk). Finally, in April 2019 the FDA called for the complete cessation of the sale and distribution of surgical mesh used for transvaginal repair of POP in the United States after the remaining manufactures were unable demonstrate reasonable safety and efficacy of these devices [55].

Also in 2019, Health Canada issued a statement that posterior compartment mesh should no longer be used and that anterior mesh should be limited to specific groups that are at high risk of recurrence or that have experienced recurrence. However, following the FDA ban in 2019, the remaining three manufacturers of transvaginal mesh also pulled out of the Canadian market so there are no longer any commercially available transvaginal mesh kits for use [39].

Australia, New Zealand, and the United Kingdom

Transvaginal mesh for POP repair has also been banned from the market in Australia (November 2017), New Zealand (December 2017), and the United Kingdom (July 2018). There has also been a complete cessation of sling mesh placement for SUI in both New Zealand and the United Kingdom [39].

European Union

In mainland Europe, with the exception of France, transvaginal mesh for POP is still in use. The European Union's position has remained unchanged since the 2015 Scientific Committee on Emerging and Newly Identified Health Risks (SCENIHR) report stated that vaginal meshes can be used in the case of POP recurrence or in cases in which the patient is at a high risk for recurrence. Additionally, the SCENIHR recommended that a certification system for implanting surgeons should be introduced, and patients should be appropriately selected and counselled prior to any mesh surgery. The rationale for continued use is that studies have demonstrated decreased

risk of recurrence rates with use of transvaginal mesh compared to native tissue repairs alone. In Germany, none of the transvaginal meshes from the FDA report are in use and they since been replaced with lighter, microporous mesh that have been shown to have lower recurrence rates [39].

Worldwide

In South America, there are currently no prohibitions on the use of transvaginal mesh. In Asia, practices are highly variable between countries, but ready-made mesh kits are available and in use in China, South Korea, Taiwan, Hong Kong, Singapore, Thailand, Malaysia, Indonesia, and India [39].

Types of Synthetic Mesh and Mesh Characteristics Used in SUI and POP Surgery

Throughout its evolution, mesh used in POP and SUI surgery has undergone various iterations, largely in response to unacceptably high complication rates that resulted from poor understanding of certain mesh characteristics. Mesh characteristics play a critical role in the risk of mesh-related complications, and most current mesh products that remain on the market today for abdominal repair of POP and SUI are Type I polypropylene mesh [27, 39]. This section will briefly outline important mesh properties such as pore size and mesh weight.

Pore Size

The most commonly used mesh classification system was introduced by Dr. Parvin Amid in 1997 with classification as follows:

Type I mesh is totally macroporous, monofilament mesh with pores of >75 μm. This large pore size allows for tissue ingrowth including macrophages, leukocytes, collagen, and blood vessels. It is much more resistant to infection than type II mesh discussed below.

Type II mesh is microporous, multifilament woven mesh with pores of <10 μm. This type of mesh is easily seeded with bacteria but the pores are too small to allow for entry of macrophages and leukocytes to clear the infection. Type II mesh has been associated with high vaginal exposure rates (up to 20–30%) along with need for complete explantation should infection occur. Historic mesh in this category includes Marlex, Dacron, and Mersilene.

Type III mesh is macroporous but contains multifilamentous or microporous components. Given microfilamentous components, it carries similar risks as type II mesh.

Mesh Weight

Mesh is often divided into the following mesh weight categories: "Ultralight" (<35 g/m^2), "Light" (≥ 35 <70 g/m^2), "Standard" (≥ 70 <140 g/m^2), and "Heavy" (≥ 140 g/m^2) [11]. In the case of mesh weights, heavier does not necessarily mean more durable. In heavy weight mesh, a phenomenon known as "stress shielding" can occur in which the stiff mesh bears undue force on tissue. This can lead to increased tissue necrosis, and therefore, increased risk of mesh extrusion and exposure [34]. Lighter weight mesh offers sufficient durability without damaging the surrounding tissue and is the reason why most mesh on the market today for abdominal repair of POP and SUI is either lightweight or ultralightweight.

In regard to light versus ultralightweight mesh, there appears to be a balance between time to prolapse recurrence and mesh-related complications. A recent study by Guigale reviewed the use of lightweight versus ultralightweight mesh for abdominal sacrocolpopexy. The authors found that while ultralightweight mesh was associated with fewer mesh-related complications (1.3% versus 5.8%, p $<$ 0.01), there was a shorter time to prolapse recurrence than with the use of lightweight mesh. Overall rates of prolapse recurrence did not differ between groups (7% overall), but the follow-up period was longer in the lightweight group [20].

Polypropylene Mesh in SUI and POP Surgery

Polypropylene mesh was developed by Dr. Francis Usher and released on the market in the 1960s. Polypropylene mesh quickly became popular for both inguinal and ventral hernia repair due to both its durability and ability to resist infection. Most mesh implants that remain on the market today for SUI and abdominal repair of POP are type I polypropylene light- or ultralightweight mesh due to the characteristics described above.

In general, use of type I polypropylene has mesh significantly reduced the risk of mesh-related complications compared to use of type II multifilament mesh. For example, many of the earliest mesh kits for POP utilized type II mesh, which resulted in significant complications. Many women required complete explant of both anterior and posterior mesh due to complications such as intractable mesh infections with associated pain, pelvic abscesses, fistula formation, and erosion into pelvic viscera [5].

Similar unacceptably high rates of vaginal exposure were seen with use of type II sling mesh for SUI, up to 17%, all of whom required surgical excision [51]. Another large retrospective cohort study reviewed outcomes of monofilament versus multifilament midurethral sling placement and found that both subjective cure and quality of life improvements were higher in the type I monofilament group. Additionally and importantly, 9.2% of women in the type II multifilament group developed mesh infection requiring complete removal versus no infections in the type I monofilament group [6]. This study did not comment on rates of vaginal mesh exposure.

Risk Factors for Mesh-Related Complications

As discussed above, mesh properties play a large and important role in the risk of mesh-related complications. The transition from type II to type I mesh has reduced, but not eliminated these complications. Surgical technique, while not an established risk factor, likely plays an important role in vaginal mesh exposures, depending on how deep or superficial the mesh is placed. Additionally, missed visceral injury to the bladder, urethra, or rectum likely increases risk of mesh exposure into these organs.

In regard to patient-related factors, one study compared women with previous history of mesh surgery with and without vaginal mesh exposure. Women with vaginal mesh exposure were slightly older and more likely to be menopausal than women without mesh exposure; however, vaginal estrogen use did not differ between the groups. Additionally, women with multiple mesh insertions were more likely to have mesh exposure [33]. History of smoking, body mass index, sexual activity, and hysterectomy status did not seem to affect risk of vaginal mesh exposure. Another study by Schimpf et al. also noted that rates of vaginal mesh exposure were higher (up to 36%) in women where mesh was inserted in multiple compartments [49].

Use and Trends of Synthetic Mesh Materials for POP

Vaginally Inserted Transvaginal Mesh for Repair of POP

Anterior Compartment Mesh

Historically, anterior compartment mesh has been the most commonly implanted type of transvaginal mesh. As discussed in the previous section, anteriorly placed transvaginal mesh demonstrated decreased risk of anatomic failure compared to use of native tissue and/or xenografts [37, 49], and women with mesh placed in the anterior compartment reported decreased awareness of prolapse, less objective prolapse on examination, and reoperation for prolapse at 1–3 years follow-up [35].

However, improved anatomic outcomes came at the cost of higher rates of complications. Vaginal exposure rates ranged from 1.4 to 19% in the anterior vaginal compartment alone, but increased to up to 36% when mesh was placed in multiple compartments [49]. Another study by Ngyuen et al. found that anterior compartment mesh was associated with the highest rate of reoperation, with 6% or women requiring repeat surgery for a mesh-related complication within 21 months of their initial operation [40].

Posterior Compartment Mesh

Overall, posterior compartment mesh has been the least commonly used type of transvaginal mesh. There are also lower rates of associated complications and reoperations for mesh in this compartment compared to both the apical and anterior compartments. The majority of complications are limited to vaginal mesh exposure and with rates of vaginal exposure around 2% [40]. Similar to apical compartment mesh, there is no significant improvement in posterior compartment POP outcomes when synthetic mesh is used [49].

Vaginal Mesh Trends

From 2005 to 2010 in the United States, the number of vaginal mesh surgeries for POP increased from 36.7 per 100,000 person-years to 60.8 per 100,00 person-years, respectively ($p < 0.001$). By 2010, 74.9% of all mesh used for POP repair was implanted via vaginal route, as opposed to abdominally instated mesh for POP [31].

Specific complications and management related to vaginally inserted mesh will be discussed in section "Management of Mesh Complications."

Abdominally Inserted Synthetic Mesh for POP

Mesh-augmented sacrocolpopexy first started in the 1970s through an open abdominal approach. This technique has continued to be refined over the years, with most of the sacrocolpopexy surgery now being performed via laparoscopic or robotic-assisted approaches, which has minimized both morbidity and length of hospital stay. With the complete cessation of transvaginal mesh for POP in many countries worldwide, sacrocolpopexy is now often considered the gold standard operation for POP.

Another important advancement in the performance of abdominal sacrocolpopexy is the transition from type II or heavier weight meshes to type 1 lightweight polypropylene mesh. One series reported outcomes of lightweight type I polypropylene mesh reported in 253 women. At 5 years follow-up, the authors reported surgical success rate of 89.3%, including both subjective and objective anatomic cure with *no* mesh-related complications [13]. This study, however, is unique because most sacrocolpopexy series document at least some complications related to mesh. For example, another recent series that utilized lightweight mesh for sacrocolpopexy noted a 5.8% rate of any mesh-related complication and a 4.0% reoperation rate for mesh-related complications [20]. Perhaps the most cited data on rates of mesh complications following sacrocolpopexy come from the long-term follow-up of the Colpopexy and Urinary Reduction Efforts (CARE) trial. Data from this study showed that the probability of a vaginal mesh exposure at 7 years was 10.5%, regardless of mesh type used [41].

When reviewing mesh complications related to sacrocolpopexy mesh, it is important to note that a large majority of both complications and complication management strategies that are reported in the literature are associated with the use of heavier weight and type II mesh. The AUGS-IUGA guideline recognizes that there is a paucity of data surrounding the management of mesh-related complications with the use of type I mesh [29].

The most common complications associated with sacrocolpopexy mesh are vaginal exposure and pain. In many cases, pain related to sacrocolpopexy mesh coincides with vaginal mesh exposure. In cases where a woman has new pain after sacrocolpopexy mesh placement but no vaginal mesh exposure, management can be more challenging. There are also a few unique and serious complications in regard to sacrocolpopexy mesh that a managing surgeon should be aware of including infection and osteomyelitis/discitis. These complications are briefly discussed below.

Unique Complications of Sacrocolpopexy: Osteomyelitis/Spondylodiscitis

Osteomyelitis/spondylodiscitis is a rare, yet serious complication of sacrocolpopexy and is less related to the use of mesh than it is to the misplacement of sutures or tacks deep into the L5-S1 disc space. A systematic review of 41 cases by Müller noted that back pain was the presenting symptom in 85% of women with osteomyelitis/spondylodiscitis so any woman presenting with persistent or worsening back pain after sacrocolpopexy should prompt further work-up. Other symptoms noted at time of presentation in their series included fever in 20 women (49%) and pain radiating to the legs in 9 women (22%). Average time to presentation after initial surgery was 76 days (range 30–165) [38].

The most common imaging modality used in evaluation is magnetic resonance imaging, which may reveal erosive changes to the bone with marrow edema and spondylodiscitis (Image). Additional work-up can include laboratory studies complete blood count (CBC) looking for leukocytosis. Inflammatory makers such as C-reactive protein and erythrocyte sedimentation rate (ESR) have also been used to aid in diagnosis. Blood cultures should be obtained in any woman presenting with fever and antibiotics initiated.

In the same series by Müller, about 1/3 of women were able to be managed conservatively with antibiotics alone, while the other 2/3 of women required surgical intervention [38]. Based on these limited data, the AUGS/IUGA guideline notes that there is insufficient evidence to advise when conservative versus surgical management is advisable in the setting of osteomyelitis/spondylodiscitis [29]. However, any woman with who presents with progressively worsening neurologic symptoms after sacrocolpopexy, such as loss of ability to walk or stand, should prompt *urgent* neurosurgical evaluation to avoid further loss of function (Fig. 1).

Synthetic Mesh Materials for Stress Urinary Incontinence

The synthetic midurethral sling was first developed for treatment of SUI in the 1990s and quickly gained popularity due to ease of insertion, short operative and convalesce times, and good

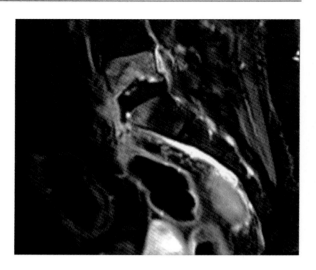

Fig. 1 Magnetic resonance imaging showing bone marrow edema at L5 and erosive osteochondrosis corresponding with progressive spondylodiscitis L5/S1 [38]. (Source: Müller et al. 2019. Open Access)

efficacy. In addition, the midurethral sling operation has demonstrated lower perioperative complication rates compared to other operations for SUI including autologous pubovaginal sling placement and colposuspension [19].

In the United States, the use of synthetic the midurethral sling remains strongly supported by the American Urological Association (AUA), the American Urogynecological Association (AUGA) and the Society of Urodynamics, Female Pelvic Medicine and Urogenital Reconstruction (SUFU). Additionally, the FDA concluded that the safety and efficacy of the midurethral sling has been well established (current as of April 2019). In a May 2019 position statement, the AUA Board of Directors stated that "any restriction of the use of synthetic polypropylene mesh suburethral slings would be a disservice to women who choose surgical correction of SUI" [4]. Most recently, AUGS and SUFU released a revised position statement in November 2021 stating "Polypropylene mesh midurethral slings are a standard of care for the surgical treatment of SUI and represent a great advancement in the treatment of this condition for our patients" [21]. Internationally, the synthetic mesh midurethral sling for SUI is still in routine use, with the exception of the United Kingdom and New Zealand, where there remains an active ban on all forms of transvaginal mesh placement [39].

In the United States, the synthetic midurethral sling is the most commonly performed operation for the indication of SUI [30, 53]. However, despite continued support of midurethral sling placement by the AUA, AUGS/SUFU, and the FDA, there has been a decline in the placement of midurethral slings following the FDA warnings. In a study by Siegal et al., the number of synthetic midurethral slings placed in the state of New York declined by 43% between 2011 and 2015, with a greater number of midurethral slings being placed by fellowship-trained Female Pelvic Medicine and Reconstructive Surgery (FPMRS) specialists [51]. Another study demonstrated a sustained decline in concomitant midurethral sling placement at the time of POP repair from 54.8% in July 2011 down to 38.9% through the end of 2015 following the FDA warning [17]. At academic medical centers, while the rates of midurethral sling placement have declined, the overall rate of treatment for SUI has remained stable, largely due to an increase in the number of autologous fascial pubovaginal slings being performed [46].

The rates of complications requiring reoperation after midurethral sling using type I mesh are generally low. One study reviewed outcomes of 3747 midurethral slings and found that at 21 months' follow-up, the rate of reoperation for voiding dysfunction, vaginal mesh exposure, and urethral exposure were 1.3%, 0.8%, and 0.08%, respectively [40]. In longer-term follow-up, two large retrospective cohort studies demonstrated that the risk of needing removal or revision of mesh for any reason after midurethral sling placement is between 3.3% and 5.3% at 9 and 10 years [8, 22].

Complications of Synthetic Midurethral Slings: Urinary Tract Infection and Voiding Dysfunction

As discussed above, the midurethral sling has demonstrated acceptably low complication and reoperation rates and remains approved for use in most countries worldwide. However, it is important for the female pelvic surgeon to be familiar with how to manage complications specific to synthetic midurethral slings.

Urinary Tract Infection after Midurethral Sling Placement: Acute and Recurrent

Development of a urinary tract infection in the short-term following midurethral sling placement (within 30–90 days) is a fairly common complication with estimated rates ranging from about 15–33% [3, 56], depending on the population studied and time frame used. Identified risk factors for developing a UTI in the postoperative period include increasing age, diabetes, and urinary retention requiring prolonged catheter use in the postoperative period [7]. Preoperative diagnosis of recurrent UTI is also associated with a post-op UTI within 6 weeks. It should be noted, however, that diagnosis of a UTI after an anti-incontinence surgery is not unique to mesh placement and is also commonly seen after colposuspension and autologous fascia pubovaginal sling placement [41].

Progression to recurrent UTI (rUTI), defined as two culture-proven UTIs over a 6-month period or three culture-proven UTIs in 1 year, is less common and ranges from 3.5 to 5.8% at 1 year [7, 23, 56]. Importantly, the most commonly identified and modifiable risk factor for recurrent UTI following midurethral sling placement is the diagnosis of rUTI preoperatively [23].

In a woman who develops de novo rUTI following midurethral sling placement, evaluation should include physical exam to assess for vaginal mesh exposure, a post-void residual measurement to ensure bladder emptying, and cystoscopy to rule out mesh exposure into the bladder and or urethra. There is little evidence to support mesh removal in a woman with recurrent UTI without mesh exposure or voiding dysfunction.

Voiding Dysfunction

Voiding dysfunction is a known complication following surgery for SUI and is not unique to synthetic midurethral sling placement. Additionally, synthetic midurethral slings are known to have lower rates of voiding dysfunction, urinary retention, and need for sling revision for these indications than with pubovaginal sling.

It's important to note, however, that unlike the pubovaginal sling which can loosen with time, obstruction or new voiding symptoms from a midurethral sling are unlikely to change with time and sling revision is often indicated. One study looked at midurethral sling revision for urinary symptoms and noted that 23.5% and 78.9% of women had complete resolution of urge urinary incontinence and of obstructive voiding symptoms, respectively. However, the authors also reported that de novo urgency incontinence and de novo SUI developed in 43.6% and 35.5% of women, respectively, with only 22.2% of women reporting that they were satisfied or very satisfied with their initial midurethral sling procedure [12].

Evaluation of Women Who Present with Mesh Complications

Any woman who presents with concern for mesh complications requires a thorough history and physical examination. Ancillary studies such as cystoscopy and imaging may be indicated and should be performed as needed to aid in evaluation and treatment planning.

History

Women who present with mesh complications may present with a wide array of symptoms including, but not limited to:

- Local symptoms: Vaginal discharge or bleeding, dyspareunia, hispareunia, vaginal pain, hematuria, dysuria, recurrent UTI.
- Regional symptoms: Groin pain, buttock pain, suprapubic pain, back pain, or pelvic pain away from known mesh placement sites.
- Systemic symptoms (rare): immunologic type symptoms such as rashes, hair loss, and diarrhea have been reported after mesh placement [1, 47].

A thorough inventory of symptoms should be documented along with the impact of these symptoms on the woman's quality of life. Additionally, it is important to understand the timing, duration, and severity of the symptoms that the woman experiencing in order to assess whether these symptoms are temporally related to mesh placement or if they could have other possible etiologies.

Finally, information should be obtained regarding what type of mesh was placed and when, along with the indication for placement. Ideally, previous operative reports should be obtained and reviewed when available. Many women may seek care from another physician other than the operating surgeon who originally placed the mesh implant [1].

Physical Examination

All women should undergo a physical exam including abdominopelvic exam to assess for abdominal of suprapubic tenderness. In the case of midurethral sling, sling entry or exit sites should be examined in either the suprapubic area or groin as there can occasionally be issues with scarring, pain, granulation, or sinus tract formation. Vaginal exam should include both visual inspection and palpation to assess for any sites of significant pain or mesh exposure. For women with a history of posterior mesh placement, a digital rectal exam is recommended [27].

While most women will tolerate an exam in the office, some women with more severe pain may require an exam under anesthesia in the operation room. This would also be an appropriate time to perform cystoscopy if indicated.

Cystoscopy

Cystoscopy is routinely recommended for any woman presenting with a mesh complication who has history of a midurethral sling or any anterior or apically placed mesh, either transvaginal or abdominally, especially if those complaints include new bladder pain, dysuria, hematuria, or recurrent UTIs. In general, cystoscopy should be performed prior to any trip to the operating room for mesh excision to allow for adequate surgical planning and counselling [47]. In a patient who cannot tolerate cystoscopy in the office, exam under anesthesia may be considered prior to definitive surgical intervention.

Imaging Studies

The decision to employ imaging studies in the evaluation of a woman presenting with mesh complications is often made on a case-by-case basis. For non-urgent complications in which adequate information can be obtained by history, physical exam, and cystoscopy alone, additional imaging is often not necessary prior to intervention. However, in cases where inadequate information cannot be obtained from the history and physical or the woman presents with more severe or urgent complaints, imaging studies should be considered and utilized as appropriate.

The type of imaging study used largely depends on the question to be answered but also what imaging modalities may be available to the

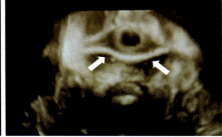

Fig. 2 Translabial Ultrasound (TLUS) demonstrating the appearance of two types of midurethral slings. (**a**) shows a retropubic sling with a more vertical trajectory. (**b**) depicts a TOT sling with a horizontal appearance headed towards the obturator canal

Table 1 Imaging Modalities used for Assessment of Mesh Complications

	Good for:	Advantages	Limitations
Translabial ultrasound (TLUS)	Assessment of vaginal orientation of midurethral slings and transvaginal mesh	Minimally invasive No contrast or radiation exposure Can be done in office	Cannot view mesh outside of the vagina Not available at many facilities
Computed tomography (CT)	Thorough anatomic assessment Assessment of stones or abscesses CT Urogram can identify ureteral involvement	Quick, can be done in an acute setting Readily available	Contrast and radiation exposure
Magnetic resonance imaging (MRI)	Soft tissue delineation including evaluation of nerve entrapment Evaluation of issues with sacrocolpopexy mesh including back pain	Provides more complete information for a pain evaluation due to improved visualization of muscle and nerves	May be less available in acute setting Patient-related factors (claustrophobia, implants) may limit ability to perform
Fluoroscopy	Assessing for fistulae related to mesh Identifying urethral obstruction from a tight sling (voiding cystourethrogram)	Can be done in office (when available) Provides real-time information	Cannot visualize mesh

evaluating physician and patient. For example, translabial ultrasound (TLUS) is a useful noninvasive tool for assessing characteristics of transvaginal mesh and midurethral slings; however not all physicians and facilities offer this modality [47, 52]. Figure 2 demonstrates the difference between a retropubic and transobturator sling seen on TLUS.

Table 1 summarizes the various types of imaging modalities that can be used in the evaluation of mesh complications along with the advantages and disadvantages of each.

Management of Mesh Complications

After completion of a thorough history and evaluation, the decision to pursue surgical intervention for mesh complications should come as the result of an informed discussion between the patient and surgeon. This section will discuss indications for mesh removal in concordance with the 2020 AUGA/IUGA "Joint Position Statement on the Management of Mesh-Complications for the FPRMS Specialist" [29].

Dyspareunia and Pain

Pelvic and vaginal pain are relatively common in women, so it is important to discern the role that a mesh implant may play in an individual's pain to help determine the appropriate intervention(s). An important aspect of this history to discern is temporality of symptoms – whether the onset of the pain occurred after mesh placement or if the patients' pre-existing pain was worsened by placement. A comprehensive pelvic exam should be performed to assess for both myofascial pain and tenderness along with specific assessment of pain with palpation over all aspects of the mesh. If a woman has a significant amount of myofascial pain, pelvic floor physical therapy can be offered. However, if the pain is more referrable to the mesh itself, there are limited data to support the role of PT in this setting, which may delay more appropriate interventions for the individual [29].

For a woman with pain that is clearly referrable to the mesh with no other abnormalities (e.g., mesh extrusion), another option includes trigger point injections with steroid and/or analgesic, but data surrounding this practice is limited. Surgical excision of the mesh can and should be considered in women with pain referrable to the mesh, especially if pain has remained refractory to conservative measures [29].

The extent of mesh to excise in a woman with pain depends on a number of factors:

1. Is the pain localized to one area or is it more diffuse over the entire mesh? If localized, it is reasonable to consider excision of a small segment to minimize morbidity of a large excision. If pain is more diffuse of regional, a more extensive removal should be considered.
2. What type of mesh is in place? In general, for localized vaginal pain for midurethral sling and transvaginal mesh, it is reasonable to excise only the transvaginal portion.
3. Are there concomitant mesh issues such as exposure or extrusion? If so, then a larger excision to treat these issues is necessary.

In counselling a woman on mesh removal for pain, it is important to note that up to one-quarter to one-half of women will still have some degree of pain despite adequate mesh removal [26].

Vaginal Mesh Exposure

Rates of vaginal mesh exposure vary due to a variety of factors including mesh composition, location of mesh placement (e.g., anterior compartment), and patient-related factors. Symptoms of vaginal mesh exposure can include local vaginal irrigation, vaginal pain, abnormal vaginal discharge or bleeding, dyspareunia, or pain for the partner (often termed "hispareunia") [1, 47].

Asymptomatic

An asymptomatic mesh extrusion occurs in an individual in whom vaginal mesh exposure is incidentally noted on exam but reports no bothersome symptoms. In the absence of symptoms, women can safely be observed regardless of mesh type (i.e., midurethral sling, sacrocolpopexy, and transvaginal meshes), and some series have reported that individuals can be safely observed with minimal complications for up to 10 years [16]. Vaginal estrogen in asymptomatic women may be offered, but its efficacy in resolution of exposures is not well established. The practice of observing asymptomatic women is supported by the AUGS/IUGA Guideline [29].

Symptomatic

In a woman with symptomatic mesh exposure, excision is the gold standard treatment. If an exposure is small, office-based trimming can be considered, although women should be counselled that the recurrence of mesh exposure is high (up to 75% in some series) and will likely require future excisions [1]. Mesh excision in the operating room is the treatment of choice for symptomatic exposures of both midurethral sling and transvaginal mesh. In general, the amount of mesh to remove is a balance of risk and benefits between recurrence of SUI or POP and preventing repeat symptomatic mesh exposures [29].

Overall, rates of recurrent vaginal mesh exposure after any partial mesh removal are not well established, as most studies only report on need for additional treatment, mostly in the form of repeat mesh excision. According to a recent systemic review, rates of repeat mesh excision after initial surgery range from 11 to 29.3% [10]. Given this risk of repeat mesh exposure, all women undergoing partial mesh removal should be counselled that there is up to a 30% risk of repeat vaginal mesh exposure that could require a repeat surgery to address.

In women with exposed sacrocolpopexy mesh, while partial excision may be performed, women should be counselled that there is an increased likelihood of repeat vaginal mesh exposure, up to 50% in some series. Quiroz et al. [45] found that no repeat vaginal mesh excisions were successful and that all cases required complete mesh excision after second or third failed vaginal mesh excision. Therefore, in the case of sacrocolpopexy mesh, repetitive trimming/excision procedures are not recommended after repeat exposure due to the risk of disrupting the integrity of the mesh which would make subsequent complete excision more challenging [29].

Infection

As discussed in the previous section on mesh types, infection was a more common occurrence with the use of non-type I mesh for both SUI and POP compared to use of heavier and multifilament meshes. Fortunately, rates of infection related to type I polypropylene mesh itself are very low in both short- and long-term settings. This is true for transvaginal, sacrocolpopexy, and midurethral sling mesh. Given that all commercially available mesh products on the market now consist of type I polypropylene mesh only, the risk of a surgeon encountering a mesh infection in the acute postoperative setting is quite low.

One case report describes management of 22 cases of infected sacrocolpopexy mesh, all of which involved concomitant vaginal mesh exposure. The management in all 22 cases involved complete mesh excision. Importantly, none of these 22 cases used type I polypropylene mesh [36].

There are only rare reports of infected type I sacrocolpopexy mesh.

Osteomyelitis/spondylodiscitis is a rare but serious complication that can occur after sacrocolpopexy and was previously discussed in section "Unique Complications of Sacrocolpopexy: Osteomyelitis/Spondylodiscitis."

While infection today remains an uncommon complication of type I mesh implants, any serious or suppurative infection requires prompt evaluation and treatment, with the expectation that all mesh may need to be removed to clear the infection.

Table 2 provides a brief summary of complications management for pain, vaginal exposure, and infection.

Visceral Injury

Mesh exposure into viscera can be one of the most devastating complications of synthetic mesh placement that often leads to significant morbidity and almost always requires surgical intervention. Surgical excision of mesh can involve a variety of techniques depending on the patient's presentation and symptoms, the surgeon's level of comfort and expertise with various surgical techniques, and the location and degree of mesh exposure.

This section describes the presentation, diagnostic evaluation, and various management strategies of women presenting with mesh exposure into the urethra, bladder, ureter, and/or rectum. This section will also cover management of visceral injuries that may occur at the time of complex mesh removal.

Bladder and Urethra

Women with mesh exposure in the bladder or urethra may present with irritative lower urinary tract symptoms that include urinary frequency, urgency, dysuria, bladder pain, recurrent urinary tract infections, and hematuria (either gross or microscopic). For mesh that has entered the urethral lumen, women may also describe voiding difficulties such as weak or intermittent stream. While many of these symptoms are non-specific for mesh exposure into the lower urinary tract, the

Table 2 Management of Pain, Vaginal Mesh Exposure, and Infection

	Pain referrable to mesh		Vaginal mesh exposure		Infection
	Vaginal	Regional	Asymptomatic[a]	Symptomatic[b]	
Midurethral sling	Vaginal excision, partial or complete	Extravaginal mesh excision +/− vaginal mesh excision	Observation	Vaginal excision of exposed mesh, partial or complete	Total mesh excision (extirpation)
Sacrocolpopexy mesh	Partial vaginal excision may be considered; will likely require total mesh excision (extirpation)	Limited data for pain only; likely require total mesh excision (extirpation)	Observation	Partial excision of exposed mesh can be considered once Total mesh excision (extirpation) if recurrence	Total mesh excision (extirpation)
Transvaginal mesh	Vaginal excision, partial or complete	Extravaginal mesh excision +/− vaginal mesh excision	Observation	Vaginal excision of exposed mesh, partial or complete	Total mesh excision (extirpation)

[a]Vaginal estrogen may be offered but limited evidence to support use in this setting
[b]Office-based trimming can be considered for all small vaginal exposures but has high rates of recurrence (up to 75%)

surgeon should maintain a low index of suspicion in women with a history of mesh placement who present with these bothersome complaints, particularly if they are recurrent or persistent after failing conservative therapy.

Cystoscopy and pelvic exam are the diagnostic modalities of choice to evaluate for mesh exposure in either the bladder or urethra. Translabial ultrasound (TLUS) can be helpful to identify the orientation, location, and extent of either midurethral or transvaginal grafts, particularly when outside operative reports are unavailable [52]. Other imaging and diagnostic modalities such as CT are MRI are generally less useful in this setting.

Table 3 summarizes management of mesh complications in the bladder and urethra.

Endoscopic Management of Midurethral Sling Exposure

In cases where midurethral sling exposure is found in the bladder and/or urethra, endoscopic management has been utilized with good success. Various techniques have been described including the use of an electrode loop with the resectoscope,

use of laparoscopic scissors, and use of the holmium laser.

A recent systematic review identified 13 case series in which 108 women underwent holmium laser excision of mesh exposure in the urethra, bladder neck, or bladder. Initial success was achieved in 72 women (67%) with a single procedure, and final success was achieved in 92% of women after one (17%), two (5.6%), or three or more (2.8%) additional endoscopic procedures. Only nine women (8%) in the series went on to require vaginal surgery to remove mesh with one patient requiring open cystolithotomy. The most notable complication was new or worsening SUI in 21% with no serious complications noted [32].

Both cystoscope and lens type along with holmium laser settings vary in the different series. A small laser fiber may be used (200–365 micron) with laser settings of 0.5 to 0.8 J at 5 to 20 Hz [25]. Some authors use the laser to fragment the mesh entirely while others use the laser to excise the mesh at the base and then extract [15]. In proper hands, holmium laser can be an effective tool for removing mesh and stones associated with mesh from the lower urinary tract.

Table 3 Surgical Management Options for Mesh Exposure in the Bladder and Urethra

	Midurethral sling – bladder	Midurethral sling – urethra	Transvaginal mesh – bladder	Sacrocolpopexy mesh – bladder
Endoscopic	Good for mesh exposure with stones. May risk leaving mesh behind increasing risk of recurrence	Good for mesh exposure with stones. Limited by adequate visualization and working space	Less described but risks leaving mesh with risk of recurrence	Could consider for stone removal or small exposure. Risk of recurrence
Transvaginal	Limited to sling exposure at the bladder neck or trigone (ureteral stent placement recommended in this scenario). Not feasible for sling arm exposure into bladder lumen	Ideal for removing all mesh in urethra	Ideal route for removing most TVM. Ureteral stent placement recommended	Not recommended due to ability to only remove part of the mesh
Abdominal (either open or laparoscopic)	Good for sling arm exposure at the anterior wall that cannot be reached via transvaginal route	Not indicated	Can consider if mesh exposure is extensive or associated with known ureteral involvement with need for reimplantation	Ideal approach to allow for good exposure and adequate bladder closure

The same review by Karim et al. also examined use of other endoscopic methods such as electrode loop with a resectoscope and use of laparoscopic scissors/forceps in 90 women. While initial success rates after a single procedure were noted to be higher than with holmium laser (80%), development of vesicovaginal fistula was seen in three women, along with two intraperitoneal and one extraperitoneal bladder injuries that required repair [32].

There is little data on use of endoscopic approaches for larger portion mesh, such as those used for anterior and apical repairs. Given the larger size of these meshes, adequate mesh excision via an endoscopic approach is less feasible and likely to result in higher rates of recurrence.

Vaginal Approaches for Midurethral Sling Exposure in the Urethra

Depending on the extent of mesh exposure in the urethra, the surgeon may opt for a transvaginal approach at mesh removal, especially if mesh exposure in to the urethral lumen is extensive.

A common technique to address mesh exposure in the urethra employs the use of an inverted U-incision to allow for creation of a vaginal flap along adequate exposure of the entire urethra and bladder neck. The urethra can then be opened to allow for complete excision of the exposed mesh. In most cases, the urethra can be closed primarily with absorbable suture followed by closure of the periurethral fascia [47]. In women with urethral exposure and concomitant urethrovaginal fistula, mesh excision can be undertaken from the fistulous tract with closure of the urethra performed. All cases of urethral repair should be performed with three layers of closure; the use of an interposition flap can be used at the discretion of the surgeon (Fig. 3).

In the case of significant urethral damage where the urethra is significantly shortened, or if there is inadequate tissue to perform primary urethral closure, the use of grafts or flaps may need to be necessary. Complex urethral reconstruction is described in more detail in ▶ Chap. 41, "Reconstruction of the Absent or Severely Damaged Urethra."

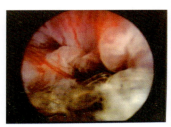
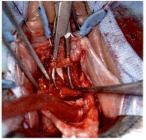
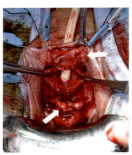

Fig. 3 Sling mesh removal in a patient with urethral exposure. (**a**) depicts cystoscopic view of mesh in the urethral lumen. (**b**) Isolation of the urethral mesh. To get this exposure, an inverted U vaginal flap was created followed by opening the periurethral fascia transversely to expose the urethra. (**c**) All urethral mesh is removed leaving the urethral lumen free of mesh. The urethra may then be closed primary using delayed absorbable suture. The periurethral fascia is closed transversely (depicted by white arrows) followed by the U-shaped vaginal flap

Vaginal Approaches for Transvaginal Mesh Exposure in the Bladder

For women with complications of transvaginal mesh with exposure into the bladder, a vaginal approach may be considered to avoid the morbidity of an abdominal operation. Temporary intraoperative ureteral stent placement should be strongly considered at the time of anterior transvaginal mesh removal to help recognize and avoid inadvertent injury to the ureter.

Operative technique may employ the use of an inverted U-vaginal flap and with exposure of the bladder and any overlying mesh. Upon entry into the bladder, care should be taken to excise all mesh and to ensure clean bladder edges prior to closure. Two-layer closure with absorbable suture is then performed, followed by the placement of a interposition flap at the surgeon's discretion. The third layer of closure is the vaginal flap [18] (Fig. 4).

Abdominal Removal of Mesh Exposure in the Bladder

An abdominal approach for mesh removal may be indicated for retropubic midurethral sling mesh exposure as the location of the retropubic midurethral sling arms, when exposed, are generally anterolateral and therefore not easily accessible from a vaginal approach. Depending on the clinical scenario, the surgeon may choose an initial abdominal approach for mesh removal based on their experience and comfort with this approach.

Sacrocolpopexy mesh exposure in the bladder tends to occur as a posterior location, and possible sites of exposure can be seen as low as the trigone ranging up the dome. Given that this mesh is placed via an abdominal approach, it is most amenable to an abdominal removal. Additionally, as discussed in section "Vaginal Mesh Exposure," partial or piecemeal removal of sacrocolpopexy mesh is generally not recommended making endoscopic and transvaginal approaches less favorable.

Both open abdominal and laparoscopic approaches to mesh removal in the bladder have been described for both midurethral sling and sacrocolpopexy mesh. One series of midurethral sling removal reported on their technique involving intraperitoneal port placement followed by taking down the bladder from the anterior abdominal wall to expose the retropubic space. The mesh can be visualized on the posterior aspect of the pubic rami, dissected free from the anterior abdominal wall, and then followed to the sites of bladder entry. The bladder can then be opened anteriorly at sites of mesh entry, mesh excised, and the bladder closed in layers using absorbable suture [44].

Ureter

It is estimated that the ureter is injured in 0.3–3% of gynecologic and pelvic floor reconstructive surgeries. While mesh involvement of the ureter at the time of mesh placement is less common, there are reports of mesh exposure into the ureter

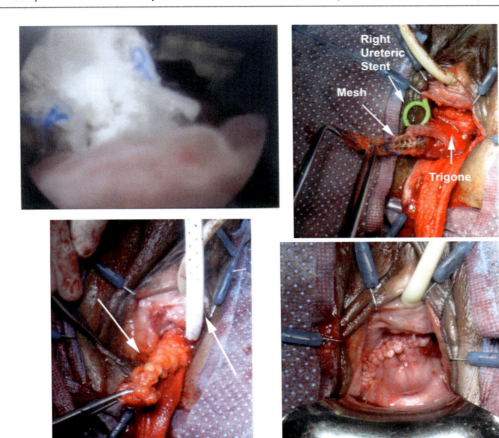

Fig. 4 Patient with history of anterior TVM presenting with urgency, frequency, pain, and recurrent UTI. (**a**) Cystoscopy demonstrates mesh at the trigone extending to the right lateral wall. (**b**) Exposure of the anterior vaginal wall is obtained and the mesh is dissected free of the trigone. A right ureteral stent was placed to aid in ureteral identification. (**c**) An in-situ labial flap is used to help cover the closure and a retropubic drain was inserted. (**d**) Anterior vaginal wall flap is advanced to cover the area of reconstruction. (Source: Raz Atlas of Vaginal Surgery. Springer. (Still awaiting Permission))

over time [47]. Additionally, the ureter may be encountered at the time of complex anterior mesh removal. As discussed in the previous section, temporary intraoperative ureteral stent placement is advisable at the time of anterior mesh removal to both help prevent ureteral injury and to better identify injury should one occur.

Ureteral Injury at Time of Mesh Removal

Small ureteral injuries may be managed with primary closure or anastomosis using absorbable suture over a ureteral stent. Larger injuries may necessitate ureteral reimplantation (ureteroneocystostomy).

Mesh Exposure into Rectum

Posterior compartment mesh is the least commonly used type of transvaginal mesh and there are lower rates of associated complications and reoperations for mesh in this compartment compared to the anterior compartment. The majority of complications related to posterior use of vaginal mesh are limited to vaginal mesh exposure, with rates of approximately 2% [40].

Vaginal discharge that is copious or foul-smelling should raise concern for mesh infection, which may be due to possible concomitant mesh exposure into the rectum. Mesh exposure into the

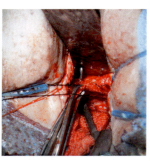
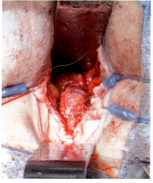
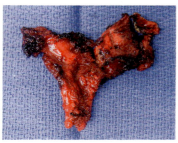

Fig. 5 Posterior mesh removal in a patient with rectal pain and vaginal mesh exposure. (**a**) depicts careful dissection of the mesh off the rectum. (**b**) The white arrow depicts the rectal wall free of mesh. The vaginal wall is retracted cephalad. (**c**) The posterior mesh removed intact

rectum itself may be associated with pain with defecation or with blood in the stool. Diagnostic evaluation in the office should involve a thorough physical exam, including both vaginal and rectal exams. Digital rectal exam should be performed to see if there is palpable mesh or suture in the rectal vault. If there is concern for rectal involvement, anoscopy may be performed to help further define the extent of involvement and aid in both diagnosis and surgical planning.

Surgical correction of vaginal mesh exposure in the posterior compartment was previously described in section "Vaginal Mesh Exposure."

For posterior mesh with concern for infection, the entirety of the mesh should be excised, particularly if the mesh is a type II multifilamentous mesh. If the mesh involves the rectal wall or if the rectal wall is entered during mesh excision, closure should be performed. For small transgressions into the rectal wall, the rectum may be closed primarily with absorbable suture with consideration of an interposition graft depending on the size and extent of the defect similar to the closure of a rectovaginal fistula [47]. For involvement of the rectal wall that requires a larger rectal excision, rectal wall advancement may be performed with advancement of the more proximal rectal mucosa to the anal verge. Additionally, depending on the surgeons' experience and level of comfort with managing and repairing the rectal injury, colorectal surgery consultation may be warranted.

In cases of more extensive exposure through the rectal wall with no vaginal wall involvement, complete transanal excision of the mesh has been described with good results [9].

Figure 5 depicts complete transvaginal removal of posterior mesh in a patient with pain and vaginal mesh exposure.

Complications After Mesh Removal

While many women experience relief and quality of life improvement after mesh removal surgery, many are left with new or recurrent pelvic floor issues that need to be addressed. Some of these issues may include recurrent SUI, recurrent POP, persistent or worsening vaginal or pelvic pain, recurrent mesh exposure, and loss of vaginal length or vaginal canal stenosis. In this section, we discuss some of these longer-term complications along with suggestions for management.

Recurrent SUI After Synthetic Midurethral Sling Removal

Recurrent SUI is common after both partial and complete mesh excisions of midurethral sling mesh regardless of the indication for mesh removal, whether it's for pain, mesh exposure, or voiding dysfunction. Therefore, all women undergoing revision should be counselled that there is a risk of recurrent SUI after sling revision and that risk appears to increase as a larger portion of the sling is excised (e.g., partial versus complete excision).

A study by Jambusaria et al. found that when midurethral slings were removed for vaginal exposure, women who had complete rather than partial mesh removal were at an increased risk of having SUI symptoms (65.4% versus 28.6%, respectively, $p = 0.01$) at 29 weeks' follow-up. The rates of having repeat SUI surgery in this same cohort were 37.2% with complete excision versus 14.3%, with only partial excision, $p = 0.09$. When mesh was removed for the indication of pain, there was a higher incidence of recurrent stress incontinence with complete sling removal at long-term follow-up (22% vs. 56%); however this finding did not reach statistical significance ($p = 0.07$) [28].

Management of recurrent SUI after mesh removal involves an informed preoperative discussion between the patient and the treating physician. In general, the options for treating recurrent SUI are similar to those of a treatment-naïve patient and can include both surgical and non-surgical options. However, depending on the indication for mesh removal and degree of morbidity from the prior mesh sling, both the patient and physician may opt for a non-mesh approach for future treatment.

Non-surgical options can include use of topical vaginal estrogen, pelvic floor muscle exercises, either with or without a physical therapist, or the use of a vaginal device such as an incontinence pessary. Non-mesh procedural options include the use of urethral bulking agents, placement of an autologous fascial pubovaginal sling, or colposuspension.

Persistent or Worsening Pain

As discussed in section "Management of Mesh Complications – Dyspareunia and Pain," many women do experience at least some, and others complete, relief of pelvic pain and dyspareunia with mesh removal. However, a significant number of women continue to experience pain despite mesh removal surgery. This has been seen after all types of mesh removal, including midurethral sling, transvaginal mesh, and sacrocolpopexy mesh. Rates of residual pain in the literature range from 11.4% to 19.5%, with 8.2% of women reporting worsening pain following mesh removal [14, 26].

Pain or dyspareunia that persists or worsens after mesh removal can be devastating for women, especially if this was their main indication for removal. It is important for surgeons seeing women with pain following mesh removal to be able to offer reassurance, compassion, and guidance of other pathways moving forward. Continued pain management strategies may involve but are not limited to:

- Pelvic floor physical therapy
- Vaginal suppositories. Agents can include diazepam, baclofen, and ketamine
- Pelvic floor trigger point injections
- Pelvic floor onabotulinum-A toxin injection
- Referral to pain management specialist for multimodal pain approach
- Referral to psychology or pain psychology to help with coping strategies
- Oral non-narcotic pain management agents within the prescriber's comfort level and scope of practice

Recurrent Prolapse

As all women undergoing POP surgery are a risk of POP recurrence, it is not entirely clear what role mesh removal plays in recurrent prolapse. A recent systematic review by Carter et al. examined the results of four studies and found that the rate of recurrent POP after transvaginal mesh removal ranged from 3.6 to 16%, which is not greater that known prolapse recurrence rates overall [10]. Regardless, any woman undergoing removal of prolapse mesh should be counselled that her prolapse may recur, or even worsen, as a result of mesh removal surgery.

At the time of vaginal mesh removal, it is reasonable for the surgeon to attempt to reapproximate/plicate what is left of the perivesical fascia anteriorly and rectovaginal septum anteriorly and posteriorly to reduce any obvious defects. If the peritoneal cavity is entered to remove mesh either vaginally or laparoscopically, uterosacral ligament plication and/or suspension or culdoplasty can be considered. At time of complete sacrocolpopexy mesh removal, some authors have reported the use of rectus fascia to perform a concomitant sacrocolpopexy with good outcomes at 9-month follow-up [43]. All decisions to address risk of recurrent prolapse at the time of mesh removal should be at discretion of the operating surgeon and should occur after an informed discussion of risks and benefits with the patient.

Following mesh removal, women should be monitored for symptom recurrence and offered treatment, should symptomatic POP recur. Treatment can include both non-surgical options such pelvic floor physical therapy or pessary and repeat surgical correction of POP at the discretion of the patient and the surgeon. Importantly, transvaginal mesh should not be used.

Recurrent Vaginal Mesh Exposure

Similar to what was previously discussed in section "Management of Mesh Complications: Vaginal Mesh Exposure," women with asymptomatic exposures can be managed expectantly with observation. In women with symptomatic recurrences, there is little guidance on what to do in the setting of repeat exposure of either midurethral sling or transvaginal meshes, so the decision of whether to proceed with additional partial versus complete mesh removal should include an in depth discussion of risks and benefits. However, for women with repeat symptomatic mesh exposure of sacrocolpopexy mesh, the AUGA/IUGA guideline recommends complete mesh removal versus another attempt at partial removal [29].

Loss of Vaginal Length or Vaginal Canal Stenosis

Loss of vaginal length or canal stenosis can result from when significant portions of vaginal skin are involved in mesh exposure requiring excision or if

there is significant scarring that results from mesh removal surgery. While significant loss of vaginal length is a relatively uncommon complication resulting from mesh removal, its effects can be devastating. Women may be left with vaginal length that is inadequate for penetrative intercourse, which can adversely affect quality of life and relationships for affected women and couples.

In a woman who has healed from mesh removal surgery but is left with either vaginal shortening or canal stenosis, a number of strategies may be offered to the patient. This section will briefly outline some of these management options, but it's important to note that most literature surrounding the management of a shortened vaginal canal comes from the vaginal agenesis population, most commonly Mayer–Rokitansky–Küster–Hauser (MRKH) syndrome and androgen insensitivity syndrome (AIS), along with post-radiation vaginal stenosis.

Vaginal Dilation

Serial vaginal dilation is the least invasive management option for both loss of length and canal stenosis. It is also associated with significantly lower rates of complication and morbidity than the more complex surgical management options discussed below. While there is limited data in the post-mesh removal patient, some authors support the early use of vaginal dilation +/− the use of a topical corticosteroid to help prevent further scarring and stenosis [2].

Increased frequency of dilation is associated with higher rates of anatomic success. Despite good rates of success, some barriers to vaginal dilation may include patient discomfort, poor understanding of the technique, poor compliance with therapy, or cost associated with purchasing dilators [42]. For physicians who are not well versed in vaginal dilation techniques and instructions, many pelvic floor physical therapists are trained in vaginal dilations and may be employed to assist in patient education, selection of dilators, follow-up, and maintenance of therapy.

Surgical Management Options

Surgical correction of vaginal shortening or canal stenosis in the form of vaginoplasty or neovagina can be considered in a woman in whom there is significant scarring not amenable to dilation or if a woman has tried and failed dilation. Any woman considering surgical revision should be counselled that vaginal dilation will likely still need to be performed at least periodically, if not regularly, even after surgery. One exception to this may be when the intestine is used for neovaginal creation and opposed to skin flaps and/or peritoneum.

Full description of these complex reconstructive techniques is outside the scope of this chapter, but it is important to be aware of various techniques that can be employed which include:

- Full or split thickness rotational skin flap placed into a dissected vaginal opening
- Surgical onlay of mobilized peritoneum cephalad to vagina caudally to extend length (e.g., Davydov procedure)
- Use of intestinal segment (usually ileum, jejunum, cecum, and sigmoid colon have been described)

Future Directions

More women are aware of mesh-related complications and may elect for mesh-free repairs even at the risk of higher rates of recurrence or increased risk of perioperative morbidity to avoid mesh-related complications later on. As surgeons who treat SUI and POP, there remains a fine balance between managing mesh-related risks, rates of surgical success, and patient expectations.

As a response to mesh-related concerns for SUI, rates of midurethral sling placement have declined with an increase in autologous pubovaginal sling placement. Other materials such as cadaveric fascia and xenografts have demonstrated low efficacy overtime so they have largely been abandoned. Regenerative medicine is an area of active research interest with investigators looking into treatment modalities such as stem cell therapy, biomaterials, and tissue engineering, along with energy-related therapies to aid in tissue regeneration. A number of trials are ongoing in these areas.

For POP, vaginal repairs using native tissue remain good options as there is little evidence to support the use of cadaveric grafts or xenografts to augment repairs. For sacrocolpopexy, cadaveric fascia lata was found to be inferior to mesh-augmented repairs at 5 years' follow-up with regard to anatomic success rates (62% vs. 93%, respectively, $p = 0.02$) [54]. More contemporary series have examined the use of autologous fascia to interpose between the vagina and the sacrum with good short-term results [50]. There have been some similar investigations into the role of biomaterials and tissue engineering for POP repair.

Conclusions

While overall rates of mesh complications have declined considerably both from the cessation of placement of transvaginal mesh, along with the use of type I polypropylene mesh for SUI and sacrocolpopexy, these rates are not zero and can lead to significant distress for women who experience these complications. All surgeons offering synthetic mesh for the correction of either SUI or POP should have a thorough understanding of these risks and be able to have a meaningful discussion of risks, benefits, and alternatives with every patient. Surgeons should be comfortable with the management of complications that may arise from placement of mesh materials, many of which were outlined in this chapter. Future research and innovation into both prevention and correction of SUI and POP will hopefully help further minimize risks to women while optimizing outcomes and quality of life benefits.

Cross-References

▶ Management of Vaginal Posterior Compartment Prolapse: Is There Ever a Case for Graft/Mesh?
▶ Open Abdominal Sacrocolpopexy
▶ Sling Operations for Stress Urinary Incontinence and Their Historical Evolution: Autologous, Cadaveric, and Synthetic Slings

► Vaginal Vault Prolapse: Options for Transvaginal Surgical Repair

References

1. Abbott S, Unger CA, Evans JM, et al. Evaluation and management of complications from synthetic mesh after pelvic reconstructive surgery: a multicenter study. Am J Obstet Gynecol. 2014;210(2):163.e1–8. https://doi.org/10.1016/j.ajog.2013.10.012.
2. Amankwah YA, Haefner HK, Brincat CA. Management of vulvovaginal strictures/shortened vagina. Clin Obstet Gynecol. 2010;53(1):125–33. https://doi.org/10.1097/GRF.0b013e3181ce8a89.
3. Anger JT, Litwin MS, Wang Q, Pashos CL, Rodríguez LV. Complications of sling surgery among female Medicare beneficiaries. Obstet Gynecol. 2007;109:707–14.
4. AUA Position Statement on the Use of Vaginal Mesh for the Surgical Treatment of Stress Urinary Incontinence (SUI). AUA Board of Directors, May 2019 (Revised). https://www.auanet.org/about-us/policy-and-position-statements/use-of-vaginal-mesh-for-the-surgical-treatment-of-stress-urinary-incontinence
5. Baessler K, Hewson AD, Tunn R, Schuessler B, Maher CF. Severe mesh complications following intravaginal slingplasty. Obstet Gynecol. 2005;106(4):713–6. https://doi.org/10.1097/01.AOG.0000177970.52037.0a.
6. Bafghi A, Valerio L, Benizri EI, Trastour C, Benizri EJ, Bongain A. Comparison between monofilament and multifilament polypropylene tapes in urinary incontinence. Eur J Obstet Gynecol and Reprod Biol. 2005;122(2):232–6. https://doi.org/10.1016/j.ejogrb.2005.01.008.
7. Berger AA, Tan-Kim J, Menefee SA. The impact of midurethral sling surgery on the development of urinary tract infections. Int Urogynecol J. 2022;33(4):829–34. https://doi.org/10.1007/s00192-021-04779-x. Published online April 2, 2021
8. Brennand EA, Quan H. Evaluation of the effect of surgeon's operative volume and specialty on likelihood of revision after mesh midurethral sling placement. Obstet Gynecol. 2019;133(6):1099–108. https://doi.org/10.1097/AOG.0000000000003275.
9. Campagna G, Panico G, Caramazza D, et al. Rectal mesh erosion after posterior vaginal kit repair. Int Urogynecol J. 2019;30(3):499–500. https://doi.org/10.1007/s00192-018-3782-4.
10. Carter P, Fou L, Whiter F, et al. Management of mesh complications following surgery for stress urinary incontinence or pelvic organ prolapse: a systematic review. BJOG. 2020;127(1):28–35. https://doi.org/10.1111/1471-0528.15958.
11. Coda A, Lamberti R, Martorana S. Classification of prosthetics used in hernia repair based on weight and biomaterial. Hernia. 2012;16(1):9–20. https://doi.org/10.1007/s10029-011-0868-z.
12. Crescenze IM, Abraham N, Li J, Goldman HB, Vasavada S. Urgency incontinence before and after revision of a synthetic mid urethral sling. J Urol. 2016;196(2):478–83. https://doi.org/10.1016/j.juro.2016.01.091.
13. Culligan PJ, Lewis C, Priestley J, Mushonga N. Long-term outcomes of robotic-assisted laparoscopic sacrocolpopexy using lightweight Y-mesh. Female Pelvic Med Reconstr Surg. 2020;26(3):202–6. https://doi.org/10.1097/SPV.0000000000000788.
14. Danford JM, Osborn DJ, Reynolds WS, Biller DH, Dmochowski RR. Postoperative pain outcomes after transvaginal mesh revision. Int Urogynecol J. 2015;26(1):65–9. https://doi.org/10.1007/s00192-014-2455-1.
15. Davis NF, Smyth LG, Giri SK, Flood HD. Evaluation of endoscopic laser excision of polypropylene mesh/sutures following anti-incontinence procedures. J Urol. 2012;188(5):1828–33. https://doi.org/10.1016/j.juro.2012.07.040.
16. Deffieux X, Thubert T, de Tayrac R, Fernandez H, Letouzey V. Long-term follow-up of persistent vaginal polypropylene mesh exposure for transvaginally placed mesh procedures. Int Urogynecol J. 2012;23(10):1387–90. https://doi.org/10.1007/s00192-012-1741-z.
17. Drain A, Khan A, Ohmann EL, et al. Use of concomitant stress incontinence surgery at time of pelvic organ prolapse surgery since release of the 2011 notification on serious complications associated with transvaginal mesh. J Urol. 2017;197(4):1092–8. https://doi.org/10.1016/j.juro.2016.11.087.
18. Firoozi F, Goldman HB. Transvaginal excision of mesh erosion involving the bladder after mesh placement using a prolapse kit: a novel technique. Urology. 2010;75(1):203–6. https://doi.org/10.1016/j.urology.2009.08.052.
19. Fusco F, Abdel-Fattah M, Chapple CR, et al. Updated systematic review and meta-analysis of the comparative data on colposuspensions, pubovaginal slings, and midurethral tapes in the surgical treatment of female stress urinary incontinence. Eur Urol. 2017;72(4):567–91. https://doi.org/10.1016/j.eururo.2017.04.026.
20. Giugale LE, Hansbarger MM, Askew AL, Visco AG, Shepherd JP, Bradley MS. Assessing pelvic organ prolapse recurrence after minimally invasive sacrocolpopexy: does mesh weight matter? Int Urogynecol J. 2021;32(8):2195–201. https://doi.org/10.1007/s00192-021-04681-6.
21. Goldman HB. Joint position statement on midurethral slings for stress urinary incontinence. Neurourol Urodyn. 2022;41(1):31–4. Published online November 22, 2021:nau.24838. https://doi.org/10.1002/nau.24838.
22. Gurol-Urganci I, Geary RS, Mamza JB, et al. Long-term rate of mesh sling removal following midurethral mesh sling insertion among women with stress urinary

incontinence. JAMA. 2018;320(16):1659. https://doi.org/10.1001/jama.2018.14997.

23. Hammett J, Lukman R, Oakes M, Whitcomb EL. Recurrent urinary tract infection after midurethral sling: a retrospective study. Female Pelvic Med Reconstr Surg. 2016;22(6):438–41. https://doi.org/10.1097/SPV.0000000000000308.

24. Haylen BT, Freeman RM, Swift SE, et al. An International Urogynecological Association (IUGA)/International Continence Society (ICS) joint terminology and classification of the complications related directly to the insertion of prostheses (meshes, implants, tapes) & grafts in female pelvic floor surgery. Int Urogynecol J. 2011;22(1):3–15. https://doi.org/10.1007/s00192-010-1324-9.

25. Hodroff M, Portis A, Siegel SW. Endoscopic removal of intravesical polypropylene sling with the holmium laser. J Urol. 2004;172(4 Part 1):1361–2. https://doi.org/10.1097/01.ju.0000139659.67173.e2.

26. Hou JC, Alhalabi F, Lemack GE, Zimmern PE. Outcome of transvaginal mesh and tape removed for pain only. J Urol. 2014;192(3):856–60. https://doi.org/10.1016/j.juro.2014.04.006.

27. Jacobs KM, Sammarco AG, Madsen AM. Historic transvaginal meshes and procedures: what did my patient have done? Curr Opin Obstet Gynecol. 2019;31(6):477–84. https://doi.org/10.1097/GCO.0000000000000587.

28. Jambusaria LH, Heft J, Reynolds WS, Dmochowski R, Biller DH. Incontinence rates after midurethral sling revision for vaginal exposure or pain. Am J Obstet Gynecol. 2016;215(6):764.e1–5. https://doi.org/10.1016/j.ajog.2016.07.031.

29. Joint Writing Group of the American Urogynecologic Society and the International Urogynecological Association. The AAGL endorses this document. The Society of Gynecologic Surgeons supports this document. Individual contributors are noted in the acknowledgment section. Joint position statement on the management of mesh-related complications for the FPMRS specialist. Female Pelvic Med Reconstr Surg. 2020;26(4):219–32. https://doi.org/10.1097/SPV.0000000000000853.

30. Jonsson Funk M, Levin PJ, Wu JM. Trends in the surgical management of stress urinary incontinence. Obstet Gynecol. 2012;119(4):845–51. https://doi.org/10.1097/AOG.0b013e31824b2e3e.

31. Jonsson Funk M, Edenfield AL, Pate V, Visco AG, Weidner AC, Wu JM. Trends in use of surgical mesh for pelvic organ prolapse. Am J Obstet Gynecol. 2013;208(1):79.e1–7. https://doi.org/10.1016/j.ajog.2012.11.008.

32. Karim SS, Pietropaolo A, Skolarikos A, et al. Role of endoscopic management in synthetic sling/mesh erosion following previous incontinence surgery: a systematic review from European Association of Urologists Young Academic Urologists (YAU) and Uro-technology (ESUT) groups. Int Urogynecol J. 2020;31(1):45–53. https://doi.org/10.1007/s00192-019-04087-5.

33. Khrucharoen U, Ramart P, Choi J, Kang D, Kim JH, Raz S. Clinical predictors and risk factors for vaginal mesh extrusion. World J Urol. 2018;36(2):299–304. https://doi.org/10.1007/s00345-017-2137-y.

34. Liang R, Knight K, Abramowitch S, Moalli PA. Exploring the basic science of prolapse meshes. Curr Opin Obstet Gynecol. 2016;28(5):413–9. https://doi.org/10.1097/GCO.0000000000000313.

35. Maher C, Feiner B, Baessler K, Christmann-Schmid C, Haya N, Marjoribanks J. Transvaginal mesh or grafts compared with native tissue repair for vaginal prolapse. Cochrane Database Syst Rev. 2016;2016(2):CD012079. https://doi.org/10.1002/14651858.CD012079.

36. Mattox TF, Stanford EJ, Varner E. Infected abdominal sacrocolpopexies: diagnosis and treatment. Int Urogynecol J Pelvic Floor Dysfunct. 2004;15(5):319–23. https://doi.org/10.1007/s00192-004-1170-8. Epub 2004 May 14. PMID: 15580416.

37. Menefee SA, Dyer KY, Lukacz ES, Simsiman AJ, Luber KM, Nguyen JN. Colporrhaphy compared with mesh or graft-reinforced vaginal paravaginal repair for anterior vaginal wall prolapse: a randomized controlled trial. Obstet Gynecol. 2011;118(6):1337–44. https://doi.org/10.1097/AOG.0b013e318237edc4.

38. Müller PC, Berchtold C, Kuemmerli C, Ruzza C, Z'Graggen K, Steinemann DC. Spondylodiscitis after minimally invasive recto- and colpo-sacropexy: report of a case and systematic review of the literature. J Minim Access Surg. 2020;16(1):5–12. https://doi.org/10.4103/jmas.JMAS_235_18.

39. Ng-Stollmann N. The international discussion and the new regulations concerning transvaginal mesh implants in pelvic organ prolapse surgery. Int Urogynecol J. 2020;31:1997–2002. Published online 2020:6

40. Nguyen JN, Jakus-Waldman SM, Walter AJ, White T, Menefee SA. Perioperative complications and reoperations after incontinence and prolapse surgeries using prosthetic implants. Obstet Gynecol. 2012;119(3):539–46. https://doi.org/10.1097/AOG.0b013e3182479283.

41. Nygaard I, Brubaker L, Chai TC, et al. Risk factors for urinary tract infection following incontinence surgery. Int Urogynecol J. 2011;22(10):1255–65. https://doi.org/10.1007/s00192-011-1429-9.

42. Oelschlager AMA, Debiec K, Appelbaum H. Primary vaginal dilation for vaginal agenesis: strategies to anticipate challenges and optimize outcomes. Curr Opin Obstet Gynecol. 2016;28(5):345–9. https://doi.org/10.1097/GCO.0000000000000302.

43. Oliver JL, Chaudhry ZQ, Medendorp AR, et al. Complete excision of sacrocolpopexy mesh with autologous fascia sacrocolpopexy. Urology. 2017;106:65–9. https://doi.org/10.1016/j.urology.2017.04.040.

44. Pikaart DP, Miklos JR, Moore RD. Laparoscopic removal of pubovaginal polypropylene tension-free tape slings. JSLS. 2006;10(2):220–5.

45. Quiroz LH, Gutman RE, Fagan MJ, Cundiff GW. Partial colpocleisis for the treatment of

46. Rac G, Younger A, Clemens JQ, et al. Stress urinary incontinence surgery trends in academic female pelvic medicine and reconstructive surgery urology practice in the setting of the food and drug administration public health notifications: SUI surgery trends. Neurourol Urodynam. 2017;36(4):1155–60. https://doi.org/10.1002/nau.23080.

47. Raz S. Atlas of vaginal reconstructive surgery. New York: Springer; 2015. https://doi.org/10.1007/978-1-4939-2941-2.

48. Read RC. Milestones in the history of hernia surgery: prosthetic repair. Hernia. 2004;8(1):8–14. https://doi.org/10.1007/s10029-003-0169-2.

49. Schimpf MO, Abed H, Sanses T, et al. Graft and mesh use in transvaginal prolapse repair: a systematic review. Obstet Gynecol. 2016;128(1):81–91. https://doi.org/10.1097/AOG.0000000000001451.

50. Scott VCS, Oliver JL, Raz S, Kim JH. Robot-assisted laparoscopic sacrocolpopexy with autologous fascia lata: technique and initial outcomes. Int Urogynecol J. 2019;30(11):1965–71. https://doi.org/10.1007/s00192-019-03884-2.

51. Siegal AR, Huang Z, Gross MD, Mehraban-Far S, Weissbart SJ, Kim JM. Trends of mesh utilization for stress urinary incontinence before and after the 2011 Food and Drug Administration notification between FPMRS-certified and non-FPMRS-certified physicians: a statewide all-payer database analysis. Urology. 2021;150:151–7. https://doi.org/10.1016/j.urology.2020.06.053.

52. Staack A, Vitale J, Ragavendra N, Rodríguez LV. Translabial ultrasonography for evaluation of synthetic mesh in the vagina. Urology. 2014;83(1):68–74. https://doi.org/10.1016/j.urology.2013.09.004.

53. Suskind AM, Kaufman SR, Dunn RL, Stoffel JT, Clemens JQ, Hollenbeck BK. Population-based trends in ambulatory surgery for urinary incontinence. Int Urogynecol J. 2013;24(2):207–11. https://doi.org/10.1007/s00192-012-1823-y.

54. Tate SB, Blackwell L, Lorenz DJ, Steptoe MM, Culligan PJ. Randomized trial of fascia lata and polypropylene mesh for abdominal sacrocolpopexy: 5-year follow-up. Int Urogynecol J. 2011;22(2):137–43. https://doi.org/10.1007/s00192-010-1249-3. Epub 2010 Aug 27. PMID: 20798922.

55. US Food and Drug Administration. FDA's activities: urogynecologic surgical mesh. Published online September 2021. https://www.fda.gov/medical-devices/urogynecologic-surgical-mesh-implants/fdas-activities-urogynecologic-surgical-mesh

56. Varasteh Kia M, Long JB, Chen CCG. Urinary tract infection after midurethral sling. Female Pelvic Med Reconstr Surg. 2021;27(1):e191–5. https://doi.org/10.1097/SPV.0000000000000890.

Vaginal Vault Prolapse: Options for Transvaginal Surgical Repair

33

Michele Torosis and Victor Nitti

Contents

Introduction 594

Anatomic Considerations 594

Indication for Vaginal Approach 597

Common Techniques for Transvaginal Native Tissue Repair 597
4a. Sacrospinous Ligament Fixation 598
4b. Uterosacral Ligament Suspension 600
4c. Comparison of Surgical Outcomes 602

Alternative Surgical Options 603
5a. Iliococcygeus Suspension 603
5b. McCall's Culdoplasty 603
5c. Augmentation with Vaginal Mesh Kits 604

Conclusion 604

Cross-References 604

References 604

Abstract

Apical compartment prolapse results from failure of the uterosacral and cardinal ligament complex. Apical prolapse should always be assessed and the need for concomitant apical repair should be considered when planning a surgery for the anterior and posterior compartment. Transvaginal repair techniques offer the most minimally invasive surgical approach. No transvaginal repair technique has been shown to be superior in regard to either anatomic or symptomatic cure. The most common transvaginal repair techniques for the vaginal apex are sacrospinous ligament suspension and uterosacral ligament suspension. Both can be performed with or without the uterus in situ. Sacrospinous ligament fixation procedure involves the fixation of the apex of the vagina to the sacrospinous ligament, typically performed unilaterally, and more commonly

M. Torosis · V. Nitti (✉)
Division of Female Pelvic Medicine and Reconstructive Surgery, Departments of Urology and Obstetrics and Gynecology, David Geffen School of Medicine at UCLA, Los Angeles, CA, USA
e-mail: mtorosis@mednet.ucla.edu;
vnitti@mednet.ucla.edu

© Springer Nature Switzerland AG 2023
F. E. Martins et al. (eds.), *Female Genitourinary and Pelvic Floor Reconstruction*,
https://doi.org/10.1007/978-3-031-19598-3_34

performed for post-hysterectomy prolapse. Uterosacral ligament suspension involves placing one or more sutures into the bilateral uterosacral ligaments. It is commonly performed at the time of vaginal hysterectomy when intraperitoneal access has already been achieved. Five-year outcome data for both techniques has shown that approximately half of patients will have some recurrent bulge symptoms and be found to have prolapse to the level of the hymen. Ten percent of patients require retreatment (pessary or surgery) and the five-year mark.

Keywords

Apical prolapse · Transvaginal repair · Uterosacral ligament suspension · Sacrospinous ligament suspension · Prolapse repair complications · Surgical technique

Introduction

Apical prolapse is the descent of the uterus, cervix, or vaginal vault. Treatment options for the management of apical prolapse include pelvic floor muscle training, pessary, and surgery. The role of pelvic floor muscle training in the treatment of prolapse appears to be limited, as it works to alleviate pelvic floor symptoms; however, there is little evidence to support that it is able to improve prolapse stage. Intravaginal pessaries are an effective option, however, and do require lifelong maintenance.

There is no specific degree of descent that mandates surgical correction. In general, stage II pelvic organ prolapse is the level of descent at which prolapse often becomes symptomatic [24]. Indications for treatment remain mostly predicated on symptom bother though recent evidence suggests that earlier treatment may result in better outcomes [17]. Resuspension of the apex may be considered with stage I prolapse, when there are other compartments involved and are being treated surgically. There is growing evidence in the literature that apical support is the key element in maintaining normal vaginal

anatomy [12]. Apical prolapse should always be assessed and the need for concomitant apical repair should be considered when planning a surgery for the anterior and posterior compartment. For example, any woman with a large anterior prolapse past the hymen, particularly in the absence of prior apical repair, should be assumed to also have some degree of apical weakness, until proven otherwise on careful pelvic exam.

The rate of apical repairs has increased as it has become apparent that missed apical defects are the cause of surgical failures. Examination of Medicare data has shown that women who underwent an anterior repair with concomitant apical suspension had significantly less prolapse recurrence than women who underwent an isolated anterior repair (11.6 vs. 20.2%) [9].

There is no consensus on the repair that offers the best combination of the most effective, safest, and most durable for the treatment of apical prolapse. And no one surgical approach is ideal for every patient. Surgical options for apical prolapse can be categorized as: restorative versus obliterative, abdominal versus vaginal versus laparoscopic/robotic approach, native tissue repair versus graft augmented, and uterine sparing versus nonuterine sparing. This chapter reviews the indications, surgical techniques, complications, and outcomes of a variety of transvaginal procedures to support the prolapsed vaginal apex.

Anatomic Considerations

Thorough understanding of the normal anatomic support and physiologic function of the pelvic musculature, vagina, and lower urinary tract is required in order to proceed with restoring normal anatomy and function. In the 1990s, DeLancey popularized the concept of levels of pelvic support. Level I support encompasses the vaginal apex and cervix which are held in place by the surrounding endopelvic connective tissue which includes the cardinal and uterosacral ligaments. Level II support refers to the mid-vagina which is supported by the lateral endopelvic fascia connections to the arcus tendinous fascia pelvis, which attaches to the levator ani. Level III support involves the distal connective tissue attachments of the urethra to the pubic bone and levator muscle support to the distal hymen [7].

Support of the vaginal apex is primarily derived from the integrity of the uterosacral and cardinal ligaments. These are not true ligaments, but rather dense connective tissue composed of condensations of the endopelvic fascia, blood vessels, nerves, and smooth muscle. The uterosacral ligament runs from the posterior cervix to sacrum and the cardinal ligament runs from lateral cervix to the obturator internus fascia. The endopelvic fascia also plays a key role in apical support. The endopelvic fascial is a supportive fibromuscular layer that underlies the vaginal epithelium. It runs the entire vaginal length, extending from the apex to the perineum. A defect in the endopelvic fascia is usually the result of its detachment from the apex, resulting in herniation and downward displacement of the affected either anterior or posterior vaginal segment. This places strain on the apex, weaking the apical support, and is a mechanism by which significant anterior or posterior compartment prolapse can lead to concomitant apical prolapse.

To rebuild apical support, understanding of two main structures used in prolapse repair is key: the uterosacral ligament and the sacrospinous ligament (SSL). The sacrospinous ligaments extend from the ischial spines on each side of the pelvis to the lower portion of the sacrum. The coccygeus muscle lies over the SSL. The body of the coccygeus muscle has a large fibrous component, within which the SSL lies. The two together are often referred to as the coccygeus-sacrospinous ligament (C-SSL) complex. The sacrospinous ligament is identified by palpating the ischial spine and tracing the flat triangular thickened ligament medial and posterior to the sacrum (Fig. 1). Above the sacrospinous ligament is the piriformis muscle and the lumbosacral plexus where the origin of the sciatic nerve is located. The sciatic nerve passes superior and lateral to the sacrospinous ligament (Fig. 2). The pudendal nerves and

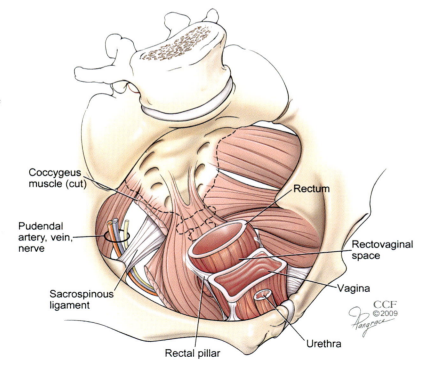

Fig. 1 Sacrospinous ligament runs from the sacrum to the ischial spine with sciatic and pudendal nerves running deep to the ligament. The coccygeus muscle lies over the sacrospinous ligament. The two together are often referred to as the coccygeus-sacrospinous ligament (C-SSL) complex

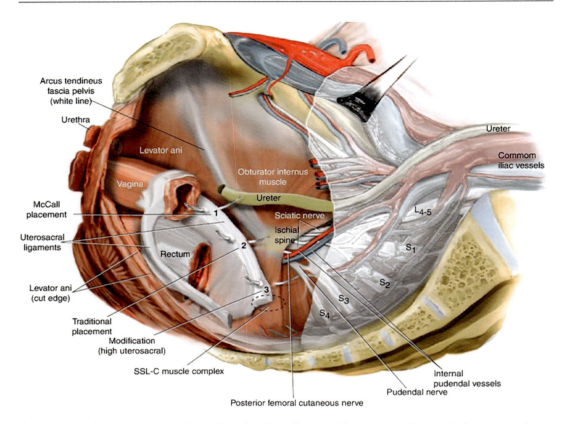

Fig. 2 The sciatic nerve passes superior and lateral to the sacrospinous ligament. The pudendal nerves and vessels and posterior femoral cutaneous nerve lie directly posterior to the ischial spine at the lateral margin of the sacrospinous ligament. The uterosacral ligament is also seen coursing on the right pelvic side wall in close proximity to the distal ureter

vessels lie directly posterior to the ischial spine at the lateral margin of the sacrospinous ligament [25].

Also, an abundant vascular supply that includes inferior gluteal vessels and hypogastric venous plexus lies superiorly. The inferior gluteal artery originates from the posterior or the anterior branch of the internal iliac artery to pass behind the sciatic nerve and the sacrospinous ligament. There is a 3–5 mm window in which the inferior gluteal vessel is left uncovered above the top of the sacrospinous ligament and below the lower edge of the main body of the sciatic nerve plexus. The main body of the inferior gluteal artery leaves the pelvis by passing posterior to the upper edge of the sacrospinous ligament and following the inferior portion of the sciatic nerve out of the greater sciatic foramen.

The uterosacral ligament runs from the posterior cervix to the anterior sacrum at the level of the S1 to S4 vertebrae. It runs lateral to the rectum and anteromedial to the ureter along the pelvic side wall. The cardinal-uterosacral ligament complex makes up the level 1 support to the uterus.

At the time of USLS, the ligament is identified posterior and medial to the ischial spine, in what is considered the midportion of the uterosacral ligament. The midportion of the USL is believed to be wider and composed of more connective tissue, making it the optimal support structure [22]. At the level of the ischial spine, the ureter is just lateral to the uterosacral ligament. The sacral plexus runs behind the uterosacral ligament (Fig. 2). Cadaver studies show that the S1, S2, S3, and S4 trunks of the sacral plexus pass under the uterosacral ligament 3.9 cm, 2.6 cm, 1.5 cm, 0.9 cm superior to the ischial spine, respectively [20].

Indication for Vaginal Approach

When planning a surgery for a quality of life disorder, such as apical prolapse, several factors need to be discussed beyond pure anatomic outcomes. This includes the woman's goals for surgery, risk tolerance for symptom recurrence and retreatment, ability to tolerate surgery, preference regarding recovery time, and concerns regarding sexual function after surgery. These preferences impact the decision to proceed with surgery via a vaginal or abdominal approach and with a native tissue repair or with synthetic mesh augmentation.

There are several benefits of transvaginal surgery over transabdominal. First transvaginal surgery has shorter operative duration and recovery when compared to abdominal procedures like abdominal sacrocolpopexy (ASC) [14]. For this reason, it is often selected by women with increased surgical risk or desire to avoid more difficult recovery.

Additionally, native tissue transvaginal repair eliminated the risk factors for mesh-related complications associated with ASC. This is particularly important in women at higher risk of mesh erosion or for patients with strong personal preferences to avoid mesh augmentation. Transvaginal surgery can also be performed without peritoneal entry making it safer for women who have had multiple prior abdominal surgeries and are at high risk for intra-abdominal adhesive disease.

Transabdominal surgery is often chosen by patients desiring the most durable repair. The most common abdominal surgery for apical prolapse is a sacrocolpopexy which can be performed laparoscopically, robotically, or via laparotomy. In clinical trials, most commonly open abdominal approaches for sacrocolpopexy have been compared to transvaginal repair techniques via SSLF [4]. A 2016 Cochrane meta-analysis evaluating 30 RCTs comparing surgical procedures for apical vaginal prolapse showed that sacrocolpopexy is associated with lower risk of awareness of prolapse, objective anatomic recurrent prolapse, and need for repeat surgery for prolapse [14]. Specifically when anatomic failure was defined as $\geq$ stage 2 prolapse, postoperative anatomic success was more likely with sacrocolpopexy compared with vaginal repair at 1–2 years (relative risk [RR] 1.89, 0.95% CI 1.33–2.70). At two years, awareness of prolapse was higher in the vaginal surgery group (RR 2.11, 95% CI 1.06–4.21). The quality of data on dyspareunia was low but did show lower rates of dyspareunia in the sacrocolpopexy group (RR 2.53, 95% CI 1.17–5.50). By contrast, a different meta-analysis reported no difference in dyspareunia in two trials and two cohort studies between the surgical approaches [20].

When considering a vaginal approach to apical prolapse repair, it is important to consider vaginal length. Transvaginal procedures ideally require sufficient vaginal length to reach the supporting ligament. In cases of significant vaginal shortening, an abdominal approach should be considered. Ultimately, the decision of route of surgery should be jointly made between patient and provider. There is no consensus opinion on gold standard prolapse repair technique, thus the factors discussed help guide decision for repair.

Common Techniques for Transvaginal Native Tissue Repair

Transvaginal apical prolapse repair is generally accomplished via uterosacral ligament suspension (USLS) or sacrospinous ligament fixation (SSLF). As will be discussed, no single transvaginal procedure has clearly been vastly superior in either anatomical or symptomatic cure. USLS potentially improves anterior vaginal wall support compared with SSLS. However, USLS relies on the integrity of the uterosacral ligament, which can be denuded or more difficult to find in older, post hysterectomy women. In contrast, the sacrospinous is a true ligament and does not get attenuated with time. While there are no rules, in general USLS is often performed at the time of concomitant vaginal hysterectomy, while SSLS is performed more commonly for post-hysterectomy prolapse repair.

4a. Sacrospinous Ligament Fixation

4ai. Surgical Technique

Sacrospinous ligament fixation is traditionally done via an extraperitoneal approach, in which the vaginal apex is suspended to the sacrospinous ligament either unilaterally or bilaterally. Although bilateral fixation allows for a more anatomic correction, unilateral fixation on the right is more commonly performed as it decreases the risk of injury to the rectum, which can occur given the proximity of suture placement. With unilateral fixation there is a slight deviation of the vaginal axis to one side.

SSLF is particularly helpful in the case of concomitant posterior compartment prolapse as it can act as support as suspension of the posterior colporrhaphy. Additionally, it is often the treatment of choice for post-hysterectomy prolapse as the procedure is performed extraperitoneally, avoiding potential intra-abdominal adhesions at the vaginal cuff. The steps in a post-hysterectomy patient will be discussed although this procedure can also be performed both at the time of hysterectomy or for hysteropexy with the uterus in situ.

SSLF does have some versatility as the ligament can be accessed via anterior or posterior approach depending on the compartments that are prolapsed. For cases of primarily anterior prolapse with a lesser apical component, the anterior approach to the ligament is particularly useful.

The steps of a sacrospinous ligament fixation are as follows:

1. The apex of the vagina is identified and grasped with two Allis clamps. The Allis clamps are elevated to the level of the sacrospinous ligament and residual posterior and anterior prolapse is assessed.
2. The SSL can be accessed through a posterior, apical, or anterior vaginal incision. In the posterior approach an incision is made in the midline posterior vaginal wall just short of the apex. If an enterocele sac is present, the sac can be dissected of the rectum and posterior vaginal wall, the peritoneum entered, and the sac closed with a high purse-string suture. Alternatively, particularly in cases of smaller enteroceles, the peritoneum can be left closed.
3. Next the right perirectal space is entered with blunt dissection through the fibroareolar tissue after mobilizing the rectum medially.
4. Once the perirectal space is entered, the ischial spine and SSL are identified. With dorsal and medial movement of the finger, blunt dissection is used to clear off the SSL so that it is easily palpated.
5. Several techniques are used for the actual passage of the sutures through the ligament. Regardless of technique, the ideal suture placement is 2–3 cm medial to the ischial spine and 0.5 cm below the superior edge of the ligament to avoid the pudendal neurovascular complex (Fig. 3). There is no consensus about suture type and a combination of delayed absorbable and nonabsorbable monofilament sutures is commonly used. Options for suture placement include:

   (a) Palpation: A Miya hook or automatic suture-capturing device like the Capio[®] device (Boston Scientific, Natick, MA) can be used to pass the suture through the ligament. The advantage of this is that it is safer and easier because the suture enters the ligament under direct palpation of distinct landmarks. The right middle fingertip is placed on the SSL just below its superior margin and guides the suture capturing device notch to the targeted area. Firm downward pressure is applied by the fingertip and the device is engaged to pass through the SSL.

   (b) Direct visualization: Three Breisky–Navratil retractors are used to expose the sacrospinous ligament, one retracting the rectum medially, another retracting the vaginal wall upward, and the third retracting laterally thus exposing the ligament. The full extent of the ligament is exposed such that the ischial spine and sacrum are palpable. Two adjacent stitches are placed through

Fig. 3 The sacrospinous ligament is reached with blunt dissection through the fibroareolar tissue, mobilizing the rectum medially. Optimal placement of the suture through the sacrospinous ligament is 2–3 cm medial to the ischial spine and 0.5 cm below the superior edge of the ligament

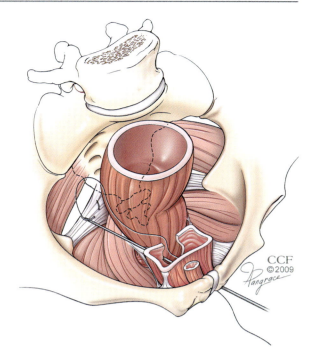

the sacrospinous ligament under direct visualization using the Deschamps needle driver. The Deschamps needle tip is typically passed from inferior to superior.

6. The stitches are then brought out to the apex of the vagina. If using delayed absorbable suture, the suture can be passed through the apex of the vagina. If permanent suture is being used, each suture is placed through the muscularis on the undersurface of the posterior vaginal epithelium.
7. If bilateral SSLF is desired the procedure is repeated on the left side, care must be taken to avoid injury to the rectum.
8. The vaginal incision is then closed with 2–0 continuous absorbable suture. The vaginal apex suspension stitches are then tied down, elevating the apex to the sacrospinous ligament.

4aii. Complications

Potential complications of the procedure include hemorrhage, nerve injury, and rectal injury. Severe hemorrhage with blood transfusion can result from overzealous dissection superior to the coccygeus muscle or ischial spine. This can result in hemorrhage from the inferior gluteal vessels, hypogastric venous plexus, or pudendal vessels. Hemorrhage from these vessels can be difficult to control. For this reason, dissection behind the sacrospinous ligament is not recommended. Bleeding extending into the retroperitoneal space can be occult and difficult to approximate in the surgical setting.

If severe bleeding occurs in the area around the coccygeus muscle, pressure and packing is the initial step to control bleeding. If this does not control bleeding, then visualization, attempted ligation with clips or sutures, and use of thrombin products should be used [16]. This area is not easily accessed transabdominally, thus exploratory laparotomy is not beneficial in this scenario.

Moderate to severe buttock pain on the side of suspension can occur immediately after SSLF. Moderate pain can be quite common and is likely due to compression of small nerves that run through the C-SSL. One retrospective review of 242 women who underwent SSLF found incidence of immediate buttock pain to be 55.4% of women [26]. Buttock pain is usually self-limiting, gradually improves, and should resolve by 6 weeks. A randomized control trial of SSLF versus USLS showed the incidence of new or worsening buttock pain at 2 weeks was 24% vs 10.5% at 4–6 weeks postoperatively in the SSLF group [2].

More severe buttock pain radiating down the posterior thigh to the foot is possible if there is an injury to the branches of the sciatic nerve. Sciatic nerve injury results from a SSLF suture placed deep and posterior to the ligament. Delay in diagnosis can result in permanent neuropathy, thus immediate removal is recommended.

Injury to the pudendal nerve is also possible given the close proximity of the nerve to the C-SSL. Pudendal nerve entrapment typically results in symptoms of unilateral vulvar pain and/or numbness and severe buttock pain. Similarly, immediate reoperation and removal of the suture is recommended.

The effect of SSLF on sexual function has not been well studied. Observational studies have reported dyspareunia in 3–10% of women who underwent SSLF [4]. In the 2013 Cochrane review, the rate of dyspareunia was 36% in pooled data from three randomized trials in which SSLS was compared with sacrocolpopexy [14].

Ureteral kinking or injury is infrequent but possible following SSLF. In a 2004 metanalysis evaluating 1922 patients undergoing SSLF the rate of ureteral kinking and difficulty in micturition was found to be 2.9% [4]. Routine cystoscopy is recommended at completion of the procedure to confirm ureteral patency.

4b. Uterosacral Ligament Suspension

4bi. Surgical Technique

Transvaginal uterosacral ligament suspension is typically performed at the time of vaginal hysterectomy since uterosacral ligament suspension is best performed intraperitoneally and the ligaments are most easily identified in this scenario. It can also be performed in post-hysterectomy prolapse and as a hysteropexy suspension technique. A benefit of USLS over SSLS is that the surgery can be tailored to the amount of prolapse that is present. In cases of more advanced prolapse the uterosacral sutures would be placed higher on the ligament, though we always attempt to place sutures above the ischial spine to reduce the risk of

ureteral kinking or injury. Additionally, this technique affixes the vaginal apex to bilateral uterosacral sutures and does not distort the anatomic axis of the vagina.

The steps of a uterosacral ligament fixation after vaginal hysterectomy are as follows:

1. The vaginal apex is opened so that the intraperitoneal contents are visible. Two moistened laparotomy sponges are placed in the posterior cul-de-sac. A Deaver is used to elevate the packs and bowel out of the operative field, exposing the uterosacral ligaments.
2. Next the uterosacral ligament is identified. There are a few options for identification and placement of the anchoring suture through the ligament. Regardless of technique, the goal is to place the suture at the level of or just proximal to the ischial spine. Suture is placed from lateral to medial to decrease the risk of incorporating the ureter within the suture. The more cephalad the sutures are placed on the USL, the more medial the sutures will be, minimizing ureteral injury. Sutures can be permanent or delayed absorbable. Note that the suture should not be too deep as to avoid injury to the sacral nerve roots (Fig. 4). Options for identification and placement of the uterosacral ligament include:
   (a) Palpation of the USL and ischial spine transrectally. A rectal finger is used to elevate the ligament off the side wall. Suture is then placed under direct visualization with a needle driver. The rectal finger helps guide the depth of suture placement and ensure there is no rectal injury.
   (b) Direct visualization of the ligament by placing an Allis on the distal uterosacral ligament at the vaginal cuff and applying traction. Under tension, the uterosacral ligament feels like a tight cord and can more easily be palpated at the level of the ischial spine. The Capio® device (Boston Scientific, Natick, MA) is used to place the suture through the ligament with direct palpation. Alternatively, a long needle driver can also be used to the place the suspension suture after appropriate visual identification of the ligament.

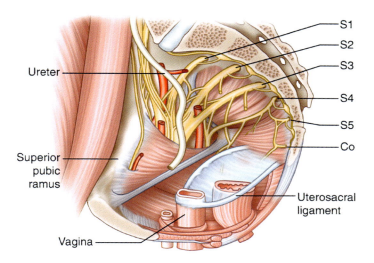

Fig. 4 Uterosacral ligament runs from posterior cervix to sacrum. The sacral nerves run in close proximity, thus when placing the uterosacral suspension sutures care should be taken as to not place the sutures too deep, reducing risk of sacral nerve injury

(c) The distal uterosacral ligament is placed on tension so that the uterosacral ligament can be visually identified. A long, curved Allis clamp is used to grasp the uterosacral ligament at the level of the ischial spine (Fig. 5). This maneuver elevates the ligament off the side wall and isolates the ligament. The Allis is then used as a guide to help in placement of the suture with direct visualization.

3. Indigo carmine, fluoresceine, or preferred ureteral efflux identification method should be employed at this juncture. Tension is place on the bilateral uterosacral ligaments and cystoscopy is performed to confirm ureteral patency prior to tying down the uterosacral sutures.
4. If delayed absorbable sutures are being used, the ends of the suture can be passed through the full thickness of the anterior and posterior vaginal cuff. If permanent suture is being used, each suture is placed through the muscularis on the undersurface of the posterior and anterior vaginal epithelium. The most caudad suture is placed laterally at the apex and the most cephalad suture is placed medially in the apex. The vaginal epithelium is closed, and the uterosacral ligament sutures are tied down thereafter, elevating the vaginal cuff (Fig. 5).
5. Cystoscopy can be performed to confirm ureteral patency an additional time after repair is complete.

4bii. Complications

The most common complication with uterosacral ligament colpopexy is ureteral compromise. The average distance from the lateral aspect of the suspension sutures to the medial border of the ureters was 14 mm in a cadaver study [28]. An observational study enrolled 15 individuals undergoing USLS. A small titanium vascular clip was applied to each base of the USLS suture and CT was performed on postoperative day 1. The right ureter was 2.1 cm from the right proximal suture and left ureter was 2.3 cm from the left proximal suture [23]. In this same study, the closest branch of the internal iliac complex was 2.6 cm from the proximal suture.

Cystoscopy should be performed routinely after placement of suspension sutures to prevent delated recognition of ureteral injury. Ureteral kinking from the uterosacral suture is found during routine intraoperative cystoscopy in up to 11% of cases [3, 15]. If there is no efflux on cystoscopy, the sutures on that side are sequentially removed from tension or removed entirely until efflux is seen. Tension on the sutures should be relieved moving distal to proximal as the most distal suture has the highest risk of ureteral kinking or injury. Often the suture can be replaced using a more proximal placement into the uterosacral ligament complex. Cystoscopy should always be performed again after replacement of suspension sutures.

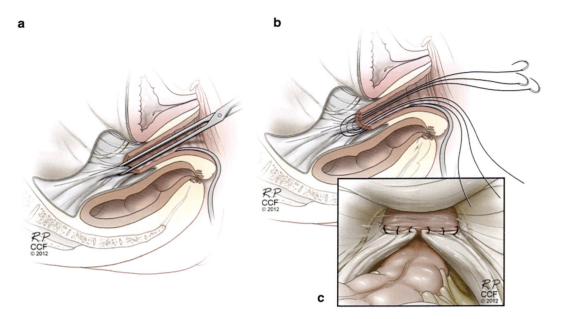

Fig. 5 (**a**) Option for uterosacral ligament to be grasped with Allis clamp at the level of the ischial spine (**b**) Two to three sutures are placed through the uterosacral ligament, typically moving lateral and superior with each placement, and brought out through the vagina. (**c**) After tying down the right and left suspension suture the vagina is elevate to the level of the ischial spine, maintaining normal vaginal axis

Sacral nerve entrapment is also a potential complication of USLS [19]. Cadaveric studies suggest a higher risk of sacral nerve entrapment when uterosacral sutures are placed using a deep, dorsal, posterior technique and suggest that sacral nerve injury may be minimized by tenting the ligament ventrally prior to placing the suture [21]. In a retrospective case series, 7 of 182 women who had undergone USLS developed sensory neuropathy and pain in the S2 to S3 dermatomes immediately postoperatively [10]. Three of these women had reduction of pain when suspension sutures were removed within four days after surgery.

4c. Comparison of Surgical Outcomes

Level 1 evidence supports that USLS and SSLF are equally effective surgical treatments with comparable anatomic and functional outcomes. The Operations and Pelvic Muscle Training in the Management of Apical Support Loss trial (OPTIMAL) [1] was a multicenter, randomized study comparing USLS and SSLF in 374 women. The primary outcome was surgical success at 2 years defined as (1) no apical prolapse beyond one-third of the vaginal length, (2) no anterior or posterior prolapse beyond the hymen, (3) no bothersome bulge, and (4) no retreatment. After 2 years of follow-up, SSLF (63.1%, 94/149) and USLS (64.5%, 100/155) showed similar success rates (adjusted odds ratio, 1.1; 95% confidence interval, 0.7 to 1.7). There was no significant difference in adverse events between the two groups. The rate of neurologic pain requiring intervention was higher in the SSLF group at 12.4% vs. 6.9%.

The five-year extension of the OPTIMAL trial [11] reported the same primary outcome and showed again no significant difference between the two groups. At five years, surgical failure was 64.8% in the USLS group and 71.2% in the SSLF group (p = 0.25). When anatomic and bothersome bulge symptoms were evaluated separately, there was still no difference between approaches (five-year anatomic failure: 51.1% vs. 59.7%, p = 0.11; 5-year bothersome bulge symptoms 42.1% vs. 47.8%, p = 0.60). Five-year retreatment rates were 11.9% for USLS and 8.1% for SSLF which did not meet statistical significance. Despite the increase in failure rate over time, patients' prolapse symptom scores in the Pelvic Organ Prolapse Distress Inventory (POPDI) remained improved throughout the follow-up period. With equal surgical outcomes, the decision between USLS and SSLF should be based on concomitant planned procedures and patient's intraoperative risks.

4ci. Impact of the Uterus

While most SSLF and USLS have traditionally been done at the time of or after hysterectomy, there is the option of doing these repairs with the uterus in situ. When performing a hysteropexy, techniques for accessing SSL and USL are similar, but the suspension sutures are placed through the posterior cervix instead of the vaginal epithelium at the cuff. In recent years, uterine preservation with hysteropexy has become increasingly popular and there is data to support equal surgical outcomes with hysteropexy compared to hysterectomy and suspension. In a multicenter randomized controlled trial of 208 women with POP, outcomes of sacrospinous hysteropexy and vaginal hysterectomy with USLS were compared. At 12 months of follow-up, hysteropexy was found to be noninferior to hysterectomy in terms of bothersome bulge, need for repeat surgery, quality-of-life measurements, or complications [8]. Hysteropexy will be discussed further in ▶ Chap. 34, "Role of Vaginal Hysterectomy in the Treatment of Vaginal Middle Compartment Prolapse."

4cii. Impact of Genital Hiatus

The size of the genital hiatus (GH) has been shown to be a risk factor for both prolapse occurrence and if uncorrected, prolapse recurrence. In a retrospective review of 260 women who underwent native tissue vaginal vault suspension composite failure (recurrent prolapse beyond hymen or retreatment) was more likely in women with GH of ≥4 cm prior to surgery which persisted at 6 weeks postoperatively [27]. The rate of recurrence in the persistently wide GH group was 51.3% versus 16.6% in women whose GH was corrected to <4 cm postoperatively. This data supports surgical correction of the genital hiatus at the time of vault suspension in women with a preoperative genital hiatus of 4 cm or greater, as there is a 4.4-fold increased odd of failure in all compartment if left uncorrected.

Alternative Surgical Options

5a. Iliococcygeus Suspension

A third option for apical support is the iliococcygeus fascia fixation. In this technique the vaginal apex is sutured to the iliococcygeal fascia over the levator plate, just below the ischial spine. The advantage of this approach is the decreased risk of injury to the pudendal nerve. This procedure is not as commonly performed thus there are no long-term studies comparing iliococcygeus suspension to other apical techniques. In a single center study at 69 months the subjective and objective cure rates were 88.6% and 84.1%, respectively [18].

5b. McCall's Culdoplasty

McCall's culdoplasty uses the proximal uterosacral ligaments to suspend the vaginal apex. It is performed at the time of hysterectomy and is ideally performed when patients are undergoing hysterectomy for nonprolapse indications and either have an increased risk for prolapse or have currently mild prolapse without significant symptoms. The benefit of this procedure is that it obliterates the posterior cul-de-sac, decreasing the risk for future enterocele formation. It is also relatively quick to perform.

The technique for the procedure involves placing a suture through one uterosacral ligament, proximal to the vaginal cuff, and then reefing across the posterior peritoneum and placing the other end of the suture through the other uterosacral ligament. When this is tied down the cuff is elevated and the posterior cul-de-sac is obliterated. The uterosacral ligaments are then closed in a full thickness fashion with the vaginal epithelium in the midline providing another layer of support. Cystoscopy should be performed at the end of this procedure to confirm ureteral patency as the ureter runs in close proximity to the uterosacral ligament at the cervical end.

The data describing the outcomes for this procedure are limited. Colombo retrospectively compared the outcomes of a modified McCall's culdoplasty with those of SSLS (n = 62 in each group) [6]. Recurrence after the McCall's culdoplasty, which was defined a Baden–Walker grade 2 or more prolapse, was 15% at 4–9 years after surgery and was not significantly different from the SSLS group.

5c. Augmentation with Vaginal Mesh Kits

As with anterior and posterior repair, the use of mesh-augmented repairs gained popularity in the early 2000s, and a number of transvaginal mesh kits became commercially available. However, complications rates were high, resulting in two safety notifications in 2008 and 2011 by the FDA. Finally, in 2019, the FDA called for the remaining manufacturers of synthetic mesh products for the transvaginal repair of POP to stop selling and distributing their products within the USA and successively Australia, New Zealand, and the UK banned the use of any transvaginal mesh for POP treatment [5]. Even when in use, the advantages of mesh augmented repairs for apical prolapse were not clear.

A 2016 Cochrane review of apical prolapse found that in 6 RCTs with 598 women comparing mesh to native tissue vaginal repair, there was no difference in prolapse awareness, repeat surgery for prolapse, or repeat surgery for SUI [13]. At this time the use of mesh augmentation for transvaginal apical repair is not recommended.

Conclusion

There are many options for apical repair, some of which have been described in this chapter. Transvaginal prolapse repair should be tailored to the individual patient, making sure to factor in the degree of prolapse, risk of recurrence, and patient expectations. At this time the literature does not support one technique as a gold standard.

Cross-References

▶ Management of Vaginal Posterior Compartment Prolapse: Is There Ever a Case for Graft/Mesh?
▶ Minimally Invasive Approaches in the Treatment of Pelvic Organ Prolapse: Laparoscopic and Robotic
▶ Stem Cell and Tissue Engineering in Female Urinary Incontinence

References

1. Barber MD, Brubaker L, Burgio KL, Richter HE, Nygaard I, Weidner AC, et al. Comparison of 2 transvaginal surgical approaches and perioperative behavioral therapy for apical vaginal prolapse: the OPTIMAL randomized trial. JAMA. 2014;311:1023–34.
2. Barber MD, Brubaker L, Nygaard I, et al. Pain and activity after vaginal reconstructive surgery for pelvic organ prolapse and stress urinary incontinence. Am J Obstet Gynecol. 2019;221(3):233.e1–233.e16. https://doi.org/10.1016/j.ajog.2019.06.004.
3. Barber MD, Visco AG, Weidner AC, Amundsen CL, Bump RC. Bilateral uterosacral ligament vaginal vault suspension with site-specific endopelvic fascia defect repair for treatment of pelvic organ prolapse. Am J Obstet Gynecol. 2000;183(6):1402–10. https://doi.org/10.1067/mob.2000.111298. discussion 1410-1. PMID: 11120503.
4. Beer M, Kuhn A. Surgical techniques for vault prolapse: a review of the literature. Eur J Obstet Gynecol Reprod Biol. 2005;119(2):144–55. https://doi.org/10.1016/j.ejogrb.2004.06.042. PMID: 15808370.
5. Clemons JL, Weinstein M, Guess MK, Alperin M, Moalli P, Gregory WT, et al. Impact of the 2011 FDA transvaginal mesh safety update on AUGS members' use of synthetic mesh and biologic grafts in pelvic

reconstructive surgery. Female Pelvic Med Reconstr Surg [Internet] 19(4):191–198. Available from: http://www.ncbi.nlm.nih.gov/pubmed/23797515

6. Colombo M, Milani R. Sacrospinous ligament fixation and modified McCall culdoplasty during vaginal hysterectomy for advanced uterovaginal prolapse. Am J Obstet Gynecol. 1998;179(1):13–20.

7. DeLancey JO. The anatomy of the pelvic floor. Curr Opin Obstet Gynecol. 1994;6:313–6.

8. Detollenaere RJ, den Boon J, Stekelenburg J, IntHout J, Vierhout ME, Kluivers KB, van Eijndhoven HW. Sacrospinous hysteropexy versus vaginal hysterectomy with suspension of the uterosacral ligaments in women with uterine prolapse stage 2 or higher: multicentre randomised non-inferiority trial. BMJ. 2015;351:h3717. https://doi.org/10.1136/bmj.h3717. PMID: 26206451; PMCID: PMC4512203.

9. Eilber KS, Alperin M, Khan A, et al. Outcomes of vaginal prolapse surgery among female Medicare beneficiaries: the role of apical support. Obstet Gynecol. 2013;122:981–7.

10. Flynn MK, Weidner AC, Amundsen CL. Sensory nerve injury after uterosacral ligament suspension. Am J Obstet Gynecol. 2006;195(6):1869–72. https://doi.org/10.1016/j.ajog.2006.06.059. Epub 2006 Oct 2. PMID: 17014812.

11. Jelovsek JE, Barber MD, Brubaker L, et al. Effect of uterosacral ligament suspension vs sacrospinous ligament fixation with or without perioperative behavioral therapy for pelvic organ vaginal prolapse on surgical outcomes and prolapse symptoms at 5 years in the OPTIMAL randomized clinical trial. JAMA. 2018;319(15):1554–65. https://doi.org/10.1001/jama.2018.2827.

12. Lowder JL, Park AJ, Ellison R, et al. The role of apical vaginal support in the appearance of anterior and posterior vaginal prolapse. Obstet Gynecol. 2008;111:152–7.

13. Maher C, Feiner B, Baessler K, Haya N, Brown J. Surgery for women with apical vaginal prolapse (review). Summary of fndings for the main comparison. Cochrane Database Syst Rev. 2016;10:1–196.

14. Maher C, Feiner B, Baessler K, Schmid C. Surgical management of pelvic organ prolapse in women. Cochrane Database Syst Rev. 2013;30(4):CD004014. https://doi.org/10.1002/14651858.CD004014.pub5. Update in: Cochrane Database Syst Rev. 2016 Nov 30;11:CD004014. PMID: 23633316.

15. Margulies RU, Rogers MA, Morgan DM. Outcomes of transvaginal uterosacral ligament suspension: systematic review and metaanalysis. Am J Obstet Gynecol. 2010;202(2):124–34. https://doi.org/10.1016/j.ajog.2009.07.052. PMID: 20113690.

16. Pahwa AK, Arya LA, Andy UU. Management of arterial and venous hemorrhage during sacrospinous ligament fixation: cases and review of the literature. Int Urogynecol J. 2016;27(3):387–91. https://doi.org/10.1007/s00192-015-2818-2. Epub 2015 Aug 19. PMID: 26282092.

17. Richter H, Sridhar A, Nager C, Komesu Y, Zyczynski H, Harvie H, Radin C, Visco A, Mazloomdoost D, Thomas S. Risk factors associated with surgical failure over 5 years in a randomized trial of sacrospinous hysteropexy with graft vs. vaginal hysterectomy with uterosacral ligament suspension for uterovaginal prolapse. Female Pelvic Medicine & Reconstructive Surgery. 2021;27(10S):S1–S129. https://doi.org/10.1097/SPV.0000000000001103.

18. Serati M, Braga A, Bogani G, Leone Roberti Maggiore U, Sorice P, Ghezzi F, Salvatore S. Iliococcygeus fixation for the treatment of apical vaginal prolapse: efficacy and safety at 5 years of follow-up. Int Urogynecol J. 2015;26(7):1007–12. https://doi.org/10.1007/s00192-015-2629-5. Epub 2015 Feb 5. PMID: 25653034

19. Siddique SA, Gutman RE, Schön Ybarra MA, Rojas F, Handa VL. Relationship of the uterosacral ligament to the sacral plexus and to the pudendal nerve. Int Urogynecol J Pelvic Floor Dysfunct. 2006;17(6):642–5. https://doi.org/10.1007/s00192-006-0088-8. Epub 2006 May 30. PMID: 16733625.

20. Siddiqui NY, Grimes CL, Casiano ER, Abed HT, Jeppson PC, Olivera CK, Sanses TV, Steinberg AC, South MM, Balk EM, Sung VW; Society of Gynecologic Surgeons Systematic Review Group. Mesh sacrocolpopexy compared with native tissue vaginal repair: a systematic review and meta-analysis. Obstet Gynecol. 2015;125(1):44–55. https://doi.org/10.1097/AOG.0000000000000570. PMID: 25560102; PMCID: PMC4352548.

21. Siddiqui NY, Mitchell TRT, Bentley RC, Weidner AC. Neural entrapment during uterosacral ligament suspension: an anatomic study of female cadavers. Obstet Gynecol. 2010;116(3):708–13. https://doi.org/10.1097/AOG.0b013e3181ec658a. PMID: 20733456.

22. Siff Lauren N, Jallad K, Hickman LC, Walters MD. Surgical Anatomy of the Uterosacral Ligament Colpopexy. Female Pelvic Medicine & Reconstructive Surgery. 2018;24(5):380–2.

23. Smith BC, Herfel CV, Yeung J, Shatkin-Margolis A, Crisp CC, Kleeman SD, Pauls RN. Uterosacral ligament suspension: a radiographic study of suture location in live subjects. Female Pelvic Med Reconstr Surg. 2020;26(9):541–5. https://doi.org/10.1097/SPV.0000000000000629. PMID: 30180050.

24. Swift SE, Tate SB, Nicholas J. Correlation of symptoms with degree of pelvic organ support in a general population of women: what is pelvic organ prolapse? Am J Obstet Gynecol. 2003;189(2):372–7.

25. Thompson JR, Gibb JS, Genadry R, Burrows L, Lambrou N, Buller JL. Anatomy of pelvic arteries adjacent to the sacrospinous ligament: importance of the coccygeal branch of the inferior gluteal artery. Obstet Gynecol. 1999;94(6):973–7. https://doi.org/10.1016/s0029-7844(99)00418-4. PMID: 10576185.

26. Unger CA, Walters MD. Gluteal and posterior thigh pain in the postoperative period and the need for intervention after sacrospinous ligament colpopexy.

Female Pelvic Med Reconstr Surg. 2014;20(4):208–11. https://doi.org/10.1097/SPV.0000000000000091. PMID: 24978086.

27. Vaughan MH, Siddiqui NY, Newcomb LK, Weidner AC, Kawasaki A, Visco AG, Bradley MS. Surgical alteration of genital hiatus size and anatomic failure after vaginal vault suspension. Obstet Gynecol. 2018;131(6):1137–44. https://doi.org/10.1097/AOG.0000000000002593. PMID: 29742664.

28. Wieslander CK, Roshanravan SM, Wai CY, Schaffer JI, Corton MM. Uterosacral ligament suspension sutures: Anatomic relationships in unembalmed female cadavers. Am J Obstet Gynecol. 2007;197(6):672.e1–6. https://doi.org/10.1016/j.ajog.2007.08.065. PMID: 18060977.

Role of Vaginal Hysterectomy in the Treatment of Vaginal Middle Compartment Prolapse

34

Luiz Gustavo Oliveira Brito, Cassio Luis Zanettini Riccetto, and Paulo Cesar Rodrigues Palma

Contents

Introduction 608

Uterine Preservation and Pelvic Organ Prolapse Surgery 608

Vaginal Hysterectomy and Pelvic Organ Prolapse 610

Prevention of Genital Prolapse in Hysterectomy Due to Benign Disease 611

Sexual Function and Uterine Management in Pelvic Organ
Prolapse Surgery 611

Conclusion 613

References 613

Abstract

This chapter discusses the general rule of removing the uterus during surgical treatment of apical prolapse, and how the correction of the apical support might influence the anterior compartment. It also discusses the reasons for

L. G. O. Brito
Division of Gynecological Surgery, Department of Obstetrics and Gynecology, Faculty of Medical Sciences, State University of Campinas – UNICAMP, Campinas, Brazil

C. L. Z. Riccetto
Division of Female Urology, Department of Surgery, Faculty of Medical Sciences, State University of Campinas – UNICAMP, Campinas, Brazil

P. C. R. Palma (✉)
Department of Surgery, Faculty of Medical Sciences, State University of Campinas – UNICAMP, Campinas, Brazil

© Springer Nature Switzerland AG 2023
F. E. Martins et al. (eds.), *Female Genitourinary and Pelvic Floor Reconstruction*,
https://doi.org/10.1007/978-3-031-19598-3_35

performing hysteropexy, the evidence regarding maintaining or not maintaining the uterus, and what data is available regarding the recommendation by some societies to perform adjuvant surgical techniques during hysterectomy to prevent pelvic organ prolapse in the future. Finally, we also discuss the sexual function after pelvic organ prolapse surgery and whether hysterectomy influences the development of genital prolapse. It is always important to listen to the patient and a shared decision-making process is recommended towards the best approach to improve women's quality of life.

Keywords

Vaginal hysterectomy · Vaginal prolapse ·
Middle compartment prolapse · Uterine

prolapse · Uterovaginal prolapse · Role of hysterectomy · Treatment of vaginal prolapse

Introduction

There are several surgical procedures to treat middle compartment prolapse involving the uterus, also termed uterine or uterovaginal prolapse. One of the most common procedures is vaginal hysterectomy. Although it is possible to surgically correct uterovaginal descensus without hysterectomy, depending on the clinical circumstances, vaginal hysterectomy is often performed for uterovaginal prolapse. Total vaginal hysterectomy for uterovaginal prolapse is a safe procedure and, when performed with the appropriate concurrent suspension of the vaginal vault, is effective for the management of uterovaginal prolapse in most cases.

Uterovaginal prolapse usually results from loss of pelvic support due to damage or weakening of pelvic support structures, including the bony pelvis. Soft tissue pelvic support systems, including the cardinal and uterosacral ligament complex and the pelvic diaphragm with its associated ani and coccygeus, and perineal membrane play a critical role in this support mechanism.

Although a detailed technical discussion of transvaginal vault suspension is not the scope of this chapter, several techniques exist for transvaginal vault suspension following vaginal hysterectomy, including the high uterosacral ligament suspension, sacrospinous ligament fixation, and iliococcygeus fascia suspension as being the most performed. Literature evidence from prospective, randomized controlled trials favoring one of these techniques over another is lacking. Therefore, there is no standard operation for supporting the vaginal cuff that can be recommended as the best one.

Uterine Preservation and Pelvic Organ Prolapse Surgery

Currently, the most commonly performed vaginal surgical procedures for the treatment of uterine prolapse are vaginal hysterectomy with uterosacral ligament suspension of vaginal vault, vaginal hysterectomy plus sacrospinous ligament colpopexy (uni or bilaterally), and two hysteropexy procedures, represented by the modified Manchester operation and sacrospinous hysteropexy (with or without mesh). These procedures are combined with corrections of simultaneous defects in the anterior or posterior vaginal wall, the first being the most frequent.

The Manchester operation was first described in 1888 and since that has become more commonly used in pelvic reconstructive surgery. Originally, the operation consisted of a combination of cervical amputation plus anterior colporrhaphy [1]. Later, the cardinal ligaments were added to the technique, by its bilateral plication and attachment to the cervical stump. The modern modified Manchester operation which has been performed by most of pelvic reconstructive surgeons also included plication of the sacrouterine ligaments. Despite the paucity of data comparing the Manchester operation to other techniques, a recent publication analyzing historical series of published cases concluded that the Manchester operation would be better than vaginal hysterectomy [2]. Moreover, a recent prospective cohort study concluded that modified Manchester operation provides proper apical compartment support and subjective results in a short-term follow-up [3]. The modified Manchester procedure is especially useful to address apical prolapse combined with cervical elongation, which, in theory, could produce better results than the sacrospinous hysteropexy. On the other hand, the modified Manchester operation could lead to stenosis of the cervical canal, recently reported in up to 11% of patients who underwent the procedure with consequent difficulty in accessing the uterine cavity for diagnostic procedures and menstrual symptoms in pre-menopausal patients [4].

The treatment of apical prolapse using uterosacral ligaments is classically performed through vaginal route but laparoscopic or robotic approaches were added more recently. Plication plus suspension of the uterosacral ligaments is one of the most widespread procedures for the treatment of apical prolapse, being generally associated with hysterectomy, which allows easy access to uterosacral ligaments by a transvaginal approach. Vault support can be obtained with non-absorbable or delayed absorbable sutures, which suspend the vaginal vault to the uterosacral ligament [5]. Laparoscopic and transvaginal uterosacral colpopexy use the natural support tissues to suspend the uterus or the vaginal vault, preventing changes in the physiological vaginal axis that may occur after other procedures. In fact, sacrospinous hysteropexy/colpopexy and sacral hysteropexy/colpopexy determine displacement of the vaginal axis in the posterior and anterior directions, respectively. Although transvaginal uterosacral hysteropexy avoids possible complications associated with hysterectomy and the morbidity associated with the use of mesh [6], one must keep in mind that sutures are applied on tissues with recognized remodeled collagen, characterized by decreased synthesis and increased degradation of its extracellular matrix metabolism [7]. That, associated with the risk of postoperative cervical stretching, can lead to higher recurrence rates and the need for reoperations and represent a major risk of vault prolapse repair based exclusively in native tissues.

Comparisons of pelvic organ prolapse repair techniques based on native tissues are particularly difficult to interpret, due to the technical variability inherent to the surgeon and other non-measurable aspects, such as the number and types of sutures used and the way each compartment defects were corrected. In 2016, a systematic review by Cochrane compared the techniques used for the treatment of apical vaginal prolapse and found that no conclusions could be made regarding the superiority of mesh hysteropexy versus other procedures including vaginal hysterectomy [8]. Although the use of transvaginal mesh procedures is still controversial, there are few high-quality, long-term data adequately compared techniques using transvaginal mesh for the treatment of apical prolapse with native tissue-based procedures. Therefore, both US FDA (Food and Drug Administration) and the UK National Institute of Excellence in Healthcare have recommended further research on procedures using transvaginal mesh [9]. More recently, a prospective multicenter randomized trial tried to compare the incidence of apical prolapse treatment failure following transvaginal hysteropexy with mesh versus vaginal hysterectomy and colpopexy with uterosacral ligament suspension. However, the results did not allow a definitive conclusion even after 3 years of patient follow-up [10].

In the OPTIMAL trial, a randomized study concluded that uterosacral ligament suspension was related to a lower rate of objective failure although the difference was not significant [11]. In another publication originated from the same dataset, a higher incidence of vascular complications associated with sacrospinous ligament fixation was described [12].

In a recent systematic review and meta-analysis, the authors concluded that uterine preservation decreased operative time and morbidities, such as vaginal exposure of the mesh, without significant worsening of the anatomical objective results of the prolapse treatment. In addition, the literature on the long-term results of prolapse treatments with uterine preservation, on the role of uterine preservation in obliterative prolapse procedures, and the risk of long-term uterine pathology are still scarce [13].

A trend for uterine preservation in pelvic organ prolapse treatments has been emerging worldwide over the years [14–19]. The change in women's attitude is well demonstrated in a study in which questionnaire surveys reveal that 60% of women prefer to spare their uterus if equal surgical efficacy can be achieved compared to concomitant hysterectomy [20]. In another research, 36% of women stated that they would prefer a uterine preservation procedure, even assuming a possible suboptimal anatomical result [21].

A classic suggested advantage of hysterectomy in the treatment of pelvic organ prolapse, especially after the menopause, is to reduce the risk of possible cervical or endometrial malignancy in the future. However, the incidence of unforeseen cervical or endometrial neoplasms in samples obtained from hysterectomy related to uterovaginal prolapse is quite low averaging 2.6% [22]. Therefore, the benefit of indistinct prophylactic hysterectomy in women with pelvic organ prolapse has been questioned, mostly due to the improvement of the screening tools, such as ultrasound scan, PAP smear, and HPV testing and vaccine, genetic biomarkers, that should be useful in identifying the best candidates for prophylactic hysterectomy.

The reasons that determine patients' desire to maintain their uterus differed from the desire to maintain fertility, raising awareness about sexuality, body image, self-esteem, quality of life, and cultural beliefs. Therefore, the discussion of uterine preservation as a surgical strategy in the correction of pelvic organ prolapse should be a fundamental step in patient-centered counseling. The patient must be explained that the uterus has a passive role in prolapse [23] and that studies have suggested that hysterectomy itself may be associated with an increased risk of prolapse in the future [24, 25]. Moreover, patients should be counselled that the supporting elements of the apex of the vagina, included in the so-called pericervical ring, are important to achieve successful outcomes after any reconstructive pelvic surgical technique and that pelvic organ prolapses are progressive degenerative diseases, which will continue to evolve, regardless of the proposed treatment [26].

Vaginal Hysterectomy and Pelvic Organ Prolapse

There has been some growing discussion on the role of vaginal hysterectomy and the need to be performed during POP surgical correction.

Hysteropexy has increased in United States in the last years, from 1.83% to 5% [27] and several factors are influencing the decision-making process such as: Patient autonomy, when the stigma related to uterus removal in some communities may weight in their own process, socioeconomic level, reproductive issues, sexual function, fear of complications, surgeon bias, and procedure costs [28]. Recently, an instrument was

developed and validated to assess how much a patient is interested to remove or not her uterus. The Value of Uterus (VALUS) instrument was tested and could differentiate by score measurement women that would like to maintain their uterus from women that did not, with a sensitivity of 100%, specificity of 76%, and accuracy of 89% [29].

There are some studies that have been published comparing hysteropexy with POP surgical correction versus hysterectomy. The SUPER trial followed for 3 and 5 years women with apical prolapse randomized into two arms: vaginal sacrospinous hysteropexy with graft vs vaginal hysterectomy with uterosacral ligament suspension. The frequency of treatment failure after the primary composite outcome (prolapse beyond the hymen, POP symptoms, or POP retreatment) had no statistical difference between groups after 3 years of follow-up [10] but with a higher failure rate in the hysterectomy group that was statistically significant after 5 years [30]. Moreover, in the 5 year follow-up, there was no difference for pelvic floor symptoms, quality of life, and pelvic pain between groups. Cost-effectiveness of hysteropexy in a Markov model has showed less expenses when compared to the hysterectomy group [31].

One might discuss whether the incidence of uterine and cervical cancer after hysteropexy would increase by maintaining the uterus. There is one study that addressed that. A retrospective cohort study with 8927 cases has found that there is 95% of certainty that the chance of cancer development after hysteropexy is smaller than 0.61% when compared to the hysterectomy group, thus indicating a small difference [32].

Biomechanically, no study was performed in cadavers and compared whether maintaining the uterus would modify the resistance of the vagina during traction after a mechanic stimulus. After increasing almost four kilos using a pulley apparatus and measuring the average distance traversed by the uterine fundus or vaginal cuff, there was no statistical difference in the distance moved by the apex between sacral hysteropexy and total hysterectomy [33].

Most of these studies are retrospective and only a few prospective, randomized studies exist. Thus, the quality of evidence of these data is low. But these data are somewhat interesting, inviting for a reflection on our own practices, perhaps as a change of paradigms. Further prospective studies are needed to know whether these data will be confirmed in a long-term period. In the meantime, a full and lengthy discussion with the patient on the most recent data available is of utmost importance.

Prevention of Genital Prolapse in Hysterectomy Due to Benign Disease

Further studies on this topic are needed as the level of evidence regarding this discussion is still low. To our knowledge, no randomized controlled trials exist to answer this question. Although a study protocol of this goal has been published, no data can be found on databases yet [34]. However, there are recommendations regarding the prophylactic prevention of vault prolapse during hysterectomy, according to the AAGL guidelines. A level B recommendation was given to McCall culdoplasty to be performed during vaginal hysterectomy to treat non prolapse-related disease in order to reduce the risk of postoperative apical prolapse for up to 3 years; moreover, uterosacral ligament suspension may be performed during abdominal (level B) and laparoscopic (level C) hysterectomy to reduce the risk of post-hysterectomy vaginal vault prolapse [35].

Another critical aspect is whether the surgical route for hysterectomy would influence the long-term risk of subsequent prolapse after surgery. A retrospective chart review assessing the risk of prolapse after abdominal, vaginal, and laparoscopic or robotic hysterectomy for up to 17 years from surgery was performed. After controlling for confounders, including surgery indication, the hazard ratio for subsequent prolapse was no different among vaginal, laparoscopic, or robotic, or open hysterectomy. Prolapse grade was similar across the three groups [36].

Sexual Function and Uterine Management in Pelvic Organ Prolapse Surgery

Pelvic floor dysfunction affects up to 24% of women [37]. Sexual dysfunction is highly prevalent among them, affecting up to 64% of women with pelvic floor dysfunction [38–40]. As female sexual function is multidimensional, in particular as they age, reported frequencies can range and the impact of interpersonal, emotional relationship, well-being, and psychological factors, in addition to biological, social, and cultural aspects can easily upset the complex equilibrium of female sexuality [41].

Both pelvic organ prolapse and stress urinary incontinence impact on sexual function. Urinary incontinence was significantly associated with low libido, vaginal dryness, and dyspareunia [42], whereas pelvic organ prolapse has an impact on a woman's feeling of femininity, which can influence desire and arousal. Moreover, prolapse can be associated with pelvic pain [43], which can affect sexual function and lead both patient and partner to avoid sexual function at a greater level among women with pelvic organ prolapse than in those with stress urinary incontinence [44]. Pelvic organ prolapse and sexual dysfunction were closely correlated, the incidence of dysfunction rising as POP worsened [45].

It would be reasonable to assume that surgical correction of prolapse would lead to improvement in sexual function, due to its importance as a physical component of sexual dysfunction in women. Nevertheless, the presence of this anatomical defect does not imply dysfunction and pelvic prolapse correction does not always improve sexual activity [46, 47]. In fact, occasionally, pelvic organ prolapse surgery can worsen sexual function in some patient subsets. The goal of pelvic surgery should be restoration of anatomic support without deleterious effects on visceral and sexual function. Data evidence are still controversial, mostly those related to different pelvic organ prolapse techniques.

Hysterectomy is among the most common major gynecological operations worldwide [48]. In most human cultures, the uterus is considered the key of female sexuality and diseases involving it are related to culture-dependent psychological effects that lead to loss of female identity and self-esteem. However, the effect of hysterectomy on sexual function is remarkably heterogeneous [49]. The goal of medical research is to identify how sexual function is affected by hysterectomy and what are the predictors for improvement or deterioration of sexual function in diseases or treatments which involve the uterus. An increasing number of women may ask for uterus preservation during pelvic organ repair. Nonetheless, pelvic surgeons need to be ready to respond to these requests and remain aware of the progress in this field.

Hysterectomy performed for treatment of most symptomatic conditions tend to improve female sexual function and quality of life, regardless of the surgical route, or whether the cervix is removed or not (level 1B evidence) [50–52]. However, there is still an assumption that women for whom uterine/cervical contractions are an important aspect of orgasm may be a subset to experience reduced sexual function after hysterectomy more commonly [53]. Pathophysiological mechanisms can also be related to the complex pelvic nerve plexus and to possible damage to the autonomic nerve endings of the cervicovaginal fascia, hence impacting on orgasm or sensation during intercourse [54, 55]. Other possible pathways for detrimental physical effects of hysterectomy include scar tissue in the vagina preventing full ballooning of the upper vagina, removed tissue reducing the capacity of vasocongestion leading to dyspareunia and hindering arousal [53].

Concomitant bilateral oophorectomy is performed in about 50% of hysterectomies [48, 56]. Although it virtually eliminates the risk of ovarian cancer, the resultant hypoestrogenism may have more detrimental effect on general women's health including their sexual function [56]. Estrogen replacement may not sufficiently improve sexual function and general health, so combined bilateral oophorectomy should be considered only in women at high risk of ovarian cancer based on an individualized risk assessment and on patient's shared decision basis.

Following hysterectomy as part of pelvic organ prolapse treatment, overall improvement in the frequency of sexual relations, dyspareunia, orgasm, vaginal dryness, and sexual desire was noted regardless of route of hysterectomy [57]. However, one should consider that distortion of pelvic anatomy can lead to dyspareunia and subsequent female sexual dysfunction. Vaginal length was not related to sexual function [58], but in women undergoing hysterectomy for prolapse or an anterior repair, vaginal length should be maintained wherever possible and excessive vaginal mucosal excision should be avoided. Moreover, a study showed that the technique for vaginal cuff closure (vertical or horizontal sutures) did not impact sexual function [59]. Most women with stage 2 or higher uterine prolapse following vaginal hysterectomy with prolapse repair experienced improvement in sexual function postoperatively, regardless of the cuff closure technique used. Although vaginal hysterectomy to treat pelvic organ prolapse improves anatomical and sexual concerns, surgery per se may have negative effects on sexual function if new-onset or worsening dyspareunia or incontinence develop [59].

Besides vault dehiscence is a rare phenomenon after hysterectomy for benign disease, affecting up to 0.4% of patients [60], it represents another drawback that can impact sexual function. Women need to be informed about this complication. Although further evidence is needed, abstinence from deep penetration may be advisable for the first three postoperative months as early resumption of intercourse was identified as a risk factor [61]. This complication has been more commonly reported in the last decade, especially after laparoscopic and robot-assisted total hysterectomy [62].

Although the impact of hysterectomy as part of pelvic organ prolapse treatment on sexual well-being is still not clearly defined, some authors showed in a prospective study that uterus-sparing surgery was associated with a greater improvement in the desire, arousal and orgasm sexual domains of the International Sexual Function Index. Moreover, they suggested that data on sexual outcome should be included in preoperative counselling and sexual evaluation, as part of the patient reported outcome, and should be included in outcome evaluation after surgery for pelvic organ prolapse [63].

Postoperative dyspareunia is reported to be between 8% and 16% after hysterectomy or hysteropexy plus sacrospinous fixation [64–66]. Combined anterior and/or posterior colporrhaphy or excessive colpectomy were identified as the most common causes of postoperative dyspareunia but vaginal narrowing and pudendal nerve injury have also been implicated [67].

In a matched case-control study comparing sacrospinous to ileococcygeal fixation, authors found no significant difference in the percentage of women who were sexually active (58% vs. 55%), who had dyspareunia (14% vs. 10%), or who had buttock pain (19% vs. 14%) [68]. It is well recognized that bilateral ileococcygeal fixation may result in shortening of the vagina so in sexually active women with vault prolapse and a short vagina, surgeons should avoid bilateral ileococcygeal fixation as it may cause severe postoperative dyspareunia.

Robot-assisted prolapse surgery is being increasingly used due to the technical advantages such as three-dimensional vision, physiologic tremor filtering, increased freedom of instrument movement, and optimal ergonomics that characterize the robot-assisted approach. These factors may help the surgeon perform a deep and precise dissection in the pelvis and anchor the mesh over the prolapsed walls as much as possible to minimize recurrence and mesh-related complications. A prospective cohort study showed improvement in sexual function 1 year after robot-assisted apical prolapse surgery (sacrocolpopexy or supracervical hysterectomy with sacrocervicopexy) in order to enhance physical and emotional scores [69]. Moreover, a study showed that sexual function after either sacrocolpopexy or sacrocervicopexy was not different in women with pelvic organ prolapse [70]. Furthermore, in another study, vaginal hysterectomy plus uterosacral ligament suspension was compared to robotic supracervical hysterectomy plus colpopexy, and authors found no difference in sexual function, despite postoperative shorter vaginal length in the vaginal hysterectomy group

[71]. Despite this, it seems that sacrocolpopexy or supracervical hysterectomy with sacrocervicopexy would be a better choice for those women with advanced uterine or vault prolapse who would like to remain sexually active postoperatively in preference to a sacrospinous fixation to preserve sexual function.

Conclusion

While vaginal hysterectomy remains a well-known and the most performed procedure in the world for uterovaginal prolapse, an increasing demand for minimally invasive including robotic surgery has been witnessed leading to a number of patients to choose uterus-preserving procedures. The main reasons for this preference include the desire to maintain future fertility, a belief that uterus excision has a negative impact on sexual function or personal identity, and potential surgical issues related to vaginal hysterectomy. When hysterectomy is necessary for uterovaginal prolapse, anatomic changes resulting from the prolapsed state must be carefully understood and accounted for intraoperatively to avoid inadvertent collateral injuries, specifically ureteric ligation, or section. The presence and degree of prolapse of other vaginal compartments in addition to the middle or apical compartment must be carefully evaluated. Transvaginal hysterectomy alone is an inefficient operation in the setting of uterovaginal prolapse, and some form of suspension of the vaginal vault should be undertaken concomitantly. The surgeon performing reconstructive surgery for apical or middle compartment organ prolapse should be able to individualize the most appropriate surgical procedure based on the individual patient's history and vaginal examination findings.

References

1. Dastur AE, Tank PD. Archibald Donald, William Fothergill and the Manchester operation. J Obstet Gynaecol India. 2010;60:484–5.
2. Tolstrup CK, Husby KR, Lose G, Kopp TI, Viborg PH, Kesmodel US, Klarskov N. The Manchester-Fothergill

procedure versus vaginal hysterectomy with uterosacral ligament suspension: a matched historical cohort study. Int Urogynecol J. 2018;29:431–40.

3. Oversand SH, Staff AC, Borstad E, Svenningsen R. The Manchester procedure: anatomical, subjective and sexual outcomes. Int Urogynecol J. 2018;29:1193–201.

4. Ayhan A, Esin S, Guven S, Salman C, Ozyuncu O. The Manchester operation for uterine prolapse. Int J Gynecol Obstet. 2006;92:228–33.

5. Haj-Yahya R, Chill HH, Levin G, Reuveni-Salzman A, Shveiky D. Laparoscopic uterosacral ligament hysteropexy vs total vaginal hysterectomy with uterosacral ligament suspension for anterior and apical prolapse: surgical outcome and patient satisfaction. J Minim Invasive Gynecol. 2020;27:88–93.

6. Aserlind A, Garcia AN, Medina CA. Uterus-sparing surgery: outcomes of transvaginal uterosacral ligament hysteropexy. J Minim Invasive Gynecol. 2020;00:1–7.

7. Zhu YP, Xie T, Guo T, Sun ZJ, Zhu L, Lang JH. Evaluation of extracellular matrix protein expression and apoptosis in the uterosacral ligaments of patients with or without pelvic organ prolapse. Int Urogynecol J. 2020;32(8):2273–81. https://doi.org/10.1007/s00192-020-04446-7.

8. Maher C, Feiner B, Baessler K, Christmann-Schmid C, Haya N, Brown J. Surgery for women with apical vaginal prolapse. Cochrane Database Syst Rev. 2016;10:CD012376.

9. Urogynecologic surgical mesh implants. US Food and Drug Administration website. https://www.fda.gov/MedicalDevices/ProductsandMedicalProcedures/ImplantsandProsthetics/UroGynSurgicalMesh/default.htm. Updated July 10, 2019. Accessed 13 Aug 2019.

10. Nager CW, Visco AG, Richter HE, Rardin CR, Rogers RG, Harvie HSMD, Zyczynski HM, Paraiso MFR, Mazloomdoost D, Grey S, Sridhar A, Wallace D. Effect of vaginal mesh hysteropexy vs vaginal hysterectomy with uterosacral ligament suspension on treatment failure in women with uterovaginal prolapse. A randomized clinical trial. JAMA. 2019;322(11):1054–65.

11. Jelovsek JE, Barber MD, Brubaker L, Norton P, Gantz M, Richter HE, Ali Weidner A, Menefee S, Schaffer J, Pugh N, Meikle S. Effect of uterosacral ligament suspension vs sacrospinous ligament fixation with or without perioperative behavioral therapy for pelvic organ vaginal prolapse on surgical outcomes and prolapse symptoms at 5 years in the OPTIMAL randomized clinical trial. JAMA. 2018;319:1554–65.

12. Jain A, Sheorain VS, Ahlawat K, Ahlawat R. Vascular complication after sacrospinous ligament fixation with uterine preservation. Int Urogynecol J. 2017;28:489–91.

13. Meriwether KV, Antosh DD, Olivera CK, Kim-Fine S, Balk EMMD, Murphy M, Grimes CL, Sleemi A, Singh R, Dieter AA, Crisp CC, Rahn DD. Uterine preservation vs hysterectomy in pelvic organ prolapse

surgery: a systematic review with meta-analysis and clinical practice guidelines. Am J Obstet Gynecol. 2018;219:129–46.

14. Maher CF, Murray CJ, Carey MP, Dwyer PL, Ugoni AM. Iliococcygeus or sacrospinous fixation for vaginal vault prolapse. Obstet Gynecol. 2001;98:40–4.

15. Wu MP, Long CY, Huang KH, Chu CC, Liang CC, Tang CH. Changing trends of surgical approaches for uterine prolapse: an 11-year population-based nationwide descriptive study. Int Urogynecol J. 2013;23:865–72.

16. Khan AA, Eilber KS, Clemens JQ, Wu N, Pashos CL, Anger JTr. Trends in management of pelvic organ prolapse among female medicare beneficiaries. Am J Obstet Gynecol. 2015;212:463.

17. Ridgeway BM. Does prolapse equal hysterectomy? The role of uterine conservation in women with uterovaginal prolapse. Am J Obstet Gynecol. 2015;213:802–9.

18. Stanford EJ, Moore RD, Roovers JPWR, VanDrie DM, Giudice TG, Lukban JC, Bataller E, Sutherland SE. Elevate and uterine preservation: two-year results. Female Pelvic Med Reconstr Surg. 2015;21:205–10.

19. de Oliveira SA, Fonseca MCM, Bortolini MAT, Girao M, Roque MT, Castro RA. Hysteropreservation versus hysterectomy in the surgical treatment of uterine prolapse: systematic review and meta-analysis. Int Urogynecol J. 2017;28:1617–30.

20. Frick AC, Barber MD, Paraiso MFR, Ridgeway B, Jelovsek JE, Walters MD. Attitudes toward hysterectomy in women undergoing evaluation for uterovaginal prolapse. Female Plevic Med Reconstr Surg. 2013;19:103–9.

21. Korbly NB, Kassis NC, Good MM, Richardson ML, Book NM, Yip S, Saguan D, Gross C, Evans J, Lopes VV, Harvie HS, Sung VW. Patient preferences for uterine preservation and hysterectomy in women with pelvic organ prolapse. Am J Obstet Gynecol. 2013;209(470):e1–6.

22. Frick AC, Walters MD, Larkin KS, Barber MD. Risk of unanticipated abnormal gynecologic pathology at the time of hysterectomy for uterovaginal prolapse. Am J Obstet Gynecol. 2010;202(4):202e1–4.

23. DeLancey JO. Anatomic aspects of vaginal eversion after hysterectomy. Am J Obstet Gynecol. 1992;166 (6 Pt 1):1717–24.

24. Forsgren C, Lundholm C, Johansson AL, Cnattingius S, Zetterstrom J, Altman D. Vaginal hysterectomy and risk of pelvic organ prolapse and stress urinary incontinence surgery. Int Urogynecol J. 2012;23:43–8.

25. Blandon RE, Bharucha AE, Melton LJ 3rd, et al. Incidence of pelvic floor repair after hysterectomy: a population-based cohort study. Am J Obstet Gynecol. 2007;197(664):e1–7.

26. Eilber KS, Alperin M, Khan A, et al. Outcomes of vaginal prolapse surgery among female Medicare beneficiaries: the role of apical support. Obstet Gynecol. 2013;122:981–7.

27. Madsen AM, Raker C, Sung VW. Trends in hysteropexy and apical support for uterovaginal prolapse in the United States from 2002 to 2012. Female Pelvic Med Reconst Surg. 2017;23(6):365–71.
28. Anglim B, O'Sullivan O, O'Reilly B. How do patients and surgeons decide on uterine preservation or hysterectomy in apical prolapse? Int Urogynecol J. 2018;29: 1075–9.
29. Chang OH, Walter MD, Yao M, Lapin B. Development and validation of the Value of Uterus instrument and visual analog scale to measure patients' valuation of their uterus. Am J Obstet Gynecol. 2022;S0002-9378(22):00483–5.
30. Richter HE, Sridhar A, Nager CW, Komesu YK, Harvie HS, Zyczynski HM, et al. Characteristics associated with composite surgical failure over 5 years of women in a randomized trial of sacrospinous hysteropexy with graft versus vaginal hysterectomy with uterosacral ligament suspension. Am J Obstet Gynecol. 2022;S0002-9378(22):00619–6.
31. Wallace SL, Syan R, Lee K, Sokol ER. Cost-effectiveness of vaginal hysteropexy compared to vaginal hysterectomy with apical suspension for the treatment of pelvic organ prolapse: a 5-year Markov model. Am J Obstet Gynecol. 2021;224(6):S736–7.
32. Kurian R, Kirchhoff-Rowald A, Sahil S, Cheng AL, Wang X, Shepherd JP, et al. The risk of primary uterine and cervical cancer after hysteropexy. Female Pelvic Med Reconstr Surg. 2021;27(3):e493–6.
33. Maldonado PA, Jackson LA, Florian-Rodriguez ME, Wai CY. Comparisons of functional apical support after sacral hysteropexy versus sacral colpopexy: a cadaveric study. Female Pelvic Med Reconstr Surg. 2020;26(11):664–7.
34. Alperin M, Weinstein M, Kivnick S, Duong TH, Menefee S. A randomized trial of prophylactic uterosacral ligament suspension at the time of hysterectomy for Prevention of Vaginal Vault Prolapse (PULS): design and methods. Contemp Clin Trials. 2013;35(2):8–12.
35. American Association for Gynecological Laparoscopy. AAGL practice report: practice guidelines on the prevention of apical prolapse at the time of benign hysterectomy. J Minim Invasive Gynecol. 2014;21(5): 715–22.
36. Gabriel I, Kalousdian A, Brito LG, Abdalian T, Vitonis AF, Minassian VA. Pelvic organ prolapse after 3 modes of hysterectomy: long-term follow-up. Am J Obstet Gynecol. 2021;224:496.e1–496.e.10.
37. Nygaard I, Barber MD, Burgio KL, et al. Prevalence of symptomatic pelvic floor disorders in US women. JAMA. 2008;300:1311–6.
38. Pauls RN, Segal JL, Silva WA, Kleeman SD, Karram MM. Sexual function in patients presenting to a urogynecology practice. Int Urogynecol J. 2006;17: 576–80.
39. Lindau ST, Schumm LP, Laumann EO, et al. A study of sexuality and health among older adults in the United States. N Engl J Med. 2007;357:762–74.

40. Roos AM, Sultan AH, Thakar R. Sexual problems in the gynecology clinic: are we making a mountain out of a molehill? Int Urogynecol J. 2012;23:145–52.
41. Lamont J. Female sexual health consensus clinical guidelines. J Obstet Gynaecol Can. 2012;34: 769–75.
42. Handa VL, Harvey L, Cundiff GW, Siddique SA, Kjerulff KH. Sexual function among women with urinary incontinence and pelvic organ prolapse. Am J Obstet Gynecol. 2004;191:751–6.
43. Zielinski R, Low LK, Tumbarello J, Miller JM. Body image and sexuality in women with pelvic organ prolapse. Urol Nurs. 2009;29:239–46.
44. Jha S, Gopinath D. Prolapse or incontinence: what affects sexual function the most? Int Urogynecol J. 2016;27:607–11.
45. Pauls RN, Berman JR. Impact of pelvic floor disorders and prolapse on female sexual function and response. Urol Clin North Am. 2020;29:677–83.
46. Zucchi A, Lazzeri M, Porena M, et al. Uterus preservation in pelvic organ prolapse surgery. Nat Rev Urol. 2010;7:626–33.
47. Pauls RN. Impact of gynecological surgery on female sexual function. Int J Impot Res. 2010;22:105–14.
48. Whiteman MK, Hillis SD, Jamieson DJ, et al. Inpatient hysterectomy surveillance in the United States, 2000–2004. Am J Obstet Gynecol. 2008;198:34–e31.
49. Radosa JC, Meyberg-Solomayer G, Kastl C, et al. Influences of different hysterectomy techniques on patients' postoperative sexual function and quality of life. J Sex Med. 2014;11:2342–50.
50. Andersen L, Zobbe V, Ottesen B, et al. Five-year follow up of a randomised controlled trial comparing subtotal with total abdominal hysterectomy. BJOG. 2014;11:1471–0528.
51. Kives S, Lefebvre G, Wolfman W, et al. Supracervical hysterectomy. J Obstet Gynecol Can JOGC. 2010;32: 62–8.
52. Lermann J, Haberle L, Merk S, et al. Comparison of prevalence of hypoactive sexual desire disorder (HSDD) in women after five different hysterectomy procedures. Eur J Obstet Gynecol Reprod Biol. 2013;167:210–4.
53. Komisaruk BR, Frangos E, Whipple B. Hysterectomy improves sexual response? Addressing a crucial omission in the literature. J Minim Invasive Gynecol. 2011;18:288–95.
54. Achtari C, Dwyer PL. Sexual function and pelvic floor disorders. Best Pract Res Clin Obstet Gynaecol. 2005;19:993–1008.
55. Thakar R, Sultan AH. Hysterectomy and pelvic organ dysfunction. Best Pract Res Clin Obstet Gynaecol. 2005;19:403–18.
56. Parker WH. Bilateral oophorectomy versus ovarian conservation: effects on long-term women's health. J Minim Invasive Gynecol. 2010;17:161–6.
57. Rhodes JC, Kjerulff KH, Langenberg PW, Guzinski GM. Hysterectomy and sexual functioning. JAMA. 1999;282:1934–41.

58. Schimpf MO, Harvie HS, Omotosho TB, et al. Does vaginal size impact sexual activity and function? Int Urogynecol J Pelvic Floor Dysfunct. 2010;21:447–52.
59. Uçar MG, Ilhan TT, Sanlikan F, Celik C. Sexual functioning before and after vaginal hysterectomy to treat pelvic organ prolapse and the effects of vaginal cuff closure techniques: a prospective randomised study. Eur J Obstet Gynecol Reprod Biol. 2016;206:1–5.
60. Drudi L, Press JZ, Lau S, et al. Vaginal vault dehiscence after robotic hysterectomy for gynecologic cancers: search for risk factors and literature review. Int J Gynecol Cancer: Off J Int Gynecol Cancer Soc. 2013;23:943–50.
61. Nguyen ML, Kapoor M, Pradhan TS, et al. Two cases of post-coital vaginal cuff dehiscence with small bowel evisceration after robotic assisted laparoscopic hysterectomy. Int J Surg Case Rep. 2013;4:603–5.
62. Ceccaroni M, Berretta R, Malzoni M, et al. Vaginal cuff dehiscence after hysterectomy: a multicenter retrospective study. Eur J Obstet Gynecol Reprod Biol. 2011;158:308–13.
63. Costantini E, Porena M, Lazzeri M, Mearini L, Bini V, Zucchi A. Changes in female sexual function after pelvic organ prolapse repair: role of hysterectomy. Int Urogynecol J. 2013;24:1481–7.
64. Colombo M, Vitobello D, Proietti F, Milani R. Randomised comparison of Burch colposuspension versus anterior colporrhaphy in women with stress urinary incontinence and anterior vaginal wall prolapse. BJOG. 2000;107:544–51.
65. Goldberg RP, Tomezsko JE, Winkler HA, et al. Anterior or posterior sacrospinous vaginal vault suspension: long-term anatomic and functional evaluation. Obstet Gynecol. 2001;98:199–204.
66. Paraiso MF, Ballard LA, Walters MD, Lee JC, Mitchinson AR. Pelvic support defects and visceral and sexual function in women treated with sacrospinous ligament suspension and pelvic reconstruction. Am J Obstet Gynecol. 1996;175:1423–30.
67. Holley RL, Varner RE, Gleason BP, Apffel LA, Scott S. Sexual function after sacrospinous ligament fixation for vaginal vault prolapse. J Reprod Med. 1996;41:355–8.
68. Maher CF, Cary MP, Slack MC, Murray CJ, Milligan M, Schluter P. Uterine preservation or hysterectomy at sacrospinous colpopexy for uterovaginal prolapse? Int Urogynecol J Pelvic Floor Dysfunct. 2001;12:381–4.
69. van Zanten F, Brem C, Lenters E, Broeders IAMJ, Koops SES. Sexual function after robot-assisted prolapse surgery: a prospective study. Int Urogynecol J. 2018;29:905–12.
70. Ko YC, Yoo EH, Han GH, Kim YM. Comparison of sexual function between sacrocolpopexy and sacrocervicopexy. Obstet Gynecol Sci. 2017;60:207–12.
71. De La Cruz JF, Myers EM, Geller EJ. Vaginal versus robotic hysterectomy and concomitant pelvic support surgery: a comparison of postoperative vaginal length and sexual function. J Minim Invasive Gynecol. 2014;26:011.

Minimally Invasive Sacrocolpopexy

35

Priyanka Kancherla and Natasha Ginzburg

Contents

Introduction	618
Patient Selection and Preoperative Evaluation	618
Surgical Technique	620
Port Placement	620
Steps of the Procedure	620
Dissection of the Sacral Promontory	620
Creation of a Sub-peritoneal Tunnel	621
Anterior Vaginal Dissection	621
Posterior Vaginal Dissection	622
Vaginal Fixation of the Graft	622
Sacral Fixation of the Graft	622
Retroperitonealization of the Graft	623
Additional Procedures	623
Outcomes	623
Complications	625
Cost	626
Future Directions	627
Cross-References	627
References	627

Abstract

Minimally invasive sacrocolpopexy is becoming a popular alternative to open vaginal vault suspension. Minimally invasive techniques aim to reproduce the excellent outcomes of open sacrocolpopexy, but with shorter hospital stays, and decreased complication rates. Appropriate patient selection and preoperative evaluation are fundamental to maximize both subjective and objective success of the procedure. Patients' expectations and quality of life goals should be considered alongside the

P. Kancherla · N. Ginzburg (✉)
Department of Urology, SUNY Upstate Medical
University, Syracuse, NY, USA
e-mail: GinzburN@upstate.edu

© Springer Nature Switzerland AG 2023
F. E. Martins et al. (eds.), *Female Genitourinary and Pelvic Floor Reconstruction*,
https://doi.org/10.1007/978-3-031-19598-3_36

surgeon's skillset when deciding on the most appropriate surgical technique for prolapse repair. Careful surgical technique, with attention payed to the essential segments of the surgery can minimize risks of complications. Patient outcomes are generally similar to open technique, and major complications are comparable. Length of hospital stay seems to be lower with minimally invasive techniques, although costs may be higher. It is important to weigh the patient's needs, goals, and potential risks when planning any surgical intervention.

Keywords

Pelvic organ prolapse · Sacrocolpopexy · Robotic surgery · Laparoscopic surgery · Prolapse repair

Introduction

Sacrocolpopexy aims to correct pelvic organ prolapse through suspension of the prolapsed vaginal vault to the sacral promontory with a bridging graft. The use of synthetic mesh as the intervening graft was first described by Lane in 1961, establishing abdominal sacrocolpopexy in the repertoire of surgical options for repair of apical pelvic organ prolapse [1]. Sacrocolpopexy re-establishes normal vaginal vault anatomy and axis and maximizes vaginal length. High success rates and durability established sacrocolpopexy as the gold standard for apical prolapse repair. Sacrocolpopexy was traditionally performed through an infraumbilical midline incision however widespread use of laparoscopy led to the first report of laparoscopic abdominal sacrocolpopexy in the early 1990s. The adoption of robotic surgery and its application to pelvic surgery led to the first report of robotic sacrocolpopexy in 2004 [2]. In this chapter, we discuss both approaches to minimally invasive abdominal sacrocolpopexy, laparoscopic and robotic, including patient evaluation, indications, surgical technique and consideration, outcomes, complications, and future directions.

Patient Selection and Preoperative Evaluation

Appropriate patient selection is paramount to maximize success and patient satisfaction and minimize risk of complications. The surgical indications for minimally invasive sacrocolpopexy are essentially identical to the open approach: symptomatic, bothersome apical pelvic organ prolapse in a woman who wishes to preserve vaginal length. Sacrocolpopexy is sometimes reserved for repair after failed native tissue repairs, depending on surgeon and patient preference.

A thorough history and physical should be performed to inform surgical decision making. Medical history can be used a basic screen to determine if the patient is a safe surgical candidate. Co-morbidities such as diabetes mellitus, connective tissue disorders, immunosuppression, and history of smoking can compromise success of repair and may represent modifiable factors to address prior to proceeding with sacrocolpopexy. Other components of a patient's medical and surgical history that are especially relevant to surgical planning are discussed later in this section.

Physical exam should include an abdominal exam with close attention paid to body habitus and prior surgical incisions and scars. Pelvic exam is directed toward evaluating the severity or stage of pelvic organ prolapse utilizing the Pelvic Organ Prolapse-Quantification System (POP-Q). Evaluation of all three vaginal compartments is important. Significant contribution of anterior and posterior prolapse may guide surgical technique and possibly necessitate additional procedure for relief of symptoms. The vaginal epithelium should be examined for evidence of vaginal atrophy. Evaluation for stress urinary incontinence including cough stress test and urethral hypermobility should be included in the pelvic exam.

Baseline voiding behavior and urinary complaints should be determined, including urinary retention, overactive bladder symptoms, and urinary incontinence. Urodynamic evaluation can be helpful in patients with bothersome baseline urinary complaints. As pelvic organ prolapse and stress urinary incontinence commonly co-exist, testing with and without reduction of prolapse can reveal those with occult stress urinary incontinence. These patients can be offered a concomitant anti-incontinence procedure. De novo stress urinary incontinence after sacrocolpopexy requires a more nuanced approach. The reported rates of de novo stress urinary incontinence after prolapse repair range widely from 10% to 80%. Two randomized, multicenter clinic trials, the Colpopexy and Urinary Reduction Efforts (CARE) and the Outcomes Following Vaginal Prolapse Repair and Mid Urethral Sling (OPUS) trials, evaluated the effect of prophylactic stress incontinence procedures at the time of sacrocolpopexy and sacrospinous fixation, respectively, in patients without baseline stress urinary incontinence [3, 4]. Both trials concluded that prophylactic incontinence procedures decreased the rate of de novo stress incontinence compared to the control group. However, this comes with the risk of overtreatment, increased complication rate, and increased cost. Therefore, the decision to perform a prophylactic anti-incontinence procedure at the time of sacrocolpopexy is at the discretion of the surgeon and should be made after appropriate counseling and discussion with the patient.

Any rectal complaints such as pain, splinting, and straining should be elicited, especially in patients with concomitant posterior prolapse. Although high quality data regarding impact of sacrocolpopexy on rectal symptoms is lacking, several studies do suggest improvement in defecatory complaints after sacrocolpopexy. Constipation should be treated preoperatively to minimize straining after surgery with gastroenterology referral in complicated cases.

Although routine preoperative radiographic studies are not standard, any existing imaging studies should be reviewed. Anatomic anomalies that may affect the surgery should be noted. A small proportion of patients may have upper tract obstruction secondary to pelvic organ prolapse with hydronephrosis on upper tract imaging. While this is unlikely to impact surgical decision making, it should be noted and followed postoperatively in order to ensure resolution of hydronephrosis. Patients with defecatory dysfunction out of proportion to the severity posterior prolapse may require further imaging with gastroenterology or colorectal surgery referral. Additionally, it may be prudent to obtain preoperative imaging in patients with a history of significant prior abdominal surgery.

Routine laboratory studies have minimal role in the evaluation of the prolapse patient. However, in anticipation of surgery a complete blood count, basic metabolic panel and coagulation profile can be obtained in the appropriate patient. Urine culture should be obtained preoperatively or in any patient with urinary complaints and confirmed to be negative.

As the majority of sacrocolpopexy cases utilize mesh grafts, patients should be counselled on mesh-associated risks and complications which will be discussed later in this text. The patient's opinion of the use of mesh in their repair will also inform discussion regarding surgical management options.

In addition to the routine evaluation and workup, several nuances must be considered when determining whether minimally invasive sacrocolpopexy is appropriate for the individual patient.

Firstly, the patient must be able to tolerate insufflation of the abdomen with carbon dioxide. Co-morbidities such as chronic obstructive pulmonary disease, congestive heart failure, ischemic heart disease, and chronic kidney disease may preclude patients from safely undergoing any laparoscopic procedure due to the effects of increased intra-abdominal pressure [5]. Additionally, minimally invasive sacrocolpopexy requires placing the patient in the Trendelenburg position. The physiologic sequelae of Trendelenburg are well-documented and affect respiratory, cardiovascular, renal, gastrointestinal, and nervous systems [6]. Patients who are at higher risk for pneumoperitoneum, or Trendelenburg, related complications should be counselled regarding this risk. A back-up plan for completing an alternative method of prolapse repair or aborting the procedure should be discussed preoperatively.

An additional caveat to patient selection includes surgical history that would impede graft fixation at the sacral promontory. This includes vascular grafts, particularly in the iliac vessels, history of pelvic renal transplant, and spinal hardware in the lumbosacral spine. Such previous surgeries can affect the surgeon's ability to safely mobilize surrounding structure to access the sacrum and placement of mesh near other implants could increase risk of complications.

Surgical Technique

The patient is placed into the low lithotomy position with arms tucked at the sides in a neurologically neutral position. Anti-slip gel or foam padding can be utilized to prevent movement toward the head of the bed in the Trendelenburg position. The patient is secured to the table. All pressure points should be padded including the elbow to prevent ulnar nerve injury and the lateral knee to prevent common peroneal nerve injury. The abdomen, pelvis, and vagina are then prepped in draped in standard sterile fashion. A Foley catheter should be placed for continuous bladder drainage. Pneumoperitoneum is establishing using standard laparoscopic techniques. In a laparoscopic sacrocolpopexy, the surgeon typically operates from the left side of the patient and the assistant operates from the right. In a robotic sacrocolpopexy, the bedside assistant is typically at the patient's right side. The robot is docked either from the patient's left, or from in between the legs. It is helpful to have access to the vagina for manipulation of a vaginal stent, so positioning of the assistant and robot should take that into consideration.

Port Placement

In a laparoscopic abdominal sacrocolpopexy, a 5 mm or 10 mm laparoscopic port is placed at the umbilicus dependent on preferred sized of laparoscopic camera. Placement of additional ports are placed under laparoscopic vision in order to avoid injury to any intra-abdominal organs. Two additional 5 mm laparoscopic ports are placed in the right and left lower quadrant, lateral to inferior epigastric artery. An additional 5 mm laparoscopic port is placed either lateral to the umbilical camera port on the left or in the midline half way between the pubic symphysis and the umbilicus.

For robotic abdominal sacrocolpopexy, an 8 mm robotic port is placed at umbilicus as the camera port. Two additional 8 mm ports are placed lateral to the camera port, each 8 cm from the camera port to prevent collision of the robotic arm. An additional 8 mm robotic port is placed in the left lower quadrant, also 8 cm lateral to and in line with the previously place left-sided port. A 12 cm assistant port is placed in the right lower quadrant, in line with the previously place right-sided port. The robot is then docked in an orientation that allows easy vaginal access. This can be either parallel or perpendicular to the patient's body, depending on the assistant's preference. Commonly used instruments include a robotic monopolar scissors introduced through the right arm, a robotic fenestrated bipolar forceps through the left arm, a robotic Prograsp forceps through the lateral left arm, but can be adjusted to surgeon preference. This description of robotic port placement and docking presumes usage of the DaVinci robotic platform. If alternate platforms are used, port placement may need to be modified (fig. 1).

Steps of the Procedure

Other than the establishment of pneumoperitoneum and port placement described above, the surgical principles of minimally invasive sacrocolpopexy are identical to the open approach. The procedure can be simplified to the following steps: (1) Dissection of the sacral promontory, (2) creation of a sub-peritoneal tunnel, (3) anterior vaginal dissection, (4) posterior vaginal dissection, (5) fixation of the graft, and (6) retroperitonealization of the graft. Each step has specific considerations related to the minimally invasive approach.

Dissection of the Sacral Promontory

Laparoscopic inspection of the abdomen is performed to identify vital visceral and vascular structures. The sigmoid colon is the retracted cranially and laterally to the left to facilitate

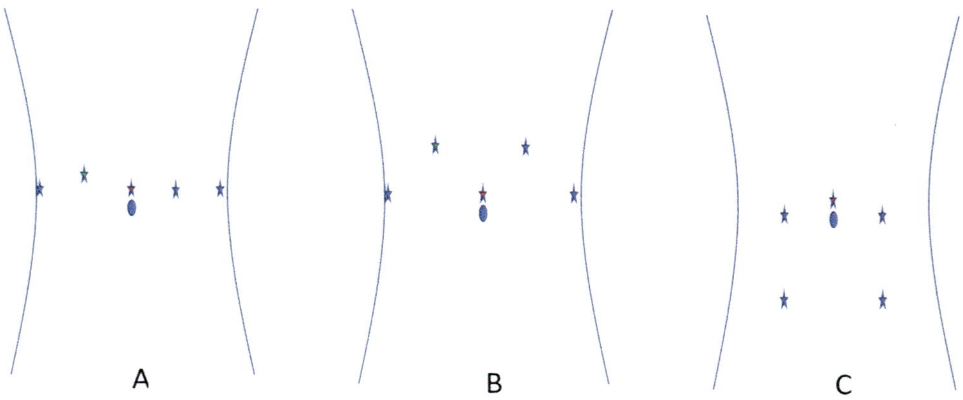

35 Minimally Invasive Sacrocolpopexy

Fig. 1 Port placement can be individualized for the surgeon; this figure depicts various options for port placement in minimally invasive sacrocolpopexy for the robotic DaVinci Xi platform (**a**), robotic DaVinci Si platform (**b**), and laparoscopic port placement (**c**). Red star indicates camera port, green indicates assistant port

identification of the sacral promontory, the superior most point of the anterior surface of the first sacral vertebrae. Surrounding vascular structures including the aortic bifurcation, iliac arteries and veins, and inferior vena cava should be identified. If mobilization of these vessels is required for adequate sacral exposure, strong consideration could be given to aborting sacrocolpopexy and pursing an alternate approach for prolapse repair. The middle sacral artery and vein should be avoided as they cross the sacral promontory. The sacral promontory can be identified using haptic feedback from laparoscopic instruments. Robotically, the surgeon lacks haptic feedback from the robotic instruments thus the bedside assistant is helpful for confirming the location of the promontory. The peritoneum overlying the sacral promontory is then opened longitudinally. The presacral space and subperitoneal fat is dissected. Care is taken here to perform meticulous hemostasis as the delicate plexus of presacral veins in encountered in this space. The periosteum of the sacral promontory and anterior longitudinal ligament are identified and a space adequate to fix the graft is cleared.

Creation of a Sub-peritoneal Tunnel

The opening in the peritoneum is extended caudally to the Pouch of Douglas, lateral to the rectum on the right side. Peritoneal flaps are raised which will be re-approximated to retroperitonealize the graft later in the case. Alternatively, a sub-peritoneal tunnel may be created through which the mesh arm is passed. The right ureter is definitively identified during this step to avoid injury.

Anterior Vaginal Dissection

A vaginal manipulator is placed in order to identify the extent of the vaginal cuff. Several commonly encountered surgical instruments as well as commercially available devices have been reported for use in this step. Sponge sticks, EEA sizers, and malleable retractors are readily available at most institutions and can be positioned within the vagina to allow identification of the cuff. Proprietary medical devices such as lighted vaginal stents are preferred by some surgeons. Still other institutions design and manufacture vaginal retractors to their desired specifications for use in this step.

Once the vaginal manipulator is placed, the peritoneum over the vaginal cuff is sharply incised. The plan between the bladder and vaginal cuff is identified. Inflating the bladder with saline may aid in identification of these structure. Dissection of the vaginal cuff may be more challenging in women with long standing, severe prolapse, or with previous vaginal repairs due to inflammation and scarring or obscured natural planes. The plane between the bladder and vagina is extended caudally approximately 4 cm, depending on the extent of any anterior defect and should not extend beyond the level of the trigone.

Posterior Vaginal Dissection

Once the anterior vaginal is dissected, the peritoneum posterior to the vagina is opened to the pouch of Douglas. The plane between the rectum and the vaginal is established and the dissection is extended caudally approximately 4 cm, depending of the extent of posterior prolapse.

The posterior dissection can be extended to the level of the perineal body so that sacrocolpoperineopexy can be performed. In these cases, the posterior mesh arm is fixed to the perineal body distally for correction of severe posterior prolapse. Alternatively, support of the posterior distal vagina can be restored using a vaginal, native tissue repair once the sacrocolpopexy is complete.

Vaginal Fixation of the Graft

Upon completion of the anterior and posterior vaginal dissection, the graft is introduced into the body. Graft options, materials, and conformations can vary and are beyond the scope of this chapter. Methods and options for graft fixation depend on surgical approach. The basic principle remains that the graft must be fixed to the anterior and posterior vagina along the length of the dissection and that upon fixation of the cranial end of the graft to the anterior longitudinal ligament at the sacral promontory, the vaginal apex is suspended from that point.

While permanent suture is typically used for sacral fixation, several studies have been conducted on the usage of permanent versus absorbable suture in vaginal graft fixation. Historically, permanent suture has been used as an additional means of reducing risk of recurrence. However, retrospective studies provided little support for the effect of suture type on mesh exposure. In effort to determine the impact of type of suture on rate of mesh exposure, a randomized-controlled trial was conducted

comparing rate of mesh and suture exposure and success rate with permanent versus delayed absorbable suture [7]. The authors find no significant difference in mesh or suture exposure rates between the two groups and no difference in success or recurrence rate at 1 year. The authors suggest that type of mesh likely impacts rate of mesh exposure more than suture type.

Suturing method for vaginal graft fixation has also been evaluated. In a randomized controlled trial, the authors compare operative time for graft fixation and anatomic outcomes between vaginal graft fixation performed with interrupted, monofilament delayed absorbable suture and running barbed delayed absorbable suture during robotic and laparoscopic sacrocolpopexy [8]. They find that the mean vaginal graft fixation time was 13 min faster using running, barbed, and delayed absorbable suture compared to using interrupted delayed absorbable suture. They found no statistical different in anatomic failure at 12 months.

Sacral Fixation of the Graft

To restore apical support, the proximal end of the graft is fixed to the sacral promontory. In a cadaveric and radiographic study of the fifth lumbar to first sacral vertebral disc space, the authors find that the most prominent structure in the presacral space is the L5-S1 disc and there is, on average, a 60° acute angle descent between this space and the sacral promontory [9]. Thus they recommend sacral fixation of the graft approximately 1.5 cm inferior to the L5-S1 disc, the average height of the disc space in this study, and to utilize the lumbosacral angle as a landmark for identification of the sacral promontory.

Consideration has also been given to the use of surgical tacks in place of suture to fix the graft to the sacral promontory. In a retrospective study of 231 patients undergoing laparoscopic sacrocolpopexy, the authors find no statistically significant difference in operative time, blood loss, complications, recurrence rate, or rate of reoperation who underwent sacral fixation of the graft with titanium surgical tacks compared to suture [10]. Particularly in laparoscopic sacrocolpopexy and depending on surgeon preference, the use of surgical tack may be beneficial due challenges associated with suturing.

When using suture of sacral graft fixation, consideration has also been given to the number and orientation of sacral sutures. In a cadaveric study the authors aim to estimate the location and orientation of sacral suture that would yield the strongest graft fixation [11]. They find that sutures placed in the anterior longitudinal ligament at or above the level of the sacral promontory are stronger than suture placed below. Horizontally placed sutures are significantly stronger than vertically placed sutures.

Retroperitonealization of the Graft

Once the graft is in position, the peritoneal flaps, previously created during creation of the sub-peritoneal tunnel, are approximated over the mesh using running delayed absorbable suture. This effectively retroperitonealizes the graft and is thought to prevent bowel obstruction, mesh erosion into bowel and adhesions of the bowel to the mesh in the event of re-operation.

Although this is an accepted step in sacrocolpopexy, consideration has been given to the need for retroperitonealization. Advocates for eliminating this step argue that closure of the peritoneum increases risk of direct or indirect ureteral injury and bleeding from additional suture placement. In a case series of 128 patients who underwent laparoscopic or open sacrocolpopexy without closure of peritoneum over the mesh graft, the authors report no bowel complications related to non-burial of the mesh and at a median follow-up time of 19 months they report a 90% success rate, defined by need for re-operation [12]. In a retrospective review of 178 patients who underwent laparoscopic sacrocolpopexy without retroperitonealization of the mesh graft, the authors aimed to determine the long terms safety and efficacy of eliminating this step [13]. They determined that three patients in their study experienced bowel complications related to intraperitoneal mesh. They determined an objective success rate of 59% at median follow-up time of 35 months. Another retrospective study compared a cohort of patient who underwent abdominal sacrocolpopexy with retroperitonealization of mesh to a cohort who did not. They report increased blood loss and operative time with peritoneal closure [14]. They find no significant difference complications between the two cohorts.

Currently available literature does not demonstrate the feared complication of ureteral injury or clinically significant bleeding with closure of the peritoneum. Published methodology for several sacrocolpopexy clinical trials allow that closure of the peritoneum over the graft is optional. Although high quality studies demonstrating risk or benefit of peritoneal closure are lacking, the recommendation is to ensure the peritoneum is closed over the graft.

Additional Procedures

After completion of sacrocolpopexy, additional procedures can be performed to ensure optimal pelvic floor support. Occasionally, the anterior support provided by the anterior arm of sacrocolpopexy mesh is inadequate. In these cases, anterior colporrhaphy can be performed vaginally to provide adequate anterior support.

In the event of significant posterior prolapse, concomitant posterior colporrhaphy and perineorrhaphy can be perform, especially if one wishes to avoid sacrocolpoperineopexy with extension of the mesh graft to the perineal body.

Incontinence procedures either via abdominal approach in the form of retropubic colposuspension or via vaginal approach with mid-urethral slings can be performed after completion of sacrocolpopexy. Indications for concomitant incontinence procedures are discussed earlier in this chapter and this textbook.

Outcomes

Historically, durable outcomes have established abdominal sacrocolpopexy as the gold standard for apical vaginal prolapse. Randomized controlled trials comparing open, laparoscopic, and robotic approaches largely demonstrate that subjective and objective cure rate are maintained independent of surgical approach and illustrate differences in other perioperative factors.

To date, three randomized, controlled trials compared outcomes of laparoscopic sacrocolpopexy to the established open approach. Freeman et al. compared objectives outcomes using point C on the POP-Q system and subjective outcomes using the Patient Global Impression of Improvement (PGI-I) questionnaire between patients undergoing open abdominal sacrocolpopexy and those undergoing laparoscopic sacrocolpopexy [15]. Objectively, significant improvement in point C was noted from baseline in both groups with no significant difference between groups at 3 month and 1 year follow-up. The subjective outcome of PGI-I score of 1 or 2 ("very much better" or "much better") was reported by 90% of patients in the open group and 80% of patients in the laparoscopic group at 1 year follow-up. These objective and subjective outcomes led the authors to conclude that open and laparoscopic sacrocolpopexy are clinically equivalent.

Cooleen et al. compare subjective, functional outcomes between open and laparoscopic sacrocolpopexy in their randomized, controlled trial [16]. The primary outcome was the Urinary Distress Inventory (UDI) questionnaire, which includes a domain for "genital prolapse," as a representation of disease-specific quality of life. No significant difference was found between the two approaches in any domains of the UDI questionnaire at 1-year follow-up. The authors do report anatomic outcome on POP-Q assessment as a secondary endpoint and find no significant difference between the two groups.

In a subsequent randomized controlled trial, Constantini et al. provided longer term outcomes [17]. Comparing open and laparoscopic sacrocolpopexy, the authors used POP-Q parameters of prolapse stage 1 or less, point C/D -5 or less and at least 7 cm total vaginal length to define cure. Based on this definition of cure, the author determined that at a mean follow-up time of 41.7 months there was a 100% cure rate and no patients had an apical recurrence. The authors did note that rate of asymptomatic anterior recurrence was higher in the laparoscopic group and the rate

of asymptomatic posterior recurrence was comparable between groups. A Kaplan-Meier analysis of these asymptomatic recurrences revealed longer recurrence-free survival for open sacrocolpopexy and significantly earlier recurrence in laparoscopic group with 83.3 recurrence occurring in first 12 months after surgery. None of these patients required re-operation during the study period. The authors conclude that clinically significant outcomes for laparoscopic sacrocolpopexy are equivalent to those of open sacrocolpopexy for apical repair however anatomical outcomes may not be for the anterior compartment.

The results of these randomized, controlled trials establish comparable short- and long-term outcomes between open and laparoscopic sacrocolpopexy.

With the growing popularity of robotic surgery, clinical trials aimed to compares outcomes of the two minimally invasive approaches. In a single center randomized trial, Paraiso et al. compared laparoscopic and robotic sacrocolpopexy [18]. While the primary outcome was total operative time, which was significantly longer in the robotic group, they also report outcomes at 1 year after surgery. Anatomically, 91% of patient in the laparoscopic group and 88% of patient in the robotic group had POP-Q stage 0–1 prolapse 1 year after surgery with no statistically significant difference between the groups. Additionally, there was no significant difference in POP-Q point measurements between the two groups at 1 year. Quality of life questionnaires also revealed no difference in subjective outcome between the two groups.

In a subsequent randomized control trial comparing laparoscopic and robotic sacrocolpopexy, Anger et al. compared surgical costs and rehospitalization at weeks as their primary endpoint and anatomic and subjective outcomes as secondary endpoints [19]. While the cost comparison will be addressed later in this chapter, the authors found no difference in POP-Q measurement and outcomes of validated symptom questionnaires at 6 month follow-up. At subsequent 1 year follow-up, both groups had sustained significant improvement in anatomic and symptomatic endpoints from baseline and there remained no significant difference between the robotic group and laparoscopic group [20].

In a single-center randomized controlled trial with the largest cohorts and longest follow-up time, Illiano et al. found compared outcomes between laparoscopic and robotic sacrocolpopexy [21]. Objective cure was defined as POP-Q parameters of prolapse stage 1 or less, point C/D -5 or less and at least 7 cm total vaginal length. At a mean follow-up of 24.06 months, objective cure was 100% in both groups. Anatomic outcomes measured by POP-Q were comparable between the two groups at all points except for C/D point which was better in the robotic cohort at -8 compared to -7 in laparoscopic cohort, a difference which reached statistical significance. There were fewer cases of asymptomatic anterior and posterior prolapse persistence in the robotic group. There were no recurrences or re-operations in either group.

The results of these trials all support the clinical equivalence of robotic and laparoscopic sacrocolpopexy. Additionally, they translate the high cure rates and durable results historically attributed to open abdominal sacrocolpopexy to minimally invasive approaches.

In addition to success and cure rates presented in the randomized trials described above, these trials also report on and compare various perioperative outcomes. Additionally, multiple comparative and retrospective studies report on outcomes larger patient cohorts.

Complications

Minimally invasive sacrocolpopexy is generally associated with decreased length of stay and fewer complications than open sacrocolpopexy [16, 22, 23]; however, the procedure is not without risks. Perioperative complications include severe bleeding (or need for transfusion), injuries to the bladder, bowel, or ureter, inability to complete procedure or need for conversion to open procedure. A number of studies have demonstrated similar rates of these complications between laparoscopic and robotic approaches [24–26]. The

rates of bowel injury range from 0.3% to 3%, while rates of bladder injury range from 1% to 7% [26–28]. Frequently, these types of injuries are identified intraoperatively, and are repaired at the time of procedure. If a bladder or bowel injury is identified during the procedure, many recommend to avoid placement of mesh to avoid risk of mesh erosion or infection. There will be some patients in whom a bowel or bladder injury is not recognized intraoperatively. These patients will most commonly present with postoperative abdominal pain or pain at port sites. A high index of suspicion warrants further investigation. Imaging with contrast enhanced computerized tomography, including oral, IV, or intravesical contrast is recommended.

Vascular injury or significant bleeding has been noted in 0.8–6.3% of minimally invasive sacrocolpopexy cases [27, 29]. Excellent visualization with careful dissection of the anterior longitudinal ligament can help to mitigate the risk of injuring the vessels in this space. Injury to the right ureter can also potentially occur, although not frequently reported.

A less common complication is infection at the sacral disc space, resulting in discitis or osteomyelitis. Patients present with lower back pain and fever, but may also have more vague symptoms of generalized malaise. Symptoms may occur in the early postoperative period but may also occur months after the surgical procedure [30]. Imaging with MRI or CT can be helpful to diagnose this. Imaging can identify findings of enhancement, edema, or abscess at the sacral disc space. Treatment may include intravenous antibiotics but may also require removal of mesh and surgical debridement.

Other complications that have been reported at long-term follow-up include port-site hernia, dyspareunia, bowel symptoms such as constipation or fecal incontinence, as well as de novo urinary symptoms. In a study published by Pacquée et al., 11.8% of patients at a mean follow-up of 85.5 months after laparoscopic sacrocolpopexy complained of dyspareunia or obstructive defecation. The number of patients with urinary problems (41.2%) was similar to that seen in other trials [31].

Mesh complications can occur in the immediate postoperative period or in a delayed fashion. Identifying the exact risk of mesh complications is difficult, possibly due to differences in reporting, surgical technique or type of mesh used. The risk of mesh complications have been reported anywhere from 0% to 27% [32], and will be discussed in more detail elsewhere in this text.

Overall, while risks of serious complications in minimally invasive sacrocolpopexy are generally low, it is important to be vigilant to their possibility.

Cost

As minimally invasive and specifically robotic surgery has been widely adopted, attention has been called to the direct cost of robotic technology compared to improvements in hospital stay length and complication rates. Multiple studies aimed to compare cost-effectiveness between apical vaginal prolapse surgeries.

In a retrospective, exploratory study, authors estimated and calculated direct and indirect costs of surgery and postoperative inpatient care and compared cost of three sacrocolpopexy approaches, open, laparoscopic and robotic, with five patients in each cohort [33]. They found that estimated direct cost for the operating room and surgical instruments was significantly lower for open abdominal sacrocolpopexy compared to robotic and laparoscopic approaches, continuing to a higher total cost for the minimally invasive approaches.

Conversely, in a separate retrospective cost-minimization analysis, the authors determine a 10% cost-savings for robotic sacrocolpopexy compared to open, despite similar operative times [34]. They do note that this savings is likely dependent on number of institutional robotic cases done annually and shorter postoperative hospital stay.

In another retrospective, single-institution review of 512 patients undergoing post-hysterectomy apical vaginal prolapse repair, the authors compared complication rates and cost between the transvaginal Mayo-McCall culdoplasty, open abdominal sacrocolpopexy and robotic sacrocolpopexy [35]. Cost was determined using a county-wide, claims-based database. The authors found a lower cost and complication rate associated with Mayo-McCall culdoplasty compared with either open or robotic abdominal sacrocolpopexy. Robotic sacrocolpopexy was associated with highest cost and complication rate and with shortest length of hospital stay.

Another retrospective study compared cost and health resource utilization between vaginal sacrospinous fixation, open abdominal sacrocolpopexy and laparoscopic sacrocolpopexy using a national, claims-based database [36]. Mean index cost, the cost associated with surgery and immediate postoperative hospital stay, was lower for sacrospinous fixation compared to open or laparoscopic sacrocolpopexy. They additionally reported follow-up costs up to 90 days and found that follow-up costs were lower for sacrospinous fixation compared to open or laparoscopic sacrocolpopexy. Re-admission rate was also lower for sacrospinous fixation. Rate of postoperative emergency room visit was lower for sacrospinous fixation compared to open sacrocolpopexy and was comparable between sacrospinous fixation and laparoscopic sacrocolpopexy.

In effort to determine long-term cost-effectiveness of vaginal apical repairs, Wang et al. constructed a Markov model to model cost of vaginal apical suspension, laparoscopic sacrocolpopexy, and robotic sacrocolpopexy over 5 and 10 years [37]. The model accounts for additional surgical repairs, recurrence, re-operative, and complications in calculating health care costs. All surgical treatment were cost-effective over expectant management with vaginal repair becoming most cost-effective over 5 years. Over a 10-year period, laparoscopic sacrocolpopexy was most cost-effective, followed by robotic sacrocolpopexy. These results add a long-term perspective to considering the cost of a surgical approach.

Although studies exploring surgical cost attempt to control for variables and biases in order to achieve generalizable conclusions, cost is just one factor in determining appropriate surgical approach. Not only does cost vary based on location, institution, and even surgeon, patient factors and surgeon experience remain paramount in surgical decision making.

Future Directions

While the widespread use of robotic surgery has decreased morbidity and recovery associated with sacrocolpopexy, future directions aim to continue improving these metrics while minimizing recurrence. Single port robotic sacrocolpopexy has been proposed as method of optimizing current surgical techniques. Single port robotic sacrocolpopexy was first reported in 2017 utilizing the da Vinci Si system with the proprietary multi-instrument single port [38]. The authors published their surgical technique and later presented a case series of 25 patients followed by a randomized control trial comparing single site robotic sacrocolpopexy to multi-port sacrocolpopexy [39]. They found longer operative times, specifically robotic console time, for the single site procedure but otherwise found comparable anatomic and patient reported outcomes at 6 months. Approved in 2018, the use of the da Vinci single port system has also been reported in sacrocolpopexy. Ganesan et al. present three cases performed using the da Vinci single port platform along with a novel magnetic retraction system, which was used applied externally and used to retract the bladder and bowel [40]. They reported no complication postoperatively or at 1 month follow-up with acceptable patient reported outcomes. Widespread adoption of single-port technology is currently limited by the availability of the single port platform. Future innovations in minimally invasive sacrocolpopexy will likely expand upon the single port system to allow for more efficient, cost-effective procedures with fewer complications.

Cross-References

▶ Open Abdominal Sacrocolpopexy
▶ Vaginal Vault Prolapse: Options for Transvaginal Surgical Repair

References

1. Lane FE. Repair of posthysterectomy vaginal-vault prolapse. Obstet Gynecol. 1962;20:72–7. https://doi.org/10.1097/00006250-196207000-00009.
2. Di Marco DS, Chow GK, Gettman MT, Elliott DS. Robotic-assisted laparoscopic sacrocolpopexy for treatment of vaginal vault prolapse. Urology. 2004;63(2):373–6. https://doi.org/10.1016/j.urology.2003.09.033.
3. Brubaker L, Cundiff GW, Fine P, Nygaard I, Richter HE, Visco AG, et al. Abdominal sacrocolpopexy with Burch colposuspension to reduce urinary stress incontinence. N Engl J Med. 2006;354(15):1557–66. https://doi.org/10.1056/NEJMoa054208.
4. Wei JT, Nygaard I, Richter HE, Nager CW, Barber MD, Kenton K, et al. A midurethral sling to reduce incontinence after vaginal prolapse repair. N Engl J Med. 2012;366(25):2358–67. https://doi.org/10.1056/NEJMoa1111967.
5. Ost MC, Tan BJ, Lee BR. Urological laparoscopy: basic physiological considerations and immunological consequences. J Urol. 2005;174(4 Pt 1):1183–8. https://doi.org/10.1097/01.ju.0000173102.16381.08.
6. Arvizo C, Mehta ST, Yunker A. Adverse events related to Trendelenburg position during laparoscopic surgery: recommendations and review of the literature. Curr Opin Obstet Gynecol. 2018;30(4):272–8. https://doi.org/10.1097/gco.0000000000000471.
7. Matthews CA, Geller EJ, Henley BR, Kenton K, Myers EM, Dieter AA, et al. Permanent compared with absorbable suture for vaginal mesh fixation during total hysterectomy and sacrocolpopexy: a randomized controlled trial. Obstet Gynecol. 2020;136(2):355–64. https://doi.org/10.1097/aog.0000000000003884.
8. Tan-Kim J, Nager CW, Grimes CL, Luber KM, Lukacz ES, Brown HW, et al. A randomized trial of vaginal mesh attachment techniques for minimally invasive sacrocolpopexy. Int Urogynecol J. 2015;26(5):649–56. https://doi.org/10.1007/s00192-014-2566-8.
9. Good MM, Abele TA, Balgobin S, Schaffer JI, Slocum P, McIntire D, et al. Preventing L5-S1 discitis associated with sacrocolpopexy. Obstet Gynecol. 2013;121(2 Pt 1):285–90. https://doi.org/10.1097/AOG.0b013e31827c61de.
10. Shatkin-Margolis A, Merchant M, Margulies RU, Ramm O. Titanium surgical tacks: are they safe? Do they work? Female Pelvic Med Reconstr Surg. 2017;23(1):36–8. https://doi.org/10.1097/spv.0000000000000340.
11. White AB, Carrick KS, Corton MM, McIntire DD, Word RA, Rahn DD, et al. Optimal location and orientation of suture placement in abdominal sacrocolpopexy. Obstet Gynecol. 2009;113(5):1098–103. https://doi.org/10.1097/AOG.0b013e31819ec4ee.
12. Elneil S, Cutner AS, Remy M, Leather AT, Toozs-Hobson P, Wise B. Abdominal sacrocolpopexy for vault prolapse without burial of mesh: a case series. BJOG Int J Obstet Gynaecol. 2005;112(4):486–9. https://doi.org/10.1111/j.1471-0528.2004.00426.x.

13. van den Akker CM, Klerkx WM, Kluivers KB, van Eijndhoven HWF, Withagen MIJ, Scholten PC. Long-term safety, objective and subjective outcomes of laparoscopic sacrocolpopexy without peritoneal closure. Int Urogynecol J. 2020;31(8):1593–600. https://doi.org/10.1007/s00192-019-04020-w.

14. Kulhan M, Kulhan NG, Ata N, Nayki UA, Nayki C, Ulug P, et al. Should the visceral peritoneum be closed over mesh in abdominal sacrocolpopexy? Eur J Obstet Gynecol Reprod Biol. 2018;222:142–5. https://doi.org/10.1016/j.ejogrb.2018.01.027.

15. Freeman RM, Pantazis K, Thomson A, Frappell J, Bombieri L, Moran P, et al. A randomised controlled trial of abdominal versus laparoscopic sacrocolpopexy for the treatment of post-hysterectomy vaginal vault prolapse: LAS study. Int Urogynecol J. 2013;24(3):377–84. https://doi.org/10.1007/s00192-012-1885-x.

16. Coolen AWM, van Oudheusden AMJ, Mol BWJ, van Eijndhoven HWF, Roovers JWR, Bongers MY. Laparoscopic sacrocolpopexy compared with open abdominal sacrocolpopexy for vault prolapse repair: a randomised controlled trial. Int Urogynecol J. 2017;28(10):1469–79. https://doi.org/10.1007/s00192-017-3296-5.

17. Costantini E, Mearini L, Lazzeri M, Bini V, Nunzi E, di Biase M, et al. Laparoscopic versus abdominal sacrocolpopexy: a randomized, controlled trial. J Urol. 2016;196(1):159–65. https://doi.org/10.1016/j.juro.2015.12.089.

18. Paraiso MFR, Jelovsek JE, Frick A, Chen CCG, Barber MD. Laparoscopic compared with robotic sacrocolpopexy for vaginal prolapse: a randomized controlled trial. Obstet Gynecol. 2011;118(5):1005–13. https://doi.org/10.1097/AOG.0b013e318231537c.

19. Anger JT, Mueller ER, Tarnay C, Smith B, Stroupe K, Rosenman A, et al. Robotic compared with laparoscopic sacrocolpopexy: a randomized controlled trial. Obstet Gynecol. 2014;123(1):5–12. https://doi.org/10.1097/aog.0000000000000006.

20. Kenton K, Mueller ER, Tarney C, Bresee C, Anger JT. One-year outcomes after minimally invasive sacrocolpopexy. Female Pelvic Med Reconstr Surg. 2016;22(5):382–4. https://doi.org/10.1097/spv.0000000000000300.

21. Illiano E, Ditonno P, Giannitsas K, De Rienzo G, Bini V, Costantini E. Robot-assisted vs laparoscopic sacrocolpopexy for high-stage pelvic organ prolapse: a prospective, randomized, single-center study. Urology. 2019;134:116–23. https://doi.org/10.1016/j.urology.2019.07.043.

22. Geller EJ, Siddiqui NY, Wu JM, Visco AG. Short-term outcomes of robotic sacrocolpopexy compared with abdominal sacrocolpopexy. Obstet Gynecol. 2008;112(6):1201–6. https://doi.org/10.1097/AOG.0b013e31818ce394.

23. Paraiso MF, Walters MD, Rackley RR, Melek S, Hugney C. Laparoscopic and abdominal sacral colpopexies: a comparative cohort study. Am J Obstet Gynecol. 2005;192(5):1752–8. https://doi.org/10.1016/j.ajog.2004.11.051.

24. Chang CL, Chen CH, Chang SJ. Comparing the outcomes and effectiveness of robotic-assisted sacrocolpopexy and laparoscopic sacrocolpopexy in the treatment of pelvic organ prolapse. Int Urogynecol J. 2021;33:297. https://doi.org/10.1007/s00192-021-04741-x.

25. De Gouveia De Sa M, Claydon LS, Whitlow B, Dolcet Artahona MA. Laparoscopic versus open sacrocolpopexy for treatment of prolapse of the apical segment of the vagina: a systematic review and meta-analysis. Int Urogynecol J. 2016;27(1):3–17. https://doi.org/10.1007/s00192-015-2765-y.

26. Pan K, Zhang Y, Wang Y, Wang Y, Xu H. A systematic review and meta-analysis of conventional laparoscopic sacrocolpopexy versus robot-assisted laparoscopic sacrocolpopexy. Int J Gynaecol Obstet. 2016;132(3):284–91. https://doi.org/10.1016/j.ijgo.2015.08.008.

27. Ko KJ, Lee KS. Robotic sacrocolpopexy for treatment of apical compartment prolapse. Int Neurourol J. 2020;24(2):97–110. https://doi.org/10.5213/inj.2040056.028.

28. Lee RK, Mottrie A, Payne CK, Waltregny D. A review of the current status of laparoscopic and robot-assisted sacrocolpopexy for pelvic organ prolapse. Eur Urol. 2014;65(6):1128–37. https://doi.org/10.1016/j.eururo.2013.12.064.

29. Vandendriessche D, Sussfeld J, Giraudet G, Lucot JP, Behal H, Cosson M. Complications and reoperations after laparoscopic sacrocolpopexy with a mean follow-up of 4 years. Int Urogynecol J. 2017;28(2):231–9. https://doi.org/10.1007/s00192-016-3093-6.

30. Gungor Ugurlucan F, Yasa C, Demir O, Basaran S, Bakir B, Yalcin O. Long-term follow-up of a patient with spondylodiscitis after laparoscopic sacrocolpopexy: an unusual complication with a review of the literature. Urol Int. 2019;103(3):364–8. https://doi.org/10.1159/000494370.

31. Pacquée S, Nawapun K, Claerhout F, Werbrouck E, Veldman J, D'hoore A, et al. Long-term assessment of a prospective cohort of patients undergoing laparoscopic sacrocolpopexy. Obstet Gynecol. 2019;134(2):323–32. https://doi.org/10.1097/aog.0000000000003380.

32. Matthews CA. Minimally invasive sacrocolpopexy: how to avoid short- and long-term complications. Curr Urol Rep. 2016;17(11):81. https://doi.org/10.1007/s11934-016-0638-7.

33. Patel M, O'Sullivan D, Tulikangas PK. A comparison of costs for abdominal, laparoscopic, and robot-assisted sacral colpopexy. Int Urogynecol J Pelvic Floor Dysfunct. 2009;20(2):223–8. https://doi.org/10.1007/s00192-008-0744-2.

34. Elliott CS, Hsieh MH, Sokol ER, Comiter CV, Payne CK, Chen B. Robot-assisted versus open sacrocolpopexy: a cost-minimization analysis. J Urol. 2012;187(2):638–43. https://doi.org/10.1016/j.juro.2011.09.160.

35. Anand M, Weaver AL, Fruth KM, Borah BJ, Klingele CJ, Gebhart JB. Perioperative complications and cost of vaginal, open abdominal, and robotic surgery for apical vaginal vault prolapse. Female Pelvic Med Reconstr Surg. 2017;23(1):27–35. https://doi.org/10.1097/spv.0000000000000345.

36. Lua LL, Vicente ED, Pathak P, Lybbert D, Dandolu V. Comparative analysis of overall cost and rate of healthcare utilization among apical prolapse procedures. Int Urogynecol J. 2017;28(10):1481–8. https://doi.org/10.1007/s00192-017-3324-5.

37. Wang R, Hacker MR, Richardson M. Cost-effectiveness of surgical treatment pathways for prolapse. Female Pelvic Med Reconstr Surg. 2021;27(2): e408–e13. https://doi.org/10.1097/spv.0000000000000948.

38. Matanes E, Lauterbach R, Mustafa-Mikhail S, Amit A, Wiener Z, Lowenstein L. Single port robotic assisted sacrocolpopexy: our experience with the first 25 cases. Female Pelvic Med Reconstr Surg. 2017;23(3):e14–e8. https://doi.org/10.1097/spv.0000000000000397.

39. Matanes E, Boulus S, Lauterbach R, Amit A, Weiner Z, Lowenstein L. Robotic laparoendoscopic single-site compared with robotic multi-port sacrocolpopexy for apical compartment prolapse. Am J Obstet Gynecol. 2020;222(4):358.e1–358.e11. https://doi.org/10.1016/j.ajog.2019.09.048.

40. Ganesan V, Goueli R, Rodriguez D, Hess D, Carmel M. Single-port robotic-assisted laparoscopic sacrocolpopexy with magnetic retraction: first experience using the SP da Vinci platform. J Robot Surg. 2020;14(5): 753–8. https://doi.org/10.1007/s11701-020-01050-1.

Open Abdominal Sacrocolpopexy

36

Frederico Ferronha, Jose Bernal Riquelme, and Francisco E. Martins

Contents

Introduction	632
Indications	633
Patient Evaluation	633
Historical Background of the Sacrocolpopexy	633
Preoperative Preparation	634
Surgical Technique	635
Postoperative Care	637
Use of Mesh	637
Outcomes	638
Complications	639
Alternative Approaches	639
Conclusion	640
References	640

F. Ferronha
Centro Hospitalar e Universitário Lisboa Central, Lisbon, Portugal

J. B. Riquelme
Urology Division, Hospital Sotero Del Rio, Santiago, Chile

F. E. Martins (✉)
Department of Urology, Reconstructive Urology Unit, School of Medicine, Hospital Santa Maria, CHULN, University of Lisbon, Lisbon, Portugal

© Springer Nature Switzerland AG 2023
F. E. Martins et al. (eds.), *Female Genitourinary and Pelvic Floor Reconstruction*,
https://doi.org/10.1007/978-3-031-19598-3_37

Abstract

Pelvic organ prolapse (POP) is a highly prevalent disorder, which decreases the quality of life of women significantly. As a result of an aging population, the prevalence of women with POP will increase notably from 3.3 million to 4.9 million over the next 40 years. Surgical treatment of vaginal apical prolapse can be achieved through a variety of vaginal or abdominal approaches. Abdominal sacral colpopexy is a well-accepted and durable repair for apical vaginal prolapse and considered the procedure of choice as symptoms of the vault prolapse are relieved and the vaginal function is maintained or restored with minimal changes to the vaginal anatomy and function. Intraoperative and perioperative complications are uncommon in the open colpopexy procedure. When comparing open sacrocolpopexy versus minimally invasive approaches, both groups demonstrated similar vaginal support and functional short-term results.

Keywords

Sacrocolpopexy · Abdominal sacral colpopexy · Pelvic organ prolapse · Vaginal prolapse · POP-Q system

Introduction

Pelvic organ prolapse is a highly prevalent disorder, which decreases the quality of life of women significantly [1]. As a result of an age-related increasing prevalence, more than 10% of women in the United States will undergo surgical treatment for this problem at least once in their lifetime [2, 3]. One in nine women who live to the age of 80 will undergo surgical therapy for pelvic organ prolapse or urinary incontinence. Also, as a result of an aging population, it is estimated that the prevalence of women with POP will increase significantly from 3.3 million to 4.9 million over the next 40 years [4]. This burden that is related to pelvic floor disorders, detriment to quality of life, and demand for pelvic floor surgical procedures is expected to rise [5].

The number of women undergoing surgical management for pelvic organ prolapse is estimated to be 400,000 every year in the United States [6]. The US Census and NHANES data estimates that the number of women with pelvic floor disorders is expected to reach 43.8 million by 2050 [4]. Although prolapse of the anterior compartment is the most common, vaginal prolapse with loss of apical support is usually present in women with prolapse that extends beyond the hymen [7–9]. Currently, it is well accepted that

effective support for the vaginal apex is fundamental for long-lasting surgical repair for patients with advanced prolapse [8, 9].

Apical suspension procedures can generally be divided into those performed by transvaginal route and those performed abdominally. Most reports suggest that the transvaginal approach is the preferred surgical option in 80–90% of the cases of apical suspension operations. The vaginal route prevents the morbidity of an abdominal incision and gives access to fixation of other coexistent support defects. This route requires fixation of the apex to several pelvic supporting structures (sacrospinous ligament, iliococcygeus fascia, and uterosacral ligaments) which may be damaged, or can often be hard to recognize, particularly in the patient with previous pelvic surgeries. Transvaginal sacrospinous ligament fixation has shorter operative time and recovery, but the vaginal apex may also be anatomically displaced [10]. Often, the vagina is relocated posteriorly after a sacrospinous ligament fixation making the anterior compartment at risk for cystocele. The vaginal sacrospinous fixation according to Richter also bears the disadvantage of vaginal length shortening, which can be dramatic in younger, sexually active patients. Additionally, other vaginal procedures may narrow and shorten the vagina by scarring [11, 12]. More recent transvaginal sacrospinous ligament fixation techniques have been shown to preserve vaginal length and provide up to a 79% cure rate for apical prolapse [13].

Abdominal sacral colpopexy is a well-accepted and durable repair for apical vaginal prolapse and considered the procedure of choice [14]. With this surgical procedure, vault prolapse symptoms are relieved, and the vaginal function is maintained or restored with minimal impact to the vaginal anatomy. This transabdominal procedure offers consistent fixation of the vaginal apex, by using a synthetic mesh and suturing it to the sacrum which constitutes an attachment less dependent on weakened points and with little displacement of the vaginal axis. In addition, the transabdominal approach allows for concomitant paravaginal repairs and urethral suspensions.

Indications

Women who are symptomatic for pelvic organ prolapse and demonstrate a Stage II–IV by pelvic organ prolapse quantification (POP-Q) examination are candidates for sacral colpopexy, via traditional laparotomy or by conventional laparoscopic or robotically assisted-laparoscopic techniques. More specifically, there must be evidence of uterine or vaginal vault descent to consider sacral colpopexy. In the absence of apical descent, compartment-specific repairs are appropriate and sacral colpopexy is not necessary. However, because of the major role of the apex to vaginal support, Hsu et al. reported that anterior and posterior vaginal repairs may fail unless the apex is adequately supported [15]. The same authors concluded that 77% of anterior wall descent can be explained by apical descent and midsagittal anterior vaginal wall length. Apical prolapse is also associated with other compartment defects (cystocele, rectocele, or enterocele) in nearly 75% of the cases.

Patient Evaluation

Initially, a detailed medical history of the patient should be obtained, including prolapse symptoms, presence of urinary incontinence and what type, and past surgical history, mainly for prior abdominal and pelvic procedures. For women with uterus, they should be counseled about concurrent hysterectomy or supracervical hysterectomy or uterus preserving sacrocolpopexy after a rigorous evaluation of any dysfunctional uterine bleeding or abnormal cervical cytology screening. Then a full abdominal and pelvic assessment is achieved in both the supine and standing position while performing a maximum Valsalva maneuver. In the abdominal examination, special attention should be taken to any incisional scars. The vaginal exam is performed to assess the presence of a cystocele, loss of apical support, enterocele, and rectocele.

Pelvic organ prolapse need to be assessed according to the International Continence Society's POP-Q system, and each compartment of the prolapse is evaluated independently (anterior, apical, and posteriorly). Urethral support and mobility must also be assessed even if incontinence is not a presenting complaint with the appropriate bladder volume. The presence of occult stress incontinence is determined only after the reduction of the pelvic organ prolapse with a pessary or a large Q-tip. If necessary, a urodynamic study (cystometry, urethral profilometry, abdominal leak point pressure, voiding pressure studies, uroflowmetry, and postvoid residual evaluation) with prolapse reduced could help in guiding and counseling regarding the concomitant anti-incontinence procedure. In grade III–IV prolapse, upper urinary tract should be further evaluated using renal ultrasound. Associated defects and their management must be considered when planning the approach and timing of vaginal vault suspension. The individual woman's surgical history and goals, as well as her individual risks for surgical complications, prolapse recurrence, and de novo symptoms favor surgical planning and choice of procedure for apical pelvic organ prolapse.

Historical Background of the Sacrocolpopexy

Restoration of apical support can be carried out through vaginal or abdominal approaches. In the beginning of the last century, the abdominal route included one of several procedures that fixed the vagina to the abdominal wall. The lower efficacy of these techniques leads to the need of more effective surgical treatments. In 1957, a method of fixating the prolapsed uterus to the anterior longitudinal ligament in the sacral promontory was first described by Arthure [16, 17].

In 1962, Lane presented the repair of the posthysterectomy vaginal vault prolapse by a transabdominal suspension to the sacral promontory using an intervening graft to prevent extreme tension. It was the beginning of the modern concept an abdominal sacrocolpopexy [18].

In 1973, Birnbaum and Feldman and Birnbaum [19, 20] in 1979 described a procedure where the mesh was fixed at the level of S3–S4 following the principle that the upper vagina is normally pointed into the hollow of the sacrum and if placed in the sacral promontory was too anterior for mesh position.

Later Sutton published a paper describing a life-threatening hemorrhage in a sacral colpopexy by lesion of the middle sacral artery during the dissection at S3–S4. This author supported anchoring the mesh upper at the S1–S2, where the middle sacral artery was more clearly detected and preserved. At the same time, this position's change to a higher level had no evident negative effect on the vaginal axis [21, 22]. Two other important modifications of the Birnbaum technique have been made: first, the patient is placed in a dorsal lithotomy (froglike position) on the operating table to allow manipulation of the vagina and uterus to facilitate the dissection and the placing of the sutures; and second, extending the presacral incision in the peritoneum down through the pouch of Douglas and up the back of the vagina, thus giving the opportunity of completely burying the mesh in a retroperitoneal location. To decrease graft detachment from the vaginal apex, Snyder and Krantz [23] extended the mesh along all the rectovaginal septum.

Addison et al. [24, 25] originally used a folded conical graft configuration to increase the surface area for implant attachment, but because of more mesh erosions, they transformed the technique and used two separate graft strips sealed with monofilament sutures. This two-strip procedure allowed different tensions on the anterior and posterior grafts, thereby potentially decreasing urinary incontinence caused when the urethrovesical angle is straightened too much or constipation when the posterior strip too tight. The abdominal sacrocolpopexy is considered by many as the most durable repair for advanced pelvic organ prolapse (POP) and has become the gold standard surgical treatment for apical vaginal defects, with long-term success rates of 78–100% [26–29].

In the last two decades, minimally invasive approaches have been widely accepted as an alternative option to abdominal sacrocolpopexy [30–32]. Laparoscopic sacrocolpopexy (LSC) was first reported in 1994 by Nezhat [33]. Robotic-assisted sacrocolpopexy (RAS) was described a decade later by DiMarco [34] in 2004.

Preoperative Preparation

Initially, a detailed medical history of the patient should be obtained, including prolapse symptoms, presence of urinary incontinence and what type, and past surgical history, mainly for prior abdominal and pelvic procedures. For women with uterus, they should be counseled about concurrent hysterectomy or supracervical hysterectomy or uterus preserving sacrocolpopexy after a rigorous evaluation of any dysfunctional uterine bleeding or abnormal cervical cytology screening. Then a full abdominal and pelvic assessment is achieved in both the supine and standing position while performing a maximum Valsalva maneuver. In the abdominal examination, special attention should be taken to any incisional scars. The vaginal exam is performed to assess the presence of a cystocele, loss of apical support, enterocele, and rectocele.

Pelvic organ prolapse need to be assessed according to the International Continence Society's POP-Q system, and each compartment of the prolapse is evaluated independently (anterior, apical, and posteriorly). Urethral support and mobility must also be assessed even if incontinence is not a presenting complaint with the appropriate bladder volume. The presence of occult stress incontinence is determined only after the reduction of the pelvic organ prolapse with a pessary or a large Q-tip. If necessary, a urodynamic study (cystometry, urethral profilometry, abdominal leak point pressure, voiding pressure studies, uroflowmetry, and postvoid residual evaluation) with prolapse reduced could help in guiding and counseling regarding the concomitant anti-incontinence procedure. In grade III–IV prolapse, upper urinary tract should be further evaluated using renal ultrasound. Associated defects and their management must be considered when planning the approach and timing of vaginal vault suspension.

The individual woman's surgical history and goals, as well as her individual risks for surgical complications, prolapse recurrence, and de novo symptoms favor surgical planning and choice of procedure for apical pelvic organ prolapse (POP).

It is not necessary to perform bowel preparation [35]. All patients need to have an anesthesia evaluation to determine the perioperative risks and should receive perioperative antibiotics and deep venous thrombosis prophylaxis [36]. Anticoagulants and antiaggregants are discontinued at the recommended times before the surgery in a patient-tailored approach and according to anesthesia consultation. All patients should be advised about the possibility of postoperative urinary incontinence de novo (occult incontinence), suture extrusion, mesh erosion, risk of pain, infection, bleeding, and damage to bowel, bladder, ureter, nerves, recurrence, and the possible need for a combined incontinence procedure at the same time [37].

Surgical Technique

The patient is placed on the operating table in in the lithotomy position. It is important to ensure that the weight of the patient's leg is borne by the heel and not the calf when positioning the lower leg into the stirrup. A Foley catheter is placed in the bladder. The abdomen is entered through a lower midline, a Pfannenstiel incision, adhesions are lysed, and bowel and omentum are packed to expose the entire pelvis. The sigmoid colon is reflected from right to left, exposing the right aspect of the sacral promontory, giving the surgeon a direct approach. A most helpful technical maneuver is to have the prolapsed vagina reduced and distended into the pelvis by placing in the vagina a retractor like a malleable valve, which is held by an assistant. With the vagina stretched, it is easier to sharply dissect the bladder from the vagina anteriorly and the rectum posteriorly and offered better stabilization of the vaginal wall during suturing. With the sigmoid colon retracted to the left, the promontory can be identified following the pelvic rim, just below the bifurcation of common iliac arteries. The peritoneum overlying the anterior sacrum is incised from just above the promontory downward in the midline and blunt dissection is used to expose the anterior longitudinal ligament at this level. Care is taken to identify critical anatomic structures, namely, the right ureter and internal iliac artery, the sacral foramina bilaterally, the middle sacral vessels, and the left common iliac vein which crosses the midline over the sacral promontory. The peritoneal incision is extended beside the colon mesentery and across the cul-de-sac to the denuded vaginal apex (Figs. 1 and 2).

There are presently two main methods to creating a groove for attachment of the proximal part of the mesh: tunneling and non-tunneling. In the tunneling technique, a tunnel under the peritoneum is created with blunt dissection from the sacral promontory distally to the level of the

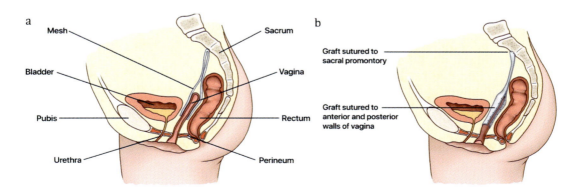

Fig. 1 Abdominal sacrocolpopexy: (**a**) mesh placed around the vagina and secured to the sacrum and (**b**) mesh sutured around the vaginal vault

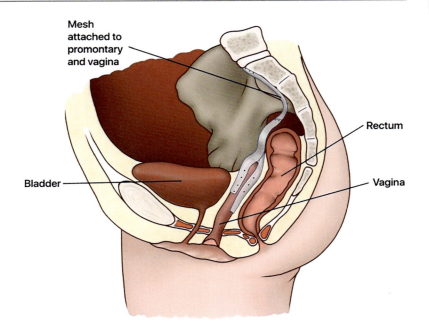

Fig. 2 Sacrocolpopexy landmarks: a synthetic graft (mesh) is used to cover the anterior and posterior surfaces of the vagina and the upper end of the mesh is attached to the sacral promontory. The mesh is then covered by peritoneum (retroperitonealization)

vaginal apex without incising the peritoneum. Alternatively, in the non-tunneling technique, the peritoneal incision is extended beside the colon mesentery and across the cul-de-sac to the denuded vaginal apex. In both approaches, careful dissection needs to be taken to avoid any injury of the right ureter. The tunneling technique is reserved normally to thin patients and allows faster retroperitonealization of the mesh but also provides a more natural curvature for mesh placement and avoids the risk of ureteral kinking (Fig. 3).

Concomitant hysterectomy (total or supracervical) or salpingo-oophorectomy is performed before the sacral dissection when indicated. Preservation of the cervical stump during hysterectomy facilitates not only suturing of the vaginal apex to ligaments but also has several advantages because is a procedure easier and safer and therefore reduces operating times and decreases the risk of mesh complications fivefold. The vesicovaginal space is entered sharply and the dissection is carried down to the level of bladder trigone. Normally the anterior dissection ranges from 5 to 10 cm in length. The right plane is usually bloodless and spreads easily.

After adjusting the vaginal manipulator to visualize the rectovaginal space, the posterior vaginal wall is dissected using blunt and sharp dissection and ideally is carried out distally up to the perineal body. If there is no uterus, it is better to leave "dome" of peritoneum intact at apex, because in doing so may cut down mesh erosion risk. If a colpotomy is performed anteriorly or posteriorly accidentally, the injured area is closed, and the dissection is continued. If a cystotomy occurs unintentionally, the injury is closed in two layers in a watertight manner.

The mesh can be cut and tailored at this point. Typically, the graft is a preformed Y-shaped implant of type 1 polypropylene mesh. The mesh can be tailored extracorporeally according to the prepared vaginal dissection measures. Additional adjustments to the mesh can be done intracorporeally if required. To secure the posterior mesh can be done in interrupted or running manner with nonabsorbable suture (2-0 Ethibond). More often is bilateral attachment to the levator ani muscle. The mesh was attached to the anterior vaginal wall with six to eight permanent sutures (2-0 Ethibond) and usually can be done before posterior fixation but depends on

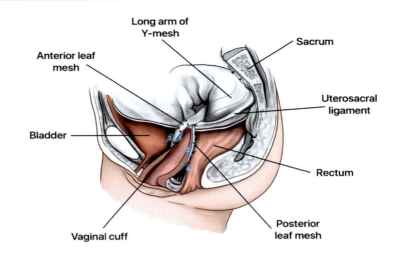

Fig. 3 Types of potential complications emerged from the anatomical relationship of the mesh: (1) vaginal mesh extrusion, (2) vaginal pain/painful intercourse, (3) mesh erosion into bladder/rectum, and (4) infection/abscess

surgeon preference. Studies have shown similar long-term outcomes with the use of absorbable sutures compared with nonabsorbable sutures for graft fixation [32].

Interrupted nonabsorbable suture (sutures of 0 Ethibond™) is used to fix the mesh, and it is important to clear the promontory completely so the mesh adheres to the ligamentum flavum (anterior longitudinal ligament) without applying tension to the vaginal attachments. When meshes are two separated strips, the anterior mesh is then attached to the posterior mesh, which is then fastened to the sacral sutures. Determining the right tension of the mesh is fundamental; the decision of how much pull the vaginal cuff depends on the maximal vaginal length. The procedure might be insufficient if the mesh is loose, and the patient may experience pain and discomfort if the mesh is placed too tight.

To help tensioning of the mesh, the surgical assistant can insert the manipulator into the vagina to measure the maximal vaginal length and pull back 1/3. The redundant mesh is trimmed away, and the previously incised peritoneum is reapproximated over it with interrupted absorbable sutures. Any other concomitant procedures can be performed as indicated like a mid-urethral sling, Burch colposuspension, culdoplasty, cystocele, or rectocele repair. Normally intraoperative cystoscopy is not performed routinely.

Postoperative Care

Patients are stimulated to ambulate some hours after the colpopexy. Clear diet is given and progress as the patient tolerates. Normally it is not necessary to do vaginal packing when there is no concomitant vaginal procedure during the surgery. The Foley catheter is removed on the first postoperative day. If there is an associated anti-incontinence surgery like a mid-urethral sling or a Burch colposuspension, special attention should be given to the voiding ability of the patient. If unable to void, women are trained to undergo a program of clean intermittent catheterization several times daily. In general, patients are discharged on postoperative day one.

Use of Mesh

The perfect material for using in a sacral colpopexy would be resilient, low-priced, easy to use, and presenting with no delayed complications as erosion, infection, carcinogenesis, or inflammation. This idyllic mesh has not still been created. Because such a material does not exist, the surgeon must take into consideration all of these characteristics. In most of the literature, the material more often used in sacrocolpopexy are synthetic meshes.

According to Amid's classification [38, 39] system, mesh "type I" is a monofilament, flexible, and lightweight graft. Therefore, these are meshes recommended for most pelvic organ prolapse surgeries because their wide pore (>75 µm) allows for tissue integration and for immune cells to scavenge bacteria. A precut Y-shaped or intraoperative tailor-made can be used in the sacral colpopexy. One option is to create a V-shaped graft using two separate pieces of polypropylene mesh for attachment to the anterior and posterior aspects of the vagina with proximal anchoring of both strips at the sacral promontory [40]. Nevertheless, different types of materials, other than synthetic meshes, can be used in sacrocolpopexy, including allograft, xenograft, and autograft meshes.

Outcomes

Outcomes for sacral colpopexy support the efficacy of the procedure as a means of supporting the vaginal apical compartment. Currently, recurrence rate of apical prolapse following colpopexy are low, ranging from 0% to 13.3% [41, 42]. However, the definition of cure in colpopexy is not always the same in the published case studies. Objective and subjective cure rates should be considered. Objective results should be based on an anatomic measurement system such as the POP-Q staging, by performing and recording preoperatively and postoperatively this examination on every patient. But not all the published studies use this evaluation anatomical scale, and many are retrospective.

Treatment failure can be described as relapse when there is >2 cm of apical descent or any leading edge beyond the hymen (Ba $= 0$ or Bp $= 0$). Some groups have advocated additional criteria such as a Ba point by POP-Q examination no greater than -1 [43]. Other groups consider surgical cures of the apex as point C being higher than one half of the total vaginal length (TVL) and no need for reoperation or pessary use for a symptomatic apical failure. Surgical cures were defined in this way to distinguish the anatomical borderlines of cure and failure. If the leading edge of the apex is at one half TVL or higher, then this would represent well less than grade II prolapse. Anterior or posterior recurrence was defined as reoperation at that compartment, pessary placement for a symptomatic cystocele or rectocele, or either Aa/Ba or Ap/Bp values that were more positive than -0.5 (prolapse grade II). The objective cure rate for all compartment was reported to be between 84–100% in some series but for apical prolapse was even higher when compared to other compartments [44, 45]. Recurrence rate was reported as 6.4% in a meta-analysis of 21 studies. The reoperation rate was reported between 2% and 26% based on long-term study results, most of those being posterior colporrhaphies [46, 47].

A review from Nygaard shows that success rates ranged from 78% to 100% for apical prolapse and 48% to 100% for prolapse in general and a reoperation rate for prolapse was 4.4% (0% to 18.2%) [47]. On the other end, subjective results are based on patients' reported measures using validated quality of life (QoL) questionnaires such as UDI-6, Likert QoL, and IIQ-7. The definitions for subjective cure rate express heterogeneity, with some publications presenting very high patient satisfaction rates changing between 90% and 100% [45, 48]. In Blanchard series, only 67% of patients in this study who experienced significant postsurgical prolapse considered their surgery successful as opposed to 100% of patients who did not experience significant prolapse [49]. The factor most predictive of decreased patient satisfaction appeared to be recurrent grade III or greater prolapse.

Regarding the results of the different surgical routes, the abdominal approach has been reported to be superior to the vaginal approach in terms of outcomes [50–52] as well as in preserving sexual activity. Since the abdominal approach has superior morbidity, many surgeons still choose the vaginal method.

In the Cochrane revision and the National Institute for Clinical Excellence (NICE, UK), the abdominal sacrocolpopexy with mesh is advocated as the optimal surgical treatment for uterovaginal prolapse [53, 54]. With these different managements of prolapses, it is mandatory to advise patients about the possible recurrent prolapse and the reoperation rates before a pelvic surgery.

Complications

Intraoperative and perioperative complications are infrequent in the open colpopexy. Most of the complications are usually minimal, namely postoperative pain, hemorrhage, infection, and mesh erosions. Wound infections generally are resolved with local wound care and antibiotics, but a major infection or dehiscence of the abdominal incision can require a prolonged hospital stay and recovery.

Pelvic floor myalgia and incisional site pain are treated with anti-inflammatory drugs, pelvic floor physical therapy, trigger point injections, and pain specialists when refractory. Bowel adhesions with subsequent obstruction are rare but if present normally requires surgical intervention with laparotomy.

Because mainly meshes that are made of synthetic material are used, they have the potential risk of causing erosion or extrusion even though extrusion into the vagina is a rare event. The most common site of mesh exposure is the posterior vaginal wall, followed by the apex. Mesh erosion into the sigmoid colon has not been witnessed; nevertheless, it is important to guarantee a space between the mesh and sigmoid. Concomitant total hysterectomy with vaginotomy, and the mesh type are risk factors for mesh erosion [45]. But some authors defend that simultaneous hysterectomy could not be clearly linked to higher erosion rates. The mesh type can also be associated with erosion rates. The best results with meshes are described with lightweight polypropylene meshes type [45]. Nygaard et al. [47] studied erosion rates in general and in series using different materials and concluded that this technique has low erosion rates, particularly when using autologous and cadaveric fascia (0%). The polypropylene mesh has also a low erosion rate (0.5%). Podratz et al. removed mesh in some patients for erosion or infection, and recurrent vaginal vault prolapse did not occur after mesh removal [55]. To prevent postoperative bowel obstruction, the posterior arm or strip of the mesh should be placed tension-free around the bowel.

The major complication of sacral colpopexy is life-threatening hemorrhage of the presacral vessels. The risk of significant bleeding has been reported from 1.2% to 2.6% and may be controlled with the use of stainless steel thumbtacks if encountered [56].

Addison et al. have modified the technique by fixing the mesh higher to the sacrum allowing to work in an area with less presacral veins seen deeper in the sacrum and therefore having less risk of bleeding from presacral vessels [57]. Other perioperative complications are bladder injuries (2–2.8%), vaginotomies (1%), and ureter and bowel injuries (<1%). Similar to other abdominal operations, postoperative ileus can occur, and laxatives can be used to resolve constipation.

Alternative Approaches

Minimally invasive sacrocolpopexy, laparoscopic or robotic, is more costly and can be more time-consuming in inexperienced hands than open colpopexy. Laparoscopic surgery has the limitation of the requirement for advanced surgical skill to dissect the presacral space and suture mesh graft to the vagina and sacrum, which many surgeons found too laborious or time-consuming to perform. In Cochrane Review, the evidence was inconclusive in comparisons of different access routes for sacral colpopexy [58]. Four trials compared access route of sacral colpopexy and importantly, in short-term results demonstrated equal anatomical outcomes between the open, laparoscopic, and robotic approaches to sacral colpopexy. The laparoscopic approach was associated with a longer operating time and reduced blood loss as compared to the open approach with similar admission time.

When the patient is unable to tolerate the Trendelenburg position, laparoscopic and robotic approaches are contraindicated, but not necessarily open abdominal sacral colpopexy. Prior abdominal surgery is not an absolute contraindication to robotic or laparoscopic approach, but this should be left to the surgeon's discretion. Long-term evidence across all surgical disciplines clearly shows that outcomes of high-volume surgeons are superior, with lower complication rates [59, 60].

Conclusion

Abdominal sacral colpopexy offers reliable fixation of the vaginal apex, usually by using a synthetic mesh and attaching it to the sacrum with minimal complications. It stands as the optimal procedure in case of vaginal vault prolapse because of the major symptomatic improvement and the durability of the cure. At the same time, this treatment maintains or restores the anatomy, the vaginal axis, and vaginal sexual function. Sacral colpopexy is associated with lower risk of awareness of prolapse, recurrent prolapse on examination, repeat surgery for prolapse, postoperative SUI, and dyspareunia than any vaginal procedure.

There are equal anatomical outcomes between the open, laparoscopic, and robotic approaches to sacral colpopexy. Sacral colpopexy should be considered for women who have failed a previous transvaginal suspension intervention and as a primary approach in young females with vaginal vault prolapse or any women with active sexual life.

References

1. Fritel X, Varnoux N, Zins M, Breart G, Ringa V. Symptomatic pelvic organ prolapse at midlife, quality of life, and risk factors. Obstet Gynecol. 2009;113(3):609–16. https://doi.org/10.1097/AOG.0b013e3181985312.
2. Wu JM, Vaughan CP, Goode PS, et al. Prevalence and trends of symptomatic pelvic floor disorders in U.-S. women. Obstet Gynecol. 2014;123:141–8.
3. Fialkow MF, Newton KM, Lentz GM, et al. Lifetime risk of surgical management for pelvic organ prolapse or urinary incontinence. Int Urogynecol J Pelvic Floor Dysfunct. 2008;19:437–40.
4. Wu JM, Hundley AF, Fulton RG, Myers ER. Forecasting the prevalence of pelvic floor disorders in U.S. women: 2010 to 2050. Obstet Gynecol. 2009;114(6):1278–83.
5. Kirby A, Luber K, Menefee S. An update on the current and future demand for care of pelvic floor disorders in the United States. Am J Obstet Gynecol. 2013;209(6):584.e1–5. https://doi.org/10.1016/j.ajog.2013.09.011.
6. Update on the Safety and Effectiveness of Transvaginal Placement for Pelvic Organ Prolapse, July 2011 [Internet]. U.S. Food and Drug Administration; 2020. Available from: https://www.fda.gov/media/81123/download
7. Brubaker L, Cundiff G, Fine P, Nygaard I, Richter H, Visco A, et al. A randomized trial of colpopexy and urinary reduction efforts (CARE): design and methods. Control Clin Trials. 2003;24(5):629–42.
8. Brubaker L, Nygaard I, Richter HE, Visco A, Weber AM, Cundiff GW, et al. Two-year outcomes after sacrocolpopexy with and without Burch to prevent stress urinary incontinence. Obstet Gynecol. 2008;112(1):49–55.
9. Visco AG, Brubaker L, Nygaard I, Richter HE, Cundiff G, Fine P, Pelvic Floor Disorders Network, et al. The role of preoperative urodynamic testing in stress-continent women undergoing sacrocolpopexy. Int Urogynecol J. 2008;19(5):607–14.
10. Boyles SH, Weber AM, Meyn L. Procedures for pelvic organ pro- lapse in the United States, 1979–1997. Am J Obstet Gynecol. 2003;188(1):108–15. https://doi.org/10.1067/mob.2003.101.
11. Given FT Jr, Muhlendorf IK, Browning GM. Vaginal length and sexual function after colpopexy for complete uterovaginal eversion. Am J Obstet Gynecol. 1993;169:284–7.
12. Carey MP, Slack MC. Transvaginal sacrospinous colpopexy for vault and marked uterovaginal prolapse. Br J Obstet Gynaecol. 1994;101:536–40.
13. Sauer H, Klutke C. Transvaginal sacrospinous ligament fixation for the treatment of vaginal vault prolapse. J Urol. 1995;154:1008–12.
14. Nygaard IE, McCreery R, Brubacker L, et al. Abdominal sacrocolpopexy: a comprehensive review. Obstet Gynecol. 2004;104:804–23.
15. Hsu I, Chen L, Summers A, et al. Anterior vaginal wall length and degree of anterior compartment prolapseseen on dynamic MRI. Int Urogynencol J Pelvic Floor Dysfunct. 2008;19(1):137–42.
16. Arthure HG. Vault suspension. Proc R Soc Med. 1949;42:388–90.
17. Arthure HG, Savage D. Uterine prolapse and prolapse of the vaginal vault treated by sacral hysteropexy. J Obstet Gynaecol Br Emp. 1957;64:355–60.
18. Lane FE. Repair of posthysterectomy vaginal-vault prolapse. Obstet Gynecol. 1962;20:72–7.
19. Birnbaum SJ. Rational therapy for the prolapsed vagina. Am J Obstet Gynecol. 1973;115:411.
20. Feldman GB, Birnbaum SJ. Sacral colpopexy for vaginal vault prolapse. Obstet Gynecol. 1979;53:399.
21. Sutton GP, Addison WA, Livengood CH 3rd, Hammond CB. Life-threatening hemorrhage complicating sacral colpopexy. Am J Obstet Gynecol. 1981;140:836–7.
22. Addison WA, Livengood CH 3rd, Sutton GP, Parker RT. Abdominal sacral colpopexy with Mersilene mesh in the retroperitoneal position in the management of posthysterectomy vaginal vault prolapse and enterocele. Am J Obstet Gynecol. 1985;153:140–6.

23. Snyder TE, Krantz KE. Abdominal-retroperitoneal sacral colpopexy for the correction of vaginal prolapse. Obstet Gynecol. 1991;77:944–9.
24. Addison WA, Timmons MC, Wall LL, Livengood CH 3rd. Failed abdominal sacral colpopexy: observations and recommendations. Obstet Gynecol. 1989;74:480–3.
25. Addison WA, Cundiff GW, Bump RC, Harris RL. Sacral colpopexy is the preferred treatment for vaginal vault prolapse. J Gynecol Technol. 1996;2:69–74.
26. Anger T, Mueller R, Tarnay R, et al. Robotic compared with laparoscopic sacrocolpopexy: a randomized controlled trial. Obstet Gynecol. 2014;123(1):5–12. https://doi.org/10.1097/AOG.0000000000000006.
27. Collins SA, Tulikangas PK, O'Sullivan DM. Effect of surgical approach on physical activity and pain control after sacral colpopexy. (Report). Am J Obstet Gynecol. 2012;206(5):438.e1–6.
28. Shepherd JP, Higdon HL 3rd, Stanford EJ, Mattox TF. Effect of suture selection on the rate of suture or mesh erosion and surgery failure in abdominal sacrocolpopexy. Female Pelvic Med Reconstr Surg. 2010;16:229–33.
29. Khan A, Alperin M, Wu N, et al. Comparative outcomes of open versus laparoscopic sacrocolpopexy among medicare beneficiaries. Int Urogynecol J. 2013;24(11):1883–91. https://doi.org/10.1007/s00192-013-2088-9.
30. Weidner AC, Cundiff GW, Harris RL, Addison WA. Sacral osteomyelitis: an unusual complication of abdominal sacral colpopexy. Obstet Gynecol. 1997;90 (4 Pt 2):689–91. https://doi.org/10.1016/s0029-7844 (97)00306-2.
31. Arbel R, Lavy Y. Vaginal vault prolapse: choice of operation. Best Pract Res Clin Obstet Gynaecol. 2005;19(6):959–77. https://doi.org/10.1016/j.bpobgyn.2005.08.
32. McDermott C, Park J, Terry C, Woodman P, Hale D. Laparoscopic sacral colpoperineopexy: abdominal versus abdominal–vaginal posterior graft attachment. Int Urogynecol J. 2011;22(4):469–75. https://doi.org/10.1007/s00192-010-1302-2.
33. Nezhat C. Laparoscopic sacral colpopexy for vaginal vault prolapse. Obstet Gynecol. 1994;84:885–8.
34. Di Marco DS, Chow GK, Gettman MT, Elliott DS. Robotic-assisted laparoscopic sacrocolpopexy for treatment of vaginal vault prolapse. Urology (Ridgewood, NJ). 2004;63(2):373–6. https://doi.org/10.1016/j.urology.2003.09.033.
35. Carlisle J, Swart M, Dawe EJ, Chadwick M. Factors associated with survival after resection of colorectal adenocarcinoma in 314 patients. Br J Anaesth. 2012;108:430–5.
36. Haya N, Feiner B, Baessler K, et al. Perioperative interventions in pelvic organ prolapse surgery. Cochrane Database Syst Rev. 2018;(8):CD013105.
37. Nygaard I, Brubaker L, Zyczynski HM, et al. Long-term outcomes following abdominal sacrocolpopexy for pelvic organ prolapse. JAMA. 2013;309:2016–24.

38. Chapple CR, Cruz F, Deffieux X, et al. Consensus statement of the European Urology Association and the European Urogynaecological Association on the use of implanted materials for treating pelvic organ prolapse and stress urinary incontinence. Eur Urol. 2017;72:424–31.
39. Amid PK. Classification of biomaterials and their related complications in abdominal wall hernia surgery. Hernia. 1997;1:15–21.
40. Winters JC, Krlin RM, Hallner B. Vaginal and abdominal reconstructive surgery for pelvic organ prolapse. In: Campbell-Walsh-Wein urology. 12th ed. Philadelphia, USA: Elsevier; 2020. p. 2776–829.
41. Fox S, Stanton S. Vault prolapse and rectocele: assessment of repair using sacrocolpopexy with mesh interposition. Br J Obstet Gynecol. 2000;107:1371–5.
42. Virtanen H, Hirvonen T, Makinen J, Kiilholma P. Outcome of thirty patients who underwent repair of post-hysterectomy prolapse of the vaginal vault with abdominal sacral colpopexy. J Am Coll Surg. 1994;178:283–7.
43. Brubaker L, Cundiff G, Fine P, et al. A randomized trial of colpopexy and urinary reduction efforts (CARE): design and methods. Control Clin Trials. 2003;24:629–42.
44. Hudson CO, Northington GM, Lyles RH, et al. Outcomes of robotic sacrocolpopexy: a systematic review and meta-analysis. Female Pelvic Med Reconstr Surg. 2014;20:252–60.
45. Serati M, Bogani G, Sorice P, et al. Robot-assisted sacrocolpopexy for pelvic organ prolapse: a systematic review and meta-analysis of comparative studies. Eur Urol. 2014;66:303–18.
46. Paraiso MFR, Jelovsek JE, Frick A, et al. Laparoscopic compared with robotic sacrocolpopexy for vaginal prolapse: a randomized controlled trial. Obstet Gynecol. 2011;118:1005–13.
47. Nygaard IE, McCreery R, Brubaker L, et al. Abdominal sacrocolpopexy: a comprehensive review. Obstet Gynecol. 2004;104:805–23.
48. Chan SSC, Pang SMW, Cheung TH, et al. Laparoscopic sacrocolpopexy for the treatment of vaginal vault prolapse: with or without robotic assistance. Hong Kong Med J. 2011;17:54–60.
49. Blanchard KA, Vanlangendonck RM, Winters JC. Recurrent pelvic floor defects after abdominal sacral colpopexy. J Urol. 2006;175:1010–3.
50. Kelleher CJ, Cardozo LD, Khullar V, Salvatore S. A new questionnaire to assess the quality of life of urinary incontinent women. Br J Obstet Gynaecol. 1997;104:1374–9.
51. Lobel RW, Sand PK. Long-term results of laparoscopic Burch colposuspension. Neurourol Urodyn. 1996;4:398–9.
52. Kotz S, Balakrishnan N, Read CB, Vidakovic B. Encyclopedia of statistical sciences. 2nd ed. Hoboken: Wiley-Interscience; 2006.
53. Kirkpatrick LA, Feeney BC. A simple guide to IBM SPSS statistics for version 20.0. Student ed. Belmont: Wadsworth, Cengage Learning; 2013.

54. Benson JT, Lucente V, McClellan E. Vaginal versus abdominal reconstructive surgery for the treatment of pelvic support defects: a prospective randomized study with long-term out- come evaluation. Am J Obstet Gynecol. 1996;175:1418–21. [discussion 1421–2].

55. Podratz K, Ferguson L, Hoverman V, et al. Abdominal sacral colpopexy for posthysterectomy vaginal vault descensus. J Pelvic Surg. 1995;1:18–23.

56. Timmons MC, Kohler MF, Addison WA. Thumbtack use for control of presacral bleeding with description of an instrument for thumbtack application. Obstet Gynecol. 1991;78:313–5.

57. Addison WA, Livengood CH, Parker RT. Vaginal vault prolapse with emphasis on management by trans-abdominal sacral colpopexy. Postgrad Obstet Gynecol. 1998;8:1–7.

58. Maher C, Feiner B, Baessler K, Christmann-Schmid-C, Haya N, Brown J. Surgery for women with apical vaginal prolapse. Cochrane Database Syst Rev. 2016;(10):Art. No.: CD012376. https://doi.org/10.1002/14651858.CD012376. Accessed 01 May 2022.

59. Mowat A, Maher C, Ballard E. Surgical outcomes for low-volume vs high-volume surgeons in gynecology surgery: a systematic review and meta-analysis. Am J Obstet Gynecol. 2016;215(1):21–33. https://doi.org/10.1016/j.ajog.2016.02.048.

60. Toomey P, Teta A, Patel K, Ross S, Rosemurgy A. High-volume surgeons vs high-volume hospitals: are best outcomes more due to who or where? Am J Surg. 2016;211(1):59–63. https://doi.org/10.1016/j.amjsurg.2015.08.021.

Management of Vaginal Posterior Compartment Prolapse: Is There Ever a Case for Graft/Mesh?

37

Olivia H. Chang and Suzette E. Sutherland

Contents

Introduction 644

Types of Surgical Repair for Rectoceles 645
Traditional Posterior Colporrhaphy with Midline Plication 645
Site-Specific Posterior Colporrhaphy 645
Graft-Augmented Posterior Colporrhaphy 645
Ventral Rectopexy at the Time of Abdominal Sacrocolpopexy 646

Surgical Outcomes: Comparative Data 647
Native Tissue Versus Augmented Posterior Colporrhaphies: Biologic Graft 647
Native Tissue Versus Augmented Posterior Colporrhaphies: Synthetic Delayed-
Absorbable Mesh 648
Native Tissue Versus Augmented Posterior Colporrhaphies: Synthetic Permanent
Mesh and Biologic Graft 648
Augmented Posterior Colporrhaphies: Synthetic Permanent Polypropylene Mesh
Versus Biologic Graft 649
Recurrent Prolapse: Native Tissue Posterior Colporrhaphy Versus Synthetic
Permanent Mesh 650
Concomitant Intussusception or Rectal Prolapse 650

Discussion 650

Conclusion 654

Cross-References 654

References 655

O. H. Chang
Division of Female Urology, Voiding Dysfunction and
Pelvic Reconstructive Surgery, Department of Urology,
University of California Irvine, Irvine, CA, USA
e-mail: ochang2@hs.uci.edu

S. E. Sutherland (✉)
UW Medicine Pelvic Health Center, Department of
Urology, University of Washington School of Medicine,
Seattle, WA, USA
e-mail: suzettes@uw.edu

Abstract

Our current literature supports a traditional native tissue repair (NTR) – posterior colporrhaphy – for the surgical management of most primary posterior compartment defects; although with the acknowledgment of limited long-term (>1–2 year) data. The concept of graft/mesh-augmented repairs was devised to increase the long-term durability of

© Springer Nature Switzerland AG 2023
F. E. Martins et al. (eds.), *Female Genitourinary and Pelvic Floor Reconstruction*,
https://doi.org/10.1007/978-3-031-19598-3_38

POP repairs: a gap that has been noted with traditional NTR. With that, global societal organizations recognize the potential durability benefits of graft/mesh-augmented POP repairs for more difficult complex POP cases such as with failed primary repair, very large complex defects, or individualized patient factors that may significantly increase the risk of subsequent surgical failure and POP recurrence. Long-term (>5 years) data is needed, as well as surgical innovation focused on improving the durability of surgical repairs.

Keywords

Rectocele · Posterior prolapse · Posterior colporrhaphy · Vaginal mesh

Introduction

Disorders of the posterior pelvic floor are associated with compromised integrity of the pelvic floor musculature. Patients with rectoceles may report vaginal bulge, constipation, straining, and/or digital splinting of the distal posterior vaginal wall or perineum to have bowel movements.

Since the early nineteenth century, surgeons have performed posterior colporrhaphies to manage tears of the posterior vaginal wall and perineum. As anatomic concepts developed, surgeons determined that the incorporation of plication of the posterior vaginal "fascia" restores the anatomic support of the vagina over the rectum without compromising functionality. The proximal vagina is supported by the endopelvic fascia attaching the vaginal walls to the aponeurosis of the levator ani muscles on the pelvic side wall. The anterior vaginal wall is attached to the arcus tendinous fasciae pelvis (ATFP), while the posterior vaginal wall is attached to the arcus tendinous fasciae rectovaginalis (ATFR). Distally, there is the perineal body which is formed by the confluence of the bulbospongiousus muscles, transverse perineii muscles, and external anal sphincter [1]. With weakening or trauma to levator ani muscles, increased abdominal straining results in the posterior vaginal wall exerting pressure on the perineal body resulting in a rectocele and perineal descent.

While the term "rectovaginal fascia" is commonly used to describe the layer between the vagina and rectum, cadaveric studies have not demonstrated evidence of fascia or a septum between the rectum and vagina [2]. Instead, what has been found is a split between the vaginal adventitia and fibromuscular layer. Hence, it is now recognized that this is not a true fascial layer. Prior researchers such as Nichols and Milley described this layer as the "rectovaginal septum" [3], and in this chapter, we refer to it as the rectovaginal muscularis.

Common techniques for posterior repair include two native-tissue approaches of posterior colporrhaphy: traditional midline plication and site-specific repair of the "rectovaginal septum." Surgical repairs for POP using native tissue have been associated with high failure rates of approximately 30% within the first 10 years [4], and the frequency of repeat surgery is higher than 50% for those who have had at least two or more procedures for prolapse [5]; admittedly, this is more commonly noted in the anterior compartment. Nevertheless, much effort has gone into the development of surgical techniques meant to increase the durability of these repairs. Grafts, either biologic or synthetic, have been developed to augment traditional rectocele repairs with the intention to improve anatomic and subjective outcomes via enhanced durability, and thereby decreasing the need for repeat surgical repair. As the adoption of grafts grew in popularity and expanded worldwide – especially that of synthetic mesh – previously unexpected complications became apparent, as did a growing awareness of the potential risks. The most commonly reported mesh-related complication is mesh exposure through the vaginal epithelium, which ranges from 4% to 19% [5]. Other risks unique to the use of synthetic mesh include mesh erosion (into an organ such as bladder or bowel) and mesh contraction, potentially leading to dyspareunia, vaginal and pelvic pain that may necessitate secondary surgery for mesh explantation.

Since the 2008 and 2011 FDA public health notifications warning the public about the concerns for transvaginal mesh, there has been much controversy throughout the world regarding the use of synthetic mesh for both SUI and POP. Major international academic urogynecology, gynecology, and urology societies have since responded with peer-reviewed recommendations in the hopes to appropriately educate providers and patients alike about the known risks and benefits of the use of synthetic mesh for vaginal procedures.

Specific to the posterior vaginal compartment, this chapter will review the outcomes of native-tissue posterior colporrhaphy relative to biologic and synthetic mesh-augmented posterior colporrhaphies as it tries to answer this question: "Is there ever a case for graft/mesh?"

Types of Surgical Repair for Rectoceles

Traditional Posterior Colporrhaphy with Midline Plication

A traditional native tissue posterior colporrhaphy is the plication of the posterior vaginal wall muscularis at the midline. Once the desired postoperative caliber of the vagina is determined, a diamond or triangle-shaped area of vaginal epithelium is excised from the posterior fourchette and perineum. The remaining vaginal epithelium is then dissected away from the perineal body and the underlying vaginal muscularis, and the dissection continues laterally towards the pelvic sidewall. Proximally, the dissection extends towards the vaginal apex. Midline plication is then performed by plicating the vaginal muscularis with delayed-absorbable sutures towards the perineal body. Any excess vaginal epithelium is trimmed, followed by re-approximation of the vaginal epithelium.

Site-Specific Posterior Colporrhaphy

According to Richardson, rectoceles are caused by a variety of breaks in the rectovaginal septum [6]. He described the most common break as a transverse separation above the perineal body,

presenting as a low rectocele. Another common fascial break was considered to result from an obstetrical tear or episiotomy that was incorrectly repaired. This midline vertical defect may involve the lower vagina and extend to the vaginal apex. Less common separations involve a lateral separation down one side of the "fascia."

The initial steps of a site-specific posterior colporrhaphy are the same as a midline plication, as described above. Once the dissection is complete, hemostasis is ensured, and irrigation may be used to attain a clean operative field to allow inspection for defects. A finger is inserted into the rectum to aid in the identification of the fascial defects. Individual defects are then repaired with delayed-absorbable sutures. The vaginal epithelium is then trimmed and reapproximated.

Graft-Augmented Posterior Colporrhaphy

The use of graft material has been suggested for recurrent prolapse [7]. The main considerations influencing the need for graft material include suboptimal native tissue to ensure a successful and durable repair, and/or the need to bridge any gaps to natural ligamentous attachments (i.e., sacrospinous ligaments) [8]. Common graft materials that have been used include synthetic permanent polypropylene mesh, synthetic delayed absorbable polyglactin mesh, and biologic grafts made of porcine acellular collagen matrix, porcine small intestinal submucosa, or bovine dermal grafts.

Below is a description of a commonly employed technique for graft use in the posterior compartment. When utilizing a biologic graft, it is first prepared for proper graft ingrowth and uptake through perforation of the graft with a hypodermic needle prior to soaking it in antibiotic solution. Following a traditional midline or site-specific posterior colporrhaphy, the graft is then laid down over the repair, oriented to match the rectocele defect, typically in a diamond or modified rectangular shape. In this way, the graft is used to "augment" the posterior plication repair. The graft must be secured with sutures (permanent or delayed absorbable) or other permanent anchoring methods: apically, in conjunction with a sacrospinous ligament fixation when apical support is also needed; dorsally, on the previously plicated vaginal muscularis; laterally towards the levator ani muscles; and distally on the perineal body. Some have described utilizing mesh under a full-thickness vaginal epithelial flap, including the underlying fascia, thereby laying the mesh directly over a manually reduced rectocele without first placing any plicating sutures. Either way, the mesh provides a new "roof" over the reduced rectum. The vaginal epithelium is then trimmed if needed and closed over the graft (see Figs. 1 and 2).

Ventral Rectopexy at the Time of Abdominal Sacrocolpopexy

If there is pelvic organ prolapse with concomitant rectal prolapse or intussusception, abdominal sacrocolpopexy and concurrent abdominal ventral rectopexy can be performed with the aid of a colorectal team. The sacrocolpopexy begins with dissection of the sacrum to reveal the anterior longitudinal ligament. The bladder is then dissected off of the anterior vaginal wall, followed by dissection posteriorly into the rectovaginal space. The posterior dissection is continued until bilateral levator ani muscles are encountered, which is as distal as the perineal body.

Synthetic mesh is sutured distally to bilateral levator muscles at the level of the perineal body using durable permanent or delayed-absorbable suture. Along the anterior rectum, additional delayed-absorbable sutures are placed to secure the mesh to the rectum. Apically, the mesh is then secured to the posterior vaginal cuff/cervix, followed by attachment to the anterior vagina, then finally to the anterior longitudinal ligament at the sacral promontory. Some colorectal

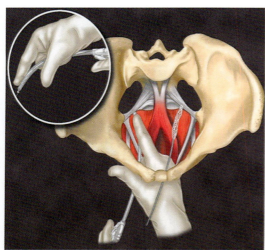

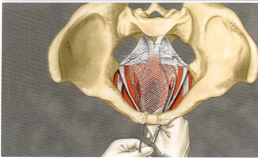

Fig. 1 Posterior prolapse mesh kit (no longer available): AMS Posterior elevate polypropylene transvaginal mesh kit. Apical bilateral sacrospinous ligament fixation anchoring method. (Lukban, J.C., Roovers, JP.W.R., VanDrie, D.M. et al. Single-incision apical and posterior mesh repair: 1-year prospective outcomes. *Int Urogynecol J* **23**, 1413–1419 (2012). https://doi.org/10.1007/s00192-012-1692-4)

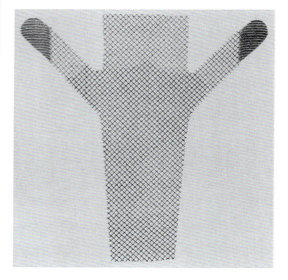

Fig. 2 Posterior prolapse mesh kit (no longer available): COLOPLAST Posterior direct fix transvaginal mesh kit. Apical bilateral sacrospinous ligament fixation suturing method

surgeons prefer using biologic graft for the rectopexy, and in this instance, a Y-shaped synthetic mesh would be placed over the vagina, and both the sacral arms of the synthetic mesh and biologic graft would be sutured to the anterior longitudinal ligament for suspension of both the vaginal vault and rectum.

Surgical Outcomes: Comparative Data

Native Tissue Versus Augmented Posterior Colporrhaphies: Biologic Graft

In the prospective randomized controlled trial (RCT) by Paraiso et al. conducted from 2002 to 2004, patients were assigned to one of three groups: (1) standard posterior colporrhaphy, (2) site-specific rectocele repair, and (3) site-specific rectocele repair with biological porcine graft augmentation [8]. All patients had a POP-Q $\geq$ stage 2 posterior vaginal wall prolapse. For the posterior colporrhaphy, 2-0 braided polyester sutures were placed in interrupted mattress stitches to plicate the rectovaginal muscularis across the midline. For site-specific rectocele repair, interrupted stitches of 2-0 braided polyester suture were placed to approximate the defects along the fibromuscularis. For the biological graft-augmented site-specific posterior repair, a 4 $\times$ 8 cm Fortagen porcine-derived graft (acellular collagen matrix) was secured superiorly to the posterior vaginal muscularis and epithelium using 2-0 delayed absorbable polydioxanone suture then attached to the vaginal muscularis with 2-0 braided polyester suture with interrupted sutures. Concurrent perineorrhaphy was performed if the patient reported splinting with defecation or if a perineal defect was noted at the time of surgery. The primary outcome was anatomic cure of the posterior vaginal wall 12 months after surgery, defined as POP-Q point Bp $\leq$ −2.

Across the three groups, there were no significant differences noted in operating time, estimated blood loss and hospital stay. For those who had porcine graft-augmentation, there were no graft exposures during the study period (12 months). Eighty-six percent of patients in the traditional posterior colporrhaphy had anatomic cure at 12 months, compared to 78% in the site-specific group and 54% in the graft-augmentation site-specific group, p $=$ 0.02. Of those with anatomic failure, 20% in the graft-augmentation site-specific group developed prolapse to or beyond the hymen compared to 7.1% in the posterior colporrhaphy group and 7.4% in the site-specific group (p $=$ 0.18).

All groups had improvement in the subscales of the Pelvic Floor Distress Inventory-20, demonstrating decreased bother from prolapse, colorectal, and urinary scales. Specifically, there was a decrease in the proportion of patients requiring to splint to defecate, to strain hard or to feel incomplete emptying across all three groups. There was no significant difference between the groups with regard to preoperative or postoperative dyspareunia, but improvement in sexual function was improved after rectocele repair, regardless of the technique used. Overall, Paraiso et al. concluded that both traditional midline plication and site-specific posterior colporrhaphies offer similar anatomic outcomes at 1 year, with no additional advantage of biological graft-augmentation seen at 1 year [8].

Another prospective RCT by Sung et al. evaluated the use of porcine subintestinal submucosal graft to augment a posterior colporrhaphy, compared to traditional native-tissue posterior colporrhaphy alone in patients with POP-Q stage 2 or greater symptomatic rectoceles [9]. For patients receiving biologic graft, a posterior colporrhaphy with either midline plication or site-specific repair was performed first, followed by augmentation with a 4 $\times$ 7 cm subintestinal submucosal graft, which was secured to the levator ani muscles bilaterally as well as to the perineal body. The primary outcome was anatomic failure of the posterior compartment at 1 year, defined as recurrent prolapse POP-Q stage 2 or greater (Ap or Bp $\geq$ −1).

A total of 160 patients were randomized, with anatomic data available for 137/160 (85.6%) patients at 12 months. In the primary repair (non-graft) group versus the biological graft-augmented group, 8.6% (6/70) and 12% (8/67) experienced anatomic failure, with a risk difference of 3.4% (95% CI -6.8% to 13.5%, p = 0.05). Subjectively, there were no statistically significant differences between the groups for improvements in bulge symptoms or defecatory dysfunction. There were no differences in postoperative dyspareunia between the groups. There were no graft exposures noted or additional surgeries required due to complications from the use of the porcine submucosal graft. When multivariable logistic regression was performed to adjust for preoperative POP-Q stage, the use of biologic graft did not decrease the odds of anatomic failure (adjOR 1.36, 95% CI 0.44–4.25). On survival analysis, the addition of graft was not associated with decreased time to anatomic failure compared to control, (adj hazard ratio 1.44, 95% CI 0.51–4.04). Overall, both groups demonstrated significant yet equal improvements in symptoms of vaginal bulge and defecatory symptoms. Sung et al. therefore concluded that augmentation with porcine submucosal graft was not superior – objectively or subjectively – to native tissue repair alone, again at 1 year [9].

Native Tissue Versus Augmented Posterior Colporrhaphies: Synthetic Delayed-Absorbable Mesh

In yet another prospective RCT by Sand et al., 160 patients were randomized to undergo traditional anterior and posterior colporrhaphies (midline plications) with (80 patients) or without (80 patients) synthetic, delayed-absorbable polyglactin 910 mesh reinforcement between 1995 and 1999. [10] Patients were included if they had a cystocele protruding to or beyond the hymen. The intervention was the placement of polyglactin mesh at the time of anterior and posterior repair at three places – below the trigone, anterior to the vaginal cuff and cephalad to the deep, transverse perineal muscles. The Polyglactin 910 mesh is a tricot knit derived from polyglactin suture yarn, which is the same composition as the suture with 90% galactoside and 10% L-lactoside. It dissolves by hydrolysis and is,

therefore, not a permanent material but acts as a temporary lattice for tissue ingrowth and granulation. The primary outcome was defined as a recurrent cystocele and rectocele to the mid-vaginal plane or beyond at 12 months. At 12 months, 43% (30/70) of patients without and 25% (18/73) of patients with polyglactin mesh had recurrent cystoceles beyond the mid-vaginal plane (p = 0.02). Evaluating the posterior compartment at 12 months, a total of 13 recurrent rectoceles were noted, with no difference seen between groups (no mesh = 10% vs. polyglactin mesh = 8%, p = 0.71). Sand et al. concluded that the use of delayed-absorbable polyglactin mesh for the posterior compartment did not result in improved outcomes compared to those with primary native tissue repair alone, again at 1 year [10].

A meta-analysis of the three RCTs above demonstrated no difference in subjective failure, defined as awareness of prolapse, in posterior colporrhaphies performed with or without biologic graft. (RR 1.09, 95% CI 0.45–2.62) [11]. With a follow-up time of 16–24 months, when evaluating for anatomic outcomes, defined as recurrent posterior vaginal wall prolapse, the risk of objective failure of native tissue repair was 130/1000 compared to 72/1000 with the use of biologic graft with a RR of 0.55 (95% CI 0.30–1.01). Looking at repeat prolapse surgery, the risk of repeat surgery after native tissue is 50/1000 compared to 30/1000 with biologic graft with a RR of 0.60 (95% CI 0.18–1.97) [10]. Overall, when the findings of the three RCTs by Paraiso, Sung and Sand were pooled, there was insufficient evidence to demonstrate a clear advantage of the use of biological or delayed absorbable graft over native tissue repair in the posterior vaginal compartment when evaluating anatomic/objective failure, subjective failure or risk of repeat surgery in the short term – at 1 year [11].

Native Tissue Versus Augmented Posterior Colporrhaphies: Synthetic Permanent Mesh and Biologic Graft

Currently, the largest study comparing synthetic mesh, biological graft, and standard posterior native tissue repair is the PROSPECT (PROlapse Surgery: Pragmatic Evaluation and randomized Controlled Trials) trial by Glazener et al. involving >1300 [12]. This was a multi-center, two-pragmatic, parallel-group RCT conducted in the United Kingdom, which included women undergoing primary transvaginal prolapse repair of the anterior or posterior compartment by 65 surgeons across 35 centers. Participants were randomized to standard native-tissue repair, or standard repair augmented with either synthetic mesh or biologic graft, and followed for 2 years. For the synthetic mesh group, a non-absorbable type 1 monofilament macroporous polypropylene mesh was used. For the biologic graft group, porcine acellular collagen matrix, porcine small intestinal submucosa, or bovine dermal grafts were used. No mesh or biological graft kits were used. The primary outcome measures were subjective assessments at 1 and 2 years and included patient-reported prolapse symptoms with the Pelvic Organ Prolapse Symptom Score (POP-SS) and a prolapse-specific quality of life (QOL) score. Two objective anatomical assessments were also done at 1 year only. Comparisons were made between groups: (1) standard native tissue repair versus synthetic mesh augmentation (Mesh Trial) and (2) standard native tissue repair versus biologic graft augmentation (Graft Trial).

At 1 and 2 years, the mean POP-SS and QOL scores did not differ within the Mesh or Graft trials. Similarly, on objective anatomical measures at 1 year, there were no significant differences noted within the two trials. Interestingly, more than 30% of the women overall (NTR, synthetic mesh or biological graft) still reported either "something coming down" or had objective prolapse extending beyond the hymen (POP-Q > 0 cm) at 2 years. More than 80% experienced at least 1 residual prolapse symptom after surgery, "highlighting the poor short-term outcomes of transvaginal anterior or posterior prolapse surgery with or without reinforcement."

Excluding mesh-related complications, there was no difference in serious adverse events during or after the surgery between the groups at 1 and 2 years, which including infection, urinary retention, dyspareunia, or other pain issues; <10% overall. Mesh-specific complications over the 2 years were 12%, most commonly seen as vaginal mesh exposure or extrusion. These were predominately deemed asymptomatic, small (<1 cm), and handled easily via partial excision with an outpatient procedure in those requiring surgical attention.

Overall, the authors of the PROSPECT trial conclude there was no perceivable symptom or QOL advantage to the use of synthetic mesh or biologic graft for augmentation of primary POP repair in the short term (1–2 years post-surgery) and therefore may pose additional unnecessary graft-related risks. They also acknowledged the need for longer-term follow-up to truly assess the potential benefits of transvaginal mesh or graft. "Given that recurrent prolapse requiring repeat repair occurs on average 12 years after a first standard repair, ongoing follow-up is essential to determining whether mesh or graft repairs might yet prove more durable in the long term, and to identify further adverse sequelae of mesh or graft insertion." [12].

Augmented Posterior Colporrhaphies: Synthetic Permanent Polypropylene Mesh Versus Biologic Graft

Utilizing a large population-based cohort, Sohlberg et al. evaluated reoperation rates for recurrent pelvic organ prolapse after biologic grafts versus synthetic mesh with a median follow-up of 2 years (745 days; interquartile range 385–1131 days). [13] Of the 14,192 women undergoing prolapse repair, 14% received biologic graft and 86% synthetic mesh. Albeit small, there were increased rates of repeat surgery for pelvic organ prolapse noted in the biologic graft group compared to the synthetic mesh group (3.6% vs. 2.5%, p = 0.01), and slightly increased rates of repeat surgery for complications in the synthetic mesh group compared to the biologic graft group (3.0% vs. 2.0%, p = 0.02). When repeat surgery for complications overall was pooled – for either prolapse recurrence or specific graft/mesh-related complications – there were no differences in the risk of repeat surgery between those who had biologic graft or synthetic mesh-augmented prolapse repair at 2 years (p = 0.79) [13].

Recurrent Prolapse: Native Tissue Posterior Colporrhaphy Versus Synthetic Permanent Mesh

A recently published secondary RCT, again by Glazener et al., utilizing 154 women from the PROSPECT trial, evaluated the efficacy of native tissue repair versus synthetic mesh (inlays or mesh kits) for subsequent treatment of recurrent POP in the same compartment. [14]. Two groups were established: Native-tissue repair (NTR) vs. mesh inlay (Mesh Inlay Trial) and NTR vs mesh kits (Mesh Kit Trial). Here again, the primary outcome was self-reported prolapse symptoms on the POP-SS at 1 year. Secondary outcomes included prolapse-specific QOL (VAS), generic QOL (EQ-5D-3L), and bladder, bowel, and sexual function improvements (PGI-I and ICIQ) at 1 and 2 years. POP-Q stage at 1 year was done for objective anatomical assessment.

Subjective improvements were seen in all groups (NTR and mesh, both inlay and kits) for all the prolapse-related symptoms and QOL outcome measures, with no discernable differences noted between the randomized groups at 1 and 2 years. Similarly, there were no statistically significant differences between the randomized NTR and mesh groups for other pelvic floor-related symptoms: urinary, fecal, vaginal, and sexual symptoms.

With "more severe prolapse" defined as beyond the hymen (POP-Q > 0), more patients with NTR (14–17%) and mesh inlay (14%) were noted with recurrence at 1 year compared to none after a mesh kit repair (0%). At 2 years, women with a mesh kit repair also reported better generic QOL scores (EQ-5D-3L). Potential advantages of mesh kits over simple inlay include reliable and secure attachments apically and laterally for enhanced durable support.

Similarly, to the initial PROSPECT trial, the overall incidence of non-mesh related serious adverse events was 10%; again, most commonly seen were infections, urinary retention, and pain. Mesh exposure at 2 years was 13% and 8% in the mesh inlay and mesh kit trials, respectively, with most reportedly asymptomatic, and only 6% (6 of 98) requiring surgical revision (all but one was $<1 \text{ cm}^2$).

The authors (Glazener et al.) concluded that, although there was an anatomical advantage with the mesh kits and a better global QOL score after repeat prolapse surgery at 1–2 years, there was not enough evidence to support the use of synthetic mesh (inlay or kits) owing to the lack of difference in prolapse symptoms between the native tissue repair and mesh repair (inlays or mesh kits). They acknowledged the limited sample size was too small to be conclusive on its own, but the information provides relevance for future meta-analysis. And again, longer follow-up is recommended, noting that "...2 years is too short a time scale to provide a definitive answer...ideally over 12 years." Ongoing follow-up for this trial is planned for at least 6 years [14].

Concomitant Intussusception or Rectal Prolapse

In the case of concurrent intussusception or rectal prolapse, considerations could be made to proceed with an abdominal repair that includes ventral rectopexy. Ventral rectopexy with permanent synthetic mesh has demonstrated significant improvements in functional outcomes, with 76% of patients reporting subjective symptom relief [15] and 78.6% reporting improvement in obstructed defecation [16]. The overall mesh-related complication rates for ventral rectopexy are notably low at 1.3–1.7%, which is lower than some reports for transvaginal mesh for POP. [15–17].

Discussion

In 2008 and 2011, the Food and Drug Administration (FDA) released a series of public health notifications with regard to the use of transvaginal mesh for female pelvic floor disorders. In 2019, the FDA requested all mesh intended for transvaginal POP repair be removed from the market. This decision was made *prior to* the maturation of the FDA-mandated 522 comparative studies between mesh-augmented and native tissue repairs. These FDA trials were designed with long-term durability and risk assessments in mind, with a minimum of 3 years follow-up, acknowledging the reportedly high rate of POP recurrence noted with traditional NTRs. The recent PROSPECT study showed that more than 30% of women who have prolapse surgery have a residual feeling of "something coming down," and more than 80% have at least one residual prolapse symptom, highlighting again the poor short-term outcomes of current transvaginal anterior and posterior prolapse surgery with or without graft augmentation. [12].

Currently, available comparative evidence in the literature does not describe a significant additional advantage with the use of graft or mesh-augmentation for posterior compartment prolapse. However, limitations associated with the published literature concerning transvaginally placed synthetic mesh for prolapse reconstruction include the use of older, heavy-weight, inflexible mesh, or use of outdated surgical techniques that require external, transobturator trocar placements. Additional limitations include postoperative follow-up of no more than 2 years. The initial design concept behind mesh-augmentation for POP was to increase the long-term durability of the repair, and thereby lead to continued POP symptom relief.

With respect to anterior and apical prolapse, there is evidence in the literature, albeit limited, that supports the use of mesh when studies were allowed to mature several years. [18–20] This more contemporary data describes transvaginal mesh POP repairs with lightweight, microporous mesh, minimally invasive, single-incision techniques, with longer-term outcomes, and notes excellent anatomical/objective, subjective patient satisfaction and QOL improvements with little to no mesh-related complications. For the posterior compartment, this durability advantage in the literature is less clear. Although most studies again are of

limited short-term postoperative follow-up of only 1 year. Further longer-term studies are needed to assess for true durability advantages of graft-augmented repairs over the traditional NTRs.

More information about anatomical POP outcomes after 2 years may help to answer the ultimate question: can graft or mesh really improve durable outcomes or not? A direct correlation between anatomical and subjective outcomes would help further our understanding about POP sequelae and longer-term recurrence rates overall.

As the largest global association focusing on women's pelvic health, FIGO's Urogynecology and Pelvic Floor Committee has reviewed and summarized the published national recommendations regarding the use of mesh (see Table 1) [5]. Current societal recommendations would advocate **against** the routine use of transvaginal mesh for POP repair, and especially in the posterior compartment where the overall published evidence remains limited in its maturity; but potential durability advantages are acknowledged, thus allowing for consideration for those who have failed prior native-tissue repairs, those with very large primary posterior prolapse and those at high risk for recurrence due to individualized patient factors (behavioral, medical comorbidities and/or connective tissue disorders, chronic cough/valsalva/straining, etc.). Overwhelmingly, there is a consensus about restricting mesh surgeries to those surgeons with appropriate training, appropriate surgical volumes, and who work in or have access to multidisciplinary referral centers. It has been well established that high-volume surgeons experience lower rates of complications overall compared to their low-volume colleagues. In the case of mesh-related complications requiring subsequent surgical intervention, the discrepancy is 3% (high volume) vs. 5% (low volume). [21] According to the American Urogynecologic Society's Guidelines Development Committee, a minimum of 30 surgical cases for POP (any route) should be performed by each surgeon each year to maintain proficiency in pelvic reconstructive surgery. [22] Various societies have also prepared peer-reviewed patient educational materials concerning the benefits and risks of synthetic

Table 1 International position statements regarding the use of synthetic mesh for the treatment of POP

Aspect	Position Statements	Associations
General		
1	In most cases, POP can be treated successfully without mesh, thus avoiding the risk of mesh-related complications	AUGS, AUA, CUA, RANZCOG, UGSA, Scottish review, Canadian Government, SCENIHR, FDA, ACOG, FEBRASGO, EAU, EUA
2	Based on the current state of knowledge, transvaginal operation (with mesh) for POP should be used only under carefully controlled circumstances	RCOG, NICE, EAU, EUA
3	Limit the amount of mesh used for all procedures where possible	SCENIHR, EAU, EUA
4	Transvaginal polypropylene mesh is not recommended as the first-line treatment for any vaginal prolapse	RANZCOG, EAU, EUA
5	Vaginal mesh can be used for the surgical treatment of POP and SUI. It is critically important to distinguish between these two uses of vaginal mesh	AUA, EAU, EUA
6	Serious complications associated with surgical mesh for transvaginal repair of POP are not rare	FDA
7	Outcome reporting for prolapsed surgical techniques must clearly define success both objectively and subjectively. Complications and total reoperation rates should be reported as outcomes	Scottish review, RCOG, Canadian Government, FDA, ACOG, JSOG, JUA, JFPFM, JPOPS, NAFC
8	Factors to consider before using surgical mesh:	FDA, ACOG
	• Surgical mesh is a permanent implant that may make future surgical repair more challenging	
	• A mesh procedure may put the patient at risk of requiring additional surgery or the development of new complications	CUA, RANZCOG, UGSA, Canadian Government
	• Removal of mesh due to mesh complications may involve multiple surgeries and significantly impair the patient's quality of life; complete removal of mesh may not be possible and may not result in complete resolution of complications, including paint	AUA, RANZCOG, UGSA, Canadian Government
	• Mesh placed abdominally for POP repair may result in lower rates of mesh complications as compared with transvaginal mesh surgery	AUGS, RANZCOG, UGSA, RCOG, FDA
9	There is no restriction on the use of transabdominal mesh used during a minimally invasive or open sacrocolpopexy	CUA, NICE
Patient selection		
1	POP vaginal mesh repair should be reserved for high-risk individuals in whom the benefit of mesh placement may justify the risk:	AUA Scottish review, SCENIHR, FDA, ACOG, IUGA, EAU, EUA
	• Recurrent prolapse where an abdominal sacrocolpopexy is contraindicated	CUA
	• Complex cases, in particular after failed primary repair surgery	SCENIHR, EAU, EUA
	• Recurrent prolapse (particularly of the anterior compartment)	AUGS, IUGA

(continued)

Table 1 (continued)

Aspect	Position Statements	Associations
	• Patients with increased risk of recurrent prolapse such as the obese, the young, those with chronically raised abdominal pressure (severe asthma, constipation), and those with stage 3 and 4 prolapse may find the risk/benefit balance of transvaginal mesh procedures acceptable	AUGS, FEBRASGO, RANZCOGJSOG, JUA, JFPFM, JPOPS
Informed consent		
1	Inform patient about the benefits and risks of non-surgical options, non-mesh surgery, surgical mesh placed abdominally, and the likely success of these alternatives vs transvaginal mesh surgery	AUGS, AUA, CUA, RANZCOG, UGSA, Scottish review, RCOG, Govern. Can, SCENIHR, FDA, ACOG, NAFC, NICE, EAU, EUA
2	For patients with postoperative symptoms that are not clearly caused by a mesh complication, removal of vaginal mesh may not improve the symptoms, and in fact may worsen their condition	AUA
3	For patients who have had vaginal mesh surgery for POP and are satisfied with their results, there is no need to take any action other than routine check-ups and follow-up care	AUA
4	Provide patients with a copy of patient labeling from the surgical mesh manufacturer if available	Scottish review, Canadian Government, FDA
Technical		
1	All gynecologist should be aware of and be encouraged to make full use of the ability to report adverse events from mesh surgery	RANZCOG, UGSA, Sottish review, Govern. Can, JSOG, JUA, JFPFM, JPOPS
2	Surgeons should undergo training specific to each device and have experience with reconstructive surgical procedures and a thorough understanding of pelvic anatomy	AUGS, AUA, CUA, RANZCOG, UGSA, Scottish review, RCOG, Canadian Government, SCENIHR, FDA, ACOG, JSOG, JUA, JFPFM, JPOPS, NAFC, NICE, SGS, EAU, EUA
	Surgeons should be able to demonstrate experience and competence in non-mesh vaginal repair of prolapse including anterior colporrhaphy, posterior colporrhaphy, and vaginal colpopexy (e.g., uterosacral or sacrospinous ligament fixation) before training in and performing vaginal mesh surgery	RANZCOG, UGSA
	Surgeons should demonstrate experience and expertise in performing intraoperative cystoscopy to evaluate bladder and ureteral integrity	RANZCOG, UGSA
Future aspects		
1	Rigorous comparative effectiveness trials of synthetic mesh and native tissue repair and long-term follow-up	ACOG, NICE
2	Outcomes and complications of transvaginal placement of surgical mesh for POP should be mentioned longitudinally, preferably using a statewide or national data collection mechanism so that peer comparison may be obtained	RANZCOG, UGSA, Scottish review, RCOG, NICE

(continued)

Table 1 (continued)

Aspect	Position Statements	Associations
3	When using the newer light-weight, transvaginal permanent meshes, consider recruiting into a clinical trial because these meshes have not been evaluated within a RCT. At minimum, extensive discussion regarding other options and referral for a second opinion should be considered. Clinical audit of all mesh procedures is encouraged	RANZCOG, UGSA, Scottish review, SCENIHR, SGS, ACOG, EAU, EUA

Abbreviations: ACOG, American Congress of Obstetricians and Gynecologists; AUA, American Urological Association; AUGS, American Urogynecological Society; CUA, Canadian Urological Association; IUGA, International Urogynecological Association; ICS, International Continence Society; EAU, European Association of Urology; EUA, European Urogynecological Association; FDA, Food and drug Administration; FEBRASGO, Federação Brasileira das Associações de Ginecologia e Obstetrícia; JSOG, Japan Society of Obstetrics and Gynecology; JUA Japanese Urological Association; JFPFM, Japanese Society of Female Pelvic Floor Medicine; JPOPS, Japanese Society of Pelvic Organ Prolapse Surgery; NICE, National Institute for Health and Care Excellence; NAFC, National Association for Continence; RANZCOG, Royal Australian and New Zealand College of Obstetricians and Gynaecologists; POP, pelvic organ prolapse; SCENIHR, Scientific Committee on Emerging and Newly Identified Health Risks; RCOG, Royal College of Obstetricians and Gynaecologists; RCT, random clinical trial; SGS, Society of Gynecologic Surgeons; SUFU, Society of Urodynamics, Female Pelvic Medicine and Urogenital Reconstruction; UGSA, Urogynaecological Society of Australasia

mesh, which outline these same recommendations for enhanced patient understanding.

On the other hand, biologic graft does not seem to improve the long-term durability of the prolapse repair but may prove helpful in other situations where additional material is needed: when there is concurrent vaginal stenosis or if there are concerns with the amount of healthy vaginal epithelium required to close over the midline plication. In these scenarios, the biologic graft can simply be inlayed to bridge the gap.

Conclusion

So…is there *ever* a case for graft/mesh for posterior prolapse repair? Maybe. Admittedly our current literature does not thus far show a clear advantage that would support the routine use of graft or synthetic mesh, especially for primary repairs, but acknowledges the limited long-term (>1–2 year) data available for review. The concept of graft/mesh-augmented repairs was first and foremost meant to increase the long-term durability of the repair: a gap that was noted with traditional native tissue POP repairs. With that, global societal organizations acknowledge the potential benefits for more difficult complex POP cases such as with failed primary repair, very large defects, or individualized patient factors that may significantly increase the risk of subsequent surgical failure. Societal consensus further recommends that mesh-related vaginal surgeries should only be done by specialty trained surgeons with high-volume practices in order to provide patients with the best possible outcomes. When using graft/mesh, patients need to be informed about the potential graft/mesh-related risks and complications, and individualized joint decision-making is always recommended. What is needed is long-term (>5 years) data involving contemporary surgical techniques and mesh to better address any potential durability advantage augmented POP repairs may offer. We also need to drive innovation to find new surgical solutions that can provide more longevity and durability to our repairs.

Cross-References

▶ Complications of the Use of Synthetic Mesh Materials in Stress Urinary Incontinence and Pelvic Organ Prolapse
▶ Etiology, Diagnosis, and Management of Pelvic Organ Prolapse: Overview

References

1. Walters MD, Karram M, Walters MD, Karram MM. Urogynecology and reconstructive pelvic surgery. 4th ed. Philadelphia: Elsevier; 2015.
2. Kleeman SD, Westermann C, Karram MM. Rectoceles and the anatomy of the posteriorvaginal wall: revisited. Am J Obstet Gynecol. 2005;193:2050–5.
3. Nichols DH, of prolapse RCLT (1996) In: Nichols DH, Randall CL, editors. Vaginal Surg. 4th ed. Ba:101–118.
4. Chapple CR, et al. Consensus statement of the European Urology Association and the European Urogynaecological Association on the use of implanted materials for treating pelvic organ prolapse and stress urinary incontinence. Eur Urol. 2017; https://doi.org/10.1016/j.eururo.2017.03.048.
5. Ugianskiene A, Davila GW, Su TH, for the FIGO Urogynecology and Pelvic Floor Committee. FIGO review of statements on use of synthetic mesh for pelvic organ prolapse and stress urinary incontinence. Int J Obstet Gynaecol. 2019;147(2):147–55.
6. Richardson AC. The rectovaginal septum revisited: its relationship to rectocele and its importance in rectocele repair. Clin Obstet Gynecol. 1993;36:976–83.
7. Hendrix SL, Clark A, Nygaard I, Aragaki A, Barnabei V, McTiernan A. Pelvic organ prolapse in the women's health initiative: gravity and gravidity. Am J Obstet Gynecol. 2002;186:1160–6.
8. Paraiso MF, Barber MD, Muir TW, Walters MD. Rectocele repair: a randomized trial of three surgical techniques including graft augmentation. Am J Obstet Gynecol. 2006;195:1762–71.
9. Sung VW, Rardin CR, Raker CA, Lasala CA, Myers DL. Porcine subintestinal submucosal graft augmentation for rectocele repair: a randomized controlled trial. Obstet Gynecol. 2012;119:125–33.
10. Sand PK, Koduri S, Lobel RW, et al. Prospective randomized trial of polyglactin 910 mesh to prevent recurrence of cystoceles and rectoceles. Am J Obstet Gynecol. 2001;184:1357–64.
11. Mowat A, Maher D, Baessler K, Christmann-Schmid-C, Haya N, Maher C. Surgery for women with posterior compartment prolapse. Cochrane Database Syst Rev. 2018; https://doi.org/10.1002/14651858.CD012975.
12. Glazener CMA, Breeman S, Elders A, et al. Mesh, graft, or standard repair for women having primary anterior or posterior compartment prolapse surgery: two parallel-group, multicentre, randomised, controlled trials (PROSPECT). Lancet. 2017;389:381–92. https://doi.org/10.1016/S0140-6736(16)31596-3.
13. Sohlberg EM, Dallas KB, Weeks BT, Elliott CS, Rogo-Gupta L. Reoperation rates for pelvic organ prolapse repairs with biologic and synthetic grafts in a large population-based cohort. Int Urogynecol J. 2020;31:291–301.
14. Glazener CMA, Breeman S, Elders A, et al. Mesh inlay, mesh kit or native tissue repair for women having repeat anterior or posterior prolapse surgery: randomised controlled trial (PROSPECT). BJOG. 2020;127(8):1002–13. https://doi.org/10.1111/1471-0528.16197. Epub 2020 Apr 6
15. Van Iersel JJ, Formijne Jonkers HA, Paulides TJC, Verheijen PM, Draaisma WA, Consten ECJ, Broeders IAMJ. Robot-assisted ventral mesh rectopexy for rectal prolapse: a 5-year experience at a tertiary referral center. Dis Colon Rectum. 2017;60:1215–23.
16. Mäkelä-Kaikkonen J, Rautio T, Kairaluoma M, Carpelan-Holmström M, Kössi J, Rautio A, Ohtonen P, Mäkelä J. Does ventral rectopexy improve pelvic floor function in the long term? Dis Colon Rectum. 2018;61:230–8.
17. Jallad K, Ridgeway B, Paraiso MFR, Gurland B, Unger CA. Long-term outcomes after ventral rectopexy with sacrocolpo- or hysteropexy for the treatment of concurrent rectal and pelvic organ prolapse. Female Pelvic Med Reconstr Surg. 2018;24:336–40.
18. Nager CW, Visco AG, Richter HE, Rardin CR, Komesu Y, Harvie HS, Zyczynski HM, Paraiso MFR, Mazloomdoost D, Sridhar A, Thomas S, National Institute of Child Health and Human Development Pelvic Floor Disorders Network. Effect of sacrospinous hysteropexy with graft vs vaginal hysterectomy with uterosacral ligament suspension on treatment failure in women with uterovaginal prolapse: 5-year results of a randomized clinical trial. Am J Obstet Gynecol. 2021;225(2):153.e1–153.e31. https://doi.org/10.1016/j.ajog.2021.03.012. Epub 2021 Mar 12. PMID: 33716071; PMCID: PMC8328912.
19. Gillor M, Langer S, Dietz HP. A long-term comparative study of Uphold™ transvaginal mesh kit against anterior colporrhaphy. Int Urogynecol J. 2020;31(4):793–7. https://doi.org/10.1007/s00192-019-04106-5. Epub 2019 Sep 16. PMID: 31529327.
20. Juliato CR, Santos Júnior LC, Haddad JM, Castro RA, Lima M, Castro EB. Mesh surgery for anterior vaginal wall prolapse: a meta-analysis. Rev Bras Ginecol Obstet. 2016;38(7):356–64. https://doi.org/10.1055/s-0036-1585074. Epub 2016 Jul 29. PMID: 27472812.
21. Kelly EC, Winick-Ng J, Welk B. Surgeon experience and complications of transvaginal prolapse mesh. Obstet Gynecol. 2016;128:65–72.
22. American Urogynecologic Society's Guidelines Development Committee. Guidelines for providing privileges and credentials to physicians for transvaginal placement of surgical mesh for pelvic organ prolapse. Female Pelvic Med Reconstr Surg. 2012;18:194–7.

Vaginal Surgery Complications

38

Jamaal C. Jackson and Sarah A. Adelstein

Contents

Introduction	657
Vaginoplasty	658
Urethrovaginal/Vesicovaginal Fistula Repair	659
Diverticulectomy	660
Urethral Prolapse/Caruncle Repair	661
Slings	661
Complications of Vaginal Mesh Surgery	663
Vaginal Hysterectomy	665
Vaginal Prolapse Repair	669
Complications of Apical Repair	669
Complications of Posterior Repair	670
Complications of Anterior Repair	671
References	672

Abstract

Vaginal surgery is the preferred approach for many extirpative and reconstructive procedures on the female genital tract. Because of the access route of these natural orifice surgical techniques, some complications of vaginal surgery are universal risks common to the approach, while others are unique to the specific procedure. This chapter will cover a review of surgical complications of vaginal surgery and management of those complications.

Keywords

Vaginal · Complications · Vaginoplasty · Fistula · Diverticulectomy · Stricture · Prolapse

Introduction

Vaginal surgery is the preferred approach for many extirpative and reconstructive procedures on the female genital tract. It is generally a less

J. C. Jackson · S. A. Adelstein (✉)
Rush University Medical Center, Chicago, IL, USA
e-mail: jamaal_c_jackson@rush.edu;
sarah_adelstein@rush.edu

© Springer Nature Switzerland AG 2023
F. E. Martins et al. (eds.), *Female Genitourinary and Pelvic Floor Reconstruction*,
https://doi.org/10.1007/978-3-031-19598-3_39

morbid and invasive surgical technique compared to open abdominal surgery. Because of the access route of these natural orifice surgical techniques, some complications of vaginal surgery are universal risks common to the approach. Others are unique to the specific procedure. This chapter will cover a review of surgical complications of vaginal surgery and management of those complications.

Vaginoplasty

Vaginoplasty procedures encompass a range of reconstructive techniques to repair or reconstruct the vagina. Common examples include repair of vaginal septa or contractures, or neovagina creation as used for congenital conditions like Meyer-Rokitansky-Küster-Hauser syndrome, or for gender-affirming surgery. The risks of vaginoplasty are not only influenced by patient factors, but the type of graft used as well. Commonly used graft materials include intestine/colon, skin, buccal mucosa, and peritoneum. Graft stenosis is one of the most common complications encountered, regardless of graft type (e.g., skin or peritoneal). Although vaginal molds are frequently used in the postoperative period, sometimes long-term dilation is needed to maintain patency. Materials utilized for vaginal molding or dilators include silicone-coated stents, hollow vulcanite molds, wood mold covered with a condom, or thermoplastic splints. Molds are typically worn every 1–3 nights for the first 3–6 months postoperatively. Removal for cleaning is recommended at least weekly to prevent infections. If uterine obstruction is not a concern, treatment of vaginal graft stenosis is optional, and only indicated when the patient desires vaginal patency. Vaginal dilators are helpful, but sometimes painful to insert into the stenotic segment. Agents such as estrogen cream, lidocaine gel, or other water- or silicone-based lubricants can ease dilation pain. Rarely, intermittent dilation under anesthesia may be required. If the stenosis is severe and unable to stretch, incision of the stenosis, Z-plasty of the stenotic segment, interposition graft with stenting and dilation, or revision vaginoplasty (possibly with an alternate graft material) may be utilized [1].

Some complications are graft-specific. There are instances in the literature detailing the incorporation of every segment of the gastrointestinal tract into vaginoplasty procedures. While many of these only serve as an historical footnote when considering contemporary methods, reported complication rates after bowel graft are generally much higher than other vaginal surgeries, with some studies estimating a rate of up to 26% [2]. Of the bowel segments, sigmoid colon has the lowest risk of graft stenosis. Other reported complications include post-operative ileus, anastomotic leak, intra-abdominal adhesions, vaginal-graft stenosis, mucosal prolapse, excessive mucosal drainage, graft polyp formation, malignancy, diversion colitis, and irritation due to de novo inflammatory bowel syndrome. Mucus drainage can be bothersome in up to 38% of patients and malodorous in roughly 21% [3]. Sigmoidoplasty tends to have copious mucus production that is most prominent within the first 6 months postoperatively [4]. This can be managed with daily saline irrigations until the drainage diminishes. Split- or full-thickness skin grafts, usually harvested from the buttocks, thigh, or groin, are often used in vaginoplasty for Mullerian agenesis. Complications specific to skin grafts, beyond stenosis, include excessive scarring at the graft harvest site and vaginal hair ingrowth. Although hair can aid in lubrication, laser hair removal may be pursued if bothersome. Buccal mucosa grafts risk graft contraction and injury to Stenson's duct, the major parotid duct allowing saliva passage into the oral cavity. Peritoneal graft is usually harvested from the Pouch of Douglas and is usually reserved for patients who have not undergone previous pelvic surgery. Complications associated with peritoneal grafts include intraoperative bowel or bladder injury, prolapse, and obliteration of the vaginal canal. The latter of which is estimated to occur in 12% of patients [5]. The use of peritoneum in vaginoplasty requires graft dilation postoperatively.

Less common complications of vaginoplasty include bleeding, prolapse, fistulas, mechanical bowel obstruction, and malignancy. Any bleeding encountered must be investigated with history, screening for STDs, and pelvic examination with or without biopsy if warranted to rule-out cancer or inflammatory colitis. Acute causes include pelvic hematoma, graft necrosis, granulation tissue, fistula, and trauma from dilation, while long-term causes include infection, carcinoma, trauma, neovaginal intestinal polyps, or inflammatory colitis. If trauma is encountered, treatment includes pelvic rest if the injured area is hemostatic and reiterating proper dilation technique. Surgery is generally reserved for cases where a laceration is noted. Colitis is common with intestinal vaginoplasty with some studies reporting an incidence up to 65% [3]. Symptoms include malodorous or excessive discharge, bleeding, and pain. Treatment includes daily sodium butyrate or 5-aminosalicyclic acid enemas over 4 weeks. Inflammatory bowel disease is a rare cause of vaginal bleeding that can also present with rectal bleeding or abdominal pain. Diagnosis is made by endoscopy of the vagina and intestines with mucosal biopsies. Treatment includes local steroid or mesalamine suppositories and systemic therapy to address the immune response. Patients should also be referred to Rheumatology. Fistulas after vaginoplasty can be rectovaginal, vesicovaginal, urethrovaginal, or ureterovaginal. The risk of formation tends to increase on subsequent vaginal surgery due to compromise of the blood supply. The use of tension-free closure and interposition flaps can lead to decreased recurrence upon repair. Urine or stool should also be diverted depending on the fistula type. Vaginal prolapse more commonly occurs with the use of bowel as the graft material. Options for surgical repair depend on several factors, including tissue quality, patient anatomy, and the type of neovagina. Mesh should be used with caution due to the higher risk of tissue breakdown. Malignancy is rare and almost exclusively reported when the sigmoid colon is incorporated [6].

Urethrovaginal/Vesicovaginal Fistula Repair

Urogenital fistulae are abnormal connections between the urinary system, most commonly the lower urinary tract structures, and the genitalia, which allows urine to leak into the genital space.

The most common etiologies in developed countries include pelvic surgeries, while ischemic injury to the bladder and vagina resulting from obstetric complications in obstructed labor predominate in developing countries [7]. The repair of urethrovaginal and vesicovaginal fistulas can be exceptionally complex due to the factors that lead to fistulae formation (i.e., tissue ischemia and inflammation). Persistence or recurrence of the fistula may occur infrequently after reconstructive surgery. When this does present, repair is recommended via transvaginal or transabdominal approach. Principles to prevent recurrent or persistent fistula include watertight closure (repair can be tested with saline or methylene blue solution) and non-overlapping suture lines. Catheter drainage is typically used during initial healing, possibly including a second drain via suprapubic cystotomy. Anticholinergics can also be used to prevent bladder spasms during the initial healing period for patient comfort, and theoretically to decrease breakdown of the repair from repeated muscle contractions. Finally, if the fistula is recurrent, or complicated by radiation history, interpositional graft (e.g., Martius labial or peritoneal) should be utilized to introduce vascularized tissue bed and prevent overlapping suture lines.

De novo stress urinary incontinence (SUI) can develop during either surgical approach if the dissection disrupts the ligamentous urethral support or the intrinsic sphincteric mechanism. Rates in the literature range from 4% to 33% when accounting for surgical intervention alone [8]. Risk factors for SUI include urethral involvement of the fistula, fistula size, diminished bladder capacity, and extensive vaginal reconstruction [9]. The propensity to develop SUI also increases in patients with urethrovaginal fistulas within the proximal or mid urethra due to being close in proximity to the urethral sphincter. Surgery to address incontinence should usually be delayed until repair of the fistula; however, if these present concomitantly, a mid-urethral sling can be considered if the dissection is not adjacent to the urethra, otherwise autologous fascia sling is usually the preferred technique for concomitant repair with fistula closure due to lower risk of fistula recurrence. The risk of developing urinary urgency is increased with any surgery involving the urethra or bladder neck. It is recommended to evaluate patients with urodynamics (UDS) prior to surgical intervention to rule of the presence of bladder outlet obstruction. When this does occur, symptoms generally tend to be most severe in the early postoperative course, but rarely persists long term after the repair. Urinary tract infection (UTI) is a common complication after fistula repair. It is important to sterilize the urine prior to surgical repair as culture-confirmed UTIs found on preoperative assessment will predispose the patient to fistula recurrence [10]. The possible role of low-dose preoperative antibiotics prior to surgery has been investigated with some studies reporting a decrease in UTI rate, edema, and tissue inflammation.

Diverticulectomy

Urethral diverticulum is a rare condition that can cause dysuria, pelvic pain, obstructive voiding symptoms, and recurrent cystitis, thought to arise from infection and obstruction of periurethral glands. Surgical excision is the mainstay of definitive management, and closure of the urethral defect is key to its success. Intraoperative complications included bleeding and urinary tract injury, but are relatively rare due to the anatomical location of the location. Recurrence of the urethral diverticulum occurs postoperatively in roughly 1–25% of patients [11]. This can present as a new diverticulum or a recurrence of the original defect. Suspicion should be raised if the presenting symptoms recur after initial resolution. Likely causes include incomplete resection of the diverticulum, inadequate urethral closure, excessive residual dead space, circumferential resection, and errors in surgical technique (e.g., excessive tension on the repair). Repeat diverticulectomy, if warranted, is usually more challenging due to distortion of the native anatomical planes and scarring. Preoperative magnetic resonance imaging (MRI) of the pelvis is useful in surgical planning to ensure complete excision; however, there remains a significantly higher rate of postoperative complications (e.g., fistula or recurrence) in the re-operative setting.

Urinary tract infections occur in as many as 31.3% of patients postoperatively [12]. Urinary incontinence can develop in 1.7–16.1% of cases as reported in the literature [12]. Stress urinary incontinence (SUI) occurs more often than urge urinary incontinence (UUI). If symptoms are identified during preoperative assessment, a full evaluation should be conducted, including urodynamic studies. Once the presence of SUI is objectively confirmed, concomitant anti-incontinence surgery can be offered. Current American Urological Association (AUA) guidelines recommend against the usage of synthetic mid-urethral slings in this setting due to the increased subsequent erosion [13]. Studies have shown good outcomes when utilizing pubovaginal autologous fascial slings [14]. In the absence of concurrent anti-incontinence surgery, de novo SUI occurs in up to 15% of cases [15]. Risk factors include diverticular size greater than 30 millimeters, proximal location, and wide surgical margins. These factors likely result from the more extensive sub-urethral dissection required in these circumstances, which can compromise the integrity of bladder neck and urethral sphincter complex. Furthermore, large proximal diverticulum can cause outlet obstruction and mask preexisting SUI. When SUI is discovered postoperatively, it should be managed conservatively for at least 4 weeks while the local inflammatory response resolves. Once it is safe to proceed with surgical intervention, any surgical approach or sling type can be applied. Consideration should be given to postoperative imaging to rule out other factors that may be contributing to the patient's symptoms. The rates of postoperative UUI are highly variable in the literature.

Uncommon complications include urethrovaginal fistula formation (0.9–8.3%), urethral stricture (0.5–2%), dyspareunia, and distal urethral necrosis [12]. The management and presenting symptoms of urethrovaginal fistula formation are largely dependent on the location of the fistula. Fistulas that form distal to the urinary sphincter may present with a split urinary stream or vaginal voiding and may not require surgical intervention if asymptomatic. Development of the fistula proximal to the sphincter (i.e., at the bladder neck or mid-urethra) will result in symptomatic urinary leakage if the patient has an incompetent bladder neck. These patients will require surgical repair with incorporation of an overlying tissue flap (e.g., Martius flap) to allow for adequate healing and prevent fistulous recurrence). The optimal timing of repair is debated, but the surgeon should allow enough time for postoperative inflammation to subside. The risk of fistula formation can be greatly decreased by implementing good surgical technique (e.g., adequate hemostasis, treating infection, creation of an anterior vaginal wall flap with preservation of vascular supply, preservation of periurethral fascia, and multilayered closure without overlapping suture lines) [15]. Dyspareunia can develop due to post-surgical changes (e.g., vaginal wall scarring/narrowing). Patients should be counseled about this risk preoperatively as it usually requires a multimodal approach to treatment. The risk of vaginal narrowing can be diminished by harvesting a wide-based vaginal flap to avoid devascularization and subsequent tissue contracture [14]. Distal urethral necrosis can rarely occur when the Spence-Duckett marsupialization procedure is utilized and results from sphincteric injury from excessive opening of the diverticulum.

Urethral Prolapse/Caruncle Repair

Urethral prolapse typically presents as a circumferential herniation or eversion of the urethral mucosa at the meatus that appears as a beefy red circular lesion surrounding the meatus. It is usually asymptomatic, but can present with bleeding, vaginal spotting, pain, and irritative voiding symptoms. This condition is usually found in postmenopausal women and prepubertal girls. Development is due to increased intra-abdominal pressure (e.g., valsalva or straining on constipation), which causes eversion of the urethral mucosa due to its loose attachment to the urethral smooth muscle. In the postmenopausal group, estrogen deficiency increases the likelihood of this phenomenon. Treatment can be medical

(e.g., topical intravaginal estrogen) or surgical (e.g., surgical excision). Complications from surgery are rare but include urethral stenosis, bleeding, and infection.

Urethral caruncle is an inflammatory lesion of the distal urethra that occurs almost exclusively in postmenopausal women. It appears as a red exophytic mass at the urethral meatus. Caruncles share a similar etiology and symptoms with urethral prolapse with voiding symptoms occurring less frequently. Surgical management includes excision. Complications are similar to those related to urethral prolapse repair except for meatal stricture, which is the most significant complication after caruncle excision. Maintaining a foley catheter for 3–5 days postoperatively can decrease the risk of stricture formation. Topical vaginal estrogen should be prescribed for postmenopausal women to facilitate healing. The surgeon should also ensure mucosal eversion of the urethral mucosa during closure.

Slings

The prevalence of female SUI is estimated at roughly 49% among the general populace [16]. Synthetic mid-urethral sling is the most commonly utilized procedure in the surgical management of SUI. Autologous fascia pubovaginal slings utilizing tissue harvested usually from the rectus abdominis fascia or fascia lata are non-synthetic alternatives for SUI surgery. Although the overall risk of slings remains low regardless of approach (e.g., transobsturator or retropubic), several complications can result. Bladder injury is relatively common and occurs at a rate of 2.7–10% in mid-urethral sling cases [17], more commonly with retropubic approach. Prior history of anti-incontinence surgery or retropubic operations also increases the risk for cystotomy [18]. Bladder injuries occur during trocar passage or vaginal dissection. Avoidance measures entail foley catheter placement at the beginning of the case to drain the bladder, and maintaining anatomic planes, meticulous vaginal dissection, and use of a metal sound/catheter guide to direct the urethra during dissection.

Vigorous use of hydrodissection when operating on the vaginal wall can assist in remaining in the right plane. Routine intraoperative cystoscopy is necessary to identify bladder perforations to allow immediate correction of trocar path and thereby prevention of delayed complications such as sling erosion, fistula formation, and infection. If the injury is on trocar passage, the sling arm should be retracted, and passage should be repeated. A foley or suprapubic catheter may be placed for 2–7 days postoperatively but is not required depending on the size and location of the defect. Urethral injuries that are missed on intraoperative cystoscopy lead to mesh erosion [19]. If intraoperative, small uncomplicated urethral injuries in healthy patients can be primarily repaired in two layers with absorbable sutures in a delayed fashion. Sling placement is often deferred in this setting due to higher risk of subsequent erosion or urethrovaginal fistula. Extensive urethral injuries or injuries in patients with poor tissue quality (e.g., prior surgeries, prior pelvic radiation, etc.) should be treated with interposition of a vascular tissue flap (e.g., Martius flap) in addition to primary urethral closure. In this setting, sling placement should be postponed until healing is complete. Distal ureteral injuries are rare and usually occur on repeat procedures. Ureter injuries can present in a delayed fashion with flank pain, fevers, wound leakage, and urinoma formation on CT imaging. When injury is suspected intraoperatively, the defect can be easily identified with a retrograde pyelogram. If signs of obstruction or kinking are noted, the sling trocar should be removed and repositioned, and a ureteral stent can be placed. Bowel injuries are rare (1% after retropubic sling), but can occur in patients with prior abdominal surgery [20]. Injury usually occurs during entry into the retropubic space in pubovaginal slings or trocar passage during mid-urethral sling placement. Initial symptoms include mild leukocytosis, malaise, ileus, progressive abdominal pain, nausea, and emesis. Prompt identification is important due to the high incidence of abscess formation, sepsis, and death in cases of delayed presentation. Situating the patient in Trendelenburg position and ensuring no increases in intra-abdominal pressure during

trocar placement can aid in avoiding this complication. When identified, urgent General Surgery consultation and computed tomography (CT) imaging are recommended. Repair requires exploratory laparotomy and bowel resection with or without fecal diversion. Other rare intraoperative complications include hemorrhage (i.e., injury to iliac, femoral, obturator, epigastric, or pelvic vessels) and osseous complications (which are rare outside of historical bone anchored sling procedures).

Urinary retention is the most common postoperative complication in urinary sling procedures. Furthermore, iatrogenic obstruction from sling surgery is the most common cause of female bladder outlet obstruction. Retention in this setting is usually transient, owing to postoperative edema of the bladder neck and urethra. Other etiologies include anxiety, trauma, local irritation, increased sympathetic response to pain, narcotic or anticholinergic use, constipation, immobility, and rarely retropubic hematoma. If postoperative void trial is unsuccessful, clean intermittent catheterization (CIC) and addressing the reversible contributing factors are the preferred initial management. Return to normal voiding tends to vary by procedure and occurs quickly after mid-urethral slings but can delay after pubovaginal sling (PVS) surgery for a few months. Routine post-void residual (PVR) should be evaluated within a few weeks of surgery. Symptoms of bladder outlet obstruction (e.g., straining, incomplete emptying) should prompt earlier follow-up with PVR assessment. Prolonged obstruction (i.e., urinary retention lasting greater than 4 weeks) occurs in 3–8% of cases with higher rates in PVS patients and women who void with minimal detrusor pressures [20]. If little to no improvement is noted within 4–6 weeks, the patient should be counseled on surgical intervention to loosen the sling. It is important to note that urethral dilation in patients with synthetic slings should be avoided due to risk of erosion. The timing of repeat surgical intervention is debated; however, historically three-month and six-week periods with catheter drainage have been used in PVS and MUS patients, respectively, as this issue resolves over that time in most patients [21]. When appropriate, surgical intervention included urethrolysis or sling incision with both having comparable efficacy. Late obstruction may occur in rare cases and should be evaluated with urodynamic studies and cystoscopy. Continence is usually maintained if urethrolysis is required. Furthermore, in cases where urethrolysis fails, which is usually due to recurrent periurethral fibrosis or retropubic scarring, repeat urethrolysis is usually effective. Recurrence of SUI can largely be avoided with appropriate patient counseling. Sexual intercourse, heavy lifting, and strenuous activity, including any activities that increase intra-abdominal pressure (e.g., squatting, bending, lunging, etc.), should be avoided for at least 6 weeks.

De novo UUI and irritative voiding symptoms may result from excess tension on the sling, unmasking of undiagnosed detrusor overactivity (DOA), or denervation secondary to surgical dissection. This occurs in 6–9% of synthetic mid-urethral sling (MUS) cases and is more common after pubovaginal sling [20]. Symptoms usually resolve within 2 weeks after MUS unless overt bladder outlet obstruction exists. Accordingly, urgency symptoms should be assessed with history, urinalysis, and culture, and post void residual within the first 4 weeks after MUS. Most patients with baseline mixed urinary incontinence report improvement in the UUI component following sling surgery [22]. Validated questionnaires (e.g., AUA symptom score) can be helpful if used pre- and postoperatively. History should focus on storage and voiding symptoms, temporal relations of symptoms to the surgery, and preoperative UDS, while the physical exam should highlight evidence of a fixed, elevated bladder neck or urethra, urethral hypermobility, SUI, worsening prolapse, or mesh erosion. Especially when UUI symptoms are chronic after SUI surgery, cystoscopy should be performed to evaluate for calculi, sling or suture erosion, or urinary tract injury or pathology. Management should follow a tiered escalation as detailed in the AUA guidelines for UUI management [23].

Recurrent UTIs develop in 4–15% of women after sling surgery [20]. Patients typically present with irritative voiding symptoms upon follow-up.

If evidence of UTI is found on evaluation, a short course of empiric antibiotics can be considered. If more concerning symptoms of ascending infection or persistent UTI, cross-sectional imaging should be added to rule-out abscess formation, upper tract obstruction, calculi, foreign bodies, erosion, or bladder pathology. Adjuncts such as UDS or PVR can be used as adjuncts to rule out further bladder-related causes. If signs of bladder outlet obstruction are identified, the obstruction should be managed, as above.

Patients with prolonged postoperative pain (>2 weeks), or pain refractory to oral medications, should be assessed for contributing etiologies (e.g., mesh extrusion, bowel or urinary tract injury, bladder outlet obstruction, adductor longus muscle or tendon perforation after transobturator MUS). Widespread pain or infection, in the absence of UTI or outlet obstruction, may be treated with mesh excision via a combined vaginal and abdominal approach. Patients should be counseled about the risk of continued pain and recurrent incontinence after mesh removal. Selected patients may also benefit from referral to a physical therapist and pain management specialist, especially in cases of preexisting pelvic pain or pelvic floor hypertonicity.

Pubovaginal slings can lead to specific complications involved in graft harvest sites. Autologous fascial slings are usually harvested from the rectus fascia or fascia lata. Rectus fascia is usually excised via a Pfannenstiel incision, which carries a low risk of incisional hernia, especially when the incision is carried lateral of the rectus sheath. Harvest of the fascia lata may cause pain on walking, incisional hernia, limping, and wound pain, but these are generally transient. Seroma development can occur in instances where there is a large suprafascial space, but this can largely be avoided with subcutaneous drain placement.

Complications of Vaginal Mesh Surgery

Synthetic mesh products have been utilized in pelvic floor surgery to augment strength and durability of prolapse repairs and continence procedures. Due to a high rate of complications, transvaginal mesh products for prolapse repair were pulled from the market in 2019 by the FDA and are now only available on research protocols.

Adherence to appropriate surgical principles is vital during transvaginal mesh placement for any means. If the dissection plane is too superficial, mesh placement may lead to vaginal wall necrosis, ulceration, mesh extrusion, dyspareunia, or pelvic pain. Avoid bunching or buckling of the mesh to decrease the risk of postoperative pelvic pain or extrusion. Furthermore, the surgeon should ensure that the mesh is not on tension which may predispose the patient to pelvic and vaginal pain. This can be accomplished by loosening the trocar arms or making a releasing incision in the mesh.

Complications from transvaginal mesh placement can occur days to years after surgery. Outlet obstruction, chronic pain, or recurrent infections can be managed with mesh revision/removal. Several steps can be taken pre- and intraoperatively to diminish the risk of postoperative complications. Topical vaginal estrogen can be initiated 4–6 weeks preoperatively to improve tissue quality in the postmenopausal patient. This should also be continued postoperatively to facilitate healing. This principle is especially important in patients who are at an increased risk for local complications (e.g., prior pelvic radiation, chronic steroid administration, chronic tobacco use, etc.). Revision operations should avoid vaginal wall trimming as this can lead to wound compromise, vaginal shortening, and dyspareunia. Postoperative foley catheter and vaginal packing may be considered.

The incidence of chronic pelvic pain syndrome is significantly higher in mesh-augmented repairs [24]. Mesh erosion occurs in 2–20% [24, 25]. Signs include persistent pain, vaginal discharge, and dyspareunia. Symptoms usually occur between 4 and 24 months postoperatively but can present several years later in some patients. Pelvic pain may also be a sign of poor positioning. Mesh placement in such a way that the fixating arms can contract and lead to reduced vaginal compliance can mimic stricture formation. Preventative measures include postoperative

resumption of sexual intercourse, local estrogen application, minimizing vaginal mucosal trimming, avoiding over-plication of soft tissue, and use of vaginal dilators, the latter of which is reserved for women who are not sexually active postoperatively. Mesh usage to augment rectocele repair is associated with a higher rate of recurrent and persistent dyspareunia, especially in patients with a history of pelvic radiation, severe urogenital atrophy, immunosuppression, active infection, heavy smoking, and certain comorbidities such as morbid obesity and poorly controlled diabetes mellitus.

Mesh erosion is an uncommon late complication. When used, mesh may erode into the vaginal, rectal, or bladder lumen. Patients with bladder erosion will present with hematuria, irritative voiding symptoms, recurrent UTIs, or chronic cystolithiasis. Clinicians must maintain a high index of suspicion and have a low threshold for cystoscopy. Mesh erosion into bowel can largely be avoided with careful mesh placement to ensure adequate space between the mesh and colon, particularly the sigmoid. When the bowel or vagina is involved, patients can develop rectal bleeding, change in bowel habits, and worsening dyspareunia months into the postoperative period. Diagnosis may require the use of rigid sigmoidoscopy as this is more sensitive than imaging alone. A DRE should be performed by the surgeon at the postoperative follow-up visit to assess any abnormalities with the repair as unrecognized bowel injuries are a common precursor to fistula formation. This complication can be managed endoscopically in selective cases, but the goal should be removal of most, if not all, of the mesh and repair of the rectal violation. Erosion rates can be affected by mesh type, surgical technique, and patient factors. Studies have shown that microporous multifilament meshes such as Gore-Tex have an 8% higher risk of erosion than polypropylene meshes [26]. The most important modifiable patient risk factor is tobacco use. This effect may be due to microvascular vasospasm leading to hypoxia and subsequent poor tissue healing. Mesh erosion rates are also elevated in procedures where graft or suture is introduced through the vagina. Well-circumscribed mesh erosions, the exposed mesh should be excised along with a 1–2-centimeter vaginal margin. The vaginal defect should be repaired in two layers with absorbable sutures. An interposition graft can also be incorporated into the repair to aid tissue healing. A vaginal approach to mesh exposure is always preferred unless there is concurrent intra-abdominal pathology to address. Lastly, the rate of de novo SUI may be higher after anterior POP repair with mesh due to more extensive dissection that may impair periurethral support or from increased hyper-suspension of the anterior vaginal axis.

Regardless of preventative measures, the risk of complications is substantially higher when undertaking mesh revision surgery after a mesh-related complication. Significant bleeding is rare, especially in transvaginal approaches. When it does occur, it is usually due to exiting the proper anatomical plane, which can be distorted from the prior surgery. Hemostasis can usually be achieved with the use of electrocautery or suture ligation with absorbable suture in a figure-of-eight fashion. Organs at risk for injury include the rectum and bladder. The repair of these should proceed as detailed in previous sections of this chapter. If organ injury occurs during mesh removal surgery, adjacent mesh should be excised prior to bladder or rectal repair to prevent further mesh erosion and/or wound infection. Vaginal mesh exposure requiring revision usually occurs due to wound separation, infection, or vaginal atrophy. If signs of infection are absent, primary closure of the separation can be attempted under local or general anesthesia. When infection is present, conservative measures can be attempted in the form of antibiotics and topical vaginal estrogen creams. Persistent infections require complete mesh excision. Delayed exposure presents after 6 weeks postoperatively and is usually due to technical error, local infection, vaginal atrophy, or wound separation in the presence of pelvic hematoma formation. Small mesh exposures can be managed conservatively with vaginal estrogen or excision of the exposed area in the occur with local anesthesia. In-office excisions should be monitored closely for re-epithelialization over the area. Mesh erosion into the bladder is usually seen at the bladder base or lateral walls where the mesh arms lie, and if missed, it can lead to stone formation as the intravesical mesh calcifies. Increased vaginal and pelvic pain can occur after revision surgery. Areas of point tenderness can be excised under general anesthesia, but the lack of anatomical landmarks can complicate intraoperative decision-making. Therefore, careful preoperative mapping of the surgical area is recommended. If pain is near the fornix and a tense, palpable area of mesh is noted, local anesthetic with epinephrine should be injected into the overlying vaginal wall. The vaginal epithelium should be incised, and the mesh arm should be exposed. The adjacent arm of mesh can then be transected to alleviate the discomfort.

Vaginal Hysterectomy

According to the American College of Obstetricians and Gynecologists, vaginal hysterectomy is the preferred minimally invasive approach for hysterectomy whenever feasible due to excellent surgical outcomes with relatively low morbidity and short recovery. It allows concurrent salpingoophorectomy as indicated. Intraoperative complications include bleeding, organ injury, and nerve injury. Average estimated blood loss for vaginal hysterectomy ranges between 215 and 278 milliliters, significantly lower than the laparoscopic transabdominal approach [27]. Risk factors for bleeding include obesity, poor exposure, distorted anatomy, uterine fibroids, surgeon's skill and experience, VTE prophylaxis, and antiplatelet therapy. Preventative measures are centered around knowledge of the anatomy. The surgeon should pay attention to staying within the avascular planes (e.g., pararectal space, paravesical space, rectovaginal septum) whenever possible. Vascular pedicles of the uterus and ovaries should be controlled, and the ureters should be identified prior to clamping the ovarian or uterine vessels. When bleeding is encountered, the priority should be improving exposure. A current type and screen should be in place with at least two units of packed red blood cells (pRBCs) on standby. In the event of significant bleeding, clotting factors should also be replaced for every four units of pRBCs administered. An attempt should be made to control the bleeding by applying direct pressure, suture ligation, hemostatic agents, and electrocautery. If this proves unsuccessful, one can resort to ligation of the anterior division of the internal iliac artery. This maneuver will decrease pelvic arterial pressure and allow for better visualization of the bleeding vessel. In rare cases where bleeding cannot be controlled, the pelvis can be packed with surgical sponges, and the patient should be transferred to the ICU for close monitoring. Consultation to Interventional Radiology for angioembolization should be considered if the patient develops hemodynamic instability. Alternatively, the surgeon may elect to return to the operating room after 48–72 hours to remove the packing and attempt to achieve hemostasis.

Ureteral injury is a rare complication that can go unnoticed in up to 66% of cases [28]. Kinking of the ureter due to adjacent suture remains the most common etiology, usually along the infundibulopelvic ligament. Risk factors include any prior history of pelvic surgery, hemorrhage, endometriosis, pelvic masses of any etiology, and obesity. Preventative measures center around identifying the ureter along the medial leaf of the broad ligament, avoiding aggressive surgical dissection of the vascular pedicles, and placing ureteral stents at the beginning of the cases with or without injection of a fluorescent contrast agent. Furthermore, it is important to assess the ureters for patency at the conclusion of the procedure with a cystoscopy. Treatment depends on the extent of the injury. Minor crush injuries can be managed with an indwelling ureteral stent, while substantial crush injuries require resection of the injured area with primary reanastomosis (or reimplantation) with ureteral stent placement. Partial transections are amenable to primary repair using absorbable sutures and ureteral stent placement. The management of complete transection is complex. When this occurs during a vaginal hysterectomy, the injury is most often isolated to the distal one-third of the ureter, which is best managed with ureteroneocystostomy. Regardless of the repair, a drain and foley catheter should be placed and maintained for at least 1 week. The ureteral stent can be removed in 6 weeks with or without CT urogram to assess the repair.

Bladder injuries occur at a rate of 0.7–4% [27]. Risk factors consist of prior anterior pelvic surgery (e.g., C-section, anterior vaginal wall repair), pelvic radiation, and pelvic inflammatory disease. Injury usually occurs intraperitoneally at the bladder dome during dissection of the vaginal wall or during the anterior colpotomy. Devascularization of the bladder wall and thermal injury can cause delayed presentation of injury. To avoid bladder injury, a foley catheter should be placed at the beginning of the case, and the drainage should be monitored for decreased output or new gross hematuria. The bladder flap should also be carefully mobilized prior to ligating the uterine artery and cervical amputation to avoid incorporation of the bladder into the resected specimen. Sharp dissection at the time of entry into the anterior peritoneum assists in mobilization of the bladder base and allows the bladder to be elevated away from the dissection. Extravasation of urine, overt laceration of the bladder, presence of the foley catheter in the surgical field, and air or blood in the foley drainage bag indicate the presence of a bladder injury. Definitive diagnosis can be made by instilling roughly 300 mL of a colored agent (e.g., methylene blue) through the foley. All injuries should be classified as full thickness or serosal, as well as intra- or extraperitoneal. Cystoscopy should be performed at the conclusion of the case. If a cystotomy is observed, mesh should not be placed near the closure as this increases the risk of mesh erosion or fistula formation. All bladder injuries should be closed in two layers using absorbable sutures and a moderately sized foley catheter should be placed. Posterior bladder injuries are best managed with an interposition graft (omental or peritoneal) due to risk of vesicovaginal fistula formation. In cases of trigonal injury, one should consider ureteral stent and suprapubic catheter (SPC) placement or large bore urethral catheter drainage. A cystogram should be obtained at 7–14 days, prior to foley removal. If a leak is observed, the foley should be maintained for an additional 2–4 weeks. Delayed injuries may present with fever, hematuria, signs of peritonitis, ileus, and/or ascites. If the ascites or pelvic fluid collection is drained, it should be sent for a fluid creatinine analysis. A urine leak should be suspected when the fluid creatinine/serum creatinine ratio greater than one is suggestive of urine leakage [29]. Bladder injury, when missed intraoperatively, can lead to fevers, suprapubic pain, pelvic discomfort, or other signs of peritonitis within the early postoperative period. Delayed cystotomies should be repaired in primary fashion with strong consideration to incorporate a Martius interposition graft or another similar technique to ensure adequate healing.

Bowel injury arises in 0.1–1% of cases [27]. Review of the literature reveals predominance by surgical approach [27]. Common signs and symptoms include fever, leukocytosis, nausea, emesis, abdominal pain, and/or distention, with or without acute abdomen in cases of perforation. Injuries can be divided into thermal, mechanical, and devascularization injuries. Thermal injuries appear as blanched spots along the bowel serosa and most often result due to use of monopolar electrocautery at the pelvic dissection due to poor visualization. These injuries can develop in delayed fashion days to weeks postoperatively, and a high index of suspicion aids in diagnosis. Mechanical injuries are the most recognizable during surgery and tend to occur during adhesiolysis. Injuries appear as denuded serosa or a full-thickness perforation of the bowel. Diagnosis can be made with CT scan of the abdomen and pelvis with oral contrast. Injuries that occur secondary to devascularization are a result of disruption of the mesenteric arteries and rarely arise during vaginal hysterectomies. Initial treatment of bowel injuries focuses on bowel rest and intravenous antibiotics. Significant bowel injury, especially thermal injuries, requires exploratory laparotomy and bowel resection. Healthy margins should be confirmed at the edges of the resected area. Bowel diversion should be performed in cases of extensive trauma with compromised blood supply, extensive infection, and history of radiation to the injured area. Regardless of the method, all repairs should be tension-free with intact blood supply.

Nerve injury is a rare complication that is almost always associated with major pelvic surgery. Injury to the femoral nerve is the most common neuropathy associated with pelvic surgery. It is usually injured along the anterior surface of the psoas muscle and inguinal canal due to compression from self-retaining retractor blades and stretch injury on hyperflexion and external rotation of the hip while in dorsal lithotomy position, respectively. The latter of which is a risk during vaginal hysterectomy. Risk of injury increases in patients with thin body habitus, prolonged operative time, use of long retractor blades, diabetes, gout, uremia, gout, alcoholism, and malnutrition. Symptoms usually present in 72 hours, such as numbness and paresthesia of the anterior thigh to anteromedial leg and medial foot. Other symptoms include dull inguinal pain, weakness of the quadriceps with inability to extend the knee and weakened patellar reflex. The diagnosis can be made by comparing quadricep strength and confirmed with an electromyogram in 2 weeks postoperatively. Of note, the axons can remain excitable for 7–11 days after the injury and can cause a false negative test. Avoidance of hip hyperflexion or excessive external rotation while in dorsal lithotomy can prevent injury to the femoral nerve during surgery. Less common neuropathies involve the iliohypogastric, ilioinguinal, and peroneal nerves. The superficial branch of the peroneal nerve can be injured when the patient is in dorsal lithotomy position. Excessive pressure from the lateral edge of the stirrup on the lateral edge of the fibular head causes compression of the nerve where it wraps around the region. Symptoms include foot drop on ambulation and burning pain in the nerve's sensory regions (e.g., the anterior and lateral lower leg, dorsum of the foot between the first and second toes). Treatment of these neuropathies consists of physical therapy, electrical stimulation, NSAIDs for pain relief, anticonvulsants (i.e., gabapentin), and the use of structural support devices (i.e., knee brace). Resolution usually occurs within days to weeks with treatment for mild neuropathies, and this condition will often resolve spontaneously in many cases.

Postoperative infection can present in many forms, including vaginal cuff cellulitis, infected hematoma, wound infection, pneumonia, and

UTI. Overall incidence after vaginal hysterectomy ranges from 9% to 13% [30]. Predisposing factors include immunocompromise, obesity, prolonged hospitalization, significant intraoperative blood loss, operative time exceeding 3 hours, malnutrition, diabetes mellitus, tobacco use, and intraoperative contamination of the surgical site. A single dose of antimicrobial prophylaxis is currently recommended for patients undergoing specific clean-contaminated genitourinary procedures [31]. Vaginal cuff cellulitis has an incidence between 0% and 8.3% and typically presents around postoperative day 4–10 [30]. Patients tend to develop fevers, purulent vaginal discharge, and pelvic, abdominal, or lower back discomfort. Physical exam will show tenderness or induration of the vaginal cuff and discharge. Patients presenting with these signs should be treated with empiric penicillin with a beta-lactamase inhibitor or a second- or third-generation cephalosporin. If symptoms persist, the regimen should be transitioned to clindamycin and gentamicin or clindamycin and metronidazole. Infected pelvic hematomas usually present after 7 days postoperatively. This complication appears in 0–14.6% of cases with symptoms of anemia, fevers, chills, pelvic pain, and rectal pressure [30]. Diagnosis can be made with use of vaginal ultrasound or CT of the pelvis. These patients should be treated with immediate IR drainage for collections over 5 cm and surgical drainage if the hematoma is difficult to access or unresponsive to minimally invasive approaches. Opening of the stitches at the vaginal cuff may be both diagnostic and therapeutic. Patients should remain on empiric gentamicin and clindamycin for at least 48 hours after drainage. Surgical wound infection occurs in 0–22.6% of cases, usually appearing after 5 days postoperatively [30]. Symptoms include cyclical fevers, increased incisional pain, purulent incisional discharge, wound erythema, and in rare cases, fascial dehiscence. The wound should be probed, and wound culture should be sent. Treatment usually consists of opening the wound, debridement of devitalized tissue, wet-to-dry dressings, possible wound vacuum placement, and empiric antibiotics (i.e., penicillin without or without vancomycin for

methicillin-resistant staphylococcus coverage). Early infections tend to result from skin flora, while late infections are usually due to staphylococcus aureus. UTIs tend to present around postoperative day 3 with the usual constellation of irritative voiding symptoms, in addition to suprapubic and anterior abdominal wall tenderness. Incidence ranges from 0% to 13% [30]. Diagnosis should center around a midstream, clean catch urinalysis and culture. Patients suspected of UTI development should be treated with a course of culture-directed antibiotics.

Uncommon complications after vaginal hysterectomy consist of vascular thromboembolic events (VTEs), vaginal cuff dehiscence, early menopause, and ovarian failure. The overall incidence of thromboembolic events in this setting is unknown, but incidence tends to be influenced by advanced age (greater than 60 years old), history of prior VTEs, duration of anesthesia, presence of lower extremity edema or varicose veins, prior radiation therapy, obesity, presence of thrombophilia, and oral contraceptive use. Any factors that may contribute to Virchow's triad should be identified preoperatively as the mainstay of preventative therapies focuses on reducing hypercoagulability or reducing stasis. A single dose of 5000 units of subcutaneous heparin should be given to all patients under 120 kg within 2 hours of the procedure. Furthermore, intermittent pneumatic compression stockings should be applied intraoperatively, and chemical deep venous thrombosis (DVT) prophylaxis in some form should be initiated postoperatively). Symptoms of VTE include hypoxia, tachycardia, and pleuritic chest pain; however, patients may also remain asymptomatic. Diagnosis can be made with the aid of lower extremity Duplex ultrasonography and chest CT with pulmonary embolism (PE) protocol or ventilation-perfusion scan if PE is suspected. Treatment should be promptly initiated with supportive care (e.g., supplemental oxygen, leg elevation, pain control) and therapeutic anticoagulation (e.g., intravenous Heparin drip) while admitted. On discharge, the patient should be transitioned to 3–6 months of warfarin, lovenox, or one of the newer oral anticoagulants. Vaginal cuff dehiscence occurs least often in

Vaginal Prolapse Repair

The transvaginal approach to prolapse repair can be performed concomitantly with vaginal hysterectomy, or independently. Many of the potential surgical complications (bowel or bladder injury, ureteral kinking, or bleeding) are similar and treated thoroughly in the preceding section. Compartment-specific concerns will be addressed here.

Complications of Apical Repair

Apical, or vault, suspension can be achieved by one of several techniques – most commonly ureterosacral ligament suspension (USLS) or sacrospinous ligament fixation (SSLF). Ureteral obstruction can occur after either repair, and is more common after USLS, and often temporary because it is usually caused by kinking the distal ureter rather than direct crush or transection

vaginal hysterectomy compared to an abdominal approach. Patients typically present in the first few weeks-to-months postoperatively with postcoital bleeding, vaginal spotting, and watery vaginal discharge [32]. Delayed presentation can occur years after the procedure and tends to be most frequent in post-menopausal women. An observational cohort study by Hur et al. showed the median time to presentation to be 6.5 years in the vaginal hysterectomy group compared to 2.5 months in other routes [32]. Preventative measures include infrequent use of electrocautery, incorporation of all vaginal layers into the final closure, closing with 1-centimeter suture margins, and maintaining adequate hemostasis. When this complication is suspected, a vaginal exam with manual palpation and inspection and an abdominal exam should be performed. CT imaging is reserved for patients suspected of bowel injury. Treatment involves initiation of broad-spectrum antibiotics, pelvic rest for small or partial dehiscence, surgical closure by vaginal approach for large and complicated cases, and inspection of the bowel for injury if evisceration is suspected.

[33]. Review of the literature reveals a 1–11% rate for ureteral injury [25]. Kinking may occur because the intrapelvic portion of the ureter is in close proximity to the uterosacral ligaments. Cystoscopy should be performed at the end of the case with or without the aid of bioluminescent dye (such as intravenously administered methylene blue or indigo carmine) to assess for ureteral injury. Sluggish or absent efflux from a ureteral orifice should raise suspicion of ureteral injury; however, the presence of bilateral efflux from the ureteral orifices does not rule out a ureteral injury. If injury is suspected, adjacent sutures should be serially cut, and the cystoscopy repeated. This resolves the blockage in many instances; however, if there is persistent concern for injury, a retrograde pyelogram should be performed with ureteral stent placement for 4–6 weeks [34]. If significant injury, such as transection or cautery injury, is suspected, the ureter should be exposed and repaired as described in above section. Delayed recognition of ureter injuries can lead to worse outcomes, including development of renal insufficiency and the subsequent need for nephrectomy. A study by Meirow et al. which found that the mean time-to-diagnosis in patients sustaining ureteral injuries during gynecologic procedures was 5.6 days [35]. Delayed injury can present with fever, flank pain, ileus, peritonitis, anuria, or continuous urinary incontinence from the vagina as a urinoma erodes through the vaginal cuff. Up to 5% of patients may be asymptomatic [36]. Diagnosis is made with CT urogram. Evidence of ureteral obstruction in the delayed setting should prompt return to the operating room for ureteral stent placement. Injuries identified in the early postoperative setting may not require further intervention, especially if absorbable suture was used for the apical suspension. In cases where open repair is required, repair has traditionally been delayed between 3 and 6 months to ensure that any local inflammation has subsided, but recent studies have shown similar outcomes with immediate and delayed repair [37].

Nerve injuries can occur with apical suspension, especially SSLF. Suture placement in SSLF should be inferomedial to the ischial spine to avoid the internal pudendal bundle and inferior to the cephalad order of the sacrospinous ligament to avoid the gluteal vessels and sciatic nerve. Adequate use of hydrodissection and remaining in the plain between the vaginal epithelium and muscularis are vital to avoid significant bleeding. Bowel injury is rare after SSLF, mainly due to its extraperitoneal nature [38]. In contrast, the risk of rectal injury remains, given the necessity to dissect the pararectal space. Use of unilateral right-sided SSLF is commonly utilized because it allows one to avoid the recto-sigmoid junction. When rectal injuries do occur, the distal anterior rectum is usually involved. A tension-free, multi-layer primary closure can be performed in most cases as the injuries are usually small (<2 cm) (72). Colorectal surgery consultation is recommended but is up to the discretion of the operating surgeon in the case of healthy patients without radiation history. Evisceration of the small bowel has been reported in rare instances after SSLF [39]. This remains a surgical emergency and requires prompt repair through a transabdominal approach. Nerve injury and subsequent chronic pain can occur in SSLF if careful suture placement is not maintained. Placement of the suture outside of the middle third of the sacrospinous ligament runs the risk of entrapment of the pudendal nerve laterally (which leads to vaginal pain) or sciatic nerves [40]. Roughly 6–14% of patients can develop buttock pain due to tension on the ligament or involvement of peripheral nerve branches, but the vast majority resolve spontaneously after 2–3 weeks [41]. Non-steroidal inflammatory drugs can be used for symptomatic control. Persistent pelvic pain should alert one to potential pudendal nerve entrapment, and the offending suture should be located and removed. Less often, USLS can injure the pudendal nerve, or sacral nerves during uterosacral suspension [42]. Uncommon complications include ileus, small bowel obstruction (SBO), recurrence of the prolapse, wound infection, dyspareunia, vaginal stricture, and SUI. Ileus presents with non-specific symptoms (i.e., nausea, emesis, bloating) and is more likely to develop in patients with advanced age. Vaginal stricture is a rare, delayed complication. These can form in various locations; however, the most common location is

the posterior wall at the level of the introitus and hymenal ring remnant. Apical stricture formation is less common. Management of the strictures involves topical estrogen cream and cauterization of the fibrous band. SUI is another rare, delayed complication.

Complications of Posterior Repair

Rectocele is a herniation of the anterior rectal wall into the posterior vagina that is estimated to effect roughly 18% of women [43]. Intraoperative complications include hemorrhage and rectal laceration. The rectovaginal septum and pararectal fascia are very well-vascularized, and vessels can retract when transected. The use of lighted retractors can improve visibility, and vasoconstrictive agents may be administered to minimize intraoperative blood loss; of note, there is a small risk of masking bleeding vessels until that agent wears off. If bleeding persists and cannot be identified, packing the vagina overnight with laparotomy sponges may prove useful. If concern for clinically significant bleeding continues postoperatively after conservative measures, return to the operating room for re-exploration or selective angioembolization with Interventional Radiology should be considered [44]. The overall incidence of rectal injury during the vaginal surgery is <1% [38]. Preoperative topical estrogen can thicken the vaginal mucosa and make tissue planes more robust. Preoperative bowel preparation can decrease the risk of gross contamination in the event of rectal injury. Serial assessment of the rectum, either by digital rectal examination (DRE) or by red rubber catheter inserted into the rectum at the beginning of the case, may aid in intraoperative assessment for injury. If an injury is identified, the area of interest should be mobilized to allow for better exposure and a tension-free repair. A two-layer closure should be performed with the first layer using delayed absorbable suture in a running fashion and the second seromuscular layer using permanent suture in a Lembert fashion. The closure should be completed with an overlying layer of fat and/or fascia incorporated. Lastly, the patient should be instructed to avoid inserting anything per rectum for at least 6 weeks.

Postoperative complications of posterior compartment repair include rectovaginal fistula, dyspareunia, defecatory pain, recurrence, constipation, UTI, and mesh erosion. Preoperative antibiotics should be administered when appropriate to avoid active infection at the time of surgery and subsequent inflammation and scarring. Constipation is the most common postoperative complication. The use of stool softeners, mineral oils, and/or fiber supplements is imperative as constipation can compromise the surgical repair if severe. Patients should be counseled to avoid excessive straining in the early postoperative period. Similarly, defecatory pain comprises the most common long-term postoperative complication. Rectovaginal fistula is an uncommon complication that can result from unrecognized rectal injuries and is more common in repairs with mesh augmentation. Presenting symptoms include foul-smelling vaginal discharge, systemic signs of infection, pelvic/perineal adenopathy, and pain. Repair of the fistula usually requires the incorporation of local tissue flaps and may rarely necessitate diverting colostomy. Dyspareunia can present with varying degrees of sexual dysfunction postoperatively. Patients should have a baseline assessment ideally, including sexual functional questionnaires such as the Female Sexual Function Index [45]. Intraoperatively, surgeons should avoid excessive tightening of the posterior vagina during the repair as well as the introitus if concurrent perineal body repair is needed. The vaginal canal should also be calibrated to 2–3 fingerbreadths. Patients should be assessed postoperatively for signs of painful intercourse and tight bands, extrusions, and tender pelvic muscles on physical examination. Conservative measures for dyspareunia include topical lubricants, vaginal estrogen, topical local anesthetics, injection of trigger points with steroid or local anesthetic, physical therapy with or without vaginal dilators, and systemic anxiolytics to help relax the pelvic floor musculature. Surgical intervention is typically reserved for refractory cases where intravaginal bands or excessive vaginal narrowing is identified.

Complications of Anterior Repair

Transvaginal repair for anterior compartment prolapse, usually cystocele, restores support to the pubocervical fascia (connective tissue between the urethra, bladder, and anterior vaginal wall). Significant intraoperative hemorrhage is rare and can occur due to dissecting in the incorrect surgical plane, scar tissue from repeat surgeries, or perforation of the endopelvic fascia when gaining access to the retropubic space. Postoperative bleeding can be largely avoided by staying in the plane between the vaginal epithelium and muscularis layer, using electrocautery during the initial dissection, and performing a tight closure to tamponade oozing vessels. Brisk bleeds should be suture ligated in a figure-of-eight fashion. Vaginal packing may be placed for a few hours or overnight if needed. Patients with suspected bleeding should be closely monitored for hemodynamic instability and may require serial hemoglobin levels. For persistent substantial bleeding, angiography with selective embolization remains an effective minimally invasive option.

Bladder, ureter, or urethra injuries are rare in the transvaginal approach to anterior POP repair. The risk of bladder injury can be decreased by decompression with a foley catheter. A cystoscopy should be performed after the reconstruction to assess for any injury. A systematic review of the literature by Gilmour et al. revealed that 95% of bladder injuries were diagnosed and repaired when using intraoperative cystoscopy, in contrast to 43% detected when cystoscopy is omitted [46]. Alternatively, 300 mL of dilute methylene blue or indigo carmine can be instilled into the bladder to assess the surgical field for leakage. Any identified cystotomies should be closed in two layers with absorbable sutures. If there is a concern for poor tissue quality, incorporation of a tissue flap can be implemented to decrease the risk of future fistula formation. Furthermore, any planned mesh placement should be aborted in this setting due to the increased risk of fistula formation. An attempt at conservative management (e.g., foley or suprapubic catheter placement) can be made in patients with delayed presentation; however, if intraperitoneal injury is suspected, surgical repair may be warranted. The rate of ureteral injury from isolated anterior compartment repair is low, estimated at 2% [47]. There is an increased risk in patients undergoing surgery for high-stage POP due to the anatomic distortion from the prolapse itself. Ureter injuries are discussed in detail in the above sections.

De novo stress urinary incontinence can occur after anterior or apical compartment repair, sometimes attributed to unmasking pre-existing SUI. The risk of postoperative SUI is higher with advanced preoperative prolapse stage. Prior to surgery, urethral kinking from the prolapse can "mask" incontinence symptoms. This is also called occult SUI. After prolapse repair, the SUI can become clinically apparent secondary to urethral hyper-suspension, intraoperative damage to the urethral sphincter, intrinsic sphincter deficiency, or compromise of the periurethral structural support. Incidence of postoperative SUI can be minimized with appropriate preoperative evaluation with history, physical examination, and cough stress testing with prolapse reduction. The latter is an office assessment that can be accomplished in the exam room, or during urodynamic testing, with the assistance of pessaries, speculums, or scopettes to reduce the prolapse and mimic post-reconstruction position of bladder and urethra to unmask occult SUI. This is performed in the standing position whenever possible. Furthermore, a concomitant anti-incontinence repair can be performed in appropriate patients and is most beneficial in women with objectively demonstrated occult SUI [48].

De novo urgency incontinence can develop in 5–7% of patients and can often be managed conservatively with behavioral modifications [49]. Medications or procedures for overactive bladder treatment can also be used as necessary. Other complications of anterior compartment repair include dyspareunia, infection, and fistula formation. The latter usually results from delayed recognition of a bladder injury. Additionally, fistula development depends on the duration of foley catheter placement postoperatively and the extent of the offending injury, and the presence of other risk factors such as radiation or foreign bodies (mesh). Treatment requires either longer catheter drainage or transvaginal fistula excision and repair.

References

1. Amies Oelschlager AM, Kirby A, Breech L. Evaluation and management of vaginoplasty complications. Curr Opin Obstet Gynecol. 2017;29(5): 316–21.
2. Callens N, et al. An update on surgical and non-surgical treatments for vaginal hypoplasia. Hum Reprod Update. 2014;20(5):775–801.
3. van der Sluis WB, et al. Diversion neovaginitis after sigmoid vaginoplasty: endoscopic and clinical characteristics. Fertil Steril. 2016;105(3):834–839 e1.
4. Bouman MB, et al. Primary total laparoscopic sigmoid vaginoplasty in transgender women with penoscrotal hypoplasia: a prospective cohort study of surgical outcomes and follow-up of 42 patients. Plast Reconstr Surg. 2016;138(4):614e–23e.
5. Willemsen WN, Kluivers KB. Long-term results of vaginal construction with the use of Frank dilation and a peritoneal graft (Davydov procedure) in patients with Mayer-Rokitansky-Kuster syndrome. Fertil Steril. 2015;103(1):220–7 e1.
6. Bogliolo S, et al. Long-term risk of malignancy in the neovagina created using colon graft in vaginal agenesis – a case report. J Obstet Gynaecol. 2015;35(5):543–4.
7. Lafay Pillet MC, et al. Incidence and risk factors of bladder injuries during laparoscopic hysterectomy indicated for benign uterine pathologies: a 14.5 years experience in a continuous series of 1501 procedures. Hum Reprod. 2009;24(4):842–9.
8. Holme A, Breen M, MacArthur C. Obstetric fistulae: a study of women managed at the Monze Mission Hospital, Zambia. BJOG. 2007;114(8):1010–7.
9. Browning A. Risk factors for developing residual urinary incontinence after obstetric fistula repair. BJOG. 2006;113(4):482–5.
10. Ayed M, et al. Prognostic factors of recurrence after vesicovaginal fistula repair. Int J Urol. 2006;13(4): 345–9.
11. Dmochowski R. Surgery for vesicovaginal fistula, urethrovaginal fistula, and urethral diverticulum. 8th ed. P.C. Walsh, Retik, A.B., Vaughan Jr, E.D., Wein, A.J. Philadelphia: Campbell's Urology; 2002.
12. Rovner ES, Jaffe WI. Urethral diverticula and other Periurethral masses. In: Zimmern PE, Norton PA, Haab F, Chapple CCR, editors. Vaginal surgery for incontinence and prolapse. London: Springer; 2006.
13. Kobashi KC, et al. Surgical treatment of female stress urinary incontinence: AUA/SUFU guideline. J Urol. 2017;198(4):875–83.
14. Romanzi LJ, Groutz A, Blaivas JG. Urethral diverticulum in women: diverse presentations resulting in diagnostic delay and mismanagement. J Urol. 2000;164(2):428–33.
15. Reeves FA, Inman RD, Chapple CR. Management of symptomatic urethral diverticula in women: a single-centre experience. Eur Urol. 2014;66(1):164–72.
16. Geelen J, Hunskarr S. The epidemiology of female urinary incontinence. Eur Clin Obstet Gynaecol. 2005;1:3–11.

17. Kuuva N, Nilsson CG. A nationwide analysis of complications associated with the tension-free vaginal tape (TVT) procedure. Acta Obstet Gynecol Scand. 2002;81(1):72–7.
18. Tamussino KF, et al. Tension-free vaginal tape operation: results of the Austrian registry. Obstet Gynecol. 2001;98(5 Pt 1):732–6.
19. Nguyen JN, et al. Perioperative complications and reoperations after incontinence and prolapse surgeries using prosthetic implants. Obstet Gynecol. 2012;119 (3):539–46.
20. Dmochowski RR, et al. Update of AUA guideline on the surgical management of female stress urinary incontinence. J Urol. 2010;183(5):1906–14.
21. Morgan TO Jr, Westney OL, McGuire EJ. Pubovaginal sling: 4-YEAR outcome analysis and quality of life assessment. J Urol. 2000;163(6):1845–8.
22. Schrepferman CG, et al. Resolution of urge symptoms following sling cystourethropexy. J Urol. 2000;164(5): 1628–31.
23. Lightner DJ, et al. Diagnosis and treatment of overactive bladder (non-neurogenic) in adults: AUA/SUFU guideline amendment 2019. J Urol. 2019;202(3):558–63.
24. Shah DK, et al. Short-term outcome analysis of total pelvic reconstruction with mesh: the vaginal approach. J Urol. 2004;171(1):261–3.
25. Amrute KV, et al. Analysis of outcomes of single polypropylene mesh in total pelvic floor reconstruction. Neurourol Urodyn. 2007;26(1):53–8.
26. Elneil S, et al. Abdominal sacrocolpopexy for vault prolapse without burial of mesh: a case series. BJOG. 2005;112(4):486–9.
27. Makinen J, et al. Morbidity of 10 110 hysterectomies by type of approach. Hum Reprod. 2001;16(7):1473–8.
28. Gilmour DT, Dwyer PL, Carey MP. Lower urinary tract injury during gynecologic surgery and its detection by intraoperative cystoscopy. Obstet Gynecol. 1999;94 (5 Pt 2):883–9.
29. Regmi SK, et al. Drain fluid creatinine-to-serum creatinine ratio as an initial test to detect urine leakage following cystectomy: a retrospective study. Indian J Urol. 2021;37(2):153–8.
30. Nieboer TE, et al. Surgical approach to hysterectomy for benign gynaecological disease. Cochrane Database Syst Rev. 2009;3:CD003677.
31. Lightner DJ, et al. Best practice statement on urologic procedures and antimicrobial prophylaxis. J Urol. 2020;203(2):351–6.
32. Hur HC, et al. Vaginal cuff dehiscence after different modes of hysterectomy. Obstet Gynecol. 2011;118(4): 794–801.
33. Lantzsch T, et al. Sacrospinous ligament fixation for vaginal vault prolapse. Arch Gynecol Obstet. 2001;265 (1):21–5.
34. Kim JH, et al. Management of ureteral injuries associated with vaginal surgery for pelvic organ prolapse. Int Urogynecol J Pelvic Floor Dysfunct. 2006;17(5):531–5.
35. Meirow D, et al. Evaluation and treatment of iatrogenic ureteral injuries during obstetric and gynecologic operations for nonmalignant conditions. J Am Coll Surg. 1994;178(2):144–8.
36. Visco AG, et al. Cost-effectiveness of universal cystoscopy to identify ureteral injury at hysterectomy. Obstet Gynecol. 2001;97(5 Pt 1):685–92.
37. Ku JH, et al. Minimally invasive management of ureteral injuries recognized late after obstetric and gynaecologic surgery. Injury. 2003;34(7):480–3.
38. Hoffman MS, et al. Injury of the rectum during vaginal surgery. Am J Obstet Gynecol. 1999;181(2):274–7.
39. Farrell SA, et al. Massive evisceration: a complication following sacrospinous vaginal vault fixation. Obstet Gynecol. 1991;78(3 Pt 2):560–2.
40. Verdeja AM, et al. Transvaginal sacrospinous colpopexy: anatomic landmarks to be aware of to minimize complications. Am J Obstet Gynecol. 1995;173 (5):1468–9.
41. Lovatsis D, Drutz HP. Safety and efficacy of sacrospinous vault suspension. Int Urogynecol J Pelvic Floor Dysfunct. 2002;13(5):308–13.
42. Schon Ybarra MA, et al. Etiology of post-uterosacral suspension neuropathies. Int Urogynecol J Pelvic Floor Dysfunct. 2009;20(9):1067–71.
43. Hendrix SL, et al. Pelvic organ prolapse in the Women's Health Initiative: gravity and gravidity. Am J Obstet Gynecol. 2002;186(6):1160–6.
44. Phillips C, Hacking N, Monga A. Super-selective angiographic embolisation of a branch of the anterior pudendal artery for the treatment of intractable postoperative bleeding. Int Urogynecol J Pelvic Floor Dysfunct. 2006;17(3):299–301.
45. Rosen R, et al. The female sexual function index (FSFI): a multidimensional self-report instrument for the assessment of female sexual function. J Sex Marital Ther. 2000;26(2):191–208.
46. Gilmour DT, Das S, Flowerdew G. Rates of urinary tract injury from gynecologic surgery and the role of intraoperative cystoscopy. Obstet Gynecol. 2006;107 (6):1366–72.
47. Kwon CH, et al. The use of intraoperative cystoscopy in major vaginal and urogynecologic surgeries. Am J Obstet Gynecol. 2002;187(6):1466–71; discussion 1471–2.
48. Brubaker L, et al. Abdominal sacrocolpopexy with Burch colposuspension to reduce urinary stress incontinence. N Engl J Med. 2006;354(15):1557–66.
49. Raz S, Klutke CG, Golomb J. Four-corner bladder and urethral suspension for moderate cystocele. J Urol. 1989;142(3):712–5.

9783031195976VOL01